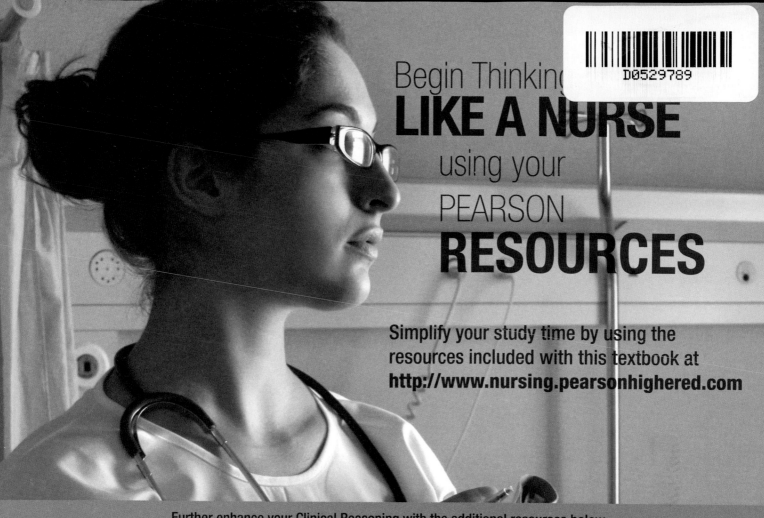

Begin Thinking
LIKE A NURSE
using your
PEARSON
RESOURCES

Simplify your study time by using the
resources included with this textbook at
http://www.nursing.pearsonhighered.com

Further enhance your Clinical Reasoning with the additional resources below.
For more information and purchasing options visit **www.mypearsonstore.com**.

Break Through
to improving results

Nursing ®

MyNursingLab provides a guided
learning path that is proven to help
students synthesize vast amounts
of information, guiding them from
memorization to true understanding
through application.

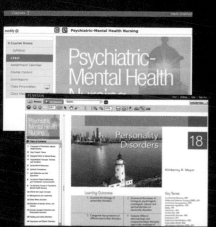

Thinking Like a Nurse in Clinical

Clinical references across the nursing curriculum!

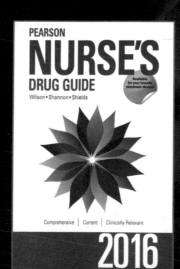

PEARSON
NURSE'S
DRUG GUIDE
Wilson • Shannon • Shields

Available for your favorite electronic device!

Comprehensive | Current | Clinically Relevant

2016

Thinking Like a Nurse for
NCLEX® Success

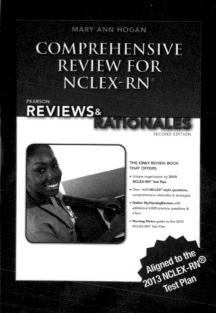

MARY ANN HOGAN

COMPREHENSIVE
REVIEW FOR
NCLEX-RN®

PEARSON
REVIEWS &
RATIONALES
SECOND EDITION

THE ONLY REVIEW BOOK
THAT OFFERS:

• Unique organization by 2010
  NCLEX-RN® Test Plan

• Over 1600 NCLEX®-style questions,
  comprehensive rationales & strategies

• Online MyNursingReview with
  additional 4,000 practice questions &
  eTest

• Nursing Notes guide to the 2010
  NCLEX-RN® Test Plan

Aligned to the
2013 NCLEX-RN®
Test Plan

ALWAYS LEARNING

PEARSON

MyNursingLab®

www.mynursinglab.com

Learn more about and purchase access to MyNursingLab.

MyNursingApp™

www.mynursingapp.com

MyNursingApp puts all the information you need in the palm of your hand.

myPEARSONstore

www.mypearsonstore.com

Find your textbook and everything that goes with it.

ALWAYS LEARNING

PEARSON

Psychiatric–Mental Health Nursing

Nursing

From Suffering to Hope

Mertie L. Potter, DNP, APRN, PMHNP-BC, PMHCNS-BC
Clinical Professor of Nursing
Massachusetts General Hospital
Institute of Health Professions
Boston, MA

Mary D. Moller, DNP, APRN, PMHCNS-BC, CPRP, FAAN
Associate Professor of Nursing
Pacific Lutheran University
Tacoma, WA

PEARSON

Boston   Columbus   Indianapolis   New York   San Francisco   Hoboken
Amsterdam   Cape Town   Dubai   London   Madrid   Milan   Munich   Paris   Montreal   Toronto
Delhi   Mexico City   São Paulo   Sydney   Hong Kong   Seoul   Singapore   Taipei   Tokyo

Publisher: Julie Levin Alexander
Executive Editor: Katrin Beacom
Development Editors: Adelaide R. McCulloch and Kim Wyatt
Program Manager Team Lead: Melissa Bashe
Editorial Assistant: Kevin Wilson
Director of Marketing: David Gesell
Senior Product Marketing Manager: Phoenix Harvey
Field Marketing Manager: Debi Doyle
Marketing Specialist: Michael Sirinides
Director, Product Management Services: Etain O'Dea
Project Management Team Lead: Cynthia Zonneveld
Project Manager: Maria Reyes

Manufacturing Manager: Maura Zaldivar-Garcia
Art Director: Mary Siener
Interior Design/Cover Design: Mary Siener
Cover Credit: Oleksiy Mark/iStock/Getty Images
Chapter Opener Images: Shane Shaw/iStock/Getty Images; Oleksiy Mark/iStock/Getty Images; mervas/iStock/Getty Images; Fuse/Getty Images; pyzata/Fotolia; ssuaphotos/Shutterstock
Full-Service Project Management: Peggy Kellar, Aptara®, Inc.
Composition: Aptara®, Inc.
Printer/Binder: RR Donnelley/Roanoke
Cover Printer: Lehigh-Phoenix Color/Hagerstown

Notice: Care has been taken to confirm the accuracy of information presented in this book. The authors, editors, and the publisher, however, cannot accept any responsibility for errors or omissions or for consequences from application of the information in this book and make no warranty, express or implied, with respect to its contents.

The authors and publisher have exerted every effort to ensure that drug selections and dosages set forth in this text are in accord with current recommendations and practice at time of publication. However, in view of ongoing research, changes in government regulations, and the constant flow of information relating to drug therapy and reactions, the reader is urged to check the package inserts of all drugs for any change in indications or dosage and for added warning and precautions. This is particularly important when the recommended agent is a new and/or infrequently employed drug.

Copyright © 2016 by Pearson Education, Inc. or its affiliates. All Rights Reserved. Printed in the United States of America. This publication is protected by copyright, and permission should be obtained from the publisher prior to any prohibited reproduction, storage in a retrieval system, or transmission in any form or by any means, electronic, mechanical, photocopying, recording, or otherwise. For information regarding permissions, request forms and the appropriate contacts within the Pearson Education Global Rights & Permissions department, please visit www.pearsoned.com/permissions/.

Many of the designations by manufacturers and sellers to distinguish their products are claimed as trademarks. Where those designations appear in this book, and the publisher was aware of a trademark claim, the designations have been printed in initial caps or all caps.

A note about nursing diagnoses: Nursing diagnoses in this text are taken from *Nursing Diagnoses—Definitions and Classification 2015–2017*. Copyright © 2014 by NANDA International. Used by arrangement with John Wiley & Sons Limited. In order to make safe and effective judgments using NANDA-I nursing diagnoses it is essential that nurses refer to the definitions and defining characteristics of the diagnoses listed in this work.

Library of Congress Cataloging-in-Publication Data
Potter, Mertie L., author.
  Psychiatric mental health nursing : from suffering to hope / Mertie L. Potter, Mary D. Moller.
  p. ; cm.
  Includes bibliographical references and index.
  ISBN 978-0-13-801558-9—ISBN 0-13-801558-9
  I.   Moller, Mary D. (Mary Denise), author. II.   Title.
  [DNLM: 1. Psychiatric Nursing.   2. Mental Disorders—nursing.   3. Nurse's Role.   4. Nurse-Patient Relations. WY 160]
  RC440
  616.89'0231—dc23
                                                                                    2014018535

10 9 8 7 6 5 4 3 2 1

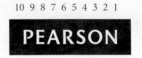

ISBN 13: 978-0-13-801558-9
ISBN 10:   0-13-801558-9

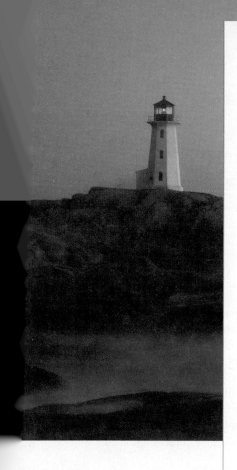

DEAR STUDENT

You are about to launch on a journey that we trust will lead you into a deeper appreciation and understanding of the suffering experienced by individuals diagnosed with mental illness and their families. Hope and recovery in mental illness are achievable and need to be fostered and encouraged in both patients and families.

Why did we title this book *Psychiatric–Mental Health Nursing: From Suffering to Hope?* During our years of nursing, we have witnessed patients and families suffer in times of emotional pain and distress as well as in times of physical illness. We also have witnessed patients make incredible recoveries as they gain hope and confidence through relationships and experiences with competent and caring nurses.

The word patient has been selected for use in this textbook due to its root meanings: 1) to suffer, undergo, or bear; and 2) to bear or endure pain. The term *patient* reminds us that nursing care focuses on relieving patient distress, as well as promoting patient health and wellness.

Caring for patients experiencing mental health challenges is rewarding for the nurse who sees patients improve, helps them learn new coping skills to meet needs, and helps them return to normal functioning. We intend for this text to assist you in providing care and compassion to patients in any clinical setting.

Throughout this text, we hope that you will learn how to:

- Promote patient empowerment using nursing interventions that alleviate patient suffering and distress and promote hope
- Find the context for patient health and recovery by recognizing how neurobiological processes, psychological factors, spiritual needs, and social networks (including family, cultural values, and beliefs) impact patient mental health
- Recognize and address needs of patients across the life span
- Engage patients in a therapeutic relationship to promote their safety and recovery

Thank you for joining us.

We are excited for you and invite you to begin…

Sincerely,

Mertie L. Potter, DNP, APRN, PMHNP-BC, PMHCNS-BC

Mary D. Moller, DNP, APRN, PMHCNS-BC, CPRP, FAAN

ABOUT THE AUTHORS

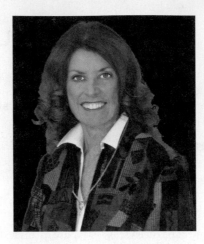

Mertie L. Potter Mertie L. Potter received her bachelor's degree from Simmons College, her master's degree from the University of Michigan, her doctoral degree from Case Western Reserve University, and her Post-Master's Certificate as a Family Psychiatric and Mental Health Nurse Practitioner from Rutgers University. She acquired common sense and a hard work ethic from working alongside her parents at Maple Leaf Farm. Her lifelong passion for helping those struggling with mental health issues piqued as a result of the family's farm property being next to a state psychiatric facility. That led to summer jobs there and observations of her parents' respect and compassion for patients at that hospital.

Dr. Potter is a Clinical Professor of Nursing at Massachusetts General Hospital Institute of Health Professions; a nurse practitioner at Merrimack Valley Counseling Association in Nashua, NH; and a nursing consultant in private practice. She is ANCC certified as a family psychiatric–mental health nurse practitioner and as a clinical nurse specialist in adult psychiatric–mental health nursing. She is abundantly blessed by her life's calling.

Dr. Potter's professional interests include group work, crisis intervention, stress management, chronic illness, pain management, suffering, grieving, spirituality, older adults, medical missions, camp nursing, and nursing theory. She has experience in education, counseling, prescribing, group work, team building, consulting, camp nursing, medical missions, and speaking/presenting. She has spoken on a number of these topics.

Dr. Potter has authored and co-authored articles, chapters, and books, one of which received an AJN Book of the Year Award. She served on the NH Board of Nursing for 5 years and had the privilege of being elected Vice-Chairperson for a number of them.

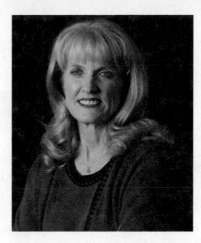

Mary D. Moller Mary D. Moller received her bachelor's degree in nursing from Mt. Marty College in Yankton, SD; her master's degree in psychiatric nursing from the University of Nebraska Medical Center College of Nursing; and her doctoral degree from Case Western Reserve University Frances Payne Bolton School of Nursing. Her doctoral research in schizophrenia received the Dean's Legacy Award in 2006. However, she attributes her real education to what she has learned from her thousands of patients and their family members encountered since 1971, when she had the privilege of becoming a registered nurse. She is dually certified as an adult psychiatric–mental health clinical nurse specialist by the American Nurses Credentialing Center and as a certified psychiatric rehabilitation practitioner by the United States Psychiatric Rehabilitation Association.

Dr. Moller was drafted rather unwillingly into psychiatric nursing in the late 1970s while teaching neurological nursing at a diploma school of nursing. Although initially she was very apprehensive, she quickly saw the parallels between neurology and psychiatry and began implementing the only kind of nursing she knew: rehabilitation nursing, working with a group of patients who had never been exposed to this kind of nursing. After seeing patients who had been experiencing catatonia respond for the first time in years, she literally fell in love with psychiatric nursing and, since 1978, has dedicated her career to improving the lives of individuals with serious and persistent mental illness and their families.

Dr. Moller is an Associate Professor of Nursing at Pacific Lutheran University in Tacoma, WA. From 2009 through 2014 she was the Coordinator of the Psychiatric Mental Health Nurse Practitioner Specialty at the Yale University School of Nursing. She is in private practice as an advanced registered nurse practitioner and conducts telemental health practicing in the specialty of telepsychiatry. Dr. Moller has an active consulting practice with an emphasis on psychiatric wellness that has taken her to China, Australia, Hong Kong, Israel, Cuba, and several other countries . Prior to returning to education, Dr. Moller founded and served as clinical director of the first APRN-owned and managed rural outpatient psychiatric clinic in the United States—the Suncrest Wellness Center, which was located in Spokane, WA, from 1992 to 2008. The experiences and relationships developed during this time in her life have blessed and continue to truly bless not only Dr. Moller, but also all those she encounters as she shares what she learned.

Dr. Moller's professional interests include psychiatric rehabilitation with people recovering from schizophrenia, bipolar disorder, major depression, PTSD, attention-deficit disorder, and personality disorders. She is the co-author of the Three R's Psychiatric Wellness Rehabilitation Program, which includes three training/participant psychoeducational manuals focusing on relapse, recovery, and rehabilitation. This program was a CMS model training program in 1996. She has also produced four videos in the award-winning Understanding and Communicating with a Person Who Is Experiencing series, which include hallucinations, delusions, mania, and relapse. She is also co-author of the Be Smart trauma recovery program, which also has both training and participant manuals. Her work centers on both individual and group therapy.

Dr. Moller has presented more than 900 research and training seminars in 49 states and 9 countries. She has published numerous articles and book chapters and received many awards, including an honorary PhD from Mt. Marty College and the Distinguished Alumnus Award from the University of Nebraska Medical Center College of Nursing. She is an active member of the American Psychiatric Nurses Association and served as President in 2009–2010. She has received the APNA Award for Clinical Excellence and the Distinguished Service Award, as well as the NAMI Professional of the Year Award.

THANK YOU!

Contributors

We extend heartfelt thanks to our contributors, who gave their time, effort, and expertise so tirelessly to the development and writing of chapters and resources. Together we have created a book that we hope will foster our goal of preparing all nursing students to work in a holistic manner to promote the principles of mental health for all patients and their families.

Joyce K. Anastasi, PhD, DNP, FAAN, LAc
Professor of Nursing
Director, Division of Special Studies in Symptom Management
New York University College of Nursing
New York, NY
Chapter 22

Barbarajo (BJ) Bockenhauer, MSN, APRN, PMHCNS-BC
Consultant
Concord, NH
Chapter 7

Bernadette Capili, PhD, NP-C
Associate Director, Division of Special Studies in Symptom Management
New York University College of Nursing
New York, NY
Chapter 22

Julie Carbray, PhD, FPMHNP-BC, PMHCNS-BC, APN
Clinical Professor of Psychiatry and Nursing
University of Illinois at Chicago
Chicago, IL
Chapter 30

Michelle Chang, MS, LAc
Division of Special Studies in Symptom Management
New York University College of Nursing
New York, NY
Chapter 22

Sylvia Durette, MS, APRN, PMHCNS-BC
Nurse Educator/Nurse Practitioner
St. Joseph School of Nursing/Merrimack Valley Counseling Association
Nashua, NH
Chapter 4

Elspeth Dwyer, MSW, MS, RN, PMHNP-BC
Psychiatric Nurse Practitioner
American University
Washington, DC
Chapter 15

Carole Farley-Toombs, RN, MSN, NEA-BC
Associate Director of Nursing
Department of Psychiatry, University of Rochester Medical Center
Rochester, NY
Chapter 11

Patrick Gagnon, APRN, CNS, BC
Cycare LLC
Bloomfield, CT
Chapter 32

Maureen Gaynor, MSN, APRN, AHN-BC, PMHCNS-BC
Assistant Professor of Nursing Education
Franklin Pierce University College of Graduate & Professional Studies
Manchester, NH
Chapter 21

Vanessa Genung, PhD, RN, PMHNP, LCSW-ACP, LMFT, LCDC
Psychiatric APRN Attending, North Texas State Hospital
Wichita Falls, TX
Chapters 3, 23

Vanya Hamrin, MSN, RN, APRN, PMHCNS-BC
Associate Professor of Nursing
Vanderbilt University
Nashville, TN
Chapter 24

Sandy Hannon-Engel, PhD, RN, CNS, PMHNP-BC
Assistant Professor of Nursing
Boston College
Chestnut Hill, MA
Chapter 15

Lora Humphrey Beebe, PhD, PMHNP-BC
Professor of Nursing
University of Tennessee
Knoxville, TN
Chapter 17

Joanne DeSanto Iennaco, PhD, PMHNP-BC, PMHCNS-BC, APRN
Associate Professor
Yale University School of Nursing
West Haven, CT
Chapters 8, 9, 25

Carla R. Jungquist, PhD, ANP-BC
Assistant Professor
University of Buffalo School of Nursing
Buffalo, NY
Chapter 12

Mary White Kudless, MSN, RN, PMHCNS-BC
Health Care Integration Consultant
Deputy Director (Retired), Fairfax–Falls Church
Community Services Board
Arlington, VA
Chapter 29

Martha Mathews Libster, PhD, APRN-CNS, AHN-BC
Professor of Nursing, Governors State University
Director, Golden Apple Healing Arts
Naperville, IL
Chapters 2, 6

Barbara J. Limandri, PhD, PMHCS-BC
Professor of Nursing, Linfield Good Samaritan School
of Nursing and Portland Dialectical Behavior Therapy
Institute
Portland, OR
Chapter 5

Pamela Marcus, RN, APRN, PMH-BC
Associate Professor of Nursing, Prince George
Community College
Clinical Specialist and Psychotherapist, Private Practice
Largo, MD
Chapters 14, 27

J. Goodlett McDaniel, MBA, EdD, PMHCS-BC, PMHNP-BC
Associate Professor and Associate Provost
George Mason University
Fairfax, VA
Chapter 31

Margaret M. McLaughlin, MSN, MS, ANP-BC
South Bay Mental Health
Worcester, MA
Chapter 16

Kimberley R. Meyer, RN, MSN, EdD
Associate Professor of Nursing, Bethel University
St. Paul, MN
Chapter 18

Betty D. Morgan, PhD, PMHCNS-BC
Associate Professor Emeritus, University of
Massachusetts–Lowell
Lowell, MA
Chapter 20

Brant Oliver, MS, MPH, PhD, FNP-BC, PMHNP-BC
Assistant Professor
MGH Institute of Health Professions School of Nursing
Boston, MA
Chapter 26

Lora Peppard, DNP, PMHNP-BC
Assistant Professor and DNP Program Director
George Mason University
Fairfax, VA
Chapter 31

Elizabeth A. Peterson, RN, DMin
Department Chair and Professor of Nursing
Bethel University
St. Paul, MN
Chapter 6

Barbara Steele, MS, APRN, PMHNP-BC
Private Practice
Concord & Nashua, NH
Chapter 19

Natasha Maynard Thomas, MSN, GNP-BC, PMHNP-BC, Esq.
Nurse Practitioner/Attorney
Stamford, CT
Chapter 10

Barbara Jones Warren, RN, PhD, APRN, PMHCNS-BC, FAAN
Professor of Clinical Nursing and Director of the
Psychiatric Mental Health Nurse Practitioner Specialty
The Ohio State University College of Nursing
Columbus, OH
Chapter 4

Donna McCarten White, RN, PhD, CNS, CADAC, CARN
Addiction Specialist, Lemuel Shattuck Hospital
MGH Institute of Health Professions
Boston, MA
Chapter 20

Christine L. Williams, RN, DNSc, PMHCS-BC
Distinguished Professor and Director of the PhD
Program in Nursing
Florida Atlantic University
Boca Raton, FL
Chapter 28

Brendan P. Wynne, DNP, PMHNP-BC
Psychiatric Nurse Practitioner
Lahey Hospital and Medical Center
Burlington, MA
Chapter 32

Reviewers

We are grateful to all the nurses, both clinicians and educators, who reviewed the manuscript of this text. Their insights, suggestions, and eye for detail helped us prepare a more relevant and useful book, one that focuses on the essential components of learning in the field of psychiatric–mental health nursing.

Diane E. Allen, MN, RN-BC, NEA-BC
New Hampshire Hospital
Concord, NH

Kim Amer, PhD, RN
DePaul University
Chicago, IL

Fredrick Astle, PhD, APRN, PMHCNS-BC
University of South Carolina
Columbia, SC

Diane Babral, MSN, RN
James Madison University
Harrisonburg, VA

Elizabeth Bonham, PhD, RN, PMHCNS-BC
University of Southern Indiana
Evansville, IN

Cynthia Bostick, PhD, RN, PMHCNS-BC
New Mexico State University
Las Cruces, NM

Nancy Buccola, MSN, APRN, PMHCNS-BC, CNE
LSU Health New Orleans
New Orleans, LA

Mary Ann Camann, PhD, RN, PMHCNS-BC
Kennesaw State University
Kennesaw, GA

Jeanette Crawford, MSN, RN
Georgia Perimeter College
Clarkston, GA

Catherine M. Dempewolf, MSN, RN
Fox Valley Technical College
Appleton, WI

Amber Donnelli, PhD, RN, CNE
Great Basin College
Elko, NV

Dianna Douglas, DNS, APRN-CNS
LSU Health New Orleans
New Orleans, LA

Sharalee Dowd, MSN, RN
Barnes Jewish College
St. Louis, MO

Chris Fasching, APRN, FNP-BC
James Madison University
Harrisonburg, VA

Leslie Folds, EdD, MSN, PMHCNS-BC, CNE
Belmont University
Nashville, TN

Diane Novack Gardner, EdD, APRN, PMHCNS-BC, CNE
University of West Florida (Retired)
Pensacola, FL

Melissa Garno, EdD, RN
Georgia Southern University
Statesboro, GA

Catherine Gilbert, EdD, RN
Armstrong Atlantic State University
Savannah, GA

Lillie F. Granger, MSN, RN
University of North Carolina–Greensboro
Greensboro, NC

Ginny Wacker Guido, JD, MSN, RN, FAAN
Washington State University (retired)
Vancouver, WA

Michele Hackney, MSN, CNE
University of Mary Hardin–Baylor
Belton, TX

Janice Harris, MSN, RN
Middle Tennessee State University
Murfreesboro, TN

Valerie Hart, EdD, APRN, PMHCNS-BC
University of Southern Maine
Portland, ME

Peggy Hernandez, EdD, APRN, PMHCNS-BC, CNE
Wichita State University
Wichita, KS

Judith Jarosinki, PhD, RN, CNE
Salisbury University
Salisbury, MD

Florence Keane, DNSc, MSN, MBA
Florida International University
Miami, FL

Dana Kemery, MSN, RN, CEN, CPEN
Drexel University
Philadelphia, PA

Sally Lehr, PhD, PMHCNS-BC, FAACS, CIRT
Emory University
Atlanta, GA

April Magoteaux, PhD, RN, CSN, NHA
Columbus State Community College
Columbus, OH

Susan Maloney, PhD, FNP-BC
Edinboro University
Edinboro, PA

Diana Marbley, RN
Milwaukee Area Technical College
Milwaukee, WI

Joan Masters, EdD, MBA, APRN, PMHNP-BC
Bellarmine University
Louisville, KY

Leslie Miles, DNP, APRN, BC
Brigham Young University
Provo, UT

Cheryl Miller, EdD, MSN, BSN
Chattanooga State Community College
Chattanooga, TN

Anna Moore, RN, MSN
J. Sargeant Reynolds Community College
Goochland, VA

Kesha Nelson, MSN/Ed, RN, CPN
Northern Kentucky University
Highland Heights, KY

Patricia O'Brien, PhD, MA, RN
Long Island University
Brooklyn, NY

Pamela Phillips, PhD, MSN, RN
Blue Ridge Community College
Flat Rock, NC

Victoria Queen, MSN, RN
Greenville Technical College
Greenville, SC

Carole-Rae Reed, RN, PhD, CNS
Stockton College
Galloway, NJ

Judy Risko, MSN, RN PMHCNS-BC
Malone University
Canton, OH

Nancy Runyan, MSN, RN
Mansfield University
Mansfield, PA

Donna Sachse, PhD, APRN, BC
Union University–Germantown
Germantown, TN

Tara Sadler, RN, BSN
South Arkansas Community College
El Dorado, AK

Nancy Scanlan, MSN, FPMHNP-BC
SUNY–Plattsburgh
Plattsburgh, NY

Barbara A. Stephens, DNP, APRN, PMHCNS-BC
Temple University
Philadelphia, PA

Gail Stern, MSN, RN
Lehigh Valley Health Network
Allentown, PA

Theresa Schwindenhammer, MSN, RN
Methodist College of Nursing
Peoria, IL

Linda Turchin, MSN, RN
Fairmont State University
Fairmont, WV

Nancy Turner, MSN, RN
West Kentucky Community and Technical College
Paducah, KY

Suzanne Urban, MS, RN, BC, CNE
Mansfield University
Mansfield, PA

Christine G. Walton, RN, MSN
Austin Community College
Austin, TX

Sheila Webster, MA, MSSA, BSN
Kent State University
Kent, OH

Cathy Weitzel, MSN, APRN, CNS-BC
Wichita State University
Wichita, KS

Shana Westerfield, PhD, MSN, MBA, MEd, RN, PMHNP-BC, CPHQ, CCM
Houston Community College
Houston, TX

Kathy Wilson, MS, RN, CRRN
Tyler Junior College
Tyler, TX

Alice B. Younce, DNP, MSN
University of South Alabama
Mobile, AL

Jaclene Zauszniewski, PHD, RN-BC, FAAN
Case Western Reserve University
Cleveland, OH

And Thanks Also To...

The authors gratefully appreciate and acknowledge the expertise and contribution of Brant Oliver, PhD, NP, MSN, MPH, to the section on QSEN in Chapter 1.

Dr. Potter gratefully acknowledges Lyndsie Ryalls, MSN, PMHNP-BC, a former graduate student for her contributions to Chapter 13.

Carole Farley-Toombs thanks the psychiatric nursing leadership team in her department for their total engagement in an empowering leadership model that makes a difference in the lives of patients every day.

Mary White Kudless thanks her mother, Margaret Sullivan White, and her husband, John M. Kudless, for their love and encouragement.

Barbara J. Limandri thanks Laura Rodgers, PhD, PMHNP-BC.

Pamela Marcus thanks her patient "Paula" for permission to share her story.

J. Goodlett McDaniel acknowledges the support of his partner, Paul Clark, PhD, LCSW.

Brant Oliver acknowledges the able assistance of Molly Jepsen, MSN, PMHNP-BC.

PREFACE

Each year, patients with mental illness enter the health care system not just for mental health care, but also for regular physical examinations and for treatment of acute or chronic medical illness. In addition, acute or chronic illness can provoke stress responses that bring on symptoms of anxiety, depression, and/or grief. As a result, nurses in all settings will encounter and have the privilege to care for patients on a continuum of mental health.

Psychiatric–Mental Health Nursing: From Suffering to Hope is designed to help nursing students recognize the signs of patient suffering and help promote hope and healing in patients across this continuum. Within its pages, nursing students will learn to recognize how the five domains of wellness—biological, psychological, sociological, cultural, and spiritual—affect and are affected by mental health and illness. Students will learn how neurobiological, genetic, and environmental constructs and familial, cultural, and spiritual values and practices affect individual wellness and inform nursing care. In addition, nursing students will learn interventions to help patients progress from high-acuity mental illness occurring at the initial onset or during a relapse through to recovery, during which patients begin to experience lower levels of acuity and learn how to manage their illness, to rehabilitation, when patients are able to return to a more normal level of functioning and engage fully in home, school, and work environments. This is particularly important because patients with mental illness can—and do—get well. To do this, they need to believe, to have hope that they can become well again, and they need to have a plan and strategies to help them on the path to wellness. Nurses in all settings need to be able to help patients navigate the health care system, manage their mental and physical health care, and believe that they can get better and reach full recovery. .

To help nursing students understand patients with mental illness and options for interventions and treatments available, *Psychiatric–Mental Health Nursing: From Suffering to Hope* is designed to:

- Provide examples of nursing interventions that will help relieve patient suffering and promote hope for recovery.

- Provide strategies nurses can use as they care for patients with mental illness, regardless of setting. These include everything from steps nurses can use to teach patients how to relax their breathing to examples of nursing interventions for patients experiencing severe anxiety, psychosis, symptoms of dementia, sleep disturbance, sexual dysfunction, and so on.

- Outline both the neurobiology and psychology of mental health to help students understand that patients with mental illness are not lying, making it up, or able to change their behavior simply because they want to.

- Present information on specific psychiatric disorders identified in the *Diagnostic and Statistical Manual of Mental Disorders* (5th ed.), published in 2013 by the American Psychiatric Association.

- Provide contexts for psychiatric illness and recovery—discussing how family members, cultural values and beliefs, and sociologic constructs affect mental illness and patient care

- Provide information relevant to nurses in the workplace: discussions of the legal and ethical issues surrounding patient care, as well as an overview of leadership and management skills that nurses need in professional health care environments.

- Address the needs of patients across the life span.

Organization

We received a number of suggestions for how to achieve the appropriate order of the chapters. Bearing in mind that faculty can assign chapters in any order they prefer, we have provided an organizational structure that we think will be accessible to a wide variety of nursing programs.

The first unit, Foundational Continuum of Psychiatric–Mental Health Nursing, presents six chapters that provide students with the scientific, theoretical, historical, and sociocultural constructs that inform psychiatric nursing practice today.

The second unit, Continuum of Psychiatric Nursing Role Development, provides nursing students with strategies and interventions they will need to provide care for patients with mental illness, including information regarding the importance of self-reflection and self-awareness in nursing practice; guidance for building the nurse–patient relationship and using therapeutic communication; an overview of the nursing process, particularly its application in psychiatric nursing; an overview of applicable ethical and legal concepts; and information on management and leadership skills and activities that promote successful nursing practice.

In the third unit, students will find information about the Continuum of Specific Psychiatric Disorders. Rather than following the organization of the DSM-5, this text introduces sleep–wake disorders and disorders of anxiety, stress, and trauma first. This is in part because an understanding of sleep disturbance and anxiety symptoms is fundamental to caring for patients with a wide variety of illnesses, both medical and psychiatric. Generalist nurses, as well as nurses considering a mental health practice, will benefit from knowing how to promote sleep hygiene, reduce anxiety, and identify symptoms of trauma early in their interactions with patients. Following these chapters, the book continues with other major categories of disorders recognized in the DSM-5. Some disorders, such as somatoform and dissociative disorders, though not prevalent, are of sufficient complexity to warrant attention. Other disorders, such as neurocognitive disorders (which include Alzheimer disease) are increasing in prevalence at disturbing rates and cause a great deal of suffering for both patients and family members.

Each chapter provides an overview of etiology and impact of the disorders through the lens of the domains of patient functioning—biological, psychological, sociological, cultural, and spiritual—as well as outlining options for the collaborative care of patients through the variety of pharmacologic and nonpharmacologic treatments shown to have a positive impact on patients with those disorders. A detailed nursing management section outlines assessment, diagnosis and planning, implementation, and evaluation of nursing care for patients diagnosed with disorders in that category. A combination of features provides nurses with meaningful strategies they can use in caring for patients. For instance, the feature "Perceptions, Thoughts, and Feelings: Validating Patient Care" gives examples of how nurses can validate their understanding of patients' concerns and help patients clarify their understanding of their mental illness and its effects on themselves and others. Evidence-Based Practice features provide examples of the implications of research on nursing practice. Nursing Care Plans assist nursing students with understanding how to develop a care plan based on a specific nursing diagnosis.

The fourth unit, Continuum of Treatments and Interventions, explores options patients have for treatment as well as nursing interventions specific to incidents critical to patient health and safety, including crisis intervention, suicide, and loss and grieving. A separate chapter on pharmacotherapy provides a basis of understanding of the role of and classes of psychotropic drugs. A chapter on complementary and alternative therapies provides an overview of both natural products and mind–body practices and their use in patients with mental illness. A chapter on group and family therapy provides an overview of working in group settings and with families experiencing mental health challenges. Finally, the unit looks at interventions for individuals in crises of different kinds, as well as interventions specific to caring for patients exhibiting suicidal ideation or behaviors and strategies for working with patients experiencing loss and grief.

The fifth unit addresses Considerations across the Continuum of Life, and includes an overview of behaviors and disorders commonly seen in children and adolescents; issues in adult transitions that affect patient mental health and care; and aspects of caring for older adults who may have been managing mental illness for a lifetime or who may be diagnosed with mental illness late in life.

Application of the Nursing Process

The nursing process is outlined in detail in Chapter 8 and throughout the chapters on the different mental disorders recognized by the American Psychiatric Association's *Diagnostic and Statistical Manual of Mental Disorders*, 5th edition (DSM-5). The heading "Nursing Management" highlights nursing assessment, diagnosis and planning, implementation, and evaluation. In addition, we feature nursing care plans throughout the text. The nursing care plans address nursing care for patients with diagnoses that are frequently seen in patients who present with the disorder that is outlined in the chapter. In most cases, the nursing care plan is built on the critical thinking feature, a longitudinal case study that describes a representative patient seeking treatment for the disorder.

Nurses today face many new challenges, among them the growing number of patients in the community who are experiencing mental illness. Changes in the workplace in response to quality improvement efforts, an ongoing nursing shortage, dramatic advances in health care knowledge, a growing population of veterans with mental health needs, and a variety of environmental disasters require skilled nurses in every setting to be prepared to work with patients with mental illness and their families. We believe that nurses are in a unique position to have a tremendous impact on their patients, families, and communities, to reduce burden levels, and to bring hope to those in need. Our goal in writing this text is to help prepare nurses with the skills and knowledge to make a positive difference for patients with mental illness and their families who are striving to maintain or regain their mental health in any and every setting in which nurses work.

Mertie L. Potter
Mary D. Moller

VISUAL GUIDE

The Visual Guide walks you through the structure and features of the text. Note that the features are color coded for ease of use.

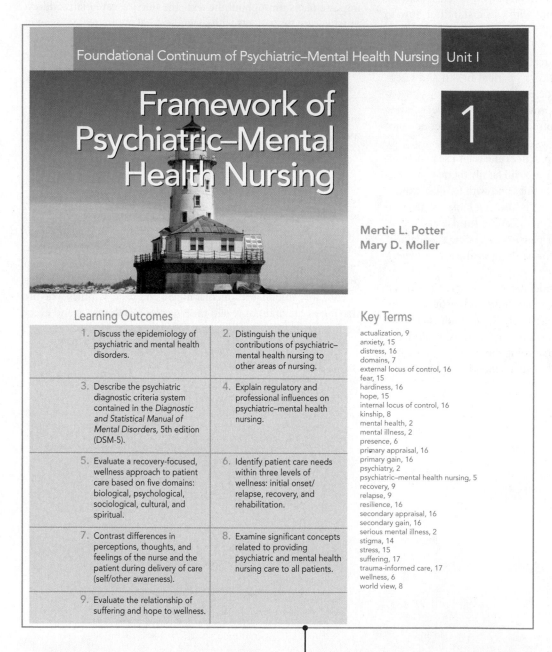

Foundational Continuum of Psychiatric–Mental Health Nursing Unit I

Framework of Psychiatric–Mental Health Nursing

1

Mertie L. Potter
Mary D. Moller

Learning Outcomes

1. Discuss the epidemiology of psychiatric and mental health disorders.

2. Distinguish the unique contributions of psychiatric–mental health nursing to other areas of nursing.

3. Describe the psychiatric diagnostic criteria system contained in the *Diagnostic and Statistical Manual of Mental Disorders*, 5th edition (DSM-5).

4. Explain regulatory and professional influences on psychiatric–mental health nursing.

5. Evaluate a recovery-focused, wellness approach to patient care based on five domains: biological, psychological, sociological, cultural, and spiritual.

6. Identify patient care needs within three levels of wellness: initial onset/relapse, recovery, and rehabilitation.

7. Contrast differences in perceptions, thoughts, and feelings of the nurse and the patient during delivery of care (self/other awareness).

8. Examine significant concepts related to providing psychiatric and mental health nursing care to all patients.

9. Evaluate the relationship of suffering and hope to wellness.

Key Terms

actualization, 9
anxiety, 15
distress, 16
domains, 7
external locus of control, 16
fear, 15
hardiness, 16
hope, 15
internal locus of control, 16
kinship, 8
mental health, 2
mental illness, 2
presence, 6
primary appraisal, 16
primary gain, 16
psychiatry, 2
psychiatric–mental health nursing, 5
recovery, 9
relapse, 9
resilience, 16
secondary appraisal, 16
secondary gain, 16
serious mental illness, 2
stigma, 14
stress, 15
suffering, 17
trauma-informed care, 17
wellness, 6
world view, 8

Each chapter begins with **learning outcomes** and **key terms.**

critical thinking

Kara Initial Onset

Kara Murphy is a 16-year-old female patient who presents for admission to a psychiatric inpatient unit. She is accompanied by her mother. When Liz, a registered nurse who works on the unit, invites Kara into a room to complete her admission assessment, Kara's mother accompanies her. Kara is casually dressed in baggy clothes, appears to be of average height and weight, and has bloodshot eyes. Her cheeks and neck appear puffy and swollen. During the assessment, Kara appears defensive, slouching in a chair with her arms crossed, and answers questions with one-word answers. Kara's mother gives answers to all questions, even those directed at Kara, while Kara continues to sit with her arms crossed and rolls her eyes and sighs heavily when her mother speaks. Kara's mother reports to the nurse that during a recent argument, Kara "told me she was going to kill herself." Kara's mother adds, "I don't know what to do with her anymore, so I brought her to the hospital."

During the assessment, Liz discovers that Kara had a prior psychiatric hospitalization for the treatment of anorexia nervosa when she was 13, and that Kara has continued to struggle with disordered eating, most recently binging and purging. Kara reports that the argument leading to her hospitalization occurred when her mother woke up late at night to find Kara binging, already having eaten a box of cereal, two large bags of potato chips, two sandwiches, and a large container of pasta salad. Kara reports that when her mother found her binging, she told Kara she was "disgusting" and then tried to physically prevent Kara from entering the bathroom to purge. Kara says at that point she became distraught and reports, "I said I was going to kill myself."

Liz learns that Kara's problems started around age 11, which her mother associates with her having started menarche early and ahead of her friends. Her mother says, "From that point on, she was just really uncomfortable in her own body." Kara's mother also reports that around this time she and Kara's father divorced and she was forced to return to work full time, having been able to stay at home with Kara (who is an only child) until that point. It was around this time that Kara began restricting food and was eventually hospitalized for anorexia at age 13 with a body mass index (BMI) of 14.5. Kara reports that since her hospitalization she has continued to have trouble; most recently, she has had episodes of binging and purging. She says, "I try to restrict what I eat, but I can't. I usually end up totally out of control and binging. Then I feel so bad, I have to try to throw it all up to stop myself from getting fat."

In addition to the ongoing problems with disordered eating, Kara reports that she experiences significant anxiety and depression. She reports she has very poor self-esteem, and constantly has negative self-thoughts about "being fat and ugly." Kara says she feels anxious most days and worries that she is going to have to stay back in school next year because her anxiety has led to her missing school and being unable to attend to her work when she is there. Kara acknowledges that all these problems have

APPLICATION

1. Address the five domains for Kara:
   a. Biological
   b. Psychological
   c. Sociological
   d. Cultural
   e. Spiritual
2. In what ways do you think Kara may be suffering? Why?
3. How would you prioritize Kara's needs at this time? Why?
4. In what way does Liz convey hope to Kara? What might you have done differently to offer hope?

Unfolding case studies portray a representative patient at the different points of wellness, from initial onset or relapse, to recovery, to rehabilitation.

DEPRESSIVE DISORDERS

Theoretical Foundations

What causes depression? Why do some individuals develop depression while others do not? Like many disease processes, depression is a multifaceted illness that is most likely due to a complex and dynamic interaction among biological, psychological, sociological, cultural, and spiritual factors. The **diathesis–stress model** postulates that individuals inherit tendencies to express certain traits or behaviors when exposed to the right conditions or stressors (Figure 16-2). Seemingly, psychological events have the ability to initiate or exacerbate a neurochemical imbalance in susceptible individuals. Thus, it would seem that under the right circumstances and given a genetic vulnerability, an individual will develop depression. However, simply having a propensity toward developing depression alone (for example, having a strong family history of depression in one or both parents) is not enough to trigger illness. An individual's diathesis (hereditary predisposition) must interact with life events to set the stage for illness. In addition, it would seem that the greater the inherited vulnerability, the less environmental stress will be needed to trigger depression. Life trauma (such as sexual abuse, physical abuse,

Biological Domain

The biological models of depression have focused on alterations in the neurotransmitters and brain structures responsible for mood regulation, as well as genetic, endocrine, and circadian factors that are responsible for depression (Warren & Lutz, 2009). These models give credence not only to the mood symptoms associated with depression, but also to its physical manifestations.

Neurotransmitters and Brain Structures

The last decade has seen exponential growth in the understanding of the complexities of the brain structures and neurotransmitters that control emotion and regulate mood. Although a full discourse of brain anatomy and physiology is beyond the scope of this chapter, an appreciation of some basic principles is essential.

When studying areas of the brain responsible for emotion and mood regulation, most research focuses on the prefrontal area, the limbic system, and the basal ganglia (Figure 16-3). Extensive functional and neuroanatomic connections exist among these structures. Of these three areas, the limbic system is the area most responsible for mood and emotion. At the base of

The section on **theoretical foundations** provides information related to current knowledge of the pathophysiology and etiology of psychiatric disorders, as well as context related to the five domains of wellness: biological, psychological, sociological, cultural, and spiritual.

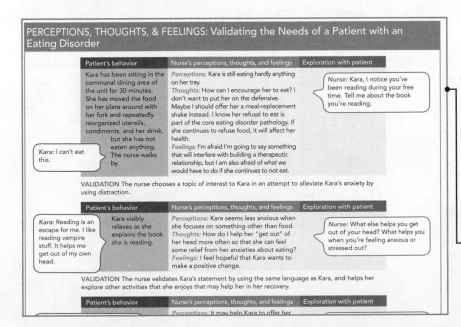

PERCEPTIONS, THOUGHTS, & FEELINGS: Validating the Needs of a Patient with an Eating Disorder

The **"Perceptions, Thoughts, and Feelings"** feature provides a sample interaction between a nurse and patient to help students build a foundation for therapeutic communication with their patients. These interactions also show how the nurse can provide validation and support to patients, even at times when the nurse is unsure of how to proceed. Rationales are provided to further validate the nurse's attempts to engage the patient.

Nurses Assisting Families

evidence-based practice

Clinical Problem

amilies struggle with their roles when caring for a family member diagnosed with mental illness. What can psychiatric nurses do to assist families as they struggle to do what is best for them and for their family member?

Evidence

Nordby, Kjønsberg, and Hummelvoll (2010) reported on results of nterviews with eight focus groups in southern Norway using a thematic analysis abstract. Focus group members were all relatives of persons with recently discovered SMI. Researchers looked at what acilitates active involvement for family members in the treatment and rehabilitation of their family member. They found that family members:

- Wanted their ill relative to be treated as a person, in addition to as a person who is ill
- Wanted staff to convey hope regardless of the circumstances, as they felt it was important for them to cope
- Needed to know what to say to their family members, how to behave with them, and what happens after discharge
- Felt their stress level decreased when they could share their concerns and receive help

n addition, researchers found that parents wanted to be involved early in their children's care and to feel that their concerns and deas were heard. Staff perceived themselves as experts on psychosis; families considered themselves experts on their family member. Family members reported mostly positive experiences from their interactions with staff. Family members and staff emphasized the importance of developing positive interactions that involved sharing information and giving guidance and support. Family members expressed a need for staff members to convey and nurture hope related to the patient's recovery and quality of life.

Foster explored the experience of being an adult child of a parent with serious mental illness and how adult children have coped with their experience. Foster analyzed 10 participants' responses using van Manen's hermeneutic method. Four themes emerged:

- Being uncertain: "You'd think this roller coaster was never going to stop."
- Struggling to connect: "We were super close and now we're not."
- Being responsible: "I think I grew up in a hurry."
- Seeking balance: "I had to be in control of the situation so awful things wouldn't happen." (Foster, 2010, pp. 3143–3151)

Foster concluded that children of parents diagnosed with mental illness experience a very chaotic family life, and adult children assume substantial caregiving roles. Relationships between parents and adult children can become strained. Professionals can help strengthen adult children's resilience and ability to cope by providing support. Nurses can give information and support to children and families in which parents have a mental illness. Focusing care on the family can enhance children's and parent's relationships and support the family's ability to cope.

Tas, Guvenir, and Cevrim (2010) performed a retrospective study with families and their adolescents who received treatment in a recently opened unit. They surveyed five areas: admission process, staff, environment/services, treatment interventions, and treatment outcome satisfaction levels of the adolescents and their families regarding service they received during their stay in the unit that were rated high. Results of the questionnaires completed by adolescents and parents revealed that availability and helpfulness of the staff and the admission process were given the highest satisfaction scores.

Implications for Nursing

Nurses are in key positions to assist families who are caring for another family member diagnosed with mental illness. Family members identify hope as important in their ability to cope and want care providers to convey hope regardless of the circumstances of their family member. Nurses can provide support and hope, which help strengthen family members' resilience and ability to cope. Patient and family satisfaction are rated high when staff are available and respond to the family's concerns.

Critical Thinking Questions

1. What strategies assisted family members in the studies cited?
2. Why do you think families identified these as helpful?
3. How might you employ any of these strategies?
4. How will you approach families differently after reading the reviews of this evidence?

Evidence-based practice features demonstrate how research informs nursing practice.

Kara—A Patient with Bulimia Nervosa

NURSING CARE PLAN

Nursing Diagnosis: Risk for injury related to suicidal ideation and uncontrollable binge–purge cycles as evidenced by patient self-report of suicidal ideation and binging and purging episodes.

Short-Term Goals *Patient will:* (include date for short-term goal to be met)	**Intervention** *Nurse will:*	**Rationale**
Remain free from self-directed harm while on the inpatient unit.	Assess for suicidal thoughts and other self-directed harm and implement suicide precautions as needed.	Priority is given to the continuous monitoring of suicidal thinking and self-directed harm behavior, which is crucial to maintaining safe treatment.
Be able to identify physical complications of binging and purging behaviors by day 3 of her admission.	Teach the patient about harmful effects of binging and purging including dental erosion, cardiac problems, and electrolyte disturbances.	Patient education and health teaching are imperative to treatment and is an integral part of the patient's understanding of the positive outcomes of healthy eating behaviors.
Identify distorted thoughts that precede episodes of binging and purging by day 5 of admission.	Provide emotional support before, during, and after meals and explore dysfunctional thought patterns.	Emotional support by the nurse helps to build therapeutic relationship. Nonjudgmental reframing of distorted thinking engenders improved communication.
Eat a reasonable amount of food without binging or purging 50% of the time by day 7 of admission to the inpatient unit.	Monitor for signs and symptoms of binging and purging behaviors including trips to the bathroom after eating, hoarding food, increased serum amylase, and swollen parotid glands.	Frequent monitoring is essential in the treatment of eating disorders. Patients are often resistant due to intense fears about gaining weight and therefore may not accurately report binging or purging behavior.
Long-Term Goal Kara will abstain from binging and purging and will have identified and used new skills for managing triggers for disordered eating behavior.	Collaborate with Kara to independently implement identified alternative stress-reduction techniques that will prevent disordered eating behavior.	Promoting patient autonomy and independence in managing life stressors is essential in the treatment of eating disorders.

Clinical Reasoning

1. What other nursing diagnoses might be appropriate for Kara?
2. What strategies or techniques might help Kara to process distorted thinking or reduce her stress level?

Nursing care plans extend the unfolding case studies to illustrate appropriate short- and long-term goals for a representative patient.

Collaborative Care

Collaborative care of patients with SSDs requires a multidisciplinary approach that typically includes treatment with antipsychotics and one or more psychosocial treatments. Health promotion and education are critical for patients with SSDs; these are discussed later, in the section on Nursing Management.

Psychopharmacology

The quality of the relationship between the care provider and the patient is critical to treatment success. Initial patient education includes medication indications, expected and adverse effects, when to report adverse effects, alternative treatments available, rationale for dosing decisions, and the likelihood of relapse if medication is discontinued.

Antipsychotics

Antipsychotic medications are the mainstay of SSD treatment. Antipsychotic medications are categorized as either typical or atypical on the basis of similarities in the mechanism of action (Chapter 23). The older, typical, or first-generation antipsychotic (FGA) medications act primarily to reduce positive symptoms by blocking dopamine receptors and increasing dopamine destruction.

Second-generation antipsychotics (SGAs) have an antagonist function against serotonin, as well as dopamine (Citrome, 2012; Stahl, 2013.). Although FGAs are still prescribed, SGAs generally are the treatment of choice based on side-effect profile and improvements in negative symptoms. In 2002, aripiprazole (Abilify), a third-generation antipsychotic, was made available. This medication has a partial agonist function for dopamine rather than an antagonist function. The medications feature provides dosage information, side effects, and nursing interventions for common SGAs and aripiprazole.

A meta-analysis of 150 double-blind studies including 21,533 the WBC > 3000 and ANC > 1500.

If the WBC is initially between 3000 and 3500 but falls to 3000 in 3 weeks or less and the ANC is >1500 mm^3, the WBC with differential should be repeated twice a week until WBC > 3500.

Extrapyramidal Symptoms

Extrapyramidal side effects (EPSs) are common in patients treated with antipsychotic medications (Veselinović et al., 2011) and involve an imbalance between dopamine and acetylcholine in the extrapyramidal system of the basal ganglia. As such, the symptoms involve the systemic motor system. Side effects may be acute or chronic. Acute EPSs include medication-induced Parkinsonism (e.g., muscle rigidity, tremors, problems with gait), dystonia (acute muscle spasms, often in the extremities), akathisia (intolerable restlessness and inability to sit still), opisthotonus (severe arching of the back), and oculogyric crisis (eyeballs rolling back into the socket). These acute side effects cause extreme distress and pain. They usually occur within the first hours, days, or weeks of treatment, are dose dependent, and are reversible if medication is reduced or discontinued. They are most common with the first generation antipsychotics that are primarily dopamine 2 receptor blockers, many of the antidepressants that effect the norepinephrine/dopamine systems, and antihistamines.

The primary chronic EPS is tardive dyskinesia (TD), which occurs after months or years of medication exposure and typically involve the oral/facial/maxillary muscles, causing uncontrollable twitching of the eyes and neck, tongue thrusting, and eye blinking. Early identification and a withdrawal or reduction of medication may be sufficient to reverse the side effects, but otherwise EPSs—in particular, TD—may be irreversible even if medication is discontinued (Adams, Holland, & Urban, 2014). In the case of acute EPS, anticholinergic/antihistamine medications can be helpful, except in akathisia, in which the treatment of choice is norepinephrine beta-blockers (Aia, Ravuelta, Cloud, & Factor, 2011).

Collaborative care sections cover pharmacologic and nonpharmacologic therapies used in the treatment of patients with psychiatric disorders.

Mood Disorders

medications commonly used to treat

Commonly Used Antidepressants

Medication	Initial Daily Dose*	Therapeutic Daily Dose Range*	Key Nursing Considerations for Medication Class
Selective Serotonin Reuptake inhibitors (SSRIs)			
citalopram (Celexa)	20 mg	20–40 mg	Instruct regarding onset of action; side effects may be minimized by starting at low doses and titrating slowly, but this may delay therapeutic onset of action. Side effects lessen with continued drug use.
escitalopram (Lexapro)	5–10 mg	10–20 mg	Discourage abrupt withdrawal or discontinuation of medication.
fluoxetine (Prozac)	10–20 mg	10–80 mg	Grapefruit juice may increase the plasma levels of some SSRIs.
fluvoxamine (Luvox)	25–50 mg	50–300 mg	Advise/monitor for common side effects of insomnia, early agitation or restlessness, sweating, GI disturbance, weight gain, sexual side effects.
paroxetine (Paxil)	10 mg	10–80 mg	Monitor for and report worsening of depression or onset of suicidal ideation.
sertraline (Zoloft)	25–50 mg	50–200 mg	
Monoamine oxidase inhibitors (MAOIs)			
isocarboxazid (Marplan)	10 mg	10–30 mg	Instruct regarding the dietary restrictions on tyramine-rich foods and drug to drug interactions; report severe headache, palpitations, chest pain or shortness of breath.
phenelzine (Nardil)	15 mg	60–90 mg	Discourage the use of caffeine.
tranylcypromine (Parnate)	30 mg	30–60 mg	Advise/monitor for common side effects of insomnia, headache, sedation, increased stimulation, dry mouth, constipation. Monitor for and report worsening symptoms or onset of suicidal ideation.
selegiline (Eldepryl, Ensam)	6 mg/24 hr patch	6–12 mg/24 hr patch	

Medications features provide an overview of medications commonly used in the treatment of different disorders.

Diagnostic Criteria for Insomnia Disorders

DSM-5

A. A predominant complaint of dissatisfaction with sleep quantity or quality, associated with one (or more) of the following symptoms:
   1. Difficulty initiating sleep. (In children, this may manifest as difficulty initiating sleep without caregiver intervention.)
   2. Difficulty maintaining sleep, characterized by frequent awakenings or problems returning to sleep after awakenings. (In children, this may manifest as difficulty returning to sleep without caregiver intervention.)
   3. Early-morning awakening with inability to return to sleep.
B. The sleep disturbance causes clinically significant distress or impairment in social, occupational, educational, academic, behavioral, or other important areas of functioning.
C. The sleep difficulty occurs at least 3 nights per week.
D. The sleep difficulty is present for at least 3 months.
E. The sleep difficulty occurs despite adequate opportunity for sleep.
F. The insomnia is not better explained by and does not occur exclusively during the course of another sleep–wake disorder (e.g., narcolepsy, a breathing-related sleep disorder, a circadian rhythm sleep–wake disorder, or a parasomnia).
G. The insomnia is not attributable to the physiological effects of a substance (e.g., a drug of abuse, a medication).
H. Coexisting mental disorders and medical conditions do not adequately explain the predominant complaint of insomnia.

Source: Reprinted with permission from the *Diagnostic and Statistical Manual of Mental Disorders*, Fifth Edition, (Copyright 2013). American Psychiatric Association.

rhythm disorders, if chronic and impairing function, are best treated by sleep specialists. Treatment usually includes supplemental melatonin 3 to 4 hours before the target time of sleep onset and early-morning bright-light therapy.

Approximately 20% of United States employees work shifts other than the traditional 9-to-5 workday (Erren, 2010). As a

Both polysomnography and the Multiple Sleep Latency Test (MSLT) confirm the loss of a normal sleep–wake pattern (American Academy of Sleep Medicine, 2001).

Several issues contribute to sleep deprivation secondary to shift work. Two main contributors to inadequate sleep in shift workers are social stressors and biological influences. Social stressors include

The **DSM-5 Diagnostic Criteria** feature provides the diagnostic criteria for a specific disorder as outlined in the *Diagnostic and Statistical Manual of Mental Disorders*, 5th edition.

Nursing Management

Nursing considerations of patients with depressive or bipolar disorders focus on safety, reducing symptom burden, and assisting the patient in returning to normal functioning. As with any patient situation, thorough assessment is needed to ensure the plan of care is based on accurate information. Patients with depressive and bipolar disorders often experience prolonged periods of despair. Nursing interventions that promote hope and help patients believe that they can return to normal functioning are essential.

Assessment

All nurses need to be versed in the evaluation and assessment of mood disorders, regardless of practice environment. The U.S. Preventive Services Task Force (2009) recommends screening children, adolescents, and adults for depression in primary care practice. A variety of standardized, easy-to-use, empirically validated assessment tools are available within the public domain and can be used with minimal burden to the patient and clinician (Table 16-6). Many of these tools also are effective measures of clinical improvement and can be used to monitor, modify, and document treatment. Nurses should familiarize themselves with several of these tools and integrate them into the evaluation to achieve optimal outcomes through the use of evidence-bas tice and standardized measures (Harding et al., 2011). The use dardized measures in clinical practice serves to inform the tr plan, improves communication between providers, and allows sonalized treatment. Once symptoms of depression or other m turbance have been identified, a complete evaluation withi domains of health should be undertaken.

Observation and Physical Assessment

Assessment of patients with depression and bipolar disorder with observation. It is through skilled observation that th gains insight into the patient's difficulties and suffering. Obse of the patient's demeanor, facial expressions, body language iors, and communication patterns provides important info that assists the nurse in formulating the nursing diagnosis and care. The nurse should consider the following critical elemen assessment of patients with depression and bipolar disorders

Biological Domain

- *Vital signs:* Obtain a complete set of vital signs, includin static vital signs in older adults and those complaining

Nursing management sections within each disorder chapter cover assessment, diagnosis, planning, implementation, and evaluation of patients with the disorder.

ACKNOWLEDGMENTS

The journey for this new and unique undergraduate psychiatric nursing textbook began in May 2008. As a first edition, much care, devotion, and oversight have gone into the "labor" and "birthing" of this project. A major highlight in this long journey has been our association with, admiration of, and appreciation for each other as colleagues and authors. We have enjoyed supporting one another's strengths and sharing in this project together. We have grown to be close colleagues through our mutual love of psychiatric nursing and our deep shared faith in God.

There are so many people to thank. First, we would like to extend deep appreciation to our development editors. Addy McCulloch has been the lifeblood of this project. Her keen insight, wisdom, wit, knowledge, and resilience have made each step of this journey truly joyous. Addy, we are grateful for and to you for being in the labor and delivery room with us. You are the star behind this project and someone we both hold dear to our hearts. "Wyatt," Kim Wyatt of California fame, has contributed invaluable insights and clarity to this endeavor based partly on her experience as a registered nurse. We are most grateful for and to you as well.

To our chapter authors, many thanks for your hard work and determination. Without you, this book would not exist.

To our reviewers, much appreciation for helping us push even harder to make this an exceptional book.

To all the others at Pearson from the editorial to production departments, we extend our deepest appreciation and gratitude for your support of us and this project and maintaining a standard of excellence throughout its production.

To our patients, former and present, who give us the privilege of bearing with them while looking for hope amidst great suffering, we thank you.

To our colleagues, thank you for the incredible work you do to help those who suffer move to a better place in their journey.

To our students, former and future, it was in hope of helping you find effective ways to bring hope and relief to your patients that we began this endeavor.

To our friends, thank you for supporting and encouraging us while we worked on this book.

To our spouses, our children, our children's spouses, and our grandchildren, we love you and want you to know how much joy you bring to our lives. Your ongoing support made the completion of this project possible. That includes for Mertie: cherished husband and best friend Fred; children Mark, Christine, & Joy; children through love—Mona, Derrick, Dave, and Stephen; grandsons—Mark, Zane, Nicholas, and Logan; granddaughters—Quinn and Lauren. For Mary, it includes her lifelong soulmate and husband Chuck and their sons and their families: Brock and Ellen and grandsons Braxton and Briggs, and Scott and Erica and grandsons Braden and Kellan.

While respecting others' views of spirituality and faith, we want to thank God for His love and kindness in sustaining us through this project and being the basis of our hope and inspiration for this book.

Mertie L. Potter
Mary D. Moller

CONTENTS

Framework of Psychiatric–Mental Health Nursing

1

Mertie L. Potter
Mary D. Moller

Learning Outcomes

1. Discuss the epidemiology of psychiatric and mental health disorders.

2. Distinguish the unique contributions of psychiatric–mental health nursing to other areas of nursing.

3. Describe the psychiatric diagnostic criteria system contained in the *Diagnostic and Statistical Manual of Mental Disorders,* 5th edition (DSM-5).

4. Explain regulatory and professional influences on psychiatric–mental health nursing.

5. Evaluate a recovery-focused, wellness approach to patient care based on five domains: biological, psychological, sociological, cultural, and spiritual.

6. Identify patient care needs within three levels of wellness: initial onset/relapse, recovery, and rehabilitation.

7. Contrast differences in perceptions, thoughts, and feelings of the nurse and the patient during delivery of care (self/other awareness).

8. Examine significant concepts related to providing psychiatric and mental health nursing care to all patients.

9. Evaluate the relationship of suffering and hope to wellness.

Key Terms

actualization, 9
anxiety, 15
distress, 16
domains, 7
external locus of control, 16
fear, 15
hardiness, 16
hope, 15
internal locus of control, 16
kinship, 8
mental health, 2
mental illness, 2
presence, 6
primary appraisal, 16
primary gain, 16
psychiatry, 2
psychiatric–mental health nursing, 5
recovery, 9
relapse, 9
resilience, 16
secondary appraisal, 16
secondary gain, 16
serious mental illness, 2
stigma, 14
stress, 15
suffering, 17
trauma-informed care, 17
wellness, 6
world view, 8

Anthony Harris Relapse Phase

You are preparing for your first day on an inpatient psychiatric unit. You learn that your assigned patient, Mr. Anthony Harris, is a 63-year-old single White male with a recent near-lethal suicide attempt in which he cut both his wrists. Mr. Harris was found by a neighbor and taken to the emergency department (ED) three days ago; he was subsequently admitted. He has suffered from bipolar disorder for more than 30 years and has had long-standing polysubstance abuse issues, but he has been sober for the past two years. Mr. Harris has had two prior suicide attempts by overdose and multiple prior inpatient stays for both manic and depressive episodes. He has several medical issues, including obesity, hypertension (HTN), hypercholesterolemia, and gastroesophageal reflux disorder (GERD). He has never married and is not close to his immediate family. He is socially isolated and has few supports aside from his professional caregivers. Mr. Harris has recently lost his construction job and is in danger of becoming homeless. He continues to feel depressed and states that his lithium is "no longer helping like it used to." Mr. Harris expresses a desire to be started on an antidepressant. There are no current psychotic symptoms. Mr. Harris's diagnoses include the following:

- Bipolar I disorder, most recent episode depressed
- Polysubstance dependence, in remission
- Avoidant personality disorder
- Obesity—weighs 312 lbs and is 5'10" tall
- HTN—BP 158/104 mmHg
- Hypercholesterolemia—HDL = 40, LDL = 200
- GERD

You are probably thinking: *Where do I possibly start in determining how to plan care for this patient? How do I begin to develop a therapeutic relationship?*

To start taking care of this patient, it is important to think in a holistic paradigm by using the five wellness domains and three phases of illness described in this text. This book identifies key aspects of nursing care that will help this patient in the recovery process.

Mental Health and Mental Illness

The principles and practices of psychiatric–mental health nursing are foundational to all aspects of patient care. All people, including nurses, have mental health needs that must be met daily. Numerous factors, such as societal and environmental influences, the amount of stress in one's life, and resources available can affect the ability of individuals to manage their mental health needs. In addition, well-being may vary on a continuum based on the combination of factors with which the individual has to cope at any given point in time. Nurses must be able to evaluate the ongoing mental health needs of each patient—regardless of medical diagnosis and site of delivery of nursing care—as well as their own mental health needs. Additionally, nurses need the skills to determine when an unmet mental health need has the potential to, or already has, become a symptom of a mental illness.

What is the difference between mental health and mental illness? The World Health Organization (2013b, paragraph 1) defines **mental health** as "a state of well-being in which every individual realizes his or her own potential, can cope with the normal stresses of life, can work productively and fruitfully, and is able to make a contribution to her or his community." In turn, the National Alliance on Mental Illness (NAMI) defines **mental illness** as a medical condition that "disrupts a person's thinking, feeling, mood, ability to relate to others, and daily functioning" that often result in a diminished capacity for coping with the ordinary demands of life (NAMI, 2013, paragraph 1). The impact and possible impairment in functioning that an individual experiences can range from mild impairment, such as difficulty sleeping the night before an important exam, to moderate impairment, such as that

associated with a major life change, to severe or serious impairment that results in dysfunction for a significant period of time in multiple areas of functioning. **Psychiatry** is the broad discipline of medicine that encompasses the diagnosis and treatment of individuals with mental illnesses, along with their family members. In the United States, mental illnesses are diagnosed based on the *Diagnostic and Statistical Manual of Mental Disorders,* 5th edition (DSM-5)(American Psychiatric Association, 2013). The DSM-5 defines a mental disorder as:

> A syndrome characterized by clinically significant disturbance in an individual's cognition, emotion regulation, or behavior that reflects a dysfunction in the psychological, biological, or developmental processes underlying mental functioning. Mental disorders are usually associated with significant distress or disability in social, occupational, or other important activities. An expected or culturally approved response to a common stressor or loss, such as the death of a loved one, is not a mental disorder. Socially deviant behavior (e.g., political, religious, or sexual) and conflicts that are primarily between the individual and society are not mental disorders unless the deviance or conflict results from a dysfunction in the individual, as described above. (American Psychiatric Association, 2013, p. 20).

Prevalence of Mental Illness

Approximately 4% of the population (12 million people) is living with what is termed **serious mental illness** (SMI). SMIs are those that create significant disability in the person's ability to achieve life goals and

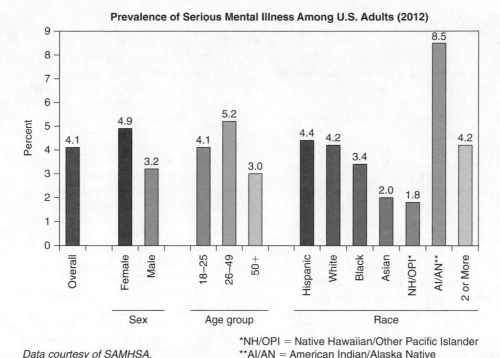

Prevalence of Serious Mental Illness Among U.S. Adults (2012)

Data courtesy of SAMHSA.

*NH/OPI = Native Hawaiian/Other Pacific Islander
**AI/AN = American Indian/Alaska Native

1-1 Prevalence of serious mental illness among U.S. adults by sex, age, and race in 2012.

include major depression, schizophrenia, bipolar disorder, obsessive–compulsive disorder (OCD), panic disorder, posttraumatic stress disorder (PTSD), and borderline personality disorder (NAMI, 2013). The World Health Organization defines illnesses by the global burden of disease, which is based on disability-adjusted life years (DALYs). DALY refers to the combination of years of life lost due to premature mortality and years of life lost due to the time lived in states of less than full health. In 2010, out of 291 diseases and injuries, depression ranked globally as the 11th most disabling illness (Murray, et al., 2012). In the United States, only about 41% of those diagnosed with *any* mental illness receive treatment (Substance Abuse and Mental Health Services Administration, 2013). See Table 1-1.

The National Institute of Mental Health (NIMH) updates the statistics on mental illness prevalence every 5 years. With more than 45,100,000 people in the United States (approximately 20% of those 18 and over) diagnosed with any mental illness (NIMH, 2010), it is certain that all nurses will encounter patients with mental illness. Mental illness knows no boundaries among sex, race, ethnicity, or socioeconomic status. See Figure 1-1.

Like patients with medical illness, patients with mental illness suffer. They also vary widely in the severity of their illness and degree of impairment, their ability to cope with their illness, their cultural and socioeconomic backgrounds, and their ability to access health care services (Box 1-1). An understanding of the key principles of psychiatric–mental health nursing will help all nurses work with patients with mental illness, give them hope, develop a recovery trajectory, and help restore them to mental health and wellness. Patients can—and do—recover from mental illness.

Classification of Psychiatric Illness
Initial attempts at classifying psychiatric diagnoses occurred because of a need to compile information on the rate of mental illness in the

Mental Health Treatment in the United States
table 1-1

Population	Number Receiving Treatment	Percentage Receiving Treatment
Adults with any mental illness	44.7 million adults / 18.6% of population	41% of those with mental illness
Adults with serious mental illness (SMI)	9.6 million adults / 4.1% of population	62.9% of those with SMI
Children ages 6–11 with any mental health disorder	5.2 million / 21% of total population	20%
Children ages 8–11 with serious emotional disorders	2.7 million / 11% of total population	53%
Adolescents ages 12–17 with any mental illness	12.5 million / 50% of total population	40%
Older adults with any mental illness	8.8 million / 20% of total population	Less than 3%

Data from Substance Abuse and Mental Health Services. (2012a). Behavioral Health, United States, 2012. Available at http://samhsa.gov/data/2012 BehavioralHealthUS/2012-BHUS.pdf; Substance Abuse and Mental Health Services Administration. (2013). Results from the 2012 National Survey on Drug Use and Health: Mental Health Findings, NSDUH Series H-47, HHS Publication No. (SMA) 13-4805. Rockville, MD: Substance Abuse and Mental Health Services Administration. Available at http://www.samhsa.gov/data/NSDUH/2k12MH_FindingsandDetTables/2K12MHF/NSDUHmhfr2012.htm#sec2-4

Facts About Mental Illness	box 1-1

In 2012, an estimated 44.7 million adults ages 18 or older in the United States had a mental illness in the preceding year. This represents 18.6% of all adults in this country. Among adults aged 18 or older in 2012, approximately 9.6 million (4.1% of all adults) suffered from serious mental illness (SMI). For that year:

- Women were more likely than men to experience mental illness (22.0% vs. 14.9%) and SMI (4.9% vs. 3.2 %).
- An estimated 9 million adults (3.9%) had serious thoughts of suicide in the past year; 2.7 million adults (1.1%) made suicide plans; and 1.3 million (0.6%) attempted suicide.
- Among adults with any mental illness, 19.2% (8.4 million adults) met criteria for substance dependence or abuse in that period, compared with 6.4% among those who did not have mental illness. Among those adults with SMI, 27.3% also had past-year substance dependence.
- Among adults with any mental illness, 17.9 million (41.0%) received mental health services in the past year, compared

with 6.0 million (62.9%) of those with SMI. Overall, 14.5% of the adult population (more than 34 million people) received mental health services during the past year.

- Among adults with both SMI and substance dependence or abuse, 64.7% received substance use treatment at a specialty facility or mental health treatment center in that period.
- More than two million youths (ages 12 to 17) had a major depressive episode (MDE) during the past year. Of those individuals, 34.0% used illicit drugs in the past year, compared with 16.3% among youths who did not experience a major depressive episode.
- Among individuals ages 12 to 17, 3.1 million (12.7%) received treatment or counseling for problems with emotions or behavior in a specialty mental health setting (inpatient or outpatient care). The most common reason for receiving services was feeling depressed (50.7%).

Source: Substance Abuse and Mental Health Services Administration. (2013). Results from the 2012 National Survey on Drug Use and Health: Mental Health Findings, NSDUH Series H-47, HHS Publication No. (SMA) 13-4805. Rockville, MD: Substance Abuse and Mental Health Services Administration. Available at http://www.samhsa.gov/data/NSDUH/2k12MH_FindingsandDetTables/2K12MHF/NSDUHmhfr2012.htm#sec2-4

United States. In 1917, the National Committee on Mental Hygiene, in combination with what became the American Psychiatric Association, created a guide for mental hospitals called the *Statistical Manual for the Use of Institutions for the Insane* (American Psychiatric Association, 2000). The first official *Diagnostic and Statistical Manual* identified 106 disorders and was published by the American Psychiatric Association (APA) in 1952. In a parallel process, the sixth edition of the International Classification of Diseases (1949) included a section on psychiatric illnesses for the first time (Grob, 1991). By the time the DSM-II and the ICD seventh edition were published in 1968, 182 disorders had been identified. In 1980, the DSM-III took a research approach to diagnosis and, after significant field trials, identified 265 diagnostic categories. The DSM-III was revised in 1987 in an attempt to reorganize categories, and named 292 diagnoses. A multiaxial approach to diagnosis emerged that addressed five separate axes:

- Axis I—Clinical disorders
- Axis II—Personality disorders and mental retardation
- Axis III—Medical conditions and physical disorders that could affect psychiatric symptoms
- Axis IV—Psychosocial and environmental factors
- Axis V—Global Assessment of Functioning (0 [low functioning]–100 [high functioning])

The purpose of the multiaxial approach was to provide a comprehensive evaluation of all aspects of a person's life that could be contributing to a psychiatric and/or mental health disorder. In 1994, the DSM-IV included clinical significance criteria and identified 297 disorders using a categorical approach. By 2000, a DSM-IV Text Revision (TR) was published to update the existing diagnoses to be more closely aligned with the ICD-9. No new diagnoses were identified.

After 20 years of research, a new version of the DSM was published in 2013 and formally adopted by the Centers for Medicare and Medicaid in 2014. The DSM-5 was designed to incorporate changes in both the International Classification of Disease (ICD-9)

criteria as well as the ICD-10, adopted by the United States in 2014. Significant changes included a change in the title from the use of Roman numerals to allow for more frequent updates, including web-based updates (e.g., 5.1), as well as removal of the multiaxial system. The multiaxial classification was eliminated to lessen stigma. All psychiatric and medical illnesses, including developmental and personality disorders (formerly Axes I, II, III), are now coded together as primary diagnoses. Axis IV, psychosocial and environmental factors impacting psychiatric and mental health conditions, is now represented through an expanded selected set of ICD-9-CM V-codes (supplementary classification of factors influencing health status and contact with health services) and from the ICD-10-CM Z-codes. Axis V (Global Assessment of Functioning) was replaced with use of the internationally adopted World Health Organization Disability Schedule, which also classifies all illnesses together (Chapter 5).

The DSM-5 is divided into three sections. Section 1 contains explicit directions for use of the manual. Section 2 comprises 20 chapters of disorders that have been reconceptualized from previous editions. Section 3 contains suggestions for future research, a potential reconceptualization of personality disorders, and various disorder-specific severity scales to assist clinicians in describing illness-specific severity, as opposed to a global assessment of functioning that was previously applied to all diagnoses (APA, 2013).

The DSM-5 is the official manual approved by the APA and the NIMH for use by all clinicians to diagnose psychiatric and mental health disorders in patients. This manual establishes standardized criteria for professionals and third-party payors to classify psychiatric and mental health disorders. As further evidence emerges, new versions will seek to clarify and classify various mental disorders according to genetics and neurobiological underpinnings. To some extent, culture will also dictate what will be considered as differences between mental health and mental illness.

As with any other medical disorder, the nurse needs to listen to the patient with a mental or emotional illness, and not just observe symptoms to categorize an illness. Providing hope is critical, and recovery is possible for many suffering with mental illnesses.

Pause and Reflect

1. *What is the difference between mental health and mental illness?*
2. *Has anyone you know been diagnosed with a mental illness? What are the symptoms? How does the illness affect the person's ability to function at home, at work, or at school?*
3. *What is most challenging for you when thinking of caring for patients diagnosed with mental illness?*

Overview of Psychiatric–Mental Health Nursing

Psychiatric–mental health nursing is a specialty within nursing. It involves helping individuals maintain mental health as well as recover from mental illness with a variety of evidence-based interventions, using a keen awareness of one's strengths and stressors to assist others in addressing theirs, and communicating professionally and effectively with patients, families, colleagues, and others at points of need validated with them.

The need for psychiatric–mental health nurses around the world is profound. Of the 3.1 million registered nurses in the United States, only 93,000 (3%) are classified as psychiatric nurses. Of those, only 12,000 (13% of all psychiatric nurses) are certified as advanced practice registered nurses (Institute of Medicine, 2010). Psychiatric–mental health nurses are employed in a variety of settings, including the following:

- General hospitals with inpatient psychiatric units
- Free-standing psychiatric hospitals
- Community mental health centers
- Crisis services, including mobile crisis vans, prisons, jails, and schools
- Primary care clinics
- Nursing homes,
- Substance abuse treatment settings
- Faith-based settings (parish nursing)

Psychiatric–mental health nurses participate in case management services, including coordination of care, assisting with obtaining medication, and consulting with community-based case managers. An important role of the psychiatric–mental health nurse is to ensure that the family is involved in the provision of care to the fullest extent possible. Work with the family includes crisis intervention, education about the illness, and referral to support groups such as NAMI. Even though not all registered nurses will become psychiatric–mental health nurses, all registered nurses must become skilled in providing mental health care and understanding the role of psychiatric–mental health nurses as a vital component of the interdisciplinary team (Figure 1-2). The art and science of mental health promotion, mental illness prevention, and the diagnosis and treatment of mental illness are essential for all nurses to understand.

Levels of Psychiatric Nursing Practice

Psychiatric–mental health nurses offer several contributions unique to the profession of nursing. These contributions strengthen the profession and help improve patient care. They include advocating for

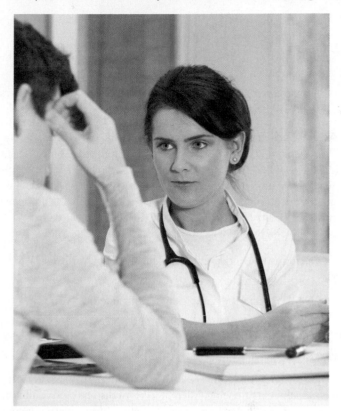

1-2 With nearly 20% of adults experiencing some form of mental illness each year, nurses in every setting will encounter patients with mental illness.

Source: Kirill Linnik/Shutterstock

and participating in an evidence base for psychiatric–mental health nursing, as well as the development and promotion of specific nursing skills. Psychiatric–mental health nurses play a vital role in early identification and treatment of mental illness. They work with individuals, families, groups, and communities.

The skills of psychiatric–mental health nursing care are applicable to all patients, specialties, diagnoses, and settings in which nursing is practiced. Registered nurses assess basic mental health needs, develop a nursing diagnosis and plan of care, implement the plan, and evaluate nursing care. By ensuring and encouraging access to effective treatment and recovery programs, nurses can enhance patient recovery and minimize impairment due to illness.

Registered Nurse (RN)

The basic level of psychiatric nursing requires that the RN demonstrate competence when providing care for individuals who have mental health challenges, problems, and/or disorders. Competence is an expected level of performance. Competence incorporates specialized knowledge, skills, abilities, attitudes, and judgment acquired through education and experience. Given the complexity of care inherent within this specialty, education at the baccalaureate level is preferred, along with credentialing from the American Nurses Credentialing Center (ANCC) (ANA, 2010a). The key tenets of care involve individualized care, partnerships, caring, nursing process, and a professional work environment (ANA, 2010a). The scope of practice and responsibilities of the psychiatric mental health registered nurse include:

- Use of the nursing process to promote health and safety, assess patient dysfunction, and assist patients in regaining health and function

- Importance of self-awareness, empathy, and personal integrity in the development of therapeutic relationships
- The roles of the nurse in a variety of clinical settings and in the development of care and treatment
- Involvement of the patient in the treatment planning process (ANA, APNA, ISPN, 2014)

Advanced Practice Registered Nurse (APRN)

The Advanced Practice Registered Nurse in Psychiatric Mental Health (APRN-PMH) is a licensed registered nurse who has received educational preparation at the master's or doctoral level in the specialty of psychiatric mental health nursing. The APRN-PMH holds advanced practice specialty certification from the ANCC as either a Clinical Specialist or Nurse Practitioner. In comparison to an RN, the APRN-PMH:

- Demonstrates a deeper and broader level of knowledge
- Performs a greater synthesis of data
- Displays increased complexity of skills and interventions
- Maintains significant role autonomy (ANA, APNA, ISPN, 2014)

Psychiatric Nursing Skills

Acquiring and developing skills to assist patients who are suffering emotionally, experiencing different levels of distress, and exhibiting various kinds of behaviors is the foundation of psychiatric–mental health nursing. The process of developing these skills can be challenging because it involves self-exploration (Chapter 7). Psychiatric–mental health nursing care is *being with* the patient more than *doing for* the patient. The nurse may or may not have a hands-on "task" to accomplish with the patient. The key skill is development of the therapeutic relationship and corresponding therapeutic use of self.

Psychiatric–mental health nursing focuses on human emotions and treating symptoms that relate to mental illness. Humans experience a range of emotions, including sadness, joy, anger, fear, and anxiety. Differentiating normal human emotions from pathology (for example, sadness versus a diagnosis of major depressive disorder) is crucial in terms of treatment planning. The latter usually requires more intensive interventions to alleviate distress and suffering. All nurses need basic psychiatric–mental health nursing skills to discern what initial interventions might best assist individuals and to determine whether additional help is necessary. Specific skills that help nurses support patients with mental illness include providing presence and therapeutic communication.

Providing Presence

The nurse first and foremost provides presence to the patient. **Presence** can be defined as being with and attending to the patient in a way that promotes a level of human engagement and interchange between the nurse and patient in a way that is meaningful to the patient. Presence may include the provision of physical comfort, therapeutic communication, active listening, and simply being with the patient. Dossey and Keegan refer to presence as communicating "whole being to whole being using all the resources of body, mind, emotions, and spirit" (2009, p. 724). In the context of the nurse-patient relationship, Hessel (2009) describes presence as a connection achieved only through a compassionate exchange of the human experience.

If the nurse is not comfortable just *being with* a patient, this can cause distress for the nurse, which may quickly turn the focus away from the patient to the nurse. Remaining focused on assessing patient needs will help the nurse maintain focus on the patient and will help the nurse become more comfortable being with the patient.

Being with a patient is key to developing the therapeutic nurse–patient relationship. Hildegarde Peplau, often called the "mother of psychiatric nursing," asserted that the nurse–client relationship is foundational to nursing (1952). Other nursing theorists who promoted the importance of presence as being vital in the nurse–patient relationship include Nightingale (Dossey, 2000), Benner (1984), and Parse (1998). Being present can promote a meaningful exchange between patient and nurse. As asserted by Parse, the nurse's presence involves "standing with [a person] during a journey" (Parse, 1999, p. 1 [a person]).

Therapeutic Communication

The therapeutic nurse–patient relationship develops through therapeutic communication. Communication involves the transmission and interpretation of both verbal and nonverbal messages. Communication between patient and nurse becomes therapeutic when the nurse listens and facilitates conversation between patient and nurse in a goal-directed manner. The nurse guides, but does not force, the communication in a direction that will be helpful for the patient. When nurse and patient engage in such communication, it can become comforting and healing (Chapter 8.)

Mental Status Examination

Assessing the patient's level of functioning can assist the nurse in differentiating whether the patient is experiencing a normal range of emotion or a pathological one. Although the patient's perception of his or her level of functioning is important, it is not the only means to determine whether pathology exists. Someone who stays up all night due to mania may be comfortable doing so. However, if the individual is not able to go to work or is causing distress to family members, more information is required to determine whether intervention is needed. Early assessment that includes a mental status examination can elicit important data that nurses and other care providers can use to differentiate symptoms and discern a patient's level of functioning. The mental status examination involves both patient report and care provider observation during the time of the interview. An in-depth description of the components of the mental status exam is found in Chapter 9.

A Wellness Domain Framework for Psychiatric–Mental Health Nursing

Wellness is a broader concept than health. It involves every aspect of living, including how people function in society. Wellness includes the interaction of biological and environmental factors, such as interpersonal relationships, spirituality, attitudes, and behaviors in a way that enables individuals to attain a satisfactory quality of life as they define it. When a person feels well, he or she is able to accomplish the tasks of everyday living and achieve desired life goals. Focusing on what can be done to achieve wellness rather than focusing on the severity of symptoms will result in better health and a higher level of wellness.

Individuals living with psychiatric illnesses have health challenges that interfere with their personal level of wellness. The stigma associated with these disorders can interfere with quality of life. It is important that individuals with psychiatric and mental health disorders establish a level of wellness that allows them to live in the environment of their choice and to do everyday activities that they enjoy.

Individuals with psychiatric and mental health concerns often find themselves diagnosed with coexisting medical conditions. In psychiatry these are referred to as *co-morbidities*. Research findings demonstrate that individuals with schizophrenia have higher rates of cardiopulmonary, metabolic, and gastrointestinal disorders, as well as higher rates of smoking, than the general population (Weber, Cowan, Millikan, & Niebuhr, 2009) and die, on average, 20 years earlier than persons who do not have the disorder (Leucht, Burkard, Henderson, Maj, & Sartorius, 2007). Additionally, the medications used to treat schizophrenia carry an increased risk of obesity, hyperglycemia, and diabetes. Individuals with bipolar disorder have, on average, 2.5 co-morbid medical conditions, including obesity, metabolic, and endocrine disorders (Kemp et al., 2010). In addition to co-morbid medical conditions, individuals with psychiatric illnesses typically experience at least two co-morbid psychiatric conditions (Weber, Cowan, Millikan, & Niebuhr, 2009). A major contributing factor to the shorter life span of individuals with mental illnesses is the lack of availability and access to primary care (Muir-Cochrane, 2006).

All nurses have a responsibility to emphasize health promotion and disease prevention in addition to actual treatment of illness. It is especially important that the care of individuals with psychiatric illnesses has a wellness focus, particularly in light of requirements of the 2010 Patient Protection and Affordable Care Act, which encourages individuals to take personal responsibility for wellness. This may sound logical, but for individuals with psychiatric illness who have compromised cognitive functioning, the ability to understand how to read food labels and to prioritize time for daily exercise is very difficult (Wildgust & Beary, 2010). Psychiatric illness often disrupts sleep, so patients may experience further impairment of daytime functioning and decreased energy (Silva, 2006; Wulff, Gatti, Wettstein, & Foster, 2010). To maximize response to treatment and improve overall health outcomes, nurses need to embrace a holistic, wellness approach to the nursing care of patients with psychiatric illnesses.

The methodology used to conceptualize an overall wellness approach to psychiatry developed for this textbook is based on the Murphy–Moller wellness model (Figure 1-3) (Murphy & Moller, 1996). Five major wellness **domains** will be used to approach the understanding and treatment of psychiatric illnesses:

- Biological (overall health)
- Psychological (attitudes and behaviors)
- Sociological (interpersonal relationships, and environment)
- Cultural (race, religion, kinship, and social support)
- Spiritual (sense of peacefulness)

The wellness model is depicted by a triangle with four of the major domains (biological, psychological, sociological, and spiritual) is balanced on three levels of functioning that rest on a base of social support composed of culture, resources, and kinship. For the purpose of this text, the base of social support is described as the cultural domain.

It is important to note that in this depiction, the wellness domains are precariously balanced because of the narrow base of social support that exists for most people experiencing an SMI. One of the important goals for nursing is to broaden the patient's base of social support by expanding resources such as housing, access to care, and decreasing stigma, as well as by increasing the kinship network through increasing social outlets and activities and providing peer support (Chapter 32).

Biological Domain

The biological domain refers to the ability of all body systems to function in a manner compatible with life and social function. The basic

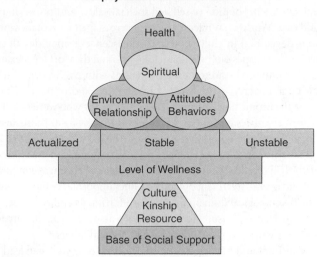

Murphy–Moller Wellness Model

1-3 The Murphy–Moller wellness model. Biological health, psychological health (which includes attitudes and behaviors), sociological health (environments, relationships), and spiritual health are supported by cultural resources. Individuals experiencing emerging mental illness (initial onset) or a relapse are considered unstable; as they move toward recovery, their mental health stabilizes. Individuals reach rehabilitation when they are able to actualize their wellness and return to full functioning.

biological (health) needs of adequate nutrition and hydration, relaxation and sleep, and exercise must be met for survival. A potential problem arises if the nurse or patient focuses on only one health need without looking at all the needs that affect each other. A high level of biological health is achieved when all body systems function in balance with one another. In psychiatry, considerable alteration in the immune, endocrine, and neurological systems contributes to increased medical co-morbidity. Biological health also includes the cognitive functions of attention, knowledge acquisition, problem solving, and decision making. Other psychiatric wellness components in this domain include good health practices such as eliminating alcohol, caffeine, street drugs, and food additives. Common psychiatric symptoms such as hallucinations, delusions, anxiety, and mood swings interfere with the ability to maintain adequate biological health.

A mnemonic to use for quick reference to general biological needs is ENERGIES:

Exercise

Nutrition

Each body system in balance

Rest

Good health practices

Information processing

Endocrine/immune

Sensory function

Psychological Domain

The psychological (attitudes/behaviors) domain consists of understanding our attitudes and behaviors as the observable outcomes of information processing systems. Attitudes are sometimes seen as the behaviors that express psychological needs. Attitudes and behaviors also include self-concept, the ability to use knowledge, moral development, and incorporation of self and societal values and norms into a world view. **World view** refers to the cognitive map or view of the world that is developed in childhood and adolescence; it includes all the learning that shapes our beliefs and feelings about the world. For example, individuals who were raised by parents with psychiatric illness; grew up in poverty; experienced abuse, trauma, and/or neglect; have lived with chronic illnesses and hospitalizations; or who were raised in war-torn countries have a very different world view from those raised without any of these negative influences. The life experiences that an individual has before experiencing a psychiatric illness can positively or negatively influence the individual's ability to actively engage in treatment and overall treatment outcomes. Other important considerations in the psychological domain include the individual's ability to tolerate pain, experience pleasure, feel worthwhile, assume responsibility for his or her own actions, and choose to love self and others.

Attitudes and behaviors help individuals to be well, can lead to the onset of illness, or can interfere with regaining wellness. It is important for patients to have hope that wellness can be increased or restored. The attitude and behavior of those who are employed in psychiatric treatment settings also affect the attitude and behavior of patients. If the staff has positive attitudes and behaviors, patients will generally do better, experience pleasure, and feel they have something to look forward to (Moller & Zausniewski, 2011). Encouraging patients with psychiatric illnesses to engage in behaviors that help them manage the challenges of life and the challenges of having a neurobiological disorder will help promote health. It is important to encourage patients to be active participants in all aspects of life.

A mnemonic for quick reference to the psychological domain is EMPOWERS:

> **E**njoy life
>
> **M**anage wellness
>
> **P**ain/pleasure
>
> **O**utlook
>
> **W**orthwhile
>
> **E**lect to love
>
> **R**esponsible for own behavior
>
> **S**uccess takes action

Sociological Domain

The sociological (environment/relationships) domain focuses on all aspects of the environment, including interpersonal relationships. Sociological needs are related to love and belonging, feeling safe in one's environment, and having sufficient economic resources to obtain adequate food, shelter, clothing, medical care, and things that bring feelings of pleasure. This domain includes evaluating the following:

- The presence of a balance of nature and the ability to get outside for fresh air every day
- Living and working conditions
- The ability to both give and receive needed services
- The people that patients talk to on a regular basis, such as family, friends, classmates, and co-workers

Feeling comfortable and accepted in one's environment is important to achieving maximum wellness. A hostile, critical environment

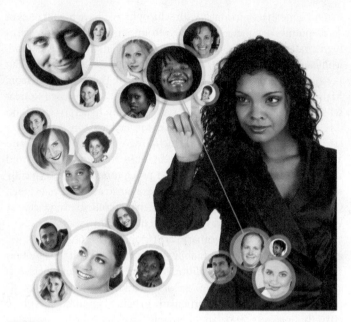

1-4   Kinship networks—networks of family, friends, and coworkers—can provide much-needed support in times of stress or illness.

Source: Luba V Nel/Shutterstock

increases the level of stress and makes it difficult to achieve wellness. When patients are around people who are negative, their personal energy diminishes. Environment includes the patient's kinship networks. **Kinship** is defined as safe and comfortable relationships with people (not necessarily relatives) who will reach out to the patient and be available for help in a time of need, as well as for social and supportive interactions (Figure 1-4).

The ability to reach out to others and to engage in meaningful conversation and to understand the requirements of illness management and health promotion requires the presence of basic communication skills. Many individuals with psychiatric illnesses have symptoms that interfere with the ability to communicate. (See Chapter 8 for further discussion of communication skills.)

A mnemonic for the sociological domain is SERVICES:

> **S**chool/work
>
> **E**njoy nature
>
> **R**esources/residence
>
> **V**alue life skills
>
> **I**nterpersonal relations
>
> **C**ommunication skills
>
> **E**conomics
>
> **S**upport

Cultural Domain

Patients seeking treatment for any mental or medical illness bring with them concerns, needs, customs, and beliefs that are rooted in their cultural background. General principles of culture include customs, beliefs, values, institutions, and language developed over time among a group of individuals who share commonalities such as race, religion, or ethnicity (Cross, Basron, Dennis, & Isaacs, 1989). Because of the increasingly diverse composition of the U.S. population, in 2001 the U.S. Department of Health and Human Services (DHHS) defined 14 National Standards on Culturally and Linguistically Appropriate Services. These standards and efforts on the part of DHHS and health care organizations such as the ANA have increased cultural competency in many areas of the health care system. Despite this growing transformation and acceptance of cultural diversity, however, access may not be equal for some cultures; furthermore, the realities of providing equal access and inclusive environments can be challenging and often stressful (Schim, Doorenbos, Benkert, & Miller, 2007).

Culture describes how individuals organize themselves socially. Language, shared beliefs, and symbols help form culture. However, shared beliefs do not always result in similar behaviors. The United States has many ethnic groups. A hallmark of U.S. culture is sharing the diversity that exists among its members (Jervis, 2006).

The ability to provide culturally competent care is critical in psychiatric nursing but is in its infancy, due primarily to language barriers between nurses and patients and lack of available bilingual and bicultural psychiatric nurses. The lack of understanding of the cultural implications of mental illness can create disparities in service delivery. Additionally, some cultures still view mental illness as demon possession or as personal weakness and failure to live up to the beliefs and practices of the individual's culture. Patients who exhibit behavior that is incongruent with their value system experience stigma and can become ostracized from their families and communities. Chapter 5 details sociological and cultural aspects of psychiatric nursing.

A mnemonic for the cultural domain is CULTURES:

Customs and actions

Understand speech and communication

Language

Thoughts and beliefs

Understand values

Race and religion

Ethnicity

Social groupings

Spiritual Domain

Spirituality is at the core of wellness and the essence of individuality. People have both a spiritual and a physical self. The spiritual self must be nourished along with the physical body. The spiritual nature strives for intellectual, moral, and spiritual enjoyments. Just as the body needs rest, food, water, and exercise, so does the spirit. Spiritual health requires faith, hope, charity, forgiveness toward self and others, values clarification, and seeking after truth. Forgiveness encompasses forgiving someone who has done wrong, as well as recognizing wrong and taking steps to turn from it and do right. Doing wrong involves harming self, others, or property. Forgiveness also includes making right the wrongs against other people as far as it is possible. Spiritual health may be maintained through faith, prayer or meditation, study, a grateful heart, integrity, service to other people, or some combination of these. Spiritual wellness results in a sense of peace, an appreciation of others, and the ability to extend love to others. (See Chapter 6 for a discussion of the spiritual domain of psychiatric nursing.)

A mnemonic for the spiritual domain is PEACEFUL:

Positive attitude

Embrace truth

Accept forgiveness

Clarify values

Express gratitude

Friendship with self and others

Understanding heart

Learn to develop insight

See Appendix A—Wellness Domains: A Quick Guide for Patients.

Levels of Wellness

As depicted in the Murphy–Moller Wellness Model, updated for this book to include "initial onset" in level 1, three levels, or phases, of wellness are used to describe symptoms and to determine the level of intensity of psychiatric patient care interventions:

- Level 1—*relapse or initial onset* of illness, in which the level of wellness is *unstable* and symptoms are acute.

- Level 2—*recovery*, in which symptoms have *stabilized.*

- Level 3—*rehabilitation*, in which symptoms, if present, no longer interfere with normal activities of daily living or regular conversation. The person is *actually* working on achieving life goals and has a future orientation.

In level 1, symptoms have become severe enough to interfere with usual activities of daily living; the patient may require emergency treatment by a mental health professional. This level of wellness is defined as unstable; the patient's overall level of functioning is compromised. The initial onset and presentation of symptoms, as well as a **relapse** (return of symptoms after stabilization), can be life threatening. This compromised level of wellness can occur when there are deficits in any one or a combination of the wellness domains. Outside intervention, frequently from a mental health care provider, may be necessary to preserve life. The goal is to stabilize the individual's level of wellness.

PRACTICE ALERT Patients must be assessed thoroughly to rule out conditions that can cause or mimic mental illness symptoms. Some medical conditions can produce psychiatric symptoms such as anxiety, depression, and psychosis. Medical rule-outs involve assessing nutrition; the brain, thyroid, and heart; attention deficit; and fatigue and sleep.

In level 2, **recovery**, symptoms are present but under control, and the individual is able to perform basic self-care. The level of wellness is defined as stable. The goal of treatment at this stage is to teach skills that will help the patient maintain a wellness lifestyle, manage symptoms, and prevent future relapse. Psychoeducation (education specific to all aspects of understanding and managing psychiatric disorders) includes providing information about diagnosis, medications, and coping with a chronic illness, and a focus on re-engaging in life goals. At this level, the person is able to resume normal interpersonal interactions. Incorporation of the SAMHSA recovery principles are essential (Box 1-2).

In level 3, rehabilitation, symptoms are in the background and the level of wellness is referred to as actualized. **Actualization** refers to establishing desired life goals and actually engaging in goal-directed activities that were common before the illness. The goal of care at this level is to assist the patient to gradually integrate back into the community. Existing community resources are accessed as needed.

The Recovery Movement

box 1-2

The psychiatric recovery movement began in the 1960s as a reflection of the civil rights movement, when patients who had been deinstitutionalized joined together to advocate for improvement in the mental health system. In 1977, the concept of psychiatric rehabilitation reached the professional level as community-based psychologists started developing formal programs addressing the needs created by deinstitutionalization (Anthony, 2000). The movement reached the federal level with the SAMHSA publication of the Consensus Statement on Mental Health Recovery (2006). This document, updated in 2012, identifies the 10 fundamental principles of mental health recovery (see list that follows) (SAMHSA, 2012b).

In 2009, SAMHSA initiated a five-year project, *Recovery to Practice*, to incorporate recovery principles into each of the core psychiatric disciplines: psychiatry, psychology, social work, and nursing, as well as substance abuse treatment programs and peer support programs. The American Psychiatric Nurses Association received the grant for psychiatric nursing and developed an introductory web-based series of modules to assist registered nurses and nursing students in becoming more recovery focused.

The recovery movement has demonstrated a major shift in the treatment of severe mental illness by promoting a collaborative approach in recovery. Consumers have been leading the way and transforming professional practice (Gehart, 2012). Psychiatric nurses are now developing tools to measure recovery-oriented practice (McLoughlin, Du Wick, Collazi, & Puntil, 2013) and are in the process of changing the focus of nursing care from illness-based care to recovery-focused nursing care (Moller & McLoughlin, 2013).

Ten Fundamental Principles of Mental Health Recovery

1. *Recovery emerges from hope.* The belief that recovery is real provides the essential and motivating message of a better future—that people can and do overcome the internal and external challenges, barriers, and obstacles that confront them. Hope is internalized and can be fostered by peers, families, providers, allies, and others. Hope is the catalyst of the recovery process.

2. *Recovery is person-driven.* Self-determination and self-direction are the foundations for recovery, as individuals define their own life goals and design their unique path(s) toward those goals. Individuals optimize their autonomy and independence to the greatest extent possible by leading, controlling, and exercising choice over the services and supports that assist their recovery and resilience. In so doing, they are empowered and provided the resources to make informed decisions, initiate recovery, build on their strengths, and gain or regain control over their lives.

3. *Recovery occurs via many pathways.* Individuals are unique with distinct needs, strengths, preferences, goals, culture, and backgrounds—including trauma experience—that affect and determine their pathway(s) to recovery. Recovery is built on the multiple capacities, strengths, talents, coping abilities, resources, and inherent value of each individual. Recovery pathways are highly personalized. They may include professional clinical treatment, use of medications, support from families and in schools, faith-based approaches, peer support,

and other approaches. Recovery is nonlinear, characterized by continual growth and improved functioning that may involve setbacks. Because setbacks are a natural, though not inevitable, part of the recovery process, it is essential to foster resilience for all individuals and families. Abstinence from the use of alcohol, illicit drugs, and nonprescribed medications is the goal for those with addictions. Use of tobacco and nonprescribed or illicit drugs is not safe for anyone. In some cases, recovery pathways can be enabled by creating a supportive environment. This is especially true for children, who may not have the legal or developmental capacity to set their own course.

4. *Recovery is holistic.* Recovery encompasses an individual's whole life, including mind, body, spirit, and community. This includes addressing self-care practices, family, housing, employment, transportation, education, clinical treatment for mental disorders and substance use disorders, services and supports, primary health care, dental care, complementary and alternative services, faith, spirituality, creativity, social networks, and community participation. The array of services and supports available should be integrated and coordinated.

5. *Recovery is supported by peers and allies.* Mutual support and mutual aid groups, including the sharing of experiential knowledge and skills, as well as social learning, play an invaluable role in recovery. Peers encourage and engage other peers and provide each other with a vital sense of belonging, supportive relationships, valued roles, and community. Through helping others and giving back to the community, one helps oneself. Peer-operated supports and services provide important resources to assist people along their journeys of recovery and wellness. Professionals can also play an important role in the recovery process by providing clinical treatment and other services that support individuals in their chosen recovery paths. Although peers and allies play an important role for many in recovery, their role for children and youth may be slightly different. Peer supports for families are very important for children with behavioral health problems and can also play a supportive role for youth in recovery.

6. *Recovery is supported through relationship and social networks.* An important factor in the recovery process is the presence and involvement of people who believe in the person's ability to recover; who offer hope, support, and encouragement; and who also suggest strategies and resources for change. Family members, peers, providers, faith groups, community members, and other allies form vital support networks. Through these relationships, people leave unhealthy and/or unfulfilling life roles behind and engage in new roles (such as partner, caregiver, friend, student, employee) that lead to a greater sense of belonging, personhood, empowerment, autonomy, social inclusion, and community participation.

7. *Recovery is culturally based and influenced.* Culture and cultural background in all of its diverse representations—including values, traditions, and beliefs—are keys in determining a person's journey and unique pathway to recovery. Services should be culturally grounded, attuned, sensitive, congruent, and competent, as well as personalized to meet each individual's unique needs.

8. *Recovery is supported by addressing trauma.* The experience of trauma (such as physical or sexual abuse, domestic

violence, war, disaster, and others) is often a precursor to or associated with alcohol and drug use, mental health problems, and related issues. Services and supports should be trauma-informed to foster safety (physical and emotional) and trust, as well as promote choice, empowerment, and collaboration.

9. ***Recovery involves individual, family, and community strengths, and responsibility.*** Individuals, families, and communities have strengths and resources that serve as a foundation for recovery. In addition, individuals have a personal responsibility for their own self-care and journeys of recovery. Individuals should be supported in speaking for themselves. Families and significant others have responsibilities to support their loved ones, especially for children and youth in recovery.

Communities have responsibilities to provide opportunities and resources to address discrimination and to foster social inclusion and recovery. Individuals in recovery also have a social responsibility and should have the ability to join with peers to speak collectively about their strengths, needs, wants, desires, and aspirations.

10. ***Recovery is based on respect.*** Community, systems, and societal acceptance and appreciation for people affected by mental health and substance use problems—including protecting their rights and eliminating discrimination—are crucial in achieving recovery. There is a need to acknowledge that taking steps toward recovery may require great courage. Self-acceptance, developing a positive and meaningful sense of identity, and regaining belief in oneself are particularly important.

Source: Substance Abuse and Mental Health Services. (2012b). The National Consensus Statement on Mental Health Recovery. SAMHSA's Working Definition of Recovery: 10 Guiding Principles of Recovery. Available at http://store.samhsa.gov/shin/content//PEP12-RECDEF/PEP12-RECDEF.pdf

This level of wellness takes time to achieve; in some ways, it is a lifelong process. Skill development is an important component. The actualized level of wellness involves incorporating a wellness lifestyle and requires setting goals, breaking the goals down into small steps, and then completing each step.

Patient progress through the levels of wellness rarely occurs in an orderly manner. Some patients may move back and forth through the levels of wellness over the course of their lifetimes (Figure 1-5).

Pause and Reflect

1. *What are the main differences between the Registered Nurse and the Advanced Practice Registered Nurse?*
2. *Which wellness domain do you think presents the greatest challenges for patient care? Why? What resources are available to help nurses develop greater knowledge and skill in working with patients on issues related to that domain?*
3. *Referring to the Critical Thinking feature: At what level/stage of wellness do you consider Mr. Harris to be? What interventions do you think will help him move toward recovery and rehabilitation? Why?*

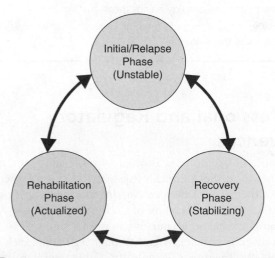

1-5 Patient progress through the levels of wellness does not always occur in an orderly manner. Some patients may move back and forth through the levels of wellness over the course of their lifetimes.

Evidence Base for Psychiatric Nursing

Patients anticipate full recovery and cure from most acute medical illnesses. *Cure* usually means complete and permanent remission. In relation to mental illnesses, cure generally is accepted to mean remission for an extended period of time. "Mental illnesses are common, chronic, and disabling," yet much of research in mental health disorders has focused on small goals or gains, such as minimization of medication side effects (Insel & Scolnick, 2006, p. 11). More emphasis needs to be placed on improved functioning, a hallmark of recovery in mental illness (Andreasen, et al., 2005). Insel and Scolnick question whether mental health care providers should be satisfied with the progress in treatment of mental disorders, such as major depressive disorder:

> In an illness characterized by intense emotional suffering, hopelessness, and suicidal ideation, should we be satisfied with treatments that require several weeks to be effective and will not lead to remission in the majority of patients? Would our colleagues in medicine be satisfied with these outcomes for an illness characterized by intense pain, high morbidity, and a 4% mortality rate? (2006, p. 13)

However, individuals experiencing their first episode of mental illness may not receive diagnosis or treatment at the first signs of symptoms. They may not seek help or may not see a provider who is skilled in diagnosing mental disorders. Furthermore, individuals at the onset of mental illness may not realize or accept that they have a chronic disorder that involves exacerbations and remissions. Complex factors and/or co-morbid conditions associated with the initial episode of mental illness, which complicate diagnosis and treatment, may be present.

Because of these factors and others, patients with mental illness and their families do not consistently and comprehensively receive evidence-based interventions. Evidence-based practice (EBP) began in the late 1900s when a British epidemiologist promoted care based on randomized clinical controlled trials (Rice, 2008). The majority of the EBP movement is directed toward developing clinical guidelines; however, much of EBP also focuses on the therapeutic relationship and clinical judgment associated with providing care. Nurses today are expected to apply EBP in their interventions to

Nurses Assisting Families

Clinical Problem

Families struggle with their roles when caring for a family member diagnosed with mental illness. What can psychiatric nurses do to assist families as they struggle to do what is best for them and for their family member?

Evidence

Nordby, Kjønsberg, and Hummelvoll (2010) reported on results of interviews with eight focus groups in southern Norway using a thematic analysis abstract. Focus group members were all relatives of persons with recently discovered SMI. Researchers looked at what facilitates active involvement for family members in the treatment and rehabilitation of their family member. They found that family members:

- Wanted their ill relative to be treated as a person, in addition to as a person who is ill
- Wanted staff to convey hope regardless of the circumstances, as they felt it was important for them to cope
- Needed to know what to say to their family members, how to behave with them, and what happens after discharge
- Felt their stress level decreased when they could share their concerns and receive help

In addition, researchers found that parents wanted to be involved early in their children's care and to feel that their concerns and ideas were heard. Staff perceived themselves as experts on psychosis; families considered themselves experts on their family member. Family members reported mostly positive experiences from their interactions with staff. Family members and staff emphasized the importance of developing positive interactions that involved sharing information and giving guidance and support. Family members expressed a need for staff members to convey and nurture hope related to the patient's recovery and quality of life.

Foster explored the experience of being an adult child of a parent with serious mental illness and how adult children have coped with their experience. Foster analyzed 10 participants' responses using van Manen's hermeneutic method. Four themes emerged:

- Being uncertain: "You'd think this roller coaster was never going to stop."
- Struggling to connect: "We were super close and now we're not."

- Being responsible: "I think I grew up in a hurry."
- Seeking balance: "I had to be in control of the situation so awful things wouldn't happen." (Foster, 2010, pp. 3143–3151)

Foster concluded that children of parents diagnosed with mental illness experience a very chaotic family life, and adult children assume substantial caregiving roles. Relationships between parents and adult children can become strained. Professionals can help strengthen adult children's resilience and ability to cope by providing support. Nurses can give information and support to children and families in which parents have a mental illness. Focusing care on the family can enhance children's and parent's relationships and support the family's ability to cope.

Tas, Guvenir, and Cevrim (2010) performed a retrospective study with families and their adolescents who received treatment in a recently opened unit. They surveyed five areas: admission process, staff, environment/services, treatment interventions, and treatment outcome satisfaction levels of the adolescents and their families regarding service they received during their stay in the unit that were rated high. Results of the questionnaires completed by adolescents and parents revealed that availability and helpfulness of the staff and the admission process were given the highest satisfaction scores.

Implications for Nursing

Nurses are in key positions to assist families who are caring for another family member diagnosed with mental illness. Family members identify hope as important in their ability to cope and want care providers to convey hope regardless of the circumstances of their family member. Nurses can provide support and hope, which help strengthen family members' resilience and ability to cope. Patient and family satisfaction are rated high when staff are available and respond to the family's concerns.

Critical Thinking Questions

1. What strategies assisted family members in the studies cited?
2. Why do you think families identified these as helpful?
3. How might you employ any of these strategies?
4. How will you approach families differently after reading the reviews of this evidence?

provide the highest standard of care (see Evidence-Based Practice: Nurses Assisting Families).

Cognitive–behavioral therapy and family psychoeducation are two evidence-based therapies that have been demonstrated to improve mental dysfunction. However, they frequently are not applied sufficiently. Providers and caregivers need to advocate for research that (1) determines the pathophysiological basis for mental disorders, (2) uses interventions to detect and prevent the severe disability that can arise from mental disorders, and (3) promotes recovery to the fullest extent possible. Psychiatric–mental health nurses must make clinical judgments and provide nursing care based on sound knowledge and existing evidence. To do so, they must be skilled in finding and applying evidence-based practices.

Professional and Regulatory Influences

Psychiatric nursing care is affected by professional influences from the ANA, the American Psychiatric Nurses Association (APNA), the North American Nursing Diagnosis Association, and the American Association of Colleges of Nursing (AACN). Psychiatric–mental health nurses also work within specific regulatory influences that are enacted through legislation, such as the 1996 Health Insurance Portability and Accountability Act (HIPAA), the 2008 Wellstone-Domenici Mental Health Parity and Addiction Equity Act, and the 2010 Patient Protection and Affordable Care Act.

The American Nurses Association

The art and science of nursing are informed by four resources published by the ANA:

- The *Code of Ethics for Nurses with Interpretive Statements* (ANA, 2008)
- The *Scope and Standards of Practice* (ANA, 2010a)
- *Nursing's Social Policy Statement: The Essence of the Profession* (ANA, 2010b)
- *Psychiatric–Mental Health Nursing: Scope and Standards of Practice* developed from the combined efforts of ANA, APNA, and the International Society of Psychiatric–Mental Health Nurses (2014).

These documents provide all psychiatric nurses with a comprehensive framework for the practice of nursing at both the RN and APRN levels.

The American Psychiatric Nurses Association

With more than 8,000 members, the APNA is the only professional nursing organization that focuses on all levels of psychiatric nursing. The core purpose is to be the unified voice of psychiatric–mental health nursing. Activities of the APNA focus on policy, education, networking with key stakeholders, and strategic outreach to members. Consisting of a board of directors, councils, and task forces, the APNA provides leadership in integrating research, practice, and education to address pressing psychiatric–mental health nursing care issues. The APNA contributes to developing the *Scope and Standards for Psychiatric Nursing* that are published every five years by the ANA.

North American Nursing Diagnosis Association International

Just as the field of psychiatry has diagnostic nomenclature, so does psychiatric–mental health nursing. *Nursing diagnoses* refer to treatment of the human response to given phenomena, such as hallucinations, psychosis, or grief and loss. The nursing diagnosis frames the desired nursing interventions and outcomes in a holistic manner. The North American Nursing Diagnosis Association International (Herdman & Kamitsuru, 2014) contains approved nursing diagnoses (Appendix B).

Quality and Safety Initiatives

In the era of health care reform and accountable care organizations (ACOs) described in Chapter 26, modern health care practice, including psychiatric nursing practice, will include a focus beyond the individual patient encounter to include a focus on the performance of systems of care (Kaiser Healthcare News, 2012). Over the past two decades, the Institute of Medicine (IOM) has documented substantive problems with quality and safety in the United States health care system, beginning with the first pivotal report, *To Err Is Human* (IOM, 1999). In mental health care, common quality and safety threats include poor treatment adherence, poor coordination of care, poor primary care service delivery, and poor safety surveillance. A common example is poor monitoring for metabolic syndrome adverse effects related to use of atypical antipsychotic medications (Newcomer et al., 2004; Internal Medicine News, 2013).

The AACN initiative Quality and Safety Education for Nurses (QSEN) represents the professional voice for quality and safety for the discipline of nursing, and has established quality and safety competencies for nursing education and practice (QSEN, 2007a). The following are the QSEN competencies:

- Patient and family-centered care
- Teamwork and collaboration (including inter-professional practice
- Safety
- Evidence-based practice
- Quality improvement
- Informatics

QSEN has developed pre-licensure and graduate-level competencies for quality and safety education in nursing (QSEN, 2007b), which are included in the AACN Essentials for undergraduate, graduate, and doctoral nursing education (AACN, 2006, 2008, 2011).

A number of organizations have examined the issue of quality improvement in psychiatric care. The Institute of Medicine (2006) has published mental health specific recommendations for improving health care quality. The APNA has established quality indicators for mental health care (APNA, 2013). The Joint Commission has published national quality indicators for psychiatric care that set specific outcome measures as a basis for reimbursement in mental health services (Joint Commission, 2013). Finally, the DHHS has established recommendations for integrating shared decision making into mental health care to improve patient-centeredness and empowerment in mental health care (U.S. Department of Health and Human Services, 2011).

Quality improvement efforts at the clinical care level have demonstrated progress in randomized controlled trials in mental health, including efforts driven by psychiatric–mental health nurses. Wells et al. (2004) demonstrated a five-year improvement in depression outcomes and reduced health outcome disparities through the use of structured quality improvement interventions. Asarnow et al. (2006) demonstrated improved depression care outcomes for adolescents after only six months of quality improvement intervention. In addition, successful interprofessional education programs targeting improved collaboration in clinical care and improved professional development in mental health clinical rotations including psychiatric–mental health nurses are described (Roberts et al., 2009). Finally, Mistler et al. (2012) have successfully applied shared decision making to populations with severe mental illness.

The IOM *Future of Nursing* report calls on the nursing profession to take a leadership role in health care improvement, asserting that nurses will have responsibility for providing safe, quality care to all patients within the health care system (IOM, 2010). In particular, the second recommendation of the report specifically calls for expanded opportunities for nurses to lead and share in collaborative improvement efforts. Nurses in all roles—from the nurse at the bedside to nurse executives—are essential to improving quality of care for individual patients in all settings. The horizon is bright with opportunities for psychiatric–mental health nurses to make a real difference in health care quality and safety, not only at the level of the individual patient encounter, but also in leading improvement in mental health care delivery systems.

Health Insurance Portability and Accountability Act (HIPAA)

First enacted in 1996, HIPAA was dramatically expanded in 2003. This law originally was passed to protect the rights of individuals with regard to their medical records when they change jobs and their health insurance and medical records transfer from one company to another. Everyone who sees a health care professional must sign a document that describes how his or her medical records will remain private. Unfortunately, this law has worked against many health care providers, as some patients wrongly interpret that HIPAA means that health care providers cannot share or exchange information about patients with other providers.

To facilitate better communication among providers serving the same patient, the U.S. government developed guidelines for protected health information (PHI). Registered nurses must be alert to refraining from discussing any aspect of patient care when in any public setting (Chapter 10).

Mental Health Parity

The 2008 Wellstone-Domenici Mental Health Parity and Addiction Equity Act (WDMHP) (Public Law 110-343) brought the needs of both individuals with mental illnesses and their family members to the forefront of the American public. The WDMHP requires that insurance companies provide mental health and substance abuse treatment at an equal rate with all other covered illnesses. This legislation went into effect January 1, 2010 and applies to businesses that have more than 50 employees. It does not extend to Medicaid and Medicare recipients, but it is a major improvement in mandated insurance coverage.

Affordable Care Act

The 2010 Patient Protection and Affordable Care Act (ACA) (Public Law 111-152, 124 Stat. 1029) was intended to provide sweeping changes for health care. It was estimated that 32 million Americans would receive health insurance for the first time, and nearly 8 million of that number would be people diagnosed with mental illness (Garfield, Lave, & Donohue, 2010). However, the actual rollout proved more difficult than anticipated by the plan's architects. At the time of this writing, it is unclear when or if these objectives will be fully realized.

Pause and Reflect

1. *What is the role of the American Psychiatric Nurses Association?*
2. *What is the role of quality improvement initiatives in psychiatric care?*
3. *How does the QSEN competency of patient- and family-centered care relate to the provision of psychiatric nursing care?*

From Suffering to Hope

Helping patients with mental illness find hope and healing presents many challenges. Patients do not operate within a vacuum—they each have families and cultural beliefs and values; think and respond differently to people, situations, and medications; and have different capacities for dealing with illness. Nurses working with patients with mental health needs and illnesses will provide better care when they do the following:

- Develop a greater understanding of significant concepts that affect every patient, regardless of the patient's level of stability and experience managing mental illness
- Help patients learn behaviors that alleviate suffering and promote hope and healing
- Gain a greater awareness of their own perceptions, thoughts, and feelings when working with patients with mental illness

Factors That Affect Patient Recovery

A number of factors can affect individuals diagnosed with mental illness, as well as their family members (Figure 1-6). The stigma that many associate with mental illness prevents many people from seeking treatment when symptoms first begin. The treatment plan may include medications with disabling side effects that dissuade the person from fully engaging in the treatment regimen. The individual may not be able to access recovery-focused services or no services at all may be available in his or her area. The individual may have lost hope, or, even more devastating, may have never experienced any sense of hope in the attempt to engage in a successful treatment process. The individual may be receiving services in a facility that has yet to adopt principles of the recovery movement.

Stigma

Stigma, which may also be referred to as discrimination, refers to the social rejection of individuals diagnosed with mental illness (Ros, Kanner, Muris, Janssen, & Mayer, 2009). Although progress has been made in the treatment of mental illness, a diagnosis of mental illness may bring an array of negative reactions, such as skepticism, fear,

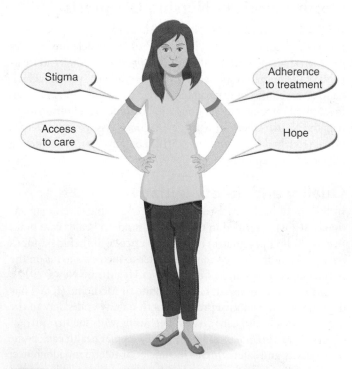

1-6   Some factors that affect patient recovery include stigma, adherence to treatment, access to care, and hope.

anger, avoidance, and rejection. These reactions may come from an individual's family, friends, and/or society and lead to prejudice and discrimination.

Stigma surrounding mental illness is complicated by the assumption that individuals with mental illness are violent, an idea perpetuated, in part, by the media. Experts examining 13 years of data on mental health and crime found that individuals diagnosed with mental illness were responsible for one in 20 violent crimes; they expressed more concern about their finding that 19 in 20 individuals who committed a violent crime were *not* diagnosed with mental illness (BBCNews, 2006).

Mental health advocates cite stigma (discrimination) as one of the reasons for lack of progress in patients with mental health disorders in contrast to those with other medical illnesses (Insel & Scolnick, 2006). Patients often identify themselves by their diagnosis rather than stating, for example, "I have an illness—schizophrenia." Likewise, professionals may refer to patients by their diagnosis, stating "the schizophrenic" rather than "the patient diagnosed with schizophrenia." Patients should not be equated with their illness. Mental illness, like other medical conditions, is a part of an individual's life, but not the sum total of his or her life.

Stigma is based on stereotypes and the belief that mental illness is a negative personal trait. Historically, mental illness was considered to indicate personal frailty. In more recent decades, it has become clear that mental illness has a biological basis. Despite this, there still are attitudes, misconceptions, fears, and biases to overcome toward mental illness and the individuals diagnosed with them (Mayo Clinic Staff, 2011).

Stigma is displayed in both direct and subtle forms. Individuals may be mocked about their mental health, discriminated against, or treated in a manner that assumes they will act in a certain way. Such treatment may cause those with mental illness to feel overwhelmed and may result in feelings of anger, frustration, denial, shame, low self-esteem, embarrassment, and withdrawal (Mayo Clinic Staff, 2011).

Adherence

Adherence to treatment is a major concern in providing care for many patients diagnosed with mental illness. Patients may not adhere to treatment for a number of reasons: financial considerations, side effects of medications, stigma, denial of illness, and difficulty accessing treatment. A fine line exists between encouraging patients to participate in a treatment regimen and coercing them into compliance. Treatment coercion is especially controversial in the provision of mental health services. In a study with 825 patients from three different states, researchers found that participants' perceived coercion scores were not associated with treatment adherence in relation to medication adherence or use of treatment services after discharge (Rain, et al., 2003).

Access

The patient's ability to access affordable and effective care can be influenced by factors that are not entirely within the patient's control. These include environmental factors, such as housing, access to transportation, and work hours (Chapter 32). Financial, geographical, and cultural hindrances to access promote disparities among those needing psychiatric–mental health care (American Nurses Association, 2014). Lack of or insufficient health insurance may also affect the patient's ability to access care. The ACA and the Domenici Mental Health Parity and Addiction Equity Act are two pieces of legislation that bring great hope in relation to resolving disparities in the treatment of mental illness.

Hope

Hope can be defined as a feeling that something an individual wants or longs for has a good chance of coming to pass. Hope is a positive and uplifting feeling. It is essential in empowering patients to work through the process of recovery to health. Optimism, a positive quality inherent in hope, is known to be a factor in the healing process and does not always require a cure (Quinn, Smith, Ritenbaugh, Swanson, & Watson, 2003).

Nurses can enhance hopeful and optimistic thinking by helping patients do the following:

- Establish positive expectations, through use of positive self-talk, making positive affirmations, visualizing health, and recognizing that mental illness is not the patient's fault.

- Embrace positive aspects of humor, friendships, volunteerism, pets, and plants.

- Appeal to a higher power (if they believe in a higher power). Spiritual wellness and the use of prayer, faith, and spiritual beliefs promote recovery from illness (Jackson, 2009).

Significant Concepts Related to Every Patient

A number of concepts apply to most patients cared for by psychiatric–mental health nurses. These include, but are not limited to, anxiety, fear, stress, and distress; coping resources; safety; and trauma-informed care.

Anxiety, Fear, Stress, and Distress

Anxiety is a foundational concept for most, if not all, mental disorders. Approximately 15% of Americans report having experienced a lifetime history of at least one anxiety disorder (CDC, 2011). **Anxiety** is a generally normal, healthy response to stress that may:

- Present as nonspecific and unidentified worry that may or may not relate to any specific event or issue.

- Exhibit as feelings of apprehension, uncertainty or tension; as an initial response to a psychic threat; as or feelings of uneasiness or dread resulting from a real or perceived threat whose actual source is unknown or unrecognized.

- Be a response to a specific stressor such as fear.

Fear is worry about a specific and identified threatening event or issue (e.g., fire, new job). Fear is determined by cognitive assessment of a situation. Fear provokes the emotional response of uneasiness, dread, or anxiety and anxious feelings.

Stress may be described in numerous ways, including as a precipitant of anxiety, a response to anxiety, or the process one goes through when feeling "anxious" or "stressed." Stress has been described as having positive, neutral, or negative influences on an individual. It has also been viewed as an event, the reaction to an event, or the outcome of an event. The most widely applied view is that **stress** relates to an individual's perception of demands being made on him or her, as well as the individual's perception of his or her ability to meet those demands; namely, a "demand-perception-response" perspective (McVicar, 2003, p. 633). Phenomena that may be associated with stress include concepts such as homeostasis (equilibrium, steady-state range), strain, distress, adjustment process, vulnerability, resistance, and resilience (Steinberg & Ritzmann, 1990).

Orlando (1961) defines an individual's response to anxiety-provoking circumstances that result in unmet needs as **distress**. Distress may arise from physical limitations, adverse reactions to the setting, and experiences that prevent the patient from communicating his or her needs (Orlando, 1961). Whether the patient is experiencing anxiety, fear, and/or stress, the common thread within all of these is the patient's subsequent response of distress. Symptoms for patients diagnosed with mental illness may increase if the patient's distress escalates rather than decreases.

For example, a hospitalized patient diagnosed with schizophrenia may have his symptom of hearing voices (auditory hallucination) in fairly good control with medication and distraction strategies. If the patient has an upsetting conversation with a family member, his anxiety level, and subsequently his distress level, may rise. The rise in distress level may trigger auditory hallucinations that provide him with some relief from the distress associated with the conversation. Working with the patient to decrease related anxiety and subsequent distress is an effective way to help the patient regain some control over his experience of the auditory hallucination.

Coping Resources

Individuals cope in numerous ways. Use of defense mechanisms is one of them (Chapter 13). Other methods of coping include a positive attitude and exercise, a well-known health-promoting activity that helps reduce the impact of stress. Another method of coping is by having an internal *locus of control*.

Locus of control relates to one's perception about causes of life events. Individuals tend to believe that outcomes of their actions occur either (1) based on what they do as individuals or (2) based on events that are beyond their control. Locus of control can be external or internal. The individual with an **external locus of control** places control of his or her life on other people and on circumstances outside the self. Those with an **internal locus of control** place such control within themselves. Patient locus of control has implications for providing care. When patients think their input makes a difference in outcomes, they are more likely to support efforts to help them take control of events in their lives. A study examining 200 patients diagnosed with epilepsy demonstrated that individuals having a greater internal locus of control had a higher incidence of controlled seizures compared with those having a lower internal locus of control (Asadi-Pooya, Schilling, Glosser, Tracy, & Sperling, 2007).

Trends have been observed related to those having a stronger internal locus of control:

- Men demonstrate a greater tendency toward internal locus of control than women.

- People tend to hold a more internal locus of control view as they get older.

- The higher one is within an organizational structure, the more likely the individual is to have an internal locus of control (Mamlin, Harris, & Case, 2001).

Coping resources may include primary and secondary gains. **Primary gain** refers to the result of an immediate benefit—specifically, relief from anxiety. **Secondary gain** occurs when an individual experiences indirect benefit from having a disorder or condition, such as financial compensation, disability benefits, personal services and attention, and/or escape from work or a difficult responsibility (Freud, 1963).

Lazarus and Folkman did pioneering work related to individuals' appraisals of their well-being and how they can cope with events that may be considered stressors. During **primary appraisal**, an individual determines whether or not the event or stressor will impact his or her well-being. During **secondary appraisal**, the individual considers what may and can be done with the coping resources available to handle the challenge, threat, or harm that is taking place (Lazarus & Folkman, 1984). An example of this follows, using the patient described in the critical thinking exercise at the beginning of the chapter:

> Mr. Harris considers a third suicide attempt. In his primary appraisal of his situation, Mr. Harris feels overwhelmed, helpless, and hopeless; he recognizes that he feels immobilized by the impact of current life stressors on his ability to function. During secondary appraisal, Mr. Harris remembers that, after his second suicide attempt, he made a "resource list" with his nurse and tells the nurse he looked at it prior to calling her. (In other words, Mr. Harris identifies what resources in the list can help him deal with feelings of being overwhelmed, helpless, and hopeless.)

Hardiness and resilience are two concepts that have significant implications for nurses. **Hardiness** refers to a group of characteristics that helps provide resistance to stressful life events. These include commitment to oneself and work, feeling control over events and outcomes, and viewing change as challenge (Ablett, 2007; Turnipseed, 1999; Kobasa, 1979). In an exploratory pilot study of graduate education, nursing administration students who rated themselves high in hardiness described having higher problem-focused coping skills (Judkins, Arris, & Keener, 2005). In another study, adults ages 85 and older demonstrated a high level of hardiness correlating positively to measures of purpose in life, sense of coherence, self-transcendence, and general mental health (Vance, Burrage, Couch, & Raper, 2008). Individuals with hardiness often have a strong internal locus of control and are proactive rather than passive when faced with changes and challenges.

Resilience is the capacity to adapt constructively to difficulty (Jackson, Firtko, & Edenborough, 2007). Nurses can increase their own resilience by fostering the following:

- Mentoring relationships

- Life balance and spirituality

- Positive emotions

- Personal growth

- Reflection (Jackson, Firtko, & Edenborough, 2007)

Nurses can promote resilience in patients as well. Knowing when patients are ready to receive information is part of patient education.

Safety

Safety is a significant priority in psychiatric–mental health nursing care. Safety in psychiatric–mental health care encompasses patients, family and significant others, and staff.

Patient safety issues may arise in relation to restraint and seclusion, medications, fall risks, milieu management, confidentiality, command hallucinations, acting-out behaviors, and others. Safety relates to both physical and psychological safety for all involved (ANA, 2007). The APNA has published position papers on workplace violence and seclusion and restraint. Additionally, the APNA has developed standards of care for use of seclusion and restraint. These standards are available on the APNA website.

Trauma-Informed Care

Many clients served by public mental health and substance abuse service systems have experienced violence, abuse, and neglect during childhood. Nurses recognize this when assessing and planning nursing care. **Trauma-informed care** is designed to inform caregivers about and sensitize them to trauma-related issues present in trauma survivors. A trauma-informed system is one that accommodates vulnerabilities of trauma survivors, avoids re-traumatization and exacerbation of symptoms for those who have been traumatized, and facilitates patient participation in treatment (Jennings, 2004; Regan, 2010).

Trauma is a key public health and policy issue for the following reasons:

- Most individuals affected by childhood trauma often have co-occuring or multiple health concerns (Waite, Gerrity, & Arango, 2010).

- Most patients in public mental health systems have experienced repeated trauma.

- Overlooking trauma has major implications for provision of services and related costs (Jennings, 2004).

Complex traumatic stress issues and problems are common in individuals having severe and persistent mental health and/or substance abuse problems. Often, these individuals are the highest users of inpatient, crisis, and residential services. Research supports trauma-based integrated treatment for these patients, and best-practice models exist that are both applicable and replicable within public health systems (Jennings, 2004). The SAMHSA has created the National Center for Trauma-Informed Care, with many publications helpful for nurses to incorporate principles of trauma-informed care (TIC) into daily practice.

Psychiatric diagnoses that are common in individuals who have experienced trauma include posttraumatic stress disorder (PTSD), borderline personality disorder, schizophrenia, depression and other affective disorders, anxiety disorders, eating disorders, dissociative disorders, addictive disorders, and sexual disorders (Jennings, 2004).

The goals of TIC are to:

- Protect patients with a history of trauma from physical harm and re-traumatization.

- Understand symptoms in the context of life experiences, history, culture, and society.

- Collaborate between provider and consumer at all phases of service delivery.

- Emphasize skill building versus symptom management.

- Understand symptoms as attempts to cope.

- View trauma as a defining experience that relates to the core of an individual's identity rather than as a single discrete event.

- Focus on what has happened to the person rather than what is wrong with the person (Hummer, Dollard, Robst, & Armstrong, 2010; Harris & Fallot, 2001; Saakvitne, Gamble, Pearlman, & Lev, 2000).

Components of TIC include the following:

- *Safety:* Is everything being done to ensure the patient's physical and emotional safety (welcome, respect, sufficient personal space, consistency)?

- *Trustworthiness:* Are expectations and interactions for everyone clear and consistent (boundaries, respect, being nonjudgmental)?

- *Choice:* Is a condition being created so individuals experience a feeling of choice and control (providing options, choices, optional program supports)?

- *Collaboration:* Is the approach one of sharing and collaboration in all interactions (learning from each other, seeking input, listening first)?

- *Empowerment:* Is there a fostering of the individual's strengths, experiences, and uniqueness for building on (recovery, hope, skill building)?

TIC speaks to shifting perspectives. Instead of asking what went wrong, the question becomes: What happened, and how do we work together?

Healing Environments

Facilities have become more aware of the need to promote healing environments. Evidence-based design indicates that these environments are therapeutic, encourage family involvement, and are efficient for staff use. Healing environments also improve safety and maintain patient privacy and dignity (Herbert & Yoder, 2008). Furthermore, they can promote a sense of connection and rapport to promote health. Color and light are two potentially energizing or calming components that can impact a patient's healing (La Torre, 2006). Many inpatient facilities are now converting at least one seclusion room to a comfort room that has comfortable furniture and a quiet atmosphere and uses color and light to promote a calming effect. Comfort rooms serve as places that patients can go to during times of stress to implement self-soothing measures. Comfort rooms can also reduce the need for seclusion and restraint in psychiatric facilities (Cummings, Granfield, & Coldwell, 2010).

Suffering

Suffering is "the condition of one who suffers: the bearing of pain or distress" (*American Heritage Dictionary*, 2006, p. 1730). It can be related to "pain, sickness, separation, abandonment, death" and can affect one physically, emotionally, spiritually, culturally, and psychologically (Gonzalbo, 2006, p. 2). Ferrell and Coyle (2008) reviewed a number of research studies related to suffering in cancer patients. They found three dimensions commonly affected by suffering:

- Physical (fatigue, pain, and side effects of chemotherapy)

- Psychological (depression)

- Social well-being (withdrawal and isolation)

They noted that these commonalities held across diverse countries and cultures.

The words "patient" and "suffering" come from similar Latin roots meaning "to bear," and to be a patient means "to suffer" (Råholm, 2008, p. 64). Suffering involves bearing some level of distress and pain and may be exacerbated through alienation and loneliness. It often is easy to recognize patients' suffering if they have chest pain or cancer or have lost a child or limb. However, it is more challenging to recognize patients' suffering when they have been ostracized by family, friends, or society because they have been diagnosed with mental illness.

Mental illness does not affect only the individual diagnosed with it. Mental illness is a shared family experience. The resulting suffering may be specific to individual family members or experienced in a relational way by the family. Marshall, Bell, and Moules describe relational suffering as "a complex, intense, human experience that involves a threat of loss to biopsychosocial–spiritual wholeness that reciprocally influences and is influenced by connection and relationship to significant others" (2010, p. 199).

Alleviating patient suffering is at the core of nursing: Wright asserts that "softening suffering is the heart, center, and essence, of nursing practice, whether it be physical, emotional or spiritual suffering" (Wright, 2008, p. 397).

Hope

Most hope theorists agree that hope is a goal-oriented thought or emotion about future expectations (Lopez, Snyder, & Pedrotti, 2003; Hammer, Mogensen, & Hall, 2009). The need for the nurse to connect with patients is critical to promoting hope, as is bearing with patients through their suffering. For example, the nurse's presence and willingness to listen to patient stories can give meaning to the experience of suffering and assist the patient through suffering (Råholm, 2008). It also can promote hope within the patient.

Morse and Doberneck (1995) devised a comprehensive model related to hope and validated it with four studies of different patient populations. They envision hope in several stages:

- Making a realistic appraisal of an event and the threat to self
- Envisioning alternative plans and setting of goals
- Bracing for negative outcomes
- Developing a realistic appraisal of personal resources and external conditions and resources
- Soliciting mutually supportive relationships
- Continuously evaluating signs to reinforce selected goals and the revision of these goals
- Determining to endure

Becoming skilled at promoting hope within clients is a great challenge for the nurse, but can make the difference in alleviating a patient's suffering and promoting healing. Nurturing self to maintain hope is equally important for nurses when experiencing or witnessing high levels of suffering.

Perceptions, Thoughts, and Feelings

The perceptions, thoughts, and feelings of the nurse can affect patient care. By making the effort to be more self-aware, the nurse may be more objective and more accepting of patients, and improve the quality of nurse–patient interactions. *Perceptions* refer to the sensory experiences of the nurse when giving care, such as what is seen, heard, smelled, and touched. *Thoughts* refer to the cognitive aspects of the way in which the nurse appraises the sensory information and makes decisions of how to interact and deliver psychiatric nursing care. *Feelings* refer to the emotional aspects of giving care to patients. Feelings often can be the catalyst for the nurse to focus on the perceptual and cognitive components of nursing care.

Experiences of the Nurse (Self-Awareness)

Self-awareness is very important when caring for and interacting with patients. When the nurse observes patient behavior, thoughts may arise based on the nurse's perception of the behavior, which, in turn, evoke feelings within the nurse (Orlando, 1961). Those feelings may be related to long-held biases, newly formed opinions, identifying with the patient, or a number of other factors. If the nurse is able to respond to those perceptions, thoughts, and feelings and validate them with the patient rather than simply reacting to them, a more helpful nurse–patient interaction may occur.

Because each nurse–patient interaction is unique, it is important for the nurse to understand what is happening during each specific interaction between the nurse and a patient and to keep the focus on the patient. As mentioned earlier, Hildegard Peplau emphasized the interpersonal relationship that takes place when a nurse and patient work together. Peplau stressed that nurses need to be aware of their own behavior. Whereas Peplau focused on the nurse–patient relationship and the stages related to such a relationship, Ida Jean Orlando focused on the nurse's meeting patient needs through a deliberative process of validating with the patient what the patient's immediate needs are and how best to meet them. Orlando's theory of deliberative nursing process assists the nurse by using the nurse's perceptions (obtained through any of the five senses), thoughts, and/or feelings to validate with the patient what the nurse and patient *together* deem is the patient's need. Orlando's theory encourages nurses to be deliberative in determining with patients what their needs are rather than assuming on their own to know what they are (Chapter 7).

Experiences of the Patient (Other-Awareness)

During a nurse–patient interaction, the nurse considers with the patient how the patient is affected, usually within one or more of the five domains of patient wellness: biological, psychological, sociological, cultural, and spiritual. The nurse validates with the patient what the nurse observes as the patient's needs.

While developing the nurse–patient relationship, the nurse is learning to *respond* to the patient rather than *react* to the patient. Observations of the patient at a certain time will be unique to the nurse observing the patient at that time. Different factors, such as location, circumstances, and time, will affect the interaction. Keeping this in mind can help the nurse respond deliberatively, rather than impulsively, and takes the focus off saying "just the right thing." *The important element within the interaction is for the nurse is to keep the focus on the patient.*

Throughout this text, nurses are encouraged to reflect on their interactions with patients; to use their perceptions, thoughts, and feelings; and to validate with patients whether their perceptions, thoughts, and feelings are accurate in relation to the interaction taking place.

Pause and Reflect

1. *What factors in your community affect patients' access to mental health care?*
2. *What aspects of trauma-informed care do you think you would find challenging as a nurse?*
3. *What resources would you use to help you provide trauma-informed care to your patients?*
4. *Can you think of a time when a professional with whom you were working failed to validate your needs? How did it make you feel? How did it make you view the professional?*

The Way Forward

Nurses who are able to assess and validate a patient's needs in each domain and level of wellness will be better able to help the patient develop strategies that alleviate distress, promote wellness, and provide hope. In addition to discussing frameworks of mental health and psychiatric nursing, the information in this text will assist students in addressing mental health and psychiatric needs of all individuals, regardless of circumstance, diagnosis, or setting.

We invite you to begin a potentially incredible growth experience—both in knowing yourself better and learning how to provide care that helps patients move from suffering to finding hope and achieving wellness. Are you ready?

Chapter Highlights

1. All nurses benefit from understanding the principles and practices of psychiatric–mental health nursing.
2. Nearly 60% of adults with mental illness do not receive treatment.
3. Recovery from mental illness is possible.
4. Psychiatric nursing care is *being with* a patient more than *doing for* a patient.
5. Wellness domains include biological, psychological, sociological, spiritual, and cultural domains.
6. Phases of psychiatric wellness include initial onset/relapse, recovery phase, and rehabilitation phase.
7. Factors that affect patient healing include stigma, adherence, access, and hope.
8. Significant concepts that impact patient care include anxiety, coping resources, safety, trauma-informed care, healing environments, suffering, and hope.
9. Hope is empowering in the process of recovery to health.
10. Providing hope can make a difference in promoting healing.

NCLEX®-RN Questions

1. The nurse is evaluating the effectiveness of education with the family of a client who has just been diagnosed with a serious mental illness. Which statement by the family indicates the need for further teaching?
   a. "Mental illness affects individuals from all socioeconomic backgrounds. There is no reason to be ashamed or believe we are responsible."
   b. "There is a relationship between substance abuse and mental illness. We understand we may need to consider treatment options that will address both."
   c. "It sounds like the percentage of persons receiving adequate mental health care is quite high. We should not have difficulty accessing care."
   d. "We never knew that one in five adults suffer from some form of mental illness. It really helps us to know that other families must be going through the same thing we are."

2. The nurse working on a medical–surgical unit is asked to participate in professional development aimed at strengthening mental health and psychosocial nursing skills. Which rationale best supports the need for the nurse to participate?
   a. Due to the relatively low proportion of psychiatric mental health nurses, nurses from other specialties need to fill an unmet need.
   b. When there are significant shortages of inpatient beds, more patients with chronic and acute mental illness present on medical–surgical units.
   c. In situations in which family members are dealing with the stress of hospitalization, the nurse is in a unique position to help them to cope.
   d. Because psychiatric nursing skills are applicable to clients across all settings, it is essential for all nurses to maintain the competency required to meet basic needs.

3. The nurse educator is preparing an in-service on the *Diagnostic and Statistical Manual of Mental Disorders*, 5th edition (DSM-5). The audience consists of baccalaureate-level nurses who are in the process of being oriented to the mental health unit. The nurse educator wants to focus on elements that are critical to the nurses' practice. Which should be included? Select all that apply.
   a. Stressing the manual's limitations in identifying the unique needs of each client
   b. Discussing the value of having standardized criteria for professionals and third-party payers
   c. Explaining how the new classification system lessens the stigma associated with mental illness
   d. Demonstrating how the nurse will use the included scales to determine the severity of the illness
   e. Describing how to go about distinguishing between psychiatric symptoms to support a specific diagnosis

4. The new nurse has just obtained a position working in an outpatient mental health clinic. Which standard of practice does the nurse recognize as distinguishing the role of the advanced practice psychiatric nurse?
   a. Collaborative partnerships
   b. Autonomous decision making
   c. Application of nursing process
   d. Use of therapeutic communication

5. The nurse is working with a patient who has been diagnosed with a major mental illness. The patient reports a childhood marked by chronic physical illness, poverty, and abuse, and states, "I don't have any reason to believe things will ever get better for me." The nurse recognizes that this statement represents a need for intervention in which wellness domain?
   a. Psychological
   b. Spiritual
   c. Biological
   d. Sociological

6. The nurse is working with a patient who has been receiving treatment for schizophrenia for two months. The patient is well groomed and organized. The nurse suspects that the patient has entered the recovery stage of wellness. Which question by the nurse would elicit the best information to support this assessment?
   a. "What are your goals for the future?"
   b. "Have you been taking your medication as directed?"
   c. "Are you still experiencing symptoms of your illness?"
   d. "How do you feel about your treatment and progress?"

7. The new nurse is assigned to care for a patient admitted to the mental health unit. After hearing the report, the nurse finds that the patient shares a history and background that are similar to the nurse's own experiences. Which action would be most appropriate for the nurse to take?
   a. Requesting a change in assignment and avoiding any future interactions with the patient
   b. Acknowledging that biases may occur and being careful to validate the patient's perceptions
   c. Ignoring the feelings of identification that are evoked and proceeding to complete assigned work
   d. Conveying a sense of empathy based on shared experiences and using the similarities to build rapport

8. The nurse is caring for a patient experiencing mental health issues. The nurse notes that although the patient does not have a diagnosis of an anxiety disorder, the patient is demonstrating many signs and symptoms associated with anxiety. Which assessment of situation is most likely to be accurate?

   The patient is:
   a. Receiving inadequate treatment for the primary disorder.
   b. Attempting to express an unmet need or unresolved feelings.
   c. Suffering from an anxiety disorder and has been misdiagnosed.
   d. Demonstrating a response common to many mental health disorders.

9. The nurse is evaluating the patient's response to interventions aimed at promoting a sense of hope in the patient using Morse and Doberneck's (1995) model. Which outcomes indicate that interventions have been effective? Select all that apply.

   The patient:
   a. Revises future goals and expectations.
   b. Prepares for future challenges and crises.
   c. Expresses belief that the illness can be cured.
   d. Focuses on mutually supportive relationships.
   e. Shifts appraisal of the situation from negative to entirely positive.

Answers may be found on the Pearson student resource site: nursing.pearsonhighered.com

Pearson Nursing Student Resources   Find additional review materials at **nursing.pearsonhighered.com**

References

Ablett, J. R. (2007). Resilience and well-being in palliative care staff: A qualitative study of hospice nurses' experience of work. *Psycho-Oncology, 16*, 733–740.

American Association of Colleges in Nursing. (2006). The Essentials of Doctorate Education for Advanced Nursing Practice. Available at http://www.aacn. nche.edu/publications/position/DNPEssentials.pdf

American Association of Colleges in Nursing. (2008). The Essentials of Baccalaureate Education for Professional Nursing Practice. Available at http://www. aacn.nche.edu/education-resources/baccessentials08.pdf

American Association of Colleges in Nursing. (2011). The Essentials of Graduate Education for Advanced Nursing Practice. Available at http://www.aacn. nche.edu/education-resources/MastersEssentials11.pdf

American Heritage Dictionary of the English Language (4th ed., new updated edition). (2006). Boston, MA: Houghton Mifflin Company.

American Nurses Association, American Psychiatric Nursing Association, & International Society of Psychiatric–Mental Health Nurses. (2014). *Psychiatric–Mental Health Nursing: Scope and Standards of Practice.* Silver Spring, MD: NursesBooks.org.

American Nurses Association. (2010a). *Nursing: Scope and Standards of Practice.* 2nd ed. Silver Spring, MD: Nursesbooks.org. Available at http://books. google.com/books?hl=en&lr=&id=N6F7_zSOQccC&oi=fnd&pg=PT4&d q=registered+nurse+standards+and+practice&ots=6hqfcNSBzt&sig=LeW MPqUsOmf9pQFzBltQKFjqAPc

American Nurses Association. (2010b). *Nursing's Social Policy Statement: The Essence of the Profession.* Silver Spring, MD: Nursesbooks.org.

American Psychiatric Association. (2000). *Diagnostic and Statistical Manual of Mental Disorders* (4th ed., Text Revision). Washington, DC: American Psychiatric Association.

American Psychiatric Association. (2013). *Diagnostic and Statistical Manual of Mental Disorders,* 5th ed. Arlington, VA: American Psychiatric Association.

American Psychiatric Nurses Association. (2013). *Quality Indicators Workgroup Report.* Available at http://www.apna.org/i4a/pages/index.cfm?pageID= 4909#sthash.KmXkAWtZ.dpbs

Andreasen, N. C., Carpenter, W. T., Kane, J. M., Lasser, R. A., Marder, S. R., & Weinberger, D. R. (2005). Remission in schizophrenia: Proposed criteria and rationale for consensus. *American Journal of Psychiatry, 162*, 441–449.

Anthony, W. A. (2000). A recovery oriented service system: Setting some system level standards. *Psychiatric Rehabilitation Journal, 24*, 159–168.

Asadi-Pooya, A. A., Schilling, C. A., Glosser, D., Tracy, J. I., & Sperling, M. R. (2007). Health locus of control in patients with epilepsy and its relationship to anxiety, depression, and seizure control. *Epilepsy Behavior, 11*(3), 347–350.

Asarnow, J. R., Jaycox, L. H., & Duan, N. (2006). Effectiveness of a quality improvement intervention for adolescent depression in primary care clinics: A randomized controlled trial. *Journal of the American Medical Association, 293*(3), 311–319.

Babal, K. (2007, October 30). Nutritional therapy for anxiety and depression. Available at http://health.discovery.com/centers/althealth/anxiety/nutrition.html

BBCNews. (2006). Mental health crime link studied. Available at http://newsvote. bbc.co.uk/mpapps/pagetools/print/news.bbc.co.uk/2/hi/health/5216836.stm

Benner, P. (1984). *From Novice to Expert: Excellence and Power in Clinical Practice.* Menlo Park, CA: Addison-Wesley.

Bost, N., & Wallis, M. (2006). The effectiveness of a 15 minute weekly massage in reducing physical and psychological stress in nurses. *Australian Journal of Advanced Nursing, 23*(4), 28–33.

Bradley-Engen, M., Cuddeback, G., Gayman, M., Morrissey, J., & Mancuso, D. (2010). Trends in state prison admission of offenders with serious mental illness. *Psychiatric Services, 61*(12), 1263–1265.

Burkhardt, M. A. (2007). Commentary on "Spirituality in nursing and health-related literature: A concept Analysis." *Journal of Holistic Nursing, 25*(4), 263–264.

Butje, A., Repede, E., & Shattell, M. (2008). Healing scents: An overview of clinical aromatherapy for emotional distress. *Journal of Psychosocial Nursing and Mental Health Services, 46*(10), 46–52.

Centers for Disease Control and Prevention (CDC). (2011). Burden of mental illness. Available at http://www.cdc.gov/mentalhealth/basics/burden.htm

Center for Substance Abuse Research. (2005, May 2). Benzodiazepines. Available at http://www.cesar.umd.edu/cesar/drugs/benzos.asp

Cooper, J., & Barnett, M. (2005). Aspects of caring for dying patients cause anxiety to first year student nurses. *International Journal of Palliative Nursing, 11*(8), 423–430.

Cross, T., Basron, B. J., Dennis, K. W., & Isaacs, M. R. (1989). Towards a culturally competent system of care. NIMH Child and Adolescent Service System Program. Available at http://eric.ed.gov/PDFS/ED330171.pdf

Cummings, K. S., Grandfield, S. A., & Coldwell, C. M. (2010). Caring with comfort rooms: Reducing seclusion and restraint use in psychiatric facilities. *Journal of Psychosocial Nursing and Mental Health Services, 48*(6), 26–30.

Cutshall, S. M., Fenske, L. L., Kelly, R. F., Phillips, B. R., Sundt, T. M., & Bauer, B. A. (2007). Creation of a healing enhancement program at an academic medical center. *Complementary Therapies in Clinical Practice, 13*(4), 217–223.

Dossey, B. (2000). *Florence Nightingale: Mystic, Visionary, Healer*. Philadelphia, PA: Lippincott, Williams and Wilkins.

Dossey, B. M., & Keegan, L. (2009). *Holistic Nursing: A Handbook for Practice* (5th ed.). Sudbury, MA: Jones & Bartlett.

Droste, T. (2007, October 30). Reiki: Hype or help? Available at http://health.discovery.com/centers/althealth/reiki/reiki.html

Edelman, C. L., & Mandel, C. L. (2006). *Health Promotion Throughout the Life Span*, 6th ed. St. Louis, MO: Mosby, Inc.

Ferrell, B. R., & Coyle, N. (2008). The nature of suffering and the goals of nursing. *Oncology Nursing Forum, 35*(2), 241–247.

Flaskerud, J. H. (2000). Ethnicity, culture, and neuropsychiatry. *Issues in Mental Health Nursing, 21*, 5–29.

Foster, K. (2010). "You'd think this roller coaster was never going to stop": Experiences of adult children of parents with serious mental illness. *Journal of Clinical Nursing, 19*(21/22), 3143–3151.

Fowler, M. D. M. (2008). *American Nurses Association Guide to the Code of Ethics for Nurses: Interpretation and Application*. Silver Spring, MD: Nursesbooks.org.

Freud, A. (1946). *The Ego and the Mechanisms of Defence*. New York, NY: International Universities Press, Inc.

Freud, S. (1963). Introductory lectures on psycho-analysis (part III). In J. Strachey (Ed. & Trans.). *The Standard Edition of the Complete Psychological Works of Sigmund Freud* (vol. 19, pp. 243–463). London, UK: Hogarth Press. (Original work published in 1925 [1924].)

Garfield, R. L., Lave, J. R., & Donohue, J. M. (2010). Health reform and the scope of benefits for mental health and substance use disorder services. *Psychiatric Services, 61*(11), 1081–1086.

Gehart, D. R. (2012). The mental health recovery movement and family therapy, part I: Consumer-led reform of services to persons diagnosed with severe mental illness. *Journal of Marital and Family Therapy, 38*(3), 429–442.

Gillespie, B. M., Chaboyer, W., Wallis, M., & Grimbeek, P. (2007). Resilience in the operating room. *Journal of Advanced Nursing 59*(4), 427–438.

Godlewski, S. (2006, September 18). Vitamins for anxiety and panic disorders. Available at http://ezinearticles.com/?Vitamins-for-Anxiety-and-Panic-Disorders&id=301888

Gonzalbo, F. E. (2006). *In the Eyes of God: A Study on the Culture of Suffering*. Austin, TX: University of Texas Press.

Griffin, M. T., Salman, A., Lee, Y., Seo, Y., & Fitzpatrick, J. J. (2008). A beginning look at the spiritual practices of older adults. *Journal of Christian Nursing, 25*(2), 100–102.

Grob, G. N. (1991). Origins of DSM-I: A study in appearance and reality. *American Journal of Psychiatry, 148*(4), 421–431.

Grohol, J. (2012). Final DSM 5 approved by American Psychiatric Association. *Psych Central*. Available at http://psychcentral.com/blog/archives/2012/12/02/final-dsm-5-approved-by-american-psychiatric-association/

Hall, C. S. (1954). *A Primer of Freudian Psychology*. New York, NY: World Publishing Company.

Hammer, K., Mogensen, O., & Hall, E. O. C. (2009). The meaning of hope in nursing research: A meta-synthesis. *Scandanavian Journal of Caring Sciences, 23*, 549–557.

Harris, M., & Fallot, R. D. (2001). *Using Trauma Theory to Design Service Systems: New Directions for Mental Health Services*. San Francisco, CA: Jossey-Bass.

Herbert, C. I., & Yoder, L. M. (2008). Creating the ultimate healing environment: Integrating evidence-based design, IT, and patient safety. *Healthcare Executive 23*(5), 16–18, 20, 22–23.

Herdman, T. H. & Kamitsuru, S. (Eds.). (2014). *NANDA International Nursing Diagnoses: Definitions & Classification 2015–2017*. Oxford, UK: Wiley Blackwell.

Hessel, J. A. (2009). Presence in nursing practice: A concept analysis. *Holistic Nursing Practice, 23*(5): 276–281.

Hermann, R. C., Chan, J. A., Provost, S. E., & Chiu, W. T. (2006). Statistical benchmarks for process measures of quality of care for mental and substance use disorders. *Psychiatric Services, 57*(10):1461–1467.

Holmes, T. H., & Rahe, R. H. (1967). The social readjustment rating scale. *Journal of Psychosomatic Research, 11*, 213–218.

Hummer, V. L., Dollard, N., Robst, J., & Armstrong, M. I. (2010). Innovations in implementation of trauma-informed care practices in youth residential treatment: A curriculum for organizational change. *Child Welfare, 89*(2), 79–95.

How to do a mental status exam. Available at http://www.psychpage.com/learning/library/assess/mse.htm

Insel, T. R., & Scolnick, E. M. (2006). Cure therapeutics and strategic prevention: raising the bar for mental health research. *Molecular Psychiatry, 11*, 11–17.

Institute for Healthcare Improvement. (2012). The Triple Aim Initiative. Available at http://www.ihi.org/offerings/Initiatives/TripleAim/Pages/default.aspx

Institute of Medicine. (1999). *To Err Is Human*. Available at http://www.iom.edu/Reports/1999/To-Err-is-Human-Building-A-Safer-Health-System.aspx

Institute of Medicine. (2006). *Improving the Quality of Health Care for Mental and Substance Abuse Conditions*. Available at http://www.ncbi.nlm.nih.gov/books/NBK19830/

Institute of Medicine. (2010). *The Future of Nursing: Leading Change, Advancing Health*. Available at http://www.iom.edu/Reports/2010/The-Future-of-Nursing-Leading-Change-Advancing-Health.aspx

Internal Medicine News. (2013). Metabolic monitoring of antipsychotics remains vital. Available at http://www.internalmedicinenews.com/single-view/metabolic-monitoring-of-antipsychotics-remains-vital/56d9778c70bcd98121c7a5e203648339.html

Jackson, D. (2009). Editorial: The importance of optimism. Available at http://www.webmd.com/mental-health/tc/mental-health-problems-and-mind-body-wellness-positive-thinking

Jackson, D., Firtko, A., & Edenborough, M. (2007). Personal resilience as a strategy for surviving and thriving in the face of workplace adversity: A literature review. *Journal of Advanced Nursing, 60*(1), 1–9.

Jaffee, L. (2007, Winter). Acupuncture for stress and anxiety. Available at http://www.acufinder.com/Acupuncture+Information/Detail/Acupuncture+for+Stress+and+Anxiety

Jennings, A. (2004). Models for developing trauma-informed behavioral health systems and trauma-specific services. Available at http://www.ct.gov/dmhas/lib/dmhas/trauma/TraumaModels.pdf

Jervis, N. (2006). What is a culture? Available at http://www.p12.nysed.gov/ciai/socst/grade3/whatisa.html

Johns Hopkins Health Alerts. (2007, May 23). The depression patch. Available at http://www.johnshopkinshealthalerts.com/alerts/depression_anxiety/JohnsHopkinsHealthAlertsDepressionAnxiety_847-1.html

Johnson, J. H., & Sarason, I. B. (1978). Life stress, depression, and anxiety: Internal-external control as moderator variable. *Journal of Psychosomatic Research, 22*, 205–208.

Joint Commission. (2013). *Specifications Manual for Joint Commission National Quality Core Measures*. Available at http://www.jointcommission.org/specifications_manual_joint_commission_national_quality_core_measures.aspx

Judkins, S., Arris, L., & Keener, E. (2005). Program evaluation in graduate nursing education: Hardiness as a predictor of success among nursing administration students. *Journal of Professional Nursing, 21*(5), 314–321.

Kaiser Healthcare News. (2012). What are ACOs? Available at http://www.kaiserhealthnews.org/Stories/2011/January/13/ACO-accountable-care-organization-FAQ.aspx?gclid=CK_ysLOR-rYCFe4DOgodmwwAdg

Kemp, D. E., Gao, K., Chan, P. K., Ganocy, S. J., Findling, R. L., & Calabrese, J. R. (2010). Medical comorbidity in bipolar disorder: Relationship between illnesses of the endocrine / metabolic system and treatment outcome. *Bipolar Disorders, 12*, 404–413.

Kessler, R. C., Berglund, P., Demler, O., Jin, R., Koretz, D., Marikangas, K. R., et al. (2003). The epidemiology of major depressive disorder: Results from the National Comorbidity Survey Replication (NCS-R). *Journal of the American Medical Association, 289*(3), 3095–3105.

Kessler, R. C., Berglund, P. A., Demler, O., Jin, R., & Walters, E. E. (2005). Lifetime prevalence and age-of-onset distributions of DSM-IV disorders in the National Comorbidity Survey Replication (NCS-R). *Archives of General Psychiatry, 62*(6), 593–602.

Kessler, R. C., Chiu, W. T., Demler, O., & Walters, E. E. (2005). Prevalence, severity, and comorbidity of twelve-month DSM-IV disorders in the National Comorbidity Survey Replication (NCS-R). *Archives of General Psychiatry, 62*(6), 617–627.

Kirmayer, L. J., & Sartorius, N. (2007) Cultural models and somatic syndromes. *Psychosomatic Medicine, 69,* 832–840.

Kobasa, S. C. (1979). Stressful life events, personality, and health: An inquiry into hardiness. *Journal of Personality and Social Psychology, 37,* 1–11.

La Torre, M. A. (2006). Creating a healing environment. *Perspectives in Psychiatric Care, 42*(40), 262–264.

Lazarus, R. S., & Folkman, S. (1984). *Stress, Appraisal, and Coping.* New York, NY: Springer Publishing Company.

LeRoy, S. (2006, October 25). What are the best natural herbs for anxiety? Available at http://ezinearticles.com/?What-Are-The-Best-Natural-Herbs-for-Anxiety?&id=337960

Leucht, S., Burkard, T., Henderson, J. H., Maj, M., & Sartorius, N. (2007). *Physical Illness and Schizophrenia.* Cambridge, UK: Cambridge University Press.

Little, N. (2006, October 19). What is hypnosis? Available at http://www.anxiety-and-depression-solutions.com/articles/complementary_alternative_medicine/hypnosis/hypnotherapy.php

Lopez, S., Snyder, C., & Pedrotti, J. (2003). Hope: Many definitions, many measures. In *Positive Psychological Assessment: A Handbook of Models and Measures.* Washington, DC: American Psychological Association, pp. 91–106.

Mamlin, N., Harris, K. R., Case, L. P. (2001). A methodological analysis of research on locus of control and learning disabilities: Rethinking a common assumption. *Journal of Special Education, 34*(4), 214–225.

Marshall, A. J. (2007). Relational suffering: A concept analysis. Unpublished manuscript, University of Calgary, Calgary, AB.

Marshall, A., Bell, J., & Moules, N. J. (2010). Beliefs, suffering, and healing: A clinical practice model for families experiencing mental illness. *Perspectives in Psychiatric Care, 46*(3), 197–208.

Mayo Clinic Staff. (2011). Mental health: Overcoming the stigma of mental illness. Available at http://www.mayoclinic.com/health/mental-health/MH00076

McLoughlin, K. A., Du Wick, A., Collazzi, C. M., & Puntil, C. (2013). Recovery-oriented practices of psychiatric-mental health nursing staff in an acute hospital setting. *Journal of the American Psychiatric Nurses Association, 19,* 152–159.

McVicar, A. (2003). Workplace stress in nursing: A literature review. *Journal of Advanced Nursing, 44*(6), 633–642.

Mental Health Problems and Mind-Body Wellness: Positive Thinking. Available at http://www.webmd.com/mental-health/tc/mental-health-problems-and-mind-body-wellness-overview

Mental Status Examination. Available at http://www.psychpage.com/learning/library/assess/mse.htm

Mistler, L. A., Brunette, M. F., Ferron, J. C., et al. (2012). Shared decision making and behavioral support interventions for people with severe mental illness and tobacco dependence. *Journal of Dual Diagnosis, 8*(2), 99–103.

Moller, M. D., & McLoughlin, K. M. (2013). Recovery in psychiatric nursing: Where are we in 2013? *Journal of the American Psychiatric Nurses Association, 19*(3), 113–116.

Moller, M. D., & Zauszniewski, J. (2011). Psychophenomenology of the post-psychotic adjustment process. *Archives of Psychiatric Nursing, 25*(4):253–268.

Morse, J., & Doberneck, B. (1995). Delineating the concept of hope. *Image: Journal of Nursing Scholarship, 27*(4), 277–285.

Moser, D. K. (2007). The rust of life: Impact of anxiety on cardiac patients. *American Journal of Critical Care, 16,* 361–369.

Muir-Cochrane, E. (2006). Medical co-morbidity risk factors and barriers to care for people with schizophrenia. *Journal of Psychiatric and Mental Health Nursing, 13*(4), 447–452.

Murphy, M. F., & Moller, M. D. (1996). The Three R's Program: A wellness approach to rehabilitation of neurobiological disorders. *The International Journal of Psychiatric Nursing Research, 3*(1), 308–317.

Murray, C. J., Vos, T., Lozano, R., Naghavi, M., Flaxman, A. D., Michaud, C., et al. (2012). Disability-adjusted life years (DALYs) for 291 diseases and injuries in 21 regions, 1990–2010: A systematic analysis for the Global Burden of Disease Study 2010. *Lancet, 380,* 2197–2223.

Mynatt, S., & Cunningham, P. (2007). Unraveling anxiety and depression. *The Nurse Practitioner, 32*(8), 28–36.

National Alliance on Mental Illness. (2013). What is mental illness: Mental illness facts. Available at http://www.nami.org/template.cfm?section=about_mental_illness

National Institute of Mental Health. (2008, February 7). Anxiety disorders. Available at http://www.nimh.nih.gov/health/publications/anxiety-disorders/complete-publication.shtml

Newcomer, J. W., Nasrallah, H. A., & Loebel, A. D. (2004). The atypical antipsychotic therapy and metabolic issues national survey: Practice patterns and knowledge of psychiatrists. *Journal of Clinical Pharmacology, 25*(5), S1–S6.

Nordby, K., Kjønsberg, K., & Hummelvoll, J. K. (2010). Relatives of persons with recently discovered serious mental illness: In need of support to become resource persons in treatment and recovery. *Journal of Psychiatric and Mental Health Nursing, 17*(4): 304–311.

Orlando, I. J. (1961). *The Dynamic Nurse–Patient Relationship.* New York, NY: G. P. Putnam's Sons.

Parse, R. R. (1998). *The Human Becoming School of Thought: A Perspective for Nurses and Other Health Professionals.* Thousand Oaks, CA: Sage Publishing.

Parse, R. R. (1999). Community: An alternative view. *Nursing Science Quarterly, 12*(2), 119–124.

Perry, P. J., Alexander, B., Liskow, B. L., & DeVane, C. L. (2007). *Psychotropic Drug Handbook,* 8th ed. New York, NY: Lippincott Williams and Wilkins.

Peplau, H. E. (1952). *Interpersonal Relations in Nursing.* New York, NY: G. P. Putnam's Sons.

Peplau, H. (1963). A working definition of anxiety. In S. Burd & M. Marshall (Eds.). *Some Clinical Approaches to Psychiatric Nursing.* New York, NY: Macmillan.

Quality and Safety Education for Nurses. (2007a). Pre-licensure competencies. Available at http://qsen.org/competencies/pre-licensure-ksas/

Quality and Safety Education for Nurses. (2007b). Graduate level competencies. Available at http://www.aacn.nche.edu/faculty/qsen/competencies.pdf

Quinn, J. R., Smith, M., Ritenbaugh, C., Swanson, K. M., & Watson, M. J. (2003). Research guidelines for assessing the impact of the healing relationship in clinical nursing. *Alternative Therapies, 9*(3), A65–A79.

Råholm, M-B. (2008). Uncovering the ethics of suffering using a narrative approach. *Nursing Ethics, 15*(1), 62–72.

Rain, S. D., Williams, V. R., Robbins, P. C., Monahan, J., Steadman, H. J., & Vesselinov, R. (2003). Perceived coercion at hospital admission and adherence to mental health treatment after discharge. *Psychiatric Services, 54,* 103–105.

Regan, K. (2010). Trauma informed care on an inpatient pediatric psychiatric unit and the emergence of ethical dilemmas as nurses evolved their practice. *Issues in Mental Health Nursing, 31,* 216–222.

Rice, M. J. (2008). Psychiatric mental health evidence-based practice. *Journal of the American Psychiatric Nurses Association, 14*(20), 107–111.

Rice, M. J. (2010). Evidence-based practice problems: Form and focus. *Journal of the American Psychiatric Nurses Association, 16*(5), 307–314.

Roberts, K. T., Robinson, K. M., & Stewart, C. (2009). An integrated mental health clinical rotation. *Journal of Nursing Education, 48*(8): 454–459.

Ros, A. E. R., Kanner, D., Muris, P., Janssen, B., & Mayer B. (2009). Mental illness stigma and disclosure: Consequences of coming out of the closet. *Issues in Mental Health Nursing, 30,* 509–513.

Saakvitne, K. W., Gamble, S. J., Pearlman, L. A., & Lev, B. T. (2000). *Risking Connection: A Training Curriculum for Work with Survivors of Childhood Abuse.* Baltimore, MD: Sidran Institute Press.

Schim, S., Doorenbos, A., Benkert, R., & Miller, J. (2007). Culturally congruent care: Putting the puzzle together. *Journal of Transcultural Nursing, 18*(2), 103–110.

Selye, H. (1956). *The Stress of Life.* New York, NY: McGraw-Hill.

Silva, J. A. C. (2006). Sleep disorders in psychiatry. *Metabolism, 55*(10 Suppl 2): S40–S44.

Stallwood, J., & Stoll, R. (1975). Spiritual dimension of nursing practice. In I. L. Beland & J. Y. Passos (Eds.). *Clinical Nursing,* 3rd ed. New York, NY: Macmillan.

Steinberg, A., & Ritzmann, R. F. (1990). A living systems approach to understanding the concept of stress. *Behavioral Science, 35*(2), 138–146.

Stephenson, P. L. (2006). Before the teaching begins: Managing patient anxiety prior to providing education. *Clinical Journal of Oncology, 10*(2), 241–245.

Substance Abuse and Mental Health Services Administration. (2006). Consensus Statement defines mental health recovery. Available at http://www.samhsa.gov/SAMHSA_News/VolumeXIV_2/article4.htm

Substance Abuse and Mental Health Services. (2012a). Behavioral Health, United States, 2012. Available at http://samhsa.gov/data/2012BehavioralHealth-US/2012-BHUS.pdf

Substance Abuse and Mental Health Services. (2012b). The National Consensus Statement on Mental Health Recovery. SAMHSA's Working Definition of Recovery: 10 Guiding Principles of Recovery. Available at http://store.samhsa.gov/shin/content//PEP12-RECDEF/PEP12-RECDEF.pdf

Substance Abuse and Mental Health Services Administration. (2013). Results from the 2012 National Survey on Drug Use and Health: Mental Health Findings, NSDUH Series H-47, HHS Publication No. (SMA) 13-4805. Rockville, MD: Substance Abuse and Mental Health Services Administration. Available at http://www.samhsa.gov/data/NSDUH/2k12MH_FindingsandDetTables/2K12MHF/NSDUHmhfr2012.htm#sec2-4

Swartz, M. S., Marvin, S., Swanson, J. W., Wagner, H. R., Burns, B. J., & Hiday, V. A. (2001). Effects of involuntary outpatient commitment and depot antipsychotics on treatment adherence in persons with severe mental illness. Journal of Nervous Mental Disease, 189(9), 583–592.

Tas, F. V., Guvenir, T., & Cevrim, E. (2010). Patients' and their parents' satisfaction levels about the treatment in a child and adolescent mental health inpatient unit. Journal of Psychiatric and Mental Health Nursing, 17(9), 769–774.

Tefera, L., Shah, A. M., & Hsu, K. (2007, May 8). Anxiety. Available at http://www.emedicine.com/EMERG/topic35.htm

Turnipseed, D. L. (1999). An exploratory study of the hardy personality at work in the health care industry. Psychological Reports 85, 1199–1217.

University of Dundee Student Services. (2007, August 31). Understanding anxiety and panic attacks. Available at http://www.dundee.ac.uk/studentservices/counselling/leaflets/anxiety.htm

U.S. Department of Health and Human Services: Substance Abuse and Mental Health Services Administration. (2011). Shared decision making in mental health care. Available at http://store.samhsa.gov/shin/content/SMA09-4371/SMA09-4371.pdf

Vance, D. E., Burrage, J., Couch, A., & Raper, J. (2008). Promoting successful cognitive aging with HIV through hardiness: Implications for nursing practice and research. Journal of Gerontological Nursing, 34(6), 22–29.

Waite, R., Gerrity, P., & Arango, R. (2010). Assessment for and response to adverse childhood experiences. Journal of Psychosocial Nursing, 48(12), 51–61.

Wanzer, M., Booth-Butterfield, M., & Booth-Butterfield, S. (2005). "If we didn't use humor, we'd cry": Humorous coping communication in health care settings. Journal of Health Communication 10, 105–125.

Weber, N. S., Cowan, D. N., Millikan, A. M., & Niebuhr, D. W. (2009). Psychiatric and general medical conditions comorbid with schizophrenia in the national hospital discharge survey. Psychiatric Services, 60(8), 1059–1067.

Wells, K., Sherbourne, C., Schoenbaum K., et al. (2004). Five-year impact of quality improvement for depression: Results of a group-level randomized controlled trial. Archives of General Psychiatry, 61(4): 378–386.

Wendling, P. (2013). Metabolic monitoring of antipsychotics remains vital. Internal Medicine News. Available at http://www.internalmedicinenews.com/single-view/metabolic-monitoring-of-antipsychotics-remains-vital/56d9778c70bcd98121c7a5e203648339.html.

Wildgust, H. J., & Beary, M. (2010). Are there modifiable risk factors which will reduce the excess mortality in schizophrenia? Journal of Psychopharmacology, 24(11 Supp 4), 37–50.

World Health Organization. (2010). Global burden of disease study. Available at http://en.wikipedia.org/wiki/List_of_countries_by_life_expectancy#List_from_the_WHO_.22GDB_2010.22_study

World Health Organization. (2013a). Disability schedule. Available at http://www.who.int/classifications/icf/whodasii/en/

World Health Organization. (2013b). Mental health: A state of well-being. Available at http://www.who.int/features/factfiles/mental_health/en/

Wright, L. M. (2008). Softening suffering through spiritual care practices: One possibility for healing families. Journal of Family Nursing, 14(4), 394–411.

Wulff, K., Gatti, S., Wettstein, J. G., & Foster, R. G. (2010). Sleep and circadian rhythm disruption in psychiatric and neurodegenerative disease. Nature Reviews | Neuroscience, 11, 1–10.

2

Past, Present, Future

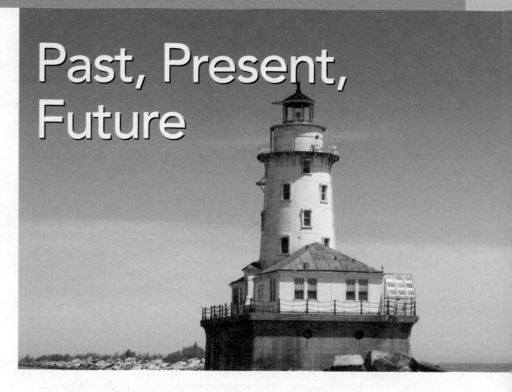

Martha Mathews Libster

Key Terms

asylum, 27
curative point, 25
healing environment, 28
history, 25
humane treatment, 27
hydrotherapy, 33
interpersonal relations theory, 33
moral therapy, 27
perseverance, 25
Vermont Study, 25

Learning Outcomes

1. Discuss the role of nurses throughout history in forming and reforming the care of individuals with mental illness.

2. Describe moral therapy, the system of care implemented by nurses in 19th-century asylums.

3. Identify social beliefs about mental illness in earlier centuries.

4. Compare historic with contemporary psychiatric science and practice.

5. Summarize what the life of individuals with mental illness was like in earlier centuries.

6. Examine the role of psychiatric nurses in health reform and social justice related to the care of individuals suffering mental illness.

7. Assess how nurses have created and cultivated healing environments that contribute to the healing of patients with mental illness.

History of Suffering and Hope

History is the record of human behavior over time. It is a documentation of individual and collective experiences from suffering to hope. The history of psychiatric mental health nursing is a story of hope. For centuries, nurses have provided support, comfort, holistic care, and an enduring presence to some of the most marginalized of society—those suffering from mental illness (Figure 2-1). The way that nurses care for the patient with mental illness has changed over time. That care is a historical reflection of any given society's decisions as to who is defined as mentally ill, what environment meets the health care needs of the patient and his or her family, and the best practices and treatments. To understand mental illness, the suffering of patients and their families, and the diversity of cares and cures over time, nurses must consider the historical context for the culture that encompasses mental illness and psychiatric mental health nursing. Studying the context for psychiatric care, past and present, can help to diminish the judgment and misunderstanding that continues to surround the history of mental illness, those who suffer from it, and the development of psychiatric mental health care over time.

This chapter highlights some of the significant events and trends in nurses' endeavors to understand and cure mental illness as well as to provide scientific and creative care within a healing environment. It focuses primarily on American history, but it also includes examples from the history of psychiatric mental health nursing care from around the globe. The purpose of this chapter is to provide nurses and nursing students with a sense of what it has been like to be a person suffering mental illness and to be a nurse to those with mental illness during the past three centuries. Even though understanding of mental illness and the corresponding way in which the efforts of nurses to care for patients with mental illness may have changed and evolved over time, there is a pattern of disease that continues. Stigma surrounding mental illness and those who suffer from it endures despite its prevalence throughout history, its common place in the human experience of suffering, and the historical presence of good nurses who provide comfort, care, and hope.

Is There a Cure?

The underlying question about psychiatric illness that has endured over the course of many centuries is quite simple: Is there a cure? The history of psychiatric care includes much discussion, dialog, and debate about defining psychiatric illness and disease, identifying acute versus chronic patterns of disease, and evaluating the effectiveness of cares and treatments—both short- and long-term—for those who suffer mental illness. There have been times when people with certain types of mental illness were shackled in chains to protect the community from what people have thought of as demonic possession. At other times, those with mental illness have been cared for in their community health care centers. Where, when, and how people are cared for demonstrates society's health beliefs at a given period in time. Historical records document those health beliefs and practices. Even though health beliefs and practices do change over time, the underlying question about the possibility of a cure—that is, the eradication of mental illness—pervades in the minds and hearts of clinicians, scientists, and clients and their families.

The research and writings of nurse–psychologist Dr. Courtney Harding exemplifies the nature of the quest and nurses' important roles in finding solutions to the question of cure. Harding's work with clients with schizophrenia, well known as the **Vermont Study** (Harding, Brooks, Ashikaga, Strauss, & Breier, 1987a, 1987b), is said to be one of the longest-running studies in American clinical medical research. This study has involved the deinstitutionalization and rehabilitation of clients with schizophrenia in their communities. Sixty-eight of 82 of the chronically mentally ill clients with schizophrenia in the study were considered to have significantly improved or recovered. They function as members of society. This evidence confronted previous beliefs about the poor outcomes of schizophrenia. Analyses comparing the outcomes of long-term studies by Harding and two others suggest that clients with schizophrenia can indeed move in the direction of improvement and recovery (Harding, 1988). However, people are still hesitant to use the word "cure" when referring to those who have learned to live with schizophrenia.

It is not surprising that Harding, a nurse, would persevere with persons suffering chronic mental illness in this way, study their suffering, help them and their families, and ultimately provide hope to persons with mental illness, their physicians, and their caregivers. **Perseverance** (the continued adherence to a course of action or path despite obstacles or resistance) is a trait that has defined nurses throughout time. Like Harding, Prudence Morrell, a nurse leader in the early Shaker community, partnered with physicians to save the lives of patients deemed incurable or destined for death by medical estimation. Sister Prudence wrote in 1849 that "the great art or skill in curing up the sick and afflicted does not always depend on the knowledge of the Physician, it some times [*sic*] partly depends on perseverance," which she went on to define as one of the acts of her "conscience" in caring for others, which "would not let her give up on them" (Morrell, 1849, preface p. 1).

The writings of Matilda Coskery, a Sisters of Charity nurse renowned for her care of the insane, add to our understanding of the details of nursing history of perseverance with the insane, the chronically ill, and the dying (Box 2-1). She, like physicians of her time, wrote about the **curative point** in the care of clients. The 19th-century term *curative point* refers to a point of view in which the patient was treated as if he or she would be cured, as opposed to given palliative care. Sister Matilda wrote in her *Advices Concerning the Sick* about the important role of the nurse in relation to the curative point:

> A small thing near the crisis of the patient, is very often the cause of death, for being at its height, & on the point of changing for better or worse, one little right matter neglected or one little wrong thing done, takes from him his last chance for recovery. This is what Drs call the curative point, and mostly rests in the hands of the nurse & attendants. (Libster & McNeil, 2009, p. 187)

Historical Context   box 2-1

Prior to the 20th century, people with mental illness were referred to as "the insane." Although insanity was not openly discussed in society, the term *insanity* was considered a descriptive, rather than derogatory, term. People with what today are referred to as developmental delays were called "idiots" or said to be suffering from "idiocy."

Her medical colleague Dr. William Stokes, physician for the insane, said of Matilda and the Sisters of Charity nurses with whom he worked closely that nurses were important to the client's convalescence particularly at "critical points":

> It is at the period of convalescence, that the services of a judicious and skillful attendant are especially needed by the insane, in order rightly to lead the returning faculties into more healthy and rational channels. There is a certain dexterity and tact, which can alone be acquired by long familiarity with insanity in all its diversified shades and phases, and which enables their possessor to accomplish much good in controlling the morbid fancies of the patient, and in properly directing his thoughts, feelings, and affections. The judicious nurse and attendant will look with watchful eye for the earliest signs of recovery, and the moment the first glimmerings of right reason display themselves, will endeavor to promote the progress of improvement thus begun. . . . If neglected, they may pass away forever, and the patient speedily glide into a darkness of mind of deeper gloom than before. Patients, therefore, at this critical period, require much delicate attention. . . . They are, at this time, particularly sensible to kind words, but easily disturbed by violent impressions or painful emotions; and it is now, when an indiscreet word, an unkind rebuke, may effectually retard recovery, that all the Physician's trust, and all his hope, rest on the judicious aid of a kind and gentle attendant. None can better appreciate than he the importance of the patient's having, at this critical moment, a nurse of intelligence and humanity. (Stokes, 1849, pp. 8–9)

Critical and curative points represent the moment in time when nurses become the instruments of hope. Nurses, with their judicious and skillful approaches and interventions, have cared for and healed people with mental illness when members of society, and even physicians, have relegated them to chains, torture, isolation, and death.

Early History of Psychiatric Nursing Care

Some of the first historical accounts of psychiatric nursing care are found in the 17th-century community records of the Daughters of Charity (DC) of Vincent de Paul in Paris, France. The Protestant Reformation had suppressed noncloistered religious life for women,

and the Tridentine decrees of the Catholic Reformation in 1563 demanded that all nuns live within convent walls. By the early 17th century, there were no Protestant communities of nurses, and Catholic leadership had denied the requests of their religious women to practice nursing. Vincent de Paul and a noblewoman named Louise de Marillac collaborated in petitioning the pope for permission to create a "confraternity" of apostolic women who, rather than residing in the cloister as nuns, would "come and go like seculars," ministering to the sick poor and insane in their homes (McNeil, 1996, p. xvii). Louise de Marillac signed the contract for their first hospital mission in February 1, 1640, at the Hôtel-Dieu in Angers (Coste & de Paul, 1985–2008a, pp. 143a, 114).

According to Vincent, the cornerstone of the DC ministry was humility, because this virtue provided a lens for the recognition and acknowledgement of both personal talents and limits (501 Vincent de Paul to Louise de Marillac 2:164 and 37 Humility 11:46 in Coste & de Paul, 1985–2008b). Vincent and Louise instructed the sisters in community life and nursing skills, which included the spiritual values essential for service to the poor. Caring for the sick poor was a tremendously difficult task. Vincent had written of the challenges of hospital ministry to the poor in particular. He described the work by saying:

> If you were to go and serve the sick, it would be in a hospital or in their own homes. If it were in a hospital, alas! Poor Brother, you would be going from the frying pan into the fire, for so many painful crosses and contradictions are encountered there that the ones about which you are complaining are nothing in comparison. The work is heavy, times of rest are short and interrupted, repugnance is certain, and reproaches and insults are frequent there. Almost all the poor grumble about things because they are never satisfied and usually complain to both the devout persons who visit them and the Administrators who are in charge of them. They even make false reports to them about those who serve them because the latter have refused them something. Those poor servants are harassed on all sides, having as many supervisors and critics as there are masters, chaplains, and persons who have some responsibility in those houses. This is what our poor Daughters of Charity find the hardest. (1537 Vincent de Paul to a Brother in the Genoa House in Coste & de Paul, 1985–2008b, p. 4:440.)

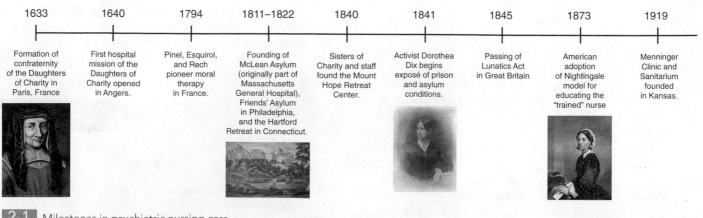

1633	1640	1794	1811–1822	1840	1841	1845	1873	1919
Formation of confraternity of the Daughters of Charity in Paris, France	First hospital mission of the Daughters of Charity opened in Angers.	Pinel, Esquirol, and Rech pioneer moral therapy in France.	Founding of McLean Asylum (originally part of Massachusetts General Hospital), Friends' Asylum in Philadelphia, and the Hartford Retreat in Connecticut.	Sisters of Charity and staff found the Mount Hope Retreat Center.	Activist Dorothea Dix begins exposé of prison and asylum conditions.	Passing of Lunatics Act in Great Britain	American adoption of Nightingale model for educating the "trained" nurse	Menninger Clinic and Sanitarium founded in Kansas.

2-1 Milestones in psychiatric nursing care.

Source: Interfoto/Alamy, McLean Hospital, Library of Congress Prints and Photographs Division [LC-USZ62-9797], E+/Getty Images.

Vincent de Paul is recognized as the "director of the first hospital in France which was devoted to the treatment of the insane" (Laignel-Lavastine and Vie as cited in Flinton, 1992, p. 136). He also cared for the insane in his congregations. His firsthand experience of the emotional pain and mental suffering of those with insanity sensitized Vincent to instructing the DC in nursing ministries, which in his day included the care of galley slaves, beggars, the homeless, prisoners, and the violent mentally ill. Although he did not make light of the challenges of caring for the insane in Paris, he also conveyed to the DC that caring for the insane was an important part of their ministry. He said, "Sisters, it is God Himself who willed to make use of the Daughters of Charity to look after those poor mental patients. What a happiness for all of you. What a great grace for those Sisters engaged in this work to have such a beautiful means of rendering service to God" (Coste & de Paul, 1985–2008b, p. 10:103).

Those in religious life were part of a small subset of society not only willing and able to help persons suffering with mental illness, but also inspired and dedicated to doing so in a more humane way than had occurred in the past. Vincent de Paul demonstrated his dedication to the **humane treatment** of the insane in caring acts such as instructing that patients be served the same food as the priests and brothers (Roman 274 in Coste & de Paul, 1985–2008b, p. 211:331). As early as the mid-1600s, the DC nurses' attention to the insane illuminated the need for vigilant social justice in regard to the care of the mentally ill.

The DC pioneered asylum-based psychiatric nursing at French hospitals such as Les Petites Maisons. **Asylums** served as a point of residential care for those with mental illness, particularly those patients who exhibited violence. They endured many of the hardships still associated today with the care of the insane, particularly the violent insane. For example, Sister Nicole Lequin (1626–1703) entered the DC community in 1649 and worked at Les Petites Maisons until her death. She was injured several times and maltreated by patients, but did not show resentment. Sister Nicole was known for her calm acceptance of patients' negative behaviors. She often expressed her hope to care for the insane until the end of her life. The brief accounts of Sister Nicole's work demonstrate the way in which she also persevered with her patients. A surgeon examined a patient abandoned by an attendant who had found the patient's condition offensive; soon, the surgeon also tired of caring for him because of the offensive odor of his infection. On observing this, Sister Nicole assumed the patient's care with great devotion and attention to him.

She used simple remedies that she had available—and he healed perfectly in very little time. Sister Nicole delighted in instructing her nurse companions and gave them practical lessons in dressing wounds and preparing herbal remedies for patients (Daughters of Charity, April 17, 1703). Some of the DC who served in the insane asylums of France "possessed profound pharmaceutical knowledge" (Jones, 1989, p. 378).

The French DC nurses' ministry and work in the 17th and early 18th centuries brought a new level of humanity and expertise to the nursing care of the insane patient. Later in the 18th century, physicians contributed greatly to that progress as well. In 1793, Dr. Phillipe Pinel ordered the release of insane "inmates" in Paris' Hôpital Général from the chains used to restrain them in their cells. He instituted a period in psychiatric care that focused on the humane treatment of patients. Until this time, French physicians and hospital administrators had considered insanity to be a social or hereditary condition, rather than an "organic" problem related to cerebral hyperemia or hardening of the nerves. Pinel and his student, Jean-Étienne Esquirol (1772–1840), who had created one of the most successful private asylums in Paris, believed that the cause of mental illness lay in the passions of the soul and that insanity did not always affect one's ability to reason. Esquirol, however, insisted on the definitive medicalization of the care of the insane. The physician was to be the principal of a lunatic hospital; it was he who should "set everything in motion. . . . The physician should be invested with an authority from which no one is exempt" (Jones, 1980, p. 386).

Henri Rech, a physician who had studied the works of Pinel and worked with Esquirol, wrote in his book *Clinique de las Maison d'Aliénés*, that the doctor was the "moral entrepreneur" within the asylum rather than the dispenser of medical therapy (as cited in Jones, 1980, p. 386). Physicians used medical therapies such as drugs for their tranquilizing or symptomatic rather than curative effect. As moral entrepreneurs, physicians applied **moral therapy,** a system of care that stressed kindness to patients and the employment of the patient in meaningful activity. Medical treatment, such as bloodletting and drugs, was considered secondary, and therefore great importance was assigned to the quality of the attendants, nurses, and supervisors who created and maintained the therapeutic environment of the asylum and administered the moral therapy.

A half century later, exploration of moral therapy continued. England's York Retreat opened as a Quaker hospital led by Daniel Tuke and George Jepson, who, following their "Inner Light" (Stewart,

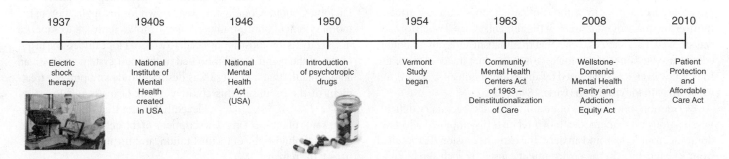

1937	1940s	1946	1950	1954	1963	2008	2010
Electric shock therapy	National Institute of Mental Health created in USA	National Mental Health Act (USA)	Introduction of psychotropic drugs	Vermont Study began	Community Mental Health Centers Act of 1963 – Deinstitutionalization of Care	Wellstone-Domenici Mental Health Parity and Addiction Equity Act	Patient Protection and Affordable Care Act

Source: Reeve Photograph Collection/Otis Historical Archives/National Museum of Health and Medicine, Karamysh/Shutterstock.

1992, p. 52), pioneered moral therapy in Britain. The York Retreat was under the control of lay therapists, rather than physicians, as was advocated by Esquirol in France until the adoption of the Lunatics Act in 1845. The Lunatics Act required that the asylum be run by a medical superintendent. Prior to 1845, Tuke and his followers believed that the "key to moral therapy lay in the quality of personal relationships between staff and patients" in Britain (Digby, 1985b, p. 57). One did not need to be a physician to implement the tenets of what had come to be known as the successful treatment of the insane, most importantly creating a **healing environment**, one in which the patient used internal and external resources to promote healing.

Creating Safe Healing Environments

In 19th-century America, moral treatment was defined as care that focused on the rational and emotional rather than the organic causes of insanity. American physicians, like many of their mentors in Europe, adopted moral therapy as essential in the treatment of the insane, particularly those whose disease was not related to organic causes such as birth trauma. "Insanity" was still the proper term in use during the 19th century to describe those with mental illness. *Insanity* was defined by the editor of the *American Journal of Insanity* as "a chronic disease of the brain, producing either derangement of the intellectual faculties, or prolonged change of the feelings, affections, and habits of an individual"(Brigham, 1847, p. 97). The term also was used when referring to "idiocy," defined as the "total want or alienation of understanding" and a "defect of development of the brain" (Andrew, 1842, p. 358). Mental diseases were generally organized into four categories: mania, melancholy, dementia, and idiocy. Hallucinations occurred in the manic or melancholic patient. Suicide and "drunkenness" or "intoxication," both of which were prevalent in 19th-century American society, were often the topic of discussions about insanity in the *American Journal of Insanity* and in professional meetings.

In his 1844 report in the *American Journal of Insanity*, Pliny Earle, superintendent physician of the Bloomingdale Asylum in New York, wrote that the causes of insanity included heredity, a predisposition in the nervous system (not in the blood, as thought by Dr. Benjamin Rush [1746–1813], whose treatment focused on bloodletting), and functional cerebral disease. Before the onset of their mental illnesses, patients were often noted to have sustained injuries or other harm from falls, masturbation (in men), fever, ill health and dyspepsia, parturition, or pregnancy and amenorrhea (in women). He also noted as possible causes of insanity chronic inflammation, such as occurred in the liver and mucous membrane of the alimentary canal when tobacco was smoked. Earle stated a belief that rheumatism and gout "undoubtedly" caused insanity due to metastasis to the dura mater of the brain. Idiocy, however, was not caused by any external influence; the person was born with the condition (Earle, 1848, p. 193).

Common moral causes of insanity included pecuniary difficulties, religious excitement, death of a relative, disappointed affection, domestic trouble, fear, and anxiety. The extreme tension that resulted from "excitements" in the environment caused by such situations as the constant shifts in population and the hectic pace of urban life, in particular, was the focus of mental health promotion and the creation of asylums such as the Mount Hope Retreat, a hospital created and administered by Sister Matilda and the American Sisters of Charity nurses, where people could live in secluded, peaceful natural surroundings. Mount Hope was landscaped with a beautiful garden, a pond, winding walkways and a meadow where patients could exercise, rest, and "forget for a time their little pains and sorrows" (Coskery, n.d., p. 32).

Resting the mind was thought key to resolving mental illness in the 19th century, just as "reducing stress" is today. Because of this belief, some thought education to be a major contributing factor in the emergence of insanity. Spending too much time *cultivating the mind* was thought to lead to excess stimulation and therefore overexcitement, a state that threatened well-being. This belief had its roots in Dr. William Cullen's (1710–1790) theory of disease. He wrote that all disease was due to excess or deficiency of excitability, the biological capacity to react to external stimuli (Bynum, 1994, p. 17). Common medical therapeutics that were considered "depletive" or draining of excess excitability included bloodletting and emetics, and those who suffered deficiency of excitability received stimulants such as opiates. Cullen was the teacher of Dr. Benjamin Rush, who took depletive therapy to the extreme in his recommendations of repeated bloodletting.

In England after 1845, moral treatment was assimilated into the area of medical expertise. The assumption of "medical monopoly over moral as well as medical treatment was a general feature of mid-nineteenth-century asylums" in Britain (Digby, 1985a, p. 13). An editorial was printed in the 1853 issue of the new *Asylum Journal* in Britain stating that the moral system of treatment could be properly carried out only under the constant supervision and continuous assistance of a physician (as cited in Digby, 1985a, p. 113).

In America there was at least one asylum, however, where moral therapy was fully implemented by nurses—the Mount St. Vincent Hospital, which a few years later became known as the Mount Hope Retreat. As stated previously, this was the asylum owned and operated by the Sisters of Charity of Vincent de Paul (SC) under the guidance of its consulting physician, Dr. Stokes. Stokes was paid $250 every quarter for his service (Daughters of Charity, 1847–1851). He also taught at medical schools and had his own practice, but was willing to serve as consulting physician to the SC for two reasons: He and the SC had a similar vision as to how to reform psychiatric care so that it was more humane, and the SC had developed an expertise in the care of the insane that he felt necessitated only a consulting rather than a resident physician, as was the case in the large state-run asylums.

Stokes and the SC believed that it was possible to care for the insane, even the violently insane, without restraint. In 1841, Stokes had visited the Hanwell Asylum in England, which was directed by Dr. John Conolly. Conolly was well known for his application of the moral system of nonrestraint treatment. Stokes returned to America in 1842 to his new post as physician to Mount Hope under "the inspiration of the grand ideas embodied in this new system and with an abiding faith, that a new era was destined to dawn upon the treatment of the insane in this country" (Our Growth and Progress, Stokes, 1880, p. 18). Stokes's Eleventh Annual Report of 1853 contains some of the most vivid descriptions of the definitions of disease, the moral philosophy of the institution, and the nurses' caring practices at the retreat.

Stokes listed the major diagnoses of patients under their care as "hereditary predisposition, family affliction and trouble, anxiety of the mind and too close application to business, ill health, intemperance, pecuniary losses and reverse of fortune, jealousy and inordinate pride, disappointment, epilepsy, and masturbation" (Stokes, 1853, p. 22).

Moral causes were more difficult to identify because people did not typically talk openly about their family member's odd behaviors. However, when the doctor and nurses at Mount Hope were called on by families and friends to help, they inspired patient confidence in their services, which Stokes stated was the "very keystone of all moral treatment" (Stokes, 1845, p. 17). Just as the name of their hospital stated, the Sisters of Charity offered people hope. They believed in the power of the healing environment, especially in the asylum created specifically for the moral management of mental diseases.

Although there are no "charts" in which the Sisters recorded daily patient care, they did keep a log that included the name and age of each patient admitted to a facility, the diagnosis, when the patient was discharged, and the outcome of care. The SC also kept community and mission records that serve as resources in the construction of historical accounts. The most lengthy and detailed of the early SC's nursing-mission records are two accounts attributed to Sister Matilda Coskery: *Cradle of Mount Hope* (Coskery, n.d.) and an instruction book for nurses titled *Advices Concerning the Sick* (Coskery, n.d. c. 1840; Libster & McNeil, 2009). These accounts provide an understanding of the human suffering that the SC and Dr. Stokes experienced firsthand, all day, every day, in the care of the insane. They left the Maryland Hospital for the Insane in 1838 to start the Mount Hope Retreat after realizing that the "whole system of treatment" of the insane at the Maryland Hospital had been "radically wrong" (Stokes, 1846–1888 11–12–39, p. 18). Stokes joined Sister Matilda Coskery and the SC, who left the Maryland Hospital in 1839 because they also were unable to influence administration to make changes the SC felt were necessary for safety of patients and themselves (Box 2-2). In the early asylums, nurses lived in the hospital with the patients. Therefore, safety was particularly important for these women healers.

Sister Matilda became the Sister-Servant (head nurse) of Mount Hope. She and the SC owned Mount Hope and administered all hospital activities—an unusual achievement for women of the period. Dr. Stokes defended not only his right to serve Mount Hope as a consultant, but also the right of the Sisters to hold administrative and clinical control within their facility. At the time, medical superintendents of state asylums had started an organization that is known today as the American Psychiatric Association. Many of the leaders thought safe and effective care of the insane equated with medical dominance (Libster & McNeil, 2009, pp. 138–148). Stokes disagreed and fully supported the Sisters' right to lead the mission of reinventing the care of the institutionalized insane entrusted to their care. Dr. Stokes wrote in an institutional report:

> We have endeavored . . . not only to keep pace with the advancing science in the treatment of the insane, but have earnestly labored to raise it to a higher and broader plane of service; and thus fulfill its great mission of benevolence and charity, with a rigor, which would increase, rather than diminish, with age. (Stokes, 1846–1888)

One of the biggest issues for the Sisters as they engaged in moral therapy and its foundational philosophy of kindness was how to safely manage violent behavior in the asylum. During the peak years of its promotion, moral treatment was aimed at engaging the mind and exercising the body. The essential components of moral treatment included removal from one's home and former associations, respectful and kind treatment in all situations, manual labor (not a cure and best applied after achieving convalescence), religious worship on Sunday, establishing regular habits, self-control, and diversion of the mind from morbid thoughts (Brigham, 1847). Patients were assigned activities appropriate to their mental and social abilities. Interventions included conversation and recreational activities, such as sewing and taking walks. The new Mount Hope facility enabled the Sisters to offer their patients a greater range of activities and allowed them to better manage patient behaviors, including the risk of patient escape.

Nursing in a 19th-Century Asylum

box 2-2

In 1833, Sisters of Charity Olympia Boyle McTaggert (1802–1869), Octavia McFadden (1813–1853), and Matilda Coskery (1799–1870) were sent to nurse the patients at the Maryland Hospital for the Insane, which was located where the present-day Johns Hopkins Hospital stands. A state inspection in 1827 had found the hospital in dire condition and in debt. Just four years after the Sisters arrived, the establishment and its equipment were partially renovated, its debts were paid, and the nursing care of the patients had improved significantly (Beam, 1837). According to the report, the SC had cared for 842 patients in 3 years. At the time of the inspection there were 74 patients and 12 "Sister-Nurses," who administered the care with the aid of two men and six assistant women.

In the 1830s, the Maryland Hospital had two areas for care. They treated diseases such as epilepsy, fever, syphilis, dysentery, typhus, gangrene, and wounds. Beginning in 1834, however, they were not allowed to admit patients with "contagious diseases." Another area at the hospital was dedicated to the care of patients with mental disorders such as mania a potu (delirium tremens), intemperance, and melancholia, as well as diseases that were referred to more generally as insanity and idiocy (Maryland Hospital for the Insane, 1834–1872, p. 1). The Sisters were also responsible for the domestic duties of the institution. The Sister-Servant collected all payments from patients and handled legal and business matters pertaining to admissions. Upon a patient's admission, she had to collect from the patient the certificate of insanity issued by the Court of Competent Jurisdiction or two physicians, except in the case of those suffering delirium tremens or drunkenness, who could be admitted as long as they furnished a certificate soon thereafter. The Sisters kept a ledger of all admissions and attended the insane under the direction of the medical attendant. They executed medical prescriptions and were to make every effort to "soothe the patient's mind." The Sisters worked with physical therapeutics, such as tea made from hops (*Humulus lupulus*), an herb that calms the nervous system. It was given hourly to patients with delirium tremens who found it hard to sleep. If the hops tea was "not sufficient to produce sleep," the Sisters might administer 40 drops of opium tincture (Medical Case Book, 1832, p. 255). The power struggles between the Sister-Nurses and the resident physician of the Maryland Hospital were not resolved; the Sisters withdrew on September 30, 1840 to forge a new path in the care of the insane, in which they would create their own place of hope: the Mount Hope Retreat.

Providing a safe, healing environment also required proper staffing. At the York Retreat in England in the 1840s, the ratio of nurses or attendants to patients was one to eight. Although this ratio was an improvement over previous conditions, it was still higher than at expensive private asylums, where the ratio was typically one nurse to two patients or even one to one (Digby, 1985b). The purpose of "coercive" treatment or use of restraints was to protect the patient and other patients and staff from violent behavior. However, the use of restraints needed to be weighed against the risk of creating excitement or irritation and, therefore, inflammation, which, as mentioned previously, was considered a significant contributor to insanity. Free motion was one way, people believed, that the body discharged its excitability. When restrained, the insane person was unable to do this. The four most common restraints in use in the 19th century were seclusion, strait-waistcoats, force, and strapping to the bed (at all four points—both hands and both feet).

The intention for the use of restraints in the Mount Hope or any facility ascribing to the philosophy of moral therapy was not to impose punishment. Restraints were a last resort to help a patient reestablish his or her self-control, that part of social conduct that was emphasized in treatment at the asylums. The Sister-Nurses at Mount Hope treated their patients as if they were rational beings; they did not reprimand them for or contradict their thoughts or feelings (Libster & McNeil, 2009). It was only when the safety of the patient, other patients, the staff, or the property was at risk that they would use coercive therapies of any kind. The Sisters were inventive when it came to using restraints and creating a safe environment for patients. In 1841, W. G. Read, who had been commissioned by the New York State Legislature to visit asylums, wrote after interviewing Sister Matilda:

> [The Sisters] never *permit the infliction of blows*, nor subject their patients to the strait-jacket, which they consider extremely harassing; and which, in one case at the Maryland Hospital, (if I remember aright), nearly caused the death of a frantic sufferer, by strangulation; the collar having, by his struggles, been drawn tightly across his windpipe, in which condition he was found by the Sisters. Neither are they partial to the 'mits,' which they consider insecure, and therefore dangerous both for patients and attendants. When they do employ them, they prefer linen ones, as less liable to stretch than leather. The Sister tells me, patients will almost always contrive to slip their hands out of the mits, when alone, and replace them when they hear some one coming. Their most usual mode of restraining the violent is, with a sort of sleeve, invented by themselves, as I understood, and which is attached to a frock body, made to lace up behind, like a lady's corset (Stokes, 1844, pp. 15–16; emphasis in original).

Patients were kept busy engaging in domestic labor, such as sewing and knitting; playing dominoes; attending vocal and instrumental music at social meetings; and reading books such as biography, travel, and history (Stokes, 1853). Manual labor was, for some patients, very important to relieve them of stagnation of mind and body. Stokes described the fatigue that the patient felt after working hard as the "best of opiates" (Stokes, 1853, p. 28). Moral treatment typically engaged convalescing patients in daily work in the asylum to prepare them for reentry to their own family life. The Sister-Nurses' focus on

a lifestyle for patients was in agreement with a number of physicians of the period, such as Edward Jarvis, who promoted the importance of exercise, occupation, and amusements to "keep patients' minds away from their delusions and vagaries, to calm their excitement, and raise them from their depression" (Grob, 1978, pp. 60–61).

By 1852, the work of Dr. Stokes, Sister Matilda, and the SC Nurses (now called Daughters of Charity) was acknowledged nationally. Just 12 years into their mission, Dorothea Dix (1801–1887), the renowned American reformer of prisons and mental health institutions, reported (despite being notably anti-Catholic) that Mount Hope was one of two successful facilities for the treatment of persons with mental illness in the state of Maryland (Dix, March 5, 1852). The Stokes–SC model of care for persons who were insane was based on a "law of humanity and kindness," for which Stokes determined the SC nurses were "peculiarly qualified" (Stokes, 1846–1888). In 1845 Stokes stated that the virtues of kindness and benevolence demonstrated by the SC nurses at Mount Hope in the care of the insane were the "direct emanations and blessed fruits of that enlightened and universal charity which they so beautifully illustrate by their lives" (Stokes, 1846–1888, p. 25).

Pause and Reflect

1. *What similarities and differences do you see between moral therapy and nursing care today?*
2. *What differences do you think use of the "curative point" might make in the provision of care?*
3. *What do you think the term "idiocy" says about 19th-century social beliefs related to mental illness?*
4. *What similarities and differences do you see between the components of care provided by the Sisters at Mount Hope and nursing care today?*

The Challenges of Providing Care

Some have judged the early nursing care of the 19th century in light of the practice of medicine at the time. Doyle wrote for the *American Journal of Nursing* in 1929, "It is reasonable to suppose that it was very simple, and was confined to procuring cleanliness, nourishment, and safety for the sick, and the administration of simple medication. Thus the work of the sisters was confined to the kitchen, the laundry, supervision of the wards, and taking care of the spiritual welfare of the patients" (Doyle, 1929, p. 781). However, the work of early nurses, such as the French DC Nurses and the American SC who followed in their footsteps 200 years later, was anything but simple. The SC created healing environments wherever they went. They cared for patients dying from cholera in makeshift "tent" hospitals without the benefit of modern plumbing. Caring for people with cholera, a disease characterized by excessive diarrhea and often rapid death, and ministering to the bereaved families of so many during an epidemic would certainly not have been "simple" physically, emotionally, psychologically, or spiritually. Caring for those with mental illness, even when surrounded by Mount Hope's natural beauty and walls of protection, was challenging, just as it had been since the 17th century.

Insanity occurred among the poor and rich alike, but the poor were more publicly visible. The destitute insane occupied the almshouses of major American cities. Many others were cared for in state asylums that often housed hundreds to thousands of inmates. The

Florence Nightingale on Invalidism and "Chattering Hopes"   box 2-3

"Chattering Hopes" may seem an odd heading. But I really believe there is scarcely a greater worry which invalids have to endure than the incurable hopes of friends. There is no one practice against which I can speak more strongly from actual personal experience, wide and long, of its effects during sickness observed both upon others and upon myself. I would appeal most seriously to all friends, visitors, and attendants of the sick to leave off this practice of attempting to "cheer" the sick by making light of their danger and by exaggerating their probabilities of recovery. The fact is, that the patient is not "cheered" at all by these well-meaning, most tiresome friends. On the contrary, he is depressed and wearied. . . . To nurses I say—these are the visitors who do your patient harm.

Source: Nightingale, F. (1860). *Notes on Nursing: What It Is and What It Is Not.* London, UK: Harrison, pp. 139–145.

19th-century American state asylum was a significant improvement on the previous options of entering the almshouse or "wandering aimlessly in community"(Grob, 1994, p. 102).

It was the reform of the state asylums and almshouses that caught the attention of women activists like Dix seeking to exercise what was socially perceived as the inherent virtues of their gender. Nurses in state and private asylums dealt with the growing national civil liberties issues surrounding commitment of an insane patient to an asylum (Applebaum & Kemp, 1982). Influential physicians of the Association of Medical Superintendents of American Institutions for the Insane promoted early hospitalization of the insane as a means of achieving better outcomes (Grob, 1966). However, there was also a growing public concern about the need for setting limits on admissions to protect the vulnerable insane, their civil liberties, and their dignity from families and physicians who would potentially misuse commitment power (Grob, "Rediscovering Asylums," in Vogel & Rosenberg, 1979, p. 140).

The responsibility for commitment of a person to an asylum in the early and mid-19th century usually rested with family and friends. Asylum care was typically sought for patients and families in crisis, when the behavior of the insane person grew beyond the capacity of the family or friends to manage. Nurses and physicians such as Sister Matilda and Dr. Stokes frequently referred to the importance of the freedom of the patients within the confines of the asylum's secure environment. They used restraint only in severe cases when it was necessary to keep patients from hurting themselves or others. Wrongful confinement, about which the public was growing increasingly concerned, was antithetical to moral therapy, the hope for healing, and the possibility of a cure.

Progress in the 19th Century

Throughout the 19th century, infectious disease and epidemics such as cholera and yellow fever, as well as social ills such as poverty and war, challenged the mental health of people and communities. Nursing care of those with emotional and mental health challenges was under development and reform in many countries. Florence Nightingale (1820–1910) of England was instrumental in introducing education for becoming a "trained" nurse to women of all classes who would care for the sick. She worked to reform care in workhouse infirmaries and change the administrative structure of the care of the insane in those workhouses and other large institutions. One example of Nightingale's health care reforms was her advocacy for the separation of the "sick, insane, infirm, & aged, incurable, imbecile, & above all the children from the usual pauper population of the

Metropolis" (Letter to Edwin Chadwick, 9 July, 1866, Nightingale, Vicinus, & Nergaard, 1990, p. 271).

Nightingale herself struggled with depression and invalidism, one of the most prevalent mental health concerns among 19th-century women (Box 2-3). Invalidism particularly affected those of higher social class, as working women could not afford to be invalids (Verbrugge, 1988). Nightingale took to her bed after leading a group of nurses to provide nursing care at the Barrack Hospital at Scutari in Turkey during the Crimean War.

Attention to the emotional and mental well-being of patients is foundational to nursing care, especially in times of great chaos such as war and pestilence. In addition to Nightingale, other women earned notoriety as nurse leaders during the chaos of the Crimean War. Mother Mary Jane Seacole (1805–1881) of Haiti raised funds for her own nursing mission to the Crimea. Clare Moore accompanied Nightingale to the Crimea as her valued assistant because of her nursing expertise in "careful nursing," a 19th-century model of nursing care developed in Ireland by Catherine McCauley and the women of the Institute of Our Lady of Mercy. Although it is not documented specifically as a model for the care of the insane as Sister Matilda's *Advices Concerning the Sick*, careful nursing was another early contribution to holistic psychiatric mental health nursing. It specifically emphasized attention to "emotional consolation provided from a spiritual perspective" as foundational to nursing care (Meehan, 2003, p. 100). The early Sisters of Mercy demonstrated the importance of "relieving the distress first" and then endeavoring "by every practicable means to promote the cleanliness, ease, and comfort of the patient" (as cited in Meehan, 2003, p. 100). Clare Moore and the Sisters of Mercy taught their tradition to Nightingale and many others.

Nightingale herself designed a training model for nurses, which was adopted in the later part of the 19th century in emerging American "training" schools. Nightingale had little formal training in nursing but did receive some mentoring in nursing from the Daughters of Charity of Vincent de Paul in Paris, with whom she stayed on two occasions prior to her trip to the Crimea. She wrote, "There is nothing like the training (in these days) which the Sacred Heart or the Order of St. Vincent gives to women" (Letter to Henry Manning, 15 July, 1852, Nightingale et al., 1990, p. 59). In addition to the instruction she received from Clare Moore and the Daughters, Nightingale was also influenced in her nursing work by a visit in 1851 to a German hospital known as the Institution of Kaiserswerth (Nightingale et al., 1990, p. 54).

A European predecessor of Nightingale, Amelia Sieveking of Hamburg, Germany, who was called to care for the sick poor in 1830, also adopted the Vincent de Paul "model for setting about her special duty" (Sieveking & Winkworth, 1863, p. 182). During the 1831 cholera epidemic, Sieveking worked in a temporary hospital. She was approached in 1837 by Pastor Fliedner of Kaiserswerth to accept a position as head nurse for his hospital. She declined, but later met with Fliedner in 1843, when she recommended one of her students for a position he was trying to fill. That student became Fliedner's second wife and a worker at the institution. Sieveking had missions in Germany beginning in 1852, and ultimately created an "Association" of nurses, which she named the Protestant Sisters of Mercy.

In 1873, the Nightingale model for creating the "trained" nurse was adopted in the United States. In 1882, a movement for the specialized training of asylum workers was led by Dr. Edward Cowles, who established a formally organized program at the McLean Asylum in Waverly, Massachusetts. Cowles is known to have removed bars from the windows and unlocked the doors of asylums. He moved the focus of nursing care from "attendance" upon the "incurable and infirm" to "nursing the sick to promote recovery" (Maranjian Church, 1987, p. 110). In the history of nursing, one way that professional nurses can be differentiated from "attendants" is by their education or training. Early formal education for nurses was vocational in nature and was conducted by the religious communities who stressed that nursing care include the spiritual as well as the physical needs of the sick, poor, and insane (Libster & McNeil, 2009). As nursing training moved away from being the sole domain of religious communities in the later 19th and early 20th centuries, it has been psychiatric nurses in particular who have continued to value the nursing tradition of providing holistic care (Tuck, Pullen, & Lynn, 1997), which includes attention to the emotional, mental, and spiritual needs of clients.

New Dimensions in Care

In the 20th century, new dimensions in mental health care, medical science, and nursing influenced plans of care. The evolution of 20th-century psychiatric nursing, as in previous centuries, paralleled the changes in medical care and society. Psychiatric care moved away from its focus on the healing environment and moral therapy toward seeking a greater understanding of the biological and chemical bases for mental health and illness.

After the Civil War in the United States, physicians and hospitals served less as consultants to the nurse educators and experts who had traditionally found strength in religious community to mentor and train nurses in their scope of practice. Hospital committees and physicians such as Cowles took it upon themselves to create or partner with emerging programs to establish programs in which the emphasis of training would often end up reflecting the needs of the institution and physicians first and foremost. Nurses, who were not part of a religious community and who wanted formalized training, participated, as they lacked organization and sociocultural power in the public sphere. In 1906, members of the American Medico-Psychological Association presented papers on the values of training asylum attendants and nurses. "Implicit in the issues was the need for involvement of the medical superintendents in the training that was offered"(Maranjian Church, 1987, p. 116). The association was first formed in 1844 as the Association of Medical Superintendents of American Institutions for the Insane. The name was changed in 1892 to the American Medico-Psychological Association and, ultimately, to the American Psychiatric Association (APA) in 1921. In 1907, the

association-appointed group of five physicians determined that the major function of the asylum nurse was "assistance to the physician in the care and treatment of the insane"(Maranjian Church, 1987, p. 118). They also deemed that the education of the nurse be the same as that of the physician but differing in "degrees," thereby negating centuries of distinct definitions of scope of practice for nurses and marking the official appropriation of control of practice of mental health nursing by the association.

Echoes of bio-medicalization of nursing could be heard in Europe as well. In Dutch asylums, psychiatrists established a new system of mental health nursing that led to the reorganization of nursing care around controlling patient behavior by somatic therapies. Psychiatrists assumed that psychiatric symptoms would vanish as a result of body-oriented treatments. Nurses spent more time in assistance in medical observation and treatment (Boschma, 1999b, p. 142). The biomedical focus on providing care that was "science-based" and the creation of physician-led specialized training for asylum nurses at the turn of the century did not serve to "give nurses their own professional identity, but rather reinforced the supremacy of medical knowledge in the care of the mentally ill"(Chung & Nolan, 1994, p. 226). Part of the reason for the strain on identity had to do with gender roles. Most nurses continued to be female and most physicians male.

When moral therapy was prevalent, attendants and nurses might be male or female. In the 20th century, as patients began to receive somatic care, many were prescribed bed rest as treatment. The change in care at asylums in the Netherlands, for example, meant that women nurses were more likely to be the providers of care (Boschma, 1999a, p. 14). Later in 20th-century America, nurse leaders stated that limitations on the role of men in nursing had "disappeared" (Peplau, 1989, p. 18). Some might disagree, but psychiatric–mental health nursing has been one field in nursing in which men have most often thrived. For example, Dr. Phil Barker, a British psychiatric nurse, is well known internationally for his professional leadership in creating the Tidal Model of care, a philosophical approach to what Barker termed "the discovery of mental health." For more information about the Tidal Model, please visit its website.

The medicalization of care and interest in psychopathology served to separate mind from body, as evidenced in the separate training programs for asylum nurses. Nursing's relationship with medicine at the time tended to pull it away from its heritage in holistic care, as represented in such models as careful nursing and moral therapy. In 1939, the *American Journal of Nursing* (*AJN*) published an article on "Modern Psychiatric Nursing" in which the author-physician wrote that many nurses, like the public, had "false conceptions that mental patients are raving maniacs, lack intelligence, are weak, stupid, or often dangerous people to be around" (Bennett, 1939, p. 397). He called for every nurse to have "some psychiatric nursing experience in order to overcome misconceptions and personal prejudices against the neurotic and mental patient"(Bennett, 1939, p. 397).

Only 30 years later, *AJN* published an article interviewing nurse leaders from the American Nurses Association's committee to establish standards for nursing practice, in which psychiatric nurse Gloria George demonstrated the strengthened role of psychiatric care in nursing and the place for advanced practice in nurse–psychotherapy. She stated that the nurse practices individual, group, and family psychotherapy and clarified that although every nurse works with families and groups, "We know that not every psychiatric nurse is going to be practicing formalized therapy"(American Nurses Association, 1969, p. 1462).

In 1913, nurse–educator Effie Taylor of the Phipps Clinic at Johns Hopkins Hospital, and later professor of psychiatric nursing at Yale University, sought to integrate mind and body once again in her nurses' training program involving general and mental health nursing. The Mental Health Act of 1946 legitimized the role of the nurse to include what is now known as psychiatric–mental health nursing and released it further from medical domination. This shift away from medicine occurred as there was a concerted effort to move care of the mentally ill from the asylum to the community. The National Institute of Mental Health was created in the late 1940s. In the same decade, members of the APA, including the Menninger brothers, who had founded the Menninger Clinic and Sanitarium in Kansas in 1919, worked to reform and reorganize psychiatry. Much of the controversy surrounding reform had to do with the role of the federal versus state government in the care of the mentally ill. In the 1940s there were a number of changes in the American health care system, including the development of the third-party payer system. The National Mental Health Act of 1946 supported research into the causes and treatments of psychiatric disorders, the training of providers, and the support of states in creating treatment facilities.

As the support for research grew in the 1950s, some believed that psychotropic medications made it more possible to modify and alleviate symptoms of severe and persistent disease, such as schizophrenia. Chlorpromazine, or Thorazine, was the first of the psychoactive drugs created. It was followed by the "tranquilizer" drugs—*Rauwolfia serpentina* alkaloids, or reserpine. The antidepressants imipramine and iproniazid emerged after that. Despite many historical references to the significant impact of the major tranquilizer medications such as Thorazine on patient outcomes, mid–20th-century nurses, as well as many psychiatrists, were not completely enthusiastic. Nursing history reveals that nurses of the time reported that the introduction of these medications did not necessarily lead to greater benefit to patients than the previous sedatives used, and they allegedly made more work for nurses (Harmon, 2005).

Nurses were engaged in many effective modalities in the care of the mentally ill. For example, **hydrotherapy,** water applications also known as "water cure" in the 19th century, was considered foundational to good nursing care for centuries, particularly in the 20th century, as care moved from an emphasis on moral therapy to more somatically based models of care (Box 2-4).

Psychodynamic care, focused on the psychological forces underlying human behavior, was popular in the 1950s when Hildegard Peplau (1909–1999) published one of the most significant works of 20th-century psychiatric nursing, *Interpersonal Relations in Nursing*. Her **interpersonal relations theory** emphasized the nurse–client relationship as *the* foundation for practice. In the book, which served as the "conceptual frame of reference for psychodynamic nursing," Peplau defined all nursing—not just psychiatric nursing—as a "significant, therapeutic process." She held two guiding assumptions: "The kind of person each nurse becomes makes a substantial difference in what each patient will learn as he is nursed throughout his experience with illness" and "Fostering personality development in the direction of maturity is a function in nursing

---

Hydrotherapy | box 2-4

Hydrotherapies—including cold wet sheet applications ("humane sheets"), continuous tub therapy, wraps, and packs found often today in healing spas and resorts—were used regularly in the care of agitated, anxious, nervous, manic, hyperactive, and "deeply disturbed" patients. Hydrotherapy was viewed as a "modern, technological alternative to sedatives, barbiturates, and the more invasive sterilizations, shock therapies, and lobotomies popular in state hospitals during the time"(Harmon, 2009, p. 493). Baths used for sedation were at skin temperature of 92°F. One nursing textbook of the time describes the effect of a tub bath: "A bath at body temperature produces no marked changes in the body, wither thermic or circulatory, but surrounds it with a medium that shields it from all external stimuli, or irritation of nerve endings from air, clothing, pressure, changes in temperature and the like. As a result, the nerve centers and the whole nervous system are protected and allowed to rest. The bath is therefore soothing and quieting in its effects and gives a chance for repair and the storage of vital energy" (Harmer & Henderson, 1939, p. 475).

---

and nursing education; it requires the use of principles and methods that permit and guide the process of grappling with everyday interpersonal problems or difficulties" (Peplau, 1952, p. xii). Peplau's work on interpersonal relations and on anxiety became foundational to nursing practice in general and psychiatric–mental health nursing in particular. More recently, some have observed that the success of generalizing interpersonal theory to all nursing in mid-century may have ultimately set the stage for challenges in differentiating psychiatric–mental health nursing as a specialty practice area (Olson, 1996).

Peplau's work was a reflection of the climate of care in nursing during the 1950s and 1960s, when the psychiatric nurse's role was expressed as "extending the therapeutic process into the ward environment by creating nurse-patient relationships that promote emotional growth"(Gregg, 1954, p. 851). During the period, there was also a "re-discovery" of moral therapy and creating a healing environment as "milieu therapy." In the 1960s, nurse reformer Esther Lucille Brown's now-historic report on patient care identified the importance of using the physical environment for therapeutic purposes and "restoring the amenities of the era of Moral Treatment"(Brown, 1961, p. 127). She also stressed the importance of the nurse's role in social therapy, discussing such interventions as taking meals with patients, a practice stressed by Sister Matilda more than a century earlier. From these historical patterns, we realize that treatments and scientific beliefs and ideas come and go over time in psychiatry and psychiatric–mental health nursing, reflecting the ebb and flow of human life. Indicative of that flow, hospitals for the mentally ill, for example, are no longer the "prisons" they were for centuries—but now, in the 21st century, hospitals for the mentally ill are closing and the burden of responsibility for care has moved back to the community and families.

Continuing today from the later 20th century, nurses have been taking the lead in their communities in the care of those with mental illness. With the support of nursing organizations such as the American Psychiatric Nurses Association, nurses are re-establishing their autonomy as demonstrated in the emergence of advanced practice nursing (APN) roles. APN roles in psychiatric nursing include the Clinical Nurse Specialist and Nurse Practitioner. Peplau reported that, by 1956, there were already 28 master's programs in advanced practice psychiatric nursing (Peplau, 1989). Today's psychiatric–mental health APNs provide therapy, medication management, and consultancy services. New models of nurse–psychotherapy care, such as brief solution-focused therapy, have been shown to be economical and effective (Montgomery & Webster, 1994). New specialties have emerged to meet societal needs, such as Sexual Assault Nurse Examiner (SANE), Forensics, and Infant Mental Health. Suffering from mental illness endures today, as does the hope for cure. What also endures is the nursing profession's commitment in communities throughout the world to bring hope to those suffering mental illness and their families through quality, holistic care.

Pause and Reflect

1. *What kinds of nursing interventions might you consider if you were to implement the Sisters of Mercy's plan of "relieving distress first"?*

2. *Why is it important for nurses to maintain a professional identity? How have nurses throughout history created their professional identity as caregivers for patients with mental illness?*

3. *What role have nurses played in creating healing environments for patients with mental illness?*

Chapter Highlights

1. Throughout history, nurses have played a crucial role in providing and improving psychiatric–mental health care. As early as the 17th century, the Daughters of Charity were pioneering asylum-based care and sought and provided more humane treatment to patients with mental illness.

2. The Vermont Study is one of the longest running studies in American clinical research. It confirms the possibility of restoring patients with mental illness—schizophrenia, in particular—to a point of wellness and functionality.

3. Perseverance is an essential trait of psychiatric mental health nursing.

4. The "curative point" refers to a point of view or attitude of treating the patient as if he or she can be cured, as opposed to providing palliative care.

5. Developed in the 19th century, moral therapy is a system of care that stresses kindness to patients and employment of patients in meaningful activities.

6. The Mount Hope Retreat stands as an early example of the power of independent nursing care and the importance of nurses in the development and reform of mental health care.

7. Florence Nightingale, an advocate for those with mental illness, was instrumental in introducing a model for educating the "trained" nurse.

8. Careful nursing was a model of nursing that emphasized "relieving the distress first" of the patient.

9. First formed in 1844, the American Psychiatric Association is responsible for establishing guidelines for care for patients with mental illness.

10. The need for nurses to have education and experience in psychiatric–mental health nursing has long been recognized and documented in the literature.

11. The introduction of psychotropic drugs and psychodynamic therapy in the 20th century are two critical advances in psychiatric–mental health care.

12. Hildegard Peplau's interpersonal relations theory emphasizes the nurse–client relationship as the foundation for practice. She defined *all* nursing practice as a "significant, therapeutic process."

NCLEX®-RN Questions

1. The nurse educator is discussing the role of the nursing profession in reforming the care of persons suffering from mental illness. Which contribution supports the use of nursing research to enhance client recovery outcomes?
   a. Harding's work with deinstitutionalized clients
   b. Dix's exposé of the conditions of asylums and prisons
   c. Coskery and colleagues' identification of curative and critical points
   d. Taylor's training of nurses at the Phipps Clinic at Johns Hopkins Hospital

2. The student nurse is researching moral therapy for a leadership project. Which historical development in this system of care best represents a major evolution in the role of nurses in caring for the mentally ill?
   a. The logging of patient information in paper records
   b. The founding of the American Psychiatric Association (APA)
   c. The administration and management of care at Mount Hope
   d. The assignment of domestic duties at the Maryland Hospital for the Insane

3. The nurse is assessing a patient with mental illness. The patient reveals a history of mental illness documented in family records dating back to the late 1800s. The client notes that certain ancestors' conditions were rarely discussed or acknowledged in family communications. The nurse recognizes which social/historical variable as most likely contributing to this finding?
   a. The shame and stigma of mental illness has endured for centuries.
   b. Mental health disorders had not yet been characterized or studied.
   c. Laws have always protected the privacy and dignity of the mentally ill.
   d. The impact of mental illness on families during that time period was not as significant as it is today.

4. The psychiatric–mental health nurse is working with patients receiving treatment for mental illness. Which contemporary interventions are comparable to those employed under principles of moral therapy? Select all that apply.
   a. Treating all patients with dignity and respect
   b. Providing activities that enable patients to remain productive and engaged
   c. Imposing coercive techniques to extinguish future violent or aggressive outbursts
   d. Treating patients in the context of their family, community, and home environments
   e. Working to ensure a safe environment through appropriate staffing ratios and restraint reduction initiatives

5. The nurse is completing a history and assessment of an older adult patient with a history of chronic schizophrenia. The nurse learns that the patient began receiving treatment in the 1960s. The nurse understands that the patient would be most likely to have been exposed to which types of psychiatric interventions common to that era?
   a. Physical therapies, "curative point" approach, convalescence
   b. Asylum treatment, depletive therapies, insulin shock therapy
   c. First-generation antipsychotics, milieu therapy, rehabilitative care
   d. Herbal remedies, palliative care, decreased emphasis on interpersonal relationships

6. The psychiatric–mental health nurse is providing education to the community about the importance of improving mental health services. A colleague questions the nurse's rationale for incorporating a historical perspective of mental illness into teaching. Which response is best?
   a. "The history of mental illness is fascinating. Providing these details may stimulate interest in the topic."
   b. "Nurses have had a key role in reforming the care of the mentally ill. Highlighting these facts will help to establish my credibility as a nurse."
   c. "The historical context of mental illness explains the culture and beliefs that surround it. Sharing this information may diminish bias and judgment."
   d. "We have come a long way in our understanding of mental illness. It is important for people to know how cures were developed for these conditions."

7. The nurse is working on the planning board of a new community mental health center. A member of the board asks the nurse why it is essential to incorporate nursing care into the client treatment model. Which response best reflects an accurate evaluation of the nursing role in the cultivation of healing environments for patients with mental illnesses?
   a. "Nurses have always been ready to care for vulnerable populations. The nursing profession is the only one that has always put client needs first."
   b. "Mentally ill clients have always required comprehensive medical care. Nurses have the technical skills to assess and respond to these needs."
   c. "Changes in reimbursement have made it possible for nurses to take on advanced practice roles. Nurse providers are likely to reduce the cost of care."
   d. "Nurses have played an essential role in the compassionate care of the mentally ill. Today's nurses have the specialized training and expertise to respond to a variety of human needs."

Answers may be found on the Pearson student resource site: nursing.pearsonhighered.com

Pearson Nursing Student Resources Find additional review materials at **nursing.pearsonhighered.com**

References

American Nurses Association. (1969). Establishing standards for nursing practice. *American Journal of Nursing, 69*(7), 1458–1463.

Andrew, T. (1842). *A Cyclopedia of Domestic Medicine and Surgery.* Glasgow, Scotland: Blackie and Son. Accessed at GoogleBooks.com

Applebaum, P., & Kemp, K. (1982). The evolution of commitment law in the nineteenth century. *Law and Human Behavior, 6*(3/4), 343–354.

Beam, R. M. (1837). *Report of the Committee on the Maryland Hospital to the Legislature of Maryland.* Maryland State Archives, Annapolis, MD.

Bennett, A. E. (1939). Modern psychiatric nursing. *American Journal of Nursing, 39*(4), 395–400.

Boschma, G. (1999a). The gender specific role of male nurses in Dutch asylums: 1890–1910. *International History of Nursing Journal: IHNJ, 4*(3), 13–19.

Boschma, G. (1999b). High ideals versus harsh reality: A historical analysis of mental health nursing in Dutch asylums, 1890–1920. *Nursing History Review: Official Journal of the American Association for the History of Nursing, 7,* 127–151.

Brigham, A. (1847). The moral treatment of insanity. *American Journal of Insanity, 4*(1), 1–15. Archives of the American Psychiatric Assocation.

Brown, E. L. (1961). *Newer Dimensions of Patient Care Part 1: The Use of the Physical Environment of the General Hospital for Therapeutic Purposes.* New York, NY: Russell Sage Foundation.

Bynum, W. F. (1994). *Science and the Practice of Medicine in the Nineteenth Century.* Cambridge, UK: Cambridge University Press.

Chung, M. C., & Nolan, P. (1994). The influence of positivistic thought on nineteenth century asylum nursing. *Journal of Advanced Nursing, 19*(2), 226–232.

Coskery, S. M. (n.d.). *Cradle of Mount Hope: Historical Account of Mt. St. Vincent Hospital/Mount Hope Retreat.* Emmitsburg, MD: Archives of the Daughters of Charity, St. Joseph's Provincial House. #11-2-39.

Coskery, S. M. (n.d. c. 1840). *Advices Concerning the Sick.* Emmitsburg, MD: Archives of the Daughters of Charity, St. Joseph's Provincial House.

Coste, P. C. M., & de Paul, V. (1985–2008a). *Regulations for the Sisters of the Angers Hospital* (Vol. 13b). New York, NY: New City Press.

Coste, P. C. M., & de Paul, V. (1985–2008b). *Saint Vincent de Paul: Correspondence, Conferences, Documents.* New York, NY: New City Press.

Daughters of Charity. (April 17, 1703). Remarks on Sister Nicole Lequin. *Circulars and Notices, 2,* 554. Emmitsburg, MD: Archives of the Daughters of Charity, St. Joseph's Provincial House.

Daughters of Charity. (1847–1851). *Mt. Hope Receipt Book.* Emmitsburg, MD: Archives of the Daughters of Charity, St. Joseph's Provincial House, 11-2-39:4.

Digby, A. (1985a). *Madness, Morality, and Medicine: A Study of the York Retreat, 1796–1914*. New York, NY: Cambridge University Press.

Digby, A. (1985b). Moral treatment at the Retreat, 1796–1846. In W. F. Bynum, R. Porter, & M. Shepherd (Eds.). *The Anatomy of Madness* (Vol. II). London, UK: Tavistock Publications, pp. 52–72.

Dix, D. (1852, March 5). Memorial of Miss D. L. Dix to the Hon. The General Assembly in behalf of the insane of Maryland. Archives of the State of Maryland website: http://www.msa.md.gov/

Doyle, A. (1929). Nursing by religious orders in the United States: Part 1, 1809–1840. *American Journal of Nursing, 29*(7), 775–786.

Earle, P. (1848). On the causes of insanity. *American Journal of Insanity, 4*(3), 185–211. Archives of the American Psychiatric Association.

Flinton, M. (1992). *Louise de Marillac: Social Aspect of Her Work*. New York, NY: New City Press.

Gregg, D. E. (1954). The psychiatric nurse's role. *The American Journal of Nursing, 54*(7), 848–851.

Grob, G. (1966). The state mental hospital in mid-nineteenth century America: A social analysis. *American Psychologist, 21*(6), 510–523.

Grob, G. (1978). *Edward Jarvis and the Medical World of Nineteenth-Century America*. Knoxville, TN: University of Tennessee Press.

Grob, G. (1994). *The Mad Among Us: A History of the Care of America's Mentally Ill*. Cambridge, MA: Harvard University Press.

Harding, C. M. (1988). Course types in schizophrenia: An analysis of European and American studies. *Schizophrenia Bulletin, 14*(4), 633–643.

Harding, C. M., Brooks, G. W., Ashikaga, T., Strauss, J. S., & Breier, A. (1987a). The Vermont longitudinal study of persons with severe mental illness, I: Methodology, study sample, and overall status 32 years later. *The American Journal of Psychiatry, 144*(6), 718–726.

Harding, C. M., Brooks, G. W., Ashikaga, T., Strauss, J. S., & Breier, A. (1987b). The Vermont longitudinal study of persons with severe mental illness, II: Long-term outcome of subjects who retrospectively met DSM-III criteria for schizophrenia. *The American Journal of Psychiatry, 144*(6), 727–735.

Harmer, B., & Henderson, V. (1939). *Textbook of the Principles and Practice of Nursing* (4th ed.). Retrieved at the University of Colorado Health Sciences Library. New York, NY: Macmillan.

Harmon, R. B. (2005). Nursing care in a state hospital before and during the introduction of antipsychotics, 1950–1965. *Issues in Mental Health Nursing, 26*(3), 257–279.

Harmon, R. B. (2009). Hydrotherapy in state mental hospitals in the mid-twentieth century. *Issues in Mental Health Nursing, 30*(8), 491–494.

Jones, C. (1980). The treatment of the insane in eighteenth and early nineteenth-century Montpellier: A contribution to the prehistory of the lunatic asylum in provincial France. *Medical History, 24*, 371–390.

Jones, C. (1989). Sisters of Charity and the ailing poor. *Social History of Medicine, 2*(3), 339–348.

Libster, M., & McNeil, B. A. (2009). *Enlightened Charity: The Holistic Nursing Care, Education and Advices Concerning the Sick of Sister Matilda Coskery, (1799–1870)*. Naperville, IL: Golden Apple Publications.

Maranjian Church, O. (1987). The Emergence of Training Programmes for Asylum Nursing at the Turn of the Century. In C. Maggs (Ed.). *Nursing History: The State of the Art*. Kent, UK: Aspen Publications.

Maryland Hospital for the Insane. (1834–1872). *Patient Register*. Maryland State Archives, Annapolis, MD, S184.

McNeil, B. A. (1996). *The Vincentian Family Tree*. Chicago, IL: Vincentian Studies Institute.

Medical Case Book. (1832). Baltimore Infirmary. *Maryland State Archives, MSA SC 4070*. Tull Collection, Annapolis, MD.

Meehan, T. (2003). Careful nursing: A model for contemporary nursing practice. *Journal of Advanced Nursing, 44*(1), 99–107.

Montgomery, C. L., & Webster, D. (1994). Caring, curing, and brief therapy: A model for nurse-psychotherapy. *Archives of Psychiatric Nursing, 8*(5), 291–297.

Morrell, P. (1849). *A Choice collection of medical and botanical receipts: Selected from experienced Physicians by whom they have been proved and found useful in the various disorders and infirmities for which they are prescribed. To which is prefixed remarks and observations for the consideration of physicians and nurses among Believers*. Winterthur Library Shaker Manuscripts, Winterthur, DE.

Nightingale, F. (1860). *Notes on Nursing: What It Is and What It Is Not*. London, UK: Harrison, pp. 139–145. Accessed at GoogleBooks.com

Nightingale, F., Vicinus, M., & Nergaard, B. (1990). *Ever Yours, Florence Nightingale: Selected Letters*. Cambridge, MA: Harvard University Press.

Olson, T. (1996). Fundamental and special: The dilemma of psychiatric–mental health nursing. *Archives of Psychiatric Nursing, 10*(1), 3–10; discussion 11–15.

Peplau, H. (1952). *Interpersonal Relations in Nursing: A Conceptual Frame of Reference for Psychodynamic Nursing*. New York, NY: G. P. Putnam & Sons.

Peplau, H. (1989). Future directions in psychiatric nursing from the perspective of history. *Journal of Psychosocial Nursing and Mental Health Services, 27*(2), 18–21, 25–28.

Sieveking, A. W., & Winkworth, C. (1863). *Life of Amelia Wilhelmina Sieveking from the German edited with the author's sanction*. London, UK: Longman, Green, Longman, Roberts, & Green. Accessed at GoogleBooks.com

Stewart, K. (1992). *The York Retreat: In the Light of the Quaker Way*. York, UK: William Sessions Ltd.

Stokes, W. (1844). First Annual Report of the Physician of the Mount Saint Vincent's Hospital for 1843. *Mount Hope Reports*. Emmitsburg, MD: Archives of the Daughters of Charity, St. Joseph's Provincial House. 11-2-39.

Stokes, W. (1845). Second Annual Report of the Physician of Mount Hope Hospital (Late Mount St. Vincent's) for 1844. *Mount Hope Reports*. Emmitsburg, MD: Archives of the Daughters of Charity, St. Joseph's Provincial House.

Stokes, W. (1846–1888). Report of the Mount Hope Institution Near Baltimore. Emmitsburg, MD: Archives of the Daughters of Charity, St. Joseph's Provincial House.

Stokes, W. (1849). The sixth annual report of the Mount Hope Institution near Baltimore, for the year 1848. *Mount Hope Reports*. Baltimore, MD: John Murphy & Co. Archives of the Daughters of Charity, St. Joseph's Provincial House. Emmitsburg, MD.

Stokes, W. (1853). The eleventh annual report of the Mount Hope Institution near Baltimore. Baltimore: John Murphy & Co. Archives of the Daughters of Charity, St. Joseph's Provincial House. Emmitsburg, MD.

Stokes, W. (1880). 38th annual report of the Mount Hope Retreat. Baltimore. Emmitsburg, MD: Archives of the Daughters of Charity, St. Joseph's Provincial House.

Tuck, I., Pullen, L., & Lynn, C. (1997). Spiritual interventions provided by mental health nurses. *Western Journal of Nursing Research, 19*(3), 351–363.

Verbrugge, M. H. (1988). *Able-Bodied Womanhood: Personal Health and Social Change in Nineteenth-Century Boston*. New York, NY: Oxford University Press.

Vogel, M. J., & Rosenberg, C. E. (1979). *The Therapeutic Revolution: Essays in the Social History of American Medicine*. Philadelphia, PA: University of Pennsylvania Press.

Biological Basis for Mental Illness

3

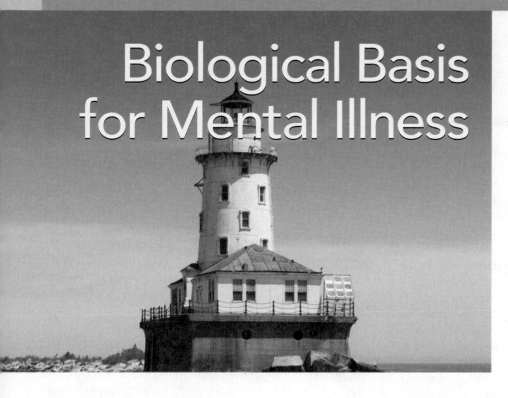

Vanessa Genung
Mary D. Moller

Learning Outcomes

1. Describe neuroanatomical structures that affect neurobiological and mental health.

2. Analyze the role of neurotransmitters in neurobiological and mental health.

3. Differentiate diagnostic techniques that elicit information on patient neurobiological status.

4. Contrast the pathophysiology of different psychiatric symptoms and disorders.

5. Examine the role of neurobiology in suffering and hope.

Key Terms

Introduction

Neuroanatomy and *neurophysiology* are terms used to refer to the structures and functions of the brain, spinal column, and nervous system. As a conductor leads musicians in a band, the brain leads the neurotransmitters (chemical substances that transmit nerve impulses across a synapse) and neuroreceptors in a series of electrical and neurochemical impulses and events in the symphony of brain activity. Neurotransmitters, receptors, various organs, brain lobes, the spine, the endocrine system, and their interconnecting neural networks all serve as musicians, interpreting the directions given by the brain as conductor, to perform the patterns of neurotransmission for the score of life. Although the process remains a mystery in many ways, advances in neurobiochemical research have revealed some of the intricate workings of the brain. This informs understanding of normal brain activity, many underlying causes of mental health issues, and changes that may occur when the brain is traumatized by injury, assault, or infection. Neurobiochemical research has also greatly influenced interventions and therapies that support patients with psychiatric illness. For example, anxiety resulting from dysregulation of the neurotransmitter serotonin may be alleviated by the introduction of a selective serotonin reuptake inhibitor, engagement in regular exercise, and/or participation in cognitive–behavioral exercises such as journaling. An understanding of the neurobiology of mental health and illness can assist nurses in helping patients determine what interventions, activities, and therapies help them alleviate symptoms that result in distress and suffering.

This chapter provides a brief overview of the structure and functions of the nervous system, neurotransmitters, and receptors involved in neurobiological and mental health; diagnostic techniques that provide information regarding the health status of the nervous system; the pathophysiology of common psychiatric disorders encountered by nurses in various settings; and a discussion of the neurobiological basis of suffering and hope.

The Nervous System

All human thoughts, feelings, and actions are initiated by activity in the brain. The brain weighs around three pounds and is 75% water. The only organ that can study itself, the brain is responsible for the display of physical behavior, as well as the expression of personality. It is the seat of intelligence and the relay system for the body's communication network. In most cases, brain development occurs in a predictable pattern (Figure 3-1). The brain processes information from the outside world through the sensory system, and organizes and coordinates the functions of all the internal body systems through the powerful and essential nervous system.

The nervous system has two divisions, the central nervous system (CNS) and the peripheral nervous system (PNS), each run by specific neurochemicals. The CNS consists of the brain and the spinal cord, and the PNS includes all ganglia and nervous structures that connect to muscles, tissues, and glands outside the skull and spinal column that connect the brain and spinal cord to the parts of the body (Figure 3-2).

Peripheral Nervous System

The **peripheral nervous system** consists of the nerves and ganglia located outside the central nervous system. It is composed of the nerves that connect the CNS to receptors, muscles, and glands. The PNS also includes the cranial nerves just outside the brain stem. The PNS is further divided into a somatic nervous system and an autonomic nervous system. The autonomic nervous system is further divided into the sympathetic nervous system and the parasympathetic nervous system (Herlihy, 2010; Guess, 2008). It is critical to understand these systems, as they form the basis for many psychiatric symptoms and act as the location of pharmacotherapy to treat these symptoms.

A great deal of attention is paid to the sympathetic nervous system and the parasympathetic nervous system because of their unique responsibilities (Figure 3-3). The **sympathetic nervous system** (SNS) innervates the thoracolumbar spine and rapidly mobilizes body systems during activity (especially during stress)—it acts in sympathy with the body. By activating adrenergic neural receptors, epinephrine (adrenaline) or norepinephrine (noradrenaline) energizes the brain and body to provide for quick thinking and fast motor response—"fight or flight" primarily in males and "tend/befriend" primarily in females. The **parasympathetic nervous system** (PSNS) innervates cranial nerves CN III, VII, IX, and X. It regulates automatic functions and is responsible for "resetting" the autonomic nervous system after activation. Because of its long neuron pathways, the PSNS is a "slow" system, conserving energy, telling the mind to relax and think clearly,

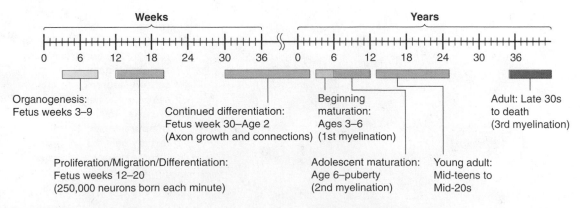

3-1   Timeline of brain development.

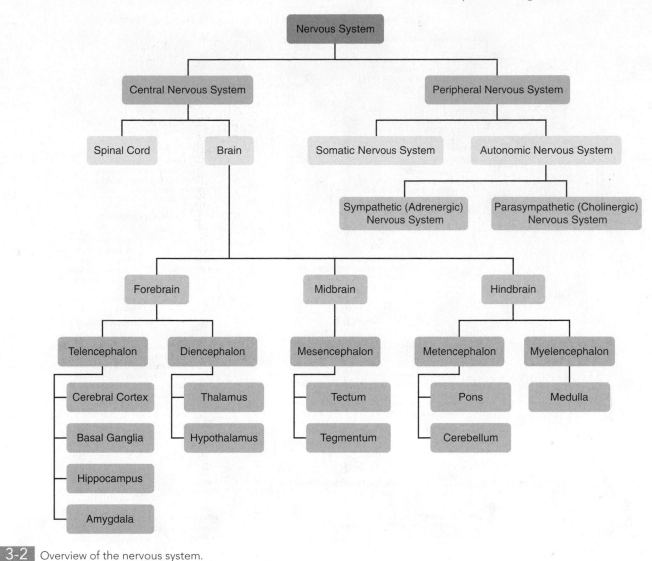

3-2 Overview of the nervous system.

and instructing the body systems to calm, restore, and "rest and digest." This system is involved in the stress response and can often function on hyper-alert in individuals who have experienced trauma. Even for those who have not experienced trauma, the ability of the PSNS to regulate the SNS is unique for each person. The actions of the PSNS explain why, after a major stressor, such as barely avoiding a car accident, it takes some individuals several hours to recover (calm down), whereas others return to feeling normal after just a few minutes.

The PSNS accomplishes communication between the body and the CNS through the spinal cord through the ascending afferent and descending efferent nerve tracts, cranial nerves, spinal nerves, and nerve cell. The difference between a neuron and a nerve is that a **neuron** is a single nerve cell and a nerve is a bundle of several neurons. The area of skin that is innervated by a single spinal nerve is referred to as a *dermatome*.

Central Nervous System

The **central nervous system** (brain and spinal cord) is responsible for integrating, processing, and coordinating sensory data and motor commands. The PNS connects the CNS to the limbs and organs of the body. The CNS decides how to respond to what happens in the world based on the information that is provided by the PNS and further relies on the PNS to send appropriate responses to the various parts of the body. The PNS does not make complex decisions, but rather acts as a relay communication network. The PNS brings in sensory information from the body. The CNS makes decisions and sends a message down the spinal cord, where the PNS sends out motor information to the body.

The CNS is contained within the brain and spinal cord and is responsible for integrating the information it receives from the PNS and for coordinating the activities of all parts of the body. This CNS executive center is protected by the bones of the skull and vertebrae and is lubricated by the cerebral spinal fluid. The blood–brain barrier (BBB) adds additional layers of protective covering for the dura mater, the pia mater, and the arachnoid membrane.

The **blood–brain barrier** involves a three-wall barrier that serves to isolate brain circulation from systemic circulation. It governs the quality of and rapidity with which substances in the blood penetrate into the brain. Water, carbon dioxide, and oxygen readily cross the barrier. The BBB rapidly escorts lipid soluble molecules into the brain and uses specific transport systems to admit water soluble molecules. Organs in the brain that have an endocrine connection

The Major Components and Functions of the Nervous System

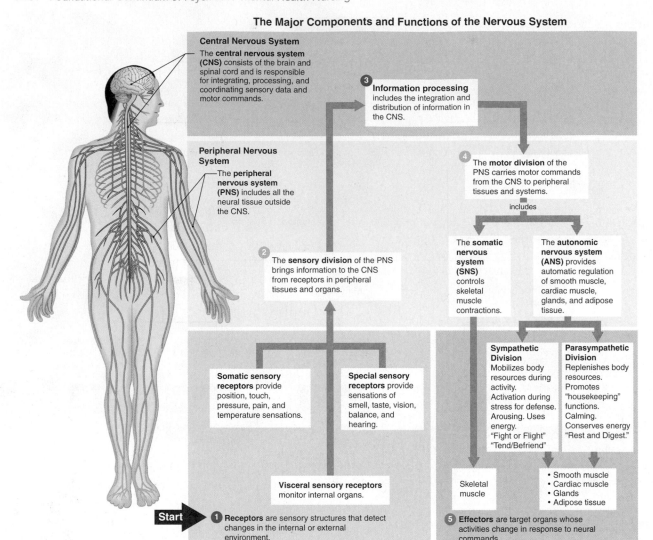

3-3   Major components and functions of the nervous system.

(such as the hypothalamus, pituitary, and pineal glands) exchange with the systemic circulation with less BBB protection to be able to have hormonal exchange. Infection and inflammation are the most common causes of BBB collapse. The BBB is intricately involved in pharmacotherapy and is more thoroughly described in Chapter 23.

Anatomy of the Brain

The brain is conceptually divided into three functioning sections: the forebrain, midbrain, and hindbrain (Table 3-1). The forebrain consists

of what is referred to as the *telencephalon* (cortex, basal ganglia, hippocampus, and amygdala), and *diencephalon* (thalamus and hypothalamus). The midbrain is referred to as the *mesencephalon* and consists of the tecum and tegmentum. The hindbrain is referred to as the *metencephalon* (pons and cerebellum) and *myelencephalon* (medulla). The tissue of the brain is composed of **white matter** (the myelinated axons of neurons) and **gray matter** (nerve cell bodies and dendrites). Gray matter is the working area of the brain containing synapses and neuronal connections. The brain is further divided into other structures.

Subdivisions of the Brain   table 3-1

Major Division	Subdivision	Structures
Forebrain (Prosencephalon)	Telencephalon	Neocortex, basal ganglia, amygdala, hippocampus, lateral ventricles
	Diencephalon	Thalamus, hypothalamus, epithalamus, third ventricle
Midbrain (Mesencephalon)	Mesencephalon	Tacum, tegmentum, cerebral aqueduct
Hindbrain (Rhombencephalon)	Metencephalon	Cerebellum, pons, fourth ventricle
	Myelencephalon	Medulla oblongata, fourth ventricle

The *cortex* is the outermost covering of the cerebrum. It is several cellular layers thick and composed of a mixture of cellular bodies and capillary blood vessels. The cortex is gray matter. It is structured with grooves and dips of wrinkles in the brain tissue that provide anatomical landmarks or reference points and serves to increase the brain's surface working area and cell communication. The small shallow grooves are called *sulci*. The deeper grooves extending into the brain are called *fissures*, and the raised tissue areas are *gyri*. Without the sulci, fissures, and gyri, the skull could not hold the brain, because the total surface area of the cortex ranges from 230 to 470 square inches.

The Cerebrum

An understanding of neurobiological processes of mental health requires a thorough understanding of the role of the cerebrum. The largest portion of the brain, the **cerebrum**, controls intelligence, motor, and sensory functions. The cerebrum is divided into two hemispheres, right and left, and the diencephalon (neural tube), which is between the two hemispheres and the brainstem. Motor impulses descend and cross in the medulla, creating what is referred to as *hemispheric lateralization*. This means that the right cerebral hemisphere controls the left side of the body and the left cerebral hemisphere controls the right side of the body. The right and left hemispheres of the brain have specific responsibilities. They communicate across the divide of the corpus callosum in the middle. The *left brain* specializes in logic, objective reasoning, and categorizing. This is where the brain possesses the ability to use and understand language and numbers and perform analytic scientific skills. It is detail oriented, mimics, and controls the right hand. The *right brain* specializes in intuition and insight, subjective reasoning, recognizing pattern, visual–spatial perception, creativity, imagination, and playfulness, as well as, generating emotional expression, art and music skills, and holistic thought; the right brain controls the left hand (Figure 3-4).

The cerebrum is further divided by fissures, creating four distinct lobes. Cerebral duties are divided among four lobes named for their overlying cranial bones: the frontal, parietal, temporal, and occipital lobes (Table 3-2). Each lobe has specific functions and responsibilities, but they also work together to coordinate, integrate, and process information.

Frontal Lobe

The **frontal lobe** is responsible for executive function and personality. It maintains focused attention, organizes thinking, planning, speech, and motor activities. It allows the individual to weigh consequences, set goals, modulate emotions, and integrate ideas, emotions, and perceptions. More specifically, it controls voluntary motor activity of muscles and coordinates movement of muscle groups. It allows for multimodal sensory input to trigger working memory, reasoning, prioritizing, sequencing, and abstraction to allow for intelligent decision making. It allows for impulse control. Broca's area, which controls the expressive, motor function of speech, is found in the frontal lobe. This is the location of the prefrontal cortex, as well as the orbitofrontal cortex, medial prefrontal cortex, and the dorsolateral prefrontal cortex. When normal frontal lobe functioning is altered, there is destabilization of emotions, a loss of impulse control, increased impulsiveness, poor decision making, poor judgment, a reduction in insight, memory loss, forgetfulness, loss of executive function such as planning and organizing, and, perhaps most notable to friends and family, a change in personality (Figure 3-5)

Parietal Lobe

The **parietal lobe** is all about body sensation impulses received from the thalamus. Its main responsibility is to regulate primary sensory areas, including pain, taste, touch, proprioception (location of the body in space), and the sensation of temperature. The processes of reading and writing also occur in the parietal lobe. It also helps maintain focused attention and processes certain motor activities, including attention and perception of spatial relations and registration of acts of aggression. Problems in the parietal lobe are recognized by sensory perceptual disturbances. The inability to recognize objects by touch or recognize parts of one's own body, and problems calculating, writing, drawing, doing familiar things, or organizing special directions all suggest problems in the parietal lobe.

Temporal Lobe

The **temporal lobes**, located just above the ears, process auditory and olfactory senses. Emotion, learning, and memory circuits are here as well. This area gives emotional tone to memories and is involved in

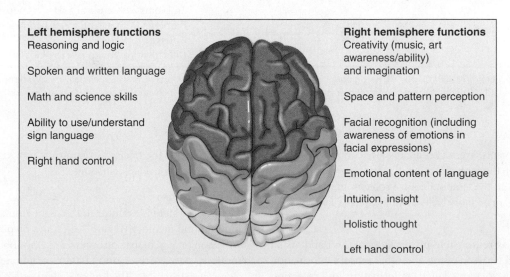

Left hemisphere functions
Reasoning and logic

Spoken and written language

Math and science skills

Ability to use/understand
sign language

Right hand control

Right hemisphere functions
Creativity (music, art
awareness/ability)
and imagination

Space and pattern perception

Facial recognition (including
awareness of emotions in
facial expressions)

Emotional content of language

Intuition, insight

Holistic thought

Left hand control

3-4 Brain hemispheres and their functions.

Selected Major Brain Structures: Functions and Dysfunction — table 3-2

Brain Structures	Functions	Dysfunction/Problems
Lobes **Frontal**	Executive function Personality Attention Organization Motivation Problem solving Sequencing Judgment Emotional control Motor integration Expressive language	Inflexible thinking Personality changes Short attention span, inattentiveness Disorganized or excessive organization Avolition or excessive drive Difficulties in problem solving, decision making Difficulty sequencing Impulsiveness, disinhibition Emotional dysregulation Motor irregularities Aphasia
Temporal	Receptive language Hearing Memory Sequencing Moral judgments Learning Emotions	Difficulty understanding Poor registration of sound Loss of short-term memory Difficulty categorizing Inappropriate behaviors Poor object recognition Aggressiveness, irritability
Parietal	Visual–spatial perceptions Motor sensations Identification or differentiation among size, shapes, colors Attention for learning	Dyslexia, right/left problems Poor visual attention Problems with eye–hand coordination Poor coordination Unawareness of body, apraxia Asterognosis, graphesthesia Poor reading/writing/math, alexia, agraphia Poor object naming, anomia
Occipital	Vision Visual memory Visual perception Perception of printed word	Alteration in visual fields, color identification Alteration in registration and recall of objects, anomia Inability to see objects move Hallucinations, illusions, visual distortions Problems identifying or recognizing words Problems reading and writing
Cerebellum	Coordination Balance, equilibrium, posture Sequential movements	Poor fine motor coordination, grasping Vertigo, tremors, tipping, unstable gait Poor proprioceptive movements
Brainstem	Alertness and arousal Automatic autonomic function regulation	Somnolence Problems with sleep and wake cycles Problems with arousal and consciousness Problems with attention and concentration Nausea, vertigo Difficulty breathing, swallowing, balance, heart rate

Based on Genung, V., & Gerardi, M. (2013, April 17). *Recognizing Target and Side Effects of Psychotropics on Brain Circuit Pathways*. Workshop presentation (Session 10) delivered at the ISPN 2013 6th Psychopharmacology Institute and International Society for Psychiatric Nurses 15th Annual Conference, San Antonio, TX.

making moral judgments. Wernicke's area is located in the temporal lobe and is involved in the comprehension of receptive speech. The hippocampus is located in the temporal lobe. Problems in the temporal lobe can lead to visual or auditory hallucinations, aphasia, and amnesia.

Occipital Lobe
The **occipital lobe** is responsible primarily for vision and visual memory. Integration between vision and other sensory information occurs in this region. Reading, language formation, and reception of vestibular, acoustic, and tactile stimuli occur here. Problems associated with the occipital region include visual field deficits, blindness, and visual hallucinations.

Limbic System
The **limbic system** is essential to the regulation and modulation of emotions and memory (Figure 3-6). It is a pivotal structure in any discussion on psychiatric disorders and emotional behaviors. Basic emotions, needs, drives, and instincts originate in this system of interactive structures. The limbic system refers to the hypothalamus, thalamus, hippocampus, and amygdala. During development,

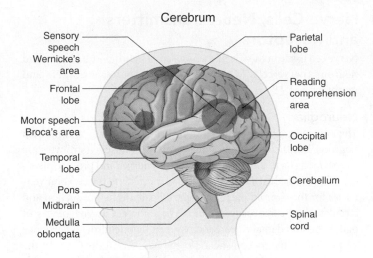

Cerebrum

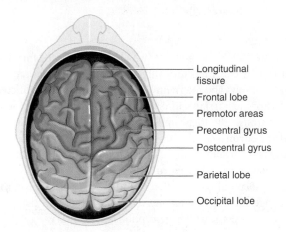

Sensory speech Wernicke's area
Frontal lobe
Motor speech Broca's area
Temporal lobe
Pons
Midbrain
Medulla oblongata

Parietal lobe
Reading comprehension area
Occipital lobe
Cerebellum
Spinal cord

Longitudinal fissure
Frontal lobe
Premotor areas
Precentral gyrus
Postcentral gyrus
Parietal lobe
Occipital lobe

3-5 Brain lobes and their functions.

the diencephalon gives rise to the thalamus, hypothalamus, as well as the pituitary and pineal glands. The limbic system is responsible for emotions, behavior, long-term memory, and olfaction.

Hippocampus

One of the primary functions of the hippocampus is memory. The hippocampus is responsible for converting short-term memory to permanent registration for recall (long-term memory), learning, and sensory integration. It also has internal sensors for temperature, osmolarity, glucose, and sodium concentration. These include steroid hormones and hormones involved in appetite control, such as leptin and orexin, as well as internal signals.

Amygdala

The amygdala is involved primarily in emotional regulation, and mediating mood, fear, anxiety, anger, social behavior, reward, and impulsive gut responses. The amygdala integrates sensory smell with emotions.

Thalamus

The thalamus acts as a relay switch to relay sensory and motor signals to the cerebral cortex and is involved in the regulation of consciousness, sleep, and alertness. It is the sensory relay station, except for the sense of smell. It modulates sensory stimulation to ensure that the cortex is not overwhelmed with sensory input. It regulates emotions, memory, and affective behaviors.

Hypothalamus

The primary responsibility of the hypothalamus is homeostasis and production of neurohormones. It also regulates hunger, thirst, temperature, and body functions and controls corticosteroid production. It contains pyramidal cells.

Other Important Structures

A number of other structures assist in the functions of the CNS.

- The *cingulate gyrus* forms a pathway from the thalamus to the hippocampus. It is responsible for focusing attention on emotionally significant events and for associating memories to smells and to pain.

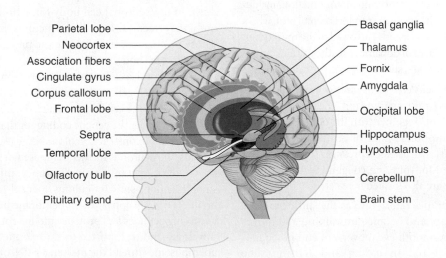

Parietal lobe
Neocortex
Association fibers
Cingulate gyrus
Corpus callosum
Frontal lobe
Septra
Temporal lobe
Olfactory bulb
Pituitary gland

Basal ganglia
Thalamus
Fornix
Amygdala
Occipital lobe
Hippocampus
Hypothalamus
Cerebellum
Brain stem

3-6 The limbic system.

- The *basal ganglia* surround the top and sides of the limbic system and are tightly connected with the cortex above them. Accommodating several smaller structures, that include the striatum (caudate nucleus and putamen), the globus pallidus, the substantia nigra, the nucleus accumbens, and the subthalamic nucleus, the basal ganglia serve as a complex feedback system to modulate and stabilize somatic and motor activity. The basal ganglia play a prominent role in the initiation and management of movement and complex motor functions. Extrapyramidal motor nerve tracks are located in the basal ganglia, allowing for repetitive behaviors, reward experiences, and focusing attention. Problems in the basal ganglia may lead to bradykinesia, hyperinesias, and dystonias. This is the location where many medication side effects occur.

- The *pineal gland* is located above and medial to the thalamus. It secretes the hormone melatonin and is associated with sleep and emotional regulation. Melatonin is secreted when the brain perceives darkness, inducing sleep.

- The *ventral tegmental area* of the brainstem (just below the thalamus) consists of dopamine pathways. It is responsible for pleasure and is referred to as the center of the reward pathway. Individuals with damage to this area tend to have difficulty obtaining pleasure in life, often turning to alcohol, drugs, sweets, sex, and/or gambling.

- The *reticular formation,* located inside the brainstem, receives input from the cortex and integrates for postsensory pathways. It innervates the thalamus, hypothalamus, and cortex. It is important in the regulation of involuntary movement, reflexes, muscle tone, and vital signs.

- The *locus coeruleus* is a cluster of neurons that initiate in the pons and fan out and innervate nearly all of the brain. It is involved in nearly every function of the brain, most importantly in the production of norepinephrine.

- The *brainstem* includes the midbrain, pons, medulla, and reticular formation, as well as the cerebellum. It also is the site of specific nuclei that produce neurotransmitters. The basic actions of all psychotropic medications begin in the brainstem.

- The *midbrain* controls many sensory and motor functions including eye movements. It contains the ventral tegmental area, which is in the very center of the brain and is involved in the reward center; the substantia nigra (area of dopamine synthesis); and centers for visual and auditory reflexes, such as moving the head and eyes.

- The *pons* contains the locus coeruleus (area of norepinephrine synthesis). It also relays information from the cerebral hemispheres to the cerebellum. Together with the pons, the *medulla oblongata* contains autonomic control centers that regulate internal body functions such as blood pressure, respiration, and digestion. Reflex centers for vomiting, coughing, sneezing, swallowing, and hiccuping are also located here.

- The *cerebellum,* sometimes referred to as the "little brain," is responsible for posture and balance in walking and movement. It is involved in smooth eye movement and in sequential movements required in eating and writing. The cerebellum controls speed and acceleration of movement, cognition and language, memory, and impulse control. Each hemisphere of the cerebellum controls the ipsilateral (same side) of the body.

Nerve Cells, Neurotransmitters and Receptors

Nerve cell tissue in the CNS is composed of neuroglia (glial cells) and neurons (nerve cells). Neurons produce neurotransmitters and receptors.

Neuroglia

The *neuroglia*, or glial cells, support, protect, insulate, and nourish neurons, but they do not conduct neural impulses. Astrocytes are star-shaped glia that bind blood vessels to nerves and provide physical support for the BBB. Ependymal glia cells line the cerebral ventricles for the choroid plexus and participate in the production and circulation of cerebrospinal fluid. Microglia act as phagocytes of pathogens and damaged cerebral tissues. Oligodendrocytes produce and maintain the myelin sheath of the neurons of the CNS. In the peripheral nervous sysem, the myelin sheath is produced and maintained by Schwann cells.

Neurons

There are 100 billion neurons, which are subdivided into 150 types that can be classified into three major groups: sensory neurons, motor neurons, and interneurons. **Sensory neurons**, or afferent neurons, carry neural signal information from the periphery (outside the body through the PNS) up to the CNS through the spinal nerves. **Motor neurons**, or efferent neurons, carry neural signal messages from inside the brain, the CNS, back out to the PNS, again through the spinal nerves. **Interneurons** are exclusive to the CNS. They connect sensory and motor (afferent and efferent) neurons in the CNS, exchange messages, interpret, communicate, and play a role in thought process, learning, perception, and memory.

Neuronal Cell Body

Neurons are responsible for communication from one cell to another. They enable the nervous system to work together as a whole in a weblike network within and between the CNS and PNS. The neuron is composed of three main parts: the dendrites, cell body, and the axon. *Dendrites* act as antennae—they look for, detect, and receive signals from another neuron, then transmit that signal down to the neuronal cell body for action. Extensions of the cell body, they resemble fingerlike structures that end in synaptic bulbs whose protein receptors receive the message to be directed to the core of the cell body.

The second section, the cell body (soma), is the largest part of the nerve cell. Together, the cell body and dendrites are gray matter (Figure 3-7A). The cell body contains the nucleus, which is responsible for containing the genetic coding for that nerve cell and contains proteins for the construction of the nerve itself. In addition to the cell nucleus, the neuron is further composed of all the normal cell materials, Golgi apparatus, polyribosomes, mitochondria, rough and smooth endoplasmic reticulums, cytosol, and neuronal cell membrane. The Golgi apparatus is membrane bound and plays a role in packaging peptides and proteins into neurotransmitters, to be placed in vesicles and transported to the axon terminals for release. The polyribosomes thread the messenger RNA that synthesizes proteins outside of the axon. The ribosomes work on the single-strand messenger RNA to make multiple copies of the same protein. The nerve mitochondria supply energy to the cell by synthesizing adenosine triphosphate (ATP) into adenosine diphosphate (ADP), which

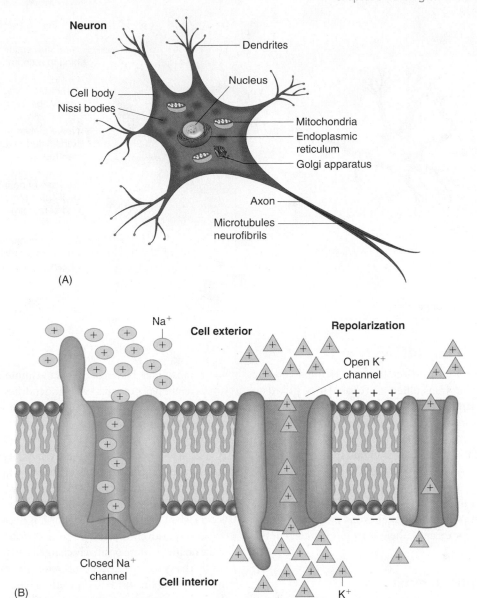

Neuron

- Dendrites
- Nucleus
- Cell body
- Nissl bodies
- Mitochondria
- Endoplasmic reticulum
- Golgi apparatus
- Axon
- Microtubules neurofibrils

(A)

Na$^+$ **Cell exterior** **Repolarization**

Open K$^+$ channel

+ + + +

− − −

Closed Na$^+$ channel **Cell interior** K$^+$

(B)

3-7 A. Neuron. B. Neuronal action potential.

fuels most of the biochemical reactions in the neuron. Neurons need a great deal of energy to do their work. Their mitochondria use oxygen and glucose to produce most of the cell's energy. The endoplasmic reticulum is a network of tubes responsible for synthesizing and transporting proteins. Cytosol is the intracellular fluid, the liquid found inside the cell. It contains water and ions (Na$^+$, K$^+$) of different concentration from the extracellular fluid, which facilitates the action potential—the electrical signaling of the cell. The neuron cell membrane is a barrier that encloses all the parts of the cell body and excludes other substances in the interstitial fluid. This neuronal cell membrane is made up of lipids (fats) and proteins (chains of amino acid peptides). It is a bilayer sandwich of phospholipids with a polar charged area that faces outward away from the cell, and a nonpolar area that faces inward toward the cell. The external face of the cell membrane contains the receptor proteins that receive the

signal. This message travels through this membrane from the dendrite, where the message is received, to the cell body for response. Together, the dendrites and cell body are gray matter.

The third section, the axon, looks like a tail. It has three parts: the axon itself, the axon hillock, and the axon terminals. The **axon** is a separate structure of the neuron and is composed of white matter. The axon is the main signal-conducting unit of the neuron cell; its responsibility is to transmit information away from the cell body. There is only one axon for each neuron, whereas there are many dendrites. The *axon hillock* is where the axon is connected to the cell body. It is from this site that electrical firing, known as action potential, occurs (Figure 3-7B). At the end of the axon are the *axon terminals*, another set of structures that look like a section of a tree root. These axon terminals have rounded terminal ends called synaptic knobs (boutons), which contain many mitochondria and the vesicles in which the neurotransmitters are stored. When discussing the

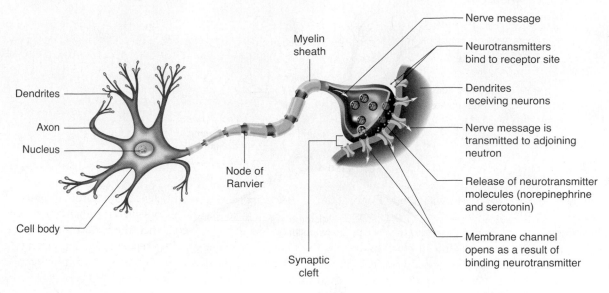

Myelin sheath

Nerve message

Neurotransmitters bind to receptor site

Dendrites receiving neurons

Nerve message is transmitted to adjoining neutron

Release of neurotransmitter molecules (norepinephrine and serotonin)

Membrane channel opens as a result of binding neurotransmitter

Dendrites

Axon

Nucleus

Cell body

Node of Ranvier

Synaptic cleft

3-8 Excitatory neuronal connection.

actual activity of neuron transmission, the axon terminals are the presynaptic site where neurotransmitters are released to be picked up by the dendritic postsynaptic receptors on the next neuron. There are three types of axons: associative, commissural, and projection. Associative axons communicate within the hemisphere through interneurons, which serve as local communicators to link sensory and motor neurons, and are limited to a specific area such as the gamma-aminobutyric acid (GABA) system. Commisural axons communicate across hemispheres via the corpus callosum and connect the two hemispheres with each other. Projection axons are long-distance axons that connect the cortex and other structures throughout the brain to the spinal cord.

Neurons and Synaptic Transmission

The dendrites at the top of the neuron are the receivers of the signal message (postsynaptic neuron site), and the axon terminals at the end of the neuron are the transmitter–senders of the signal message (presynaptic neuron site). The **synapse** is the junction where one bulb of the presynaptic axon terminal makes contact with the postsynaptic dendrite receptor membrane site of another nerve. The synaptic cleft is the narrow, fluid-filled space between the presynaptic neuron and the postsynaptic neuron.

Nerves are activated at the synapse by electrical and neurochemical signal messages. First, an electrical signal or impulse is conducted from the axon hillock, along the axon, instantaneously to the next cell. This is caused by the movement of positive sodium (Na^+) and potassium (K^+) ions across the membranes. This ion signaling typically is bidirectional, meaning that the ions can flow both ways. Second, the neurochemical signal refers to the transmission of impulses from one neuron to another neuron through neurotransmitters. There are two types of neurotransmitter neurochemical junctions. Type 1 is an excitatory synapse typically found on postsynaptic dendrites receiving neurotransmitter signaling from glutamate, a major excitatory transmitter (Figure 3-8). Type 2 is an inhibitory synapse generally found on the cell body, receiving neurotransmitter signaling from gamma amino butyric acid, a major inhibitory

neurotransmitter. Different neurotransmitters are released at these two different types of synapses. The dendrites of individual cell bodies are capable of receiving impulses from many different neurotransmitters at once. The strength of the given neurotransmitter will determine if the overall result is excitatory or inhibitory.

Action potential refers to the series of steps that occur to change the nerve from a polarized–resting state with a negative (–) charge, to a depolarized–activated state with a positive (+) charge, and back to the repolarized–resting state negative charge again. Polarization occurs when the inside of the neuron is negatively charged and the outside is positively charged. Depolarization occurs when the inside of the neuron is more positively charged and the outside is more negatively charged. Repolarization is returning the neuron to the negative charge on the inside and positive charge on the outside resting state. This is accomplished by adjusting ion concentrations by moving Na^+ and K^+ ions in and out of the cell. In the resting, depolarized state, the inside of the cell is more negative and the outside more positive. Potassium ion (K^+) is the chief intracellular positively charged ion (cation), along with several negatively charged ions (anions). During the resting, depolarized state, K^+ diffuses, or leaks, out of the cell, taking its positive charge and leaving the negative anions inside the cell to negatively charge the inside of the cell. The ATP-driven pumps force K^+ back into the cell, restoring the positive charge on the inside of the cell. The exchange of Na^+ in the cell occurs by the process of diffusion. Na^+ is the chief extracellular cation. When the cell membrane is stimulated, Na^+ is allowed to leak (diffuse) back inside the cell. This increases the inside of the cell's positive ionic concentration and charge. The cell quickly detects this imbalance and tries to redistribute by stopping Na^+ diffusion in, and allowing K^+ to leak out. The cell is designed to have greater concentrations of Na^+ on the outside of the cell and K^+ inside the cell, so the cell tries to rectify the imbalance by stopping the Na^+ from coming into the cell, thereby increasing the Na^+ concentration outside the cell, where it belongs. It also allows K^+ to leak out until a balance is achieved, at which time the cell receives an ATP charge, forcing the K^+ out of the cell, and the process begins again.

A wave of action potentials is propagated along the presynaptic axon cell membrane, arriving at the synaptic knob in the axon terminal, where the neurotransmitters are being held in the vesicles. Calcium ion (Ca^{++}) voltage-gated channels in the synaptic knob open in response to depolarization of the cell membrane, and calcium ions flow from the extracellular fluid into the synaptic knob. This increase in calcium concentration causes the vesicles holding the neurotransmitters to drop down and fuse with the membrane of the synaptic knob, at which time they release the neurotransmitter into the synaptic cleft via exocytosis, and the calcium voltage-gated channel is closed. This is a one-way process from presynaptic axon terminal release of neurotransmitter to the postsynaptic dendrite or cell body of the postsynaptic cell. The communication in neurotransmission can occur in one of three ways. The fastest method and the predominant method is **classic neurotransmission**, in which, as described, the neurotransmission signal travels from one neuron directly to the next neuron. For example, delegating a task to someone is a one-way conversation. This is the case with most neurotransmissions. The second method is referred to as **retrograde neurotransmission**, in which the postsynaptic cell communicates with the presynaptic neuron. Neurotransmitters using this method include endogenous cannabinoids, nitrous oxide, and nerve growth factor. This two-way conversation is rare in neurotransmission. The third method is **volume neurotransmission**, in which the neurotransmission occurs (without a synapse) to an adjacent neuron by process of diffusion. Volume neurotransmission occurs when nearby receptors pick up the neurotransmitter and perform a weaker signal. Volume neurotransmission can be compared to having a conversation with a friend when someone nearby, who is engaged in a different conversation, overhears your conversation.

Neurons, receptors, and neurotransmitters (ligands) allow communication between the neuronal cells in the CNS and with the outside world via the PNS. A **receptor** is a protein molecule that receives and responds to a neurotransmitter ligand, a drug ligand (or medication), or other substances such as hormones and antigens. A **neurotransmitter** is a chemical that is synthesized (created) in, and released from, a vesicle in a presynaptic neuron. Once released from the presynaptic neuron, the neurotransmitter waits in line in the synaptic cleft (space between presynaptic neuron and postsynaptic neuron) for a turn to take a seat on a specific receptor embedded in a postsynaptic nerve. The neurotransmitter's mission is to elicit a specific response from the postsynaptic neuron. They fit together like lock (receptor) and key (neurotransmitter). The neurotransmitter unlocks the receptor. The neurotransmitter's responsibility is to either excite the postsynaptic nerve cell or inhibit and stop the cell action once it opens the receptor door to the postsynaptic nerve cell.

After the neurotransmitter has relayed its message to the receptor of the postsynaptic cell, it is released back into the synaptic cleft and picked up by a reuptake scoop (reuptake transporter) on the presynaptic neuron. From there it is stored for later, recycled for re-release to be used again in the cycle as described, or metabolized by enzymes in the presynaptic neuron and inactivated. Monoamine oxidase (MAO) is the enzyme that is typically responsible for this duty.

Monoamine oxidase inhibitors (MAOIs) are medications that prevent this enzyme from breaking down the neurotransmitters. A deficit in the neurotransmitters means inadequate activation of the receptors, which may lead to mental health issues such as depression and anxiety. An excess in the neurotransmitters means additional activation of receptors, which may lead to other mental health issues, such as bipolar disorder, psychosis, and schizophrenia. Medications (drug ligands) exert their effects by inhibiting the reuptake scoop on the presynaptic neuron or by engaging (sitting on) the postsynaptic neuron and either activating the cell (agonists) or inactivating the cell (antagonists) (Chapter 23).

Receptors

Receptors are proteins embedded in the dendrites and neuron cell membrane of the cell body. Receptors are the door into the cell. Receptors are activated (opened) by neurotransmitters, hormones, growth factors, and sensory signals and then turn around and activate the effector (cell). When the neurotransmitter or hormone binds to the receptor, the receptor changes its protein shape. There are four types of receptors. Two are neurotransmitter receptor types: ligand-gated receptors (ionotropic) and G protein-coupled receptors (metabotropic). The other two receptor cell types are tyrosine kinase receptors and nuclear receptors. *Ligand-gated receptors* contain an ion channel and can be excited by neurotransmitters (ligands) such as glutamate and aspartate, nicotinic acetylcholine, and serotonin$_3$, or inhibited by neurotransmitters such as GABA and glycine. *G protein-coupled receptors* (GPCR) are neither excitatory nor inhibitory, but rather modulate neurotransmitter activity. They are called G coupled proteins because of their ability to bind the guanine nucleotides guanosine triphosphate (GTP) and guanosine diphosphate (GDP) (Schatzberg & Nemeroff, 2009). Most neurotransmitters are GPCRs that work by transmitting an information signal to the appropriate "effector," second messengers within the cell. Receptors that use the GPCR include catecholamines, serotonin, acetylcholine, peptides, and sensory signals such as light and odorants.

Ionotropic receptors direct electrical activity by regulating movement of ions across membranes. Ionotropic receptors contain four or five subunits that open when the neurotransmitter binds to them, allowing ions to flow into the cell (Na^+, Ca^{++}, Cl^-), or out of the cell (K^+), thereby generating synaptic action potential. Some neurons can be specific and dedicated for one receptor system, whereas others can have multiple types of receptors on them.

For definition purposes, *autoreceptors* are located on neurons that produce the endogenous (from within) ligand for that particular receptor (for example, a serotonin receptor on a serotonin neuron). *Heteroreceptors* are receptor subtypes that are present on neurons but do not contain an endogenous ligand for that particular receptor subtype (such as a serotonin receptor located on a dopamine neuron). The third type of receptor is the *tyrosine kinase receptor*, which is used for cell growth factors such as neurotrophic factors and cytokines. The fourth type of receptor is the *nuclear receptor*, which is used for genetic transcription and regulates the expression of target genes in response to steroid hormones and other such ligands, such as glucocorticoids, gonadal steroids, and thyroid hormones.

In the *cholinergic* (parasympathetic) brain circuit pathway, the postsynaptic receptors are muscarinic, nicotinic, and histaminic. The neurotransmitters for that system are *acetylcholine, nicotine,* and *histamine*. In the *adrenergic* (sympathetic) pathway, the receptors are alpha and beta and the catecholamine neurotransmitters are *epinephrine* and *norepinephrine*. In the *serotonergic* pathway, the receptors are serotonergic and the indoleamine monoamine neurotransmitter is serotonin. In the *dopaminergic* pathway, the receptors are dopaminergic and the catecholamine monoamine neurotransmitter is dopamine. There are several subsystems within each major neurotransmitter system.

Neurotransmitters and Target Receptors

Some neurons synthesize only one specific neurotransmitter, whereas others make two or more different types of neurotransmitters. Most neurotransmitters are derived from amino acids in the diet. Some neurons modify these dietary amino acids to form an "amine" neurotransmitter (acetylcholine, serotonin, norepinephrine, dopamine). Other neurons combine the amino acids to form peptide chain neuromodulators (endorphins, enkephalins, dynorphins). The primary neurotransmitters of the nervous system include the following:

- Cholinergic neurotransmitters (acetylcholine [ACh] and histamine)
- Serotonergic indoleamine serotonin (5HT) neurotransmitters
- Adrenergic catecholamines norepinephrine (NE) and epinepherine (EPI)
- Dopamine (DA) neurotransmitters
- Gabaergic neurotransmitters GABA and glycine
- Glutamanergic neurotransmitters (glutamate/aspartate)

The nervous system's primary opioid peptide neuromodulators include β-endorphins, met-enkaphalins, leu-enkaphalins, and dynorphins. These systems perform checks and balances on each other. The sympathetic and parasympathetic systems work together for balance in the autonomic system, whereas the catecholamines and indoleamines (such as serotonin) work together to establish balance in the sympathetic nervous system.

Cholinergics

Acetylcholine (ACh) is a neurotransmitter formed from choline that is derived from the amino acids in red meats in the diet. Coenzyme A is involved in the synthesis of ACh, which is found in both the brain (forebrain, pons, cortex, hippocampus) and the spinal cord of the CNS and also in the PNS, most particularly at the neuromuscular junctions of the skeletal muscles. It initiates in the basal ganglia nucleus and projects broadly throughout the cerebral cortex to the septal area (rostral to the hypothalamus) to the hippocampus. ACh targets the nicotinic ($N_{(1-4)}$) and muscarinic ($\mu_{(1-5)}$) cholinergic receptors. (The subscripts indicate the number of different types of receptors.) Nicotinic nerve (Nn) receptors serve all the autonomic nervous system. Nicotinic neuromuscular (Nm) receptor junctions are found at the skeletal muscles. Muscarinic (μ) receptors are found in all parasympathetic target organs—eye, heart, lung, bladder, GI tract, sweat glands, sex organs, and blood vessels. ACh mediates cognitive functioning directly, and plays an important role in learning, memory, wakefulness, attention, and movement (Table 3-3). It contributes to circadian rhythm. It is implicated in nicotine dependence and contributes to excessive arousal of thought with the use of cocaine and amphetamine. It has also been implicated in dementias, owing to decreased ACh secreting

neurons, and myasthenia gravis, related to muscle weakness due to reduced ACh receptors.

Histamine is another cholinergic neurotransmitter involved in several systems in the body. CNS histaminic cholinergic receptors (H_1, H_2, H_3, H_4) are found in the hypothalamus, projections in cerebral cortex, limbic system, hypothalamus, and mast cells.

- H_1 is found in smooth muscles and endothelial cells and is related to acute allergic responses.
- H_2 is located in gastric parietal cells and is related to secretion of gastric acid.
- H_3 is responsible for modulating CNS neurotransmission.
- H_4 is located in mast cells, eosinophils, T-cells, and dendritic cells regulating immune responses.

In general, histamine is involved in allergic responses, control of gastric secretions, smooth muscle control, cardiac stimulation, stimulation of sensory nerve endings, and alertness. The role of histamine in the CNS is elusive, but it is known to modulate the neurotransmission in addition to its role in the allergic response. The exact mechanism is not yet known. Psychotropic medication blockage of

Neurotransmitter Functions	table 3-3

Neurotransmitter	Function
Norepinephrine (NE)	EXCITE Fright–flight–fight Awake, alert, energized Vigilance, interest Concentration, attention Memory, learning
Dopamine (DA)	MODULATE Promotes well-being Pain–pleasure, reinforcing Motivation–drive Reward-seeking behavior Creativity, imagination Clear thinking, memory Evaluation of reality
Serotonin (5HT)	MODULATE Mood, affect Sleep, appetite, sex Interest, learning Executive function Impulse control
Gamma-aminobutyric acid (GABA)	INHIBIT Balances activating neurotransmitters Calming, quieting, relaxing Pain reduction
Acetylcholine (ACh)	MODULATE Calm Rest–digest–restore Activates calm in PSNS Antiexcitatory in SNS

histamine often results in weight gain, sedation, and hypotension. Nonetheless, since histamine is found to play a significant role in many of the side effects of psychotropic medications, alerting prescribers to the fact that there are cholinergic receptors for histamines throughout the central and peripheral nervous systems.

Adrenergics: Indoleamines

Serotonin monoamine targets the family of serotoninergic receptors with many subtypes ($5HT1_{ABDEF}$, $5HT2_{ABC}$, 5HT3, 5HT4, 5HT5, 5HT6, 5HT7), and is derived from dietary amino acids that are metabolized into tryptophan. The serotonin neuronal pathway initiates in the midbrain and broadly projects throughout the cortex, the hypothalamus and thalamus of the limbic system, and the cerebellum, brainstem, and spinal cord. Serotonergic receptors are found in the brain, spinal cord, guts, and platelets. This brain circuit pathway is most likely to be involved in temperature regulation, pain perception, sleep, appetite, sexual interest, fear, depressive and anxious mood mental health disturbances, delusions and hallucinations, and vomiting. Most antidepressants have at least some effect by blocking the reuptake of serotonin. This leaves more of the neurotransmitter available for longer periods of time in the synapse, resulting in improved mood. Lysergic acid diethylamide (LSD) and 3,4-methylenedioxy-*N*-methylamphetamine (ecstasy) have their primary effects in the serotonin pathways; however, cocaine, amphetamine, alcohol, and nicotine also affect serotonin transmission.

The process of reuptake transporter activity is about the same for all neurotransmitters (Figure 3-9). Using serotonin (5HT) for example, termination of the 5HT effects are brought about by the serotonin transporter system (SERT/5HTT). After release into the synapse, 5HT either attaches to a postsynaptic 5HT receptor and activates the cell and is released back to the synaptic cleft, or it just sits in the synaptic cleft, waiting. The next step is that 5HT is taken back up into the presynaptic dendritic terminal by the SERT/5HTT,

where it is metabolized by the enzyme MAO or sent to the secretory vesicles by the vesicle monoamine transporter (VMAT). The transport process using the SERT/5HTT and VMAT is said to occur through the Na^+/K^+ pump. The transporter binds the monoamine (neurotransmitter) and co-transports it with Na^+, while K^+ is translocated across the membrane to the outside of the cell (Schatzberg & Nemeroff, 2009).

Adrenergics: Catecholamines

Norepinephrine monoamine (noradrenaline) is the most prominent neurotransmitter in the nervous system. It is derived from tyrosine. The noradrenergic receptors are found in the locus coeruleus, projecting broadly throughout the brain to the lateral tegmental area, the pons, and medulla. Projections are widespread in the cortex, forebrain, hypothalamus, thalamus, cerebellum, brainstem, and spinal column. The norepinephrine reuptake transporter (NET) is dependent on extracellular Na^+/Cl^- driven as previously described. NE is responsible for the response to stress. It regulates awareness of environment, attention, learning, memory, sleep, and arousal. Cocaine and amphetamines affect the transmission of NE and contribute to the stimulating and pleasurable effects of these drugs. Tyrosine is biosynthesized to L-dopa, then to dopamine, to norepinephrine, and then to epinephrine. Epinephrine (EPI) (adrenaline), the derivative of NE, has a limited presence in the brain. It is found mostly in the central tegmental area, and contributes to "fear–fight–flight" responses in the PNS. The adrenergic receptor subtypes include $\alpha1_{a,b,c,d}$, located in the eye, arterioles, veins, male sex organs, and bladder; $\alpha2_{a,b,c,d}$, located in the presynaptic nerve terminals; $\beta1$, located in the heart and kidneys; and $\beta2$, located in the arterioles, bronchi, uterus, and liver skeletal muscle. The neurotransmitter EPI has affinity for $\alpha1,2$ and $\beta1,2$. The neurotransmitter NE has greatest affinity for $\alpha1,2$ and $\beta1$ (Schatzberg & Nemeroff, 2009). Because of all these subreceptors, psychiatric medications can affect every body system, resulting in a number of side effects. This is the path most likely activated in mental health issues such as attention-deficit/hyperactivity disorder, depressive and anxiety disorders, memory loss, and social withdrawal. Some antidepressants work by inhibiting the MAO that would break down NE, whereas others block the reuptake of NE neurotransmitters, allowing more to be available to the receptors to provide to the effector cell area.

Dopamine, a neurotransmitter found primarily in the brainstem, is well distributed throughout the brain and is also derived from tyrosine (a dietary amino acid). Again, tyrosine is biosynthesized to L-dopa, then to dopamine, to NE, and then to EPI; therefore, it is structurally related to NE and EPI. The dopaminergic receptors initiate in the ventral tegmental area and project to the amygdala, nucleus accumbens, striatum, and substantia nigra. There are five dopamine receptors (D1, D2, D3, D4, D5) and a dopamine transporter (DAT). Dopamine receptors have been grouped as D1,5 and D2,3,4 based on their specific properties. D2 is the targeted receptor for antipsychotic medications. The DAT functions as a NA^+/K^+ pump to clear DA from the synaptic cleft.

The different dopamine receptors are found on four dopamine pathways in the brain: the mesocortical (cortex), mesolimbic (limbic), nigrostriatal (basal ganglia), tuberoinfundibular (pituitary), and the mysterious fifth (thalamus) (Stahl, 2013). The mesolimbic

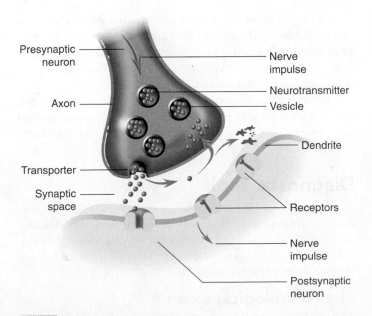

Presynaptic neuron

Axon

Transporter

Synaptic space

Nerve impulse

Neurotransmitter

Vesicle

Dendrite

Receptors

Nerve impulse

Postsynaptic neuron

3-9 Neurotransmitter reuptake activity.

DA pathway projects from the midbrain ventral tegmental area to the nucleus accumbens and through the limbic system. This is considered the reward path and is activated by most substances of abuse. This also is the path most likely to be activated in mental health issues such as mania, psychosis, and the schizophrenias. Increased DA in this pathway is a cause of positive symptoms of psychosis.

The mesocortical DA pathway projects from the midbrain ventral tegmental area to the dorsolateral prefrontal cortex (which mediates cognitive symptoms) and the ventral medial prefrontal cortex (which mediates affective symptoms). This is considered the pathway of executive function. This is also the path most likely to be activated in mental health issues such as depression, catatonia, decreased attention or concentration, mania, and schizophrenia. Decreased DA in this pathway is a cause of negative symptoms of mood and psychosis.

The nigrostriatal DA pathway projects from the substantia nigra to the basal ganglia to the ventral tegmentum, the extrapyramidal system, and striatum. This pathway is a prominent site for ACh as well as DA. Because of the ACh presence in the basal ganglia striatum, this is considered the pathway of motor control. This is the path considered the most likely to be activated in mental health issues such as Parkinson disease, extrapyramidal side effects (EPSE) from psychotropic medications, movement disorders, and choreas. When dopamine levels drastically drop in this pathway, there is an ACh increase, which can cause EPSE (akathesis, dystonia, tardive dystonia, or pseudoparkinsonism).

The tuberoinfundibular DA pathway projects from the arcuate hypothalamus to the anterior pituitary and is considered an endocrine pathway involved in issues such as hyperprolactinemia, sexual dysfunction, weight gain, and demineralization of bone. All D2 antagonist antipsychotics work by decreasing dopamine in the tuberoinfundibular pathway, but because this is also a hormone pathway, it is saturated with prolactin receptors. When dopamine levels drastically drop in the anterior pituitary, there is a release of prolactin. When prolactin levels rise, the individual may experience gynecomastia (breast enlargement), galactorrhea (breast milk secretion), or amenorrhea (irregular menstrual periods).

The mysterious fifth DA pathway arises from multiple sites, including the periaqueductal gray (PAG), ventral mesencephalon, hypothalamic nuclei, and lateral parabrachial nucleus, and it projects to the thalamus. Its function is not yet known (Stahl, 2013). The DA pathways are discussed in greater detail in Chapter 23.

In summary, DA is involved in complex motor movement, learning, memory clarity, judgment and insight, executive functioning, pleasure, and motivation. DA is implicated in mental health issues such as mood states, addictive behaviors, psychosis, Parkinson disease, and schizophrenia.

Other Neurotransmitter Categories

Glutamate (Glu) is an excitatory neurotransmitter found throughout the brain. It is the most abundant neurotransmitter in the body; glutamate receptors can be found on most dendrites to stimulate the neuron. Glu is derived from proteins in the diet. Glu is essential in hippocampal functioning and thus is important in learning and cerebral information flow. In excess, it can have neurotoxic effects due to its excitation of the neurons. Hallucinogens such as phencyclidine (PCP) act on the Glu N-methyl D-aspartate (NMDA) receptors. Glu has been implicated in brain damage caused by stroke,

hypoglycemia, sustained hypoxia, ischemia, and degenerative diseases such as dementias.

Gamma-aminobutyric acid (ā-aminobutyric acid, or GABA) is an inhibitory neurotransmitter derived from glutamate and is found in intrinsic feedback loops and interneurons of the cerebrum that are widely distributed throughout the nervous system. It is responsible for slowing the activity of nerve cells. Neurons fire primarily when the Glu input outweighs the GABA input. The inhibitory effect of GABA may be involved in anxiety, agitation, and seizures and is involved in the sedative effects of benzodiazepines, barbiturates, and alcohol. GABA has been implicated in dementia, schizophrenia, and anxiety disorders.

Glycine is an inhibitory neurotransmitter. It extends primarily from the spinal cord and brainstem. Projections are limited, but are found prominently in the auditory system and olfactory bulb, with some projections to the medulla, midbrain, cerebellum, and cortex. It is responsible for decreasing the excitability of spinal motor neurons, but not cortical neurons. Glycine functions within the glutamate system.

Neuropeptides

Neuropeptides connect chains of amino acids; 200 or more have been identified in the brain. Opioid peptides, primarily endorphins, are the body's natural pain killers.

Neuropeptides manage food and water intake regulation and play a role in modulating anxiety, pain, reproduction, and the pleasure of food and drugs. Heroin and morphine bind to receptors used by these endogenous neuropeptides.

Endogenous opioid peptide receptors (OPs) such as mu (μ), delta (ä), and kappa (ê) Â-endorphins, met- and leu-enkephalins, and dynorphins, suppress pain, modulate mood, and reduce stress. These have implications in reward and addiction. Some OPs regulate pituitary hormone release.

Melatonin, secreted in the dark and suppressed in light, helps regulate the sleep–wake cycle as well as other biological rhythms. It is produced in the pineal gland, which has wide neuron projection within and through the CNS.

Cholecystokinin is a primary intestinal hormone involved in satiety, also involved with control of anxiety and panic. It is found predominately in the ventral tegmental area of the midbrain. It is widely distributed within and outside the CNS. Projections are in the frontal cortex where it is co-localized with DA.

Substance P is involved in pain transmission, movement, and mood regulation. It is found widespread in the raphe system and spinal cord, projects into the cortex and brainstem, and is associated with sensory neurons.

Diagnostic Tools

The complexities of the nervous system make it challenging to diagnose nervous system and psychiatric disorders successfully. A variety of diagnostic tools assist in the assessment and diagnosis of these disorders. Neurological exams, laboratory diagnostics, and neuroimaging techniques are part of the available diagnostic arsenal.

The Neurological Exam

As part of every initial psychiatric assessment, all registered nurses are expected to be able to complete and document a thorough neurological exam. Remembering that a cardinal rule in psychiatric evaluation is to rule out medical causation of symptoms, an accurate and thorough neurological exam is critical. The neurological exam is a specialized examination conducted to assess sensory–motor and vestibular functioning of the 12 cranial nerves and the 31 major spinal nerves: 8 cervical, 12 thoracic, 5 lumbar, 5 sacral, and 1 coccygeal. The cranial nerves are referred to as the *facial* or the *cranial segment*. The cervical, thoracic, lumbar, sacral, and coccygeal nerves are referred to as the *spinal dermal segment* or *dermatomes*. The following 10 functions are to be assessed: orientation, eyes, face, hearing, swallowing, tongue, sensory perception, muscle strength and tone, reflexes, and balance and coordination.

Sensory Perception

The testing of sensory perception involves testing pain, pressure, position (proprioception), and the sensation of temperature.

- To assess pain, use the end of something fairly sharp, such as the end of a safety pin or the wooden end of a cotton swab. Do not break the skin. A soft touch will elicit a response. To elicit movement using peripheral pain, apply pressure to the nail bed.

- To assess pressure, use the soft end of a cotton-tipped swab, brush it against the skin, and ask the patient to identify where you touched him or her.

- To assess proprioception, have the patient touch thumb to each finger of the same hand or have the patient close his or her eyes as you grasp the index finger and move it side to side and up and down, asking the patient to identify its location. The great toe is another digit to complete this test on, as well.

- To assess temperature, hand the patient or touch the patient with something metal or mildly chilled, such as a test tube or tube of ice, or the metal of the reflex hammer.

Other sensory tests include stereognosis, graphesthesis, two-point discrimination, extinction, and point locations (Box 3-1). These can

---

Selected Sensory Tests — box 3-1

Stereognosis: Place a common object (such as a paperclip, pencil, or coin) in the patient's hand and ask the patient to identify it.

Graphesthesis: Draw a number or a letter in the patient's palm and ask the patient to identify it. The patient may be told if the object is a letter or a number. For both of these assessments, try each hand separately.

Two-point discrimination test: Simultaneously apply two pricks to the skin surface using the blunt end of a cotton swab. Start with the two separated at a distance and continue applying them in closer proximity until the patient indicates that he or she can feel only one. The fingertips are the most sensitive for recognizing two point differences, whereas the back, thighs, and upper arms are the least sensitive. In the case of extinction, simultaneously touch the same place on the opposite sides of the body. The patient should feel two separate stimuli.

Point location: Touch a point in the body and ask the patient to touch the same place. A lesion will impair a patient's ability for extinction and point location.

---

be done on the cranial nerves as well as the dermatomes for assessment of sensory relay.

Glasgow Coma Scale

As discussed in Chapter 1, a mini mental status exam (MMSE) may be used to assess mental functioning in patients in a variety of settings. The **Glasgow Coma Scale** is the universally accepted method for assessing a patient's level of consciousness and to measure or predict the progression of the patient's condition (Table 3-4). To elicit movement on comatose patients using central pain, apply deep pressure to the trapezius muscle (trapezius pinch), or to the supraorbital ridge (supraorbital pressure), or knuckle pressure to sternum without rub (sternal rub pressure).

Cranial Nerve Assessment

Assessing the cranial nerves assists in assessing hearing, speech, vision, movement, coordination, balance, mental status, mood, and behavior. Components of a cranial nerve neurological assessment include the interview and vital signs, assessment of level of consciousness, pupils, cranial nerves, motor and sensory function, muscle tone, and cerebral function. The interview between the nurse and the patient is critical in setting the tone to gather data, provide information, make referrals, develop rapport with the patient and the family, and initiate the development of a patient specific plan of care.

A rule of thumb in neurological assessment is to compare the left to the right sides and the head to the feet. First, identify whether the patient is right or left handed, as the patient's dominant side will be stronger. Establish the patient's level of arousal (eyes open or closed) and the patient's awareness of self, you, and the environment, focused and intact or otherwise. Once this is done, move to the assessment of level of consciousness. Is the patient fully conscious and awake, confused, lethargic, obtunded, stuporous, or comatose? Next, assess the patient's speech and language patterns, fluency, and word usage. Can the patient follow one- or two-step commands (such as "Fold the paper and place it on the table")?

Next, assess speech. Can the patient name common objects and their uses (for example, show the patient a cup or a pencil and ask him or her to name the object and say how it is used)? *Aphasia* is a disorder in processing language, *apraxia* demonstrates a problem in the programming of speech, and *dysarthria* is a problem in the mechanics of speech itself. Two areas of the brain in particular are involved. Problems in Broca's area will be reflected in the individual's difficulty in converting thoughts to speech, using few words. Problems in Wernicke's area will be reflected in a lack of fluency of speech, increased perseveration, or incorrect word substitution (spoken or written).

If a swift assessment is required to determine the severity of neurological compromise, a good screening technique is to ask the patient, "Do you know where you are and how you got here?" Then ask the patient to close and open the eyes, stick out the tongue, and touch the left ear with the right hand. Patients who are able to complete this brief assessment sucessfully are neurologically stable for the moment. For further clarification, ask the patient a question with a recognizable contradiction, such as, "Do you walk on water or swim on land?" or "Do you drive a bike or ride a car?" If the patient is able to discriminate or laugh at the absurdity, the patient is demonstrating higher cortical functioning.

Cranial nerves are the next to be assessed. It is important that this be done in an orderly fashion, but not necessarily in numerical

Glasgow Coma Scale (GCS)   table 3-4

The GCS is a universally accepted method to record a patient's level of consciousness and measure or predict the progression of the patient's condition. There are three parameters: Patients' *eye opening* response spontaneously, to sound, or to pain; patients' *verbal articulations*, what they say and how they say it; and *motor responses* to follow commands or in response to pain.

Each category is scored from the most robust response to the least active response. Select only the highest response score from each of the three categories. The lowest score for each category is 1 and the total possible score for all categories is 15. The possible score range is 3 to 15, with 3 being the lowest and 15 being the highest possible scores.

Eye opening (E)	Score	Total E
Spontaneous eye opening	4	Max possible = 4
To sound	3	
To pain	2	
No eye opening	1	

Verbal response (V)	Score	Total V
Oriented	5	Max possible = 5
Confused conversation	4	
Inappropriate words	3	
Incomprehensible sounds	2	
No verbal response	1	

Motor response to pain (M)	Score	Total M
Obeys commands	6	Max possible = 6
Localizes pain	5	
Normal flexion (withdrawals to pain)	4	
Abnormal flexion (decorticate)	3	
Abnormal extension (decerebrate)	2	
No response to pain	1	

Outcome	Total Score
13–15 = minor injury	(E + V + M = GCS)
9–12 = moderate injury	Max possible = 15
4–8 = severe injury	**GCS=_____**
3 = No response/coma (No eye opening, or no verbalization, or motor response to pain). The patient in a coma does not open eyes, respond to commands, or utter understandable words.	

Source: Teasdale, G., & Jennett, B. (1974). Assessment of coma and impaired consciousness: A practical scale. *Lancet, 2*(7872), 81–84.

order. The cranial nerves can be grouped by similar areas (Table 3-5). Bolek (2006) devised a mnemonic to help clinicians remember the twelve nerves: *On Old Olympus, Tiny Tots, a Finn, and German View Some Hops.*

Assessment of Motor Functioning

Next is the assessment of motor functioning. Conducting a cerebellar–motor exam involves checking the motor–neuronal tracks from the frontal lobe and cerebellum to the eighth cranial nerve and the dermatomes of the body for muscle tone, strength and equality, coordination, gait, balance, and control. If the patient cannot perform due to pain, this exam is not considered valid. The following are assessed in a motor exam: muscle size; symmetry; movement against gravity; strength against resistance; and proper coordination and control. Cerebellar–motor assessment includes examining the patient's coordination, gait, balance, and muscle control. Assessing motor functioning requires that the patient be able to understand the instructions, cooperate, and move on command.

1. Have the patient stand with eyes closed and put both arms straight out in front of him or her. Look for sway and balance of both arms in position. With the patient's eyes open, then with the eyes closed, hold your index finger up and have the patient touch your finger with his or her index finger and then touch the patient's nose. Move your index finger to another position and have the patient repeat the process (*finger to finger test*). With the patient's eyes closed, have the patient extend both arms and alternate touching the nose with a finger from each arm (*finger to nose*). The movements should be accomplished smoothly and accurately.

2. Have the patient stand and slide the heel of one foot, from knee to ankle, down the shin of the other foot. This should be accomplished smoothly, accurately, and without tremors. The *Romberg test* for balance is also a cerebellar–motor assessment tool, as is *tandem walking*, which is having the patient walk heel to toe in a straight line.

3. Next evaluate muscle size, symmetry, movement against gravity, strength against resistance, control, and reflex. Observe the body positioning during movement and at rest. Look for similarity in size, proportions, and equality of strength when comparing muscles on the right and left sides of the body. The

Overview of Cranial Nerve Assessment

table 3-5

Cranial Nerve(s)	Assessment	Nursing Implications
Smell **I – Olfactory nerve** **Controls sense of smell**	• Provide patient different scents to smell, such as coffee and soap. • Have the patient, with both eyes closed, close one nostril and gently inhale to smell the scent. • Remember to do both nostrils.	• Typically done with patients who present with facial trauma.

Vision
 	
II – Optic nerve
 	
Controls central and peripheral vision
 	
III – Oculomotor nerve
 	
Controls pupil constriction
 	
IV – Trochlear nerve
 	
Moves eyes downward to nose
	• Instruct patient to:
	  – Read from a card with one eye at a time.
	  – Look straight ahead and tell how many fingers you are holding up.
	• Dim the room lights and use a penlight; move it from the outside periphery to the center of each eye and observe the pupillary response.
	• Instruct patient to follow your finger while you move it down toward the patient's nose.
		• Report any indication of difficulty with visual acuity or ability.
		• Describe pupil size: Pupils should be equal, reactive, and respond with a blink with a threat.
		• Check whether there is ptosis of the eyelid by noting where it falls on the eye.
		• Note any difficulties and abnormalities.

Face and mouth **V – Trigeminal nerve** **Controls forehead, cheek, jaw**	• Instruct patient to open mouth and jaw, moving against your slightly resistive pressure. • Ask the patient to close eyes. Then touch face with cotton and ask patient to report where touch was felt.	• If you suspect problems with nerves VI and VII, check the corneal reflex with a cotton wisp while you are at this part of the exam.
Vision **VI – Abducens nerve** **Eye movements to the side**	• Have the patient look toward each ear. • Then take one finger and instruct patient to track it moving the eyes (not head) up, down, right, left, in six directions, and then to the nose.	• Observe the patient for any eye twitches or nystagmus (fast and uncontrollable eye movements).
Facial movements and expression; taste **VII – Facial nerve** **Corneal reflex, eyelid and lip closure** **Anterior 2/3 of tongue**	Instruct patient to: • Smile; pucker lips; show teeth; puff out cheeks. • Raise eyebrows, wrinkle forehead. • Keep eyelids and lips closed while you try to open them. Have a sugar packet and a salt packet available to test for taste.	• Observe for symmetry—both sides of the face should move the same. • When the patient smiles, observe for weakness or flattening. • If the patient complains of lack of taste, ask to identify sweet and salty.
Hearing and balance **VIII – Acoustic nerve**	To test hearing: • Use a tuning fork and count the number of seconds the patient can hear the tuning fork's sound as it diminishes. Hold it first to the patient's skull until the patient can no longer hear it, and then near the ear until the patient indicates he or she can no longer hear it. • Rub your fingers near the ear and ask what the patient can hear. • Whisper a word or phrase peripherally away from the ear and ask what the patient heard. To test balance: • Use the Romberg test—have the patient (eyes open) stand with arms at side and feet together. If this is successful (no sway), have the patient do it with eyes closed.	• Controls acoustic hearing and vestibular balance. • Observe for any abnormalities or difficulties.
Speech, taste, swallowing **IX – Glossopharyngeal nerve**	• Instruct patient to swallow. Watch for the "Adam's apple" of the throat to move. • Gently touch the back of the throat with a sterile tongue depressor to assess gag reflex. • Assess sense of taste on the back of the tongue.	• This nerve innervates the tongue (pharynx) and throat (larynx), which are checked together. • This assessment also checks for CN X. • Innervates the posterior third of the tongue.

(continued)

Overview of Cranial Nerve Assessment (*continued*)

table 3-5

Cranial Nerve(s)	Assessment	Nursing Implications
Speech **X – Vagus nerve**	• Ask the patient to open his or her mouth and say "aah"; observe the uvula. • Check that it lies centrally and does not deviate on movement. • Asking the patient to speak gives a good indication to the efficacy of the muscles.	• This nerve controls the muscles of speech. • This nerve is involved in most aspects of digestion. • Also controls heart rate and glandular function.
Neck and shoulder **XI – Spinal accessory nerve** **Head and shoulder movement** **XI – Spinal accessory nerve**	• Ask the patient to raise shoulders while you push down. • Ask the patient to turn head against your hand. • Instruct patient to turn the head from side to side and shrug the shoulders (one at a time) against your mild pressure resistance.	• Observe for any abnormalities or difficulties. • Responsible for head rotation and shoulder elevation.
Tongue **XII – Hypoglossal nerve**	• Have patient stick out tongue and touch inside of each cheek with tongue. • Assess articulation of speech. • Ask for problems with eating, swallowing, or speaking.	• Controls gagging, swallowing, taste, tongue movement, speech. • Check this nerve when you check IX and X.

Based on Bolek, B. (2006). Facing cranial nerve assessment. *American Nurse Today, 1*(2), 21–22.

following muscle movement behaviors would be considered abnormal: athetosis, chorea, dystonia, fasciculations, myoclonus, tics, tremors, spasticity, paratonic (gegenhalten) posturing, decerebrate or decorticate posturing, or seizure activity (Wherrett, 2008). If involuntary movements are noted, observe their location, quality, rate, rhythm, amplitude, and setting. Inspect muscle bulk for contours. Muscle tone is assessed for resistance to passive and active movement and stretch. Muscle tone assumes full active and passive range of motion (ROM) (Box 3-2). Observe for a pattern in any detectable muscle weaknesses, which may indicate lower motor neuron lesion affecting a peripheral nerve or nerve root.

4. Finally, an examination of reflexes, which are the innate stimulus–response mechanisms that allow for basic defenses, is completed by evaluating reflexes side to side, top to bottom, and above and below the foramen magnum (the "great hole" in the skull through which the spinal cord exits the cranium). Reflex assessment is of the deep tendon reflexes, superficial reflexes, and brainstem reflexes. The scale on which the reflexes are graded includes 0 = absent, no response; 1+ = diminished, below normal; 2+ = normal, average; 3+ = brisker than normal; 4+ = very brisk, hyperactive (clonus) (Figure 3-10).

Laboratory Tests

Laboratory tests can be ordered as part of a regular checkup to provide general, baseline information or to identify specific health concerns that have an impact on brain function. Screening of the blood, urine, kidneys, liver, and thyroid, as well as peak and trough levels of medications, may be ordered by the prescriber. For example, blood

Grading Muscle Movement and Strength

box 3-2

Muscle movement tone is graded using the following scale: 1 = normal, 2 = rigid, 3 = spastic, 4 = abnormal flexion, 5 = abnormal extension, 6 = flaccid or atonic. Muscle strength is graded against gravity and resistance to pressure. Muscle strength is graded using the following: 0 = no movement–paralysis, +1 = slight weak movement, +2 = able to move with gravity (ROM), but not lift, +3 = able to move (full ROM), but not against resistance, +4 = full ROM, but weak against resistance, +5 = full ROM, full strength against resistance.

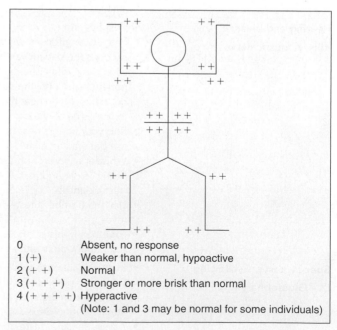

0	Absent, no response
1 (+)	Weaker than normal, hypoactive
2 (+ +)	Normal
3 (+ + +)	Stronger or more brisk than normal
4 (+ + + +)	Hyperactive
	(Note: 1 and 3 may be normal for some individuals)

3-10 A stick-figure scale for recording reflex activity.

PET Scan

box 3-3

A **positron emission tomography (PET) scan** is very similar to a SPECT scan and often done in conjunction with a CT scan. It is a radioactive, computer imaged, scan of any part of the body that produces a 3D image of the glucose uptake of the tissue area scanned. The procedure involves inhalation, ingestion, or IV injection of a short-lived radioactive tracer isotope and a 30- to 60-minute wait for the radioactive tracer molecule, fluorodeoxyglucose, a sugar, to be absorbed and concentrated into tissue. The patient is then placed awake on a table and inserted into the machine, which will record the gamma ray and positron emission decay (positive beta decay) that occurs as the antiparticle of the electron with the opposite charge is discharged (Fischbach & Dunning, 2012). As the radiographic compound that travels into the brain circulates, it displays various physiologic functions of the brain, such as glucose metabolism, blood flow, and neurotransmitter receptor activity through three-dimensional imagery. The procedure can take 2 to 3 hours, is painless, and is relatively risk free. Patients should be advised not to eat anything for 4 to 6 hours before the scan. They may drink

water. If they are claustrophobic, they may need a preprocedure sedative. Medications, including over-the-counter medications and neutraceuticals, as well as pregnancy and breastfeeding, should be assessed. Blood sugar or insulin levels can interfere with the glucose metabolism readings. Radiation is eliminated from the body in 2 to 10 hours (Dugdale, 2012). Disadvantages include radiation exposure (although it is in small, quickly wasted amounts, and too little to affect the normal process of the body), and the high cost of equipment and procedure.

Several radioligand tracers have been developed for PET for specific neuroreceptor types: dopamine (D2/D3), serotonin reuptake transporters (SERT 5HT1A, 5HT2A), opioid receptors (μ), and enzyme substrates. PET scans are used to differentiate dementias or observe amyloid plaques; show blood flow, diseased tissue, or tumors; measure cellular and/or tissue metabolism; and evaluate seizure disorders, memory disorders, and brain changes following injury or drug abuse (National Institute of Neurological Disorders and Stroke, 2011).

---

tests such as a complete blood count (CBC) may be ordered to monitor for infections, toxins, preexisting conditions, or responses to medications such as agranulocytosis, changes in white blood count, neutrophils, or anemias, thrombocytopenia, or neutropenia (Fischbach & Dunning, 2012; Genung, 2011; Weiner & Levitt, 1978). Therapeutic levels of medications may be ordered to monitor for medication effectiveness ranges and to prevent drug toxicity. Common medications requiring frequent blood level testing include lithium, valproic acid, and carbamazepine. Metabolic testing of the blood—such as basic metabolic panel (BMP), comprehensive metabolic panel (CMP), or individualized chemistry studies—may be ordered to identify preexisting conditions or monitor side effects to medications such as elevated cholesterol or blood glucose levels; alterations in electrolytes (sodium, potassium, calcium, chloride, magnesium, and phosphate); and metabolic end products such as ammonia, bilirubin, blood urea nitrogen (BUN), and creatinine. Additional tests may be ordered to assess for hormone levels, liver enzymes, and thyroid function (Fischbach & Dunning, 2012; Stern et al., 2008). Urinalysis can reveal pregnancy, diabetes, proteins, or drug abuse.

Neuroimaging Techniques

Neuroimaging is becoming increasingly vital to assessing and diagnosing the presence of neurological conditions. Patients will have many questions about recommended procedures and can be referred to several reputable Internet sources, such as the National Institute of Neurological Disorders and the National Institute of Health. Although neuroimaging alone is not used to define a psychiatric diagnosis, contemporary electrographs, radiographs, and neuroimaging techniques provide helpful information about structural contributions to mental health issues. There are three categories of technologies available to visualize or observe brain activity (Table 3-6) (Schatzberg & Nemeroff, 2009; Stern, et al., 2008; & Guess, 2008):

- *Structural imaging* identifies specific anatomical structures. Structural imaging includes computed tomography (CT),

computed axial tomography (CAT) scan, magnetic resonance imaging (MRI), and various radiographs, such as X-ray, cerebral angiogram, and myelogram.

- *Functional imaging* images parts of the body during activity. Functional imaging includes electroencephalography (EEG), magnetoencephalography (MEG), single photon emission computed tomography (SPECT), and positron emission tomography (PET) (Box 3-3).

- *Combined structural–functional imaging* images both the structure and functioning of various body parts during selected activities. Structural–functional imaging includes functional MRI (fMRI), magnetic resonance spectroscopy (MRS), and three-dimensional event-related (3D ER) fMRI.

Pathophysiology of Mental Illness

As discussed in Chapter 1, mental health is a delicate balance between genetics and environment, between the internal world and the external world. Understanding the pathophysiology of how areas of the brain function during mental illness and the neurobiological changes that occur provides another approach to helping patients resolve mental illness challenges and improve their overall quality of life. The following section describes major mental health conditions and their neurological causes.

Mood and Affect

Depressive disorders involve marked changes in affect, mood, cognition, and behavior. *Affect* refers to the emotion a person expresses at any given moment, and normally is fluid throughout the day, changing in response to different circumstances. *Mood*, on the other hand, is an individual's subjective feeling state. Mood is expected to remain stable, representing how the individual feels most of the time. A depressed mood is not the same as a passing irritability or grief, nor is it a sign of personal weakness, a transient mood that can be willed away. Changes in affect, irritability, hormones, and events, or the

Neuroimaging Techniques

table 3-6

CATEGORY	Procedure Technique	Exposure	Application	Nursing Action
Structural Radiographs				
	X-Ray X-ray picture film	Low radiation	• Bone injuries, erosions • Tumors	• Assess pregnancy, child risks
	Lumbar Puncture Needle in subarachnoid space	Local anesthetic	• Intracranial pressure, infection, inflammation, bleeding, cancer • Inject spinal anesthetics, chemotherapy	• Assess for pregnancy, history of headaches, current medications—especially OTC blood thinners such as aspirin—latex, and/or dye sensitivity • Encourage lying flat and provide hydration post-procedure
	Myelogram X-ray or CT	Contrast dye	• Spinal nerve injury • Herniated discs • Fractures • Pain • Tumors • Inflammation • Stenosis	• Assess medication and allergy history, especially iodine • Assess for seizures, pregnancy, anticoagulant therapy
	Ultrasonography Transducer wand	High-frequency sound waves	• *Adult* Locate brain mass during surgery • *Pediatric* Evaluate cranium while fontanels are open	Noninvasive
	Transcranial Doppler (TCD) Transducer probe	High-frequency sound waves	• View arteries of neck and head • Emboli • Stenosis • Vasospasm	Noninvasive
Structural Neuroimaging				
	CT or CAT scan X-ray 2D, 3D visualized computer image	With or without contrast dye Radiation	• Acute bleeding • Tumors • Abscesses • Organics • Lesions	• Assess allergy to dye, iodine, seafood • Assess pregnancy status
	MRI scan Magnetic field and radio waves	With or without gadolinium dye	3D views of all brain anatomical structures and tissues	• Assess allergy to dyes, iodine • Assess pregnancy status • No metal on patient when in machine • Machine is loud
Functional Electromagnetic				
	EEG Electrode patches or small wires to scalp	No dyes No radiation	• Intracranial electrical activity • Seizures • Tumors • Traumatic brain injury (TBI) • Inflammation • Headaches • Alcholism • Metabolic and degenerative diseases • Sleep disorders • Confirmation of brain death	• Avoid caffeine and medications that affect CNS prior to procedure

CATEGORY	Procedure Technique	Exposure	Application	Nursing Action
	EMG, ENG, ENoG Electrode patch	No dye No radiation	• Nerve and muscle dysfunctions • Spinal cord diseases • Paralysis • Neurological conditions • Coma • Brain death	Avoid ASA, NSAIDs, caffeine, nicotine, and medications that affect nervous system before procedure.
	MEG Similar to CT and MRI scans	No dye No radiation Large helmetlike head scanner	• Dementias • Schizophrenia • Alcoholism • Facial pain • Tumors • Seizures	• Noninvasive • Painless
Functional Neuroimaging				
	SPECT 2–3D visualized computer imaging of brain functioning	Gamma radioisotope gallium Radiation exposure	• TBI • Dementia • Clogged blood vessels • Seizures • Encephalitis • Thyroid • Bone issues	• Assess medications, allergies, especially dye • No metals • Contraindicated with pregnancy, breastfeeding
	PET 3D visualized computer imaging of brain functioning	Gamma radioisotope tracer fluoro-deoxyglucose Radiation exposure	• Dementias • Blood flow • Diseased tissue tumors • Metabolism • Seizures • Memory disorders • TBI	Same as SPECT
Structural-Functional Neuroimaging				
	fMRI Same as MRI with more functional measures	Same as MRI	• Greater functioning imaging • TBI • Neurodegenerative diseases • Neurological conditions • Cerebrovascular accident (CVA) • Tumors	Same as MRI
	NMR/MRS Magnetic resonance	Same as MRI	• Determining concentration of brain metabolites • Tumor • Metabolite levels	Same as MRI

Note. Computed axial tomography (CT or CAT) scan; magnetic resonance imaging (MRI); electroencephalography (EEG); electromyography (EMG); electronystagmography (ENG); electroneuronography or electroneurography (ENoG); magnetoencephalography (MEG) scan; single photon emission computed tomography (SPECT); positron emission tomography (PET) scan; functional magnetic resonance imaging (fMRI); nuclear magnetic resonance spectroscopy (NMR or MRS).

presence of an illness, all can account for brief (less than two weeks) changes in mood. Changes in mood beyond a short period, especially if combined with anhedonia, may indicate a depressive disorder and require further evaluation (Chapter 16).

Mood, cognition, and resulting behaviors influence each other. Thoughts, mood, and affect are a function of neurotransmitter activity; behavior is the external expression of that activity. Any situation that carries potential to have an impact on neurotransmitter activity—certain medications, acute or chronic illnesses, adverse life events, and drug and alcohol abuse—may impact mood and affect. Some individuals may experience a change in mood and affect without any precipitous event due to genetic predisposition or a deficiency or dysregulation in some aspect of neurotransmission.

There is no unified hypothesis regarding pathophysiology and etiology of depression, in part because patients demonstrate individualized responses to treatments. The course of illness varies considerably among individuals and among different types of depressive disorders. Molecular neurobiology and functional brain imaging have provided support for a biogenic amine hypothesis of depression, suggesting a dysregulation or reduction in the neurotransmitters 5HT, NE, and DA (Hasler, 2010; Nemeroff, 2008). Increased attention is being given to the preeminent role of the CNS dopamine activity circuits. This arises from well-documented, suboptimal therapeutic responses to selective serotonin reuptake inhibitors and serotonin–norepinephrine reuptake inhibitors.

Another line of thought is that there is a change in the post synaptic receptor sensitivity and decreased receptor binding (Hasler, 2010). Evidence suggests reduced activity of serotonergic neurons, reduction in the number of serotonin transporter (SERT) binding sites (midbrain and amygdala), and reduced $5HT_{1A}$ receptor density in both presynaptic (in the midbrain) and postsynaptic (in the meso-temporal cortex) serotonin neurons contribute to the development of depression (Stahl, 2013; Hasler, 2010; Nemeroff, 2008). As previously discussed, each neurotransmitter has a responsibility. When there are sufficient neurotransmitters (e.g., DA, NE, SE, ACh) in the synaptic cleft for the postsynaptic neural receptor to acquire the neurotransmitters, then regulation of certain mood and behaviors may be achieved (Figure 3-11). When there are insufficient neurotransmitters, mental health issues such as depression are expressed. When there is an excess of a neurotransmitter, other mental health issues, such as bipolar disorder and psychosis, may result (Table 3-7).

Major depressive disorder is associated with impairments of cerebral structural plasticity and neuronal cellular resilience. Additionally, a reduction in CNS volume and reduction in numbers and sizes of glia and neurons in the prefrontal cortical, striatal, and limbic systems has been noted (Stahl, 2013; Hasler, 2010). PET scans have revealed abnormalities in cerebral blood flow and glucose metabolism in these regions (Hasler, 2010; Manji, Drevets, & Charney, 2001). Associated changes in neuroendocrine functions in individuals with depression also include reduced binding sites and hypersecretion of the stress hormone corticotrophin releasing factor (CRF), which functions as a neurotransmitter in extrahypothalamic areas and also modulates secretion of ACTH (Hasler, 2010). CRF production is increased in the hypothalamic areas, locus coeruleus, and amygdala. Furthermore, genetic differences make some individuals more vulnerable than others to the effects of early life stress (such as child abuse and neglect) (Nemeroff, 2008).

Anxiety

Anxiety is a generally normal, healthy response to stress that may manifest as worry or feelings of apprehension or dread. Perception of stress, anxiety, or fear is individualized and is determined by the individuals' perception of the event or stressor (real or imagined) and their expectations, coping skills, and available resources (Genung, Cruz, & Epperson, 2013). The bioamine theory suggests that excessive levels of serotonin and norepinephrine in the hypothalamus, thalamus, basal

DOPAMINE (DA)

DA Regulation
Pleasure-Reward
Motivation-Drive
Pain Avoidance
Moderation
Creativity-Imagination
Clear Thinking
Clear Sensory Perceptions
Inner/Outer Reality Awareness

DA Dysregulation
Anhedonia
Avolition
Impaired Judgment
Addiction
Excess Imagination
Delusions
Hallucinations
Psychosis

DA-5HT Regulation
Balanced Memory
Clear Thinking
Mood Stability
Good Problem Solving
Achievement Satisfaction
Moderation of
     "Appetites"

DA-5HT Dysregulation
Forgetful
Confusion
Aggression
Uncertainty-
     -Poor Insight
Satisfaction Distortions
Obsession-Compulsion-
     -Addiction

DA-5HT-NE Regulation SCHEME
Sensory Stability
Cognitive Stability
Habits & Appetites Stability
Energy Stability
Mood Stability
Evaluation of Inner-Outer Worlds Balanced

DA-NE Regulation
Energetic
Motivated
Novelty Seeking

DA-NE Dysregulation
Impulsive
Risk Taking
Reward Dissatisfaction

5HT-NE Regulation
Normal Sexual Responses
Social Activity
Calm
Alert
Awake

5HT-NE Dysregulation
Impotence-Sexual Dysfunction
Social Disinterest
Anxiety-Fatigue
Inattentive
Insomnia-Somnolence-Hypersomnia

5HT Regulation
Relaxed
Food Satiation
Impulse Control
Rational Self-talk
Executive Functions

5HT Dysregulation
Irritable
Eating Disorders
Compulsory Acts
Negative Self-Appraisal
Ruminations-Obsession

NE Regulation
Alert
Vigilant
Interested
Energized
Socialization
Concentration

NE Dysregulation
Distracted
Ritualized
Disinterested
Fatigued
Withdrawn
Inattentive

SEROTONIN (5HT)   **NOREPINEPHRINE (NE)**

3-11 Neurotransmitter regulation and dysregulation effects.

Neurotransmitter Functions and Symptoms

table 3-7

NT	Function	Deficit	Excess	Associated Disorders
NE	EXCITE Fright–flight–fight Awake, alert, energized Vigilance, interest Concentration, attention Memory, learning	Avolition Thought confusion Distraction Disinterest Inattentiveness, forgetfulness Fatigue, depression Loss of sex drive	Anxiety Panic Hyperactivity Tremors Agitation Aggression Mania	ADHA OCD Mood disorder Anxiety disorder

DA	MODULATE
	Promotes well-being
	Pain–pleasure reinforcement
	Motivation–drive
	Reward-seeking behavior
	Creativity, imagination
	Clear thinking; memory
	Evaluation of reality
		Anhedonia
		Emptiness
		Joylessness
		Pain
		Confused thought
			Euphoria
			Exhilaration
			Super-confidence
			Excitement
			Rumination
			Obsession
			Expansiveness
				Addictions
				Psychosis
				  Hallucinations
				  Delusions
				OCD
				Schizophrenias
				Parkinson disorder
				EPS

5HT	MODULATE Mood, affect Sleep, appetite, sex Interest, learning Executive function Impulse control	Impulsiveness, jitters Hyperactivity Suspicion, anxiety Insomnia Depression, irritability Compulsiveness Ritualistic behavior	Pain sensitivity Hyperactivity Agitation Aggressiveness Expansiveness	Sleep disorder Eating disorder Anxiety disorder Depression Autism Hallucinations OCD Pain
GABA	INHIBIT Balances activating NTs Calming, quieting, relaxing Pain reduction	Anxiety Stress Agitation, aggression Potential for seizure Pain sensitivity	Disinhibition Loss of sensation Sedation CNS depression	Addictions
Ach	MODULATE Calm Rest–digest–restore Actives calm in PSNS Antiexcitatory in SNS	Dulled thinking Inattentiveness Memory problems Slowed movement	Robust memory Excitability Movement tics, tremors	Delirium Dementia Movement disorder Myasthenia Gravis Parkinson disorder EPS Nicotine dependence

ganglia, and overall limbic system, and diminished levels of serotonin in the prefrontal cortex, may be involved (Ishibashi, 2010). Disruption of the GABA system, the primary inhibitory neurotransmitter system, is also implicated. A high density of GABA benzodiazepine receptors are found in the hippocampus, amygdala, and orbital frontal cortex and decreased levels of GABA appear in the cortex and limbic systems of individuals with anxiety (Shelton, 2004).

Recent advances in neuroimaging have made it possible to visualize the structural and functional changes in the brain. The limbic system seems to be overactivated in stress responses that become chronic anxiety. The hypothalamus and thalamus link the CNS to the endocrine system. During stress, the thalamus and hypothalamus secrete a corticotropin-releasing hormone, which, in turn, stimulates the pituitary to stimulate the adrenal cortex. Collectively, these structures are referred to as the *HPA axis*. The amygdala communicates with several brain stations to modulate emotion. The insula is the link to conscious motor control and physical expression of anxiety.

The hippocampus encodes and consolidates memory—the way in which the individual recognizes or remembers the source of the anxiety. The anterior cingulate cortex regulates the autonomic functions such as heart rate and respiration, which are increased in times of stress. The prefrontal cortex interprets the incoming sensory and emotional experience, provides a definition and interpretation of afferent sensory stimulation, and sends efferent messages instructing how to act in response to the stress (Genung, Cruz, & Epperson, 2013). It is posited that anxiety arises from the amygdala, which has received an afferent sensory message of alarm. The amygdala registers the incoming signal and the hippocampus then stores it in emotional memory. The efferent pathways from the central nucleus of the amygdala send messages to the parabrachial nucleus, resulting in dyspnea and hyperventilation. The dorsomedial nucleus of the vagus nerve activates the PSNS, and the lateral hypothalamus results in the activation of the SNS. At the same time, the amygdala is also messaging the medial prefrontal cortex to interpret and respond to the stimulus, which, in turn, responds with a lack of inhibition of the unwanted thoughts and impulses, provoking rituals in an attempt to remove the anxiety (Stahl, 2013; Stern et al., 2008).

Psychosis

Psychotic symptoms create an enormous disturbance in an individual's life and that of his or her family members and community cohorts. This is in part because of the individual's inability to distinguish between internal and external stimuli. Most people are able to hear sounds or voices in their heads—such as a song that pops into their head or a phrase often used by a family member—and sort this type of internal experience from the external, recognizing the source of the experience. However, when an individual begins to misinterpret internally produced sensory experiences (voices, visions, taste, touch, or smell) inaccurately as information from the external real world, then the individual is experiencing psychosis. After a hallucination (the mislabeling of the source of sensory information) occurs, a delusion (a self-drafted, fixed false belief) often forms that allows the individual to explain the context of the hallucination. This occurs, in part, because of the brain's natural function of collecting, processing, and interpreting information from the external world to return a behavior that reflects this consideration in appropriate reality.

Symptoms of psychosis are classified within four categories (Chapter 17) (Stahl, 2013; Schatzberg & Nemeroff, 2009; Stern et al., 2008; Sadock & Sadock, 2007):

- *Positive symptoms:* hallucinations, delusions, paranoia, thought disorganization
- *Negative symptoms:* affective flattening, impoverished speech, ambivalence, anhedonia
- *Mood symptoms:* dysphoria, anxiety, agitation, suicidality
- *Neurocognitive symptoms:* distractibility, learning deficits, memory deficits, impaired abstract thinking

Factors that can influence the expression of psychosis include birth trauma, older age, metabolic diseases that deteriorate the brain, viral or bacterial infections that cross the BBB, dementia, depression, sleep disturbance, cognitive impairment, personality disorders, alcohol and drug abuse, traumatic events, traumatic brain injury, and genetics (Stern et al., 2008; Sadock & Sadock, 2007; Zahodne & Fernandez, 2008). The structures involved in psychosis have been reported to involve enlarged cerebral ventricles, smaller hippocampus, smaller superior right medial temporal and lateral temporal lobes, small medial diencephalon, smaller inferior frontal gyrus, smaller cingulate cortex bilaterally, and denser cell packing in the dorsal lateral prefrontal cortex (Stern et al., 2008). The neurotransmitters most often reported to be involved in the expression of psychosis are in the dopamine pathways, prominently the mesolimbic and the mesocortical dopamine pathways, via the neurotransmitters DA, 5HT, and glutamate. The evidence to support this comes predominantly from observing a reduction of psychotic symptoms with the use of medications that target these neurotransmitters and pathways, or the observation of an exacerbation of symptoms when exposed to medications or illicit drugs that supercharge the expression of these neurotransmitters.

Dementia

Dementia is a term used to describe an array of symptoms associated with the degeneration of the neurological systems of the brain. There are several types of dementia, many stemming from neurocognitive disorders such as Alzheimer disease, Lewy body disease, and Parkinson disease. Each form of dementia has a different cause and course of cognitive decline. Some causes include degeneration of nerve cells (Alzheimer, Parkinson, Huntington diseases); stroke or arterial infarcts (vascular dementia); toxic reactions (drug and alcohol abuse); nutritional deficiencies (vitamin B_{12} and folate); and infections that invade the CNS (AIDS, Creutzfeldt–Jakob disease). Other types of infections, tumors, and traumatic brain injury may also result in dementia (National Institutes of Health, 2011; Stern et al., 2008, Sadock & Sadock, 2007). Damage to neurotransmitters interferes with the ability of different regions of the brain to perform their functions and communicate with one another. Different types of dementia are associated with particular types of brain cell damage in specific regions. The region that experiences the damage accounts for the symptoms expressed by the individual. For example, the hippocampus, in the telencephalon of the forebrain, is the center for learning and memory. Memory loss is often a first sign of dementia. Forgetfulness and confusion are often early signs of dementia, but they may be caused by other variables. Thorough assessment of the individual who presents with confusion is necessary to determine and treat the underlying source of the confusion (Table 3-8).

Although each type of dementia has a different onset, most brain changes that cause dementia involve permanent decline in mental functions such as thinking, memory, reasoning, personality, mood, and behavior severe enough to interfere with a person's daily functioning, and worsening over time. Neurobiologically, it is posited that an imbalance in the production and/or clearance of beta amyloid (Aβ), a small amyloid precursor amino acid peptide protein, results in accumulation of Aβ as plaques or oligomers. This triggers a cascade of events wherein Aβ collects extracellularly and intraneuronal neurofibrillary tangles develop, initiating inflammation, tau protein hyperposphorylation, neuronal dysfunction, neurotransmitter deficits, neuronal death, loss of gray matter, dementia, and, eventually, death (Christensen, 2007; Stahl, 2013). "The amyloid plaques consist of an insoluble, aggregated core of Aβ surrounded by dystrophic axons, dendrites, activated microglia, and reactive astrocytes. Neurofibrillary tangles are made up of hyperphosphorylated tau protein that destroys cellular architecture and aggregates into paired helical filaments in the cytoplasm of the limbic and cortical neurons" (Christensen, 2007, p. 114). The outcome is cortical shrinkage, enlargement of the cerebral ventricles, and shrinkage of the hippocampus, until neuronal damage becomes so severe that life cannot be supported. Treatment is available to slow down the progression of dementia after early recognition, but no treatment is available to stop the progression of the disease (Chapter 21).

Impulsive and Aggressive Behavior

Expression of impulsive and aggressive behaviors can be found in the normal range of human responses. The context and frequency of expression of these behaviors is what is considered significant. Defensive aggression is viewed as normal in protection of oneself or a significant other. Impulsive aggression and premeditated (predatory) aggression, on the other hand, are considered pathological and a cause for concern (Coccaro & Siever, 2002). Individual motivations, stressors/triggers, meditators, and expressions of impulsive and aggressive behaviors vary significantly (Chapter 25). Understanding the mechanisms responsible for creating a predisposition to aggression and violence is pivotal to the discussion on how to assist the individual to cease or change the behavior. The relationship between

Causes of Confusion — table 3-8

Domain	Cause
Epileptic	Postictal state
	Complex partial status epilepticus
	Absence status epilepticus
Infectious and inflammatory	Meningitis
	Encephalitis
	Vasculitis
	Abscess
Metabolic	Hypoxia
	Hypoglycemia
	Uremia
	Hepatic disease
	Thiamine deficiency
	Electrolyte imbalance
	Endocrine imbalance
Neoplastic	Deep midline tumor
	Increased intracranial pressure
Postsurgical	Preoperative atropine
	Hypoxia
	Analgesics
	Electrolyte imbalance
	Fever
Toxicity	Prescription drugs
	Nonprescription drugs
	Drug withdrawal or overdose
	Polypharmacy
Traumatic	Concussion
	Traumatic brain injury
Vascular	Stroke
	Subarachnoid hemorrhage

Based on Weiner, H. L. & Levitt, L. P. (1978). *Neurology for the House Officer.* Baltimore, MD: Williams & Wilkins; Genung, V. (2011a, April 8). *Medicine in Psychiatry: Diagnosis and Treatment of Hematologic,Hepatic, Renal, and Electrolyte Abnormalities.* Poster presentation delivered at the 25th Annual Psychiatric Nursing Symposium, Arlington, TX.

aggression and anxiety or fear is regulated by the amygdala, anterior cingulate cortex, and regions of the prefrontal cortex that control neural circuits that trigger defensive, aggressive, or avoidant behavior (Pavlov, Chistiakov, & Chekhonin, 2012). Excessive amygdala reactivity, along with inadequate prefrontal regulation, serves to increase the likelihood of aggressive behavior. Prefrontal neuronal development is not complete until young adulthood; therefore, a young person does not have the advantage of prefrontal input to deescalate amygdala fear and anxiety.

Neurogenomics is the pathway from genes to behavioral expression. It is suggested that there is a link for genetic control of aggressive behavior. Protein synthesis related to the 5HT neurotransmitter system belongs to a group of genes that modulate aggressive behavior in three distinct ways: (1) the effect of the knockout of MAO-A, the principle enzyme in 5HT degradation; (2) genes encoding pivotal enzymes in 5HT metabolism (TPH and MAO-A), 5HT transporter, $5HT_{1A}$, and $5HT_{1B}$ receptors; and (3) imbalances in testosterone/5HT (increased testosterone and reduced 5HT) and imbalances in testosterone/cortisol (increased testosterone and reduced cortisol levels) (Pavlov, Chistiakov, & Chekhonin, 2012; Popova, 2006; Stahl, 2013).

Serotonin facilitates prefrontal inhibition. An inverse correlation has been observed between amounts of 5HT in cerebrospinal fluid (CSF) and history of aggression. A life history of impulsivity, aggression, and defiance of authority is associated with diminished levels of 5HT (Coccaro & Siever, 2002; Lesch & Merschdorf, 2000; Sadock & Sadock, 2007; Stern et al., 2008). Similarly, inverse correlations have been observed between decreased noradrenergic and dopaminergic activity with increased impulsive and aggressive violent aggression (Coccaro & Siever, 2002). Increased androgens (testosterone, progesterone) are positively correlated with aggressive behaviors in that more aggression is seen in individuals with excessive androgens (Coccaro & Siever, 2002).

Limbic dysmodulation theory proposes that some individuals experience a lower threshold for limbic reaction or interference with the frontal lobe, resulting in intermittent explosive disorder (IED), which manifests as extreme emotions combined with impulsivity (Coccaro, 2012). It has been suggested that IED could be a brain electrical disorder. Although IED does not produce any epileptiform seizure-type features on an EEG, it can be measured by event-related potential EEG.

In addition to the neurochemical changes that may result in impulsive and aggressive behavior, human development may also play a role. *Domestication* is the transformation of the wild into the relatable and attached. The main feature of domestication is to have contact without fear or threat, to associate with others with trust. Children raised in families that provide sufficient security, love, and trust may be more resilient to developing impulsive and aggressive behaviors. However, factors such as early childhood abuse and trauma, exposure to impulsive and aggressive behaviors (via a parent who exhibits these behaviors, for example), and exposure to mature media content may affect neurotransmitter expression, increasing the risk for developing impulsive and aggressive behaviors.

Addictive Behavior

All addictive behaviors follow the same neurological pathways of engagement and reward, which are discussed in detail in Chapter 20. A basic principle of nature is to seek pleasure and avoid pain. Either can become pathological when practiced to excess or to the exclusion of the other. In the brain there are two motivating neurological systems that signal pleasure and pain, or reward and punishment and lead to the ultimate behavioral expression of either approach or avoidance, and a third neurobehavioral system that leads to passivity. The neocortex and the limbic system are the two cerebral structures that are involved in addictive behaviors. The primary neurotransmitters that regulate pleasure (and which are involved in drugs of abuse by mimicking these neurotransmitters) include DA, primarily, and 5HT, NE, GABA, and phenylethylamine (Stahl, 2013; Genung, 2011; Genung, White, & Moceo, 2011; Stern et al., 2008).

There are several areas of the brain whose activation can have gratifying effects, but it is the stimulation of the dopamine pathways that produces the most intense pleasure. The nerve fibers for this reward circuit are a substructure of the medial forebrain bundle, whose axons originate in the reticular formation, cross the ventral tegmental area, pass through the lateral and ventromedial nuclei of the hypothalamus, and continue on into the nucleus accumbens, amygdala, septum, and prefrontal cortex (Stahl, 2013). When the cortex receives a stimulus indicating pleasure, it sends a signal announcing this to the ventral tegmental area in the midbrain. The receipt of this pleasure signal acts to engage reward signaling by increasing the dopamine transmission in the ventral tegmental area, releasing dopamine to the nucleus accumbens, the amygdala, the prefrontal cortex, and parts of the thalamus. The hypothalamus then acts on the ventral tegmental area and signals the pituitary endocrine gland to activate autonomic and endocrine functions. Near the ventral tegmental area is another dopamine pathway, the nigrostriatal dopamine pathway in the substantia nigra of the basal ganglia. Here the dopamine axons project into the corpus striatum and influence movement. This dopaminergic mesocortico–mesolimbic system allows the body to focus attention (prefrontal cortex) and physically make efforts to acquire (substantia nigra) whatever caused the signaled pleasure (ventral tegmental area to nucleus accumbens) (Genung, 2012; Moceo, White, & Genung, 2011; Stahl, 2013; Stern, et al., 2008). Repetition of the gratifying action strengthens the associated pathway. In psychological behavioral terms, this is the pathway of positive reinforcement. Other parts of the reward circuit use other neurotransmitters (5HT, GABA) to reinforce behaviors.

The brain is all about balance. Where there is a pleasure–reward–"repeat this" center, there is an aversive–punishment–"avoid this" center as well. When an aversive stimulus provokes the fight or flight response, the brain's punishment circuit is activated to enable the individual to cope with something unpleasant. In 1962, DeMolina and Hunsperger hypothesized that the periventricular punishment pathway innervates the hypothalamus, thalamus, and the central gray substance surrounding the aqueduct of Sylvius, with additional centers in the amygdala and hippocampus (Institute of Neurosciences, Mental Health Addiction, n.d.). It involves the cholinergic and adrenergic nervous systems. Acetylcholine stimulates the secretion of adrenocorticotropic hormone (ACTH), which, in turn, stimulates adrenal glands to release adrenaline for action. Stimulation of the periventricular punishment circuit can inhibit the reward circuit, supporting the notion that fear and punishment can override pleasure. The medial forebrain bundle and periventricular motivation systems encourage individuals to suppress impulses and avoid painful experiences. Positively reinforced behaviors are engaged in and repeated because they elicit a subjective or objective experience of pleasure. The behavioral inhibition system was first identified by Laborit in the early 1970s (Institute of Neurosciences, Mental Health Addiction, n.d.) and is associated with the septo-hippocampal system, the amygdala, and the basal nuclei. The system receives input from the prefrontal cortex and transmits its outputs via the noradrenergic fibers of the locus coeruleus and the serotonergic fibers of the medial raphe nuclei. It is activated when both fight and flight seem impossible and the only remaining option is to submit passively. The pathological consequence to this behavioral inhibition is demonstrated when there is no longer an effort by the patient to stop a harmful behavior or no attempts to remove a particular harmful stimulus. Hence, the meaning the patient may attribute to behaviors and situations, not the actual stimulus, may pose the real problem.

A working understanding of the pathophysiology of certain mental processes and disorders informs nurses' understanding of patient symptomatology, provides information necessary for initiating assessment protocols, and indicates what therapies and treatments may be beneficial. Careful assessment allows nurses

and other clinicians to provide appropriate, individualized care regardless of the setting, recognizing that patients in all settings may present with anxiety, depression, and other symptoms of mental illness. As discussed in chapters 4 and 23, both psychotherapy and pharmacotherapy may work to change both brain structure and function, alleviating distressing symptoms and promoting patient coping.

Neurobiological Basis of Suffering and Hope

Experiences of pain and pleasure direct most human behaviors. The human disposition is typically to move away from or avoid things that lead to pain and move toward or seek things that bring pleasure. Both pain and pleasure are perceptual experiences that arise from a combination of neurochemical reactions that occur as the brain tries to interpret internal and external environmental stimuli. The terms *suffering* and *pain* often are used interchangeably. However, *pain* can more specifically be applied to the physical and sensory experience, whereas *suffering* better describes bearing the mental, emotional, psychological, or spiritual burden of pain. Both physical pain and mental suffering hurt.

Pathophysiology of Pain and Suffering

The experience of perceived physical sensory pain is based on nociceptor sensory input, neurochemical structural response, mood, attention and expectation, genetics, and prior experiences. Pain detection occurs in two paths: ascending afferent neuropathways from the bottom up (body to brain), and descending efferent neuropathways, from the top down (modulation by cognitive processes to determine source and severity). Once a pain signal is received from the specialized afferent free peripheral nerve endings (nociceptors), the brain begins to interpret the signal. "Where does it hurt?" is discriminated by the lateral thalamus and the somatosensory cortex. "How much does it hurt?" is processed by the medial thalamus, anterior cingulate cortex (ACC), insula, prefrontal cortex (PFC), and the amygdala (Higgins & George, 2013).

The affective motivational element of suffering is determined by the medial thalamus, amygdala, ACC, and PFC areas typically associated with mood, attention, and fear (Higgins & George, 2013). Automatic emotional regulation occurs through the limbic system's amygdala, thalamus, ventral striatum, and hippocampus. Cortices of the prefrontal cortex (dorsal lateral PFC, ventral lateral PFC, medial PFC, and dorsal ACC) provide both voluntary and automatic emotional reactions in general, and, in particular, reactions to fear and stress.

Pain or suffering input from the prefrontal cortexes, ACC, insular cortex, hypothalamus, and amygdala, when descending, will converge on the periaqueductal gray (PAG). The PAG is composed of gray matter surrounding the third ventricle and cerebral aqueduct in the midbrain. At this juncture, analgesia occurs. Rather than sending the message directly on to the dorsal horn as occurs in other efferent signaling, the PAG defers and projects out to intermediaries such as the rostral ventral medulla (RVM).

Relief, Reinforcement, and Reward

A pathway of particular interest in the discussion of pain is that of the opioid-mediated pain modulation circuit. **Opioid peptide receptors** (OPs) are heavily concentrated in the PAG, RVM, and dorsal horn;

these receptors have a significant pain modulating and relief effect. The OP can also be found in the skin, muscles, and joints, and throughout the body. The discovery of the body's natural endogenous opioid peptides (β-endorphin, met- and leu-enkephalins, and dynorphins) was monumental. These are neuromodulators that modify the action of neurotransmitters and are naturally designed by the body to relieve pain, affect perception of pain, enhance feelings of well-being, produce pleasurable feelings, lift mood, promote tissue regeneration, and enhance immune system, allowing the individual to continue functioning without being overcome by circumstances (International Union of Basic and Clinical Pharmacology, 2013).

Along with the body's natural endogenous OPs, serotonergic, noradrenergic, and dopaminergic neurons respond down to the upcoming peripheral afferent nerve, causing a reduction in the afferent signal coming up to the brain (Higgins & George, 2013). The result is a dampening down or descending inhibition of hurt signaling being sent to the brain. The serotonin, noradrenergic, and dopaminergic pathways play a role in communication of pain and suffering and of mood. Patients who report mood dysregulation often also report symptoms of aches and pains (Chapter 16).

As serotonin is a major player in mood and norepinephrine in energy, the neurotransmitter dopamine is largely responsible for the brain's experience of pain and pleasure. It exercises this role through its activity in the PAG, ACC, thalamus, basal ganglia, and spinal cord. The greatest density of dopamine neurons in the brain are found in the ventral tegmental area. These project to the mesocortical dopamine pathway, which targets the prefrontal cortex and insular cerebral cortex, modulating emotions, executive thought processes, and high-level decision making. Here the individual decides if a stimulus is pain or pleasure or if the reward outweighs the punishment of an activity (for instance, playing in the big game despite a minor injury, or continuing to use alcohol or drugs). The dopamine neurons project to the mesolimbic pathway, which targets the nucleus accumbens and limbic structures, modulating emotions, motivation, desire and pleasure. What feels best? What do I want? What will reward me the most? These questions related to motivation are processed and answered here. The dopamine neurotransmitters also project to the nigrostriatal pathway to target muscle movements. Here the individual gets the charge to move in the direction of the decision made. When the individual's experience is perceived as enjoyable, more dopamine is released from the ventral tegmental area to the nucleus accumbens and prefrontal cortex. This then triggers an arousal, joy, and a motivation to repeat the experience. This is the reward pathway.

Defining Expectations of Pain and Suffering

Pain and suffering are highly influenced by psychosocial expectations. Reports in medical literature, sensational media coverage, campaign ads by famous persons, dramatization of reality shows and televised coverage of news and court proceedings, invitations offered by litigation attorneys' commercials, and pharmaceutical advertisements all serve to define entitlements and incite extremes of dissatisfaction, bringing on a great suffering in our current society. Expectation of disability; family history of coping methods; personal history of coping methods; attribution of symptoms; societal and personal definitions of pain, process, recovery, rights, and expectations; perspective; attitude; and expectation of gains are all important determinants of how suffering and hope are defined, and therein, the

definition of overcoming untoward circumstances. These defining expectations of what may be gained offer insight into the significant psychological motivators for patients reporting symptoms of pain and suffering.

These gains fall within three categories. **Primary gain**, which falls within the individual's internal motivations, feeds the ego, bringing attention, sympathy, or reinforcement that results in immediate benefit to the individual. **Secondary gain** occurs when an individual experiences indirect benefit from having a disorder or condition; indirect benefits may include financial compensation, disability benefits, personal services and attention, and/or escape from work or a difficult responsibility. **Tertiary gain** refers to gains achieved by someone other than the patient as a result of the patient's illness. For example, a caregiver may benefit from the additional income that results when a patient with schizophrenia qualifies for disability.

Hope and Renewal

Defining what constitutes suffering and whether that suffering is inevitable or optional goes a long way in helping individuals direct their recovery. Helping patients define what the experience means to them, what they want to happen, and what resources they have to accomplish what they consider success is paramount in how patients define their own suffering. Sometimes suffering occurs as a process toward a goal. A distressful experience is an effort to accomplish an outcome, a means toward an end. For example, a patient may continue to abuse a substance to achieve brief euphoria despite the unpleasant effects that follow, or a patient may engage in hand washing to the point of skin damage in order to alleviate anxiety. Some patients will regard the process with great expectation of good outcome. Some will not expect a good outcome, but regard the process as worthy to experience. Those who have negative perspectives on the process and the outcome experience greater suffering. The road to hope is in the belief that success can be achieved, things can get better, and that challenges serve a purpose. Some believe that this involves spiritual practices or a rite of passage; some view this as psychological mental exercises; others may view their suffering as being for the greater good (such as the mother who neglects her own well-being in the care of her family) or may not attribute any meaning to their suffering at all. Regardless of how individuals view their suffering, the mental processes involved are accomplished as neurotransmitter functions in the brain structure interactions with the neurotransmitter–receptor, neuromodulator–receptor functions discussed in this section. Thoughts are neurochemicals. Feelings are neurochemicals. Changing thinking changes feelings and can offer hope. Changing expectations can create optimism. Exercise releases neurotransmitters to help healing. All of these are accomplished by dopamine, serotonin, norepinephrine, GABA, glycine, glutamate, and the body's own opioid peptides, endorphins, enkephalins, and dynorphins.

Research into psychology and psychotherapy has increased our understanding of how to heal the mind. Nurses who are able to develop an understanding of the neurochemical processes involved in thought processes, feelings, and behaviors will be better able to assess their patients and plan and implement care that promotes healing and hope. By assisting patients to understand their emotions, triggers, and behaviors, nurses can assist them to reduce distressing symptoms and begin to restore function and enjoy life.

Chapter Highlights

1. All human thoughts, feelings, and actions are initiated by activity in the brain.

2. The structures that make up and support the central and peripheral nervous systems affect neurological and mental health.

3. The central nervous system is responsible for integrating, processing, and coordinating sensory data and motor commands.

4. The peripheral nervous system brings in sensory information to the body, where the sympathetic nervous system mobilizes body systems during activity or stress.

5. The parasympathetic nervous system regulates automatic functions and is responsible for "resetting" the autonomic nervous system after activation.

6. The limbic system is essential to the regulation and modulation of emotions and memory.

7. Neurons produce neurotransmitters and receptors. Receptors receive and respond to a variety of substances (such as hormones, antigens, and medications).

8. Neurotransmitters are chemicals that relay messages to receptors of postsynaptic neurons.

9. Tools for assessing and diagnosing impairment of the nervous system include the neurological examination, laboratory tests, and neuroimaging techniques such as X-rays and PET scans.

10. Impairment in neurotransmission may result in psychiatric symptoms.

11. Pain describes the physical and sensory experience of hurt, whereas suffering describes the mental, emotional, psychological, or spiritual burden of pain. Pain and suffering are highly influenced by psychosocial expectations.

NCLEX®-RN Questions

1. The nurse is caring for a patient who has had a head injury. The patient has been having difficulty with attention, organization, and problem solving. Based on an understanding of the neuroanatomy of the brain, the nurse suspects that the patient most likely experienced trauma to which brain lobe?
   a. Frontal
   b. Occipital
   c. Parietal
   d. Temporal

2. The nurse is preparing to administer a selective serotonin reuptake inhibiter to a patient experiencing depression. The nurse reads that the mechanism of action is believed to result in increase of extracellular serotonin. Based on an understanding of neurotransmitters in neurological and mental health, which conclusions by the nurse are correct? Select all that apply.
   a. The reuptake of serotonin may have a negative impact on extracellular neurotransmitter function.
   b. Neurotransmitters such as serotonin are not necessary for proper intracellular function.
   c. Serotonin is the only neurotransmitter implicated in the development of mood disorders.
   d. Depression is the result of an imbalance in neurotransmitters unrelated to external events or experiences.
   e. Insufficient serotonin in the synaptic cleft may play a significant role in the neurobiology of depression.

3. The nurse has provided education to a patient scheduled for a positron emission tomography (PET) scan of the brain. Which statement by the patient indicates that teaching was effective?
   a. "I may require anesthesia to reduce pain associated with the test."
   b. "I should avoid food and only have clear liquids prior to the exam."
   c. "This test is limited to detecting structural abnormalities in my brain."
   d. "I will need to allow several hours for the procedure to be completed."

4. The nurse is admitting a patient to the acute care setting following surgery. The nurse notes that the patient also has a diagnosis of a major mental health disorder. Which best describes the implications of the co-morbid disorder with respect to the provision of appropriate nursing care?
   a. The patient's needs are likely to exceed that which can be addressed in this setting.
   b. The nurse will need to obtain assistance from an experienced mental health nurse.
   c. Patient interventions will be limited to addressing the primary reason for admission.
   d. The nurse will need to provide care that is informed by an understanding of both conditions.

5. The nurse is helping the patient with depression to understand the neurochemical processes contributing to the disorder. Which evaluation finding supports the effectiveness of this intervention?
   a. The patient recognizes that she does not have control over the biological processes contributing to the disorder.
   b. The patient understands the limitations of treatment interventions that are aimed at addressing psychosocial factors.
   c. The patient verbalizes an accurate understanding of the variables underlying her emotions, triggers, and behaviors.
   d. The patient acknowledges that pharmacological interventions will be necessary to correct neurochemical dysfunction.

Answers may be found on the Pearson student resource site: nursing.pearsonhighered.com

References

Bolek, B. (2006). Facing cranial nerve assessment. *American Nurse Today, 1*(2), 21–22.

Christensen, D. D. (2007). Alzheimer's disease: Progress in the development of anti-amyloid disease modifying therapies. *CNS Spectrums, 12*(2),113–123.

Coccaro, E. F., & Siever, L. J. (2002). Pathophysiology and treatment of aggression. In Davis, K. L., Charney, D., Coyle, J. T., & Nemeroff, C. (Eds). *Neuropsychopharmacology: The Fifth Generation of Progress (1709–1723)*. Philadelphia, PA: Lippincott, Williams, & Wilkins for American College of Neuropsychopharmcology.

Coccaro, E. F. (2012). Intermittent explosive disorder as a disorder of impulsive aggression for DSM-5. *American Journal of Psychiatry, 169*, 577–588.

Dipak, K. S., Sengupta, A. A., Zhang, C. C., Boyadjieva, N. N., & Murugan, S. S. (2012). Opiate antagonist prevents μ- and δ- opiate receptor dimerization to facilitate ability of agonist to control ethanol-altered natural killer cell functions and mammary tumor growth. *Journal of Biological Chemistry, 287*(20),16734–16746.

Dugdale, D. C. (2012). PET scan. *Medline Plus U.S. National Library of Medicine. National Institute of Health.* Available at http://www.nlm.nih.gov/medlineplus/ency/article/003827.htm

Dugdale, D. C., & Jasmin, L. (2010). Electromyography. *Medline Plus U. S. National Library of Medicine. National Institute of Health.* Available at http://www.nlm.nih.gov/medlineplus/ency/article/003929.htm

Ekstrom, A. (2010). How and when the fMRI BOLD signal relates to underlying neural activity: The danger in dissociation. *Brain Research Reviews, 62*, 233–244.

Fischbach, F. T., & Dunning, M. B. III (2012). *A Manual of Laboratory & Diagnostic Tests* (8th ed.) Philadelphia, PA: Lippincott Williams & Wilkins.

Georgopoulos, A. P., Karageorgiou, E., Leuthold, A. C., Lewis, S. M., Lynch, J. K., Alonso, A. A., et al. (2007). Synchronous neural interactions assessed by magnetoencephalography: A functional biomarker for brain disorders. *Journal of Neural Engineering, 4*(4), 349–355.

Genung, V. (2011a, April 8). *Medicine in Psychiatry: Diagnosis and Treatment of Hematologic, Hepatic, Renal, and Electrolyte Abnormalities.* Poster presentation delivered at the 25th Annual Psychiatric Nursing Symposium, Arlington, TX.

Genung, V. (2011b, April 8). *Neurobiology of Addiction: Biologic Treatments for Drug and Alcohol Dependence.* Poster presentation delivered at the 25th Annual Psychiatric Nursing Symposium, Arlington, TX.

Genung, V. (2012). Understanding the neurobiology, assessment, and treatment of substances of abuse and dependence: A guide for the critical care nurse. *Critical Care Nursing Clinics of North America, 24*(1), 117–130.

Genung, V., Cruz, E., & Epperson, B. (2013). Neuroimaging advances in the neurocircuitry of post-traumatic stress disorder (PTSD). In A. Costa & E. Villalba (Eds.), *Horizons in Neuroscience Research* (Vol. 12). New York, NY: Nova Publications.

Genung, V., Ellington, E., Cruz, E., Kropp, D., & Munholland, J. (2011, October 20–21). *Behavioral Health Consultation by the Psychiatric APRN in the Emergency Department: Management of Acute, Chronic, and Recurrent Pain Patients.* Poster presented at the 25th Annual American Psychiatric Nurses Association Conference, Anaheim, CA.

Genung, V., & Gerardi, M. (2013, April 17). *Recognizing Target and Side Effects of Psychotropics on Brain Circuit Pathways.* Workshop presentation (Session 10) delivered at the ISPN 2013 6th Psychopharmacology Institute and International Society for Psychiatric Nurses 15th Annual Conference, San Antonio, TX.

Genung, V., White, G., & Moceo, V. (2011, October 22). *Psychiatric APRN Role in Alcohol and Substance Abuse Evaluation in the Emergency Department: DAWN-ing of a New Day.* Podium presentation #4012, delivered at the 25th Annual American Psychiatric Nurses Association Conference, Anaheim, CA.

Grosheva, M., Wittekindt, C., & Guntinas-Lichius, O. (2008). Prognostic value of electroneurography and electromyography in facial palsy. *Laryngoscope, 118*, 394–397.

Guess, K. (2008). *Psychiatric–Mental Health Nurse Practitioner Review and Resource Manual* (2nd Ed.). Silver Spring, MD: American Nurses Credentialing Center.

Haas, H. L., Sergeeva, O. A., & Selbach, O. (2008). Histamine in the nervous system. *Physiological Reviews, 88*(3), 1183–1241. Available at www.physrev.physiology.org/content/88/3/1183full#ref-235

Hasler, G. (2010). Pathophysiology of depression: Do we have any solid evidence of interest to clinicians? *World Psychiatry, 9*(3), 155–161.

Herlihy, B. (2010). *The Human Body in Health and Illness* (4th ed.). St. Louis, MO: W. B. Saunders Co.

Higgins, E. S., & George, M. S. (2013). *The Neuroscience of Clinical Psychiatry.* Philadelphia, PA: Lippincott Williams & Wilkins.

Husney, A., & Schaff, H. (2011). Myelogram. *WebMD.* Available at http://www.webmd.com/back-pain/myelogram-16147

Institute of Neurosciences, Mental Health Addiction (INMHA). (n.d.). *The Brain From Top to Bottom! An Interactive Web Site on the Human Brain and Behavior.* Canadian Institutes of Health Research (ICIHR), www.cihr-irsc.gc.ca. Available at www.thebrain.mcgill.ca

Ishibashi, K. (2010). 210-C5-Pathophysiology anxiety disorders. Available at www.my-pharm.ac.jp/~kishiba/2010-C5%20anxiety.pdf

International Union of Basic and Clinical Pharmacology (IUPHAR). (2013). Opioid receptors: introduction. Available at http://www.iuphardb.org/DATABASE/FamilyIntroductionForward?familyId-50

Lesch, K. P., & Merschdorf, U. (2000). Impulsivity, aggression, and serotonin: a molecular psychobiological perspective. *Behavioral Sciences and the Law, 18*, 581–604.

Lord, J. A. H., Waterfield, A. A., Hughes, J., & Kosterlitz, H. W. (1977). Endogenous opioid peptides: Multiple agonists and receptors. *Nature, 267*, 495–499.

Manji, H. K., Drevets, W. C., & Charney, D. S. (2001). The cellular neurobiology of depression. *Nature Medicine, 7*(5), 541–547.

Mayo Clinic Staff (2012). Lumbar puncture (spinal tap). Available at http://www.mayoclinic..com/health/lumbar-puncture/MY00982

Moceo, V., White, G., & Genung, V. (2011, September 15). *DAWN-ing Trends: Alcohol and Substance Abuse Evaluation.* Poster presented at the 34th Annual Fall Conference of the Texas Society of Allied Health Professionals, Dallas, TX.

Montez, T., Poil, S. S., Jones, B. F., Manshanden, I., Verbunt, J. P. A., van Dijk, B. W., et al. (2009). Altered temporal correlations in parietal alpha and prefrontal theta oscillations in early-stage Alzheimer disease. *Proceedings of the National Academy of Sciences of the United States of America, 106*(5), 1614–1619.

National Institutes of Health (NIH). (2011). Dementia. U.S. National Library of Medicine, National Institutes of Health (NIH). Available at http://www.nlm.nih.gov/medlineplus/ency/article/000739.htm

National Institute of Neurological Disorders and Stroke (NINDS). (2013). Neurological diagnostic tests and procedures. National Institute of Neurological Disorders and Stroke (NINDS)–National Insitutes of Health (NIH). NIH Publication No. 05-5380. Available at http://www.ninds.nih.gov/disorders/misc/diagnostic_tests.html

Nemeroff, C. B. (2008). Recent findings in the pathophysiology of depression. *Focus, 8*, 3–14.

Pavlov, K. A., Chistiakov, D. A., & Chekhonin, V. P. (2012). Genetic determinants of aggression and impulsivity in humans. *Journal of Applied Genetics, 53*(1), 61–82.

Poinier, A. C. & Chalk, C. (2010). Electroencephalogram (EEG). *WebMD.* Available at http://www.webmd.com/epilepsy/electroencephalogram-eeg-21408

Popova, N. K. (2006). From genes to aggressive behavior: The role of serotonergic system. *BioEssays 28*, 495–503.

Qureshi, J. (2012). Skull X-ray. National Institutes of Health. Available at http://www.nlm.nih.gov/medlineplus/ency/article/003802.html

Radiological Society of North America (RSNA). (2012). Cranial ultrasound/head ultrasound. *RadiologyInfo.Org.* Available at http://www.radiologyinfo.org/en/info.cfm?pg=ultrasound-cranial

Richter, P. (2008). Pathophysiology and clinical biochemistry (PAT331H/PMH330Y) faculty of pharmacy. University of Toronto, Anxiety Disorders Clinic, CAMH. Available at www.pharmacy.pixelfactor.ca/files/2008/phm330panic2008.ppt.

Romito, K. & Schaff, H. (2010a) Angiogram of the head and neck. *WebMD.* Available at http://www.webmd.com/stroke/angiogram-of-the-head-and-neck/

Romito, K. & Schaff. H. (2010b). Cranial ultrasound. *WebMD.* Available at http://www.webmd.com/brain/cranial-ultrasound/

Rosmarin, D. H., Bigda-Peyton, J. S., Kertz, S. J., Smith, N., Auch, S. L., & Bjorgvinsson, T. (2013). A test of faith in God and treatment: The relationship of belief in God to psychiatric treatment outcomes. *Journal of Affective Disorders, 146,* 441–446.

Sadock, B. J., & Sadock, V. A. (2007) *Kaplan & Sadock's Synopsis of Psychiatry* (10th ed.). New York, NY: WoltersKluwer Lippincott Williams & Wilkins.

Schatzberg, A. F., & Nemeroff, C. B. (2009). *Psychopharmacology* (4th ed.). Washington, DC: American Psychiatric Publishing, Inc.

Shelton, C. I. (2004). Diagnosis and Management of Anxiety Disorders. *Journal of the American Osteopathic Association,* Supplement #3, *104*(3), 52–55.

Staudacher, T., Shi, F., Pezzagna, S., Meijer, J., Du, J., Meriles, C. A., et al. (2013). Nuclear magnetic resonance spectroscopy on a (5-nanometer)^3 sample volume. *Science, 339* (6119), 561–563.

Stahl, S. (2011). *The Prescriber's Guide* (4th ed.). New York, NY: Cambridge University Press.

Stahl, S. (2013). *Stahl's Essential Psychopharmacology. Neuroscientific Basis and Practical Applications* (4th ed.). New York, NY: Cambridge University Press.

Stern, T. A., Rosenbaum, J. F., Fava, M., Biederman, J., & Rauch, S. L. (2008). *Comprehensive Clinical Psychiatry.* Philadelphia, PA: Mosby Elsevier.

Suthana, N., & Fried, I. (2012). Percepts to recollections: Insights from single neuron recordings in the human brain. *Trends in Cognitive Sciences, 16*(8), 427–436.

Tarapore, P. E., Tate, M. C., Findlay, A. M., Honma, S. M., Mizuiri, D., Berger, M. S., & Nagarajan, S. S. (2012). Preoperative multimodal motor mapping: A comparison of magnetoencephalography imaging, navigated transcranial magnetic stimulation, and direct cortical stimulation. *Journal of Neurosurgery, 117*(2), 354–362.

Teasdale, G., & Jennett, B. (1974). Assessment of coma and impaired consciousness: A practical scale. *Lancet, 2*(7872), 81–84.

Thompson, E. G., & O'Donnell, J. (2010). Lumbar puncture. *WebMD.* Available at http://www.webmd.com/brain/lumbar-puncture/

Weiner, H. L., & Levitt, L. P. (1978). *Neurology for the House Officer.* Baltimore, MD: Williams & Wilkins.

Wherrett, J. R. (2008). The role of the neurologic examination in the diagnosis and categorization of dementia. *Geriatrics and Aging, 11*(4), 203–208. Available at www.medscape.com/viewarticle/579827

Zahodne, L. B., & Fernandez, H. H. (2008). Pathophysiology and treatment of psychosis in Parkinson's disease: A review. *Drugs and Aging, 25*(8), 665–682.

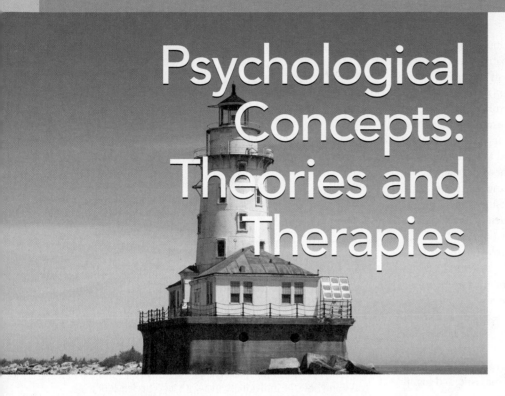

Psychological Concepts: Theories and Therapies

4

Mertie L. Potter
Sylvia Durette
Barbara Jones Warren

Learning Outcomes

1. Apply developmental theories that inform nurses' understanding of patient development.

2. Discuss humanistic theories that contribute to nurses' understanding of patients' abilities to direct and manage their lives.

3. Illustrate cognitive and behavioral theories that help nurses understand patients' thought processes and behavior patterns.

4. Compare components from psychoanalytic, behavioral, humanistic, and cognitive theories.

5. Summarize contributions of relevant nursing theories to the nurse–patient relationship.

6. Describe psychological and biomedical therapies used in the care of patients with psychiatric illness.

Key Terms

accommodation, 72
adaptation, 72
anal stage, 68
assimilation, 72
behavior modification, 73
behavioral theory, 73
classical response, 73
cognitive theory, 72
cognitive–behavioral therapy, 80
countertransference, 69
ego, 68
equilibrium, 72
fixation, 68
genital period, 68
humanistic theory, 70
id, 68
latency period, 68
Maslow's hierarchy of needs, 70
nursing theory, 75
oral stage, 68
phallic stage, 68
psychiatric nursing theory, 68
psychoanalytic theory, 68
psychosocial theory, 69
self-efficacy, 73
schemas, 72
social cognitive theory, 72
superego, 68
theory, 68
transference, 69

Introduction

This chapter highlights selected theories that formulate the evidence-based approaches that nurses use in the care of patients in a variety of settings, as well as specific therapies helpful in the treatment of patients with mental illness. A **theory** is a group of interconnected concepts, definitions, and/or models that help explain why a series of incidents occur (Kail & Cavanaugh, 2012; Tusaie & Fitzpatrick, 2013). Nursing theories present an organized, analytic approach to the solving of problems that are uniquely related to the discipline of nursing. In particular, **psychiatric nursing theory** systematically identifies, assesses, and solves issues within those areas that are uniquely related to psychiatric mental health nursing (American Psychiatric Nurses Association, International Society of Psychiatric Mental Health Nurses, American Nurses Association, 2014).

It is important that nurses understand the role that theory plays within their practice settings, as theory guides development and implementation of evidence-based education and practice regarding the care of patients with mental illness (Institute of Medicine, 2010). Theories also help nurses understand human behavior and symptomatology in the context of mental health, wellness, and illness (Kail & Cavanaugh, 2012; Tusaie & Fitzpatrick, 2013). Nursing theories, including psychiatric–mental health nursing theory, evolved from psychoanalytical, developmental, behavioral, humanistic, and cognitive theoretical perspectives (Kail & Cavanaugh, 2012; Tusaie & Fitzpatrick, 2013). This chapter includes a discussion of these theories and presents ideas for consideration that address theoretical perspectives within psychiatric–mental health nursing.

Theories of Human Development

As previously mentioned, it is important that psychiatric–mental health nurses understand the role of theory regarding human development. Theories help define the interrelated concepts involved within human developmental stages. Assessment of an individual's developmental stage provides context regarding that person's state of mental health, wellness, and illness. Some broad categories of developmental theories include psychoanalytic, psychosocial, humanistic, cognitive, and moral. This section discusses various theories with select examples and integrates significant and historical developmental theories as appropriate. Interestingly, some theorists emphasize negative aspects and weaknesses in relation to abnormal personality development, whereas others focus on positive aspects and strengths in relation to normal personality development.

Psychoanalytic Theory

Psychoanalytic theory proposes that personality develops in a progressive manner grounded in psychosexual stages (Freud, 1953; Kail & Cavanaugh, 2012). Sigmund Freud, considered the founder of psychoanalysis, used a combination of hypnosis, dream analysis, and free association to identify concepts that created pathological outcomes related to human development (Freud, 1953; Kail & Cavanaugh, 2012). Freud did not focus on mental health and wellness. However, his theory was pivotal in systematically identifying components associated with the development of mental distress and illness. Nurses in a variety of settings often incorporate selected components of Freud's developmental theory in assessment of patients based on the patients' developmental stage and presence of symptoms.

Freud's Components of Personality — table 4-1			
Example	**Id**	**Ego**	**Superego**
Needing money	"I will take whatever money I need from whomever I can."	"I will have the money that I have earned."	"I will never take money from someone else. That is wrong."
Taking a ride with strangers	"I will take a ride with this stranger because I want to."	"Taking rides from strangers is not wise or safe."	"Mom and Dad said never to take a ride with strangers."

Freud hypothesized that all human behavior emerges out of a person's unconscious motivation and struggle between societal prohibitions and primitive sexual (libido) and aggressive drives. Freud theorized that the unconsciousness functions in three states of being: (a) the **id**, which seeks self-gratification; (b) the **superego**, which functions as a moral compass; and (c) the **ego**, which serves as the referee between the id and the superego (Table 4-1) (Freud, 1953). Central to this struggle is anxiety and how the individual copes with it (Wheeler, 2008).

From responses to similar situations, it becomes clear that when the id dominates in making decisions, impulsive and perhaps reckless behavior may result. When the ego is able to supersede the id's wishes, more tempered approaches are available for the individual to use, and the individual can delay gratification. When the superego controls decision making, the individual is able to make decisions using a value system. Freud asserted that individuals have the capacity to function on all three levels. He postulated that all human personality is developed between the ages of birth and 7 years and that behavior occurring later in life is based on the initial 7 years and how the individual resolved (or failed to resolve) the three primary psychosexual stages (oral, anal, and phallic). Freud asserted that positive and progressive development of an individual's personality depends on the quality of care that is provided by the caretaker, primarily the mother (Freud, 1953).

According to Freud (1953), each stage encompasses development of sensitivity within erogenous areas within the body. The **oral stage,** birth to 18 months, emphasizes sensitivity and pleasurable achievement of sucking and biting within the mouth, lips, and tongue zones. The **anal stage** encompasses ages 18 months to 3 years and involves the anus, rectum, and bladder zones. Sensitivity areas for this stage include initially expelling and then retaining feces. The **phallic stage,** ages 3 to 7 years, involves the sensitivity area of the genitals and pleasure associated with masturbation. Freud (1953) developed two additional areas of development later in his career, although he considered these of lesser importance. The **latency period** occurs during middle childhood. During this period, sexuality is suppressed and play is associated with either female or male perspectives. Puberty causes sexuality needs to re-emerge in the **genital period,** which is characterized by emotional turmoil, infatuation, and the need to development satisfying sexual associations (Freud, 1953; Kail & Cavanaugh, 2012).

Freud's (1953) theory claimed that a child may develop **fixation** in any stage, meaning that the child may not be able to work through unconscious motivations involved within that stage. He further indicated that specific behaviors were noted when an individual was

Freud's Stages of Psychosexual Development

table 4-2

Stages	Age	Task	Behavior Indicating Resolution	Behavior Indicating Fixation
Oral stage	0–18 months	Oral satiation	Hunger, thirst met	Smoking, overeating and drinking, nail biting
Anal stage	18 months–3 years	Environment exploration and bladder/bowel control	Able to be with others, toilet trained	Hostility and defiance, difficulty relating to authority, preoccupation with rules, rigidity
Phallic	3–6 years	Identify with same-sex parent, develop sexual identity	Able to identify gender, maintain mutual, favorable relationship with same-sex parent	Sexual problems, inability to manage relationships
Latency	6–12 years	Focus on same-sex peers	Able to have good relationships with peers	Struggles with relationships
Genital	13–20 years	Focus on opposite-sex relationships	Able to have relationships with peers of both sexes	Adolescents direct sexual urges onto opposite-sex peers; primary focus of pleasure is the genitals

Based on Freud, S. (1953). Three essays on the theory of sexuality. In J. Strachey, A. Freud, A. Strachey, & A. Tyson (Eds.). *The Standard Edition of the Complete Psychological Works of Sigmund Freud.* London, UK: Hogarth Press, pp. 135–248; Kail, R. V., & Cavanaugh, J. C. (2012). *Human Development: A Life-Span View* (6th ed.). Belmont, CA: Wadsworth Cengage Learning.

locked or fixated at a certain level. An individual who develops fixation in a stage becomes stuck in the pleasurable sensations within that stage (Table 4-2).

Freud identified two important concepts that may occur and create negative outcomes within the therapist–patient interaction. **Transference** occurs when the patient attributes feelings regarding another person in his or her life to the therapist (Kail & Cavanaugh, 2012). The patient might say, "You remind me of my sister," and begin to react to the therapist as if the therapist were the patient's sister. **Countertransference** occurs when the therapist attributes feelings regarding someone within the therapist's life to the patient. The therapist may be thinking, "This patient is so like my father," and the therapist begins to react to the patient as if the patient were the therapist's father instead of responding to the patient as an individual. Nurses working with patients with mental illness must be able to assess whether transference and countertransference are present within their interactions with patients. Failure to recognize, interpret, and interrupt the feelings and reactions associated with these concepts will negate the therapeutic alliance within the nurse–patient relationship, which leads to negative patient outcomes (Wheeler, 2008).

Finally, Freud proposed that mental distress is produced when a person's unconscious thinking process creates conflicts and fixations. Thus, treatment must be directed to resolving conflicts and fixations within a person's unconscious (Freud, 1953; Kail & Cavanaugh, 2012).

Freud noted that these conflicts cause an individual to use certain mental defense mechanisms to cope with the resulting anxiety; his daughter, Anna Freud, expanded on the idea of defense mechanisms (Chapter 13).

Critics of Freud's theory indicate that his theory is not applicable for general populations, as it was grounded out of his work with adults and focused, for the most part, on unhealthy behaviors. Using the benefit of hindsight, they say, Freud designated developmental stages and outcomes for infant, child, and adolescent behaviors and actions. Moreover, Freud's theory focuses on men's developmental processes and ignores those related to women (Kail & Cavanaugh, 2012). Although some critics argue that Freud's theory blames women for the development of others' psychological problems, some psychiatric–mental health experts think that Freud's concepts of the id, ego, and superego have great applicability to an individual's state of mental health, wellness, and illness (Wheeler, 2013).

Object Relations Theory

Much of borderline personality disorder is based on an understanding of object relations theory, which asserts that positive and negative dyad experiences occur during development. An internalized experience of self becomes linked to an internalized experience of another, usually the infant's caregiver. These attachment styles and experiences become set in the inner self and determine future relationship patterns and triggered responses (Mahler, 1975). It is thought that those with borderline personality disorder internalize negative dyadic experiences in which needs do not get met by the caregiving "other," often a parent, so the individual becomes frustrated and views both the needy self and the depriving other negatively (Yeomans & Levy, 2002).

Psychosocial Theory

Erik Erikson (Erikson, 1969) altered and extended the stages of development that were postulated by Freud. His **psychosocial theory** focuses on the achievement and mastery of life challenges that occur within certain time periods, as opposed to Freud's focus on pathology in developmental stages. The expected outcome for mastery of the stages is a healthy personality. Failure to master each stage results in a person's altered personality development and an inability to deal with reality. For example, if a baby fails to develop trust, he or she cannot develop autonomy and/or move on to the other developmental stages. The same issue may evolve at any juncture of developmental stage if the favored outcome does not occur. Erikson's stages begin at infancy with trust versus mistrust and continue until the end of physical life, with despair versus hope and faith (Table 4-3).

Jane

Jane is in a session with her therapist. She begins to get angry at what her female therapist says because it reminds her about interactions Jane had with her mother as she grew up. Jane always saw her father as being supportive of her, whereas she saw her mother as being unsupportive and hyper-critical of anything Jane wanted to do. The therapist is unaware of why Jane is reacting to her as she is. Consequently, the therapist ignores Jane's anger and moves on to talk about another issue within Jane's therapy. Jane becomes increasingly unresponsive and uncommunicative during the session and refuses to make another appointment with the therapist.

APPLICATION

1. What could the therapist do to address the feelings of anger that Jane is expressing?

2. Describe the response that may be taking place between Jane and the therapist.

3. Can you think of any one that ever reminded you of someone else—either positively or negatively? Did that affect how you responded to the person?

Erikson maintains that an individual's personality develops based on interactions between social norms and biological drives with others (Fonagy & Target, 2009); it is up to the individual, not the primary caretaker, to solve the crises that are present in each developmental stage. Crises present an opportunity for persons to grow and become stronger. Unlike Freud, Erikson contended that a human being's personality continued to develop and evolve over the life span instead of being formed only during the first 6 to 7 years of life. Erikson's theory is applicable for psychiatric nursing in that he stresses the mastery of life and the continuation of that mastery throughout an individual's entire life. This is a holistic and positive approach to life that stresses the role of the individual in moving forward. This is a recovery-based concept that also stresses resilience factor within individuals.

Humanistic Theory

Humanistic theory is a holistic perspective that concentrates on the ability of humans to control their everyday events and determine what they want to accomplish in the future. Maslow and Rogers are the developers of humanistic theory (Table 4-4).

Abraham Maslow

Abraham Maslow focused on a **hierarchy of needs**, in which individuals prioritize needs in five areas: physiological needs,

Erikson's Developmental Stages   table 4-3

Stage	Years of Stage	Desired Outcome for Stage
Trust vs. mistrust	Birth–1 year of age	Trust in self, parents, and world
Autonomy vs. shame and doubt	2–3 years of age	Self-control without losing self-esteem
Initiative vs. guilt	4–5 years of age	Direction and purpose in activities
Industry vs. inferiority	6 years–puberty	Mastery and competence
Identity vs. identity confusion	Adolescence	Sense of self and ego identity
Intimacy vs. isolation	Early adulthood	Intimacy with another and work toward career development
Generativity vs. stagnation	Middle adulthood	Concern for next generation
Integrity vs. despair	Late adulthood	Satisfaction from examining the past
Despair vs. hope and faith	Late 80s and beyond	Self-care and sense of wisdom

Adapted from Davis, S. G., Palladino, J. J., & Christopherson, K. M. (2013). Psychology (7th ed.). Boston, MA: Pearson Education, Inc.

Humanistic Theorists   table 4-4

Theorist	Components	Outcomes Associated with Theory
Abraham Maslow (1921–1970)	• Focus on health • Holistic, interactive approach • Needs and self-actualization	• Person-centered motivation to grow and develop in a healthy way.
Carl Rogers (1902–1987)	• Patient to client focus • Human potential for goodness • Use of empathy and positive regard	• Therapist is not to provide advice. • Therapist clarifies client feelings.

Maslow's Hierarchy of Needs

table 4-5

Category of Needs	Description
Physiological	Air, food, water, sleep, shelter *Example:* Individuals in a state of altered physiological homeostasis (e.g., dehydration, starvation) are unable to attend to higher-order needs.
Safety and security	Includes emotional and physical security in home, neighboring, and work environments; also includes available resources (including financial) *Example:* An individual who is homeless or unemployed likely will be unable to meet higher-order needs (and may also not be able to meet some or all physiological needs).
Love and belonging	Capacity to maintain loving, meaningful connections with others—friendships, family, working relationships *Example:* An individual feels close to a number of individuals within his family unit but has low self-esteem and belittles himself frequently.
Self-esteem	Ability to reflect and review accomplishments, respect others and earn the respect of others; positive self-regard associated with increased confidence and ability to adapt to stressors. *Example:* Individuals who accept themselves and manage life amidst various stressors.
Self-actualization	Individuals who achieve this level exhibit creativity, capacity for harmony with and ability to focus on others, and comfort being alone or with others. Not all individuals achieve this level of functioning. *Example:* People who achieve what they are able to become. Mother Teresa was comfortable with being known for her joy in meeting others' needs.

Based on Maslow, A. (1970). *Motivation and Personality* (rev. ed.). New York, NY: Harper & Brothers.

requirements for safety and security, needs for love and belonging, self-esteem, and self-actualization (Figure 4-1). According to Maslow, individuals must meet their basic physiological needs for food, water, and shelter before they can progress to higher-order needs (Table 4-5). Once individuals are healthy, safe and secure, strengthened by loving relationships and a sense of belonging, they are able to achieve a healthy self-esteem and then begin to reach their fullest potential, known as *self-actualization* (Maslow, 1970). Achievement of self-actualization helps individuals become more self-directed, happy, and focused on achievements within life.

In developing humanistic psychology, Maslow focused on the more positive qualities of people. This represented a major shift in the field of psychology. In particular, Maslow became intrigued with the personal behaviors of some of his peers—notably, anthropologist Ruth Benedict and Gestalt psychologist Max Wertheimer. It was through studying the work of Benedict and Wertheimer that Maslow developed his hierarchy of needs. Maslow did much to emphasize mental health and the individual potential of all humans.

With theories such as these, it is important to keep in mind the sample on which the theory was formed. Maslow's work was done with Americans. Different cultures demonstrate other needs as more pressing. For example, Korean culture values interdependence, whereas Western culture values independence. Talk therapy is valued by Western culture but not by Japanese culture. In general, basic-level needs, such as physiological and safety needs, take precedence over higher-level needs, such as love and belonging, self-esteem, and self-actualization. Determining at what level an individual may be can assist the nurse in determining how best to help the individual.

Carl Rogers

Carl Rogers preferred the use of the term "client" in his client-centered theory. Rogers stressed the good within individuals and the importance of fostering health versus focusing on illness. According to Rogers, the use of empathy and unconditional positive regard (a deep and genuine respect of the client by the therapist) facilitates an individual's psychotherapeutic development and growth (Rogers, 1980). The clinician uses these concepts in all verbal and nonverbal interactions with the patient or client. In addition, the clinician focuses on clarifying the client's feelings and avoids giving advice. Critics of Rogers's theory indicate that this nondirective approach never facilitates changes that clients may need to make to alleviate stress and manage symptomatology within their lives.

Moral Theory

Lawrence Kohlberg is best known for his theory of moral development (Kohlberg, Levine, & Hewer, 1983). He theorized that morality—the knowledge of right and wrong behavior—develops or is stymied depending on various elements that are either internal or external to the individual. Kohlberg investigated how individuals are able to grow out of their egocentricity and perform tasks meant to help the

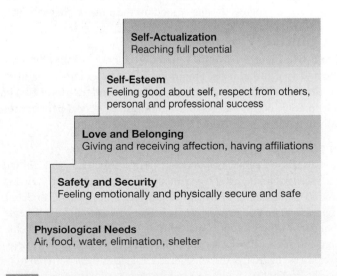

4-1 Maslow's hierarchy of needs.

Kohlberg's Stages of Moral Development   table 4-6

Stage	Level	Moral Development
Pre-conventional	Obedience and punishment orientation	Avoidance of punishment; deference to power.
	Individualism and exchange	Reciprocity is key: You take care of me and I will take care of you.
Conventional	Good interpersonal relationships	Approval earned by being nice.
	Maintaining social order	Doing one's duty to keep social order.
Post-conventional	Social contract and individual rights	Legal point of view with an ability to change laws if necessary for the social good.
	Universal principles	Abstract principles that guide the conscience in decision-making— for example, the Golden Rule: Do unto others what you would want them to do unto you.

Based on Kohlberg, L. (1973). Continuities in childhood and adult moral development revisited. In P. Baltes & K. W. Schaie (Eds.). *Lifespan Development Psychology: Personality and Socialization.* San Diego, CA: Academic Press; Ciccarelli, S. K., & White, J. N. (2013). *Psychology.* Upper Saddle River, NJ: Pearson Education, Inc.

community. For example, he asserted that individuals are able to put aside their own self-gratifying needs when others may benefit.

Kohlberg went on to describe three stages of moral development (Table 4-6). The first stage is the pre-conventional stage. During this stage, young children develop and express their morality in terms of themselves. They want to be liked; they want people to think they are good. Therefore, they act to please others. Kohlberg included obedience and punishment orientation, as well as individualism and exchange, in this category.

The second stage is the conventional stage. This phase is marked by reasoning based on social rules and norms. Kohlberg postulated that individuals adhere to rules because they exist. The development of good interpersonal relationships and ability to understand and maintain the social order occurs during the conventional stage.

The third and last phase is the post-conventional stage. It is important to note that Kohlberg did not see this category as fully attainable for all individuals. He maintained that individuals could enjoy a moral life without attaining the level of morality defined during this stage. During the post-conventional stage, individuals develop an understanding of social contract and individual rights and universal principles. One can see the progression of inclusivity as individuals develop their morality. They start with what is important for them and progress to what is good for the universe they inhabit.

Cognitive Theory

Cognitive theory focuses on the internal knowing and thinking processes of individuals. Cognitive theorists examine cognitive development—how perception, organization, and transformation of information occur. Piaget's and Bandura's theoretical perspectives inform modern understanding of cognitive development.

Jean Piaget

Jean Piaget's theory explains components that suggest how children and adolescents think, learn, and become aware of themselves and the world around them (Piaget, 1932; Piaget & Inhelder, 2000; Wadsworth, 2005). His was the first theory to recognize that children's and adolescents' thought processes are very different from those of adults, and that children and adolescents are very interactive and contextual in their cognitive processing (Kail & Cavanaugh, 2012). Piaget's theory evolved from his observations of children and adolescents within their everyday life experiences. His theory does not focus on pathological behaviors. Intel-

lectual components of development include the following (Kail & Cavanaugh, 2012; Piaget & Inhelder, 2000):

- **Adaptation:** the modification of behaviors to meet environmental needs
- **Assimilation:** taking new information and interpreting it to confirm to already existing information
- **Schemas:** cognitive ways of dealing with the environment
- **Accommodation:** changing schemas to meet life reality
- **Equilibrium:** the balance between taking in new information (assimilation) and changing schemas to meet life reality (accommodation)

Piaget connected his stages of cognitive development to the biological growth of children and adolescents. He thought that all the stages needed to be achieved in a sequential manner (Piaget & Inhelder, 2000). However, he did contend that the stages could occur more quickly or slowly based on teaching and life experience. The stages include sensorimotor, preoperational, concrete operational, and formal operational (Table 4-7).

Piaget's theory has implications for nurses who work with children and adolescents, as it informs assessment of behavior and symptomatology as well as care planning. Being able to identify normal development and its associated outcomes helps nurses better understand what children and adolescents may need if they are experiencing symptoms of mental distress or impairment in physical health.

PRACTICE ALERT   Medical illness can create a variety of stressors to children, adolescents, and their families. Careful assessment of stress and coping is needed for patients and their families who require care for acute and chronic medical illness. By providing care that is age and developmentally appropriate, nurses can instill confidence, reduce anxiety, and promote hope in young patients and their families.

Albert Bandura

Albert Bandura extended Piaget's theory by focusing on the role of self-efficacy. Bandura's **social cognitive theory** indicates that the level of self-efficacy is a critical component for the ability to effectively manage occurrences within everyday functioning (Bandura, 2001). Bandura contended that an individual not only reacts to a stimulus

Piaget's Cognitive Theory of Development

table 4-7

Name of Stage	Developmental Activity	Nursing Considerations
Sensorimotor Birth–2 years of age	• Children learn to discern themselves from their environments. • Exploration primarily involves sensations and motor behaviors. • *Object permanence*, the understanding that something exists even when it is out of sight, develops toward the end of the first year of life.	• Promote maternal bonding through skin-to-skin contact. • Hold infants to comfort them during hospital visits and procedures. • Use crib mobiles, manipulative toys to provide interesting stimuli and comfort, and to distract during procedures and assessments. • Provide consistency of caregiver; address stranger anxiety.
Preoperational Ages 2–7	• Children are learning language ahead of logic development. • Understanding of cause-and-effect relationships tenuous. • Children continue to be self-involved into the preschool years.	• Provide opportunity to touch or play with medical equipment prior to assessments and procedures. • Offer explanations of assessments and procedures. • Clearly explain child is not responsible for situation/illness. • Listen to children's feelings. If child is unable to verbally express feelings, providing opportunities to draw or express feelings with dolls or stuffed animals may be helpful.
Concrete operational Ages 7–11	• Rational and logical thinking begins: Children are able to understand when concrete items are used in explanations. • Children learn *conservation*, the concept that matter does not change when its form is altered, at this stage.	• Give clear information regarding treatment. • Show the child items or equipment that will be used in treatment. • Assess for and encourage the child to participate in favorite activities.
Formal operational 11 years and older	• Adolescents are able to engage in abstract thinking, can consider a range of possible outcomes or alternatives.	• Provide clear and complete information, in both verbal and written form. • Recognize and respect adolescents' need for increased privacy. • Promote interaction with peers.

Based on Piaget, J., & Inhelder, B. (2000). *The Psychology of the Child*. New York, NY: Basic Books; Ball, J., Bindler, R., & Cowen, K. (2012). *Principles of Pediatric Nursing: Caring for Children* (5th ed.). Upper Saddle River, NJ: Prentice Hall.

but also has the ability to adapt and reinforce positive, healthier responses to the stimulus (**self-efficacy**). Nurses can be instrumental in helping patients of all ages to develop, strengthen, and use self-efficacy to maintain or regain their mental health and wellness.

Behavioral Theory

Behavioral theory focuses on elements that reinforce and maintain maladaptive behaviors. Ivan Pavlov and B. F. Skinner are the leading behavioral theorists. They focused on how individuals learn and how responses to stimuli are involved in learning.

Pavlov and Classical Response

Pavlov's theory involved his work with animals, specifically dogs. Pavlov conducted a series of experiments, ringing a bell just prior to feeding a dog. After a while, the dog would immediately start to salivate when the bell rang, even when food was not presented. In this experiment, the bell was the *stimulus* and the *response* was the salivation. Pavlov referred to this outcome as a **classical response**, a conditioned response to a recurrent stimulus (Pavlov, 1928). Pavlov's theory has been adapted to humans. For example, imagine a 6-year-old child whose father regularly yells at and then spanks the child, after which the child experiences stomach pain and nausea. The child goes to school, hears a male teacher raise his voice, and experiences stomach pain and nausea in response. The child now responds to any male

voice (stimulus) with these symptoms (responses), even though the teacher is not yelling at or spanking him (Kail & Cavanaugh, 2012; Tusaie & Fitzpatrick, 2013).

It is important that nurses understand that the behavior of their patients may be contingent on the patients' involvement with negative stimuli that provoke a classic conditioned response. In these cases, the nurse can help patients work through the idea that the stimulus response does not mean that the negative outcome will occur. This promotes change by helping patients realize that the stimulus does not have to lead to the physiological response. This is called *operant conditioning*, and it replaces the classical response.

Skinner and Behavior Modification

B. F. Skinner sought to extend Pavlov's work by examining human responses to stimuli. Skinner's theory proposes that there is a connection between punishments and rewards to the reaction a person has to stimuli (Kail & Cavanaugh, 2012; Tusaie & Fitzpatrick, 2013). Techniques of **behavior modification** can be used to facilitate changes in an individual's behavior patterns. Skinner's theory involves four responses to facilitate change in behavior (Ciccarelli & White, 2013):

• Adding something desired to encourage positive behavior

• Adding something unpleasant as a consequence of negative behavior

- Removing or avoiding undesired reinforcement of negative behavior
- Removing something desired as a consequence of negative behavior

Behavior modification can be used in a number of situations. As an example, consider the child who keeps interrupting her parents when they speak with others. The tendency for many parents is to stop talking and ask the child what she wants. Skinner might suggest that the parent ignore the child's interruptions as a strategy to extinguish the negative behavior. In this approach, the child does not receive reinforcement of the interrupting behavior. Another approach might be to provide positive reinforcement: The parent may say, "I will speak with you as soon as I am done talking with my friend, as long as you do not interrupt again." In yet a third approach, the parent might count to five with the expectation that the child will cease interrupting or else receive some type of discipline, such as withdrawal of screen time.

Interpersonal Theory

Interpersonal theory was developed by Harry Stack Sullivan and Adolf Meyer. The basic premise is that interpersonal relationships and mood affect each other and can cause, maintain, or buffer depression. Interpersonal theory and Bowlby's attachment theory form the foundation for interpersonal psychotherapy (IPT) (Ciccarelli & White, 2013; Interpersonal Psychotherapy for Children, 2012).

Harry Stack Sullivan laid the foundation for interpersonal theory by focusing on interpersonal relations—specifically, the patterns in which individuals interact with others (Rioch, 1985). Sullivan also valued the roles of society and culture in personality development and psychpathology (Evans, 2005). He challenged Freud's psychosexual theory, especially regarding infantile sexual drives as being central to personality development and psychopathology. Sullivan has been cited as influential in the development of both group therapy and family systems theory. It also has been noted that even though he rarely referred to "love" in his work, his work indicated that love between humans assisted individuals in being free (Evans, 2005).

Change Theory

Kurt Lewin is considered to be the father of social psychology in that his work furthered understanding of group dynamics and change. Social psychology emphasizes the impact of the environment on the individual's personality development and investment in community.

Lewin was interested in studying how people interact with each other, examining the reasons behind how a group of people functioned together. For example, he would have been interested in why one group of nursing students is able to complete a project easily, whereas another group is unable to agree on a time to meet, much less complete the project. Lewin was the first to coin the phrase "group dynamics" in 1939. He is also the founder of *change theory*, proposing that change occurs for people within three distinct stages: unfreezing, changing, and freezing (Cummings & Worley, 2009) (Table 4-8).

Lewin theorized that for an individual to consider a change, he or she must first release or "unfreeze" old unhealthy patterns or "encounter" forces, feelings, or thoughts within himself or herself that cause the individual to think about a change, either by encouraging change or by restraining change. Forces that cause individuals to halt or reconsider change are called *restraining forces*. For example, if a patient is overweight, the patient may start to think about some weight loss measures. The patient's thinking may start to shift as a result of unhealthy laboratory values or other factors that motivate change. As the patient contemplates the change, thinking about restraining forces (for instance, avoiding friends who do not engage in healthy eating) may immobilize the individual. Lewin refers to this immobilization as a state of equilibrium, in which the push and pull of differing ideas results in no change at all.

For example, during the unfreezing stage, the individual considering weight loss may consider that even though multiple weight loss programs have not worked previously, there still is one out there that might. This state of unfreezing is done systematically, in a series of three steps: The first is to increase the driving forces by listing, visualizing, or thinking about the benefits for the change. The second is to decrease the opposing or restraining forces to make the goal seem more attainable. In the third stage, the individual is able to manage both driving and restraining forces, always working at keeping things in perspective.

Lewin's second stage is the changing stage. It is during this stage that a strategy or a new relationship can become a catalyst for change, and the individual begins to look at things differently.

As the new behavior becomes more of a habit, the behavior becomes part of a "refreezing." If the individual does not get some reward or relief by changing behavior, then the refreezing does not occur. It is at this point that the individual may resort to previous behaviors. For example, the individual who is working to lose weight may stop exercising and counting calories and resort to previous, unhealthy behaviors.

Prochaska, DiClemente, and Norcross (1992), in their theoretical work on how individuals change addictive behaviors, identified a five-stage model of change (Box 4-1). This model can assist nurses and clinicians in identifying a patient's readiness for change, as well as appropriate interventions.

▍Pause and Reflect

1. *Where do you think you are on Maslow's hierarchy?*
2. *Why might an individual move from a more self-actualized category to a "lower" category on Maslow's hierarchy?*

Lewin's Stages of Change		table 4-8
Stages	**Process**	**What Does It Look Like?**
Unfreezing	Reduce forces to maintain behaviors	Give information that helps individuals see discrepancies between how things are and how they might be.
Changing	Shift old behaviors to new behaviors	Help develop new behaviors, values, and attitudes.
Freezing	Reinforce new state	Provide supports, such as culture, rewards, and structures.

Based on Cummings, T. G., & Worley, C. G. (2009). Organization Development and Change (9th ed.). Mason, OH: South-Western Cengage Learning. Available at http://books.google.com/books?id=rdjtPTfkWG8C&printsec=frontcover&source=gbs_ge_summary_r&cad=0#v=onepage&q&f=false

Stages of Change

box 4-1

The stages of change model developed and subsequently studied over time by Prochaska, DiClemente, and Norcross (1992) recognizes five stages of change (Figure 4-2) through which individuals may move that reflect their willingness to admit a need to change a behavior or situation and their ability or readiness to make a change. Individuals may move back and forth among the stages, and some individuals who reach the maintenance stage will relapse.

In the *precontemplation stage*, the individual is unaware or unable to admit that a problem exists. The individual typically either minimizes or denies the problem. At this stage, the individual has no intention of making any changes. At this stage, nurses avoid confronting the problem behavior, instead helping patients identify possible stressors and working with them to decrease exposure to stress and improve communication skills. At this stage, nurses help patients identify techniques to reduce stress, which patients may identify as helpful without directly addressing or confronting behaviors that require change.

In the *contemplation stage*, an individual acknowledges that a problem exists and begins to seriously think about making a change. Nursing interventions at this stage are similar to those attempted in the precontemplation stage, with the addition of helping patients identify the pros and cons of changing behaviors. At this stage, nurses and other clinicians begin offering information regarding therapies and treatment options.

In the *preparation stage*, individuals may plan to make changes or may begin making attempts to reduce problem behaviors. Interventions at this stage include those appropriate for early stages, with the addition of working with the patient to identify alternative coping methods. During the preparation stage, it often is appropriate to work with patients to identify factors that contribute to problem behaviors or that may affect treatment, such as co-occurring medical illness or friends or family members who enable or promote negative behavior patterns.

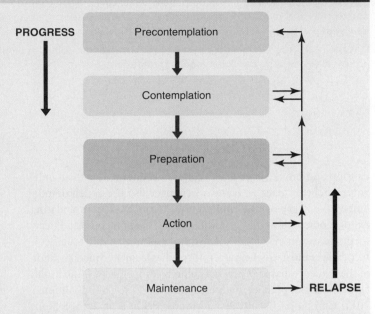

4-2 The five stages of change: precontemplation, contemplation, preparation, action, and maintenance.

During *the action stage*, individuals make changes in their behaviors, experiences, and/or environments. They are accepting of interventions such as medical treatment, pharmacotherapy, and psychotherapy.

In the *maintenance stage*, individuals work to continue on the path of wellness and to avoid relapse. Ongoing interventions focus on continuing therapy, support, and stress reduction.

Based on Prochaska, J. O., DiClemente, C. C., & Norcross, J. C. (1992). In search of how people change: Applications to addictive behaviors. *American Psychologist, 47*(9), 1102–1114. Available at http://www.ncbi.nlm.nih.gov/pubmed/1329589; Prochaska, J. O., Norcross, J. C., & DiClemente, C. C. (2013). Applying the stages of change. *Psychotherapy in Australia 19*(2), 10–15. Available at http://www.psychotherapy.com.au/fileadmin/site_files/events/pdfs/APPLYING_THE_STAGES_OF_CHANGE_JOHN_NORCROSS.pdf

Psychiatric Nursing Theory

Nursing theory focuses on aspects of nursing care, helping explain behavior and nursing roles by identifying and defining components that are relevant. Most nursing theories have four key components: person, environment, health, and nursing.

For most nursing theorists, the primary concept is the *person*—the patient or client. Nursing theorists define the person as the individual(s) receiving care from the nurse and needing to be viewed holistically: encompassing body, mind, and spirit. The next concept is the *environment*—the internal and external factors that affect an individual. The third concept is that of *health*, the continuum of wellness and illness and where the individual's well-being falls on the continuum in relation to the context of the individual's physiological, psychological, social, spiritual, and cultural factors. The fourth concept is that of *nursing* itself, the process by which nurses help individuals meet their needs. This section will briefly delineate several theories and concepts relevant to nursing care of individuals with mental illness (Table 4-9).

Nightingale's Environmental Theory

Florence Nightingale viewed the nurse as a component within the concept of person, as the individual who acts on the *person* (that is, the patient). Nightingale also recognized that the environment affects the person, and that the environment is composed of physical, psychological and social foundational issues (Nightingale, 2010). According to Nightingale, the health of a patient depends on the nurse's use of the patient's abilities and factors in the environment (such as fresh air, nutrition, and rest). Nightingale's concepts are relevant to the psychiatric nursing care in that she stresses the internal strength of patients as well as the role of the nurse in promoting and maintaining health and wellness.

Leininger's Transcultural Care Theory

Madeline Leininger examined the role and universality of culture in the development of health, wellness, and illness within individuals (Leininger, 2006). Leininger theorized that the role of the nurse is to

Luis

You are the nurse working in an outpatient clinic. Luis is a 41-year-old male client who makes frequent phone calls and requests numerous office visits. You suspect that Luis is using the calls and visits to deal with a very high level of anxiety that is causing him to have many somatic complaints.

Luis has had 3 tests done in the past 2 months for various somatic complaints. None of the tests have revealed any medical condition requiring treatment.

> ### APPLICATION
> 1. What does psychiatric nursing theory say about how you should care for Luis?
> 2. How would you assess Luis's readiness for changing using Lewin's stages of change?

develop and provide care that is culturally congruent with an individual's beliefs, values, and norms. Leininger also stressed the importance of preserving patients' cultural nuances, accommodating cultural practices, and re-patterning health care practices and treatments based on evidence-based strategies and the individual's cultural beliefs and needs. Leininger's theory has facilitated incorporation of the evidence-based process of cultural competence within health care education, practice, and research settings (Warren & Broome, 2011; Campinha-Bacote, 2007; Munoz, Primm, Ananth, & Ruiz, 2007; Warren, 2009).

Peplau's Theory of Interpersonal Relations

As discussed in Chapter 1, Hildegard Peplau's theory provides an essential foundation for psychiatric–mental health nurses, informing the education and care they provide for individuals, groups, communities, and populations. Peplau examined the interactions and relationships among the patient, nurse, and the therapeutic encounter to promote or re-establish mental health and wellness (Peplau, 1952). Peplau emphasized that it is the psychiatric nurse's responsibility to establish, maintain, and move forward the therapeutic relationship. Problem solving, anxiety reduction, and the forward movement of the client's health state are components of Peplau's theory. Peplau also noted that the psychological care of clients needs to include the assessment and treatment of the physiological and spiritual components. Peplau's theory is congruent with the idea of recovery and the use of evidence-based approaches within nursing education and practice (Forchuk, 1991; Hamric & Deering, 2012; Lusk & Melnyk, 2011; Melnyk & Fineout-Overholt, 2012; Moran, Burson, & Conrad, 2014).

Orlando and the Deliberative Nursing Process

Ida Jean Orlando (1961) described the task of nursing as the nurse validating and meeting the patient's perceived needs. She emphasized nursing's responsibility to assess the patient's needs in such a way that a patient's needs are made known. Orlando assumed that each patient and each nurse–patient interaction is unique, calling on nurses to be ready to change their approaches to patients as needed.

Orlando theorized that nurses' relationships with patients are ever changing. As a result, nursing is dynamic and must be fluid in its approach to patients. Without this fluidity, nurses are unable to assess their patients' levels of distress accurately. Orlando focused on several important components:

Distress involves the concerns and worries of the individual patient. This is an important distinction, as it clarifies the importance of the patient's actual concerns, as opposed to the concerns of the nurse or the health care team. For example, a nurse may see a patient with hypertension or a high level of anxiety, and may want the patient to begin a course of medication to combat the hypertension or a medication to relieve the anxiety. Instead, the patient presents with a primary concern of being cold. Orlando's work emphasizes the importance of assessing and validating the patient's concern.

Perceptions refer to any observation the nurse makes related to senses—namely, what is seen, heard, smelled, or touched. *Thoughts* follow from the nurse's perceptions, and the nurse may then experience *feelings* based on those perceptions and feelings. Orlando encourages nurses to respond to the patient by reflecting or sharing their perceptions, thoughts, and/or feelings as appropriate to determine together the best course for the patient.

Orlando defined *deliberative nursing* as the ability to assess and perceive the immediate needs of the patient. At each step of the relationship, the nurse validates his or her perceptions of the patient and the patient's concerns in a deliberative, careful manner. Nursing actions are defined as the interventions that the nurse validates and confirms with the patient that help meet the patient's needs. The goal is to deliver interventions that result in therapeutic outcomes. For Orlando, outcomes may be changes in a patient's behavior or reports of relieved distress. A positive outcome would be noted when a patient is able to convey a change in mood or behavior that positively affects the quality of his or her life.

Neuman's Systems Model

Betty Neuman (1995) used a holistic, or systems, approach to patient care. She emphasized that nurses should assess the patient's status related to both actual and potential stressors. Some of the basic assumptions of this theory are that individuals are to be viewed as unique entities. Nurses should view patients as the unique individuals they are and treat them holistically. Neuman asked nurses to be cognizant of the potential responses that individuals have to their stressors: Each individual has the opportunity to respond to stressors in different ways and at different times as the stressors present themselves. Neumann stated that homeostasis is a goal of the individual.

Some key aspects of Neuman's systems theory are:

- Central core
- Normal line of defense

Relevant Nursing Theories

table 4-9

Theorist	Theory	Components/Explanation of Theory
Florence Nightingale	Environmental theory	• Person • Environment • Health • Nursing Health problems are created by an unclean environment. Environment is composed of ventilation, light, warmth, "effluvia" (foul odors), noise.
Madeline Leininger	Transcultural care theory	• Cultural congruence • Universality • Preservation • Accommodation • Re-patterning Health, wellness, and illness development and treatment are grounded in the connection between client's and nurse's cultural beliefs, values, and norms.
Hildegard Peplau	Interpersonal relations theory	• Nursing as a psychodynamic process • Nurse's understanding of self • Nurse's understanding of patient needs The nurse is responsible for the development, maintenance, and forward movement of the client–nurse therapeutic relationship in order to re-establish and/or maintain health and wellness.
Ida Jean Orlando	Deliberative nursing process	• Patients' immediate needs • Use of perceptions, thoughts, and feelings • Validation with patients • Every nurse–patient interaction is unique. Nurses must validate with patients, by using the nurse's perceptions, thoughts, and/or feelings, what their immediate needs are and whether the nurse's interventions are meeting them.
Betty Neuman	Systems model	• Each individual has a central core. • Individuals have lines of defense to protect the core from illness. • Primary, secondary, and tertiary prevention. Nursing's role is to assist the client system to attain, maintain, or regain system homeostasis.
Dorothy Orem	Self-care deficit theory	• When self-care needs exceed the individual's ability to provide self-care, nursing is required. • Emphasizes the interrelationship of self-care, self-care deficit, and nursing systems. Nurses need to provide care for individuals who are unable to provide that care for themselves.
Martha Rogers	Science of unitary human beings	• Humans are considered integral with the universe. • Energy field is central to the theory. • Humans and the environment constantly exchange energy. Nursing focuses on wholeness versus disease; interventions are creative.
Jean Watson	Theory of transpersonal caring	• Caring for the purpose of healing. Nursing emphasis is on spiritual and mental growth for the nurse and others more through being than doing as an agent of change.
Various	Tidal Model—an interdisciplinary approach	Emphasizes patients' involvement in their own care. Ten commitments: • Voices of patients and providers • Respect patient's story • Develop curiosity • Become the student • Use the patient's story • Determine recovery steps • Give time • Help patient see progress • Expect change • Be transparent in explanations Nurses focus on helping individuals make their own discovery of what needs to be done.

Based on George, J. B. (2011). *Nursing Theories: The Base for Professional Nursing Practice* (6th ed.). Upper Saddle River, NJ: Pearson Education, Inc; Tidal Model: http://currentnursing.com/nursing_theory/Tidal_Model.html

- Flexible line of defense
- Primary, secondary, and tertiary nursing prevention

The *central core* of the individual includes the physiological, psychological, sociocultural, spiritual, and developmental variables that make up this person. Objective data within a person's core includes vital signs, genetic makeup, and illnesses to which the individual is predisposed. It also includes the level of organ functioning, ego structures, and personal value systems. Additionally, Neuman stressed the importance of the individual's spirit as a component of the core.

Neuman refers to lines of defense that help the patient preserve wellness. The *normal line of defense* is the individual's normal state of wellness next to the core. The *flexible line of defense* is the outermost boundary to the central core of the individual. The more energy an individual has and the more stressors are under control, the stronger the line of defense that protects this central core.

The lines of resistance offer further protection for the individual as the stressors become stronger than the endurance of the central core. An individual not experiencing a disease state or one who is feeling in control of functioning will have lines of resistance that can ward off the effects of the stressors more readily than an individual who is consumed by illness or feelings of helplessness. Neuman went on to define three major categories of stressors:

- *Intrapersonal:* Stressors related to the individual's thoughts and feelings, more personal or within the person.
- *Interpersonal:* Stressors between individuals. These stressors could be with family members or peers, or between the patient and the health care provider.
- *Extrapersonal:* Stressors emanating from the environment. These stressors could be from school, work, or community.

Neuman also examined the importance of primary, secondary, and tertiary prevention. Primary prevention includes a list of possible risk factors that an individual may encounter. During the period of primary prevention, nurses are able to help patients reduce those risk factors. During the secondary prevention phase, patient symptoms are evident as responses to stressors. The nurse's role is to prioritize the nursing interventions to help reduce the effect of the stressors. The tertiary prevention phase includes activities that patients could accomplish to help them get their status back to the primary prevention phase.

Orem's Self-Care Deficit Theory

Dorothy Orem's theory is known as the *self-care deficit theory* (Foster & Bennett, 2002; Orem, 1971). This theory focuses on the role of the nurse, optimal patient health, and successful patient outcomes in consideration of the patient's perspective. More specifically, the role of the nurse involves the nurse as provider of care, manager of care, and member of the profession. These roles depend on professional standards and state and national laws and statutes. Optimal patient care includes the nurse assisting patients to maintain, regain, or obtain optimal health levels based on the patient's level of ability to provide self-care. Patient outcomes relate to a safe environment for the patient, the patient's ability to return to a premorbid level of functioning, and the nurse's ability to help the patient reach the patient's optimal level of health.

Tidal Model

The Tidal Model is a model of care developed by both psychiatric patients and psychiatric nurses; it is practiced more widely in countries outside of the United States, notably England, Australia, and Canada. In England, the Tidal Model was developed and furthered by Dr. Phil Barker and Poppy Buchanan-Barker (Barker & Buchanan-Barker, 2005). The Tidal Model represents an interdisciplinary approach to patient care and is informed by the work of Harry Stack Sullivan and Hildegard Peplau.

Significant to this model is the involvement of patients in their own care. This involvement starts immediately with the first nurse–patient encounter, no matter how severe the patient's symptomatology. Barker and Buchanan-Barker emphasized that regardless of severity, patient involvement in care and recovery should be initiated. For example, as soon as a patient is admitted to a medical–surgical unit, the interdisciplinary team engages the patient in the provision of care, including mental health care, and begins planning for discharge.

Practitioners of the Tidal theory work with patients on both individual and group levels. At each level, patients are encouraged to relate their stories. The Tidal Model lists ten commitments made between patients and providers. They include:

1. *Value patient and provider voices.* Providers commit to using the same words a patient uses to describe symptoms and emotions.

2. *Respect the patient's language.* Providers should not modify a patient's story for the sake of the record. Spelling errors, words used out of context, and word choices make each patient's story authentic. Respecting the patient's words can assist in the patient feeling respected by the care team.

3. *Develop genuine curiosity.* Genuine curiosity in the patient's well-being is accurate to successful assessment and care. For example, a provider who is interested only in prescribing medications to alleviate symptoms may miss the message of the patient's entire story and miss an opportunity to provide more appropriate care.

4. *Become the apprentice.* Nurses and health care providers who recognize the importance of this commitment become the students in learning about the patient's response to illness.

5. *Use patient-based experiences and practice.* Nurses and other clinicians need to focus on the patient's past experiences and present story to help move the patient forward toward recovery.

6. *Determine next steps in recovery.* Along with the patient, the health care provider determines the steps needed to attain the next level of recovery.

7. *Give patients time.* The model emphasizes that one of the greatest things to give patients is time. Providing time to listen to patients' stories demonstrates respect for them and their concerns.

8. *Reveal personal wisdom.* This encourages nurses and clinicians to use the patients' knowledge to help them on their journey to recovery. For example, the patient with asthma may communicate that a certain drug elevates his heart rate, which increases his anxiety level. The patient shares that another, similar drug carries a lower side effect profile for him as an individual patient. Thus, the patient's own knowledge and experience of his condition may be used to inform the plan of care.

9. *Change is inevitable.* Health care providers help patients note their progress as they continue on their journey.

10. *Provide transparency.* Health care providers constantly and consistently explain the reasons for some things and use terminology familiar to the patient, allowing the patient to be an active participant in the plan of care.

Knowledge of a variety of theories can assist nurses in understanding the thoughts and behaviors of their patients to help them better plan nursing care that meets the needs of individual patients. A working knowledge of these theories is also necessary, as many of these theories inform current psychiatric therapies and treatments.

Pause and Reflect

1. *Which nursing theory most appeals to you? Why?*
2. *Describe how you would use two aspects from one of the nursing theories to help Jane and Luis (described in the critical thinking features).*
3. *Give an example of how you have experienced or observed a nurse use two aspects of interpersonal theory with you or someone else.*

Psychiatric Therapies

Psychiatric therapies are used to assist individuals with varied mental health issues. Individuals of all ages usually are able to participate in some form of therapy or treatment. Therapies are provided by licensed providers who have special education, training, and certification. Examples of qualified providers include advanced practice mental health nurses, mental health counselors, licensed clinical social workers, licensed addiction specialists, psychologists, and psychiatrists. Typically, each therapist or provider works with a specific population, such as children and adolescents or couples, or in a specific subject area, such as eating disorders or substance abuse. Certifications and specific educational programs that combine theory with evidence-based practice are available to assist practitioners in learning skills and techniques to provide the best possible care to their patients. Although therapies can be categorized a number of ways, this chapter examines psychological and biomedical therapies, as well as the concept of recovery. Psychological therapies include what are customarily described as the "talk" therapies. Biomedical therapies include pharmacotherapy (discussed in Chapter 23), brain stimulation, electroconvulsive therapy, and psychosurgery.

Psychological Therapies

The Recovery Model is depicted by the recovery-based Wellness Recovery Action Plan (WRAP) in this chapter. Psychological or "talk" therapies are based on the major theories of psychology described earlier: psychoanalytic, psychosocial, humanistic, interpersonal, behavioral, and cognitive theories. The goal of talk therapy is to assess the patient's mental illness and to engage in a therapy mode that will assist the patient in decreasing symptoms and increasing function. The approach to the treatment plan differs according to the tenets of the theorist on which the therapy is based and the needs of the patient. The patient and therapist work together within the process specified by the form of therapy being used.

Each type of therapy requires establishing a therapeutic alliance with the patient and establishing goals of therapy. In some cases, specific time frames must be established; these may be designated by the type of therapy or program or by the individual's health insurance provider. Just as care of the patient with a physical disorder is constrained by financial regulations, care of patients suffering with mental health issues also is regulated. It is important to note that some providers adhere to more than one theoretical approach or may use more than one type of therapy with a single patient. Psychodynamic psychotherapies based on psychoanalysis have their beginnings in the work of Sigmund Freud and his personality theory. The therapist who adheres to Freud's theory may use free association, hypnosis, and dream analysis to better understand the patient's thoughts. This therapist likely will delve into the patient's past to explore the patient's relationship with parents and siblings. Freud asserted that patterns developed during childhood have the potential to contribute insight into the patient's suffering. The therapist will analyze the patient's patterns of thought and dream content in the quest to understand a patient's emotional discomfort.

Some therapies can be brief in nature. Brief psychotherapy and crisis intervention last between six and 12 sessions. Brief psychotherapy does not work well for clients unable to identify their symptoms or are unable to communicate their feelings and thoughts.

Behavioral Therapy

The basis of behavioral (or behavior modification) therapy usually is the maladaptive behavior exhibited by the patient. The therapist works with the patient to identify behavior that is not meeting the needs of the patient and helps the patient learn new patterns of behavior or coping. This type of therapy has more success alleviating stressful symptoms when the patient is able to identify the behaviors or thoughts that are causing distress. For many patients, behavioral therapy assists them in getting back some control of their lives.

In behavioral therapy, both patient and therapist work together to identify the stressors that may be causing the behavior. Together, they discuss and agree on strategies. The therapist spends time educating the patient about strategies that might reduce distressing symptoms. Behavioral therapists also assist patients in building new skills. Role playing may be used to identify some of the patient responses to stressors or practice new responses to replace old behaviors.

Behavioral therapy is useful for patients across the life span. Children, especially, respond well to behavioral therapy that uses a rewards system. Sticker charts, lists of responsibilities that can be checked off, and other strategies can help reinforce appropriate behaviors.

Systematic desensitization and breathing exercises are some other behavioral techniques that may be used during behavior therapy. Examples include the following (Davis, Palladino, & Christopherson, 2013):

- *Systematic desensitization* is the reduction of an individual's negative behavior by exposure to a feared object or situation paired with an activity designed to offset the resulting anxiety. For example, if a person fears public speaking, learning stress management breathing may be helpful. The individual might practice breathing techniques while thinking about the event, prior to going into the event, and during the event to help decrease anxiety.

- *Aversion therapy* involves exposing an individual to painful or obnoxious stimuli that is paired with something the individual desires. A classic example is the administration of disulfiram (Antabuse) to someone who desires to stop drinking alcohol. The individual taking disulfiram will become nauseated and vomit if he or she is exposed to strong odors of alcohol or ingests alcohol.

- *Modeling* is particularly useful with phobias. Modeling offers the patient the opportunity to observe someone else handling the feared situation appropriately and to be guided by that example.

- *Extinction* is the withdrawal of reinforcement for a negative behavior. For example, a parent stops addressing temper tantrums with comforting behavior and instead ignores them.

- *Punishment* is the withdrawal of positive reinforcement or the application of negative reinforcement in response to negative behavior. This form of treatment can be controversial and must be examined in terms of ethics. For example, the use of restraints in response to negative behavior may not be ethical.

- *Token economies* use tokens to reinforce positive behaviors. This treatment modality was used years ago when state psychiatric facilities had large populations. This methodology is the basis of reward systems used for children, such as accumulation of stars and stickers toward a goal of accumulating a certain number to earn a prize or reward (the token).

Cognitive Therapy

Cognitive therapy (CT) was developed by Aaron Beck. Beck asserts that individuals who are depressed tend to think negatively in relation to their perceptions of the world, themselves, and their future (Beck, 1967). CT encourages individuals to rethink or reframe negative, pessimistic thoughts. CT does not address issues from the patient's past but looks at the present and what is not working (Davis, Palladino, & Christopherson, 2013).

Some cognitive distortion categories are:

- Arbitrary inference (someone thinks he has been snubbed, but the other person did not hear him)

- Selective abstraction (a nursing student makes a medication error and concludes nursing is the wrong profession for him)

- Overgeneralization (an individual gets abdominal pain on two occasions after eating fish and concludes she has a fish allergy)

- Magnification/minimization (a student does well on an exam and tells everyone she is the smartest individual in the class; a student receives a scholarship but tells her parents that it is not "such a big deal" because other students in the university received a scholarship as well) (Wade, Tavris, & Garry, 2014)

With CT, a patient expressing negative assumptions, beliefs, and thoughts is encouraged to challenge beliefs against evidence. For example, a patient thinking that someone does not like her might be asked, "What makes you think the person doesn't like you? Did the person do something that makes you feel that way?" (Davis, Palladino, & Christopherson, 2013).

Cognitive–Behavioral Therapy

Albert Ellis developed rational therapy (RT), a form of cognitive therapy in the mid-1950s. His form of therapy has evolved into rational emotive therapy (RET). and eventually rational emotive behavioral therapy (REBT), which combines techniques from both cognitive and behavior therapies; hence, the term *cognitive–behavioral therapy* (CBT) (Ellis, 1994).

Cognitive–behavioral therapy is one of the most effective psychotherapies and may be used to treat a wide variety of mental disorders. As the name implies, it helps patients examine and reframe negative thinking patterns as well as identify negative behaviors and replace them with more constructive behaviors. Some studies indicate that CBT changes brain activity, helping individuals improve brain function. In many cases, CBT has been shown to be as effective as using medication alone (Spielmans, Berman, & Usitalo, 2011). CBT usually is short in duration, occurring weekly or biweekly for between 15 and 25 sessions. It generally involves some type of homework: Patients may be given readings about their disorders, stories about other people with their same disorders, and/or questionnaires and logs to use to record their symptoms. Logs or journals assist patients in identifying and writing down their thoughts, which can help patients and therapists identify negative thought patterns and the stressors or situations that trigger or exacerbate them.

Historically, CBT was not recommended for patients with psychosis, but research examining the use of CBT with this patient population has shown much success. Morrison et al. (2004) worked with 58 individuals who were at high risk for first episode of psychosis and found that cognitive therapy significantly reduced the likelihood of their moving to psychosis. Other findings in this study revealed reduced likelihood of antipsychotic medication, less chance of being diagnosed with a psychotic disorder, and significantly improved positive symptoms of psychosis over a12-month period (Morrison, et al., 2004). (See Chapter 17, Schizophrenic Spectrum Disorders).

Biomedical Therapies

Biomedical therapies involve treatment modalities such as psychotropic medications, transcranial magnetic stimulation, electroconvulsive therapy, and psychosurgery. Psychotropic medications are discussed in detail in Chapter 23. An overview of TMS, ECT, and psychosurgery follows.

Obtaining informed consent is critical with all therapies but especially with more invasive treatments, such as the biomedical therapies. Informed consent is obtained by the provider performing the treatment procedure. The nurse's role often involves witnessing the patient's signature on the consent form.

Transcranial Magnetic Stimulation

Transcranial magnetic stimulation (TMS) is a non-invasive therapy that involves the placement of a large coil on the left prefrontal cortex (near the forehead). The electromagnet causes electric currents to stimulate nerve cells that affect mood and depression. Individuals with severe depression have benefited from this treatment, but more research is needed to provide necessary statistics related to its efficacy (Wade, Tavris, & Garry, 2014).

Nurses help reassure patients that there is no pain involved with TMS, which is usually administered in an outpatient setting. TMS does not require any anesthesia, surgery, or electrode implantation. During the procedure, the patient reclines in a chair with a treatment coil placed on the scalp. Brief magnetic pulses are sent by the coil to stimulate pre-selected areas of the brain. Generally, treatments last 40 minutes. Five treatments are given weekly for up to six weeks (Rosedale, 2009).

Electroconvulsive Therapy

Electroconvulsive therapy (ECT), sometimes referred to as *shock therapy*, is used for treatment of severe depression and suicidality or refusal to eat, but it is especially indicated for individuals who have not responded to other treatments for depression. The electric current applied to the brain causes an individual to experience a mild seizure. Placement of electrodes is either unilateral (on the right side

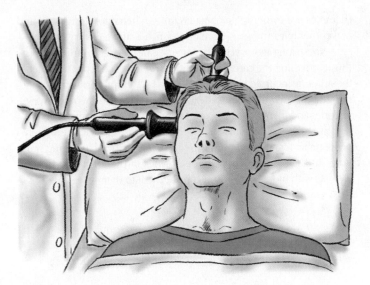

4-3 Electroconvulsive therapy (ECT) may be used for treatment of severe depression and suicidality or refusal to eat, especially in patients who have not responded to other treatments for depression. The electric current applied to the brain causes the individual to experience a mild seizure. Unilateral placement of the electrodes (shown here) generally results in less post-treatment confusion.

of the head and on top of the head) or bilateral (on both sides of the head). Unilateral placement generally results in less post-treatment confusion (Figure 4-3). Muscle relaxants and anesthesia prevent the individual from thrashing during the current-induced convulsion. The number of treatments ranges from 4 to 20, but the average is 6 to 12 (Kellner, 2013).

Patients needing special consideration include those with diabetes (no food or drink after midnight prior to the morning of treatment), pregnant women (effects on fetal heart rate), those with cardiac or hypertensive issues (temporary elevated blood pressure during treatment), and those with glaucoma (increased pressure issues) (Reti, 2013).

Nursing care before, during, and after ECT includes:

- *Providing education and support:* Assure patients that no pain will be experienced; instruct patients who smoke not to smoke on the morning of the procedure, as smoking may interfere with the treatment; inform patients that electrodes will be placed on the head for the ECT and electrodes will be placed on the chest to monitor heart rhythm; inform patients that short-term memory loss, confusion, and extreme fatigue are common right after treatment; advise that mood usually begins to lift after two to four treatments; make sure the patient does not drive after treatment and make arrangements for a driver if the patient needs to drive somewhere.

- *Performing pretreatment assessments:* Ensure removal of contact lenses and dentures; offer opportunity to use the bathroom; confirm that the patient has not eaten or smoked; insert a needle for intravenous medications (muscle relaxant to minimize muscle reaction to seizure and anesthesia to induce sleep).

- *Monitoring the procedure:* Monitor blood pressure, oxygen administration, and oxygen measurement with pulse oximeter.

- *Observing and interpreting post-treatment patient responses:* Monitor vital signs until the patient stabilizes; remind the patient not to make any major decisions right after treatments (Kellner, 2013).

Psychosurgery

Psychosurgery involves surgically severing or disabling parts of the brain. The first psychosurgery was performed in 1891 by Gottlieb Burkhardt on six clients diagnosed with mental illness as well as severe aggression and dementia. The results were diverse. In 1937, Egas Moniz performed the first prefrontal lobotomy. In this procedure, termed psychosurgery, two holes were drilled into the patient's prefrontal lobes in an attempt to control behavior. Since that time, the acceptance of psychosurgery by the medical community and the public has been inconsistent (Cosgrove & Rauch, 2005; Davis, Palladino, & Christopherson, 2013; Wade, Tavris, & Garry, 2014).

Psychosurgery is reserved for patients with refractory psychiatric illness who experience no periods of remission. However, these procedures occur in only a small number of medical facilities so their use is very restricted. Different parts of the brain have been targeted, but the limbic system appears to be the area most beneficial for patients who have severe mood dysregulation disorders that have not responded to other treatments.

The two most often used psychosurgeries today are cingulotomy and capsulotomy. Both procedures involve using heat or gamma radiation to sever nerve bundles that are implicated in obsessions and compulsions (Davis, Palladino, & Christopherson, 2013).

Nursing care during any psychosurgical procedure would be based on specific hospital protocols for brain surgeries, as well as monitoring symptoms being treated, such as severe obsessive–compulsive behaviors. Many patients often require ongoing behavioral and medication therapy post-psychosurgery (Psychosurgery, 2008).

Recovery Model

As discussed in Chapter 1, the recovery model supports the potential of an individual to recover from mental illness and/or substance abuse. The Substance Abuse and Mental Health Services Administration (SAMHSA) posted an official definition in 2011: "A process of change through which individuals improve their health and wellness, live a self-directed life, and strive to reach their full potential" (SAMHSA, 2011).

One particular recovery-based model is the Wellness Recovery Action Plan (WRAP), which was developed by individuals experiencing mental illness difficulties. WRAP is included in the SAMHSA registry of evidence-based programs and practices. Results have been positive, with recovery and long-term stability occurring. Advocated by researcher and author Mary Ellen Copeland, the purpose of WRAP is to help individuals identify, develop, and access their own wellness resources to successfully manage their mental illness. The goals of WRAP are:

- Use the concepts of recovery (hope, personal responsibility, education, self-advocacy, and support) daily.

- Determine wellness tools—activities to feel better when struggling with mental health challenges.

- Develop an advance directive that involves family members or supporters when unable to take correct actions on one's behalf.

- Formulate an individualized post-crisis plan for use as the mental health difficulty subsides, thus supporting return to wellness (WRAP, 2013).

From Suffering to Hope

Theories and evidence-based data that support them help inform nursing care of patients with mental illness. Developmental theories provide guidelines to assess individual development and potential need for intervention. Nursing theories impart conceptual foundations and frameworks to direct practice. Nursing theories can help provide best practices when the theories demonstrate evidence-based data through research.

There is a wide variation of therapies for those suffering with mental illness. Quite often an *eclectic* approach is taken—namely, a therapist employs various features from several therapies. Older therapies are evolving (such as cognitive–behavioral therapy) and newer therapies are being developed (such as the recovery model).

Not so long ago, psychiatric nursing care was determined solely by those providing the care. Currently, more hope is offered for relief of the suffering incurred with mental illnesses by empowering those diagnosed with such illnesses to be actively involved in their recoveries. Theories and therapies can be used to help patients reframe patterns of negative thinking, examine cognitive distortions, and learn new, appropriate behaviors to use in response to stressors and challenging situations. In the recovery model, hope comes in the form of providing patients with more voice in and commitment to their recovery.

Chapter Highlights

1. Theories are interrelated concepts, definitions, and/or models that help explain why series of incidents occur.

2. Theories guide development and implementation of evidence-based psychiatric–mental health nursing education and practice.

3. Freud's psychoanalytical theory provided the foundation for today's psychotherapy.

4. Humanistic theories help nurses' understanding of how patients view their needs and their ability to direct their lives.

5. Cognitive and behavioral theories inform nurses' understanding of patients' thought processes and behavior patterns.

6. Peplau's theory of interpersonal relations influences much of psychiatric nursing today.

7. Change theory assists in our understanding of patient readiness for change.

8. Nursing theories usually address four major areas: person, environment, health, and nursing.

9. Psychological therapies and biomedical therapies may be used independently or in combination in the care of patients with mental illness.

10. Cognitive–behavioral therapy has proven effective in the treatment of a wide variety of psychiatric disorders.

NCLEX®-RN Questions

1. The nurse is documenting an admission assessment on a 78-year-old adult patient. The patient reveals being consumed with regret about the way that he has lived his life. Which entry is most appropriate for the section asking about the patient's developmental status?
   a. Patient lacks a sense of self and ego identity.
   b. Patient is struggling with the achievement of integrity.
   c. Patient has never achieved industry and competence.
   d. Patient has not met the need to contribute in some way.

2. The nurse is assigned to the care of a patient who has dementia. How would the nurse anticipate the patient benefiting from the theoretical approaches developed by Carl Rogers and Abraham Maslow?
   a. Self-efficacy can be achieved by encouraging independence.
   b. Quality of life can be promoted by focusing on holistic needs.
   c. Cognitive schemas can be adjusted through reality orientation.
   d. Behavior can be modified as a result of positive reinforcement.

3. The nurse is applying principles of operant conditioning with a patient who was a victim of abuse. The patient becomes anxious and diaphoretic each time she hears a radio. The nurse learns that the perpetrator would turn on the radio prior to abusing the patient. Which evaluation finding best indicates that the nurse's approach has been effective?
   a. The patient no longer experiences anxiety and diaphoresis in response to the radio.
   b. The patient learns to develop strategies to avoid any exposure to the negative stimulus.
   c. The patient acknowledges that listening to the radio is a positive experience for most people.
   d. The patient recognizes that the anxiety and diaphoresis do not mean that danger is present.

4. The nurse is comparing theoretical approaches to determine their appropriateness for the care of patients diagnosed with mental illness. Which conclusions by the nurse are accurate? Select all that apply.
   a. Lewin's theories may be applied to improve organizational function as well as assist patients to achieve therapeutic goals.
   b. Erikson's theories are useful in adapting teaching to meet the cognitive abilities of developing children and adolescents.
   c. Skinner's theories help nurses recognize complex psychodynamic forces underlying the modification of behavior patterns.
   d. Maslow's theories can provide nurses with a framework for determining which patient problems should be addressed first.
   e. Freud's theories can be used to understand the strong feelings that are evoked in the context of therapeutic relationships.

5. The nurse educator is preparing a poster presentation for nurse's week. The focus of the poster is on the unique contributions of nurse theorists to psychiatric care. Which statement best describes the nature of these contributions?
   a. Care comprises environmental modifications, elimination of psychological and physiological alterations and illnesses, and redefining patient needs.
   b. Care is based on correcting the patient's physiological and psychological imbalances, teaching healthy behaviors, and restoring previous levels of functioning.
   c. Care is composed primarily of complementary and alternative interventions, addressing intrapersonal aspects of health, and fostering spiritual health.
   d. Care is focused on internal and external factors that affect an individual, achieving the greatest level of functional capacity, and partnering with patients to meet their needs.

6. The nurse is providing patient teaching about electroconvulsive therapy (ECT). Which statement by the patient indicates the need for further teaching?
   a. "It is important not to eat or drink prior to the procedure."
   b. "I should not experience any pain during the procedure itself."
   c. "I will be able to resume normal activities after the treatment."
   d. "In general, effects of ECT are expected after 6 to 12 treatments."

Answers may be found on the Pearson student resource site: nursing.pearsonhighered.com

Pearson Nursing Student Resources Find additional review materials at **nursing.pearsonhighered.com**

References

American Psychiatric Nurses Association, International Society of Psychiatric Mental Health Nurses, & American Nurses Association. (2014). *Psychiatric-Mental Health Nursing: Scope and Standards of Practice*. Silver Spring, MD: American Nurses Association.

Anthony, W. A. (1993). Recovery from mental illness: The guiding vision of the mental health services in the 1990s. *Psychiatric Rehabilitation Journal, 2*(3), 17–24.

Ball, J., Bindler, R., & Cowen, K. (2012). *Principles of Pediatric Nursing: Caring for Children* (5th ed.). Upper Saddle River, NJ: Prentice Hall.

Bandura, A. (2001). Social cognitive theory: An agentic perspective. *Annual Review of Psychology, 52*, 1–26.

Barker, P. & Buchanan-Barker, P. (2005). *The Tidal Model: A Guide for Mental Health Professionals*. New York, NY: Brunner-Routledge. Available at http://books.google.com/books?id=99KDXMEbG1QC&printsec=frontcover&dq=tidal+model&hl=en&sa=X&ei=7sy8UZXKL--x0QG3sYCQDA&ved=0CC8Q6AEwAA

Beck, A. T. (1967). *The diagnosis and management of depression*. Philadelphia, PA: University of Pennsylvania Press.

Campinha-Bacote, J. (2007). *The Process of Cultural Competence in the Delivery of Healthcare Services: The Journey Continues*. Cincinnati, OH: Transcultural CARE Associates.

Ciccarelli, S. K., & White, J. N. (2013). *Psychology*. Upper Saddle River, NJ: Pearson Education, Inc.

Copeland, M. E. (2013). Mary Ellen's Bio. Available at http://wraparoundtheworld.com/about/mary-ellens-bio/

Copeland, M. E. (2014). What is a Wellness Recovery Action Plan (WRAP) and how do I use it? Available at http://www.mentalhealthrecovery.com/

Cosgrove, G. R., & Rauch, S. L. (2005). Psychosurgery. Available at http://neurosurgery.mgh.harvard.edu/functional/psysurg.htm.

Cummings, T. G., & Worley, C. G. (2009). *Organization Development and Change* (9th ed.). Mason: OH: South-Western Cengage Learning. Available at http://books.google.com/books?id=rdjtPTfkWG8C&printsec=frontcover&source=gbs_ge_summary_r&cad=0#v=onepage&q&f=false

Davis, S. G., Palladino, J. J., & Christopherson, K. M. (2013). *Psychology* (7th ed.). Boston, MA: Pearson Education, Inc.

Ellis, A. (1994). *Reason and emotion in psychotherapy: Comprehensive method of treating human disturbances: Revised and updated*. New York, NY: Citadel Press.

Erikson, E. H. (1969). *Childhood and society*. New York: Penguin Books.

Evans, B. F., III. (2005). *Harry Stack Sullivan: Interpersonal Theory & Psychotherapy*. New York, NY: Routledge.

Fonagy, P., & Target, M. (2009). Theoretical Models of Psychodynamic Therapy. In G. O. Gabbard (Ed.). *Textbook of Psychotherapeutic Treatments*. Arlington, VA: American Psychiatric Publishing, Inc.

Forchuk, C. (1991). Peplau's theory: Concepts and their relations. *Nursing Science Quaterly, 4*(2), 54–60.

Foster, P. C., & Bennett, A. M. (2002). Self-care deficit theory. In J. B. George (Ed.), *Nursing Theories: The Base for Professional Nursing Practice* (5th ed.). Upper Saddle River, NJ: Prentice Hall.

Freud, S. (1953). Three essays on the theory of sexuality. In J. Strachey, A. Freud, A. Strachey, & A. Tyson (Eds.). *The Standard Edition of the Complete Psychological Works of Sigmund Freud*. London, UK: Hogarth Press, pp. 135–248.

George, J. B. (2011). *Nursing Theories: The Base for Professional Nursing Practice* (6th ed.). Upper Saddle River, NJ: Pearson Education, Inc.

Hamric, V., & Deering, C. G. (2012). Mental health assessment of children and adolescents. In M. A. Boyd (Ed.). *Psychiatric Nursing: Contemporary Practice* (5th ed.). Philadelphia, PA: WoltersKluwer, Lippincott Williams & Wilkins, pp. 661–678.

Interpersonal Psychotherapy for Children. (2012). Available at http://effective-childtherapy.com/content/interpersonal-psychotherapy-depression

Institute of Medicine (IOM). (2010). *The Future of Nursing: Focus on the Scope of Practice*. Washington, DC: Institute of Medicine.

Kail, R. V., & Cavanaugh, J. C. (2012). *Human Development: A Life-Span View* (6th ed.). Belmont, CA: Wadsworth Cengage Learning.

Kellner, C. (2013). Patient information: Electroconvulsive therapy (ECT) (beyond the basics). Available at http://www.uptodate.com/contents/electroconvulsive-therapy-ect-beyond-the-basics

Keltner, N. L., & Vance, D. E. (2011). Introduction to psychotropic drugs. In N. L. Keltner, C. E. Bostrom, & T. McGuinness (Eds.). *Psychiatric Nursing* (6th ed.). St. Louis, MO: Mosby, pp. 142–154.

Kohlberg, L. (1973). Continuities in childhood and adult moral development revisited. In P. Baltes & K. W. Schaie (Eds.). *Lifespan Development Psychology: Personality and Socialization*. San Diego, CA: Academic Press.

Kohlberg, L., Levine, C., & Hewer, A. (1983). *Moral stages: A current formulation and a response to critics*. Basel, NY: Karger.

Leininger, M. M. (2006). Culture care diversity and universality theory and evolution of the ethnonursing method. In M. M. Leininger & M. R. McFarland (Eds.). *Culture Care and Universality: A Worldwide Nursing Theory*. Boston, MA: Jones & Bartlett Publishers, pp. 1–41.

Lusk, P. & Melnyk, B. M. (2011). COPE for the treatment of depressed adolescents. Lessons learned from implementing an evidence-based practice change. *Journal of the American Psychiatric Nurses Association, 4*, 297–309.

Mahler, M. S., Pine, F., Bergman, A. (1975). *The psychological birth of the human infant: Symbiosis and individuation*. New York: Basic Books.

Maslow, A. (1970). *Motivation and Personality* (rev. ed.). New York, NY: Harper & Brothers.

Mayo Clinic (2013). Transcranial magnetic stimulation. Available at http://www.mayoclinic.org/transcranial-magnetic-stimulation/?mc_id=comlinkpilot&placement=bottom

Melnyk, B. M., & Fineout-Overholt, E. (2012). *Evidence-Based Practice in Nursing & Healthcare: A Guide to Best Practice.* Philadelphia, PA: Lippincott, Williams & Wilkins.

Moran, K., Burson, R., & Conrad, D. (2014). *The Doctor of Nursing Practice Scholarly Project: A Framework for Success.* Burlington, MA: Jones & Bartlett Learning.

Morrison, A. P., French, P., Walford, L., Lewis, S. W., Kilcommons, A., Green, J., et al. (2004). Cognitive therapy for the prevention of psychosis in people at ultra-high risk: Randomized controlled study. *British Journal of Psychiatry, 185,* 291–297.

Munoz, R., Primm, A., Ananth, J., & Ruiz, P. (2007). *Life in Color: Culture in American Psychiatry.* Munster, IN: Hilton Publishing Company.

National Association of Cognitive Behavioral Therapists (NACBT). (2008). History of cognitive behavioral therapy. Available at http://nacbt.org/historyofcbt.htm

National Association of Mental Illness. (2012). Cognitive-behavioral therapy. Available at http://www.nami.org/Template.cfm?Section=About_Treatments_and_Supports&Template=/ContentManagement/ContentDisplay.cfm&ContentID=141590

Neuman, B. (1995). *The Neuman Systems Model* (3rd ed.). Norwalk, CT: Appleton & Lange.

Nightingale, F. (2010). *Notes on Nursing* (revised original edition). Seattle, WA: Pacific Publishing Studio.

Nursing Theories. Available at http://currentnursing.com/nursing_theory/

Orem, D. (1971). *Nursing: Concepts of practice.* New York: McGraw-Hill.

Orlando, I. J. (1961). *The Dynamic Nurse–Patient Relationship: Function, Process and Principles.* New York, NY: G. P. Putnam's Sons.

Pavlov, I. P. (1928). *Lectures on conditioned reflexes.* (Translated by W.H. Gantt) London: Allen and Unwin.

Peplau, H. (1952). *Interpersonal Relations in Nursing.* New York, NY: Putnam.

Piaget, J. (1932). *The moral judgment of the child.* London: Kegan Paul, Trench, Trubner and Co.

Piaget, J., & Inhelder, B. (2000). *The Psychology of the Child.* New York, NY: Basic Books.

Prochaska, J. O., DiClemente, C. C., & Norcross, J. C. (1992). In search of how people change: Applications to addictive behaviors. *American Psychologist, 47*(9), 1102–1114. Available at http://www.ncbi.nlm.nih.gov/pubmed/1329589

Prochaska, J. O., Norcross, J. C., & DiClemente, C. C. (2013). Applying the stages of change. *Psychotherapy in Australia 19*(2), 10–15. Available at http://www.psychotherapy.com.au/fileadmin/site_files/events/pdfs/APPLYING_THE_STAGES_OF_CHANGE_JOHN_NORCROSS.pdf

Psychosurgery. (2008). Available at http://medical-dictionary.thefreedictionary.com/psychosurgery

Reti, I. M. (2013). Electroconvulsive therapy today. Available at http://www.hopkinsmedicine.org/psychiatry/specialty_areas/brain_stimulation/images/DepBulletin407_ECT_extract.pdf

Rioch, D. M. (1985). Recollections of Harry Stack Sullivan and of the development of his interpersonal psychiatry. *Psychiatry, 48*(2), 141–158.

Rogers, C. (1980). *A Way of Being.* Boston, MA: Houghton Mifflin.

Rosedale, M. (2009). Transcranial magnetic stimulation (TMS): An entirely novel form of treatment in psychiatry and a groundbreaking opportunity for psychiatric mental health nursing. *Journal of the American Psychiatric Nurses Association, 15:* 299–302.

Spielmans, G. I., Berman, M. I., Usitalo, A. N. (2011). Psychotherapy versus second-generation antidepressants in the treatment of depression: A metaanalysis. *Journal of Nervous and Mental Disorders, 199,* 142–149.

Substance Abuse and Mental Health Services Administration (SAMHSA). (2011). SAMHSA announces a working definition of "recovery" from mental disorders and substance use disorders. Available at http://www.samhsa.gov/newsroom/advisories/1112223420.aspx

Tidal Model. Available at http://www.tidal-model.com/and http://currentnursing.com/nursing_theory/Tidal_Model.html.

Tusaie, K. R., & Fitzpatrick, J. J. (Eds.). (2013). *Advanced Practice Psychiatric Nursing: Integrating Psychotherapy, Psychopharmacology, and Complementary and Alternative Approaches.* New York, NY: Springer Publishing Company.

U.S. Department of Health & Human Services (USDHHS). (1999). *Mental Health: A Report of the Surgeon General.* Washington, DC: USDHHS.

U.S. Department of Health & Human Services (USDHHS). (2001). *Mental Health: Culture, Race, and Ethnicity: A Supplement to Mental Health: A Report of the Surgeon General.* Washington, DC: USDHHS.

Wade, C., Tavris, C., & Garry, M. (2014). *Psychology* (11th ed.). Upper Saddle River, NJ: Pearson Education, Inc.

Wadsworth, B. J. (2004). *Piaget's theory of cognitive and affective development: Foundations of constructivism.* London: Longman Publishing.

Warren, B. J. (2009). Teaching the fluid process of cultural competence at the graduate level: A constructionist approach. In S. D. Bosher & M. D. Pharris (Eds.). *Transforming Nursing Education: The Culturally Inclusive Environment.* New York, NY: Springer Publishing Company, pp. 179–206.

Warren, B. J. (2010). Cultural competence in psychiatric nursing. In N. L. Keltner, L. H. Schwecke, & C. E. Bostrom (Eds.). *Psychiatric Nursing* (6th ed.). St. Louis: Mosby, pp. 164–172.

Warren, B. J., & Broome, B. (2011). CNE Series: The culture of adolescents with urologic dysfunction: Mental health, wellness, and illness awareness. *Urologic Nursing, 31*(2), 95–104.

Wellness Recovery Action Plan (WRAP). (2013). Available at http://nrepp.samhsa.gov/ViewIntervention.aspx?id=208.

Wheeler, K. (2013). *Psychotherapy for the Advanced Practice Psychiatric Nurse.* St. Louis, MO: Mosby.

Yeomans, F. E., & Levy, K. N. (2002). An object relations perspective on borderline personality disorder. *Acta Neropsychiatrica, 14,* 76–80.

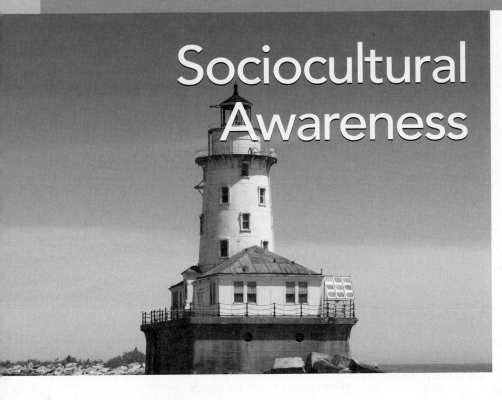

Sociocultural Awareness

5

Barbara J. Limandri

Learning Outcomes

1. Explain common terminology used when discussing the role of culture in providing psychiatric nursing care.

2. Compare theoretical frameworks that can assist nurses in providing culturally competent care.

3. Contrast variations in culture that may affect how individuals view and approach health care.

4. Summarize physical and mental health problems commonly seen in different cultures.

5. Apply principles of cultural sensitivity when working with patients and staff in mental health settings.

6. Evaluate the impact of societal influences on individual mental health and illness.

7. Plan culturally sensitive nursing care for patients with mental illness.

Key Terms

Lamont Clemmons Initial Onset

Lamont Clemmons is a 15-year-old high school student who was referred to the clinic because he was expelled from school after fighting with other students and bringing a handgun to school. Lamont's parents divorced when he was 5 years old; he lives with his father and stepmother and their three younger children. Lamont's father is a Caucasian man who grew up in rural Arkansas and married a Haitian woman he met through work. Although Lamont's father is over six feet tall, Lamont has his biological mother's slight stature and dark skin, which contribute to considerable bullying from other kids at Lamont's school. In the interview with the psychiatric nurse, Lamont explains that he took a handgun to school to show the bullies at school that he was "no sissy" and they needed to fear him. The nurse inquires about Lamont's heritage. Lamont responds aggressively by saying, "Don't you call me Black." He adds that he hates his mother and hopes "she goes back to that place she came from." He has refused to visit with his mother when she comes for court-approved visitations. He has reported to teachers that his mother beats him and denies him food when she has him stay with her; however, several investigations have failed to substantiate this accusation. Following the initial assessment and discussions with both Lamont and his father, Lamont is assigned to work with an advanced practice psychiatric nurse (APRN) named Claire McGill.

> ### APPLICATION
>
> 1. What are your concerns about Lamont at this time?
>
> 2. What additional assessment information do you think would be helpful in determining Lamont's needs?
>
> 3. What sociological or cultural factors are important for the nurse working with Lamont to consider?

Introduction

People differ in shapes, sizes, color, and scents based on their ethnicity and genetics. Languages, dialects, and accents vary even within the same nation. For example, in the United States, someone from Buffalo, New York, may find it difficult to understand an individual from Kecoughtan, Virginia, even though both are speaking English. Furthermore, when people move from one location to another, they may find a different way of life. The United States is a nation of immigrants to such an extent that its complexion has changed remarkably, as evidenced by current census data (Table 5-1).

In addition to general diversity, mental illness superimposes a layer of difference that frequently is associated with stigma. Those with mental illness, especially those with disorders of a persistent nature, have customs, institutions, and norms that distinguish them from others, adding to the challenge of recovery. To be effective, the nurse needs to understand and respect this culture and engage patients relative to their way of living. Therefore, it is important for the student to first be a sharp observer of the lifestyles and customs of patients while withholding judgment.

Defining Culture

Identifying an individual's culture entails more than knowing the person's race or nation of origin. A simplistic definition of culture is that it is the way of life for a group of people with specific shared values, beliefs, and traditions. However, culture is more complex than that. As stated in Chapter 1, the definition of culture specifies an integrated pattern of behavior. To expand on this, UNESCO defines **culture** as "the set of distinctive, spiritual, material, intellectual, and emotional features of society or a social group . . . that encompasses in addition to art and literature, lifestyles, ways of living together, value systems, traditions, and beliefs" (UNESCO, 2001). Both these definitions portray culture as learned, intergenerationally transmitted and transformed, and dynamic. Although the people in the group may share a common race, national origin, religion, and so forth, they might not have any of that in common and instead share a sense of purpose, status, and attitudes (Eshun, 2009). Culture extends beyond national origin and race and includes how any designated group of people share common values that must be considered relevant to their holistic health state. For example, nurses may compose a

Population by Race in the United States: 2000 and 2010   table 5-1

Race	2000		2010		Change 2000–2010	
	Number	Percentage of total population	Number	Percentage of total population	Number	Percent
American Indian and Alaska Native	2,475,956	0.9	2,932,248	0.9	456,292	18.4
Asian	10,242,998	3.6	14,674,252	4.8	4,431,254	43.3
Black or African American	34,658,190	12.3	38,929,319	12.6	4,271,129	12.3
Hispanic or Latino Origin or Race	35,305,818	12.5	50,477,594	16.3	15,171,776	43.0
Native Hawaiian or other Pacific Islanders	398,835	0.1	540,013	0.2	141,178	35.4
Some Other Race	15,359,073	5.5	19,107,368	6.2	3,748,295	24.4
White	211,460,626	75.1	223,553,265	72.4	12,092,639	5.7

Sources: U.S. Census Bureau, *Census 2000 Redistricting Data (Public Law 94–171) Summary File*, and *2010 Census Redistricting Data (Public Law 94–171) Summary File*.

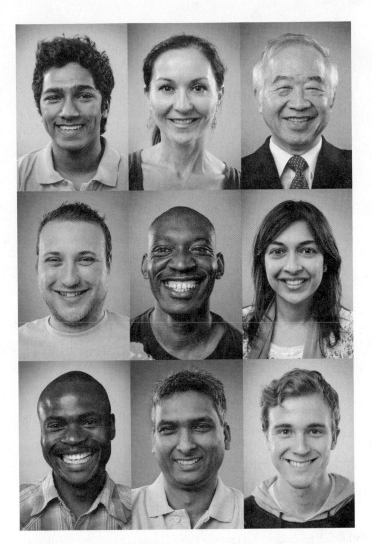

5-1 The population of the United States is becoming more diverse. Are you ready to work with patients from different backgrounds? Races? Cultural views? Spiritual beliefs?

Source: Warren Goldswain/Fotolia

cultural group that internally demonstrates a conflict of caring for others and caring for self. It is not at all uncommon to see nurses extending their physical and mental capabilities to accommodate others at their own expense.

The U.S. Census Bureau reports population distribution by categories of ethnicities that are generally recognized in this country, including the term "Hispanic," which is used to refer to people who are "of Cuban, Mexican, Puerto Rican, South or Central American, or other Spanish culture or origin" (Humes, Jones, & Ramirez, 2010). However, there are people who were born in Mexico who do not have Spanish origin; that is, they were indigenous to Mexico before Spain occupied it. As a result of historically large numbers of immigrants from Western Europe, a large percentage of the U.S. population is considered White: approximately 72%. According to the 2010 census, a percentage that reflects a net decrease from the 2000 census by 5.7%. By contrast, Asian and Hispanic/Latino populations in the United States have increased by 43% each. Other than those of indigenous and White Americans, the percentages of all racial and ethnic groups in the total population of the United States have increased over the past 10 years (Figure 5-1). Texas, the District of Columbia, Hawaii, and New Mexico have a majority–minority; that is, their state populations have a majority of people of the nondominant White culture (Humes, Jones, & Ramirez, 2010).

Culture becomes an issue of dominance when one group of people determines policies, practices, and societal patterns regardless of the views of people who are fewer in number. Dominance may become accepted as normal and reasonable simply because it is common. A timely example is that the American culture has different beliefs about marriage. Some hold that marriage should be between a man and a woman only. Some hold that marriage may also be between two men or between two women. Others believe that marriage may involve multiple partners and multiple relationships within the marriage. The topic of marriage in American culture brings a great deal of emotional charge with it because individuals view marriage from the perspective of their own individual belief systems.

Culture, therefore, introduces conflict because our identities, strong beliefs, and perceptions are based on culture. In a pluralistic society such as that of the United States, these identities are likely to clash. It becomes important for nurses to understand culture in general and examine their own cultural background as it influences their practice. This is especially true in mental health nursing. The DSM-5 introduced a cultural formulation interview (discussed in detail later in this chapter) in which the clinician can assess the role culture plays in the mental health and illness of patients from both the patient's perspective and that of a caregiver or close informant. The interview guide helps the nurse focus on important aspects of culture with minimal cultural bias.

Terminology Related to Culture

What is culture and how is it related to mental health nursing and people with mental health issues? Culture is a way of life that shapes perceptions, thoughts, lifestyle, pace of life, attitudes, and beliefs. It is largely influenced by ecology in that the natural surroundings and climate shape skin color and texture, words in the language, and awareness of what is normal and abnormal. Those who live in Arctic climates have multiple words for snow and cold, for example, and because their skin is rarely exposed to the elements, it has a texture indicative of that. Similarly, those who live in sub-Saharan climates have dark skin and different sweat gland distribution to manage the heat, sun intensity, and dry air. So what happens when an individual from Kenya moves to Antarctica? Does his or her skin acclimate? No, because an individual's body responds to his or her ecology. Culture is also generationally determined and shared with successive generations, both deliberately and unconsciously. In this way, cultural responses are learned.

Cultural competence is defined as "[h]aving the capacity to function effectively as an individual and an organization within the context of the cultural beliefs, behaviors and needs presented by consumers and their communities" (U.S. Department of Health and Human Services, Office of Minority Health, 2013, p. 138). In reality, nurses and health care providers probably can never achieve full cultural competence, but instead are constantly striving to acquire knowledge about different cultures. Through that knowledge comes greater awareness, skill, and sensitivity. Chapter 1 introduced the National Standards on Culturally and Linguistically Appropriate Services (CLAS), in which the first standard is that "[h]ealth care organizations should ensure that patients/consumers receive from all staff members effective, understandable, and respectful care that is provided in a manner compatible with their cultural health beliefs and practices and preferred language" (U.S. Department of Health and Human Services, Office of Minority Health, 2013, p. 56). By federal mandate, all mental health services need to provide services that include multicultural and multilingual staff and appropriately trained interpreters who not only translate the patient's words but also the cultural meaning conveyed. Nurses and other staff need to be adequately prepared in different cultural practices to understand each individual.

Because culture involves race and ethnicity, it is important to distinguish between these concepts. **Race** is based on genetically determined and geographically based characteristics. Often, but not always, it is apparent through skin color, which is a biological adaptation to the geography that may vary as groups of people migrate and intergenerate. **Ethnicity** includes race in that it describes how a group of people share common characteristics, such as nationality, religion, language, and cultural heritage. For example, an individual with olive-toned skin may be Caucasian by race and Italian by ethnicity, or an individual with dark skin may be African American by race and Southern American by ethnicity.

To comprehend and be competent in all aspects of culture requires nurses to have **cultural humility**—that is, to recognize the limitations of their own culture and be motivated to learn about other cultures (Dayer-Berenson, 2011). Being open to how individuals behave and respond to their environment, asking questions rather than assuming meaning, and engaging in discussion about how culture influences the patient's response to illness demonstrates cultural competence and humility.

Pause and Reflect

1. *What is your own cultural background? To what extent do you practice customs or hold values due to your cultural background?*
2. *In what ways does your cultural background, values, or customs influence how you view or treat others?*
3. *How motivated are you to learn about other cultures? Why?*

Theoretical Foundations

Given the complexity of culture, it is clear that the nurse working in a multicultural society needs to be competent in caring for others in a culturally sensitive way. A number of theories and conceptual frameworks can guide nurses in this process.

Leininger's Transcultural Nursing Theory

In 1995, Madeleine Leininger introduced the term **transcultural nursing**, which she defined as the caring practice of helping individuals achieve and maintain health or reach death in a culturally relevant way (Leininger & McFarland, 2006). Leininger received her doctorate in anthropology during a time when nurses were going to other disciplines that are foundational to nursing to build the knowledge base of the discipline. She recommended that nurses learn about the cultures of patients to better understand and anticipate behavior and provide sensitive care (Dayer-Berenson, 2011). Leininger coined the phrase **cultural pain** in describing the incongruency between the patient's cultural needs and the nurse's inappropriate response or lack of response. The theory of culture care provides both a basis for holistic practice and a mechanism for theory-based research. Leininger's theory was not only the first nursing theory proposed to guide nursing development, practice, and education, but also has been the most enduring broad-based theory.

Leininger's Sunrise Enabler Model

The Sunrise Enabler Model depicts the interrelationships among world view; the dimensions of cultural and social structures; and the influences on care expressions, patterns and practices, and holistic health/illness/death within the contexts of folk care, nursing care, and general professional care. These, in turn, provide the basis for transcultural care decisions and actions contributing to health care preservation/maintenance, accommodation and negotiation, and re-patterning and restructuring care (Leininger, 2002). In essence, the model guides the nurse to listen carefully and nonjudgmentally to patients as individuals, families, or communities, both in clarifying the issues the patients are dealing with as well as the world view in which the patients experience the issues. The nurse needs to include in the assessment the ways the patient addresses self-care and encourage the patient to freely offer what might improve his or her health. If the patient includes the cultural practice of coining (an Asian traditional practice of firmly rubbing a lubricated coin on the skin to relieve certain ailments), for example, the nurse needs to include this in the assessment and plan of care, even if the nurse does not fully comprehend or endorse this practice. Additionally, the nurse advocates for the patient with other health providers to sustain culturally relevant care.

Giger and Davidhizar's Transcultural Assessment Model

Initially, Giger and Davidhizar (2002) developed their model from Leininger's general theory and then substantiated the elements through research by others over time. The model specifies six dimensions of culture that are essential in nursing assessment, with an underlying assumption that every patient is culturally unique. Because culture is consistent and intergenerationally transmitted, there are commonalities that can help focus assessment (Figure 5-2, Table 5-2). These dimensions are communication, space, social organization, perception and use of time, environmental context, and biological variations (Giger and Davidhizar, 2002):

- *Communication* entails both verbal and nonverbal language and frequently contributes to misunderstanding patients and misinterpreting cues that influence nursing diagnosis. Assessing communication must include determining what the patient conveys through both speech and nonverbal communication.

- *Space* includes the proxemics that individuals maintain in relation to others. For example, Americans frequently require more physical distance between each other in conversation, whereas Arabs tend to require much less distance (Yassim, 1981).

- *Social organization* refers to kinship structures, roles, and beliefs. This includes the closeness of nuclear and extended family members, how the family treats elder members, and the roles members assume in relation to each other and the family as a unit.

- *Perception and use of time* are highly culturally determined. Some cultures show more polychronic orientation with a sense of fluidity and flexibility, whereas other cultures have more linear, monochronic orientation with expectations of single tasks and

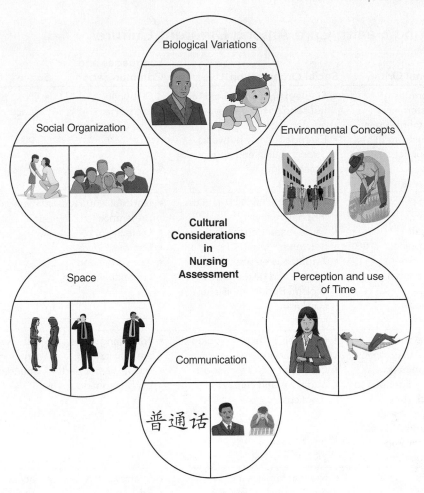

5-2   Giger and Davidhizar's Transcultural Assessment Model.

being exactly on time for appointments. In the polychronic orientation, the individual views time in relative terms and may be the one who is always late for events, whereas the individual with monochronic orientation views time in absolute terms—that is, for example, 9 a.m. means exactly 9 a.m. Time also includes present, past, and future orientation that may influence a person's health care and disease prevention activities.

- *Environmental context* influences sense of self-control, such as the awareness of having control over one's fate and outcomes as opposed to being at the mercy of the environment. This can be especially relevant with patients who are confined for long periods of time in hospitals or forensic settings. Without a sense of autonomy, the individual may be more prone to behavioral outbursts as a way to reassert his or her sense of self. Similarly, crowded conditions and nonstimulating interior structures frequently seen in forensic settings may elicit emotional responses that are not usually acceptable in specific cultures (Parish, 2013; Riemer, 2009).

- *Biological variations* reflect genetic and physical responsiveness. For example, genetic and ethnic variations occur in the cytochrome p450 system and the ability to metabolize food and drugs. Such variations need to be included in an assessment, as some individuals may respond to much smaller doses of medication than are usually seen as therapeutic. African Americans,

for example, frequently are given first-generation antipsychotic medications at larger doses than they can tolerate (Hudson, Cody, Armitage, Curtis, & Sullivan, 2005).

The benefit of Giger and Davidhizar's model is that it offers a practical and efficient template for nurses to incorporate into their thinking process when assessing patients. It carries forth Leininger's theoretical approach in a thoughtful manner and is based on solid research. One controversial aspect of both approaches is that they can contribute to stereotyping because they are based heavily on applying knowledge about a culture in general to an individual in particular. **Stereotyping** can be defined as overgeneralizing group characteristics that reinforce societal biases and distort individual characteristics (Grandbois & Sanders, 2012). No individual can be expected to represent an entire culture faithfully, and there is wide individual variation in how a group of people manifests a culture. This leads to the third theoretical framework, proposed by Campinha-Bacote, who addresses the issue of cultural competency in nursing care.

Campinha-Bacote and Culturally Competent Care

Campinha-Bacote emphasizes that cultural competence is a process rather than an endpoint and requires five elements: awareness, knowledge, skill, encounters, and desire (Campinha-Bacote, 2002). Each of these elements is essential and contributes to each other.

Variations Affecting Health Care Among Different Cultures | table 5-2

	National Origin	Social Organization	Languages and Communication	Space	Time Organization
African American	• Countries of Western and Southern Africa • Dominican Republic • Haiti • Jamaica	• Single-parent households and households headed by women are common • Extended family networks • Strong church and community organizations	• National languages • Use of dialects	• Close personal space	• Present over future
Asian and Pacific Islanders	• China • Japan • Hawaii • Philippines • Vietnam • Asian India • Korea • Samoa • Guam	• Hierarchical family structures emphasize loyalty • Large, extended family networks • Tradition is emphasized • Established religions include Taoism, Buddhism, Islam, Hinduism	• National language preference • Dialects • Use of silence • Nonverbal and contextual cueing	• Prefer no contact	• Present
American Indian and Alaskan Native	• More than 500 American Indian nations are indigenous to North America. • Native Alaskans include Aleuts and Eskimo populations.	• Emphasis on family—biological and extended • Children taught to respect traditions and cultural practices	• Tribal languages are maintained. • Use of silence and body language	• Space is important and has no boundaries	• Present
Latino/Hispanic	• Spain • Cuba • Mexico • Central & South America • Puerto Rico	• Nuclear families are emphasized as well as extended family networks. • Strong church and community affiliations	• Spanish • Portuguese	• Tactile relationships • Touch, handshakes, embracing	• Present
White/European Americans	• Countries of the United Kingdom • Germany • Some Mediterranean countries • Scandinavian countries • Former Soviet Union countries	• Nuclear and extended families are emphasized. • Judeo-Christian religions • Community social organizations	• Many early immigrants valued learning English over using native language • Verbal more than nonverbal	• Northern European more aloof & distant • Southern European closer contact & touch	• Future over present

Source: Based on Spector, R. (2013). Cultural Diversity in Health and Illness (8th ed.). San Francisco, CA: Pearson.

Cultural awareness begins with the nurse's self-examination and continual reflection on his or her own roots, biases, and prejudice. By the very nature of culture, all individuals have strong beliefs and identities that influence their ways of being with others. Without full awareness of their own cultural background, nurses may respond to others blindly with possible ethnocentrism. By seeking **cultural knowledge**—information about other cultures and ethnic groups—nurses can widen their perceptions to be more inclusive and use this knowledge to employ **cultural skill** to assess others and provide care that incorporates cultural knowledge. Cultural awareness

also assists nurses to seek out diverse **cultural encounters**—conversations and exchanges with individuals of other cultures—that further validate, refine, and expand the nurse's own beliefs and values about culture. Finally, cultural competence involves a **cultural desire**—a personal motivation to be culturally competent and not just meeting some external requirement. It is the juncture of all five elements that contributes to cultural competency (Campinha-Bacote, 1999).

Incorporating Campinha-Bacote's model into tools for assessment allows the nurse to engage with the patient in a culturally relevant manner. A mnemonic, ETHNIC, guides the nurse in patient assessment and development of culturally sensitive interventions:

- **Explanation:** Ask the patient what the patient believes caused the problem and what started it. Determine what the patient calls the problem.

- **Treatment:** Ask the patient what kind of treatment he or she thinks would be helpful and what the patient hopes to experience from treatment.

- **Healers:** Ask the patient who has helped with the problem now and in the past. What did that person do for the patient that was helpful?

- **Negotiate:** Ask what the patient believes will work the best in recovering from the problem, and how the nurse can help the patient at this time.

- **Intervene:** Engage in culturally sensitive nursing interventions based on the assessment and negotiation with the patient.

- **Collaborate:** Work with the patient, family, and other healers and providers to achieve the best outcome for the patient (Campinha-Bacote, 2011).

In using Campinha-Bacote's model, the nurse can develop a better understanding of the patient and therefore provide care that meets the patient's needs holistically. Each of these encounters with culturally diverse patients further expands the nurse's cultural competency.

Pause and Reflect

1. *How might cultural social organization affect individual mental health or perception of mental illness?*

2. *Why does Campinha-Bacote view cultural competence in nursing as a process? What implications does this have for the individual nurse? For you?*

Sociological and Cultural Influences

Environment and culture often interact on a number of levels. Sociological needs of love and belonging, safety, and economic survival are often met through the individual's interactions in both the sociological and cultural domains. Within the context of the sociological domain, family structures and practices greatly influence individual mental health and illness. The specific interplay of family in mental health and illness is discussed throughout this text, with treatment of family dysfunction through therapy discussed in detail in Chapter 24. Another sociological factor that has implications for patients with mental health issues and psychiatric disorders is the concept of stigma.

Culture, Society, and Family

Because culture is manifested in the social organization, the family is the primary vehicle for cultural transmission. The family has not only general traditions and legacies, but also specific health practices that are passed on through the generations, overtly and covertly. The famous "chicken soup cure" for common illnesses is an example of a cultural health practice embedded in family life. Such practices do not have to make sense or meet criteria for evidence-based practice for them to be worthwhile in maintaining traditions in families. In one family, when a child is cranky and not sleeping or eating as well as usual, it is time for an enema. Another family may assert avoiding swimming when a young woman is having her menstrual period.

Even consumption of large amounts of vitamin C in tablet form or through foods to prevent or treat the common cold can be a hard-fought battle against science. Some mothers insist that sugar causes children to become hyperactive and maintain practices to reaffirm this belief, in total disregard for scientific evidence that says otherwise.

Family structures are similarly important in health care. Often, in many cultures, the mother makes significant decisions about health care. The family expects the mother to make appointments for health care and maintenance; when the mother is not available or able to carry out this function, the family struggles to meet health needs. There may also be strong beliefs related to mental health that serves as a challenge in maintaining health. For example, many cultures believe that emotional and behavioral issues should remain in the family only and not be discussed among strangers, including mental health professionals. In a psychiatric interview, the mental health nurse may struggle to elicit a family history of mental health issues because the family does not share this type of information publicly. The cultural heritage of the family may dictate that mental illness is the consequence of evil or misdeeds and, therefore, must be kept secret and tolerated in private. Families who consider mental illness related to evil or misbehavior are not likely to consider seeking help or using community health to address symptoms of depression or psychosis (Saechao et al., 2012; Ungar, 2010).

Culture, Mental Health, and Stigma

The most obvious effect of culture on mental health is stigma. Regardless of the cultural background, mental illness and treatment for mental health issues is fraught with misconceptions and stereotypes, resulting in stigma. The notion of stigma conveys shame and humiliation, something to conceal and hide (Idemudia & Matamela, 2012). It can come from society in general through stereotypic messages about people with mental illness, humor about "crazy people," and even indirectly through media depictions of those with mental illness in fact or in fiction (for example, the movie *One Flew Over the Cuckoo's Nest*). This is referred to as **enacted stigma** (actual discrimination or mistreatment related to having a stigmatizing condition) and can be exquisitely painful (Idemudia & Matamela, 2012). A timely example of stigmatization is the public discussion about gun violence and associations to people with mental illness. Even though someone with a mental illness can perpetrate violence, such acts are equally likely in those without mental illness. When an individual who suffers from depression or schizophrenia or has a close relative with a mental illness reads reports that associate violence with people who are mentally ill, he or she may feel ashamed or fearful or doubt himself or herself. Imagine how difficult it would be for this individual then to seek services for his or her illness. This becomes **internalized stigma**, in which the individual accepts the stigma as a characteristic of self that contributes to self-hatred (Idemudia & Matamela, 2012).

Stigma affects health professionals as well, because all health professionals are a product of their culture and experience the same societal messages as the lay public. Nurses and staff in general areas of a hospital and in emergency departments have frequent contact with patients who have psychiatric illnesses. Research indicates that these patients have reported being isolated in the emergency department and left for hours without services or monitoring beyond in-room cameras or occasional visits. Their illnesses are not always taken seriously in primary care or when they are hospitalized for acute medical problems (Shim & Rust, 2013). Primary care and behavioral health have had to compete for scarce resources instead of collaborating to provide quality care for patients, regardless of the origins of their illnesses. Consequently, such health care stigmatization contributes to poor health outcomes; for example, patients with schizophrenia die up to 25 years earlier than those without schizophrenia (Shim, 2013). Several studies have identified the persistent public stigmatization not only of those with mental illness, but also of those who care for them (Pescosolido, Medina, Martin, & Long, 2013; Halter, 2008). Guilt by association contributes to psychiatric nurses seen as "not real nurses" or that caring for those with mental illness entails "just talking." Not only might this pull skilled nurses and other health professionals away from psychiatric care, it may also diminish how patients who need these services value psychiatric care.

Psychiatric diagnoses may be distorted by culture, for example, there are culture bound syndromes that would be considered an illness if viewed out of the cultural context. Consider the following clinical example:

> Family members brought their school-age boy to the emergency department of a small urban hospital because he had a high fever and was lethargic and confused. When the nurse undressed the child, he observed bruising over the child's back in a distinctive pattern of 3-cm circles. Thinking this was abuse, the nurse wanted to call in the social worker to interview the child and parents. The nursing assistant, who also was present in the room, recognized the bruising pattern as the practice of coining to draw out illness. She explained it to the nurse. The nurse was relieved that he had not called in the social worker and learned a valuable lesson of not jumping to conclusions before trying to understand common health practices used by some Asian families to try to treat various illnesses.

Pause and Reflect

1. *Think about recent events and how they have been portrayed in the media. How does the media portray events in ways that may promote the stigmatization of individuals with mental illness?*
2. *What concerns you when you hear reports of patients with mental illness being isolated and practically ignored in acute care settings? Why is it important to prioritize care for these patients as you would any other patient with an acute illness?*

Providing Culturally Competent Care in Psychiatric Nursing

Providing culturally competent care for patients with psychiatric disorders involves more than learning stereotypical characteristics of different ethnic and racial groups. It involves a process of learning about one's own cultural heritage and respecting that legacy. It involves allowing all patients to provide information about their culture and listening intently to how they view health and illness: What does this illness mean to the patient and to the family? What would the patient do to heal from this illness or these symptoms, and who would the patient want to help him or her?

Nurses incorporate these perspectives and practices into the overall care they provide. They involve the family members by asking them to explain what this illness means to them, and how it affects each family member. In partnering with the patient and family, the psychiatric nurse is both the student and the teacher for the patient. The nurse learns about the cultural beliefs and practices of the patient and integrates additional knowledge about illness and health into the patient's knowledge.

Culturally competent care is person-centered and based on the recognition that the patient has autonomy and personal knowledge that is as powerful as the clinician's knowledge. The two forms of knowledge need to be blended together in equal proportions. The patient and family become active members of the treatment team and not people added after the staff has conceptualized the problem. The nurse may need to bring in a culture broker to help with this integration of knowledge. This may be someone from the patient's community who can provide knowledge and resources about the culture, and may include a consumer advocate to provide an understanding of the culture of being a psychiatric patient.

The culturally competent psychiatric nurse acknowledges the disparity in mental health services and seeks to distribute care in a more equitable manner. This will require more than the individual nurse's effort and will involve organized nursing prompted by nurses' associated efforts. It is evident that mental health care is different for those who are White, well-educated, and employed with health benefits. Research shows that people of color are much more often diagnosed with psychotic conditions and less often with depressive or anxiety disorders; are more frequently medicated with first-generation antipsychotics that are less expensive but have serious side effects; are more likely to be overmedicated, even with the knowledge of differential pharmacokinetics affecting dosage effects; and typically receive shorter treatment appointments (Carpenter-Song et al., 2011; Williams, 1986). People from Asian cultures frequently are misdiagnosed with physical problems without receiving treatment for mental health problems such as depressive and anxiety disorders. Mental health providers may not recognize the cultural transitions and strain experienced by immigrants and refugees or not allow enough time and support for these individuals who are settling into a new cultural environment (Sonethavilay et al., 2011). Cultural competency involves more than having sufficient interpreters available for communicating with patients. The DSM-5 includes **culture-bound syndromes,** or disorders, found among different cultural groups; however, these are to be considered with caution, as they may evoke a stereotypic view of behavior as much as an enlightened perception. Table 5-3 summarizes some common health problems attributed to different cultural beliefs.

Vulnerable and At-Risk Populations

Although all individuals experience anxiety and symptoms of sadness or fear from time to time, some populations are more vulnerable to experiencing mental illness than others. Vulnerability may be related to race/ethnicity, ability status, age, gender, sexual orientation, geography, or socioeconomic status. Social determinants of health are those circumstances shaped by economics and politics of where individuals grow, live, and work. They include poverty, unemployment, underemployment, educational opportunities, and health disparities of race, ethnicity, and stigma about mental illness. These

Common Physical and Mental Health Problems of Different Cultural Groups

table 5-3

	Physical Problems	Mental Health Problems
African American	*Mal puesto*, hex, root-work, or voodoo involves unnatural deaths. Unnatural diseases and death result from the power of people who use evil spirits.	*Boufée delirante:* sudden outburst of agitation and aggression, confusion, or hallucinations *Falling out:* sudden collapse without warning in response to trauma *Zar:* altered state of consciousness in which the person is possessed by a spirt and may shout, weep, laugh, bang head against the wall, or sing *Brain fog:* physical and mental exhaustion, difficulty concentrating, memory loss, irritability, and sleep and appetite disturbances
Asians and Pacific Islanders	*Koro:* sensation that the penis is retracting into the abdomen and, when it disappears, death will result. *Wind/cold illness:* fear of wind and cold contributing to weakness and susceptibility to illness when the natural elements are imbalanced. *Karoshi:* death by overwork.	*Latah:* startle reaction with imitative fearful and defensive behaviors beyond control and compliant to suggestions of others *Amok:* sudden outburst of aggression followed by apathy and withdrawal *Sinking heart:* sensation in the chest and heart that resemble both cardiovascular disease and depression caused by excessive heat, exhaustion, worry, or social failure
American Indian and Alaskan Native	*Ghost sickness:* weakness and dizziness caused by a curse by evil forces and ghosts of deceased members.	*Wacinko:* feelings of anger, withdrawal, mutism, and suicide in response to interpersonal disappointment and rejection *Windigo/witiko:* intense urge for cannibalism with disgust for ordinary food and feelings of depression and anxiety that may lead to homicide, suicide, or death by starvation
Latino/Hispanic	*Fatigue:* asthma-like symptoms. *Pasmo:* paralysis-like symptoms in face or limbs. *Empacho:* food forms into a ball and clings to the stomach, causing pain and cramps. *Mal ojo:* sudden unexplained illness in a usually well person, attributed to the evil eye. *Wind/cold illness:* fear of wind and cold contributing to weakness and susceptibility to illness when the natural elements are imbalanced. *Mal puesto*, hex, root-work, or voodoo involves unnatural deaths. Unnatural diseases and death result from the power of people who use evil spirits.	*Susto/espanto:* sudden fear of losing one's soul causing shock, weight loss, excessive thirst, and possibly death *Ataque de nervosa:* screaming, falling to the ground, wildly moving arms and legs, intense crying resulting from the evil eye

Based on Spector, R. (2013). *Cultural Diversity in Health and Illness* (8th ed.). San Francisco, CA: Pearson; Tseng, W. (2006). From peculiar psychiatric disorders through culture-bound syndromes to culture-related specific syndromes. *Transcultural Psychiatry, 43*(4), 554–576.

factors overlap and contribute to greater vulnerability. The following are a few examples:

- The individual with hearing impairment who has schizophrenia may not be able to adequately communicate his distress or receive sufficient therapeutic engagement.
- The rural preteen who is discovering her attraction to girls may risk being disowned by her family or experience severe depression that places her at high risk for suicide.
- The farm worker who immigrated from Mexico worries that he cannot support his immediate and extended family without leaving them for long periods of time, and perceives discussing these worries with psychiatric providers as weakness and family betrayal.

All these individuals are vulnerable to severe mental illness and face barriers to access to care.

Working with populations who are vulnerable requires innovative and culturally sensitive means of reaching out and inviting individuals to receive care in a way that is relevant to them. This can require creativity, and nursing students and professional nurses alike can share in efforts to serve these populations. For example, nursing students in a health promotion class attended a mobile health clinic for migrant farm workers, where they provided blood pressure and depression screenings. They were prepared with discount coupons for follow-up appointments with local mental health providers and primary care clinics. Another group of students provided a sex education class in an urban alternative high school for pregnant teens, in which they also

Cultural Formulation Interview

box 5-1

The Cultural Formulation Interview (CFI) may be used by any clinician, including the nurse, to elicit a patient's cultural understanding of a mental health issue and to clarify the role of social and cultural influences on the patient's health status. Aspects of the CFI include questions to:

- Assess the patient's view of the presenting problem and priority concerns.
- Determine the patient's perceptions of how others (e.g., family, friends) view the presenting problem.
- Assess the patient's social supports and stressors.
- Assess key aspects of the patient's identity or background that affect the patient's well-being.

- Assess coping mechanisms and sources of help.
- Elicit information about barriers the patient has experienced to mental health or to accessing treatment in the past.
- Elicit and address patient concerns about the therapeutic relationship, treatment, and other aspects of health care.

It is important to remember that patient perspectives on mental health and illness can be influenced by world view, upbringing, and both personal and cultural values and beliefs. These are of great importance to providing nursing care. In particular, patients benefit when their help-seeking patterns and preferences for traditional, alternative, or complementary care are incorporated into the care plan.

Data from the *Diagnostic and Statistical Manual of Mental Disorders*, Fifth Edition, (Copyright 2013). American Psychiatric Association.

---

discussed family violence and gender dysphoria. For National Depression Screening Day, held annually in October nationwide, providers in a community near several large military bases targeted National Guard members and veterans for depression and suicide screening. Positive screenings resulted in private, brief counseling to refer the individual for follow-up with providers specially trained in war trauma.

Caring for Patients of Different Cultures

The logical starting point for caring for patients is the assessment process. Elsewhere in this text are general mental health assessment tools and guides. The DSM-5 has introduced some useful assessment measures in Section III of the manual that are available online.

The WHO Disability Assessment Schedule (WHODAS 2.0) is a tool that all students should review and learn to administer and score. It is a 36-item self-report that can be provided at intake of new patients in the hospital or mental health clinic with follow-up reassessment to evaluate progress. Using this tool in conjunction with a recovery-oriented plan provides a way to assess the patient's starting point and level of commitment for change. The nurse can then engage the patient in motivational interviewing to design a plan of care to help the patient reduce his or her level of disability. Re-administering the

WHODAS periodically also provides an objective means of demonstrating outcomes of treatment (World Health Organization, 2012).

Another important tool for the nurse to use in assessment is the Cultural Formulation Interview (CFI), which explores four domains: cultural definition of the problem; cultural perceptions of the cause, content, and support; cultural factors affecting self-coping and past help-seeking; and cultural factors affecting current help-seeking (Box 5-1). This tool helps the nurse clarify patients' cultural identity and description of distress from their cultural perspective. It also identifies stressors that place patients at risk and their level of resilience. Finally, the CFI allows the nurse to identify features of culture that influence the relationship between the patient and the clinician. Using this tool early in the relationship with the patient establishes the cultural context of the relationship and demonstrates to the patient that the nurse seeks to provide culturally relevant care.

In the practical sense, nurses need to expand their cultural awareness not just by reading about different cultures, but also by experiencing them. Campinha-Bacote states that nursing care is culturally sensitive when there is an interaction on the part of the nurse with cultural awareness, cultural knowledge, skill, encounters with multicultural situations, and a desire to explore beyond one's own

---

Lamont Recovery Phase

critical thinking

During several weeks of therapy with Claire McGill, the APRN, Lamont is sullen, refuses to talk, does not do his therapy homework (for instance, keeping track of his emotions during the week, practicing some emotion regulation skills), and misses several sessions of the skills group he was required to attend. In one session, Claire asks Lamont to draw a picture of himself and is surprised to see that he draws an image of a tall, muscular, light-skinned person with a semiautomatic rifle in each hand and a mean facial expression. His explanation of the picture is that he is "the meanest SOB alive." Underneath the meanness, though, he agrees that he hates the "little Black boy" he sees in the mirror. At the end of that session, Lamont threatens Claire. He is transferred to Scott Weber, a male APRN.

Again, after several sessions, Lamont becomes aggressive and threatening. This time, however, Scott takes him to a gym and the two of them work out together using the elliptical equipment and working with a punching bag. Scott works with Lamont to increase Lamont's time engaged in physical activity and exercise. Within a few more months, Lamont is able to discuss his self-hatred verbally with Scott and practice his verbal skills in group. Lamont begins to develop a muscular physique and begins playing soccer with a team. Other teens admire his skills on the soccer field and ask him to teach them some of his moves.

Eventually, Lamont is able to return to regular high school and begins to read about his Haitian heritage. He has not been able to reunite with his mother, though, because she returned to Haiti and relinquished custody to Lamont's father and stepmother.

APPLICATION

1. How does Lamont's aggressive behavior relate to his cultural identity?

2. What might have made the difference in the two APRNs' work with Lamont?

3. How might family affect Lamont's identity? What concerns do you have for Lamont related to his family?

cultural experiences (Campinha-Bacote, 2011). Students who have the opportunity for international travel courses return with a new-found, deeper understanding about culture and recognize the significance of being outside the dominant culture. These experiences help students and nurses become empowered to care for people of all cultures in individualistic and person-centered ways. This is the essence of recovery in caring for those with mental disorders and distress. When nurses treat patients with respect, and honor their cultures of heritage, their family values, and their beliefs, they help patients open themselves to the therapeutic alliance and help them believe that there is hope for recovery and rehabilitation.

Pause and Reflect

1. *Why do you think racial disparities exist in the treatment of mental illness? What is the nurse's responsibility to patients at risk for receiving disparate or differential treatment?*

2. *How do social determinants affect individual health and well-being? What are some of the barriers that prevent individuals with mental illness from accessing care and treatment?*

3. *Now that you have read this chapter, what steps do you need to take next to continue in the process of developing cultural competence as a nurse?*

Chapter Highlights

1. Culture may be defined as a set of distinctive features of a society or social group that encompasses a way of living together, value systems, traditions, and beliefs.

2. Culture extends beyond national origin and race and includes how any designated group of people share common values relevant to their holistic health state.

3. Leininger's theory of transcultural nursing defines nursing as the caring practice of helping individuals achieve and maintain health in a culturally relevant way.

4. The transcultural assessment model emphasizes six dimensions of culture that are essential to assessing the unique cultural perspective of every patient: communication, space, social organization, perception and use of time, environmental context, and biological variations.

5. Campinha-Bacote emphasizes that cultural competence is a process that requires five essential elements: awareness, knowledge, skill, encounters, and desire.

6. Although some culture-bound syndromes such as wind/cold illness, ghost sickness, or *ataque de nervosa* have been identified among people from specific cultures, nurses must consider these with caution to prevent stereotyping.

7. Caring for patients from different cultures requires nurses to be competent in conducting culturally sensitive assessments. The WHO Disability Assessment Schedule and the Cultural Formulation Interview can assist nurses and other clinicians in assessing an individual's cultural values, beliefs, perceptions, and health-seeking behaviors.

NCLEX®-RN Questions

1. The nurse is caring for a patient from another culture. Which of the following best demonstrates an understanding and application of cultural competence?
   a. The nurse strives to incorporate an awareness of cultural behaviors and needs when providing care.
   b. The nurse recognizes the need to adhere to the patient's cultural practices regardless of safety outcomes.
   c. The nurse demonstrates the full capacity to exercise culturally informed care in a variety of situations and circumstances.
   d. The nurse modifies care according to the body of literature that explains the practices of individuals within various cultures.

2. The nurse is attempting to provide care for a patient who is receiving treatment for a mental health condition. When selecting a theoretical framework, the nurse recognizes that the selection of which model(s) has the potential to lead to overgeneralizing group characteristics?
   a. Leininger only
   b. Giger–Davidhizar only
   c. Leininger and Giger–Davidhizar
   d. Leininger and Campinha-Bacote

3. The nurse is caring for a patient from another culture who is chronically late for appointments. After discussing the issue with the patient, the nurse learns that the patient has difficulty understanding why Americans are so focused on strict schedules. The nurse recognizes that the patient's views are most likely the result of which culturally mediated factor?
   a. Proxemics
   b. Social organization
   c. Environmental context
   d. Polychronic orientation

4. The nurse is conducting a psychoeducation group for patients experiencing anxiety. The focus of the session is on mindfulness and awareness of the moment. Based on knowledge of sociocultural norms, which patient would the nurse anticipate having the most difficulty with these concepts?
   a. The Alaskan Native patient
   b. The Latino Hispanic patient
   c. The White European patient
   d. The patient from the West Indies

5. The nurse is using the Cultural Formulation Interview (CFI) to assess a patient presenting with mental health issues. The nurse recognizes that this tool offers which advantages? Select all that apply.
   a. Is available in a self-administered version
   b. Elicits health seeking patterns and preferences
   c. Can be used to measure progress across domains
   d. Assists in identifying the patient's priority concerns
   e. Provides information about relationships with providers

6. The nurse is evaluating the impact of societal influences on a young adult patient presenting with a major mental illness. The nurse understands that which factor is most likely to bias providers to the diagnosis of a psychotic disorder?
   a. The patient is uneducated.
   b. The patient is a person of color.
   c. The patient has a very stressful job.
   d. The patient comes from a rural area.

7. The nurse is providing care to the patient from another culture. The patient requests that the nurse assist the patient to carry out a complementary healing practice, with no known therapeutic value, that the nurse does not endorse. Which initial action is appropriate?
   a. Carry out the patient's request.
   b. Determine whether the practice is safe and feasible.
   c. Gently explain that the practice has no benefits.
   d. Teach the patient about more effective treatments.

Answers may be found on the Pearson student resource site: nursing.pearsonhighered.com

Pearson Nursing Student Resources Find additional review materials at: **nursing.pearsonhighered.com**

References

American Psychiatric Association. (2013). *Diagnostic and Statistical Manual of Mental Disorders* (5th ed.). Washington, DC: American Psychiatric Publishers.

Bernstein, K., Park, S., Shin, J., Cho, S., & Park, Y. (2011). Acculturation, discrimination and depressive syndrome among Korean immigrants in New York City. *Community Mental Health, 47*, 24–34.

Campinha-Bacote, J. (1999). A model and instrument for addressing cultural competence in health care. *Journal of Nursing Education, 38*(5), 203–207.

Campinha-Bacote, J. (2002). The process of cultural competence in the delivery of healthcare service. *Journal of Transcultural Nursing, 13*(3), 181–184.

Campinha-Bacote, J. (2011). Delivering patient-centered care in the midst of a cultural conflict: The role of cultural competence. *Online Journal of Issues in Nursing, 16*(2), 1.

Carpenter-Song, E., Widley, R., Lawson, W., Quimby, E., & Drake, R. (2011). Reducing disparities in mental health care: Suggestions from the Dartmouth-Howard collaboration. *Community Mental Health Journal, 47*, 1–13.

Davis, R. (2000). Cultural health care or child abuse? The Southeast Asian practice of Cao Gio. *Journal of the American Academy of Nurse Practitioners, 21*(2), 112–114.

Dayer-Berenson, L. (2011). *Cultural Competencies for Nurses: Impact on Health and Illness*. Sudbury, MA: Jones and Bartlett.

Eshun, S. A. (2009). *Culture and Mental Health: Sociocultural Influences, Theory, and Practice*. Chichester, West Sussex, UK: Wiley & Sons.

Giger, J. N., & Davidhizar, R. (2002). The Giger and Davidhizar transcultural assessment model. *Journal of Transcultural Nursing, 13*(3), 185–188.

Grandbois, D. M., & Sanders, G. F. (2012). Resilience and stereotyping: The experiences of Native American elders. *Journal of Transcultural Nursing, 23*(4), 389–396.

Halter, M. (2008). Perceived characteristics of psychiatric nurses: Stigma by association. *Archives of Psychiatric Nursing, 22*(1), 20–26.

Hansson, L., Jormfeldt, H., Svedberg, P., & Svensson, B. (2013). Mental health professionals' attitudes towards people with mental illness: Do they differ from attitudes held by people with mental illness? *International Journal of Social Psychiatry, 59*(1), 48–54.

Hudson, T., Cody, M., Armitage, T., Curtis, M., & Sullivan, G. (2005). Disparities in use of antipsychotic medications among nursing home residents in Arkansas. *Psychiatric Services, 56*(6), 749–751.

Humes, K., Jones, N., & Ramirez, R. (2010). *Overview of Race and Hispanic Origin: 2010*. (U. D. Commerce, Ed.) Washington, DC: U.S. Census Bureau.

Idemudia, E. S., & Matamela, N. A. (2012). *The role of stigmas in mental health: A comparative study. Curationis, 35*(1), E1-E8.

Jones, A. A. (2012). Shame and acute psychiatric care. *Mental Health Practice, 16*(4), 26–27.

Leininger, M. (2002). Culture care theory: A major contribution to advance transcultural nursing knowledge and practices. *Journal of Transcultural Nursing, 13*(3), 189–192.

Leininger, M. M., & McFarland, M. (2006). *Culture Care Diversity & Universality: A Worldwide Nursing Theory* (2nd ed.). Sudbury, MA: Jones and Bartlett.

McFarling, L., D'Angelo, M., Drain, M., Gibbs, D., & Olmsted, K. (2011). Stigma as a barrier to substance abuse and mental health treatment. *Military Psychology, 23*, 1–5.

Parish, C. (2013). Change ward culture to cut violence and aggression. *Mental Health Practice, 16*(10), 6–7.

Pescosolido, B., Medina, T., Martin, J., & Long, J. (2013). The "backbone" of stigma: Identifying the global core of public prejudice associated with mental illness. *American Journal of Public Health, 103*(5), 853–860.

Riemer, D. (2009). Creating sanctuary: Reducing violence in a maximum security forensic psychiatric hospital unit. *On the Edge, 15*(1), 1–8.

Saechao, F., Sharrock, S., Richertert, D., Livingston, J., Aylward, A., Whisnant, J., et al. (2012). Stressors and barriers to using mental health services among diverse groups of first-generation immigrants to the United States. *Community Mental Health Journal, 48*, 98–106.

Shim, R., & Rust, G. (2013). Primary care, behavioral health, and public health: Partners in reducing mental health stigma. *American Journal of Public Health, 103*(5), 774–776.

Sonethavilay, H., Miyabayashi, I., Komori, A., Onimaru, M., & Washio, M. (2011). Mental health needs and cultural barriers that lead to misdiagnosis of Southeast Asian Refugees: A review. *International Medical Journal, 18*(3), 169–171.

Spector, R. (2013). *Cultural Diversity in Health and Illness* (8th ed.). San Francisco, CA: Pearson.

Tseng, W. (2006). From peculiar psychiatric disorders through culture-bound syndromes to culture-related specific syndromes. *Transcultural Psychiatry, 43*(4), 554–576.

U.S. Department of Commerce. (2011). *United States Census Quick Facts*. United States Census Bureau: Available at http://quickfacts.census.gov/qfd/states/00000.html

U.S. Department of Health and Human Services. (2010). *The Registered Nurse Population: Initial Findings from the 2008 National Sample Survey of Registered Nurses*. Health Resources and Services Administration. Washington, DC: U.S. Department of Health and Human Services.

U.S. Department of Health and Human Services, Office of Minority Health. (2013). Culturally competent nursing care: A cornerstone of caring. Available at https://ccnm.thinkculturalhealth.hhs.gov/

UNESCO. (2001). *Universal Declaration on Cultural Diversity*. Available at UNESCO: www.unesco.org/confgen/press_rel/021101_clt_diversity.shtml

Ungar, M. (2010). Families as navigators and negotiators: Facilitating culturally and contextually specific expressions of resilience. *Family Process, 49*, 421–435.

Williams, D. (1986). The epidemiology of mental illness in Afro-Americans. *Hospital and Community Psychiatry, 37*(1), 42–49.

Wilson, D. (2010). Culturally competent psychiatric nursing care. *Journal of Psychiatric and Mental Health Nursing, 17*, 715–724.

Yassim, M. A. (1981). Arabs communicating: A sociolinguistic approach. *The Incorporated Linguist, 20*(3), 96–99.

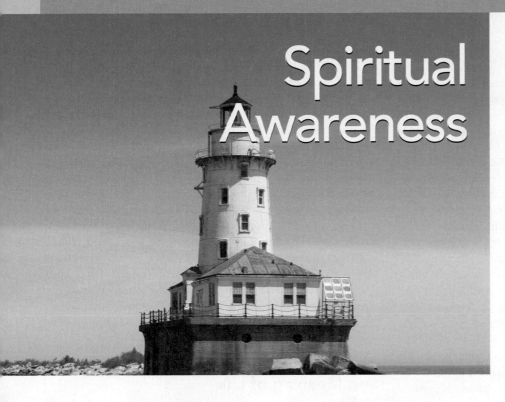

Spiritual Awareness

6

Martha Mathews Libster

Learning Outcomes

1. Discuss how different world views attempt to answer the major questions about life.

2. Compare the differences and similarities between the terms *spirituality* and *religion*.

3. Identify a process for assessing a patient's spirituality.

4. Discuss how and when spirituality can bring comfort to patients in distress.

5. Describe possible nursing diagnoses relating to a patient's spirituality.

6. Evaluate nursing interventions in relation to a patient's spiritual domain.

7. Plan evidence-based nursing care for patients with mental illness that takes their spiritual domain into account.

Key Terms

positivism, 101
postmodernism, 101
presence, 104
religion, 99
spirituality, 99
transcendent, 98
world view, 98

Perspectives on the Spiritual Domain

Understanding the spiritual domain is one of the most important—and yet most challenging—aspects of psychiatric nursing. It is important because an individual's spiritual beliefs and practices relate to the very nature of personhood, but it is challenging because there are many difficult, and sometimes controversial, issues to consider in relation to this domain. This challenge occurs for several reasons. First, there are many different perspectives about the nature of the spiritual domain across cultures and disciplines. Second, each patient has a different **world view**: the set of beliefs that individuals hold about the basic makeup of the world (Sire, 2004). Third, because patients possess different world views or beliefs, the spiritual domain is complicated to understand and to define, making both assessment and identification of appropriate interventions challenging. Finally, it can be difficult to determine the difference between a patient's spiritual and psychiatric experiences, causing some practitioners to be unsure about what might be appropriate nursing interventions. This chapter highlights some different perspectives regarding the nature of the spiritual domain and introduces different world views. This is followed by a discussion of nursing assessment and intervention in the spiritual domain, including discussion of situations in which it is difficult to determine the difference between the spiritual and psychiatric experiences of the patient.

Spirituality and Mental Health and Illness

Nursing students often find that practitioners have very different perspectives on the spiritual domain. Some choose to ignore it, some see it as a cause of their patient's difficulties, and others see it as an important strength of the patient. The following example illustrates what a particular group of nursing students experienced.

> A group of nursing students were interacting in an inpatient psychiatric unit with a male patient who was experiencing auditory hallucinations and delusions. He heard voices telling him to tell the students that they should repent because the world was coming to an end, and he believed that God was speaking to him through his MP3 player. When he finished talking to the students, he walked over to the window, looked out at the cross on a church across the street, crossed himself, genuflected, and walked away. The staff nurse who watched all this take place turned to the students and said, "I wish they would take down that cross. It makes our patients crazy."

This statement raises an important question for discussion: Is having religious beliefs a cause of or a solution to mental illness?

Even though some practitioners still have questions about the role of religion in their patients' health and wellness, there is a growing body of evidence to support a positive relationship between faith and mental health for many individuals. For example, evidence suggests that aspects of life such as coping, having hope, finding meaning and purpose in life, the ability to forgive, and an overall quality of life are related to having a religious faith (Koenig, 2005). Additional studies have found an association between intrinsic religiousness and greater life satisfaction (Salsman, Brown, Brechting, & Carlson, 2005); that religious individuals may have some protection against the physiological consequences of stress (Tartaro, Luecken, & Gunn,

2005); that spirituality is a predictor of better outcomes in schizophrenia and schizoaffective disorders (Mohr et al., 2011); and that religion may instill hope in individuals with schizophrenia (Mohr, et al., 2010). However, it is still very difficult to find definitive evidence about the relationship between religious beliefs and mental health and illness. Part of the reason for this is that researchers are still trying to define the terms that are important to understanding this relationship and to determine how to measure them.

Another reason why the relationship between religion and mental health and illness has been challenging to determine is that, historically, mental health professionals and representatives of various faith traditions have often been critical of one another or have sometimes simply ignored one another (Koenig, 2005). Part of the reason for these misunderstandings is that both groups are attempting to answer some of the major questions about life, but they are doing it from very different perspectives, and many times from different world views. This also is true of patients, who have different perspectives about the nature of life and how it relates to mental health and illness. Understanding some of these varying perspectives may help the nurse become more effective in assessing and providing intervention in the spiritual domain.

The Search for the Nature and Meaning of Life

The history of philosophy records centuries of attempts to answer questions about the nature and meaning of life: What is the nature of reality? What is good? How do I know what I know? (Magee, 1998). Most people probably express those questions in a much less formal way, such as: How do I find hope when things are going bad? How do I forgive myself or someone who has hurt me? What is true? For most people it is necessary to find some kind of answers to these questions to make sense out of life. How individuals answer these major questions reflects their world views and beliefs about the nature and meaning of life.

Probably the most basic question about the nature and meaning of life is whether one believes in something that is **transcendent**—that there is something (e.g., nature) or someone (e.g., a supreme being) that goes beyond the physical and material and beyond that which can be understood by human knowledge (McKim, 1996). Some people reject the notion of transcendence, believing only in what they have personally experienced. Others believe only in what can be proven by science. Of those who embrace the idea of the transcendent, some talk about a belief in a natural force or power, such as the universe. Others believe in a supreme being or God. There are also those who believe in many gods, and others who describe a combination of several beliefs. How an individual incorporates the belief in the transcendent into his or her own belief system will affect how he or she answers most of the other major questions about life. For example, if a person has a belief in the transcendent, then determining the right thing to do in a situation might involve choosing an action that causes one to be in harmony with, or even being obedient to, this transcendent belief. It might also mean that failing to live in harmony or obedience to the transcendent may be viewed as a personal moral failure and cause significant guilt.

This desire to live in harmony with the transcendent, the need to answer questions about life that go beyond that which we encounter directly, the need to recognize something that is bigger than ourselves, and how these are recognized, defined, or not recognized by an individual are components of individual spirituality. **Spirituality** refers to "the inherent quality of all humans that activates and drives the search for meaning and purpose in life. It involves all aspects of the individual as lived in relationships with self, others, and a transcendent dimension" (Hermann, 2006, p. 737). In the nursing literature, spirituality is often associated with discovering one's meaning and purpose in life, finding a way to accept one's own or others' failures, experiencing love and connectedness, and having hope (Carson, 1989; Burkhart & Hogan, 2008). Some authors suggest that religion and spirituality are two different entities that have little or nothing to do with each other. However, by first recognizing that most people ask basic questions about the nature of life even though they may do it in different ways, it becomes clear that religion and spirituality are terms that both represent ways to answer these very same questions. Spirituality is actually a broader term, whereas the term **religion** represents a formalized, and often structured, way of answering questions about the nature of life. This formalization may include structured ways of worship or spiritual practices, such as specific prayers said for specific purposes; sacred texts that outline instructions for daily living; and/or a hierarchy of leadership.

This means that some people may answer questions regarding the meaning and purpose of life by relying on beliefs outlined by a formalized religion, whereas others may formulate their own system of beliefs. It is also important to understand that even individuals who espouse a particular religious belief may not believe or practice every tenet of their religion and may, in fact, have their own individual answers to questions about life.

Pause and Reflect

1. *How would you define the term* spirituality?
2. *Why might it be true that an individual's belief about the transcendent affects how he or she answers most of the other major questions of life? Do you agree?*
3. *How does your own spirituality affect your decisions about your own health or mental health?*

Organized Belief Systems

For much of history, people have believed in something that transcended the physical reality and have ordered their lives around this belief. Karen Armstrong provides examples of this from the ancient world. She describes people such as South Sea Islanders, Latins, and Arabs, all of whom spoke of mysterious forces, spirits, or gods, and frequently regarded nature as the manifestation or embodiment of these forces (Armstrong, 1993). Armstrong suggests that not only did the ancients want to figure out the characteristics and expectations of these mysterious forces so they could please or be in harmony with them, but they also wanted to admire and revere these forces. As a result, it is common to find descriptions of mysterious forces, such as the god of thunder or the god of the sun, in their literature or art. Although this thinking was common among early societies, there are still people today who continue to believe in mysterious forces or spirits, often manifested through nature, that are to be worshiped, satisfied, or appeased. Examples of these religions include Wicca, which involves worship of goddess figures, observance of festivals, and use of magic (Warwick, 1995); and shamanism, which involves the belief in spirits that have power to affect people and the role of the shaman in working with those spirits to promote health and maintain equilibrium within the community (Stutley, 2003).

Over time, some societies and groups defined and organized their beliefs into a more systematized fashion. The Greeks and the Romans had extensive beliefs about the gods who influenced both their society and individual lives. Formalized religions, such as Hinduism, Buddhism, Judaism, Islam, and Christianity, also grew and developed over time (Tables 6-1 and 6-2). These various religious traditions formulated very different answers to the basic questions about the nature of life, but they shared the common belief that there was more to life than just the physical and material. As formalized religions developed, they often had teachers or prophets who were considered authorities about the nature of life. In some religions, these individuals were believed to speak for God—such as Moses in

Major World Religions

table 6-1

Religion	Beliefs	Comments
Buddhism	• Emphasizes that things appear one way but are really another. • All of life is impermanent. • Suffering is the result of not understanding the way things really are. Everyone must live with the results of suffering. • Karma (see Hinduism) is a part of the life cycle. • Meditation is important to cleanse the mind of greed, hatred, and delusion. • Death leads to rebirth after rebirth until greed, hatred, and delusion are removed. • In rebirth, one needs to remove the cause of suffering, such as being self-centered or craving for possessions. • Nirvana is the end of suffering and rebirth.	• The Buddha was a historical individual, but the term "Buddha" means "enlightened one." • Buddhism emphasizes the teachings of the Buddha, not him as a person.
Christianity	• God is Creator and Lord over everything, and humans have been made in the image of God. • Humans have rebelled against God and deserve to be punished, but God is merciful. • Jesus Christ is the unique son of God, who came to earth as a human being. This was necessary so that he could die to take the punishment for the people. He did not stay dead, but came back to life and is now in heaven.	• Although Christianity is declining in growth in Europe, it is growing in areas such as Latin American and Africa. • Christianity developed from Judaism.

(continued)

Major World Religions (continued)

table 6-1

Religion	Beliefs	Comments
	• The Bible comes from God and thus has authority to guide behavior and to serve as the basis for belief. • Suffering can be a challenge to Christianity because it seems to challenge the idea that God is love. Suffering is an inevitable part of life, but will not be present in heaven. Jesus Christ chose to experience suffering and, consequently, can comfort humans in their suffering.	
Hinduism	• Hindus believe in karma, that actions of the past have consequences in the present, and actions in the present have consequences for the future. • Each individual needs to act with integrity. • The universe has no beginning and no end. • There are three paths to spiritual fulfillment: knowledge, insight, and wisdom; action; and ecstatic devotion. • People experience reincarnation, which is endless rebirth based on past behavior. The process of reincarnation is characterized by suffering. • Liberation from the suffering of life is obtained though spiritual knowledge, right action, and devotion, and often detachment from the experience of suffering. • Humans should pursue four goals: worldly wealth and success; pleasure; virtue and morality; and spiritual liberation, which involves a release from suffering and rebirth.	• Hinduism has many diverse beliefs. • Some experts refer to Hindu religions rather than the Hindu religion.
Islam	• God, Allah, is one. • Allah is both merciful and all-powerful, and controls the events of life. • On the last day, Allah will judge people based on what they have done and assign them to either heaven or hell. • Allah expects people to be generous. • Major practices involve worship and prayer; giving to the poor; fasting (during the month of Ramadan); and making a pilgrimage to Mecca. • Devoted Muslims (followers of Islam) emphasize intimacy with Allah through spiritual purification. • The Qur'an is Allah's word in written form. • Suffering can be a challenge to Islam because it seems to challenge the idea that Allah is all-powerful. Muslims view suffering as part of the purposes of Allah. Consequently, suffering may serve as a test of faith and as a path of growth.	• Islam began in Mecca around 610 AD with Muhammad, the prophet, who believed that Allah spoke to him with messages for the people. • Islam has two basic groups: the Sunni and Shi'a. The two groups formed over a disagreement about who should be Muhammad's successor. • Islam is the fastest growing religion worldwide.
Judaism	• God the Creator made a covenant with the people, especially Israel. This covenant involved lists of obligations and rewards for the people. • God is all-powerful and all-knowing, a transcendent creator who is actively involved in the world. • God can be brought into the world through everyday actions and interactions. Humans are partners with God. • Suffering is a part of human growth and change, but God does not test people beyond what they are able to bear. • The Torah is a sacred text; many consider the commentaries made by rabbis about the Torah to be sacred as well.	• There are three main branches of Judaism today. One of the main differences between the groups involves how closely they interact with and are influenced by contemporary culture. • Kabbalah is a Jewish mystical tradition that emphasizes the meaning of letters in the Hebrew alphabet, as well as philosophy.

Based on Partridge, C. (2005). *Introduction to World Religions.* Minneapolis, MN: Fortress Press; Bowker, J. (1970). *Problems of Suffering in Religions of the World.* Cambridge, UK: Cambridge University Press.

Judaism; Muhammad in Islam; and Jesus, who is believed to be the son of God, in Christianity. Some formalized religions have collated the teachings of their prophets into texts that summarize their teachings and that outline the tenets or beliefs of the religion—for example, the Qur'an in Islam, the Torah in Judaism, the Bhagavad-Gita in Hinduism, and the Bible in Christianity. A major function of these texts was, and still is, to provide guidance about how individuals should live. Depending on the tradition, some of these texts were regarded as authoritative; that is, containing directives about how followers should live their lives.

The Age of Reason

In the West, a major shift in thinking known as the Enlightenment, or the Age of Reason, took place in the 17th and 18th centuries. Until that time, most people relied primarily on their religious beliefs to answer questions about the nature of life. The Enlightenment emphasized human reasoning as the source of answers for these questions and, as a result, the authority of organized religion decreased, especially among the intellectually elite (Magee, 1998). An even greater challenge to religious thinking and authority occurred with Auguste

Major Religious Traditions in the United States

table 6-2

Religious Tradition	% Among all Adults
Christian	**78.4%**
Evangelical Protestant	26.3
Catholic	23.9
Mainline Protestant	18.1
Historically Black Churches	6.9
Mormon	1.7
Jewish	**1.7**
Buddhist	**0.7**
Muslim	**0.6**
Unaffiliated	**16.1**

Source: Pew Research, Religion and Public Life Project Religious Landscape Survey, 2008. Available at http://religions.pewforum.org/affiliations

Comte's philosophical perspective known as **positivism** (Alexander, 1982). Those promoting positivism maintained that the only real "truth" was found in observable, scientific facts, and basically rejected the transcendent and religion as sources of truth. The result of this perspective was that science was elevated to being the primary source for determining valid answers about the nature in life. Because things that were physical and material were the primary—and sometimes exclusive—interest of science, interest in the transcendent as the source of answers about life declined significantly, again especially among the intellectually elite. This change in thinking had a direct impact on the understanding and treatment of mental illness.

Sigmund Freud, considered the father of modern psychiatry, was a product of this new thinking. He not only attempted to find scientific explanations for mental illness, but also suggested that a reliance on religious thinking might be a manifestation of mental illness.

> Freud was convinced that religion had no objective validity, that one could find no evidence of a transcendent reality, and therefore religious beliefs and experiences derived solely from human needs and desires. . . . Given his philosophical background, Freud's application of psychoanalytic theory to religion could only conclude that religious experience, ideas and rituals were the result of a perverted attempt to resolve internal conflict and deflect unconscious drives. (Blazer, 1998, p. 67)

Freud's growing influence in the treatment of mental illness and training of psychiatrists, coupled with growing emphasis on neurobiological explanations for mental illness, further widened the divide between psychiatry and transcendent world views. On the one hand, the biological, scientific approach to psychiatry had many positive outcomes, including the development of psychotropic medications. On the other hand, it dismissed the importance of religion or spirituality to patients who found a spiritual perspective helpful to answering questions about the nature and meaning of life and to guide their personal decision-making processes.

In the early 20th century, another major change in thinking among intellectuals occurred. This new perspective, known as postmodernism, represented a rejection of the thinking and values of the Enlightenment. **Postmodernism** is characterized by many ideas,

including (1) an affirmation of diverse perspectives; (2) a rejection of the idea of absolute truth or broad explanations about the nature of reality, such as those contained in both science and religion; (3) a skepticism toward absolute distinctions such as male and female and good and bad; and (4) an emphasis on community (Grenz, 1996). Postmodernism helped provide the intellectual climate for the more holistic views of personhood, as well as the emphasis on mental wellness and the interest in spirituality that we see in contemporary nursing practice.

Even though there have been dramatic changes in thinking throughout history regarding the role of science, spirituality, and religion in explaining issues related to mental health, religious groups have often been involved in the care of the mentally ill, and in many cases set standards of care that continue to be reflected in current practice (Chapter 2).

Before turning to a discussion of spirituality and the practice of nursing, it is important to review important points on world view perspectives. To make sense out of "life," answering questions about the nature of life may be helpful. This includes questions such as:

- Is there something that goes beyond the physical or material?
- How do we decide what is the right thing to do?
- Is there such a thing as truth?
- How do we make sense out of life, especially when things are difficult?

These questions may seem abstract, but they have real influence on how people make decisions in the real world. *How do we decide what is the right thing to do?* Imagine the challenges facing the parents of a teenager with mental illness, as they confront both the illness and difficult choices for treatment. *Is there such a thing as truth?* Imagine the challenges for patients who have trouble with reality testing and orientation in time and space. *How do we make sense out of life?* Imagine the grief of the mother who has lost her child. How individual patients interpret these questions and their answers can have direct bearing on their decisions regarding mental health, mental illness, and treatment.

As previously discussed, different people answer these questions differently. In summary, the basis for an individual's beliefs about the meaning and purpose of life may be rooted in one of four broad categories:

- A transcendent force related to nature or mysterious forces, spirits, or nature gods
- A belief system defined through an organized religion
- Scientific, material, or physical (observable) explanations
- An eclectic, unorganized, often self-determined explanation

It is worth repeating that individuals may hold strong beliefs and yet choose not to follow one or more beliefs specific to their spiritual or religious world view. For example, a woman may take birth control pills even if she practices a religion that prohibits the use of birth control. Another example might be that of a patient from a belief system that recognizes faith healers, as some Native American tribes do, yet who may agree to take prescribed medication. These personalized exceptions make it especially important that nurses do not make assumptions about patients' beliefs related to spirituality and religion, but instead assess each patient to determine what role spirituality plays in the patient's beliefs about his or her wellness or illness status and decisions about health care.

Pause and Reflect

1. *What are the beliefs that underlie your answers to the major questions of life?*
2. *Think about someone who has very different beliefs from your own. What are the similarities in your beliefs and what are the differences?*
3. *What might it be like for you to work with a patient whose beliefs are very different from your own? To support a patient's decisions regarding treatment that are contradictory to your own belief system?*

Spirituality and Nursing Practice

With all the discussion about differences in thinking and world views, it would be easy to decide that assessing and intervening in the spiritual domain are just too complicated, especially with the time constraints of nursing practice. However, ignoring the spiritual domain of a patient with mental illness means that the nurse is ignoring a significant aspect of the patient that may be able to provide him or her with a means of understanding his or her life situation and a source of hope for the future. The importance of the spiritual domain is described by the nursing theorist Betty Neuman: "Through careful assessment of client needs in the spiritual area, followed by purposeful intervention, such as fostering hope that affects the will to live, the relation between the spiritual variable and [the patient's] wellness may be better understood and utilized as a source of energy in achieving client change" (Neuman & Fawcett, 2002, p. 16).

Assessment

Once the nurse understands that assessing a patient's spirituality is really learning how he or she answers questions about the meaning in life, accepts his or her own or others' failures, and experiences connectedness with others, including the transcendent, then assessment of a patient's spiritual domain actually becomes less complex. The goal of assessment is to learn how the patient answers these questions and how satisfied he or she is with those answers. To accomplish that, assessment involves a process that begins on admission and continues throughout the time that the individual is receiving services. Sometimes nurses wonder whether a spiritual assessment is not the role of the chaplain or the religious advisor. Certainly, it is important to recognize and use these individuals' expertise, but nurses need to have information about the patient's spiritual domain to provide holistic care.

Lorraine Wright, a nurse–family therapist, suggests that nurses form relationships with patients and their families to promote health and decrease suffering. She further suggests that when patients experience illness and suffering, it leads into the spiritual domain of nursing practice (Wright, 2005). Mental illness in itself is a source of suffering. When mental illness is coupled with struggles that relate to the basic questions of life, such as *why am I even alive?*, patients' suffering is often dramatically increased. For example, a patient who is depressed and angry because his business partner embezzled money from the business may be dealing not only with the symptoms of depression, such as a loss of energy and an inability to concentrate, but also with questions about forgiveness and why something like this could happen to him. A college student who has her first psychotic episode may be dealing not only with the fear of having another episode, but also with questions about what kind of a future she can hope for.

The initial assessment of a patient's spirituality usually begins on admission and involves basic questions about a patient's spiritual or religious practices and what, if any, assistance the patient needs in carrying them out. This primarily involves closed questions, such as:

- Do you have a religious preference?
- Are there any spiritual or religious practices that are important to you?
- Would you like for us to contact your clergy member or religious advisor?

These questions are important because they provide minimum baseline information that is important in planning care and are examples of the kinds of questions that are suggested for spiritual assessment by the Joint Commission (formerly the Joint Commission on Accreditation of Health Care Organizations [JCAHO]). For example, the admissions assessment may indicate that a woman who has had multiple abortions also is a practicing Catholic, or that a man who was arrested for being with a prostitute is a follower of Islam. Knowing these patients' religious preferences may alert the nurse to the possibility that they might be experiencing guilt because of a failure to follow their chosen religion's ideologies. As another example, the admission assessment may reveal that a patient wants only a specific religious advisor representing his church or denomination, or a credentialed religious advisor, such as a chaplain, to talk to him about his spiritual concerns. It is equally important to know if a patient has no religious beliefs or interest in religion, so a visit from a religious advisor might not be suggested as an intervention. Examples of assessment questions are found in Box 6-1.

Even though these preliminary admission questions are important, they rarely are sufficient to help a nurse understand how a patient is answering or struggling with the questions of life and suffering. To accomplish that, the nurse needs to ask more focused and

---

Spirituality Assessment Questions   box 6-1

Do you have a religious preference?

Are there any spiritual or religious practices that are important to you?

Do you wish us to contact your clergy member or religious advisor?

How do you make sense out of what has happened to you?

In what ways has your illness affected your view of yourself or of others or your faith?

What is your source of support or meaning in this experience?

How do you decide what you should do next?

What kind of support do you have?

What is your source of hope?

open-ended questions over time, as the nurse–patient relationship develops. This involves asking the patient about how he or she answers life questions and his or her perspective about how effective these answers are. This aspect of a spiritual assessment is not intended to be carried out using a checklist, or even with a set of predetermined, standard questions. Instead it requires careful listening and responsive questioning in the context of a nurse–patient relationship.

In addition to asking a patient how he or she answers life questions, it also is important to ask the patient how well these answers are working, to provide understanding for his or her situation in life. Sharon Parks (1986), who has done significant work with young adult spiritual formation, suggests that one of the most important aspects of a belief system is that it is based on a foundation that is strong enough to handle the changes and challenges of life. Many times life experiences that precede the onset or exacerbation of mental illness can cause a patient to question whether previous answers to the questions of life still are satisfactory. Consider the example of Mr. Foster, a middle-aged man with depression who is alienated from his wife and children and states, "I thought that by being a good provider, I was doing what I was supposed to be doing in life. Look where it got me. So, what in the world do I do with my life now? I'm no good to anyone." Other patients may express distress differently, such as Mrs. Kline, a woman nearing the end of her life who has just lost her husband and has difficulty finding comfort or purpose in religious beliefs she has held for years. She asks, "Why did God do this to me?" or "What did I do to deserve this?" Although the patients in each of these examples express spiritual distress very differently, both examples convey that discovering with patients their thoughts about the effectiveness of their own answers to life questions is a very significant part of assessment, because that perspective may become a major component in determining appropriate intervention.

Nursing Diagnoses

Probably the most common nursing diagnosis used in relation to the spiritual domain is *spiritual distress*. Spiritual distress is the disruption of an individual's capacity to assimilate or find meaning and purpose in his or her life by connecting with self, others, the arts, nature, and/or a higher power (Wilkinson, 2005). Characteristics of spiritual distress include expressions of a lack of hope or meaning and purpose in life, feelings of alienation from others, feelings of being abandoned by or being angry with God, or indicating the presence of suffering. Another diagnosis that might be appropriate is *powerlessness*, defined as the belief that one has no control over circumstances or outcomes (Wilkinson, 2005). Powerlessness is characterized by expressions of

having little or no control over one's life situation and outcome, feelings of anger, guilt, or difficulty expressing one's feelings. A third diagnosis is *hopelessness*, a state in which an individual feels restrained (without choices or alternatives) and immobilized (Wilkinson, 2005). Characteristics of hopelessness are decreased affect, lack of initiative, passivity, and lost belief in transcendent values or God (Wilkinson, 2005). The DSM-5 also includes a code for *religious* or *spiritual problems* described as "distressing experiences that involve loss or questioning of faith, problems associated with conversion to a new faith, or questioning of spiritual values that may not necessarily be related to an organized church or religious institution" (APA, 2013, p. 725).

One of the major criticisms of both the DSM-5 and NANDA-I nursing diagnoses classification systems is that they are problem focused and, consequently, negative. Although patients certainly can have problems in the spiritual domain, such as the patient with schizophrenia who may suffer from religious hallucinations, for some patients their spirituality may be their primary source of hope, or meaning and purpose, or self-esteem. In other words, their spirituality is a strength, not a problem or weakness. Karen Stolte (1996) recognized this limitation with many diagnostic categories, and suggested a way to reword the diagnostic labels to fit with a wellness approach. Thus, in the area of spirituality, she suggests several possible alternative diagnoses: *progressive religious faith, maintaining strong spiritual foundation, maintaining hope and trust in higher power, progressive ability to forgive self and/or others, continued belief in meaning and purpose of life,* and *at peace with self and/or health status.*

Intervention

In psychiatric nursing, it can be difficult to determine where assessment ends and intervention begins. This is especially true in the spiritual domain, which is why it is absolutely essential that nursing interventions be based on a thorough assessment. Listening is, of course, one of the most important interventions carried out by psychiatric nurses; this is true in the spiritual domain as well. Encouraging patients to think through how they answer life questions may help patients to reaffirm their beliefs or to decide to make life choices that are more consistent with their beliefs. It may help them look for different or additional beliefs that provide them with the answers to facilitate coping and promote healing.

Intervention in the spiritual domain also includes assisting patients with religious practices that are important to them (Box 6-2). Providing the patient with a quiet place to read religious books such as the Bible or the Qur'an may assist that person in coping and identifying goals for the future, and may promote peace of mind. For

Comfort in Ritual   box 6-2

Rituals can change how individuals perceive or value events or circumstances (Halvorson, 2013). Spiritual rituals often provide comfort and assist individuals in placing certain events or circumstances in perspective. Illness may cause individuals to become stronger in their beliefs, challenge their beliefs, be drawn back to their beliefs, or find beliefs that help them make sense of what they are experiencing through the illness.

Patients who subscribe to a specific core system of beliefs or an organized religion may find comfort in following daily rituals, especially if they have followed these prior to

the onset of mental illness. Nurses must be alert to the needs of these patients and help them to schedule treatments, such as therapy sessions, around practices that must be conducted at specific times. A common example is the Muslim practice of praying at specific times during the day. Ensuring that patients are able to access prayer rugs, prayer books, and Bibles or other sacred texts, and have access to ritualized objects that bring comfort, such as a cross or a statue of a religious figure (such as an angel), can promote comfort and healing.

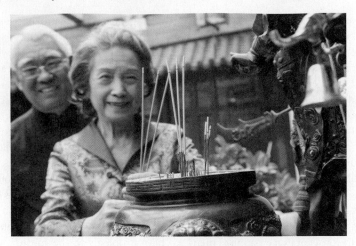

6-1 Many patients may take comfort in spiritual or religious rituals. Here, a couple offers incense at their local temple. How would you help patients in a hospital or inpatient setting observe rituals that are important to them?

Source: Xixinxing/Fotolia

some patients, being able to follow routines related to prayer and meditation can be very important (Figure 6-1). Nurses can promote individual religious practices by scheduling activities around designated prayer times or ensuring that items needed for prayer, such as a rosary or prayer book, are made available to patients who need them. Sometimes a patient may wish to meet with a chaplain or a religious advisor from his or her own faith. The nurse can help to arrange this or, if available, the chaplain may assist with this. It is important to provide for as much privacy as possible when a patient meets with the chaplain or religious advisor. It may also be helpful to patients to encourage them to contact other members of their faith community for support and assistance as they face their illness.

In addition to these rather general interventions, some interventions relate specifically to the spiritual domain: instilling hope and helping the patient to find meaning in suffering. There are no simple interventions or approaches for any of these issues, but they are often very important aspects of mental illness. Patients frequently experience hopelessness, especially when they recognize that they have a chronic illness. Sometimes, encouraging them to use their beliefs to deal with their feelings of hopelessness can be helpful. A study of 270 patients with depression found that having religious beliefs was a significant predictor of decreased hopelessness and depression, in part because religious beliefs provided patients with a cognitive framework or way to think about their illness. The results imply that incorporating the patient's religious beliefs into treatment might help to prevent or decrease hopelessness (Murphy, Ciarrocchi, Piedmont, & Cheston, 2000). An example of this might be to ask a patient to talk about how his or her beliefs help in thinking about the future or his or her worth as a person (see Perceptions, Thoughts, and Feelings: Listening to a Patient's Spiritual Concerns).

Connectedness

In some cases, connectedness and being a part of a group can help to increase hope. Often this happens by receiving support from others living with mental illness or by confronting unhealthy ideas or ways of living. One study used a structured group to help individuals with mental illness address issues of stigma and dysfunctional beliefs.

Although the authors advise that further research is needed, they found that, after attending the group, a majority of participants (72%) indicated that they experienced an increase in hope (Roe et al., 2010). Two other researchers also developed a spiritual issues group for patients with serious mental illness. These were patients who considered themselves "very religious," "religious," "very spiritual," or "moderately spiritual." In that group they talked about spiritual resources and struggles, hope, and forgiveness. At the end of the 7-week group, participants indicated that they wanted the group to continue because they found the emphasis on spiritual issues to be often neglected in mental health settings. They also expressed appreciation for the nonjudgmental atmosphere of the group, and the opportunity to connect with others in the group and to hear their perspectives on spiritual beliefs and interests (Phillips, Lakin, & Pargament, 2002). Starting such a group or suggesting that patients participate in a support group that focuses on spiritual issues might be a helpful intervention to increase hope.

Meaning in Experience

Helping patients to find meaning in the experience of the suffering of mental illness is another important intervention. As indicated earlier, Wright (2005) maintains that suffering leads people into the spiritual domain as they face questions about the nature of life. If that is true, then nurses need to be willing to enter into the patient's process of facing those questions. The nurse does not need to answer the questions for the patient or to expect that the patient will have well-formulated answers. Instead, most of the time, it is necessary only for the nurse to be present and to listen. Schaffer and Norlander (2009) suggest that **presence** as a nursing intervention involves attentiveness to the concerns of the patient; accountability to what is good for the patient; sensitivity to the needs and concerns of the patient; and being active. The goal of this intervention is to help patients use their own religious or spiritual resources to find meaning in their current experience. Mattis (2002) found that religion or spirituality can be a significant aspect of finding meaning in adverse situations. She interviewed African American women and discovered that religion or spirituality helped them to both question and accept reality, to face and move beyond limitations, to ask hard questions about life, to find purpose and destiny, to experience personal growth, and to trust in transcendent sources of knowledge and wisdom. All these are outcomes that come from patients' using their own spirituality as a resource and can help as they work through issues relating to a diagnosis of mental illness.

It is also important to be sure that both nursing assessment and interventions regarding the patient's spiritual domain are documented in the patient's medical record so other health care providers can follow the same plan of care.

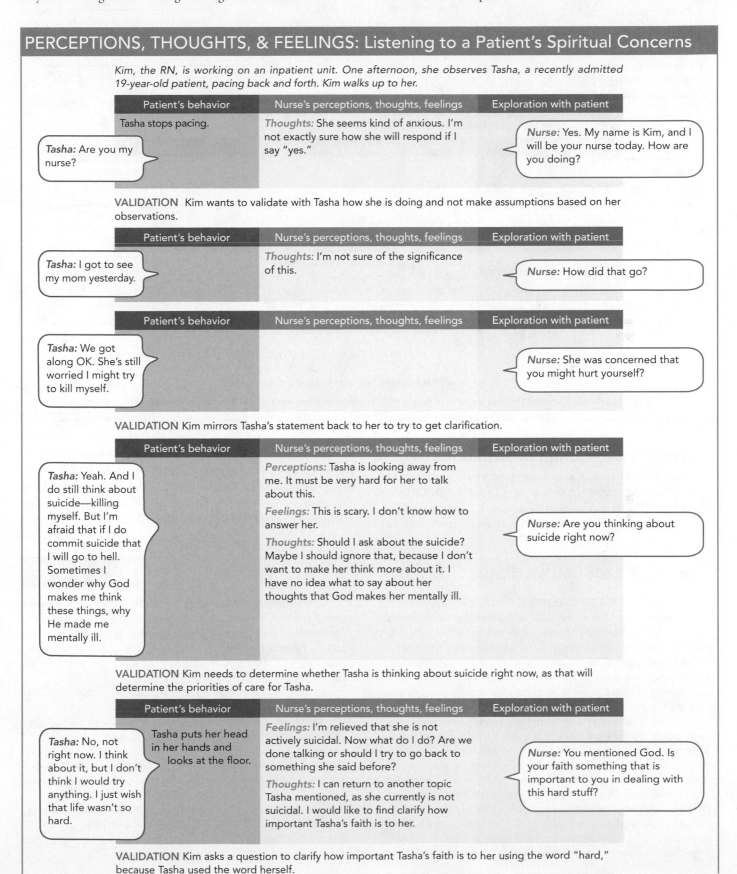

PERCEPTIONS, THOUGHTS, & FEELINGS: Listening to a Patient's Spiritual Concerns

Kim, the RN, is working on an inpatient unit. One afternoon, she observes Tasha, a recently admitted 19-year-old patient, pacing back and forth. Kim walks up to her.

Patient's behavior	Nurse's perceptions, thoughts, feelings	Exploration with patient
Tasha stops pacing. Tasha: Are you my nurse?	Thoughts: She seems kind of anxious. I'm not exactly sure how she will respond if I say "yes."	Nurse: Yes. My name is Kim, and I will be your nurse today. How are you doing?

VALIDATION Kim wants to validate with Tasha how she is doing and not make assumptions based on her observations.

Patient's behavior	Nurse's perceptions, thoughts, feelings	Exploration with patient
Tasha: I got to see my mom yesterday.	Thoughts: I'm not sure of the significance of this.	Nurse: How did that go?

Patient's behavior	Nurse's perceptions, thoughts, feelings	Exploration with patient
Tasha: We got along OK. She's still worried I might try to kill myself.		Nurse: She was concerned that you might hurt yourself?

VALIDATION Kim mirrors Tasha's statement back to her to try to get clarification.

Patient's behavior	Nurse's perceptions, thoughts, feelings	Exploration with patient
Tasha: Yeah. And I do still think about suicide—killing myself. But I'm afraid that if I do commit suicide that I will go to hell. Sometimes I wonder why God makes me think these things, why He made me mentally ill.	Perceptions: Tasha is looking away from me. It must be very hard for her to talk about this. Feelings: This is scary. I don't know how to answer her. Thoughts: Should I ask about the suicide? Maybe I should ignore that, because I don't want to make her think more about it. I have no idea what to say about her thoughts that God makes her mentally ill.	Nurse: Are you thinking about suicide right now?

VALIDATION Kim needs to determine whether Tasha is thinking about suicide right now, as that will determine the priorities of care for Tasha.

Patient's behavior	Nurse's perceptions, thoughts, feelings	Exploration with patient
Tasha: No, not right now. I think about it, but I don't think I would try anything. I just wish that life wasn't so hard. Tasha puts her head in her hands and looks at the floor.	Feelings: I'm relieved that she is not actively suicidal. Now what do I do? Are we done talking or should I try to go back to something she said before? Thoughts: I can return to another topic Tasha mentioned, as she currently is not suicidal. I would like to find clarify how important Tasha's faith is to her.	Nurse: You mentioned God. Is your faith something that is important to you in dealing with this hard stuff?

VALIDATION Kim asks a question to clarify how important Tasha's faith is to her using the word "hard," because Tasha used the word herself.

PERCEPTIONS, THOUGHTS, & FEELINGS (continued)

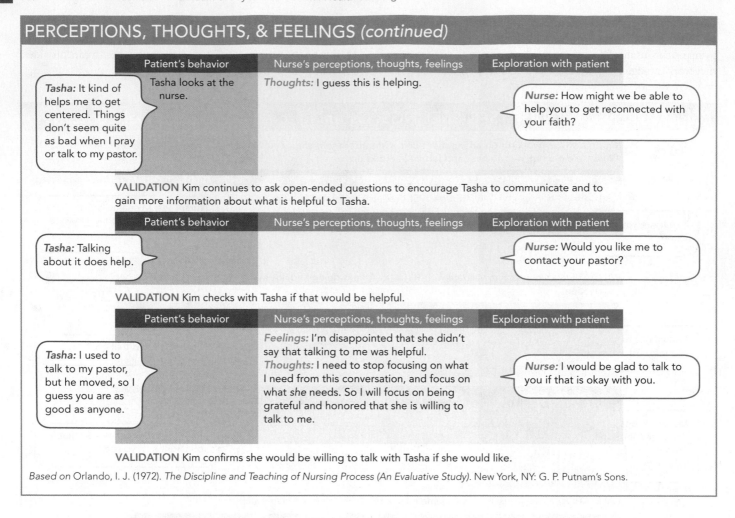

Patient's behavior	Nurse's perceptions, thoughts, feelings	Exploration with patient
Tasha: It kind of helps me to get centered. Things don't seem quite as bad when I pray or talk to my pastor. Tasha looks at the nurse.	**Thoughts:** I guess this is helping.	**Nurse:** How might we be able to help you to get reconnected with your faith?

VALIDATION Kim continues to ask open-ended questions to encourage Tasha to communicate and to gain more information about what is helpful to Tasha.

Patient's behavior	Nurse's perceptions, thoughts, feelings	Exploration with patient
Tasha: Talking about it does help.		**Nurse:** Would you like me to contact your pastor?

VALIDATION Kim checks with Tasha if that would be helpful.

Patient's behavior	Nurse's perceptions, thoughts, feelings	Exploration with patient
Tasha: I used to talk to my pastor, but he moved, so I guess you are as good as anyone.	**Feelings:** I'm disappointed that she didn't say that talking to me was helpful. **Thoughts:** I need to stop focusing on what I need from this conversation, and focus on what *she* needs. So I will focus on being grateful and honored that she is willing to talk to me.	**Nurse:** I would be glad to talk to you if that is okay with you.

VALIDATION Kim confirms she would be willing to talk with Tasha if she would like.

Based on Orlando, I. J. (1972). The Discipline and Teaching of Nursing Process (An Evaluative Study). New York, NY: G. P. Putnam's Sons.

Intervention in Complex Situations

At times, a patient's spiritual beliefs or practices seem to have a more negative than positive effect on the patient. This can manifest in different ways. Sometimes it may involve someone from the patient's religious group using his or her religious authority to unduly influence the patient. It may also be seen when a patient's beliefs or practices become closely tied to manifestations of mental illness, such as when a mother believes that God has told her to kill her children. Other times patients may refuse to take medications and believe, instead, that they should trust God to make them well (Box 6-3).

Spiritual Beliefs and Medication Therapy   box 6-3

Patients, even those with mental illness, have the right to refuse medications most of the time, so it is important to respect that right. However, it is also important that patients have adequate information to make that decision. Sometimes patients who decline medications believe that the medications will alter their ability to think clearly or that the medications will take away their ability to make choices. This may be due, in part, to the fact that many psychotropic medications do make people sleepy initially, and can make them feel like they are "sleepwalking" until the dose is properly regulated. Some patients do feel as though they cannot think clearly when that happens. In some situations, providing those patients with more information about the temporal nature of some of these medication side effects may help to ease their concern. Other times it may be helpful to suggest that there are people of faith who take medications to help them deal with their illness and to be more engaged in life. For example, Lewis Smedes, a theologian, writing about his experience with depression, shared this observation:

"I must, to be honest, tell you that God comes to me each morning and offers me a 20-milligram capsule of Prozac. With this medication he clears the garbage that accumulates in the canals of my brain overnight and gives me a chance to get a fresh morning start. I swallow every capsule with gratitude to God" (Smedes, 2003, p. 133).

Some patients simply need the reassurance that they are not abandoning their faith by taking medications.

There are also situations in which patients may start taking medications but then discontinue them because they are doing well and believe that they have been healed. In those situations, the nurse needs to listen carefully to the concerns and disappointment of the patient, review the nature of his or her illness and the action of the medications, and help the patient explore feelings about not being healed as the patient expected and hoped. For some patients, it may take a relapse (or even several relapses) for them to realize that they do need their medications to function successfully and prevent a relapse.

Arterburn and Felton (1991) describe a phenomenon known as *toxic faith*, which occurs when an individual's beliefs interfere with his or her health and relationships with others. They suggest that experiences such as extreme guilt or isolation, difficulty maintaining relationships with others, believing that thoughts of suicide or homicide that come from God, or thinking that God is regularly communicating in an audible voice may be examples of toxic faith. Because not all beliefs are health producing, it is important that nurses assess whether patients' beliefs seem to interfere with or enhance their growth and well-being.

Researchers asked a group of psychiatric nurses what criteria they used in evaluating their patients' spiritual-type experiences. Because this kind of evaluation is frequently complicated by the fact that patients may have differing cultural or religious beliefs that may not be understood by or be a part of the world view of the nurse, this was an important question. The nurses interviewed believed that spiritual beliefs were an indication of illness when they were similar to common symptoms of illness, had negative content, the patients posed a risk to themselves or others, there was a negative emotional outcome or grandiosity of the beliefs, or individuals close to the patient expressed concern. The nurses also held that spiritual beliefs were indications of well-being when those indicators were not present, when they were somewhat congruent with the patient's beliefs in the past, and when the patient showed good functioning at work and in relationships (Eeles, Lowe, & Wellman, 2003).

Situations in which the patient's spiritual beliefs seem deeply entwined with his or her symptoms of mental illness, such as with the patient with schizophrenia who believes that God speaks to him through the television or who hears God's voice telling him to kill himself, can be very challenging. Certainly, in these situations nurses need to use their knowledge of appropriate interventions for patients who are experiencing hallucinations or delusional thinking, but it is also important not to ignore the spiritual aspect of these symptoms. In situations such as this, one of the challenges for practitioners is to figure out the difference between someone who is very zealous in his or her faith and someone who is actually manifesting illness. What often happens is that practitioners try to do this based on the *content* of what the patient is saying. The problem with this is that other people who do not have a mental illness may express the same ideas. For example, it is not unusual for someone with schizophrenia to express the belief that the world is coming to an end. At the same time, there are religious groups that have predicted that the world was coming to an end and have rearranged their whole lives according to that belief. We would want to be very cautious, though, before suggesting that everyone in groups such as those has a mental illness. However, that leaves questions about whether a strongly held religious belief is just that, or if it is a religious delusion. One group of researchers suggests that the more a belief (1) is unlikely or does not seem to have an explanation, (2) is strongly held, (3) is not shared by other people, (4) causes distress in the person, and (5) seems to take over the person's whole focus and perspective on life, the more likely it is to be a delusion (Freeman et al., 2007). These criteria can be useful in helping the nurse to understand the complexity of working with a patient whose delusions are religious in nature. Because of this complexity, however, nurses sometimes forget that the patients' spiritual beliefs can still be a resource to them, even when they are experiencing religious delusions or hallucinations. This idea is illustrated by another group of researchers who interviewed patients about their spirituality. They interviewed a man with paranoid schizophrenia who told them, "I am anxious about meeting people, so beforehand I pray that everything will be OK. Then I am confident in the situation." They also described a woman with undifferentiated schizophrenia who shared, "When I feel despair, prayer helps me find peace, strength, and comfort." This certainly suggests that for some patients, spirituality may continue to be a source of strength for them even though they manifest symptoms of mental illness. Tapping into spiritual resources also has the potential to provide individuals, regardless of their diagnoses, with meaning, comfort, and hope.

Pause and Reflect

1. *What might it take to increase your comfort level in assessing the spiritual domain within patients?*
2. *How might you incorporate a patient's faith into his or her plan of care?*
3. *How might you respond if a patient asks you what your belief system is?*

Elizabeth

APPLICATION

1. What information do you have about the five domains for Elizabeth?

2. What assessment questions would you ask Elizabeth to gain more understanding of her spiritual domain?

3. In what ways might Elizabeth's faith and her church friends be a support to her? In what ways might it make her recovery more challenging?

Elizabeth is a 35-year-old woman who immigrated to the United States from West Africa 10 years ago. She was recently hospitalized on a psychiatric unit for depression and suicidal ideation. She is married and has four children between the ages of 2 and 12. She is a student at the local community college and works as a dietary aide in another hospital. Her husband is not living in the home, and she is the sole economic support for the family. During the admissions interview, she told the nurse that she became depressed and suicidal because her husband was having an affair with another woman and that he no longer provides the family with any money. She has told the staff that she is currently not feeling suicidal. When asked about personal resources, Elizabeth indicated that she has many friends from her home country and that the people in her church are very supportive. When the nurse commented that it sounded as though her faith and her church community were important to her, she responded, "I just need to get out of here so that I can pray. I have to trust God to make a way. They want me to take medicine, but I don't need medicine. I need a miracle." Elizabeth also shared that a friend had told her that someone had placed a spell on her husband and that consequently he was unable to resist having this affair.

critical thinking

Chapter Highlights

1. Patients have different world views—sets of beliefs they hold about the basic makeup of the world.

2. Patients' world views inform how they understand the nature and meaning of life.

3. Spirituality refers to the inherent quality that drives the search for meaning and purpose in life. It involves lived experience in relationship with others.

4. Religion represents a formalized, and often structured, way of answering questions about the nature of life. This formalization may include structured ways of worship or spiritual practices, sacred texts that outline instructions for daily living, and/or a hierarchy of leadership.

5. Assessment of the spiritual domain begins with forming a therapeutic relationship and involves asking basic questions about spiritual or religious practices and what, if any, assistance the patient needs in carrying them out.

6. As the nurse–patient relationship develops, open-ended questions and careful listening may help patients answer life questions. Encouraging patients to answer these types of questions may help patients reaffirm their beliefs or decide to make life choices that are more consistent with their beliefs.

7. Nursing diagnoses may be used to identify patients' struggles with spirituality. More positive wording put forth by Stolte—such as *at peace with self and/or health status* (Stolte, 1996)—may help nurses view spirituality from a wellness approach.

8. Encouraging patients to make connections with those who can provide support—family, friends, therapy groups—is an important nursing intervention.

9. Patients may find meaning, comfort, and hope in their spirituality even when struggling with serious mental illness.

NCLEX®-RN Questions

1. The nurse is caring for a patient who states that she belongs to an organized religion. The patient reports participation in weekly services at a local house of worship. Which assumption about the patient's spiritual orientation can be made based on this information?

   The patient:
   a. Adheres to all the tenets of the identified religion.
   b. Organizes aspects of her life around religious activity.
   c. Rejects the notion that there is a scientific explanation for illness.
   d. Satisfies her need to answer to questions about the purpose of life.

2. The nurse is attempting to meet the diverse needs of a patient in the mental health setting. Which activity best indicates that the nurse is addressing the patient's spiritual needs?
   a. Determines the particular sect of the religion that the patient follows
   b. Checks to ensure that kosher meals meet the patient's satisfaction
   c. Notes the religion of the patient in the chart and provides information about pastoral services
   d. Encourages the patient to examine how his belief system can be used to make sense of the experience

3. The nurse is assigned to care for a patient being admitted to the mental health unit. Which method is most likely to be effective in assessing the patient's spiritual needs?
   a. Asking open-ended questions over time and in the context of a therapeutic relationship
   b. Requesting an assessment consult from a pastor or chaplain familiar with the patient's religion
   c. Conducting a comprehensive literature review on the religion with which the patient is affiliated
   d. Providing a quiet space for the patient to complete a questionnaire about religious preferences

4. The nurse is reviewing the progress of a patient diagnosed with mental illness with members of the interdisciplinary team. A team member questions the value of allowing the patient to spend time in his room praying out loud because the patient has a history of religious grandiosity. Which response by the nurse best supports allowing this practice to continue?
   a. "Talking to a higher power is the only way for patients to make sense of their pain. Everyone can benefit from the power of prayer."
   b. "A family member confirmed that this behavior is acceptable in their culture. We should let it continue unless it makes others uncomfortable."
   c. "The patient finds comfort in taking time in his room to meditate and pray. We have noticed that he is less anxious when we don't interfere with this activity."
   d. "I can understand your concern due to the fact that the patient has a history of becoming disorganized. Unfortunately, it is illegal to prevent patients from praying."

5. The nurse is counseling the parents of a patient who has been diagnosed with a major mental illness. The parents state that they feel there is nothing they can do to help their child because they believe it is a punishment for not following religious principles. Which nursing diagnosis best addresses the parents' needs at this time?
   a. *Spiritual distress* related to abandonment of faith
   b. *Hopelessness* related to circumstances that test their faith
   c. *Powerlessness* related to the perception that they cannot affect an outcome
   d. *Ineffective denial* related to inability to accept the reality of the illness

6. The nurse is working with a patient who has experienced a spiritual crisis as a result of illness and hospitalization. Which outcomes best indicate that the patient has re-established a healthy sense of spiritual well-being? Select all that apply.

   The patient:
   a. Reaches out to connect with others.
   b. Expresses a sense of hope in the future.
   c. Finds meaning in day-to-day challenges.
   d. Embraces more mainstream religious beliefs.
   e. Adheres to beliefs that provide absolute truths.

7. The nurse manager is evaluating the use of evidence-based practice (EBP) with regard to spirituality on a mental health unit. Which observations demonstrate consistency with EBP? Select all that apply.
   a. Positivism is encouraged as a means of seeking meaning and truth.
   b. Staff make every effort to accommodate religious and spiritual rituals.
   c. Patients are encouraged to embrace more holistic, transcendental beliefs.
   d. Spirituality is discouraged only in patients with delusions or hallucinations.
   e. Nurses assess and respond to spiritual needs as part of their role function.

Answers may be found on the Pearson student resource site: nursing.pearsonhighered.com

Pearson Nursing Student Resources Find additional review materials at **nursing.pearsonhighered.com**

References

Alexander, J. (1982). *Positivism, Presuppositions, and Current Controversies*. Berkeley, CA: University of California Press, pp. 5–15.

Ameling, A., & Povilonis, M. (2001). Spirituality: Meaning, mental health, and nursing. *Journal of Psychosocial Nursing and Mental Health Services, 39*(4), 16–19.

American Psychiatric Association. (2013). *Diagnostic and Statistical Manual of Mental Disorders* (5th ed.). Washington, DC: American Psychiatric Publishers.

Armstong, K. (1993). *A History of God*. New York, NY: Ballantine, pp. 1–5.

Arterburn, S., & Felton, J. (1991). *Toxic Faith: Understanding and Overcoming Religious Addiction*. Nashville, TN: Thomas Nelson.

Blazer, D. (1998). *Freud vs. God: How Psychiatry Lost Its Soul and Christianity Lost Its Mind*. Downers Grove, IL: InterVarsity Press, p. 67.

Bowker, J. (1970). *Problems of Suffering in Religions of the World*. Cambridge, UK: Cambridge University Press.

Burkhart, L., & Hogan, N. (2008). An experiential theory of spiritual care in nursing practice. *Qualitative Health Research, 18*(7), 928.

Carson, V. B. (Ed.). (1989). *Spiritual Dimension of Nursing Practice*. Philadelphia, PA: Saunders, pp. 14–21.

Eeles, J., Lowe, T., & Wellman, N. (2003). Spirituality or psychosis—an exploration of the criteria that nurses use to evaluate spiritual-type experiences reported by patients. *International Journal of Nursing Studies, 40*, 197–206.

Freeman, D., Pugh, K., Green, C., Valmaggia, L., Dunn, G., & Garety, P. (2007). A measure of state persecutory ideation for experimental studies. *Journal of Nervous and Mental Disorders, 195*(9), 781–784.

Grenz, S. (1996). *A Primer on Postmodernism*. Grand Rapids, MI: Eerdmans, pp. 39–59.

Halvorson, H. G. (2013). New research: Rituals make us value things more. Available at http://blogs.hbr.org/2013/12/new-research-rituals-make-us-value-things-more/

Hermann, C. (2006). Development and testing of the spiritual needs inventory for patients near the end of life. *Oncology Nursing Forum, 33*(4), 737.

Koenig, H. (2005). *Faith and Mental Health*. Philadelphia, PA: Templeton Foundation, pp. 26, 48–66.

Magee, B. (1998). *The Story of Philosophy*, New York, NY: D.K. Publishing, pp. 7–9, 68–70.

Mattis, J. (2002). Religion and spirituality in the meaning-making and coping experiences of African American women: A qualitative analysis. *Psychology of Women Quarterly, 26*, 309.

McKim, D. (1996). *Westminster Dictionary of Theological Terms*, Louisville, KY: Westminster John Knox Press, 285.

Mohr, S., Borras, L., Betrisey, C., Brandt, P., Gillieron, C., & Huguelet, P. (2010). Delusions with religious content in patients with psychosis: How they interact with spiritual coping. *Psychiatry, 73*(2), 158–172.

Mohr, S., Perroud, N., Gillieron, C., Brandt, P. Y., Rieben, I., Borras, L., & Huguelet, P. (2011). Spirituality and religiousness as predictive factors of outcome in schizophrenia and schizo-affective disorders. *Psychiatry Research, 186* (2–3), 177–182.

Murphy, P., Ciarrocchi, J., Piedmont, R., Cheston, S., & Peyrot, M. (2000). The relation of religious belief and practice, depression and hopelessness in persons with chronic depression. *Journal of Consulting and Clinical Psychology, 68*(6), 1105.

Neuman, B., & Fawcett, J. (2002). *The Neuman Systems Model*. Upper Saddle River, NJ: Prentice Hall, p. 16.

Orlando, I. J. (1972). *The Discipline and Teaching of Nursing Process: An Evaluative Study*. New York: G. P. Putnam's Sons.

Parks, S. (1986). *The Critical Years: The Young Adult Search for a Faith to Live By*. San Francisco, CA: Harper and Row, pp. 12–13.

Partridge, C. (2005). *Introduction to World Religions*. Minneapolis, MN: Fortress Press.

Pew Research, Religion and Public Life Project Religious Landscape Survey. (2008). Available at http://religions.pewforum.org/affiliations

Phillips, R., Lakin, R., & Pargament, K. (2002). Development and implementation of a spiritual issues psychoeducational group for those with serious mental illness. *Community Mental Health Journal, 38*(6), 493–494.

Roe, D., Hasson-Ohayon, I., Derhi, O, Yanos, P., & Lysaker, P. (2010). Talking about life and finding solutions to different hardships. *Journal of Nervous and Mental Disease, 198*(11), 807–812.

Salsman, J., Brown, T., Brechting, E., & Carlson, C. (2005). The link between religion and spirituality and psychological adjustment; the mediating role of optimism and social support. *Personality and Social Psychology Bulletin, 31*(4), 522–535.

Schaffer, M., & Norlander, L. (2009). *Being Present: A Nurse's Resource for End-of-Life Communication*. Indianapolis, IN: Sigma Theta Tau International, pp. 5–7.

Sire, J. (2004). *Naming the Elephant: Worldview as a Concept*. Downers Grove, IL: InterVarsity Press, 19.

Smedes, L. (2003). *My God and I: A Spiritual Memoir*. Grand Rapids, MI: Eerdmans, p. 133.

Stolte, K. (1996). *Wellness: Nursing Diagnosis for Health Promotion*. Philadelphia, PA: Lippincott-Raven, pp. 57–59.

Stutely, M. (2003). *Shamanism*. London, UK: Routledge, pp. 6–7.

Tartaro, J., Luecken, L., & Gunn, H. (2005). Exploring heart and soul: The effects of religiosity/spirituality and gender on blood pressure and cortisol stress responses. *Journal of Heath Psychology, 10*(6), 753–766.

Warwick, L. (1995). Feminist Wicca: Paths to empowerment. *Women and Therapy, 16*(2), 122.

Wilkinson, J. (2005). *Nursing Diagnosis Handbook*. Upper Saddle River, NJ: Pearson Prentice Hall, pp. 247–249, 386–388, 507–509.

Wright, L. (2005). *Spirituality, Suffering, Illness*. Philadelphia, PA: F.A. Davis, p. xviii.

7

Self-Reflection and Self-Awareness

Barbarajo Bockenhauer

Key Terms

Learning Outcomes

1. Define self and the dimensions and function of self-concept.

2. Describe the contribution of philosophy to understanding the concept of self.

3. Demonstrate use of the process of reflection in developing self-awareness and self-growth.

4. Examine the relationship between Maslow's hierarchy of basic human needs and theories of psychological development and understanding of self.

5. Distinguish authentic use of self in the nurse–patient interaction.

6. Compare strategies that support the nurse's use of self.

7. Discuss how the nurse's therapeutic use of self can provide support to patients with mental illness.

Introduction

The Scope and Standards of Practice developed through the collaboration of the American Nurses Association, the American Psychiatric Nurses Association, and the International Society of Psychiatric–Mental Health Nurses references the use of self with purpose as part of psychiatric nursing practice (2014). Each area of nursing has its own specialized practice—specific techniques nurses develop in order to care for patients of different ages, influenced by different cultures and different social and geographic environments. The theories of human behavior are the universally applied lens of developmental stages and basic human needs through which the nurse evaluates each patient against the norm. Each area of nursing practice directs that the nurse deliberately put into service, or "purposefully use," certain skills essential to the technical tasks of that specialty. In psychiatric nursing practice, an essential skill is the use of **self**, "the union of elements (body, emotion, thoughts, and sensations) that constitute the individuality of a being, as well as the consciousness of one's own being" (Arnold & Boggs, 2011, p. 63).

Hildegard Peplau described use of self as an "integral tool" of practice (Peplau, 1952). A tool, such as a stethoscope, is standardized and can be continually evaluated and refined to ensure that it is the optimal design for its purpose. Directions for its use are explicit. The nursing student can practice and receive expert, objective examination of his or her technique before using the tool with a "real" patient. Correct and incorrect use can be recognized; inadequate or defective tools can be replaced. Peplau acknowledges that the nurse's self as a tool of psychiatric–mental health nursing practice can be recognized only as it is reflected in the behavior of the nurse. She challenges the student of psychiatric nursing to attend with "unflinching self-scrutiny and total honesty in assessment of this behavior in interaction with patients" (Peplau, 1997, p. 162). No stethoscope comes with *that* message in its directions for use.

Patricia Benner declared, "Any nurse who is unfamiliar with both the patients and the tools required to provide patient care must be considered a 'novice' and will remain a novice until those conditions change" (Benner, 1984, p. 20). Benner acknowledges the learning goals of the novice. She indirectly references the shared goal of *all* nurses in support of the development of the "tool" of psychiatric nursing: to reflect, understand, and support the growth of self (Box 7-1). Although using the tool of one's self may be more complex than using any other nursing tool, its use is, as Nightingale foretold, fundamental to *all* nursing (LaSala, 2009). As cited in LaSala, Nightingale believed that the nurse achieves "the moral ideal" when using "the whole self" to establish a caring relationship with "the whole of the person receiving care" (LaSala, 2009, p. 423).

This chapter provides the student with an understanding of the central importance of the self of the nurse in caring for the patient with a mental illness through integration of theory as applied to clinical examples. The organizing framework is the simple elegance of Ida Jean Orlando's directive that the nurse use self as manifested in the nurse's reaction (perceptions, thoughts, and feelings) to the patient's behavior. Early nursing theorist Martha Rogers (1970) contended that we are in a state of constant change and evolution. As such, the student of psychiatric nursing will reflect on an endlessly evolving self. This evolution will occur *while* the nurse is participating in a therapeutic interpersonal relationship with the patient who lives with a psychiatric illness, a disease that affects behavior and mood rather than organ or system function. The student will evaluate the patient's suffering, as it is both witnessed and reflected upon. Theories of human development should explain the conditions and characteristics that support or interfere with the *development* of self. Orlando's nursing theory will provide a framework within which the self *conceptualizes* a plan to provide nursing care. It is important to understand that theories alone cannot precisely design specific interventions that assist the nurse to master the use of self; the nurse's experiences provide the *opportunity* to do so.

The practice of **self-reflection** provides an opportunity for nurses to examine their own actions and motivations and feelings. It helps nurses make sense of their actions within the context of their relationships with patients and develop creativity in nursing practice (Asselin, 2011).

Self as Art versus Self as Tool

box 7-1

Like art, the self is highly personal and unique. Pieces of art may reflect a similar color scheme, technique, or subject, much as the self reflects a general physiological and psychological pattern common to *all* selves. However, both art and self have intrinsic qualities that differentiate one from any other. Art conveys different meanings at different times in one's life, a quality of evolution and change that mirrors the constant evolution of the individual's self. As with art, the use of self can be powerfully influential with both individuals and groups.

Although the use of self is integral to the practice of psychiatric nursing, a "practice self" is not provided in the psychiatric–mental health nursing simulation lab. No precision instrument measures how much, or what type of, self is needed or has been delivered. A template self cannot be downloaded, nor can a spare self be borrowed from a roommate. The self being "used as art" is the same self that is continually:

- Learning the theories of human behavior, with the consequent and constant changing that learning promotes.

- Filtering perceptions, thoughts, feelings, and behaviors in new experiences through consciously remembered or unconsciously incorporated previous experiences of life.
- Witnessing, supporting, accompanying, and helping an individual who is experiencing the suffering associated with the loss of part of self.

Critical Thinking Questions

1. Reflect on your own self as a work of art. What size and shape are you? What colors and textures make up your self? Is the image calm and cool, or energetic and warm? Is the image completely organized and able to be seen, or are there parts of your self that overlap or are crumpled into a tight ball so that they are not visible to you?

2. Do you think your self is the same in the morning and the evening? When you are with friends or alone? When you are tired? Frustrated?

3. What are you feeling as you reflect on your self?

Julie and Steve	journal exercise 1

Introduction

Harrison and Fopma-Loy (2010) developed and pilot-tested journal prompts with students of psychiatric–mental health nursing. The prompts were based on Goleman's domains of emotional intelligence and the competencies associated with those domains. The authors noted that the prompts, used progressively over the duration of the course, were an effective tool with which to introduce and stimulate growth of the student's emotional intelligence. The authors also noted that students found completing a response to the prompt to take considerable time and emotional energy, as did faculty in providing feedback to the student responses. The students needed time to integrate and comment on the experience as well as time and a "safe" environment with the faculty member to explore thoughts and feelings identified in the response. In this chapter and on the companion website, journal prompts are provided that can be used or modified for use by students and faculty. For some prompts, sample journal entries for "Julie" are provided in text or on the website; sample entries for "Steve" are provided on the companion website. Each sample entry comes with critical thinking questions for use in classroom discussions.

Julie and Steve, Journal Exercise 1

Julie and Steve are nursing students who have been assigned, on different days, to the same clinical placement for their psychiatric–mental health nursing rotation—the day hospital of the crisis center affiliated with the local community mental health center. The day hospital offers patients a safe environment, medication adjustment and monitoring, and an opportunity to participate in intensive individual and group therapies until the crisis is resolved. Peer counselors play an active role at the day hospital, which is also staffed by an Advanced Practice Registered Nurse, primary nurses, a psychologist, a social worker, an occupational therapist, and clinical mental health counselors. Whether those they serve are identified as consumers, clients, or patients, all are supported in meeting individualized clinical goals. Julie and Steve will "shadow" Kelly, one of the primary nurses, and be assigned to patients in her caseload. Their clinical instructor is Shawn Wilson, APRN, a Naval Reserve officer who recently returned from a reactivation tour in Afghanistan. In addition to the journal prompts that are standard for each clinical experience, students are asked to begin a self-reflective journal, starting with the direction to "think about your self—what defines you and makes you an individual? How would your best friends or family describe you? How do you imagine who you are will have an impact on the patient with whom you work?"

Julie's Entry: I'm Julie. I think I'm mostly defined as a single parent, a part-time nursing assistant, and a full-time student. I'm a returning senior but should have graduated this past spring. I'm in the top of my class, but I had to withdraw for a semester because my pregnancy got very complicated. Ben is 18 months old now, and we are both healthy, although I haven't lost my pregnancy weight. I am renting a room in my parents' house until I graduate and get a full-time nursing job. Ben stays with my parents while I'm at school and work; my mom says she enjoys being a stay-at-home grandmother even more than she enjoyed being a stay-at-home mom, but she needs to get a part-time job. My dad is disabled and my mom and I both need to work at least part time to cover our bills while I am in school. My younger brother is in the Army and is going to Iraq next month.

My school friends all graduated last year, but my current classmates would probably describe me as "driven" because I don't join in their activities. I just don't have a minute to relax. My instructors have always said I excel at critical thinking, but may not be as comfortable "connecting" with patients. I believe that a patient would rather have a nurse who knows what to do than one who just knows how to hold hands. I have my final preceptorship in an emergency department. The ED Manager said he might have a job for me after graduation ". . . if you survive your psych rotation." I am a little worried about that comment, but I only have to get through 14 clinical days. My brother's friends say that some of their buddies go "psycho" when they get back from combat. My dad's been in AA for years and always makes a point of saying that an alcoholic can stop drinking but "a crazy person can't stop being crazy." All I know about mental illness is what I've read in the newspaper or seen in movies and heard in class. I have to say I'm not really looking forward to spending time with people who are unpredictable and sometimes dangerous.

Critical Thinking Questions

1. What aspects of self does Julie reveal in her initial entry?
2. What similarities do you see between yourself and Julie? What differences?

Based on Harrison, P. A., & Fopma-Loy, J. L. (2010). Reflective journal prompts: A vehicle for stimulating emotional competence in nursing. Journal of Nursing Education, 49(11), 644–652. Steve's entry may be found on the Pearson student resource site nursing. pearsonhighered.com

Self-Reflection, Awareness, and Growth

"I wonder if I've been changed in the night? Let me think: Was I the same when I got up this morning? I almost think I can remember feeling a little different. But if I'm not the same, the next question is 'Who in the world am I?' Ah, THAT'S the great puzzle!"

(Carroll, *Alice's Adventures in Wonderland*, 1865, 1990)

It is unlikely that students of psychiatric–mental health nursing will be quite as puzzled as Alice when she went through the looking glass.

However, the *process* of reflecting that is being proposed is not dissimilar to Alice's, and the *result* of reflection is the same—a change of self. The interest in reflective practice in nursing grew from a recognition that the highly technical aspects of nursing education appeared to develop students who focused on and valued the "'hands-on skills' . . . while overlooking the human being for whom they are caring" (Harrison & Fopma-Loy, 2010, p. 44). Psychiatric–mental health nursing, in contrast, has no technical skills on which to focus, and it is the self of the nurse that is characterized as an integral tool in the care of the suffering psychiatric patient. The student of

Process of Reflection

table 7-1

Stage 1—*What?*	• Willingness and openness to perform self-assessment • Focus on thoughts, beliefs, and feelings related to experiences • Struggle between comfort and discomfort • Thinking about a situation prior to having to deal with it
Stage 2—*So What?*	• Critical analysis and exploration of alternatives • Determination of strengths and areas for development • Thinking about the situation in the moment using self-awareness, existing knowledge, and previously learned knowledge
Stage 3—*Now What?*	• Judgment concerning different or same actions in future • Commitment to change if necessary • Formulation of action plan • Thinking about the situation after it happens and processing to make sense of it in order to improve future decisions

Based on Atkins & Murray, as noted in Freshwater, D. (2008). Reflective practice: The state of the art. In D. Freshwater, B. Taylor, & G. Sherwood (Eds.). *International Textbook of Reflective Practice in Nursing*. Oxford, UK: Blackwell, pp. 1–18; Borton, T. (1970). *Reach, Teach and Touch*. London: McGraw Hill; Jasper, M. (2007). Using reflective journals and diaries to enhance practice and learning. In C. Buhlman and S. Schultz (Eds.), *Reflective Practice in Nursing* (4th ed.). Chichester, West Sussex, UK: Blackwell Publishing, Ltd., pp. 163–188; Sherwood, G. D., & Horton-Deutsch, S. (2012). *Reflective Practice: Transforming Education and Improving Outcomes*. Indianapolis: Sigma Theta Tau; Greenwood, J. (1998). The role of reflection in single and double loop learning. *Journal of Advanced Nursing*, 27, 1048–1053.

psychiatric–mental health nursing must attend to learning the qualities and capacities of self.

Reflection, in the context of learning, is defined as the thinking and feeling behaviors that are used to both create and clarify the meaning of an event (Mezirov, 1990). The process of reflection is subjective, involving a conscious focus and attention to exploration and understanding of the thoughts and feelings that are in one's conscious awareness (Horton-Deutsch & Sherwood, 2008). Reflection also involves developing and comparing an objective understanding of self that may have been experienced subjectively and without understanding (Harrison & Fopma-Loy, 2010; Freshwater, 2008). By focusing on one's own beliefs, attitudes, values, and the meaning one attaches to experiences and people, reflection provides a vehicle to access a greater understanding of one's own convictions and values (Freshwater, 2008). The nurse measures the effect of reflection in increased self-understanding and, potentially, in changes in his or her own thoughts and behavior. Table 7-1 outlines the process of reflection.

The process of reflection requires preparation. More than simply participating in an intellectual process, the nurse must actually *want* to reflect. As such, reflection is grounded in an attitude of openness and eagerness to turn one's focus *in*, rather than *out*, and to become *aware* of and *think about* the feelings and ideas that are being uncovered (Asselin, 2011). As described, the process of reflection offers an opportunity for change. The nurse regulates this transformative potential by choosing *what* and *how much* to reflect. This choice also reflects level of energy and personal courage, because reflection may involve emotional risk (Asselin, 2011; Harrison & Fopma-Loy, 2010; Freshwater, 2008). Additionally, the process involves discomfort as an inescapable, yet essential, element in the recognition and the process of deciding *whether* to change, as well as the *act* of change itself (Freshwater, 2008).

Self-awareness is the capacity to actively identify, process, and collect information about one's internal mental state and public behaviors, including general physical appearance (Morin, 2004). Morin acknowledges the development of the self as noted by developmental theorists, but also suggests that the self develops as a function of self-awareness in which the individual reflects on self and "speaks" to self (2004). Morin's work affirms that of Johnson and others (2002) that the task of self-awareness can be recognized by increased brain activity, primarily in the prefrontal lobes.

Awareness develops through examining one's own behavior and also through receiving feedback about that behavior. A model to understand the different methods of increasing self-awareness, including feedback as well as self-disclosure, was first presented in diagram format, called a Johari window, by Luft and Ingham (1955). See Figure 7-1.

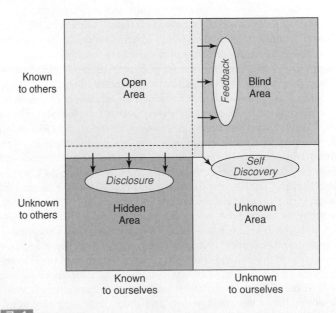

7-1 Johari window.

According to the Johari window, the larger the area known to self and others, the more elements of the self that are available through which to filter, interpret, and cope with the feedback provided by the environment. The environment includes direct verbal feedback as well as nonverbal feedback (for example, a shrug or a smile), but it also includes the feedback received from one's own body in response to stress or changes in health. The blind area is reduced through the process of seeking and receiving feedback from others and the environment. Self-disclosure is a strategy to decrease the hidden area of self. Taking risks in new experiences provides the individual with an opportunity to learn new, previously unknown, information about the self.

The requirement to constantly enrich *and* use the self can be both energizing and exhausting (see Evidence-Based Practice: Compassion Fatigue). Crigger and Godfrey suggest that a particular attitude is integral to self-reflection: "As a critical part of the process, being humble becomes the prerequisite for true reflection on self and one's orientation within the professional world" (Crigger & Godfrey, 2010, p. 314). The nurse's humility is demonstrated by acknowledging that his or her current understanding is inadequate or faulty. Associated with that possibility is the nurse's awareness that he or she may not be able to achieve accurate understanding without the assistance of others. This realization may create a certain degree of anxiety. As the psychiatric–mental health nurse participates in self-reflection, the dissatisfaction with elements of the current self may be experienced as a form of suffering that is resonant with the suffering of the patient.

Pause and Reflect

1. *Why is the nurse's use of self so essential to psychiatric– mental health nursing practice?*
2. *How does self-reflection help nurses in their daily practice?*
3. *In what ways do we receive feedback about our behavior?*

Compassion Fatigue

evidence-based practice

Clinical Question

How is the psychiatric nurse to avoid compassion fatigue if use of self is one of the major factors in its development?

Evidence

Working with patients in crisis can be stressful for nurses, in part because of the requirement that nurses engage in the use of self. As a result, nurses are susceptible to burnout and compassion fatigue. Hooper et al. (2010) reference Maslach's original description of *burnout* as the emotional exhaustion, reduced sense of accomplishment, and distancing associated with prolonged emotional engagement in stressful relationships and situations. Compassion fatigue may be understood as a form of burnout that is experienced by those in caregiving professions, especially nurses. In their concept analysis, Coetzee and Klopper contend that **compassion fatigue** in nursing—the inability to sustain a compassionate and nurturing attitude—is "the final result of a progressive and cumulative process that is caused by prolonged, continuous and intense contact with patients, the use of self and exposure to stress" (2010, p. 237). Their model proposes a gradual evolution of compassion fatigue, starting with compassion discomfort and progressing through compassion stress to eventual compassion fatigue, a state in which the nurse cannot restore the energy that has been expended and is unable to recover a compassionate self. Think of their model on a continuum.

Compassion discomfort is characterized by weariness, diminished enthusiasm and ability, weakening attention, and increasing impatience. The nurse who is unable to overcome this discomfort using appropriate self-care measures (including rest, nutrition, and exercise) may develop *compassion stress*. According to Coetzee and Klopper (2010), compassion stress manifests in a number of ways, including physical discomfort and loss of strength. Irritability, inability to concentrate, and a diminished capacity for empathy— an inability to share in the patient's suffering—may also appear. These combined effects typically result in reduced output and performance. If the nurse is unable to counter this level of stress, *compassion fatigue* results. The nurse experiencing compassion fatigue will be more prone to accident and error, feel apathetic and indifferent to his or her environment, and show poor judgment in the clinical setting (Coetzee & Klopper, 2010).

A study of mindfulness-based stress reduction (MBSR) examined the qualitative and quantitative effect of an 8-week stress-reduction program on nurses' experience of burnout and compassion fatigue (Cohen-Katz, Wiley, Capuano, Baker, & Shapiro, 2004, 2005a, 2005b). The study was designed as a true experiment; subjects were exposed to a pretest and posttest with randomization and a wait list control group. Instruments included the Maslach Burnout Inventory (MBI); the Brief Symptom Inventory (BSI), a measure of psychological distress; the Mindfulness Attention Awareness Scale (MAAS); and, for the experimental group, an evaluation tool. Both groups were tested prior to the intervention (T1); immediately following the test group's completion of the intervention (T2), which coincided with a second cohort's starting the intervention; and at 3 months post-intervention (T3). Nurses were recruited to the study during a one-hour informational program, through articles in the in-house magazine, and at information tables at hospital sites. No cost or payment was associated with the study, other than the cost of a CD set containing guided instruction.

Of the 14 subjects in the experimental arm of the study, 12 completed testing prior to (T1) and immediately following (T2) the intervention, and 10 completed the evaluation. The 12 subjects in the control group completed T1 and T2.

No significant differences were found between groups at T1. Significant differences were found at T2: decreased emotional exhaustion ($P = 0.050$) and increased feelings of personal accomplishment ($P = 0.014$), and increased mindfulness ($P = 0.001$) and a trend toward significance in decrease in feelings of depersonalization ($P = 0.063$). The qualitative results highlighted the impact of participation on relationships, with quotes such as "As a result of this course, I've more to give to others. That 'more' is patience, presence and caring" (Cohen-Katz et al., 2005b, p. 82).

Critical Thinking Questions

1. Does this study provide an answer to the question of how nurses can avoid compassion fatigue?
2. This study included psychiatric nurses, but was not limited to *only* psychiatric nurses. Would you expect the results to be the same or different with different populations of nurses? Why or why not?
3. What other factors may have been affecting the subjects?

Theoretical Foundations

Evidence of interest in the self precedes modern psychological theory by approximately 2500 years: "Know thyself" was carved on the forecourt of the Temple of Apollo at Delphi in the 6th century BCE. In the 4th century BCE, Socrates considered self as the "essential" element of man. His students and their students speculated on the relationship between self and the mind—the center of will, self-motivation and knowing, as well as the source of the development of personal insights into one's desires and feelings (Plato [429–347 BCE] in Ekroth-Bucher, 2001). In an exercise to develop his *own* sense of knowing, 17th-century French mathematician and philosopher René Descartes spent months systematically questioning and doubting all the elements of life that he had previously assumed to be fact (Skirry, 2008). Descartes ultimately arrived at an absolute that could not be doubted—his own existence. In addition to his insight that one's awareness of oneself as a sentient being confirmed one's existence—*I think, therefore I am*—he also proposed that the body was controlled by the mind, which, in turn, received information from the body's interaction with the environment. This mind/body/environment connection supported a holistic focus in psychological and psychiatric theory that would be confirmed, centuries later, by empirical data (Johnson et al., 2002).

Johnson and his colleagues (2002) proposed to identify the anatomical location of the process of conscious reflection on the "self"—examining brain activity as measured by increased blood flow during response to questions that encompass a sense of self—questions about participants' own attitudes, abilities, and traits. Adult subjects were asked to evaluate themselves on a series of statements intended to stimulate thoughts about their mood, social interaction, and cognitive and physical abilities while undergoing functional magnetic resonance imaging (fMRI). In this small study, the investigators confirmed the activation of the anterior medial prefrontal cortex and posterior cingulate cortex during response to self-evaluative, but not factual, knowledge statements. How the self develops in interaction with the mind/body/environment continues to be a focus of psychiatric clinicians and provides the organizing framework for developmental theorists.

Abraham Maslow

Abraham Maslow's description of a hierarchy of human needs evolved from his thoughts on motivation (Maslow, 1970). As discussed in Chapter 4, his contention was that the individual would not seek need fulfillment at the highest level—self-actualization—if basic human needs such as food, water, and shelter were not met. Freedom from immediate danger was essential to being able to belong to a group and establish close friends. Building from that level, the individual would be able to seek and accept recognition and develop self-confidence. From a confident position, the individual is ready to self-actualize.

Self-actualization is not one-dimensional. An example of cognitive self-actualization is an attitude of seeking and accepting learning for the sake of learning, rather than to avoid a bad grade or to ensure inclusion in a social group. Self-actualization also includes an aesthetic element of comfort with one's own self and one's life meaning. Each of these supports the well-being commonly associated with self-actualization: knowing who one is, understanding one's purpose in life, and having a sense of how to accomplish (or how one has accomplished) that purpose. Applied to developmental theory, Maslow's hierarchy suggests that the individual will not be reasonably

motivated to seek and successfully achieve the developmental milestones if basic needs are unmet. The developmental theories that follow are predicated on the individual having met physiological, safety, social, and esteem needs on at least the basic level.

William James

In his classic text, *Principles of Psychology*, American philosopher and psychologist William James defines a "self" that includes both "I" and "me," establishing the framework for modern psychology and psychiatry that attends to the person as both one who experiences *and* is aware of the process of experiencing (James, 1890). James's seminal work conceptualized the "I-self" as the self that acts in order to learn, the "self as knower." This is the part of self that takes initiative to seek experiences and understanding (James, 1890). The "me-self" was the "self as known." This is the part of the self that the person has access to and is composed of consciously known elements. James speculated that the number of different aspects of "self" was directly proportional to the number of individuals whose opinion mattered to the person. By this expansive definition of the "self," James included all the people, things, and characteristics in which the individual has an emotional investment. James's self is dynamic and fluid, changing in response to the environment and completely unique to the individual (James, 1890).

James's definition of self explains the sense of loss of self that is experienced when moving from a well-loved community, losing a meaningful job, or even breaking a treasured trinket. Each holds meaning and helps define the individual's self. The emotional investment and meaning in each of these are part of the self of the person and begin to characterize what has been described as **self-concept**, that part of self that lies within the conscious awareness. Self-concept encompasses those perceptions, thoughts, and feelings as well as values and ideals that are part of the self (Arnold & Boggs, 2011).

Harry Stack Sullivan

Twentieth-century psychiatrist Harry Stack Sullivan built on the work of James and Freud with his emphasis on the impact of the *interpersonal* experience on the *intrapsychic* development (Sullivan, 1953). Sullivan's interpersonal theory proposes that development of the self is dependent on one's reflection from the "others" with whom one interacts. He described a "self-system" made up of the self-images reflected from interactions with one's environment, the "good me," the "bad me," and the "not me." The child instinctively seeks out opportunities to define self positively through rewarding and validating interactions. Consider the baby's smile that is rewarded with the comforting tactile stimulation of a hug. The child adds the characteristic "one who is safe and cared about" to his or her good sense of self, the smiling "good me." The anxiety associated with defining self negatively is stimulated by the punishing, disapproving, or invalidating experiences of self—the "bad me." The behavior of pulling the cat's tail and sustaining the resultant scratch provides support for the characteristic of self as naughty, as "one who should experience pain." The "not me" is defined as that intensely anxiety-inducing situation experienced as overwhelming and destructive of self. Sullivan contended that it was the failure to be able to avoid this destructive anxiety that was a source of serious psychiatric illness.

Sullivan proposed that the effective self-system serves three purposes: (1) self-definition, by supporting the individual's development of a consistent sense of self; (2) protection, by providing a barrier to anxiety; and (3) connection, by establishing the characteristics that ensure security in interpersonal relationships (Sullivan,

1953). Sullivan considered that self-development occurred simultaneously with physical maturation, and was essentially complete by late adolescence. In acknowledging the commonality, rather than differences, between those in need of care and those who provide the care, Sullivan reminds the nurse that that we are all "much more simply human than otherwise." (Sullivan, 1953, p. 4).

Carl Rogers

Psychologist Carl Rogers used a systems theory perspective to describe the self as consisting of a pattern of conscious perceptions and values of the "I" or "me" (Rogers, 1952). Rogers agrees that the self develops through a process of interaction with the environment, noting that this interaction may result in the unconscious incorporation of others' ideas and values into one's own self (Rogers, 1952). Rogers noted that the self seeks internal consistency and drives the individual to engage in actions that are consistent with the internal self. The comment "that's not like him" captures our recognition that this consistency has been violated. Rogers predicts the relative infrequency of these violations by pointing out that experiences that are not consistent with the self are perceived as threats and are avoided. Rogers does not propose a timeline for change, as do Freud, Sullivan, and other theorists, but he does acknowledge that the self changes as a result of maturation and learning.

Erik Erikson

Erikson conceptualized a maturational process that was likely mediated by the naturally occurring physiological changes of progressive brain myelinization as well as the impact on that physiology from the social/emotional influences of interpersonal interactions (Erikson,

1968). In Erikson's developmental model, the individual must successfully and sequentially meet physiological and psychosocial challenges roughly corresponding to a chronological age in order to be prepared to meet the challenges of the next stage. Failure to manage the tasks of one stage may result in a reduced capacity to meet the challenges of the next stage and become an area of continuing weakness (Erikson, 1968). By analyzing observed behaviors, the nurse can hypothesize the level at which developmental challenges were experienced. The model purports to describe a developmental process that continues through old age until one's death.

Vaillant examined Erikson's work in a longitudinal study of two samples of inner city dwelling men. As a result of his findings supporting Erikson's stages, Vaillant proposed two additional developmental "tasks" associated with the healthy transition of the adult through old age (Vaillant & Milofsky, 1980). Between intimacy and generativity, Vaillant added *career consolidation*—a stage in which men must achieve some reasonable sense of meaning and purpose in their career. Vaillant also proposed a stage that is a variation on generativity—the *keeper of the meaning*. In this stage, the individual feels responsible to think and act beyond the small confines of family to ensure that the culture and way of life persists after the individual ceases to do so.

Table 7-2 demonstrates the relationship between Freud's psychosexual stages, Erikson's psychosocial development (Chapter 4), and its variation as a result of the work of Vaillant (including ego strengths and overall goals), the behaviors associated within each stage that reflect age-appropriate successful resolution of the state, and behaviors that the nurse could recognize as reflective of effective resolution of the developmental stage.

Stages of Development of the Self   table 7-2

Theorist/Developmental Stage	Ego Strength/Goal	Behaviors Indicating Resolution of Developmental Tasks	Stage Stressors
Freud: Oral—focus on mouth, dependency **Erikson:** Trust vs. mistrust *Corresponding age:* 0–2 years	Hope To get, to take	• Appropriate attachment behaviors; social smiling; eating successfully; exploring textures and objects with mouth • Gives and listens to information related to self and health • Shares opinions and experiences easily • Demonstrates judgment in deciding whom and how much to trust	• Unfamiliar environment • Inconsistency in care • Pain • Lack of information • Unmet needs • Losses at critical times or accumulated loss • Significant or sudden loss of physical function
Freud: Anal—focus on control of elimination; self-control and obedience **Erikson:** Autonomy vs. shame and doubt *Corresponding age:* 2–4 years	Willpower To hold on, to let go	• Bowel and bladder control • Expresses opinions freely and able to incorporate polite behaviors • Delays gratification • Accepts reasonable rules • Regulates own behaviors • Makes age-appropriate decisions	• Overemphasis on unfair or rigid regulation • Cultural emphasis on guilt and shaming as a way of controlling behavior • Limited opportunity to make choices • Limited allowance for individuality
Freud: Phallic—focus on sexual organs; sexual identity **Erikson:** Initiative vs. guilt *Corresponding age:* 4–6 years	Purpose To make, to "make like" (to play or pretend)	• Sexualized play • Develops realistic goals and initiates actions to meet them • Makes mistakes without undue embarrassment	• Significant or sudden change in life pattern that interferes with role • Loss of a mentor, particularly in adolescence or with a new job • Lack of opportunity to participate in planning of care

Theorist/Developmental Stage	Ego Strength/Goal	Behaviors Indicating Resolution of Developmental Tasks	Stage Stressors
		• Curious about body and environment, willing to recognize health care as part of self-care needs • Develops fantasies as well as constructive, reality–based plans • Works to achieve goals	• Overinvolved parenting that seriously limits experimentation • Hypercritical authority figures
Freud: Latency—Calm **Erikson:** Industry vs. inferiority *Corresponding age:* 6 years–puberty	Competence To make things, to make things together	• Experiences meaning and sense of accomplishment in school, play, or work • Achieves pattern of satisfactory balance between work and play activity • Plays/works effectively with others, including teachers and staff • Completes tasks and self-care activities in line with age-appropriate capabilities • Describes personal strengths and challenges accurately; has realistic self-evaluation	• Limited opportunity to learn and master tasks • Illness, circumstance, or condition that compromises or eliminates opportunity for usual activities • Lack of cultural support or opportunity for learning/training
Freud: Genital—Sexuality, intimacy development completed **Erikson:** Identity vs. identity diffusion *Corresponding age:* Post-puberty (13–19 years)	Fidelity To be oneself, to share oneself	• Establishes friendships with peers • Asserts independence and dependence needs realistically • Accepts self-image, including physical characteristics, personality • Expresses and acts on personal values • Self-perception congruent with observations of significant others, nurse	• Lack of access to peer group • Overprotective, neglectful, or inconsistent parenting • Sudden or significant change in appearance, health, or status • Lack of role models
No Freudian stage **Erikson:** Intimacy vs. isolation *Corresponding age:* Young adulthood (20–30 years)	To lose oneself and find oneself in another	• Establishes strong reciprocal interpersonal relationships • Identifies available support system • Open to feeling cared about by others • Establishes stable, harmonious, fulfilling relationships with family and friends	• Competition • Communication that includes a hidden agenda • Projection of images and expectations onto another person • Lack of privacy • Loss of significant others at critical points of development
Vaillant: Career consolidation *Corresponding age:* Middle adulthood	Finding purposeful activity that reflects value to others	• Finds contentment, compensation, competence, and commitment in a work activity • Establishes collegial relationships that provide support and companionship	• Physical, psychological, or social challenges to accessing meaningful work
Erikson: Generativity vs. stagnation and self-absorption *Corresponding age:* Middle adulthood and beyond	To let be and to make be, to take care of	• Engages in age-appropriate activities • Realistically assesses own contributions to society • Maximizes productivity • Provides care for what one has created • Shows concern for others and a willingness to share ideas and knowledge • Healthfully balances work, family, and self demands	• Aging parents, separately or concurrently with adolescent children • Obsolescence or layoff in career • "Me generation" attitude • Inability to function as previously • Children leaving home • Forced retirement

(continued)

Stages of Development of the Self (continued)			table 7-2
Theorist/Developmental Stage	**Ego Strength/Goal**	**Behaviors Indicating Resolution of Developmental Tasks**	**Stage Stressors**
Vaillant: Keeper of the meaning *Corresponding age:* Late adulthood	Conservation and preservation of the collective products of mankind	• Provides "care" for the culture in which one lives and its institutions	• Psychological challenges to this attitude • At-risk culture
Erikson: Integrity vs. despair *Corresponding age:* Late adulthood	To face not being	• Satisfied with personal lifestyle • Acceptance of growing limitations while maintaining maximum productivity • Acceptance of death; satisfaction with one's contributions to life	• Rigid lifestyle • Loss of significant other • Loss of physical, intellectual, and emotional faculties • Loss of previously satisfying work and family roles

Based on Arnold, E. C., & Boggs, K. U. (2011). Interpersonal Relationships: Professional Communication Skills for Nurses. St. Louis, MO: Elsevier Saunders; Erikson, E. H. (1950, 1963). Childhood and Society. New York: W.W. Norton; Erikson, E. H. (1968). Identity, Youth and Crisis. New York, NY: W.W. Norton; Freud, S. (1955, 1971) The Psychopathology of Everyday Life. New York, NY: W.W. Norton; Vaillant, G. E. (2003). Mental health. American Journal of Psychiatry, 160(8), 1373–1384; Vaillant G. E., & Milofsky, E. (1980). Natural history of male psychological health: Empirical evidence for Erikson's model of the life cycle. American Journal of Psychiatry, 137(11), 1348–1359.

The developmental process fits well into what has been described as "scaffolding"—a passive, natural process by which the abstract and less-understood concepts are mapped onto understood skills and concepts, while retaining the character of the original (Williams, Huang, & Bargh, 2009). This phenomenon is noted most easily when interacting with an individual with whom one has had a close relationship since childhood. The energetic and interpersonally sensitive child can still be recognized in the developmentally mature high power and highly effective sales manager. Although the individual may be relatively unaware of his or her original "scaffold," it remains a factor in his or her additional development or understanding. The process of reflecting on one's own "scaffold" provides information about self that leads to understanding and growth (Jack & Miller, 2008; Vandemark, 2006).

Pause and Reflect

1. *Do you know people whose basic needs are not met? How does this affect their ability to learn? To care for others? How does it affect their daily functioning?*
2. *How might interaction with the environment result in the unconscious incorporation of others' ideas and values? Have you ever observed this in yourself or others?*
3. *What implications do Vaillant's stages of career consolidation and keeper of meaning suggest for nursing care of older adults?*

Nursing Theories

The theories of human behavior provide the science for psychiatric–mental health nursing. The fields of psychology, psychiatry, and counseling all reference the theories that have been described. However, it is the nursing theorists that are integral to understanding the art of nursing.

Hildegard Peplau

Hildegard Peplau (1952) noted that the self of the nurse is used to evaluate or confirm that the work done with the patient is, in fact, therapeutic. Peplau (1997) incorporates Sullivan's thoughts on the development of the self as a result of interactions within the interpersonal environment. She identifies the therapeutic significance of what happens between the nurse and the patient, and recognizes that the nurse is involved in a continual process of developing self within that relationship. Peplau asserts that the psychiatric nurse's development also includes acquiring an ability to trust others and become comfortable with dependency, to delay satisfaction, and to develop what she refers to as "participatory skills" (1997). In the current nursing environment, this last task would likely be described as learning how to act as a member of a clinical team. Peplau did not suggest that these tasks were sequential, although they clearly reflect elements of development explored by Erikson, Sullivan, and Freud. Her work is particularly influenced by Sullivan's interpersonal focus (Peplau, 1997).

Ida Jean Orlando

Orlando's focus on the self is implied in her directive that the nurse use any part of his or her *reaction* to the patient as the starting point to begin to validate the patient's experience of distress and plan interventions to reduce that distress (Orlando, 1961, 1987). Her definition of the nurse's reaction includes perceptions, or cues picked up by any of the five senses; thoughts that are stimulated by the perceptions; and feelings, the emotional responses to the thoughts that had been generated. *Although the nurse may be an expert on a particular physiologic condition, the patient is the expert in the lived experience of that condition.* The nurse's ability to be genuine and focused on the patient "in the moment" is essential to the effectiveness of this approach. Orlando contends that the nurse *depends* on the patient to verify (1) the presence of the patient's distress, (2) the possible source of that distress, (3) the plan for management of the distress, and (4) the evaluation of the effectiveness of that plan. To do so, the nurse must be aware of what parts of the reaction to the patient are, in fact, a reaction to a part of the nurse's own self (Potter & Bockenhauer, 2000). By validation of perceptions, thoughts, and/or feelings, the nurse confirms what the patient needs and deliberatively meets that need. The process of checking or validating engages the nurse's genuine self. Figure 7-2 illustrates the constant process of validation (V) of perceptions (P) and/or thoughts (T) and/or feelings (F) that result in deliberative nursing (DN). This process of validation can be illustrated through **process recording**, a written record of an interaction between two or more individuals, in this case the nurse and the patient. Journal Exercise 2 provides an illustration of use of this model.

$$\frac{P +/- \ T +/- \ F}{V} = DN$$

Pause and Reflect

1. *Why does the process of developing the self continue through the therapeutic nurse–patient relationship?*
2. *Why is it important to recognize the patient as the "expert in the lived experience" of his or her illness?*

7-2   Deliberative nursing is a constant process of validating perceptions, thoughts, and feelings.

Julie—Focus on Judgment   journal exercise 2

Julie is given the assignment to journal about a situation she encounters in her clinical rotation, in which she is asked to detail a situation in which she felt she was being judged and a situation in which she judged someone else. She is to journal about her feelings, how the judging may have affected her or the other person's sense of self, and how it affected her subsequent behavior.

PERCEPTIONS, THOUGHTS, & FEELINGS: A Patient with Schizophrenia

Dan Porter is a 42-year-old man who was diagnosed with schizophrenia, paranoid type, at age 26. He hasn't been hospitalized since 2000 and is stable on a combination of olanzapine, an antipsychotic, and depakote, a mood stabilizer. He sees his advanced practice nurse once every three months, or more often if needed. He is tall and thin (BMI = 19), and today is dressed in wrinkled but clean-looking clothes and worn sneakers. He is clean shaven, with several small cuts on his jaw and neck that have been blotted with bits of toilet paper; his hair is long and wet and pulled back into a ponytail. He comes to the clinic once each week to participate in a group program in which members discuss their individual wellness plans. Dan has been working on being more careful with his grooming so that he can again use the public library. He had been asked to leave because his body odor and general appearance were disturbing to the library's other users.

Perceptions	Thoughts and feelings	Action	
Standing, shifting weight from foot to foot, in front of appointment desk. Sign on appointment desk says "I'll be back in five minutes; please take a seat."	*Thoughts:* Is he having akathisia? Does he know how to read the sign? Is he confused about what to do or is he ambivalent about whether to sit down or remain standing? *Feelings:* Mildly anxious Eager to establish a therapeutic relationship with him	Approach patient, introduce myself, smile and attempt to make eye contact.	**Nurse:** Hi. I'm Julie, a nursing student. Would you like to talk with me for a bit?
Turns slightly to look at me, makes brief eye contact, says "Hi," then turns away.	*Thoughts:* Able to focus, not responding to auditory hallucinations at this time *Feelings:* Less anxious	I pointed out the area designated as the "quiet conversation" corner.	**Nurse:** Can we meet each Tuesday that I am here, at 10 a.m. in this lobby? We can sit in that corner.
Dan: You're a student?	*Thoughts:* Attending to the here and now experience, seeking orientation. Is he having disorganized thoughts? *Feelings:* I need to orient D.P. to my role.	Elements of therapeutic contract	**Nurse:** Yes, I am a nursing student. I'll be here every Tuesday for the next seven weeks and I'd like to plan to meet with you each Tuesday at 10 a.m. Is that OK?
Dan: What college?	*Thoughts:* Is he too disorganized in his thinking to keep track of all the pieces of information that I was giving him? *Feelings:* Concerned about boundaries	OK to disclose personal information that is not private	**Nurse:** I go to State, like my badge says. So, can we plan to meet each week?

Julie—Focus on Judgment (continued)

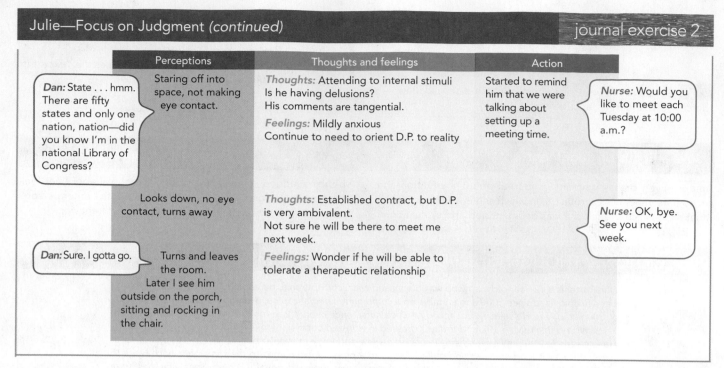

	Perceptions	Thoughts and feelings	Action
Dan: State . . . hmm. There are fifty states and only one nation, nation—did you know I'm in the national Library of Congress?	Staring off into space, not making eye contact.	**Thoughts:** Attending to internal stimuli. Is he having delusions? His comments are tangential. **Feelings:** Mildly anxious. Continue to need to orient D.P. to reality.	Started to remind him that we were talking about setting up a meeting time. **Nurse:** Would you like to meet each Tuesday at 10:00 a.m.?
	Looks down, no eye contact, turns away	**Thoughts:** Established contract, but D.P. is very ambivalent. Not sure he will be there to meet me next week.	**Nurse:** OK, bye. See you next week.
Dan: Sure. I gotta go.	Turns and leaves the room. Later I see him outside on the porch, sitting and rocking in the chair.	**Feelings:** Wonder if he will be able to tolerate a therapeutic relationship	

Julie's Journal Entry

When I spoke with Kelly, the primary nurse, about working with D.P., I told her my concerns about boundaries and that I thought D.P. was experiencing delusions. She said that D.P. had a doctoral degree in history and wrote a book that was indeed catalogued in the Library of Congress. Then we talked about the difference between concrete thinking and delusions. She also mentioned that D.P. tends to bring up his book as a self-esteem boost. When she said that, I wondered if she thought I had not been attentive to this need when I was talking with D.P. I actually felt sick to my stomach that she would think that of me. Later I went back to her and apologized for not doing a better job with D.P. She looked a little surprised and said that she respected my using her to help figure things out and that she enjoys working with students. I thought she was judging me, but maybe she wasn't. Even thinking she was felt awful. As I read over my process recording, I think I might have been judging D.P., too. I thought I understood what symptoms he was having and judged his comments to be part of his illness, rather than meaningful information.

Critical Thinking Questions

1. Consider Maslow's hierarchy of needs. What need does Julie express in this journal entry?
2. How do you think engaging in self-reflection is helping Julie in her growth as a nurse?
3. What emotion is she able to recognize in her patient? In herself?

Based on Harrison, P. A., & Fopma-Loy, J. L. (2010). Reflective journal prompts: A vehicle for stimulating emotional competence in nursing. Journal of Nursing Education, 49(11), 644–652; Orlando, I. J. (1972). The Discipline and Teaching of Nursing Process (An Evaluative Study). *New York: G. P. Putnam's Sons.*

Characteristics of Self

Characteristics of self that inform who we are include our perceptions, thoughts, and feelings. Our senses, cognitive abilities, and feelings all play a role in both the development and the use of self.

Perceptions, Thoughts, and Feelings

Orlando (1971) suggests that perception is the primary element in the nurse's initial reactive response to the behavior of the patient. **Perception** includes the capacities of the five senses and is the primary cognitive process by which an individual collects sensory data and clusters it into a pattern (Arnold & Boggs, 2011; Lotto, 2010). Naming the pattern and remembering its name relies on other elements of self—cognition, in particular. The development of perceptual ability is dependent on the physiological *and* social environment (James & Swain, 2011). James and Swain provide empirical evidence of the importance of self-generated action in establishing the sensory–motor systems in the

developing brain. They found greater learning to be associated with visual and tactile stimulation involving the object being learned.

The infant begins learning relevant visual and auditory and tactile patterns at birth, building neural pathways to being able to recognize people, toys, and letters. Rather than functioning precisely, like a camera or recording device, the patterns created are those that conform to patterns that have previously been evaluated as relevant (Lotto, 2010) or to those that one has greater motivation to see (Balcetis & Dunning, 2006; Chabris & Simons, 2010)). Simply put, individuals see and hear that which has proved useful to see and hear, and are relatively inattentive to stimuli with which they have no experience or do not think that they need.

In research with undergraduates, Chabris and Simons (2010) used the term *attentional blindness* to refer to the process of seeing what is important and paying relatively little attention to the rest of the visual stimulation. In their classic study, college-age subjects were asked to count how many times people in a videotape passed a

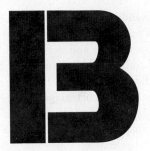

Attentional blindness: B or 13?

basketball among themselves. Fully 40% of subject "counters" failed to see a person dressed in a gorilla suit walk slowly into the middle of the group who were passing the basketball, turn to the camera, beat its chest, and then walk out. The subjects were motivated to focus on the basketball and not the figure of the gorilla, despite its obviousness.

Balcetis and Dunning (2011) used sophisticated ocular tracking processes to confirm that individuals' motivation will affect what their senses actually respond to. When showed the same ambiguous figure and told that if it were the number "13" it would direct them to the group that would sample a tasty-looking drink, whereas if it were a "B" it would direct them to the group that would be sampling an unappealing drink, subjects interpreted the figure to direct themselves to the group that would receive the more appealing drink (Figure 7-3). The figure itself did not change; the motivation of the subjects defined their perception of the figure (Box 7-2).

Cognition
Cognition, or thought, is described as the more complex process of creating order and meaning from experiences. Piaget's definitive research in the area of cognitive development is based on extensive observational study of children and provides a template from which to compare functional levels (1952). Piaget hypothesized that infants are born with schemes operating at birth, which he called "reflexes." In other animals, these reflexes control behavior throughout life. However, as the infant uses these reflexes to adapt to the environment, the reflexes are quickly replaced with constructed "schemes"— behaviors organized and planned though a cognitive process.

Piaget described two processes used by the individual in the attempt to adapt: assimilation and accommodation. Both of these processes are used throughout life as the person increasingly adapts to the environment in a more complex manner. *Assimilation* is the process of using or transforming the environment so it can be placed in preexisting cognitive structures (understood in relationship to existing knowledge). *Accommodation* is the process of changing cognitive structures to accept something from the environment. Both processes are used simultaneously and alternately throughout life. An example of assimilation would be an infant's use of touching and grasping activity to explore new things, an ability developed by previously using the hand to explore familiar people and objects. An example of accommodation would be the child's modifying the touching behavior to one that would be successful for patting a dog.

Emotions
The affective responses—our feelings or emotions—are believed to arise as a reaction to the meaning ascribed to perceptions and thoughts. As feelings are an integral element of the self, recognizing what one feels is highly relevant to nursing practice. Goleman has popularized the concept that one's ability to recognize and control the expressed feelings—one's social and emotional behaviors—actually reflects a separate type of intelligence: emotional intelligence, or EQ (1995). In contrast to intellect or IQ, **emotional intelligence** is a measurement of interpersonal phenomena and includes the following:

- Accurate conscious perceptions and monitoring of one's own emotions
- Modification of one's emotions so that their expression is appropriate; managing one's own anxiety and sustaining hope in the face of adversity
- Accurate recognition of and response to emotions in others
- Skill in negotiating close relationships with others
- Capacity for channeling emotional energy to goal achievement—delaying gratification and diverting impulses (Goleman, 1995)

Becoming aware of how one is feeling provides insight into the particular emotional filters that one may be applying in a situation.

Empathy
Awareness also provides the opportunity to plan to understand and control the behavioral manifestations of a feeling and is a factor in the ability to use empathy. **Empathy** can be defined as understanding and experiencing the feelings, thoughts, and experience of another from the other's perspective—connecting with and feeling what the other person is feeling. Sympathy, in contrast, is fundamentally an affirmation of separateness from another's painful experience. It does not involve experiencing what the other person is thinking or feeling. Although sympathy may motivate one to provide invaluable assistance,

---

Motivation and Perception   box 7-2

Emily, a 60-year-old executive director of an investment firm, has been struggling with the symptoms of a major depressive episode for the past month and is considered to be at risk for suicide. Her husband, Cliff, a retired civil engineer, has accompanied her each week as she checks in with Susan, an Advance Practice Registered Nurse, and attends a cognitive–behavioral group session. Cliff greets Susan with a smile and pulls her aside to report that Emily is "back to reading her finance journals all day already. I think she probably doesn't even need that medication." Susan observes that Emily is neatly dressed and groomed. The finance magazine that she is holding, which completely blocks her face from view, is upside down.

Critical Thinking Questions
1. What is Emily's husband motivated to see?
2. What is Emily's APRN motivated to see?
3. What strategies might you use to improve your "sight"?

it does not engage the core functions of the nurse. There may actually be two separate systems for empathy: an emotional system that supports our ability to empathize emotionally, and a cognitive system that involves cognitive understanding of the other's perspective (Shamay-Tsoory, 2011).

It appears that any rigid boundaries among perceptions, thoughts, and feelings are artificial; thoughts, feelings, and perceptions are likely neurochemically linked and influence one another (Balcetis & Dunning, 2006; Lotto, 2011; Picard et al., 2004; Shamay-Tsoory, 2011). This phenomenon has been clinically reflected in nurses' work with psychiatric patients. Consider the individual who is depressed and who looks in the mirror and sees a body that is *almost* thin enough, whereas the anxious clinician sees a gaunt and critically malnourished patient. Both the patient and the clinician perceive a pattern that provides meaning and reflects the influence of their emotions as well as their thoughts.

Self-Concept

Commonly correlated to self-esteem, **self-concept** is broader in scope and reflects, in addition, body image, emotional status, role performance, life goals, sense of identity, spirituality, and the relationship between one's "real" self and one's "ideal" self (Prescott, 2006). The term refers, simply, to how one characterizes oneself—including the thoughts, attitudes, feelings, and beliefs one has about the nature of one's personality and how it is organized (Cunha & Goncalves, 2009). Arnold conceptualizes a holistic self-concept consisting of physical, cognitive, emotional, and spiritual aspects (Arnold, 2011). An individual's self-concept is both unique and dynamic—reflecting the effects of the individual's interaction with the environment as well as the creation of the character of that interaction. The unique aspects of each interaction assist the individual's self-concept to continue to develop and differentiate.

Body image can be described as how one views one's own body in relation to one's own perceptions of what is valuable or beautiful, as well as in relation to how one views others' perceptions. The degree of importance and characteristics of body image may vary according to developmental stage and/or culture. For example, the toddler is unaware of his or her protruding belly and unmanageable hair, but the adolescent is totally consumed by thoughts of exactly those characteristics. Similarly, individuals may focus intensely on reducing the appearance of skin that has lost elasticity or hair that has lost its original color. These body image standards are highly culture-dependent. As an example, in African culture, extra weight is interpreted as a sign of wealth and health, whereas Westernized culture puts a greater value on thinness.

Another element associated with self-concept and grounded in culture is **body space**, the amount of distance that provides a sense of comfort in social situations (Figure 7-4). Hall (1966) did the original work in this area and, through rigorous testing in American

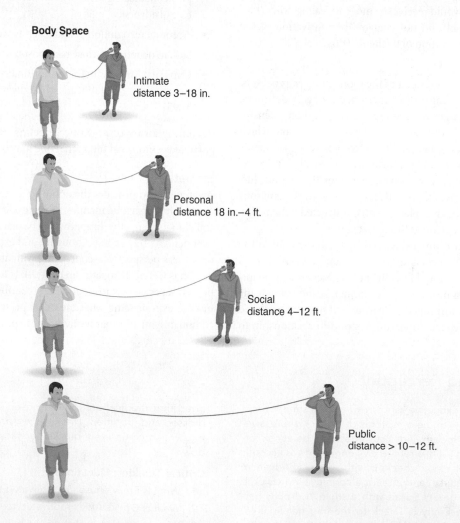

Body Space

Intimate
distance 3–18 in.

Personal
distance 18 in.–4 ft.

Social
distance 4–12 ft.

Public
distance > 10–12 ft.

7-4 Body space.

culture groups, identified four "body spaces"—intimate, personal, social, and public. The parameters of body space often affect how individuals perceive an interaction. For example, one individual may be more comfortable when speaking in close proximity to a complete stranger; another person may require more space to feel comfortable having the same discussion. How one uses body space is referred to as **proxemics**.

Social roles also contribute to self-concept. Roles can be chosen or acquired without voluntary decision making. Although gender and gender identity typically are acquired social roles, an individual may choose not to disclose gender identity. The student role is likely a choice, as is how the student acts in that role—whether, for instance, as one who plans to graduate with honors or one who does not. Leader, follower, boss, and employee are all social roles that could be described as chosen.

Toman, in his classic examination of family constellation, suggests that certain social roles are predictable, based on the individual's position in the family. In his studied population of former and current patients, he found that the oldest sisters of brothers are likely to be highly organized, comfortable with managing and nurturing, and highly pragmatic (Toman, 1969). He found that the youngest brother of brothers is often somewhat flighty and highly dependent on a peer group to help him make decisions. Toman found that an 8-year age difference between the closest siblings would predict a youngest child behaving not completely as a socially motivated "youngest," but more like an "only" child—more tolerant of being alone and acting in a leadership role. He also noted the impact of early parental loss on social roles.

Self-esteem is a personal judgment of self-worth, based on the amount of overlap that exists between **ideal self**—the self one should or would like to be—and what one believes to be true about the actual self. Self-esteem has been identified as a factor in exercise program achievement, surgical outcome, academic testing, and social performance (Arnold & Boggs, 2011). Individuals with high self-esteem are generally able to perform a task equally well with or without observations, possess a positive perception of themselves and their abilities, have strong social support systems, and respond assertively to criticism. In contrast, individuals with low self-esteem view themselves and their abilities negatively, do not perform well under observation, lack a strong support system, and respond poorly or defensively to criticism (Arnold & Boggs, 2011).

Self-concept contains elements that do not seem coherent and are discordant with the whole. Consider the schoolteacher who is gentle with her kindergarten class but vicious on the soccer field, or the brilliant financial manager who cannot write up a shopping list for a simple meal. Individuals define self-concept as the answer to the question "Who am I?" and look for experiences that affirm their self-identity. Although self-concept is clearly rooted in the individual's past experiences and the appraisals of others, it also includes a future orientation (Lee & Oyserman, 2009). A hopeful, positive self-perception may have as much influence on a positive outcome as objectively positive data (Blazer, 2008).

Death of a parent, dysfunctional parenting, inadequate opportunities for education, and a low level of parental education have been shown to have a negative impact on self-concept. Stability of living environment, supportive parental figures and mentors, as well as structured sports activities and the opportunity to be praised for one's successes support the development of positive self-concept (Vaillant, 2003; Vaillant & Milofsky, 1980). A healthy self-concept reflects attitudes, emotions, and values that are realistically consistent with meaningful purposes in life and satisfying to the individual (Arnold & Boggs, 2011). An effective self-concept supports the nurse's ability to engage in a reciprocal relationship with the patient.

Julie   journal exercise 3

Prompt

Experience: Describe a situation in which you did not meet your personal expectations for your clinical performance.

Reflection: Thinking about it now, were your expectations realistic or unrealistic? Explain. Were your expectations healthy or unhealthy? Explain. How might you respond to a peer who voiced these expectations for himself or herself? What are the similarities and differences between how you might respond to a peer and the way in which you responded to yourself (your self-talk)?

Implications: What might be the overall health implications for you if you repeatedly engage in the self-talk you described so it becomes a pattern?

Julie's Journal Entry

I had to use my process recording with D.P. (Dan Porter; see patient description in Journal Exercise 2) because I realized that I was thinking about it a lot, actually losing sleep over it. I kept thinking about how far off I was with him. I expected that by doing the reading and analyzing what he said that I would show you that I understood psychiatric–mental health nursing concepts. But I felt like I completely failed at understanding my patient. I've never "failed" like that. I also realized that I was the only one calling it failure. It's interesting to think about how I would react to one of my classmates, because I think of myself as the "mom" of the group. I give pep talks and try to help out—I'd never call anyone a failure if they did what I did. It may not be like irrigating g-tubes, but this is definitely something that takes learning. Feeling like a failure isn't healthy, but I sure don't feel successful here.

Critical Thinking Questions

1. What roles does Julie assume?
2. What changes to her EQ does she experience?

Based on self-awareness and self-management prompt by Harrison, P. A., & Fopma-Loy, J. L. (2010). Reflective journal prompts: A vehicle for stimulating emotional competence in nursing. *Journal of Nursing Education, 49*(11), 644–652.

Pause and Reflect

1. *What implications do you think the cognitive processes of assimilation and accommodation have for nursing practice?*
2. *What is the relationship between emotional intelligence and empathy?*
3. *Why is it important for nurses to demonstrate behavior consistent with their own personal values and character?*

Use of Self in Nursing Practice

Caring for a patient with a mental illness presents the nurse with the experience of suffering that extends beyond the symptoms of the disease itself. The stigma, or discrimination, associated with mental illness has a profound impact on the patient and family and is considered to be major factor in failure to seek treatment (U.S. Department of Health and Human Services, 1999). Mental illness, as well as the *treatment* of mental illness, causes suffering (Lindholm & Eriksson, 1993; Leete, 1989). Lindholm and Eriksson (1993) also recognize that individuals who have a mental illness are not exempt from the normal life experiences that involve suffering. The nurse has an opportunity to positively influence the provision of care directly, as well as indirectly through modeling and teaching caregivers and family members.

Råholm (2008) suggests that the patient's narrative may be both the source of suffering and the point at which growth and development of potential begin. She confirms the message given by noted psychiatric–mental health nursing and suffering theorists—the patient guides the nurse's response to his or her suffering.

Morse (2001) defines the nurse as the "caretaker of suffering." She contends that the suffering individual fluctuates between a state of *enduring*—experienced as suppressing painful emotions—and the state of emotional release associated with active "suffering." She notes that the individual's choice to engage in the emotional release of suffering is paradoxical in that this release is likely to cause distress in the individual who is responding empathically, thus actually increasing suffering. The individual may choose to conceal the suffering by enduring.

Patients' efforts to conceal suffering also are motivated by the shame and stigma associated with mental illness. Mental health consumer activist Judi Chamberlin (1998) wrote poignantly of being cautioned by other hospitalized patients to avoid looking sad or crying, as staff would think she was depressed and prescribe more medication or delay discharge. Typical human emotional responses—disappointment, anger, longing—were interpreted as pathology if experienced by an individual receiving treatment for a mental illness. In their small, hermeneutic study of caring conversations between patients and nurses, Frederiksson and Lindström (2002) found that the suffering and shame associated with mental illness restricted patients' willingness to risk being open to care. The façade created by the patients with psychiatric illnesses to protect themselves from these painful feelings interfered with their ability to engage with both their illnesses and with their caretakers. The authors suggest that the nurse can influence the resolution of the façade and work toward the patient's self-actualization by engaging in a caring conversation with the patient. In this conversation, the nurse helps the patient reconnect on an interpersonal level, establishing an "interpersonal bridge." It is crucial that the nurse be cognizant of the façade in place and sensitive to its purpose. The nurse creates time and space for the patient to share his or her story and assists in interpreting as needed to help the patient answer the question "Why?" related to the experience of suffering. The authors confirm the *patient's*

role in directing the pace of the process. Respect for this role demands the patience of the nurse (Frederiksson & Lindström, 2002).

Nurses may employ a variety of strategies to connect with patients and promote the strength and hope they need to begin the hard work of recovery. Strategies related to the use of self include authenticity, mindfulness, and presence. Additional strategies, including therapeutic communication, are discussed in Chapter 9.

Authenticity

Nursing theorist Ida Jean Orlando references the importance of the nurse using any part of his genuine, authentic reaction to the patient's behavior as a starting point for a deliberative nursing action (Orlando, 1987). Starr (2008) characterizes **authenticity** in nursing as the nurse's awareness of genuine personality, character, and values, as well as the nurse's demonstrated behavior that is consistent with that awareness, despite pressures to behave otherwise. Starr found that nurses who are authentic people, who demonstrate congruence among ideals, values, and actions, are inherently trustworthy. If the authentic nurse's ideas and values are to promote authenticity in the patient, the nurse may be able to help the patient both realize and act on the patient's potentials (Starr, 2008). Here lies the *art* of nursing.

Shattell, Starr, and Thomas (2007) conducted a secondary analysis of data from a phenomenological study originally designed to explore mental health patients' experience of being understood. Participating patients recognized and acknowledged the importance of the clinician's open, genuine (authentic), nonjudgmental attitude. Patients reported seeking out authentic providers who "said it like it was" and were "real," "straight-up," and "honest."

Reflecting Orlando, Munhall describes authenticity as the nurse being "knowingly" present in his or her own life and interacting "with *full unknowingness* about the other's life" (Munhall, 2004, p. 100, emphasis in original). Munhall acknowledges that the nurse needs to interact genuinely with the patient in order to answer the questions "Who are you? How can I help?"

An authentic existence is one in which the individual is fully aware of the present moment, chooses how to live life in the moment, and takes responsibility for that choice (Corey, 1982). A defining element in the act of choosing is that the decision is based not on following others, but on critically assessing the available options and making choices that reflect the true self (Corey, 1982). As each self is personal and unique, being authentic is necessarily unconventional and anxiety inducing (Thompson, 2005). Nurses who seek increased authenticity do so when they are dissatisfied with some aspect of their lives and decide to face the problem despite the anxiety induced.

The nurse's authenticity is reflected in how the nurse directs energy toward getting to know the patient as the patient is, in the patient's world (Porr, 2005). It may be interesting to consider whether the electronic health information system's software is currently configured to translate that knowing into meaningful data for use in planning and providing care. Consider the change-of-shift report that describes a patient as "quiet, somewhat isolative, attended groups but did not participate"—a description of the patient's behavior from the perspective of the world of the nurse. The report does not describe the patient's response to the different authentic nursing strategies used to try to understand his or her behavior. The report does not describe the conditions of "isolative" behavior in a way that adds to the knowledge of the next shift. Does the patient avoid loud stimulation or choose a particular space at a particular time? What pattern is present? Absence of this information leads the next shift to repeat the same, ineffective approaches.

Rogers's model of authenticity also acknowledges the consistency between one's actual physiological state, emotions, and cognitions and the *awareness* of that experience and the behavioral and emotional expression of that state as reflective of authentic living (Wood et al., 2008). The authentic life is part of and responsive to external influences, rather than alienated or resistant to them. Questions the nurse can ask to examine authenticity include:

- What behaviors do I use that convey trustworthiness? What behaviors do I engage in that come across as less than trustworthy?

- What behaviors do I engage in that communicate sensitivity to others? Do any of my behaviors express insensitivity in some way?

- How good am I at communicating with others clearly? Do I use any behaviors that interfere with my ability to communicate clearly?

- Am I able to see the world from the point of view of my patient? Am I able to understand the patient's values and beliefs?

Mindfulness and Presence

Mindfulness is a form of self-awareness that may be described as a state of being in the present moment and accepting things for what they are without judgment. The "mindful" state is one in which the individual is aware in the current moment but not reacting automatically. The individual is responsive and deliberately aware of the con-

Mindfulness Exercise	box 7-3

1. Pause for a moment before sitting down with a patient or seeking a patient to talk with.
2. Set aside any concerns regarding the past or the future.
3. Gently close your eyes or focus on a neutral space or wall.
4. Breathe deeply and slowly.
5. Repeat to yourself, "I am here for the greater good of this patient. I give my full attention to the here and now."
6. Direct awareness to the area around your heart, bringing to mind something or someone that evokes your feeling of caring and compassion.
7. When connected with that feeling of caring and compassion, repeat, "I am present in the moment."

scious decision to respond (Box 7-3). The mindful state is consistent with Orlando's concept of deliberative nursing action.

Presence refers to a condition in which all of one's attention and energy are focused *in the* moment *on the* purpose of that moment (Figure 7-5). When one is fully present, one feels completely alive and energized. Holistic practitioners suggest that the nurse can learn to achieve this state, regardless of the activity being undertaken, providing the opportunity to experience this level of energy in any work or life experience. The hypothesis is that the more present we are, the more meaningful our entire lives become. Ferrell and Coyle (2008) suggest that the primary way in which the nurse provides a response to suffering is by presence. The nurse's ability to convey the message of mindful presence, willingness to go where the patient leads (rather than leading), and ability to convey

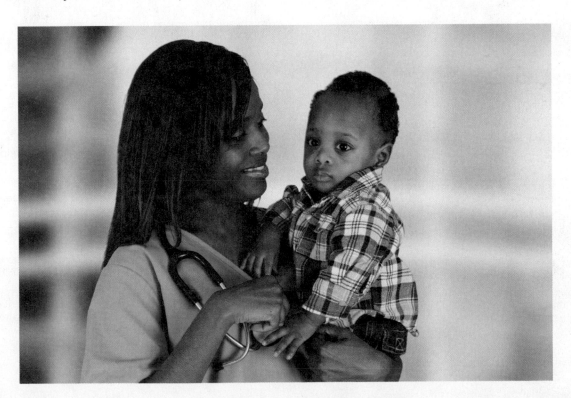

7-5 In what ways is the nurse conveying presence? How might the therapeutic use of self differ when working with a child versus working with an adult?

Source: Rob/Fotolia

courage may provide the patient with a message that his or her experience of suffering can be safely shared.

> **PRACTICE ALERT**   To use the self effectively and consistently, the nurse must ensure care for his or her self. The specific strategies to care for self are individual and based on the nurse's own needs. Those strategies that ensure a healthy body—good nutrition, regular exercise, adequate sleep, and relaxation—also are strategies that support the self. Specific interventions in support of replenishing or focusing the self include meditation, mindfulness, and presencing. The nurse integrates self-care, self-responsibility, and reflection as an essential part of nursing practice.

Pause and Reflect

1. *How can nurses use self-awareness to care for patients who are reluctant to discuss their illness?*
2. *Why do you think presence is so important to caring for patients who are suffering?*

From Suffering to Hope

The structural elements of the self include anatomic and physiologic components, such as our systems of function (e.g., cardiovascular, gastrointestinal) and form (e.g., bone structure, weight distribution). These elements are relatively comparable across cultures and also relatively stable along a recognizable evolutionary trajectory. Individuals are born, develop physiologically and socially, and establish relationships and purposeful action. Different degrees of function of these elements do not diminish the *presence* of self, despite the inclination to think otherwise. Individuals in wheelchairs win Nobel prizes for science; people with mental illness have insights and the capacity to love and be loved. The environment essential to the self's development is not structural and may not be in the awareness of the person—the thinking, knowing, and feeling experienced in interaction with the world. It is these elements of the self that are both tools to support the development of the "self" and part of the "self" being developed. Every interaction creates a tension of exploring what is "self" and what is "not self" in a process that continually serves to shape the self-concept—everything one knows, feels, believes, and values about his or her self (Arnold & Boggs, 2011).

It is the human brain and nervous system's **neuroplasticity**—its incredible ability to change structurally and functionally as a result of input from the environment—that may form the basis for the individual's ability to recover from trauma, an impoverished early environment, or the experience of suffering. Learning and practicing new cognitive and emotional skills likely have the same effect on the brain as exercise has to strengthening muscles (Cloninger, 2009; James & Swain, 2011; Williams, Huang, & Bargh, 2009). The skills practiced in an interaction—such as attention, organization of thought, comparison, and impulse control—are examples of "exercises" that the psychiatric–mental health nurse uses to build skills—of the nurse as well as the patient. The self that the nurse reflects on and develops awareness of and that grows and changes is not, fundamentally, different from the self of the patient. What is different is the responsibility that the nurse has to use this self. As Peplau notes, "Being able to understand one's own behavior, to help others to identify difficulties, and to apply principles of human relations to the problems that arise at all levels of experience—these are functions of psychodynamic nursing" (Peplau, 1952, p. xiii).

Chapter Highlights

1. The purposeful use of self is essential to psychiatric nursing.
2. The practice of self-reflection provides an opportunity for nurses to examine their actions, motivations, and feelings.
3. Awareness of self develops through examining one's own behavior and receiving feedback about that behavior.
4. As early as the time of Socrates, philosophers were examining the idea of the self.
5. Maslow posited that individuals cannot engage in self-exploration until more basic needs (e.g., food, shelter, safety) are met.
6. Freud's stages of psychosexual development are one of the first attempts at describing a sequential development of personality.
7. Carl Rogers observed that the self develops through interaction with the environment, and that the self seeks to engage in actions that are consistent with the internal self.
8. In Erikson's developmental model, failure to master essential developmental tasks may result in a reduced capacity to master the next stage and may become an area of weakness.

9. Peplau recognized that the nurse is involved in a continual process of developing self within the therapeutic relationship.
10. Orlando's process of deliberative nursing helps the nurse engage in self-reflection and helps validate the patient's expressions of need.
11. Attentional blindness refers to the process of seeing only what the individual perceives as important.
12. Emotional intelligence includes accurate recognition of and response to emotions of others.
13. Self-concept reflects an individual's emotional status, life goals, body image, sense of identity, and relationship between the "real" and the "ideal" self.
14. Authenticity in nursing is the nurse's awareness of his or her own genuine personality, character, and values as well as demonstrated behavior consistent with his or her awareness.

NCLEX®-RN Questions

1. The nurse is asked to consider variables that may influence his or her ability to provide effective care to patients with mental illness. Which question is least likely to relate to the "use of self" as a tool?
   a. "What experiences have shaped my approach to patient care?"
   b. "How can I get others to recognize my authority and expertise?"
   c. "How do I feel when I am with patients experiencing mental illness?"
   d. "What are my values and beliefs with regard to patients with mental illness?"

2. The nurse is explaining the historical context of the concept of self-knowledge during a Nurses' Day presentation. Which statement regarding the evolution of related theories and philosophies is accurate?
   a. Nightingale spoke of the use of the whole self as fundamental to nursing.
   b. Martha Rogers contended that the state of self generally remains constant.
   c. Philosophical interest in the relevance of self emerged in the late 19th century.
   d. Patricia Benner declared that the nurse's use of self is reflected in the behavior of the psychiatric nurse.

3. The nurse manager is evaluating the progress of a nurse in the novice stage of practice. The new nurse has been asked to use self-reflection as a tool for learning. Which barrier would the manager recognize as having the greatest potential to limit the new nurse's growth?
   a. The nurse did not learn how to self-reflect in nursing school.
   b. The nurse is concerned about the risks involved in the process.
   c. The nurse experiences anxiety while considering aspects of self.
   d. The nurse is unwilling to explore his thoughts, feelings, and values.

4. The nurse is evaluating the patient's readiness to explore aspects of self that are necessary to grow and develop. Which outcome is least likely to indicate that the patient is ready to shift goals?
   a. The patient obtains a job.
   b. The patient's physiological needs are met.
   c. The patient establishes a safe living environment.
   d. The patient effectively manages self-care activities.

5. The mental health nurse is attempting to establish a therapeutic relationship with a new patient. Which behaviors by the nurse demonstrate authenticity in interactions? Select all that apply.
   a. Being present and listening to the patient
   b. Ensuring that feedback is consistently positive
   c. Concealing intentions for the benefit of the patient
   d. Demonstrating congruence between words and actions
   e. Describing patient behaviors through the lens of one's own perspective

6. The nurse is using Orlando's theory of nursing and "focus on the self" during an encounter with a patient. What does the nurse identify as the primary objective of this approach?
   a. Determining the patient's willingness to embrace change
   b. Prioritizing based on a structured model of patient needs
   c. Using the nurse's expertise to respond to a particular condition
   d. Verifying the nurse's understanding of the patient's experiences and needs

7. The mental health nurse is working to improve the ability to respond effectively to the needs of patients with mental illness. Which aspect of self-awareness does the nurse recognize as essential to responding to the patient's suffering?
   a. Insight
   b. Experience
   c. Motivation
   d. Mindfulness

Answers may be found on the Pearson student resource site: nursing.pearsonhighered.com

Pearson Nursing Student Resources Find additional review materials at **nursing.pearsonhighered.com**

References

American Nurses Association, American Psychiatric Nursing Association, & International Society of Psychiatric-Mental Health Nurses. (2014). *Psychiatric–Mental Health Nursing: Scope and Standards of Practice*. Silver Spring, MD: NursesBooks.org

Arnold, E. C. (2011). Self-concept in the nurse-client relationship. In E. C. Arnold & K. U. Boggs (Eds.), *Interpersonal Relationships: Professional Communication Skills for Nurses*. St. Louis, MO: Elsevier Saunders, pp. 62–82.

Arnold, E. C., & Boggs, K. U. (2011). *Interpersonal Relationships: Professional Communication Skills for Nurses*. St. Louis, MO: Elsevier Saunders.

Asselin, M. E. (2011). Reflective narrative: A tool for learning through practice. *Journal for Nurses in Staff Development, 27*(1), 2–6.

Balcetis, E., & Dunning, D. (2006). See what you want to see: Motivational influences on visual perception. *Journal of Personality and Social Psychology, 91*(4), 622–625.

Beauvais, A. M., Brady, N., & O'Shea, E. R. (2011). Emotional intelligence and nursing performance among nursing students. *Nurse Educator Today, 31*(4), 396–401.

Benner, P. (1984). *From Novice to Expert: Excellence and Power in Clinical Nursing Practice*. Menlo Park, CA: Addison-Wesley.

Beck, C. T. (2011). Secondary traumatic stress in nurses: A systematic review. *Archives of Psychiatric Nursing, 25*(1), 1–10.

Blazer, D. G. (2008). How do you feel about...? Health outcomes in late life and self-perceptions of health and well-being. *Gerontologist, 48*(4), 415–422.

Borton, T. (1970). *Reach, Teach and Touch*. London: McGraw Hill.

Burtson, P. L., & Stichler, J. F. (2010). Nursing work environment and nurse caring: Relationship among motivational factors. *Journal of Advanced Nursing, 66*(8), 1819–1831.

Carroll, Lewis. (1865, 1990). *Alice's Adventures in Wonderland*. Available at http://www.literature.org/authors/carroll-lewis/alices-adventures-in-wonderland/chapter-02.html

Chabris, C., & Simons, D. (2010). *The Invisible Gorilla and Other Ways Our Intuition Deceives Us*. New York, NY: Crown Publishing.

Chamberlin, J. (1998). Confessions of a noncompliant patient. *Journal of Psychosocial Nursing, 36*(4), 49–52.

Cloninger, C. R. (2009). Evolution of human brain functions: The functional structure of human consciousness. *Australian and New Zealand Journal of Psychiatry, 43*, 994–1006.

Coetzee, S., & Klopper, H. C. (2010). Compassion fatigue within nursing practice: A concept analysis. *Nursing and Health Sciences, 12*(2), 235–243.

Cohen-Katz, J., Wiley, S. D., Capuano, T., Baker, D. M., & Shapiro, S. (2004). The effects of stress reduction on nurse stress and burnout: A quantitative and qualitative study. *Holistic Nursing Practice, 18*(6), 302–308.

Cohen-Katz, J., Wiley, S. D., Capuano, T., Baker, D. M., & Shapiro, S. (2005a). The effects of stress reduction on nurse stress and burnout, Part II: A quantitative and qualitative study. *Holistic Nursing Practice, 19*(1), 26–35.

Cohen-Katz, J., Wiley, S. D., Capuano, T., Baker, D. M., & Shapiro, S. (2005b). The effects of stress reduction on nurse stress and burnout, part III: A quantitative and qualitative study. *Holistic Nursing Practice, 19*(2), 78–86.

Corey, G. (1982). *Theory and Practice of Counseling and Psychotherapy.* Monterey, CA: Brooks/Cole.

Crigger, N., & Godfrey, N. (2010). The importance of being humble. *Advances in Nursing Science, 33*(4), 310–319.

Cunha, E., & Goncalves, M. (2009). Commentary: Accessing the experience of a dialogical self: Some needs and concerns. *Culture & Psychology, 15*(3), 120–133.

Daniel, L. (1998). Vulnerability as a key to authenticity. *Image—The Journal of Nursing Scholarship, 30*(2), 191–192.

Davidson, R. J. (2000). Affective style, psychopathology and resilience: Brain mechanisms and plasticity. *American Psychologist, 55*, 1196–1214.

Detmore, D. and Gabriele, L. C. (2011). Don't just do something, stand there: Responding to unrelieved patient suffering. *Journal of Psychosocial Nursing, 49*(4), 35–38.

Dunn, D. J. (2009). The intentionality of compassion energy. *Holistic Nursing Practice, 23*(4), 222–229.

Ekroth-Bucher, M. (2001). Philosophical basis and practice of self-awareness in psychiatric nursing. *Journal of Psychosocial Nursing and Mental Health Services, 39*(2), 32–39.

Ekroth-Bucher, M. (2010). Self-awareness: A review and analysis of a basic nursing concept. *Advances in Nursing Science, 33*(4) 297–309.

Erikson, E. H. (1950, 1963). *Childhood and Society.* New York, NY: W.W. Norton.

Erikson, E. H. (1968). *Identity, Youth and Crisis.* New York, NY: W.W. Norton.

Fejes, A. (2008). Governing nursing through reflection: A discourse analysis of reflective practices. *Journal of Advanced Nursing, 64*(3), 243–250.

Ferrell, B. R., & Coyle, N. (2008). The nature of suffering and the goals of nursing. *Oncology Nursing Forum, 35*(2), 241–247.

Fisher, S., & Greenberg, R. P. (1977). *The Scientific Credibility of Freud's Theories and Therapy.* New York, NY: Basic Books.

Forneris, S. G., & Peden-McAlpine, C. (2007). Evaluation of a reflective learning intervention to improve critical thinking in novice nurses. *Journal of Advanced Nursing, 57*(4), 410–421.

Frederiksson, L., & Lindström, U. A. (2002). Caring conversations—psychiatric patients' narratives about suffering. *Issues and Innovations in Nursing Practice, 40*(4), 396–404.

Freshwater, D. (2008). Reflective practice: the state of the art. In D. Freshwater, B. Taylor, & G. Sherwood, (Eds.). *International Textbook of Reflective Practice in Nursing.* Oxford, UK: Blackwell, pp. 1–18.

Freud, S. (1955, 1971) *The Psychopathology of Everyday Life.* New York, NY: W.W. Norton.

Goleman, D. (1995). *Emotional Intelligence.* New York, NY: Bantam.

Greenwood, J. (1998). The role of reflection in single and double loop learning. *Journal of Advanced Nursing, 27*, 1048–1053.

Hall, E. T. (1966). *The Hidden Dimension.* New York, NY: Anchor Books, Doubleday.

Harrington, R., & Loffredo, D. A. (2010). Insight, rumination and self-reflection, as predictors of well-being. *Journal of Psychology, 145*(1), 9–57.

Harrison, P. A., & Fopma-Loy, J. L. (2010). Reflective journal prompts: A vehicle for stimulating emotional competence in nursing. *Journal of Nursing Education, 49*(11), 644–652.

Hessel, J. A. (2009). Presence in nursing practice: A concept analysis. *Holistic Nursing Practice, 23*(5), 276–281.

Hooper, C., Craig, J., Janvrin, D. R., Wetsel, M. A., & Reimels, E. (2010) Compassion, satisfaction, burnout, and compassion fatigue among emergency nurses compared with nurses in other selected inpatient specialties. *Journal of Emergency Nursing, 36*(5), 420–427.

Horton-Deutsch, S., & Sherwood, G. (2008). Reflection: An educational strategy to develop emotionally-competent nurse leaders. *Journal of Nursing Management, 16*, 946–954.

Huitt, W., & Hummel, J. (2003). Piaget's theory of cognitive development. *Educational Psychology Interactive.* Valdosta, GA: Valdosta State University. Available at http://www.edpsycinteractive.org/topics/cognition/piaget.html

Jack, K., & Miller, E. (2008). Exploring self-awareness in mental health practice. *Mental Health Practice, 12*(3), 31–35.

James, K. H., & Swain, S. N. (2011). Only self-generated actions create sensory-motor systems in the developing brain. *Developmental Science, 14*(4), 673–678.

James, W. (1890). The self and its selves. In C. Lemert, (Ed.). (2010). *Social Theory: The Multicultural Readings.* Philadelphia, PA: Westview Press, pp. 161–166. Available at http://mills-soc116.wikidot.com/james-self-and-its-selves

James, W. (2000). Stanford, http://plato.stanford.edu/entries/james/. Retrieved July 14, 2011.

Jasper, M. (2007). Using reflective journals and diaries to enhance practice and learning. In C. Buhlman and S. Schultz (Eds.), *Reflective Practice in Nursing* (4th ed.). Chichester, West Sussex, UK: Blackwell Publishing, Ltd., pp. 163–188.

Johnson, S. D., Baxter, L. C., Wilder, L. S., Pipe, J. G., Heiserman, J. E., & Prigatano, G. P. (2002). Neural correlates of self-reflection. *Brain, 125*, 1808–1814.

Kilpatrick, L. A., Suyenobu, B. Y., Smith, S. R., Bueller, J. A., Goodman, T., Creswell, J. D., et al. (2011). Impact of mindfulness-based stress reduction training on intrinsic brain connectivity. *Neuroimage, 56*(1), 290–298.

Landeweer, E. G., Abma, T. A., & Widdershoven, G. A. M. (2011). Moral margins concerning the use of coercion in psychiatry. *Nursing Ethics, 18*, 304–316.

LaSala, C. (2009). Moral accountability and integrity in nursing practice. *Nursing Clinics of North America, 44*(4), 423–434.

Lee, S. J., & Oyserman, D. (2009). Expecting to work, fearing homelessness: The possible selves of low-income women. *Journal of Applied Social Psychology, 39*(6), 1334–1355.

Leete, E. (1989). How I perceive and manage my illness. *Schizophrenia Bulletin, 8*, 605–609.

Lindholm, L., & Eriksson, K. (1993). To understand and alleviate suffering in a caring culture. *Journal of Advanced Nursing, 18*, 1354–1361.

Lotto, R. B. (2011). Lotto Lab Studio: Deepening our understanding of perception and human behavior. Available at http://www.lottolab.org/

Luft, J., & Ingham, H. (1955). The Johari window, a graphic model of interpersonal awareness. *Proceedings of the Western Training Laboratory in Group Development.* Los Angeles, CA: UCLA.

Maslow, A. H. (1970). *Motivation and Personality* (2nd ed.). New York, NY: Harper & Row.

Mayer, J. D., Salovey, P., & Caruso, D. R. (2004). Emotional intelligence: Theory, findings and implications. *Psychological Inquiry, 15*(3), 197–215.

Morin, A. (2004). A neurocognitive and socioecological model of self-awareness. *Genetic, Social and General Psychology Monographs, 130*(3), 197–222.

Morse, J. M. (2001). Toward a praxis theory of suffering. *Advances in Nursing Science, 24*(1), 45–79.

Munhall, P. (2004). "Unknowing": Toward another pattern of knowing. In P. G. Reed, N. C. Shearer, & L. H. Nicoll, (Eds.). *Perspectives in Nursing Theory.* Philadelphia, PA: Lippincott Williams & Wilkins, pp. 239–245.

Orbanic, S. D. (1999). The Heideggerian view of person: A perspective conducive to the therapeutic encounter. *Archives of Psychiatric Nursing, 13*(3), 137–144.

Orlando, I. J. (1971). *The Dynamic Nurse-Patient Relationship.* New York, NY: National League for Nursing.

Orlando, I. J. (1987). Nursing in the 21st century: Alternate paths. *Journal of Advanced Nursing, 12*, 405–412.

Peplau, H. E. (1952). *Interpersonal Relations in Nursing.* New York, NY: G. P. Putnam & Sons.

Peplau, H. E. (1997). Peplau's theory of interpersonal relations. *Nursing Science Quarterly, 10*(4), 162–167.

Piaget, J. (1952). *The Origin of Intelligence in Children.* New York, NY: International Universities Press.

Picard, R.W., Papert, S., Bender, W., Blumberg, B., Breazeal, D., Cavallo, D., et al. (2004). Affective learning—A manifesto. *BT Technology Journal, 22*(4), 253–269.

Plowman, E. K., & Kleim, J. A. (2010). Motor cortex reorganization across the lifespan. *Journal of Communication Disorders, 43*(4), 286–294.

Porr, C. (2005) Shifting from preconceptions to pure wonderment. *Nursing Philosophy, 6*(3), 189–195.

Potter, M., & Bockenhauer, B. (2000). Implementing Orlando nursing theory: A pilot study. *Journal of Psychiatric Mental Health Nursing, 6*(2), 457–468.

Prescott, A. (2006). *The Concept of Self in Medicine and Health Care.* New York, NY: Nova Science Publishers, Inc.

Rae, G. (2010). Alienation, authenticity and the self. *History of the Human Sciences, 23*(4), 21–36.

Råholm, M. (2008). Uncovering the ethics of suffering using a narrative approach. *Nursing Ethics, 15*(1), 62–72.

Rogers, C. (1952). *Client-Centered Therapy.* Cambridge, MA: Riverside Press.

Rogers, M. E. (1970). *An Introduction to the Theoretical Basis for Nursing.* Philadelphia, PA: F. A. Davis.

Shamay-Tsoory, S. G. (2011). The neural bases for empathy. *Neuroscientist, 17*(1), 18–24.

Shattell, M., Starr, S., & Thomas, S. (2007). "Take my hand, help me out": Mental health service recipients' experience of the therapeutic relationship. *International Journal of Mental Health Nursing, 16,* 274–284.

Sherwood, G. D., & Horton-Deutsch, S. (2012). *Reflective Practice: Transforming Education and Improving Outcomes.* Indianapolis: Sigma Theta Tau.

Sigma Theta Tau. (2007). Reflective practice. Available at http://www.nursingsociety.org/aboutus/PositionPapers/Documents/resource_reflective.pdf

Sinnot, J. D. (2009). Complex thought and construction of the self in the face of aging and death. *Journal of Adult Development, 16*(3), 155–165.

Skirry, J. (2008). Rene Descartes (1596–1650): Overview. *Internet Encyclopedia of Philosophy.* Available at http://www.iep.utm.edu/descarte/

Starr, S. S. (2008). Authenticity: A concept analysis. *Nursing Forum, 43*(2), 55–61.

Sullivan, H. S. (1953). *Interpersonal Theory of Psychiatry.* New York, NY: W.W. Norton.

Thompson, M. (2005). The way of authenticity and the quest for personal integrity. *European Journal of Psychotherapy, Counseling and Health, 7*(3), 143–157.

Toman, W. (1969). *Family Constellation.* New York, NY: Springer Publishing Co., Inc. Universal Digital Library, call number 1533.

U.S. Department of Health and Human Services. (1999). Mental Health: A Report of the Surgeon General—Executive Summary. Rockville, MD: U.S. Department of Health and Human Services, Substance Abuse and Mental Health Services Administration, Center for Mental Health Services, National Institutes of Health, National Institute of Mental Health.

Vaillant, G. E. (2003). Mental health. *American Journal of Psychiatry, 160*(8), 1373–1384.

Vaillant, G., & Mukamal, K. (2001). Successful aging. *American Journal of Psychiatry, 158,* 839–847.

Vaillant, G. E., & Milofsky, E. (1980). Natural history of male psychological health: Empirical evidence for Erikson's model of the life cycle. *American Journal of Psychiatry, 137*(11), 1348–1359.

Vandemark, L. M. (2006). Awareness of self and expanding consciousness: Using nursing theories to prepare nurse-therapists. *Issues in Mental Health Nursing. 27*(6), 605–615.

Westermeyer, J. F. (2004). Predictors and characteristics of Erikson's life cycle model among men: A 32-year longitudinal study. *International Journal of Aging and Human Development, 58*(1), 29–48.

Williams, L. E., Huang, J. Y., & Bargh, J. A. (2009). The scaffolded mind: Higher mental processes are grounded in early experience of the physical world. *European Journal of Social Psychology, 39,* 1257–1267.

Wood, A. M., Linley, P. A., Maltby, J., Baliousis, M., & Joseph, S. (2008). The authentic personality: A theoretical and empirical conceptualization and the development of the authenticity scale. *Journal of Counseling Psychology, 55*(3), 385–389.

Yoder, E. A. (2010). Compassion fatigue in nurses. *Applied Nursing Research, 23,* 191–197.

8

The Nurse–Patient Relationship and Therapeutic Communication

Joanne DeSanto Iennaco

Key Terms

Learning Outcomes

1. Describe key principles that influence the development of relationships with patients.

2. Define empathy and differentiate features of empathic communication.

3. Compare and contrast features of therapeutic and social relationships.

4. Identify the stages of the nurse–patient relationship and evidence of movement between stages.

5. Examine factors important to setting and maintaining boundaries in the therapeutic relationship.

6. Summarize features of nonverbal, verbal, and meta-communication and how they affect processes of communication.

7. Distinguish features that indicate use of active listening techniques.

8. Discriminate therapeutic from nontherapeutic communication techniques.

9. Evaluate tools used to aid the nurse in better understanding therapeutic interactions and the therapeutic nurse–patient relationship.

Chuck Malloy

APPLICATION

APPLICATION

1. What are some of the feelings you had as you read a little bit about Chuck's history?

2. What are some of the challenges you would face as a nurse working with Chuck?

Chuck Malloy is a 29-year-old man who has a long history of alcohol and drug abuse. He was admitted to your inpatient dual diagnosis unit after what he describes as an "accidental overdose" of heroin in combination with alcohol and use of alprazolam (Xanax) he obtained on the street. He has a history of many arrests for possessing and selling narcotics. He has a 5-year-old son who was found with a bag of drugs in his backpack at school last month, and the news story went viral. His son is now in the custody of the Department of Children and Youth Services. Chuck tells you that this is a devastating loss for him, and that the event led to his recent increase in drug use, as he has lost his reason to try to kick his addictions.

Introduction

In the field of psychiatric–mental health nursing, nursing intervention primarily takes place through nurse–patient interaction, making communication and development of nurse-patient relationships essential. The idea of communicating therapeutically as a means of helping others is not a new one: Antiphon of Athens (480–411 BCE) suggested the idea of therapeutic communication when he discussed the "art of solace," and Plato identified the importance of catharsis as a way to "purify the soul" (Watzlawick, 1978, pp. 7–8). **Therapeutic communication,** the communication that takes place between patient and nurse, is the primary tool used by clinicians to help patients in the mental health setting. Nurses develop a therapeutic relationship with patients founded on the principles of respect, dignity, unconditional positive regard, and a focus on fostering patient growth and healing. From this foundation, nurses use communication skills to help people. Given that communication is more than the words spoken, nurses need to understand all the other elements and processes involved in communication. It is true that "it isn't only what you say, but also how you say it." Unfortunately, not all communication is helpful or of a kind that promotes patients' well-being. Communication problems can arise not only from the words spoken, but also from the tone, gestures, facial expressions, and behaviors that accompany the words. For this reason, nurses must understand different modes of communication. The development of therapeutic relationships and use of therapeutic communication skills are the foundation to helping patients heal.

Some basic tenets are important for clinicians to consider as they pursue work in the field of psychiatric–mental health nursing. Some universal principles include a desire to help others achieve better physical and mental health, having unconditional positive regard (Rogers, 1961) for patients and families, involving patients and families as equal partners in care, and awareness of self. Even though individuals may have distinctly different views on how each term is specifically defined, there is commonality in the general conception of each principle that is typically shared by those who work in this field. Rogers (1957) asserted that to help patients change, nurses are required to have unconditional positive regard and empathic understanding that they communicate to the patient. These universal principles were part of the qualities identified by Dziopa and Ahern (2009b) in a recent review of research on the therapeutic nurse–patient relationship. Other qualities of the nurse they identified included accepting individuality, providing support, being available, being genuine, promoting equality, demonstrating respect, having self-awareness, and maintaining clear boundaries.

Principles that are considered universal to caring for patients with mental health needs, including unconditional positive regard, active listening, patient-centered care, and the use of empathy, are reviewed in this chapter, followed by information about the development of therapeutic nurse–patient relationships and use of therapeutic communication skills.

Essential Ingredients of a Therapeutic Relationship

How nurses develop a therapeutic relationship with any patient, especially patients suffering from mental illness, as well as their families, has a great impact on the quality of care. Essential to the development of the relationship are the nurse's view of health and mental health, an attitude of unconditional positive regard for the patient and family, and an emphasis on patient-centered care, in which the patient is an equal partner in the provision of nursing care. These factors provide a solid foundation to the development of the therapeutic relationship, to successful communication with patients, and, as a result, to alleviating suffering and promoting hope in patients and their families.

View of Health and Mental Health

How each nurse views the concepts of *health* and *mental health* significantly impacts how he or she understands, relates to the world, and performs his or her role as nurse. Health is a concept that is part of the nursing paradigm, and nursing theorists readily define the concept as part of the world view that frames nursing theory. World view refers to the way a person thinks about the world. Hildegard Peplau defines health as the forward movement of personality and human process in a direction of "creative, constructive, productive, personal and community living" (1992, p. 12). However, *health* is most typically conceived of as the state of being without illness. This definition is problematic in that it suggests that those with a diagnosed illness, such as heart disease or depression, cannot possibly be healthy. In reality, though, many individuals with a variety of illnesses adapt in such a way that they would be considered healthier than some individuals without any illness. The nursing conception of health tends to include a holistic view that is inclusive of all aspects of an individual's life. In this sense, health might be considered in relationship to one's physical, emotional, environmental, social, interpersonal, and spiritual well-being. Health may also be considered in light of the roles individuals take in life (such as student, parent, friend) and their ability to function in these roles.

Aspects of life to consider in assessing physical and mental health may include quality of life in relation to both physical and mental health. How individuals choose to spend their time and focus their attention, and the reasons they make choices in these areas, are important to how they understand the health of others. Nurses attempt to assist individuals in moving toward better health, but many have different conceptions of what "better" would be. It is the nurse's responsibility to learn the goals patients have for their own health and to provide information and other kinds of care to help them attain their goals.

Mental health is another concept that is often difficult to define. Qualities often mentioned include having a sense of purpose and meaning in life, flexibility, the ability to give and receive love, the ability to take in and consider information or input, the ability to experience emotions without distress, the ability to organize and convey one's thoughts and desires to another, and the ability to make important decisions about one's life. Embedded in these qualities are the ideas that human beings are thinking and feeling individuals with interpersonal, family, and community relationships.

Unconditional Positive Regard

An important concept in developing therapeutic relationships with others is the idea of offering unconditional positive regard to those who seek nursing care (Rogers, 1961). Nurses use **unconditional positive regard** when they meet patients in a positive, accepting manner and treat them with respect and dignity. A provision in the Code of Ethics for Nurses (American Nurses Association, 2010) is that the nurse respects the worth, dignity, and rights of the patient, including the right to patient self-determination. This means that the nurse suspends judgment or approval. This holds true regardless of the patient's story, history, symptoms, or behaviors. This may seem difficult at times, such as when caring for someone who has committed a violent or socially unacceptable act. However, it is important that nurses suspend their own judgment and regard the individual as they would anyone who approaches them for care.

As nurses prepare to meet with patients, they consider not only the words they will use, but also how to communicate active interest and positive regard. Research suggests that several aspects of nonverbal communication, including physical proximity, good eye contact, leaning slightly forward, and orienting to face the person all communicate a positive attitude toward the patient (Mehrabian, 1969, 1970). Having awareness of how nonverbal communication adds to the understanding of verbal communication is important in developing relationships with patients. In relating unconditional positive regard to providing patient care, Peplau said, "Unconditional interest and acceptance on the part of the nurse is an essential part of observation which leads the nurse to a basis for understanding the patient and for fostering his growth" (1991, p. 206).

Patient-Centered Care

The idea that nurses and patients are equal partners in care is important in the sense that individuals should make decisions about and determine the course of their care. As stated earlier, patient self-determination or autonomy, which is part of the Code of Ethics for Nurses, means that patients should be involved in planning for their care to the extent that they desire and are able (American Nurses Association, 2010). It is easy for a professional to abuse power within relationships, given the professional's knowledge about and roles of authority in the health care system. Because of the potential for imbalance of power,

nurses must use care to partner with their patients and actively engage them in their own care. Although a part of the nurse's role may be to act as a guide to better health, the driving force for care should be directed by those seeking help. As professionals, nurses are trained to evaluate situations, identify and prioritize needs, and develop plans of care. If this is done without consultation and direction from the individual requiring care, the nurse develops a strict "nursing care plan" rather than a plan driven by the patient's needs and goals.

The first step in determining the direction of care should be based on the reasons and needs for treatment identified by the patient. **Patient-centered care** means that patients determine the direction of their treatment and goal identification starts with the individual patient. Many theorists have embraced the idea of a patient-centered approach to care, including Rogers (1980), Hart (2010a), and nursing theorists Neuman and Young (1972).

Rogers (1980) described a person-centered approach as one that views people as having the capacity and resources to understand themselves and to alter their attitudes and behaviors if they have a climate that facilitates growth. Rogers identifies three conditions of this growth-enhancing climate: genuineness or congruence, unconditional positive regard, and empathic understanding. Rogers identifies genuineness as the therapist being himself or herself versus wearing a façade in the relationship, suggesting that the therapist is transparent within the relationship in terms of his or her feelings and attitudes experienced, and these may be communicated if appropriate. Neuman and Young (1972) identified a model of patient-centered care in nursing that embraces collaboration with patient and family, with the nurse actively seeking participation in all aspects of care. Oriented toward a holistic view of the patient, the model emphasizes both the patient's and the nurse's perceptions of stressors and collaborative negotiation of goals and outcomes (Neuman, 1997). Similar to the ideas of Rogers, this process requires communication skills, use of empathy, and an ability to respond helpfully with emotions expressed by the patient.

Hart (2010a) discusses how the nurse might use a patient-centered approach by seeking to understand the patient's perceptions of the illness, the patient's view of why he or she has an illness, the feelings and fears of the patient, and the patient's expectations of the provider. This leads to a better understanding of the meaning and impact of health problems on the patient's life. In addition, this encourages the nurse to focus on the patient's experience as opposed to categorizing individuals into particular diagnostic groupings or categories. Use of this approach has led to improved outcomes, including better patient communication, improved patient satisfaction, and improved provider satisfaction (Hart, 2010a). Other studies suggest improved health outcomes in chronic disease with greater patient involvement and communication (Kaplan, Greenfield, & Ware, 1989).

Pause and Reflect

1. *How does it feel to consider communication a primary tool for work in this field? What are your strengths in communicating? Do you have areas of communication that you find difficult?*

2. *Referring to the critical thinking exercise at the beginning of the chapter, how will you offer unconditional regard to patients like Chuck who act in ways that you or society find unacceptable?*

3. *What are some ways in which a nurse can engage patients as equal partners in care?*

Therapeutic Use of Self

The tool nurses in the psychiatric–mental health setting use is the *self* (Chapter 7). Because nurses use communication and their relationships with patients to assist patients to move toward a healthier state, nurses must pay close attention to the processes involved in how they communicate and develop relationships with their patients. As with preparing and being very careful to maintain a sterile field while performing a dressing change or surgical intervention, the nurse prepares to be a therapeutic tool in a relationship by maintaining self-awareness and actively maintaining a nonjudgmental or neutral stance during interactions with patients. This process requires nurses to be aware of their own feelings, opinions, and desires, yet maintain focus on patients and their healing. Using a variety of communication skills and techniques, nurses help patients work through difficult experiences and negative patterns that have gotten in their way in the past. This is done without consideration of the nurse's own personal thoughts, feelings, or behaviors.

Therapeutic Neutrality

Nurses set aside their own "self" interests and work to focus on the individual and to understand that person's thoughts, feelings, and needs, without indulging in mutually sharing emotions or personal experiences. By setting aside his or her own reactions and feelings for a later time, the nurse allows the moment to belong to the patient, and encourages openness and depth of sharing so the experience might allow for some release of emotions and feelings that are difficult to contain. If the nurse were to disclose his or her own difficulties or problems in the same area or share a similar experience, the nurse would move the focus of the interaction from the patient to the nurse. Setting aside the self is a key difference between developing a therapeutic relationship and a personal relationship or friendship. Research shows that clinicians who are able to acknowledge their own emotional experience and to be free from their own psychological disturbance are able to respond in more helpful ways to their patients (Gurman, 1972).

One term for this idea is **therapeutic neutrality**, which was originally identified by Freud (1915) and is the idea of a clinician allowing the individual exposure to experiences and emotions without imposing judgment. It is impossible, as a human being, to be completely free of all opinions, ideas, or beliefs. The nurse has not "failed" if some aspect of his or her own belief or opinion is shared. However, the nurse must carefully consider whether this does occur, so that he or she does not unwittingly prevent or inhibit patient sharing, and to ensure that the patient does not feel judged based on the opinions or beliefs shared by the nurse. In this sense, it is important for the nurse to be an authentic human being in the therapeutic nurse–patient relationship while at the same time maintaining neutrality, thereby allowing patients to share freely and fully, form their own opinions, and make their own decisions unbiased by the nurse's views or preferences.

The idea of therapeutic neutrality implies that the nurse interacts not based on his or her own opinions or desires, but rather with a focus on the patient's views and desires. Humphries (1982) discusses how difficult it is to follow through on the idea of not influencing the patient. He also suggests that it is appropriate for each clinician to acknowledge that he or she is a person with particular views, but that the patient is encouraged to draw his or her own conclusions regardless of the clinician's viewpoint or frame. Nurses must maintain self-awareness and be open about their own beliefs, while actively introducing or acknowledging that multiple views exist. Katz discusses the use of therapeutic neutrality and the debate about whether this is actually possible, and points out that, in reality, one cannot be completely neutral but that "relative neutrality" is possible (2010, p. 314). In this sense, neutrality is important and occurs when the clinician starts with recognizing and keeping in check his or her own issues and views, allowing patients to share their unique perspectives to explore new ideas without interference or direction based on the clinician's preferred view or bias.

Centering

The nurse clinician can use the technique of **centering** to assist in both identifying important thoughts and feelings that are present, and in clearing the mind of the extraneous reactions, allowing a neutral stance and clear frame for starting an interaction with a patient. The idea of centering is that nurses spend some time acknowledging their own feeling states. Centering suggests that nurses focus inside themselves and identify the processes they are currently experiencing. It involves attending to the events of that day and identifying the feelings associated with them.

The identification of feelings of happiness, sadness, anger, or fear will help nurses to understand their emotional states and to set aside these feelings for the present time, allowing a neutral stance or frame for interacting with the patient. Some clinicians journal about their insights from centering exercises, whereas others use their colleagues or team members to ventilate regarding the emotional debris, whether from personal experiences or from the prior patient interaction (Chapter 7). Generally, the centering exercise is closed with additional cleansing breaths to help clear the current feeling state and achieve a state of relaxation before coming back to full attention and awareness. See the scripted centering exercise available on the student resource site at nursing.pearsonhighered.com.

Empathy

Empathy is a quality or tool nurses use to better understand others' experiences. **Empathy** can be defined as sensing the perceptions or feelings of an individual and one's relationship to the individual's situations and experiences (feeling what the other person is feeling), and communicating and validating or adjusting them based on feedback from that person. In the patient setting, the nurse employs empathy in such a way that he or she has a sense of the patient's experience and the patient realizes that the nurse understands. Research validates the importance of the presence of three elements in this process: sensing the patient's world, communicating this to the patient, and the patient's perception of being understood (LaMonica, 1981). Sabo (2006) identifies empathy as having components of both perception and interaction; more than a quality or characteristic, it is also a communication tool that validates the experience of the patient. Empathy is an essential quality in the field of psychiatric–mental health nursing, given that the nurse's role is to help others with their emotional experiences.

In using empathy as a tool, nurses must clear their own experiences, feelings, and reactions from their consciousness and try to fully engage in others' experiences in an attempt to get a sense of how the patient is feeling at that moment in time. Rogers identifies that evidence indicates that "a high degree of empathy in a relationship is possibly *the* most potent . . . in bringing about change and learning" (1975, p. 3). Haase and Tepper (1972) studied the contribution of verbal and nonverbal communication to empathy and found that the nonverbal aspects, including eye contact, leaning, distance and body orientation, had twice the effect of the verbal message expressed. For these reasons it is important that nurses carefully consider not only their words, but also their nonverbal behaviors, in preparing themselves to communicate empathic understanding.

Empathy is a difficult skill to master; it develops over time as nurses learn how to clear themselves of current thoughts, ideas, and feelings and fully tune in to what the other person presents. If nurses have difficulty managing or understanding their own feelings, they may unwittingly close themselves off to others. It can be difficult to empathize with others; as the nurse learns how to empathize and develop the therapeutic relationship, it can be easy to feel overwhelmed by the emotions of the patient until the nurse becomes more skilled at this process. Because it can be difficult to disengage from others' feelings and experiences, nurses may find it difficult to separate the patient's experiences from their own. Given the range of possible experiences, it may be helpful to think of empathy as being on a continuum, where on one side one has only limited ability or willingness to understand another's felt experience, while on the other end, one feels another's pain too strongly. The empathic understanding exercise (Box 8-1) is one tool nurses can use to separate the experience of patients from their own experience, as it involves requesting feedback (which requires the nurse to withdraw slightly from the felt experience), and then to reframe their perspective based on the feedback provided. This can assist nurses and clinicians to move out of the feeling state and recognize whether they moved into their own "similar experience" or whether they are actually sensing what the patient feels.

Setting aside one's own perspective can be especially difficult when the nurse has had a personal experience similar to the one being described. When this happens, nurses must be careful to remind themselves that there are multiple ways to experience the same situation. It is important to seek to understand how the patient actually feels, and not to expect the patient to have the same or similar feelings as the nurse. Otherwise, the patient may view the nurse as failing to understand or respect the patient's feelings.

One way to prevent misinterpretation of the patient's feelings is for nurses to check their perceptions with the patient (see Perceptions, Thoughts, and Feelings: Empathic Understanding). This might be most easily done by asking how that situation made the patient feel. In some ways, experiencing empathy for another seems to be "sensing" emotions of others or learning to read the emotions of others. Another way to validate whether the nurse is really in tune with the patient is to say something like, "Many people might feel ____ when faced with a situation like that. How did you feel?" This allows the nurse to share the feeling impression he or she picked up on without prescribing how that patient feels. In addition, it identifies that that the nurse is interested in that person's experience regardless of whether the nurse's perception was accurate.

At times, individuals are unable to identify or express the feelings they are experiencing. In these situations, nurses may pick up on the feeling tone expressed and ask for clarification. One way to do this is by saying something such as, "As you were talking about your engagement to your boyfriend, you were talking about what is usually a happy moment, but you sounded almost angry as you described it," and then seeing whether the patient can further clarify the emotions involved. This kind of clarification may help the nurse to discover exactly the feeling that the patient experienced. When this occurs, patients are far more likely to feel deeply understood and relieved of some suffering.

New clinicians describe feeling overwhelmed at times with the emotional residue of their interactions with their patients. The active work of empathizing with patients requires that nurses listen very deeply and intently and truly allow others' experiences to wash over them. Nurses must be aware of how others' feelings affect them. For example, if the patient is feeling sad and hopeless, a nurse may feel the depth of sadness, pain, and anguish the patient is experiencing. New clinicians may also find they relate so deeply to the patient that they lose their ability to be objective and see things only from the patient's perspective. When this occurs, it can be difficult to be helpful to the patient. It is important to take a step back from the patient at these times so some perspective on the experience can be maintained (Box 8-2). There are many ways to do this and, as nurses gain skill, they are able to maintain their own perspective and objectivity while also allowing the feeling state of the patient to clearly come through. It is often helpful for nurses to discuss experiences using empathic skills with a peer, mentor, or supervisor or to use supervision to best understand how they are reacting to the patient.

Empathy and Empathic Understanding

box 8-1

Rogers's originally defined empathy or being empathic as: "to perceive the internal frame of reference of another with accuracy and with the emotional components and meanings which pertain thereto as if one were the person, but without ever losing the 'as if' condition. Thus it means to sense the hurt or the pleasure of another as he senses it and to perceive the causes thereof as he perceives them, . . . but if this 'as if' quality is lost then the state is one of identification" (Rogers, 1959, pp. 210–211). Later, Rogers identified empathy as a process rather than a state, describing empathy as "entering the private perceptual world of the other and becoming thoroughly at home in it" (1975, p. 4). Rogers went on to explain that the empathic individual is able to sense changes in the other's emotions and to express care and concern for the other. The nurse or therapist who employs empathic understanding does so successfully in part by setting aside his or her own self, views, and values. As discussed throughout this chapter, this requires a great deal of self-awareness.

Empathic Understanding Exercise

Try this exercise: In your next interaction with a patient, after actively listening to the patient presenting a feeling or experience, respond by trying to offer a sentence or two in which you try to get exactly at the meaning of that experience or situation for that person. Present that sentence this way: "As you described [briefly restate situation], it sounded like you felt . . . [provide your sentence or two]. Is that what it was like for you?" Then listen intently for the patient's response. The patient either will validate that you did capture what he or she was trying to convey or what he or she experienced, or will tell you that you were not on target. If you are not on target, then you could say, "Help me better understand what that was like for you," or request clarification in some other way. This will help you to get a better idea of the experience and will allow you to adjust your understanding. Then repeat the first statement, substituting a new try at what your sense of the experience was.

Stepping-Back Exercise   box 8-2

Patients suffering mental illness must often overcome a traumatic experience in order to begin the healing process. As part of the therapeutic process, patients often need to share their traumatic experiences with the nurse. These experiences can be highly emotional (for example, abuse in childhood, death of a family member, witnessing violence), and at times may be very similar to the nurse's own experiences. Even the most experienced nurse can become overwhelmed with the experience of empathic understanding of emotion.

This exercise is intended to help the nurse who is feeling inundated or overwhelmed by an exchange with a patient and who is unable to regain perspective to assist the patient in a helpful way. The idea of this exercise is to provide the nurse with a series of potential ways to step back enough to disengage personally from the emotions or experiences that have been activated in you to regain the ability to communicate therapeutically.

Steps

1. Validate the feeling experience with the patient. *Rationale:* It is important for the patient to recognize that you are a genuine, authentic human being. This does not mean that you have to share why the experience moved you so deeply if it is of a personal nature, but you should identify how you think it may have felt to the patient.
2. Bring the discussion of the patient's feeling or experience to the here and now, or, if it is a current situation, ask the patient to reflect on any other situations in the past that have been similar.

3. Follow up the response with either identification of possible coping strategies the patient has used in the past, or problem-solve regarding possible coping to use currently to manage those feelings.

Nurse Experience of Empathic Understanding	Response to Return to Therapeutic Neutrality
Tears up or begins to cry while listening to patient	"Your experience strikes a chord with me in terms of how sad [or whatever feeling] that really was for you. What helps you to manage the sadness?"
Experiences sense of helplessness or powerlessness and inability to imagine how things could ever get better, change, or improve in the patient's life	Identifies own experience of helplessness and reflects back to patient seeking validation if that is accurate (brings discussion to process patient's feelings).
	Brings patient to how that experience affects him or her in the here and now.
	Suggests brainstorming together to develop some options for how to cope when that experience or feeling recurs again.

PERCEPTIONS, THOUGHTS, & FEELINGS: Empathic Understanding

Hector is a 20-year-old, single Cuban man who is a student at the local community college. He is currently a patient on the inpatient psychiatric unit after going to the police to request protection from the FBI, whom he believed to be tracking him through his cellphone because his family was involved in a plot to kill Cuban leader Fidel Castro. Hector grew up in a very traditional family, and his parents were immigrants who struggled to make ends meet. He is the youngest of five siblings and describes growing up as chaotic, as his father was always working and his mother tried to hold things together at home. The following is an example of an interaction between Hector and a nurse working on the unit.

Patient behavior	Nurse's perceptions, thoughts, and feelings	Nurse's exploration with the patient
Hector: Yes, all the time we were getting into trouble. When I was like 6 or 7, my mother thought I tried smoking—all my brothers smoked but me. She was so mad . . . she used to really scream at me! Hector is sitting quietly on the couch, very neatly dressed and groomed.	*Thoughts:* What a busy household, with just his mother to manage. I want to get a sense of what his life was like growing up.	*Nurse:* She screamed at you a lot?

PERCEPTIONS, THOUGHTS, & FEELINGS (*continued*)

Patient behavior	Nurse's perceptions, thoughts, and feelings	Nurse's exploration with the patient
Hector: My brothers blamed me so they didn't get in trouble. It always bothered me . . . but I wasn't the best kid—I probably deserved the punishment. I was always getting punished for something.	*Thoughts:* So his brothers picked on the youngest one. He seems sensitive; interesting that it sounds like he thinks he deserved punishment. I wonder if he was physically punished. *Feelings:* I feel sad that he was picked on by his brothers and he seems to believe he deserved punishment.	*Nurse:* How were you punished?

Patient behavior	Nurse's perceptions, thoughts, and feelings	Nurse's exploration with the patient
Hector: That time she thought I was smoking, she stood me in the corner and I had to hold a hot pepper in my mouth for like an hour as punishment. That was pretty typical. She didn't believe in physical punishment.	*Thoughts:* I can imagine this little boy standing in the corner with his mouth burning. I think this was very abusive and mean. I wonder if he realizes that is pretty severe. *Feelings:* I feel so sad for him. And I feel angry about the severe way chosen to punish a child.	*Nurse:* What was that like as a punishment?

Patient behavior	Nurse's perceptions, thoughts, and feelings	Nurse's exploration with the patient
Hector: I don't know. You just sort of cope with it, I guess. My mouth would burn for hours after it. But it could have been worse.	*Thoughts:* He makes it sound like a mild punishment. I need to pull back a little bit here. *Feelings:* I feel so bad for the little boy who was treated this way, I am starting to tear up hearing about it.	*Nurse:* I'm imagining you as a little boy. It makes me feel sad to think you were treated this way. This was a pretty severe punishment.

Patient behavior	Nurse's perceptions, thoughts, and feelings	Nurse's exploration with the patient
Hector: I never even thought about it. I guess it was pretty hard to stand there. I used to try to hold my breath so it wouldn't hurt so much. Hector tears up. *Hector:* I don't think she meant to hurt me that way. Hector tries to compose himself.	*Thoughts:* Wow, he really has normalized this. I don't think he has ever processed any of these events. *Feelings:* I feel sad to see his pain, and it is hard to see him start to lose composure.	*Nurse:* I can see how hard it must have been for you.

VALIDATION In this interaction, the nurse has made an empathic connection with the patient. To manage the overwhelming emotions, the nurse identified how she was feeling and then made a statement to present reality regarding the statement, which brings the patient from describing the experience to processing the experience.

Based on Orlando, I. J. (1972). The Discipline and Teaching of Nursing Process: An Evaluative Study. New York: G. P. Putnam's Sons.

Active Listening

Active listening is another tool that helps nurses achieve full presence with the patient; it is a central tool of therapeutic communication and helpful in building the nurse–patient relationship. **Active listening** is more than just hearing what someone says. It involves carefully attending to the patient during an interaction. The nurse using active listening is alert to cues given by the patient. In addition, the nurse demonstrates interest in what is being said both verbally and nonverbally. Ways to demonstrate interest include short statements such as "uh-huh," and "go on," as well as nonverbal cues such as nodding, making direct eye contact, and leaning slightly forward, showing attention to what the patient is saying. The nurse makes active attempts to understand or interpret meaning. Therapeutic communication techniques used to convey active listening and interest include affirming statements, reflecting back ideas or emotion, and summarizing or repeating back what the patient says. These techniques identify that the nurse has heard the patient and validates the meaning or interpretation of the communication.

Pause and Reflect

1. *When you are interacting with someone, how intensely do you "sense" what that person has experienced or is describing? Have you ever had trouble either with sensing someone's feelings or with getting too immersed in those feelings? What has helped you most in either allowing the feelings in or separating from and regaining your own sense of experience?*

2. *Describe the active listening skills you use. What do you look like, do, and say to indicate you are listening intently or deeply? Now, ask your roommate or a friend to describe the active listening skills you use. To what extent do your descriptions match or differ?*

Developing the Therapeutic Nurse–Patient Relationship

The **therapeutic relationship** is a critical connection between patient and nurse. It is a planned, goal-directed relationship that exists for the purpose of the nurse to assist the patient to progress toward goal attainment. The relationship developed between the nurse and the patient is significant in all areas of nursing. In a study of the nurse–patient relationship in palliative care, Mok and Chiu (2004) found that the relationship was essential to both patients' and nurses' well-being. Findings included that the development of trust in the relationship enhanced the nurses' ability to provide holistic care and improved understanding of patient suffering, and that the reciprocity achieved in the relationships had a positive effect on the patients' physical and emotional needs as well as the nurses' degree of job satisfaction. The Registered Nurses' Association of Ontario (2006) developed a best practice guideline to developing nurse–patient relationships that identifies, in addition to requisite knowledge, capacities the nurse must have to establish a therapeutic relationship. These capacities include self-awareness, self-knowledge, empathy, and an awareness of ethics, boundaries, and limits of the professional role. Because the main tool and interventions used in psychiatric settings involve communication, nurses working in these settings must carefully develop the therapeutic relationship and use it to the greatest benefit of the patient. The relationship involves a structure or therapeutic frame with boundaries and specific roles of both the patient and therapist (Smith & Fitzpatrick, 1995).

Therapeutic relationships differ from social relationships; in part, this is because the therapeutic relationship uses the process of interaction as a tool. It is one of the few healthy relationships in which one party helps another or acts in the best interest of another without expectation that the other person will return the action. In addition, the therapeutic nurse–patient relationship is one-sided in terms of the depth with which both parties get to know one another. The nurse or therapist maintains boundaries that ordinarily are not maintained in personal relationships. The therapeutic frame has structural elements including explication of time, place, and cost, as well as the content of what transpires (Smith & Fitzpatrick, 1995). Regardless of type of therapy provided, the principles identified by Smith and Fitzpatrick include that the clinician does not seek satisfaction of his or her own needs, maintains focus on the patient agenda, maintains therapeutic neutrality, and promotes patient autonomy and independence. This structure offers a safe therapeutic alliance within which the therapist works to promote the best interests of the patient.

A difficulty that commonly occurs in therapeutic relationships is that newcomers to this type of relationship (both nurses and patients alike) do not know how to respond, and they often fall back on relationship skills learned in friendships, family relationships, or other personal relationships (Table 8-1). This can lead to the patient asking questions about the nurse's personal life and to the nurse answering them simply out of habit because most other interpersonal experiences involve this kind of give and take. Without identification of the core difference in the relationship when developing it with a patient, the nurse often finds the patient treating the nurse as he or she would treat a friend. If the nurse does not maintain professional boundaries, he or she may find herself sharing personal information, opinions, or feelings, thereby taking the focus off the patient. For this reason, the nurse must attend to development of the therapeutic relationship and reflect on interactions to better understand the interpersonal dynamics. The attention paid to monitoring the relationship is important to maintaining its therapeutic nature.

Therapeutic Alliance

The **therapeutic alliance** is achieved when the patient is able to freely discuss concerns and needs and work to achieve goals. This alliance develops from the safe, neutral space provided through the successful development of the therapeutic relationship and is based on the trust that the nurse establishes with the patient over time. Evidence shows that the therapeutic alliance is an important factor in accounting for treatment outcomes regardless of therapy type (Fluckiger et al., 2012). For example, Beck, the founder of cognitive behavioral therapy, discusses factors important to any therapy, including "genuine collaboration" (1976, p. 220), and discusses the need for patient and therapist to come to a consensus on the goals of therapy and ways of reaching that goal. In addition, Beck identifies research by Rogers (1951) and Truax (1963) that identifies important qualities of the therapist which lead to successful therapeutic outcomes—genuine warmth, acceptance, and accurate empathy. In interpersonal psychotherapy (IPT), Weissman, Markowitz, and Klerman (2000) identify the importance of the relationship to understanding how the patient may experience and relate in other important relationships. Positive relationship qualities, from the perspective of both the clinician and patient, have been found to be associated with improved patient outcomes (Berry et al., 2012; Bressington et al., 2011; Forchuk et al., 2001; Gilburt, Rose, & Slade, 2008). Huckshorn (2007) identifies the importance of all mental health workers being able to rapidly create therapeutic alliances.

An important consideration in the therapeutic relationship is the patient's experience of being in that relationship with the nurse. Experiences within the relationship are useful in understanding how the patient relates to others and to provide experience with learning

Differences Between Social and Therapeutic Relationships   table 8-1

	Social or Personal Relationship	Therapeutic Relationship
Purpose	Enjoyment, pleasure, meet mutual needs	Goal-directed to meet needs and goals of patient
Role	Friend	Counselor, educator, caregiver
Power	Equal	Nurse has power and authority in health care system; unequal access to information about patient, to resources, to providers
Time frame	May be lifelong	Limited to episodes of care
Activity and behavior	Spontaneous, based on interests, values	Specific to meeting patient goals, guided by ethical and professional standards
Context or environment	Variable, not defined or confined to one place or location	Based in health care setting or area of practice only
Sharing	Mutual, equal	One-sided and focused on a single person (patient) Unequal sharing; patient shares more than nurse
Reciprocity	Equal between both parties	Unequal: Nurse acts for benefit of patient without expectation of return
Meeting needs	Offers to loan things, gives gifts, freely offers opinion or advice about actions to be taken: e.g., "I have some extra socks at home, I'll bring them in for you tomorrow."	Assists in problem solving to meet needs or identifies resources available at hospital for all patients to use to meet needs. May help to identify list of options to solve problems.
Verbal communication	Casual or colloquial language Shared confidences Intimate disclosures	Careful, purposeful, professional use of language

how to approach situations that are difficult. Similar to the description of the therapeutic nurse–patient relationship in IPT, the therapist is expected to be warm and friendly, although not engaging in a social relationship, and the focus is on the patient's needs, not those of the therapist (Weissman, Markowitz, & Klerman, 2007).

Theoretical Foundations

Many theorists, including Hildegard Peplau, Carl Rogers, and Harry Stack Sullivan, have carefully developed models of how therapeutic relationships should develop. The basic tenets of the therapeutic relationship are the basis for many therapeutic interventions, including psychodynamic psychotherapy, interpersonal therapy, motivational interviewing, and cognitive behavioral therapy. Peplau's examination of the roles of the nurse and the phases of the nurse–patient relationship (1952) was influenced heavily by her work with Harry Stack Sullivan, MD, during World War II. (Sullivan published his ground-breaking *Interpersonal Theory of Psychiatry* in 1953.) The three phases of the therapeutic nurse–patient relationship are *orientation, working,* and *resolution* (Table 8-2). The working phase is further divided into two subphases, *identification* and *exploitation.* The phases of the relationship are sequential, but they also have overlapping tasks or goals. A critical part of any phase is a reflective evaluation of (1) the relationship between the nurse and patient; (2) the problems and goals mutually identified as needing intervention; and (3) the movement or progress in meeting the goals of the relationship and the patient's treatment.

Studies have identified factors in the therapeutic nurse–patient relationship that are important to patients (Box 8-3). Forchuk and Reynolds (2001) found that patients view factors such as closeness, genuine liking, and trust as important. They also found that even

when the nurse was seen as friendly, the nature of the relationship was not that of a friendship and that patients clearly delineated the nonsymmetrical nature of the relationship. Characteristics of caring identified by patients included sensitivity and accurate perception, consistency, confidentiality or trust, neutrality, respect for patients, and active listening. Other studies have identified the importance nurses place on attributes of the nurse's role, such as being equal partners in caring and developing a structured relationship with boundaries and goals focused on the patient (Dziopa & Ahern, 2009a).

Phases of the Therapeutic Relationship

The development of the therapeutic nurse–patient relationship has been examined; phases have been identified that outline characteristics of the changing relationship over time, as well as activities commonly engaged in by patient and nurse in each phase.

Orientation Phase

The **orientation phase** of the relationship refers to the initial meeting of the nurse and patient. This phase often begins prior to their actual introduction. This is referred to as the **pre-orientation phase** because both nurse and patient enter the relationship with some prior knowledge or perception of one another. For example, the nurse frequently has some information about the patient, whether from another clinical setting, from a report given by another professional, or from those who made the initial appointment or initially greeted the patient on arrival. It is important that nurses reflect on this initial information for many reasons. The information may inform the nursing assessment that follows. It is important for the nurse to consider any data prior to the patient meeting and carefully decide how this information relates to the reality or truth of the current experience of that

Phases, Actions, and Goals of the Therapeutic Nurse–Patient Relationship   table 8-2

Phase	Goal	Actions (Nurse)	Actions (Patient)
Pre-orientation	• Gathers information and materials required to meet and begin process of caring for a patient.	• Is aware of conditions in the setting that may affect patient or relationship. • Reviews any history or reports available to aid in preparation for patient. • Identifies and collects materials and resources likely to be used at the initial meeting.	• Identifies a felt need and seeks help for that need. • Anticipates/expects what setting of care and caregivers will be like. • Considers other caregivers and prepares self for current level of care. • Informs support system of plan for care. • Financial arrangements are made for care.
Orientation	• Develops trust. • Signals to patient interest in and welcomes patient to share concerns. • Meets the patient and gains understanding of needs, concerns, and goals of care. • Completes formal assessment of health. • Gathers information about care needs.	• Identifies purpose of relationship and associated structure (when and where meetings will occur, confidentiality expectations and limits). • Seeks patient's perceptions about care needs. • Assesses needs, symptoms, strengths, and limitations. • Helps patient better understand the health problem.	Active participant: • Provides information about self and health needs. • Clarifies own needs and goals of treatment. • Provides information on interventions that have helped or not in past to build on in current situation.
Working	• The "work" of treatment occurs.	• Plans for sessions, accounts for inter-session work done by patient. • Nurse is consistent and reliable.	• Engages in relationship with nurse, identifies and pursues treatment goals.
Identification	• Identify problems that can be worked on in the relationship. • Characterized by interdependence between nurse and patient.	• Clarify patient's expectations for care. • Seeks goals of patient for treatment. • Defines plans for care with patient. • Accepts patients as they are.	• Responds to those offering help. • Learns how to use the nurse–patient relationship to meet goals and needs. • Begins to engage in problem solving, adopts feelings of hope and ability instead of helplessness. • May participate interdependently, isolate from nurse, or dependently on nurse.
Exploitation	• Makes use of resources available to achieve goals and meet needs. • Identifies and plans for discharge needs to sustain progress.	• Assists patient to problem solve, learn and integrate new methods of coping; provides information needed by patient to work towards and achieve goals.	• Takes advantage of services available. • Acts to use help and services; gains independence in coping, problem solving, and learning to meet own needs. • Works to strike a balance between need for dependence and independence.
Resolution	• Movement toward independent management of needs. • End of nurse–patient relationship.	• Review and identification of goal achievement. • Engages in review of relationship. • Assists with discharge planning to meet future care needs.	• Identifies changes and progress that have been achieved. • Actively engages in planning for next steps in own growth.

Based on Peplau, H. E. (1952). Interpersonal Relations in Nursing: A Conceptual Frame of Reference for Psychodynamic Nursing. New York, NY: Putnam.

Research on the Therapeutic Nurse–Patient Relationship   box 8-3

Peplau (1992) describes the genesis of her theory of interpersonal relations in nursing as derived from work by Harry Stack Sullivan (1953), who was grounded in psychoanalytic theory but used social science theory to develop this model. Although her original work was based on Sullivan's model, in 1948 Peplau began to explicate her concepts based on her own data from clinical work with psychiatric patients. Peplau identified the purpose of the relationship being to further the personal development of the patient and the importance of the nurse replacing social communication with "the responsible use of words if this process is to be productive" (1960, p. 964). From her work, the main elements of the nurse–patient relationship were defined, including that four components were required: "two persons, professional expertise, and client needs" (p. 964). In describing the relationship, Peplau defines phases that each have a purpose, and that this relationship is both "time-limited and has an end-point" (p. 964). Forchuk has done several studies of Peplau's theory—in particular, to better understand the development of the nurse–patient relationship (Forchuk, et al., 2000) and to understand the developments in the orientation phase of the nurse–patient relationship (Forchuk, 1994).

In 1994, Forchuk prospectively studied a total of 124 newly formed nurse–client dyads (pairs) to better understand how preconceptions, levels of anxiety, and positive feelings in the relationship affect progress in development of therapeutic relationships. Instruments to identify the development of the nurse–patient relationship included the Relationship form and the Working Alliance Inventory. Anxiety was measured using the Beck Anxiety Inventory and preconceptions were measured by a seven-point scale, ranging from good to bad, on descriptions of the nurse and the patient. Results of correlations between preconceptions and weeks in orientation indicated that preconceptions were predictive of length of time in the orientation phase, although in adjusted models only the client's preconceptions

remained significant. Anxiety was not found to be significant to the evolving relationship studied.

Pounds (2010) describes the verbal and nonverbal communication between a psychiatric clinical nurse specialist and patients with schizophrenia. A problem in schizophrenia is social cognitive dysfunction, which can have a negative impact on facial and vocal recognition and social skills and result in difficulties with interpersonal interaction. From a community mental health center, Pounds videotaped three medication monitoring sessions with three patients diagnosed with schizophrenia; these patients had been part of the nurse's caseload that met inclusion criteria. Videotapes were analyzed with attention to the interaction as a whole and to nonverbal communication (including changes in facial features and areas of "disconnect" between verbal and nonverbal communication). The nurse was observed to lean forward and decrease the distance between nurse and patient, as well as to smile and nod at appropriate times. In addition, the nurse displayed changes in facial and vocal cues that appeared to improve the connection between nurse and patient, resulting in patient eye contact with the nurse. This study offers one method of using videotaped interactions to better understand the effects of schizophrenia on the communication patterns in a therapeutic nurse–patient relationship.

Peplau encouraged use of data from the work of the therapeutic nurse–patient relationship, including actions of the nurse and response of the patient to physical care, teaching, and counseling interventions, stating: "As nurses help patients in these ways to articulate and know more about their reactions to their illness experiences, nurses also gain invaluable data for advancement of the nursing profession. Study of such data later can help enlarge and enrich nursing's body of knowledge through publications about the phenomenology of human responses to disease and health concerns" (1997, p. 164).

patient. For example, a patient may have been brought by law enforcement or emergency personnel to the emergency department (ED) after an altercation at home. The evaluation at the ED may indicate that the patient requires inpatient admission. In such a case, nursing staff at the psychiatric inpatient unit will receive information and a narrative about the patient, his or her history, and the current situation that has been interpreted by several others, such as family members, law enforcement, and the ED staff. It is easy to imagine how events might become distorted in this "tag team" communication about the patient and his or her history. This sometimes explains why initial expectations of a patient being hard to manage never come to fruition.

In considering information that is made available prior to the initial meeting with a patient, nurses must acknowledge that various labels and scenarios that are part of the description of a patient may trigger reactions that have nothing to do with the current patient, but that are residual feelings from nurses' own past relationships and experiences. When seen in clinicians, this experience is called **countertransference**; in patients, it is called **transference.** These terms refer to the reaction of individuals to others that occur when attitudes or ideas are attributed to others based on some prior relationship or experience. Most important is for the nurse to recognize

the presence of some feelings and reactions to a patient whom he or she has never met so that the nurse may return to this and reflect on it later. It is important for the nurse to **bracket** this experience, acknowledging that it is occurring but setting aside the reaction for examination and reflection on how it might be interfering with the actual relationship developed with the patient. Clinicians often make the mistake of believing that it is a bad thing to have these reactions, and to deny or avoid recognition of them. However, these reactions are only human. The key is to acknowledge and reflect on them so this information is in one's conscious awareness and does not negatively affect the development of the current relationship. As nurses begin to approach and build the therapeutic relationship, it is important to consider the prior experiences patients may have had in this and other settings, with nurses and other health care professionals in the past, including experience with treatment. Just as nurses' prior experiences affect how they feel about and perceive the world, this same process occurs with patients. It is thus helpful to consider patients' prior experience.

The orientation phase continues with the nurse meeting the patient for the first time. At this initial meeting, it is important that the nurse signal that he or she is receptive and interested in the patient's concerns; otherwise, the nurse may prevent the development of a helpful working relationship (Peplau, 1997). In addition to conveying interest and unconditional positive regard, it is important in this first meeting for the nurse to identify the nature and expectations of the relationship with the patient. Often, it is in doing this that the nurse makes clear to the patient that the relationship he or she is entering is one of helping, rather than that of a friendship (see Table 8-1). Identifying the purpose of the relationship conveys an important boundary that may reduce the common problem of the patient asking personal questions about the nurse. The meeting with the patient is a goal-directed one, as the nurse seeks to have the patient identify the goals that he or she has for treatment in the current setting. In listening carefully to the patient's needs, goals, and expectations, the nurse begins to develop rapport and build trust with the patient, and clearly identifies that the patient's goals are a priority in treatment. The nurse uses this initial meeting to assess patient strengths and assets as well as needs, symptoms, and limitations that interfere with the patient's ability to function in daily life. During this phase, the nurse learns about the patient and engages in mutual planning with the patient to support the patient's goals for treatment. While obtaining information about the patient, the nurse integrates the data obtained with the prior reports and clarifies information by asking the patient about differences in history as needed.

As the nurse gathers information, he or she may identify difficulties through assessment and assist the patient in understanding the relationship of identified problems and goals that the nurse sees as important, but that the patient has not identified or cannot yet identify. For example, if the nurse is working with an acutely suicidal individual, the patient's perception is often that life is not worth living and death is the only solution. Clearly, this is important information to understand about the patient and how severely upset he or she is; however, the nurse will seek to engage in treatment planning around a shared goal that supports the patient's safety in treatment. In this phase, the nurse may also find that the patient challenges aspects of the relationship with the nurse or with the clinical setting. This testing of limits may be part of a process in which the patient is determining the integrity of both the nurse and the treatment setting, and is an important aspect to attend to in the relationship.

Peplau (1992) identifies the importance of the orientation phase because it sets the foundation for future intervention (p. 14). It is wise for the nurse to reflect on the process of this initial phase of the relationship, as it may offer insights into the relationship and treatment that otherwise would not be noticed, including information about the interpersonal skills of the patient.

Forchuk et al. (2000) studied nurse–patient dyads and found that the nature of the therapeutic relationship was evident for relationships that progressed through the phases as identified by Peplau. Some relationships studied did not progress from the orientation phase; these were marked by inconsistency, unavailability, negative feelings of the nurse, and unrealistic expectations. The movement from orientation to the working phase has been studied; patients indicated that factors facilitating movement to the working phase included the perceived attitude of the nurse and the nature of therapeutic interactions with the nurse, whereas barriers included unavailability of either party, a sense of inequality or distance between nurse and patient, values differences, and mutual withdrawal (Forchuk, Westwell, Martin, Bamber-Azzapardi, Kosterewa-Tolman, & Hux, 1998). These findings suggest that the nurse plays an important role in patient progress and that reflection, self-awareness, and clinical supervision can help the nurse actively engage so that the therapeutic

nurse–patient relationship can progress and patients can work toward and achieve goals.

Working Phase

Once mutual understanding is reached about the patient's presenting problems and goals, the relationship shifts from the orientation to the working phase. The **working phase** of the therapeutic nurse–patient relationship begins as the nurse and patient identify problems and begin to develop trust. This initial step in the process has been called the *identification subphase* and includes identification of steps that can be taken to meet the goals that were identified during the orientation phase. These discussions lead to another part of the working phase, the *exploitation subphase*, in which the patient engages actively in the helping process and works toward meeting goals. The working phase includes activities such as the provision of physical care, teaching, counseling, and interviewing (Peplau, 1997). Part of the exploitation phase is the implementation of the interventions or action plan to attain the goals identified. Throughout both parts of the working phase, the nurse reflects with the patient about needs previously identified as well as needs that emerge through the course of treatment and require interventions incorporated into the plan. There is an overlapping process of the phases; for example, discharge planning begins in the working phase and is also a part of the resolution phase of the relationship (Peplau, 1997).

Resolution

In the **resolution phase,** goals that could be attained in the setting have been met and, as the patient moves forward toward discharge or the next stage of care, the relationship with the nurse comes to an end. This phase has also been called the *termination phase*, as it involves summarizing and providing closure to the relationship (Peplau, 1997). This phase is marked by reflection and validation of steps taken toward meeting goals and by identification of potential goals for future growth, whether the patient remains in treatment or not. Planning and intervention revolve around communication, discharge planning, and outreach to the community so the patient has adequate supports and services in place to sustain progress. Health promotion is an important aspect of this phase of the relationship, as the nurse assists the patient to better understand the current episode of illness and recognize risk factors and warning signs for future episodes of illness, with a focus on intervention to prevent recurrence or limit severity of symptoms in the future. Successful resolution of the therapeutic relationship also rests on the nurse and patient reflecting together on the process of the relationship so that interpersonal gains in both communication and problem-solving skills can be transferred to relationships in the patient's life. In this way, the patient gains from the interpersonal interactions that were a part of the therapeutic relationship and their broader treatment in the clinical setting.

Developing and Maintaining Boundaries

Boundaries can be difficult to manage in interpersonal relationships, and therapeutic relationships are no different in this regard. The nurse maintains many types of boundaries, including limiting self-disclosure, not engaging in social or personal relationships with patients, and not behaving in a way that exploits the therapeutic nurse–patient relationship. Unfortunately, boundary management is a very difficult skill to learn, as it requires clinical judgment and insight that develop gradually over time. Nightingale refers to nurses maintaining boundaries in the Nightingale pledge, as does the American Nurses Association (ANA) Code of Ethics, which identifies that the nurse recognizes and maintains boundaries and limits in relationships with patients (Holder & Schenthal, 2007). In the psychiatric setting, in particular, it is expected that the nurse maintain professional boundaries with patients at all times. Some identify the creation and maintenance of boundaries in the nurse–patient relationship as the most important competency in the field of psychiatric–mental health nursing (Hectornelj-Taylor & Yonge, 2003).

One key to maintaining boundaries is for the nurse to be intentional in developing the therapeutic relationship with a patient. For example, a nurse meeting a patient for the first time introduces himself or herself as a professional involved in the patient's care, rather than informally telling the patient his or her name and making a comment about the weather, the patient's appearance, or a topic unrelated to patient care. Although there is nothing wrong with having informal interactions or being friendly with a patient, doing so gives the patient a different message than a statement that clearly identifies the nurse's role and purpose. If the relationship has a clear therapeutic frame from the start, nurses tend to have less need to clarify boundaries over time.

At times, patients will attempt to test boundaries. When this occurs, the nurse must keep in mind the inherent imbalance in power between the nurse and the patient. Despite efforts to involve patients fully in their care, patients are at their most vulnerable when they require help from the nurse, and they expect that the nurse will use his or her power to encourage growth and meet the goals of treatment (Hectornelj-Taylor & Yonge, 2003). This is an important responsibility of the nurse, regardless of patient requests for boundaries to change.

Several areas deserve consideration as nurses proceed to develop therapeutic relationships with appropriate professional boundaries. Nurses must be careful to focus on meeting patient needs, and not focus on meeting their own personal needs. This is of importance whether the nurse's need is a simple one, such as the need to be liked or gain approval, or whether the need is a more serious one, such as being sexually attracted to a patient. The relationship must be focused on meeting the patient's needs; this often requires careful self-awareness and reflection by the nurse to be certain that the patient's needs are the focus. Self-disclosure is a difficult area in the nurse–patient relationship, as sharing about self may or may not be appropriate, and what is shared appropriately may vary by individual patient, setting, or circumstance. Peplau's view on self-disclosure was very clear; she states that the patient "does not need information about the personal life of the nurse" (1997, p. 164). For example, by sharing a similar experience of loss and identifying how distressed and hopeless he or she felt, the nurse may lead a patient to wonder whether the nurse is capable of helping the patient or if the patient should try to care for the nurse.

The use of touch is another area of the therapeutic relationship in which boundaries must be established. Again, if the nurse is motivated to touch a patient, the nurse should first consider whose needs would be met by the touching, as often impulsive touching or hugging meets the needs of the nurse more than those of the patient (Hectornelj-Taylor & Yonge, 2003). In particular, nurses must be careful with touch when working with patients with mental illness, given the frequent history of physical or sexual abuse and trauma in these patients, and given the potential for misinterpretation of that touch.

Problems with boundaries in therapeutic relationships lie on a continuum, from minor acts that have little negative effect on patients to major acts that have serious effects on patients or result in severe injury. Acts could be classified into those that are boundary crossings and those that are boundary violations. Boundary crossings are considered less severe than boundary violations. The National Council of State Boards of Nursing defines **boundary crossings** as decisions to deviate from a boundary for a therapeutic purpose, such as appointment changes, disclosing personal bits of information, or the giving or receiving of small gifts. These are small breaches with a likely return to expected limits of the professional relationship. Unfortunately, minor boundary crossings can lead to more serious acts that can be harmful or abusive to the patient (Smith & Fitzpatrick, 1995). Even trivial boundary crossings may progress to boundary violations. **Boundary violations** might include holding dual roles with a patient (such as that of nurse and friend), inappropriate self-disclosure or touching, or sexual misconduct (Hectornelj-Taylor & Yonge, 2003).

There are many strategies nurses can use to better understand how to manage professional boundaries in the therapeutic nurse-patient relationship (Table 8-3). Hectornelj-Taylor & Yonge (2003) suggest that the nurse actively pursue a variety of activities such as self-care, self-awareness, monitoring of needs and relationships, involving team members or peers in debriefing, and seeking clinical supervision. For example, the nurse must plan to have personal needs met in personal relationships so these needs do not unwittingly drive behavior in the therapeutic nurse–patient relationship.

In general, it is wise to clarify the goals and focus of the therapeutic relationship nurses develop with patients. As discussed previously, in daily life it is unusual to develop a therapeutic relationship of the kind developed by mental health clinicians. For this reason, developing a therapeutic relationship may seem foreign and may result in either the nurse or patient relying on knowledge and skills on how relationships work from other kinds of interpersonal relationships, including friendships and family relationships. Those relationships, however, may not have provided good modeling of effective interpersonal boundaries. Therefore, it is important for the nurse to be attentive and intentional in development of the therapeutic relationship and to seek to be aware of his or her own verbal and nonverbal communication. If these aspects of communication are unexamined, the nurse may inadvertently convey that the relationship is other than professional and therapeutic. For this reason, it is very important for mental health nurses to learn as much about themselves and their interpersonal styles of communicating as is possible.

Peplau (1997) discussed challenges that occur in the therapeutic relationship that can test the integrity of the nurse. Some of these challenges may also be considered boundary crossings, such as using the patient's time to talk about the nurse's experiences, and avoiding rather than managing the anger or annoyance of the patient. For example, if the patient asks the nurse for personal information (about the nurse), and the nurse shares that information in an effort to seem more socially acceptable and/or avoid angering the patient, the nurse avoids maintaining a boundary. Even seemingly minor exchanges may lead unwittingly to a role reversal, with the patient becoming confidant of the nurse. It is only through self-awareness and ongoing work to maintain an understanding of our

Cues to Boundary Crossings and Violations   table 8-3

Cues That Indicate Boundary Crossings and Violations	Appropriate Nurse or Supervisory Responses

• Strong feelings about a patient (positive or negative)
• Extending sessions
• Providing "special services"
• Treating patient differently from most other patients
• Feeling a "special relationship" with patient
• Inappropriate communication
• Off-hours phone calls or messaging (e-mail, texting)
  – Frequency
  – Timing (late at night, on weekends)
  – Immediacy of responses
• Providing personal information
• Gift giving
• Accepting gifts from patients
• Overdoing
• Overprotecting
• Overidentifying
• Keeping secrets with patient
• Loans to or from patients
• Bartering
• Sale of goods to patient
• Purchase from patient
• Self-disclosure of clinician
• Touching
• Comforting
• Sexual attraction to patient
• Sexual contact with patient
• Allowing patient to think that relationship may continue after discharge
	• Avoid "solo" involvement in caregiving:
	  – Regular treatment team reviews of patients
	  – Discuss in supervision
	  – Use clinical supervision for case review
	• Maintain regular supervision schedule with ability to have "consults" as needed
	• Identify prior relationship with or to patient:
	  – To supervisor
	  – To treatment team
	• Limit or exclude engagement in care
	• Use "on call" service rotation
	• Identify policy on gift giving and acceptance
	• Reflect regularly on care giving
	• Compare quality of relationship across patients
	• Be aware of therapist feelings about patient
	• Maintain therapeutic boundaries
	• Avoid other roles or relationships:
	  – Business services
	  – Customer
	• Evaluate actions based on:
	  – Contributing to therapeutic relationship
	  – Consistency with plan of care
	  – How colleagues or supervisor would respond
	• Seek consultation from supervisor or mentor

Based on Walker, R., & Clark, J. J. (1999). Heading off boundary problems: Clinical supervision as risk management. *Psychiatric Services, 50*(11), 1435–1439; Wright, L. D. (2006). Violating professional boundaries. *Nursing, 36*(3), 52–54.

own behavior that we manage relationships and avoid exploiting the vulnerability of the patient.

There are many other behaviors that are considered boundary violations in the nurse–patient relationship. These include developing a social or intimate relationship with a patient, using confidential health information to benefit the nurse, and giving or accepting gifts from patients (College of Registered Nurses of Manitoba, 2011). Friendships and intimate relationships are violations of boundaries, given that the nurse has a position of power and that these may result in the patient not acting freely, as well as in the nurse having information about the patient that normally the patient would disclose only within a friendship or intimate relationship. It is generally expected that a nurse would decline gifts from patients, but if the situation arises, it is wise to carefully consider the implications of the gift and discuss the situation with a supervisor. Some examples of appropriate responses in situations that carry the potential for boundary crossings or violations are given in Box 8-4.

Self-Disclosure

Self-disclosure is an important consideration in understanding relationship boundaries. Individuals who self-disclose frequently to many people might be considered as having very permeable or open boundaries. Those who rarely self-disclose could be described as having very closed boundaries. Most people are somewhere in the middle of this

continuum. Sharing information that is designed to further develop rapport or help the patient meet health care goals may be useful; however, there must be some clear benefit consistent with the patient's plan of care that supports the use of self-disclosure. In a therapeutic relationship, self-disclosure of a personal nature is never acceptable if it is lengthy or irrelevant to the patient's treatment or of a deeply personal or intimate nature (College of Registered Nurses of Manitoba, 2011). If an action or behavior oversteps normal professional boundaries to meet the nurse's needs, then this is considered a boundary violation (National Council of State Boards of Nursing, n.d.). Key to understanding interpersonal relationships, self-disclosure, and boundaries is one's own level of self awareness about interaction. These qualities, combined with experience and good judgment, determine how boundaries are set in interpersonal relationships. One way to consider these qualities is to consider the Johari window, a model of the process of human interactions that offers one way to analyze and better understand information sharing with others.

Johari Window

As discussed in Chapter 7, the **Johari window** is a model developed by Joseph Luft and Harrington Ingham (combining their names to form Johari) to describe the process of interaction and the relationship of self awareness to interaction (Luft & Ingham, 1955; Luft, 1969). It is important to remember that the areas of each window are considered

Avoiding Boundary Crossings or Violations box 8-4

When called on to respond to a request from the patient that crosses the line between professional and personal, the nurse must consider the patient, the setting, and the context, as well as the meaning of the request. One consideration is to evaluate whose needs would be met by the crossing (Holder & Schenthal, 2007). Although being genuine or authentic within the nurse–patient relationship is important, it is also important for the nurse to carefully consider the potential implications of such

requests. Unfortunately, as with many things related to work of an interpersonal nature, there are no black or white, right or wrong rules. However, the potential for boundary violations is present in every professional and varies based on the context as well as the presence of risk factors for boundary violation, such as the work setting, type of patients, and experience (Holder & Schenthal, 2007). The following table provides examples of appropriate responses to common types of patient requests.

Patient Statement	Appropriate Nurse Response
"I was admitted from the emergency department and don't have any socks. Here's $20, could you buy me some and bring them in tomorrow?"	"Rather than give me your money, let's ask the social services department for help; they have extra supplies for purposes like this."
"You have been such a wonderful helper to me while I've been here, I'd like to give you something to show my appreciation."	"I appreciate the compliment, but we don't accept gifts for the work we do. If you really felt you wanted to do something special, you could give some small gift to the unit or the clinic."
"You're about my age and you seem to understand me better than anyone else in my life. If you aren't dating someone, maybe we could get together after I leave this place and have coffee?"	"Thanks, but the relationship we have is specific to this setting. It wouldn't be right for me to continue our relationship after you left here."
"My brother died last month and I just can't seem to get over it. Have you ever lost someone close to you?"	"Losses are often difficult to deal with. I'm here to talk with you about *your* experiences. Tell me more about your brother's death."

dynamic in this model and their configuration may vary based on the person or context considered. For example, upon meeting a new person, the window might be much smaller, and as the relationship develops the window gets larger as more information is shared.

The combination of whether something is known or unknown to self and whether it is known or unknown to others defines the four quadrants of the window. Luft and Ingham describe this as how individuals' personality traits influence their behavior (Luft, 1969). In the first quadrant is the free or open information about self. These are things individuals recognize about themselves and that others know about them, such as their name or height. In the current electronic age, it may also relate to information the individual shares through social media, such as thoughts, feelings, or behaviors. The second quadrant is considered a "blind" area, in that information here is not known to the self but is known to others. Examples include forgetting to remove a nametag at the end of a conference or having a piece of food stuck between one's teeth. Although these are rather obvious examples, consider also the nuances of communication and body language. For example, think of times someone has said to another, "You look tired," or "You look anxious," and the individual is not aware of this until someone points it out.

The third or "hidden" quadrant contains awareness that is known to self, but not known by others. This may include things individuals do not feel comfortable sharing with others. It may be a wide variety of things that are hidden, for a variety of reasons. The configuration of the window relates to the relationship or setting involved. For example, when starting a new job, most people do not disclose much information initially about their political, religious, or other beliefs or opinions. Once they get to know their co-workers and develop trust in the situation, however, they may be comfortable disclosing this information. As trust develops in relationships, more personal or intimate details are shared between individuals or groups. Because the quadrants all relate to one another, as one is enlarged, the corresponding quadrants change in size as well.

The final quadrant is that of the "unknown," in which neither party is aware of certain behaviors or motives. Over time, individuals may become aware of these aspects as they become known to self, others, or both. For example, an individual may realize she is reacting unusually to a new person in her life, perhaps feeling angry with that person for no reason at all. On reviewing the situation, she may begin to realize that there is a quality the person has that is reminiscent of some other experience or time, and may discover feelings that were there all along but never acknowledged. By doing so, the individual may bring knowledge of self into the known to self region and potentially, if shared with others, into the "known to others" arena as well.

Self-awareness and self-disclosure are processes that occur both intentionally and unintentionally. As trust develops in relationships, there is a tendency to disclose more fully with greater levels of trust. In general, self-awareness and self-disclosure are considered facets of mental health. The ability to relate to others, to know about one's self, and to safely share with others is important in our relationships and our lives. The Johari window is one way to picture how the components of self-awareness and self-disclosure interact and affect relationships (Figure 8-1).

Pause and Reflect

1. *What is your general tendency in terms of self-disclosure? Are there differences based on the kind of information? For example, do you share information on the types of music you like more readily than you share information about your family? How do you decide what you will disclose to whom?*

2. *Reflect on how boundaries are different for you in your role of nurse versus in your role of friend or family member. Can you give examples of how your boundaries are different when acting in the role of friend compared with the role of family member?*

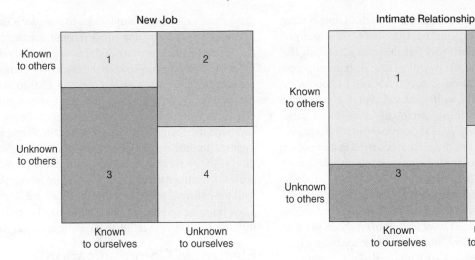

8-1 Johari window showing differences in quadrants between "new job" and "intimate relationship": (1) Known to others, (2) unknown to others, (3) known to ourselves, (4) unknown to ourselves.

Forms of Communication

Communication is the way that people share information and meaning with one another. It is the way we let others know what is going on in our thoughts and emotions, or the way we make external our internal experience. In any interaction between two or more individuals, there are several forms of communication at work. **Verbal communication** consists of the actual words chosen. **Nonverbal communication** includes gestures, posture, and appearance, as well as other factors. **Meta-communication** refers to those involved in the interaction (who is sending the message and who is receiving it), how the message is sent (in person, over the telephone, or through e-mail, for instance), the context of the message (for example, nurse and patient in a clinical setting, supervisor and employee in a workplace, friends in a restaurant), and other factors. Each form of communication has important implications for the success of the interaction.

Verbal Communication

Verbal communication is the words that people use when they speak. As seen earlier in Box 8-4, the words the nurse chooses can clearly differentiate the nurse's role as a professional, even when the patient challenges the nurse to cross professional boundaries. Particularly in the context of psychiatric mental health nursing, words carry power. Words can empower and support, or dismiss and disrespect. The verbal communication of a nurse—the words that he or she chooses—has a great impact on a patient's ability to achieve understanding about his or her illness, to believe in the ability to improve his or her own mental health status, and to begin to have hope that his or her suffering will improve.

Nonverbal Communication

Clearly, language is not the only way in which individuals convey internal experiences to others. Posture, tone, volume, eye contact, gestures, dress, and other external modes may also be used to convey these experiences. Nonverbal communication consists of all the other components of the communication that are not spoken; nonverbal communication can account for more than half of what an individual communicates at any given time. Nonverbal communication includes tone of voice, facial expression, eye contact, body language, gestures, touch, and other aspects of communication with others. In addition to the verbal and nonverbal communication used, communication is interpreted within a cultural context. Types of communication can vary greatly from culture to culture. For example, in many cultures a smile indicates happiness, but in some cultures smiling also can be used to hide sadness or embarrassment.

Types of nonverbal communication include the following:

- Body language
- *Oculesics,* which consists of eye gaze and eye contact
- *Proxemics,* which involves interpersonal distance or use of space and changes in body position (discussed further in Chapter 7)
- *Kinesics,* or actions and positions of the body, head, and limbs
- Touch
- Vocal cues
- *Chronemics,* or use and meaning of time
- Appearance
- Physical environment and objects
- Smells

Argyle hypothesized that verbal communication or spoken words communicate information about external events, whereas nonverbal communication functions to establish and maintain relationships (Argyle et al., 1970; Argyle, 1988). Argyle concluded that there are five primary functions of nonverbal communication: to express emotion, to convey interpersonal attitudes, to manage interaction cues between speakers and listeners, to present one's personality, and for rituals such as greetings. *Immediacy behaviors* are ways that individuals communicate interpersonal closeness and include actions such as touching, eye contact, and smiling (Argyle, 1988). An important aspect to consider is the agreement among different types of communication used. Body language is the use of parts of the body such as facial expressions, hand movements, and posture to convey meaning to others. Oculesics (eye contact) may involve direct staring into other's eyes, avoiding another's eyes, or gazing down. In some cultures, gazing down may imply respect, whereas in others it may convey insincerity.

Use of space relates to the distance individuals maintain when they are interacting with others. Sommer (1959, p. 247) discusses personal space, reviewing early efforts to define the term, identifying that von Uexküll (1957) made the analogy of personal space to people "surrounded by soap-bubble worlds." Stern is credited by Sommer as identifying the personal world with a natural center, about which everything else extends with those "personally near" as an "aura" around the person (Stern, 1938, p. 248). Sommer (1959) did studies on personal space, and found that differences occurred in terms of use of personal space and choice of seating arrangements for interactions in terms of gender as well as for participants with schizophrenia, who tended to sit distant from others and would face away from others and not speak. Sommer also found that women sit closer to other women than to men and that men tended to sit farther from others of either sex. From these studies and others, limits that define space have been developed (See Chapter 7, Figure 7-4). Culture also plays an important role in the distance used in communication with others. Use of touch varies greatly by culture, with some cultures using a great deal of touching within social conversation and others using very little touch. Consider even a handshake as an element of communication that can convey a lot of information between individuals.

Facial expression was noted by Darwin (1872) as important to development and well-being. He identified that the first forms of communication between mother and child are enacted through smiling and other expressions. In addition, Darwin suggested that expression reveals information about the thoughts and intentions of others, whereas words may not be as truthful. Facial expressions might be seen as a window on feelings or emotions that are experienced. Similar also are posture, gesture, and movement in their ability to provide information about communication.

Many aspects of speech are nonverbal, including volume, rate of speech, tone, and tempo. Laughing, burping, or yawning are also nonverbal aspects of speech. Use of time is another important part of communicating; for example, consider how arriving early or late for an appointment may be interpreted by others. In addition, time may relate to considering whether one speaker dominates a conversation, whereas another may interrupt others. Use of time also is an important consideration from a cultural standpoint.

Appearance includes dress or clothing choices, actual physical features of one's body, and hair and skin color, as well as piercings or tattoos. Smell is also a property of communication, conveying a message and possibly relating to hygiene, use of perfume, and spice. The physical environment relates to considering the area or location of an interaction, the size of the area, its appearance, and its accessibility. Finally, the degree to which verbal, nonverbal, and behavioral cues are congruent should be considered when interpreting the meaning of communication (Figure 8-2).

Meta-Communication

Meta-communication is communication about the communication. It refers to information about the communication, such as who is sending and receiving the message, how the message was sent, the context of the message, and whether the meaning is supported by both verbal and nonverbal communication or whether there are aspects that are contradictory or incongruent. Reade and Smouse (1980) discuss the importance of congruence of the clinician's verbal and nonverbal communication with the patient. For example, the literal interpretation is the meaning of the words, but meta-communication involves the nonverbal elements that offer information about how to interpret the communication. This may include information about the relationship of those communicating. A similar idea to consider is the idea of content (the words) and process (information communicated about the words).

In psychiatric–mental health nursing, communication is the primary tool used to help patients. It is a very complex process and requires that clinicians carefully consider all aspects of their own and the patients' communication. The nurse uses communication in a careful and mindful way to assist patients to better understand and cope with their symptoms and problems. In planning to interact with a patient, the nurse plans for an appropriate setting, space, and time to meet with the patient. In addition, the nurse considers the patient's goals for treatment and helps to structure interactions so that time with the patient is well spent and goal directed. The nurse uses both active listening and therapeutic communication techniques to engage with the patient in a positive, therapeutic, and goal-directed way.

Electronic Communication

Many changes in communication have occurred with the invention of various technological devices. Some have suggested that there are negative consequences to this trend in communication, and that individuals will need interaction and face-to-face relationships like those developed in psychiatric–mental health nursing to provide an outlet for the lack of others able to actively listen or process

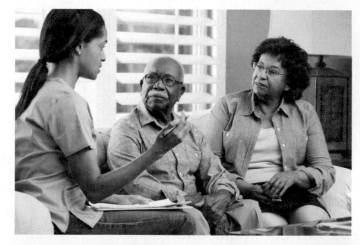

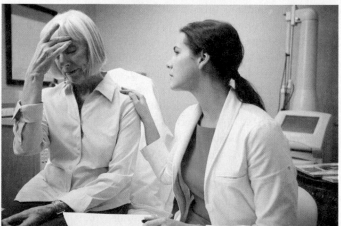

8-2 A. What does the nonverbal communication used by the nurse and the patient and his wife suggest about the therapeutic relationship? B. What does the posture of the patient (on the left) suggest to you? What are your thoughts about how the nurse is responding?

Source: Monkey Business/Fotolia

experiences (Hart, 2010b). Today, many individuals use electronic or digital media as a primary form of interaction. Often friends, family, colleagues, and acquaintances stay in communication or contact via texting, e-mail, and social networking sites. The question, of course, is whether the convenience of these avenues of interaction has any downsides. New terms, such as *Internet addiction*, as well as health problems associated with the accompanying passive and inactive lifestyle are beginning to emerge in response to growing use of the Internet and digital media.

A clear benefit of technology and electronic communication to patients is the access to support systems that are available around the clock. As with other forms of interaction, there are ways to structure or control the forms of interaction using these methods. Rather than dismissing these important avenues of support, clinicians and clinical organizations may be wise to discuss and provide guidance on helpful versus nonhelpful methods of electronic communication, how to discern quality of information available, and developing secure sites that offer a way to connect and communicate safely.

Much of work life has been transformed by e-mail, Internet access to information, tweeting, and text messaging. Clinical services and settings likewise are changing through the use of technologic innovations. The health care industry has been undergoing change in preparation for electronic medical records that will be available across systems of care. Tele-health programs are offering clinical services, including psychiatric care, to patients in rural areas where caregivers are not readily available. Nurses in many settings are using technology in many aspects of their profession, including interdepartmental communications and patient care. As with any transformative change, there are positive and negative aspects to consider.

The positive aspects of electronic communication include their ease and immediacy. Sending an e-mail or text message is instantaneous and does not involve any other resource than an Internet or wireless connection. Today, the use of Skype allows clinicians to actually "see" their patients during long-distance conversations. Tele-health programs are using video feeds to enable clinical evaluation and intervention. Some clinicians have used website forums, discussion boards, and e-mail successfully to provide therapy and suggest that this is an effective mechanism despite the lack of face-to-face connection. These methods allow a patient or clinician in an established therapeutic relationship to continue treatment with geographic moves or time away from the formal office setting. Interactive forums and websites offer patients with common concerns or needs a place to interact with others, although these may be most successful when used as a support group rather than as a substitute for direct therapy. Internet forums and websites may be especially helpful for those with rare or very specific conditions.

The negative aspects of electronic communication include the limited amount of information and limited range of emotions that can be shared with text-based communications such as e-mail, texting, or tweeting. As a result, it is very easy to misinterpret innocuous electronic messages as critical, negative, or insensitive to emotional needs. Unfortunately, it is very easy to hit "send" without reviewing a message carefully and considering any potential ambiguities. This creates the possibility of misinterpretation of motive, intent, tone, and other nuances normally available in a combination of verbal and nonverbal communication. Another problem with electronic communication is with expectations regarding the clinician checking e-mail and with awareness or communication regarding safety issues. For example, what if a patient who is used to electronic access communicates suicidal thought or intent, but the message is not retrieved and read immediately?

Another point to consider is that the electronic medical record has resulted in nurses and other professionals typing information into a computer or tablet while interacting face to face with a patient. Depending on how this is done, a patient could feel that the nurse is focusing on the screen rather than on the patient. Confidentiality of communication is another important issue to consider with use of electronic communication. With text-based or Internet communication, there is the potential that information could be seen by others unexpectedly. Safeguards must be provided to prevent breaches of confidential information and to ensure that HIPAA requirements are met. Nurses must know the policies regarding electronic communication in the settings in which they work. The American Nurses Association has provided guidelines for the appropriate use of social media in the health care environment (Larson, 2011).

Pause and Reflect

1. *Think about the last time you had a heated discussion with a friend. How much of the message would you estimate was conveyed by the words alone? (Try to come up with a percentage: 10%? 30%? 50%? 80%?) Identify the key elements of nonverbal communication used by you and your friend. Include space, time, touch, posture, and rate and volume of speech.*

2. *If you had that same conversation but both of you were blindfolded, what would have been different? If the words from each of you were read out loud by the same computerized voice in a monotone, what would have been similar and different? What aspects of the communication or interaction would be different, and how?*

Therapeutic Communication Techniques

A variety of techniques are used in therapeutic communication. Some of these have been discussed previously, such as active listening skills and unconditional positive regard. Equally as important are methods of communication that are nontherapeutic. These include social responding and giving advice or approval. Nurses working in psychiatric settings in particular must be knowledgeable about skills and behaviors that both promote and discourage therapeutic communication.

Therapeutic Communication Skills

Table 8-4 identifies many techniques that promote therapeutic communication and provides examples of how they might be used in the therapeutic nurse–patient relationship. Each technique can be used for a variety of purposes in communication, but for ease of presentation and learning, they are presented here in groups of related skills. The groups include active listening skills, qualities present in or conveyed by the nurse, unconditional positive regard, assessment skills, insight-oriented techniques, and interventions. Nurses typically use multiple techniques in combination, often without thinking about them. Methods of purposeful therapeutic communication that employ multiple strategies also can be helpful. Motivational interviewing is one such technique.

Motivational interviewing (MI) is a collaborative, person-centered prescribed set of interviewing strategies based on the work of Carl Rogers (Chapter 4) and the stages of change (Prochaska,

Therapeutic Communication Skills

table 8-4

Active Listening Skills

Therapeutic Technique	Definition	Example
Active listening	Focuses full attention on another's communication both verbally and nonverbally, excluding all distractions, while engaging to encourage further communication.	Nonverbal/body language: faces person, makes good eye contact, nods, leans forward toward speaker. Verbal: Uses sounds and statements that encourage further explication, such as "Uh-huh, hmmm, yes, tell me more. . ."
Broad opening	Begins communication with a lead that allows the person to move in a direction of his or her choice.	"Tell me what led to you making an appointment here today."
Eye contact	Uses enough eye contact to indicate engagement and involvement in the interaction without "staring down" the patient or causing discomfort.	
Incomplete sentences	Provides some information to cue direction of discussion in desired direction.	"In the house?" "Any family members affected?" "Then what?"
Observing	States unsaid or nonverbal communication.	"When you talked about Sam taking your keys, you looked like you had tears in your eyes." "You are sitting upright and looking very tense."
Open-ended questions	Provides opening to discussion and allows patient to choose focus or direction of discussion.	"Tell me how that situation made you feel." "Tell me about the kinds of jobs you have held."
Paraphrasing	Summarizes patient statements in own words. Concisely identifies what has been stated or discussed.	[". .. and that is the story of how I came to be named Joseph."] "So you were named after your father." "Since your emergency surgery, your family has watched you carefully and is worried about your physical health?"
Restating	Repeats back what was shared.	"You are worried that you've been out of school too long to go back?"
Use of silence	Allows silences and pauses during conversations without needing to "fill space."	

Qualities Present In or Conveyed by the Nurse

Therapeutic Technique	Definition	Example
Empathy	Puts oneself in another's place to understand felt needs and experiences.	"When you described your teacher punishing you, it sounded like you felt humiliated and angry at the same time. Is that what it was like for you?"
Neutrality	Maintains nonjudgmental or objective perspective. Accepts information without showing approval or disapproval. Allows patient to try out feelings, behaviors, affect without interjecting opinion.	"After you were arrested, did you have to serve any time in prison?" "After the accident and DUI charges, what was the end result?" "You shared that you have had several abortions, and you prefer not to use birth control. Tell me more about that."
Offering of self	Identifies availability and willingness to listen and support the patient.	"I am available to talk with you this afternoon, if you would like that." "I am the nurse caring for you today. If I can help you in some way, please let me know."
Self-disclosure	Shares information about personal experience, reactions, opinions, or feelings.	"I decided to return to school because I wanted to learn more about psychology." "I enjoy watching football too."
Suggesting collaboration	Encourages patient to engage with team members and other supports to advance towards meeting goals.	"Perhaps if you and your sister both find yourselves feeling lonely in the evening, you could plan to do something together you both enjoy." "Have you identified your needs and concerns with your teacher?"

Unconditional Positive Regard

Therapeutic Technique	Definition	Example
Accepting	Identifies willingness to engage and hear concerns regardless of content, agreement, or values.	"I hear how difficult it was for you to be fired from your job. Destroying files was a reaction you wouldn't normally do, but in difficult moments we sometimes behave in ways that we normally wouldn't."
Acknowledging	Expresses recognition of or validates the existence of something.	"I am glad you came to group today. I know how hard it is for you to drive on the highway to get here."
Affirming	Positively acknowledges another, or characteristics of another.	"It sounds like you clearly and logically explained your concerns to the store manager."
Giving recognition	Identifies the presence of traits, qualities, actions, or behaviors.	"The way you handled that situation shows how thoughtful and kind you are to your sister."
Validation	Seeks to have the patient confirm information that has been shared.	"Would I be correct in saying that you feel anxious and fearful when you walk in the city because you think your enemies might be looking to harm you?"

Assessment

Therapeutic Technique	Definition	Example
Clarification	Identifies information not clear to listener and requests further information.	"Earlier you said you lived with your mother and father, but you just mentioned that your father lives in a different state. Help me understand that."
Directing	Moves discussion to a different topic or area, or identifies or instructs what is to occur next.	"I appreciate you sharing your family history with me, but I need some further information about your health. Have you ever had any hospitalizations or procedures for a health problem?" "The group will meet in the dining area; please come with me and join us."
Exploring	Encourages the patient to discuss more fully an experience or situation, to better identify thoughts, feelings, and dynamics associated with it.	"You mentioned an exchange of eye contact with your husband that had some meaning for you. Tell me more about that."
Focusing	Requests further elaboration of pertinent topics; organizes identification of information for use in assessment.	"You mentioned losing your job. Tell me what led up to that happening."
Giving leads	Directs flow of interaction to topics of importance or to obtain clarification.	"Did you grow up and go to school in town?"
Placing events in time sequence	Validates sequence of events described by patient.	"After you left high school, you joined the army—is that when you moved to North Carolina?"
Seeking information	Requests information or feedback.	"How many children were in your family?" "What kinds of jobs have you held in your life?"
Summarizing	Provides a review of what the patient discussed, to aid in reflection, moving forward in the discussion, or to validate understanding.	"So about three months ago, after you broke up with your girlfriend you began to feel sad and hopeless and felt more irritable. These depression symptoms have bothered you since and most recently you have had insomnia and trouble concentrating at work."

Insight-Oriented Techniques

Therapeutic Technique	Definition	Example
Encourage comparison	Encourages reflection on similarities and differences of current situation with others in the patient's life experience.	"Have you ever had a similar reaction?"
Encourage description of perceptions	Tries to more fully understand how the patient is experiencing a situation.	"Tell me exactly what you thought and felt when your sister yelled at you."

(continued)

Therapeutic Communication Skills *(continued)*

table 8-4

Insight-Oriented Techniques

Therapeutic Technique	Definition	Example
Identify themes	Shares observations of patterns, common aspects to patient interaction or difficulty/problems presented.	"You have mentioned loss as a problem that has repeatedly been part of your life in the past year." "It seems that losses keep coming up and they cause great difficulty for you."
Present reality	Identifies real experience, truth of situation that is commonly accepted by society.	"I realize you thought the red light in the ceiling was a listening device, but it is actually the fire alarm." "The notes I took during our meeting were about the changes in symptoms you identified this week. You can see them if you would like. They show the progress you are making in meeting your goals."
Reflection	Considers or thinks about an experience or situation to gain greater perspective on it, or attain a new understanding. A technique to encourage the patient to reconsider his or her experience by reviewing some aspect.	May be done quietly or through writing or review of an experience with others. "You described your reaction to your father as confused, but your voice and body position seemed angry."
Reframing	Understands and interprets a situation or experience from a different perspective.	"I know you described your choice to quit your job as 'wimping out,' but maybe it was an example of you taking better care of yourself."
Translating into feelings	From discussion, identifies possible feeling states described by the patient and seeks confirmation or clarification.	"It sounds like you felt very sad and disappointed when you found out your score on the test."
Verbalizing the implied	States the indirect message behind the patient's statements.	"Once your mother remarried and had your stepsisters and stepbrother, it sounds like you felt left out and different from the rest of the family."
Voicing doubt	Identifies and tests statements that go beyond the evidence presented.	"Getting a 60 on one exam does not mean you aren't smart."

Interventions

Therapeutic Technique	Definition	Example
Giving information	Provides information important to the focus of interaction; supplies information about processes, norms, rules of the setting.	"The information we discuss as part of your admission is used to help your team plan for your care and to meet the goals of your treatment here."
Hope	Identifies positive change that has occurred, can occur, or will occur in future.	"Most people who take this medication have improvement in their symptoms." "With treatment, people often feel they are making progress toward their goals."
Humor	Joins patient in seeing humor in day-to-day and sometimes difficult situations; lightens tone of discussion to relieve tension, connect with patient.	[After patient spills her drink all over the carpet during a group meeting] "That's OK, Pam, we've been hoping to replace that carpet; maybe it'll happen sooner now."
Planning	Assists patient to identify goals for the future and to sequence activities to accomplish goals.	"You said you would like to find a new job. If this is your goal, what steps are you planning to take toward accomplishing that?"
Suggesting options	Assists patient in identifying possible actions that can be taken.	"While your car is broken down you might consider the bus, train, or even a rental car. What things are you considering?"

DiClemente, & Norcross, 1992). MI was formalized and manualized by Rollnick and Miller in 1995. The focus of MI is the development of a therapeutic relationship for the specific purpose of identifying readiness for and facilitating change in health-related behaviors. It is not a psychotherapy, but rather a formalized conversational way of implementing therapeutic communication techniques. MI is both an assessment strategy and an intervention that is most effective when the patient is ambivalent about any aspect of treatment.

The guiding principles for the nurse using motivational interviewing are summarized in the acronym RULE:

- *Resist the reflex to be right.* The change that is desired in the patient needs to be the patient's idea, not that of the nurse.

- *Understand the patient's motivation for engaging in a specific health-related behavior.* For example, a patient may choose to go off his or her medication because of sexual side effects, but may not be comfortable in talking about it to the nurse.

- *Listen to the patient.* This is done through conveying empathy and sincere interest. It is helpful for the nurse to actually make guesses about what the patient is saying; that way, the patient will clearly see that actively listening is taking place.

- *Empower the patient to explore ways in which he or she can make a difference in his or her own health.* This lies at the heart of patient-centered care.

To be successful in using motivational interviewing, nurses and clinicians learn to "roll with resistance"—to adjust to patient resistance rather than opposing it directly and to avoid argument and direct confrontation, especially when the patient is in denial and interrupts. As the session progresses, the nurse begins to develop the discrepancy between the patient's goals or values and current behaviors. By recognizing, eliciting, and reinforcing change talk (e.g., "I wish I could stop making my mom mad"), the nurse can assist the patient in finding motivation for change. The spirit of MI is collaborative yet honors the autonomy of the patient, as the patient is the one to ultimately decide he or she is ready to change.

There are four fundamental phases to the entire MI process: (1) patient engagement; (2) guiding the conversation to a strategic focus related to change; (3) transitioning to MI techniques by selectively eliciting (evoking), responding, and summarizing once the patient is questioning his or her ambivalence; and (4) planning, which includes negotiating a change plan and consolidating commitment.

In the *engagement phase*, patient-centered counseling skills are depicted by the acronym OARS, which include the following therapeutic communication techniques:

- **O**pen-ended questions
- **A**ffirmations
- **R**eflections
- **S**ummaries

In the *guiding phase*, an agenda for change is selected based on patient desire. In the *transitioning phase*, the patient is using what is referred to as "change talk" ("I want, I wish, I need to, If I only could. . ."). In this phase, it is very important for the nurse to listen carefully with a goal of understanding the dilemma. For example the nurse can say, "On a scale of 1 to 10, how important is it for you to make this change?" A 10 indicates that a key problem has been identified. The nurse should next ask, "On a scale of 1 to 10, how hard to you think it is going to be to make this change?" If the patient also answers 10 to this question, then the nurse knows that the problem is important, but the chance of success is going to be slim at first. In the *planning phase*, a goal and plan are selected and commitment to the plan is elicited. The entire process can be achieved in one session. Table 8-5 provides an example of using MI to help a patient who needs to quit smoking.

Nontherapeutic Communication Skills

There are many types of communication that block or create barriers to effective communication (Table 8-6). Many can be grouped into common categories: social responding, giving advice or opinions, challenging, and judging or giving approval or disapproval. These categories are presented to help to structure your thinking about the kinds of communication that can result in barriers to nurse–patient communication. In addition, problems with boundaries and attending to the patient may present barriers.

Social responding refers to responses at the level of usual social interaction versus therapeutic interaction. It may involve unwittingly devaluing a patient's experience by implying that the patient's feelings are so commonplace as to be insignificant, such as saying, "That's normal, everyone feels that way." Use of clichéd, stereotyped responses and giving false reassurance refer to the use of "pat" responses that do not promote the individual nurse–patient relationship.

Giving advice involves directly suggesting or telling the patient what to do. Even though giving an opinion may be less direct, it also involves the nurse identifying his or her own personal thoughts, experiences, or views and placing them above or projecting them onto the patient's situation or concerns.

Challenging refers to several different barriers, including direct questioning of the patient by using questions that begin with "Why?" Peplau (1960) discussed the intimidating quality that "why" questions can have and encouraged the nurse to ask or encourage the patient to further describe the what, where, when, or who of the experience to encourage more sharing and open communication.

Judging involves responses to patients or comments that suggest that the nurse has cast judgment on the patient and rendered a verdict. This can include moralizing, in which particular values or beliefs of the nurse are encouraged in the patient. Attending problems relate to behaviors in which the clinician is not actively listening, or not attending to the needs presented by the patient. Finally, boundary problems include seeking information not needed to provide care or behaving in a way to meet the nurse's personal needs.

When using communication as a primary mode of intervention, it is difficult to communicate "perfectly." Anyone can easily slip into using techniques that may block communication. The important thing is that the nurse works to be aware of the communication techniques he or she uses and to manage communication skills so that the balance tips more and more to use of techniques that encourage open sharing by patients and away from statements that inhibit progress and the process of patient goal achievement. Several techniques are available to help the nurse be more aware of communication patterns and bad habits that need to be changed. They include use of individual or peer supervision, taping or recording interactions with patients for analysis, and use of process recordings to increase awareness and promote change to more helpful communication techniques.

Context of Communication

Many factors can be considered part of the context of communication, including the characteristics of the setting, space, and time. *Setting* refers to the place or purpose of the place where caregiving is occurring. The setting might include an inpatient unit, a private office, an outpatient clinic, or the patient's home. For nurses who

Example Motivational Interview

table 8-5

Patient	Nurse	MI Phase and Strategy
John, age 43, is diagnosed with depression and is in the moderate stage of emphysema from smoking two to three packs of cigarettes a day. He doesn't believe it is a problem because his grandfather lived to 90 and smoked every day.	The nurse introduces herself. After a few preliminary questions, she says, "I understand that the doctor suggested you stop smoking immediately. How do you feel about that?"	Engagement Begin OARS using open-ended questions
"It really upset me. Why should I have to quit smoking? There's nothing wrong with me! Smoking is the only thing that makes me feel better when I get super-depressed."	"I'm understanding that you don't think your current level of smoking is a problem, and in fact, it makes you feel better than your medications."	Engagement—affirmation/reflection
"That's exactly right. It sounds like you understand what the doctor doesn't."	"I am trying to understand. The major problem right now for you is that there are some serious changes in your lungs caused by the smoking, and you will have to go on oxygen in the near future. I'm wondering if that was explained to you."	Engagement—giving information
"No, it wasn't. If I have to go on oxygen, that would really change my lifestyle. I thought I would be like my grandfather and get to smoke forever. Nothing relaxes me like a good smoke."	"It has to be very hard to think about changing a major habit. But I'm glad I was able to sit down and chat with you about it. It seems like you're beginning to realize how serious a problem this is."	Engagement—summarize
"I don't even know how to even begin to think about quitting."	"Let me see if I can help. On a scale of 1 to 10, with 1 being not important, how important do you now think quitting smoking is?"	Guiding
"I guess I need to quit, I just don't have a clue how to. All my friends smoke."	"Let's talk about that. On a scale of 1 to 10, with 1 being easy and 10 being hard, how hard do you think it will be to quit?"	Transition to MI
"10"	"It sounds like to me that you are willing to think about quitting, and that you know it will be hard. You don't have to stop today, but I can give you a phone number and you can get help quitting right over the phone. "Here's something else. Did you know that quitting smoking will help make your antidepressant medication work better?"	MI Roll with resistance
"No. That sure gives me something else to think about."	"I know this is a lot to take in, but you're doing a really good job."	
"Do I have to give you an answer today? I would like some time to think about it. I guess I'm going to have to really think about quitting."	"How about coming back to see me in another week so I can answer some more questions. Would that work out your schedule?"	Planning Goal and plan
"Yes I can do that. What was the phone number you mentioned earlier?"	"Great, you can make an appointment with the receptionist. The phone number is 1-800-QUIT-NOW, 1-800-784-8669."	Planning Goal and plan
"Thank you, I will call that number and see what they have to say."		Commitment to change

work with the homeless or as members of Assertive Community Treatment (ACT) teams, the setting might be a park bench or a coffee shop. Inherent to the setting of care is information about the severity or nature of problems the patient presents with, and the culture of that setting. Structured settings typically involve a variety of rules and regulations that are commonly followed.

There are several considerations important to the physical space where interactions or communication takes place. Safety is a critical consideration for interactions between the nurse and a patient or patients. When the nurse is seated in a private room with a patient, there should be equal access of both persons to the door so that, if needed, the nurse can safely exit the room or the patient can leave freely (Figure 8-3). In many settings, doors contain glass windows so occupants can be easily seen from outside the room and situations that are of concern can be monitored. If the nurse is threatened or believes there is an imminent risk of danger, there

Blocks to Therapeutic Communication

table 8-6

Social Responding

Barrier	Definition	Example
Automatic responses	Responds in a general, routine, or rehearsed way rather than specific to the situation.	"Just rest quietly and sleep will come." "Everybody always wants more coffee here."
Devaluing	Implies that experience or feelings shared are common or not as significant as the patient feels that they are.	"Everyone gets nervous sometimes."
False reassurance	Attempts to set at ease or be positive despite evidence to the contrary.	"As soon as you return home. your friends will support you again." "Now that you're in treatment. staying off drugs will be much easier."
Social responding/ cliches	A commonplace or overused statement or comment.	"Everything will be OK."
Stereotyped comments	Response that is rote or overused and does not have direct personal meaning.	"It's for your own good."

Advice Giving

Barrier	Definition	Example
Advice giving	Suggests what should be done.	"If I were you, I would sue that doctor."
Giving opinions	Provides personal thoughts or ideas about situation or topics.	"I think you should leave your husband—he doesn't treat you well."

Challenging

Barrier	Definition	Example
Arguing	Disagrees with, disputes what is said; engages in conflict or struggle.	"You can't leave the hospital—you have been detained by the police." "I don't belong here." "You need to stay because you aren't safe to leave."
Ask for explanations	Requests or demands reasons for thoughts, or behavior. Requires others to justify themselves.	"Why did you say that?"
Challenging	Directly questions patients thoughts, feelings, behaviors.	"Why did you . . ."
Testing	Evaluating, determining, or asking for proof of thoughts, ideas, abilities.	"What is today's date?" "Tell me again who was with you when that happened."

Judging

Barrier	Definition	Example
Approval/disapproval	Renders judgment on, endorses, or condemns actions, behavior, or ideas.	"I agree with you—you should tell your friend you are moving out." "It's a bad idea to withdraw from school now."
Defensiveness	Responds or reacts to negate what was said. Supports without consideration of information or evidence to contrary.	"The doctor is very good." "Your therapist would never lie to you."
Judging	Provides opinion or evaluation of what is correct.	"You should get back to work to support your family."
Moralizing	Provides opinion or evaluation of what is right or wrong.	"If you used birth control, you wouldn't need an abortion."
Rejecting	Refuses to accept or rebuffs negatively.	"You shouldn't feel that way," "I don't want to hear that you . . ."

Attending Problems

Barrier	Definition	Example
Changing the subject	Turns discussion to other topics.	"By the way . . ." "Your story reminds me that . . ."
Interrupting	Does not allow others to finish verbalizing their thoughts or ideas.	"After that my wife suggested…" "Did you get weighed earlier today?"

(continued)

Blocks to Therapeutic Communication *(continued)*   table 8-6

Boundary Problems

Barrier	Definition	Example
Asking personal questions	Inquires about information that is not needed for safe treatment.	"I know you work at the manufacturing plant; do you work with John Strong?" "I heard you won the lottery ten years ago; how much money do you have in the bank?"
Probing	Delves into topic or information not freely offered, presses patient to explain or tell information.	"You need to tell me more about . . ."

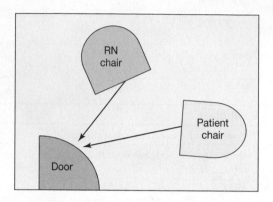

8-3 Safe room arrangement.

should be a way for the nurse to summon help. Many settings have an alarm button or phone button that can be pressed to summon others for assistance. In some settings, staff members have personal alarms or use or carry some other system of calling for help, such as a two-way radio device. Privacy is also a very important consideration for settings; patients need to feel comfortable that the information they share will be confidential to the nurse or treatment team involved, and not overheard by other patients, uninvolved staff members, or visitors.

Pause and Reflect

In turn, imagine yourself as the nurse and then the patient in interactions in the following scenarios. How would you feel?

1. *The nurse sits beside the patient in a crowded day room where at least three or four other patients sit within a few feet of them. The nurse starts to assess the patient's symptoms and medication side effects.*
2. *The nurse brings the patient to a quiet private room and performs an assessment of symptoms and medication side effects.*

Consider what each scenario conveys or communicates regarding respect, dignity, privacy, and power.

Making Sense of Interactions

Important to the work of psychiatric nurses is making sense of interactions with patients. In many settings, the nurse uses members of the interdisciplinary team to discuss, further understand, and make sense of interactions. This occurs formally in change-of-shift reports and in team meetings where individuals report in on interactions

with patients, including providing assessment of symptoms and behaviors. The nurse may suggest interpretation of meaning and seek feedback from other team members to make sense of these experiences. Communication among team members should be frequent so all workers have important information about the patients whom they share. This communication also is important as a way for team members to debrief from the often emotional and sometimes difficult interactions that can occur in the psychiatric setting.

In addition to interactions with other team members and colleagues, there are several tools that can help clinicians increase their own self-awareness in interactions as well as in learning how to interact in a therapeutic way. Common tools include journaling (discussed in Chapter 7), process recordings, audio and/or videotaping, and use of individual or group supervision. Other possibilities include interpretive groups, a process similar to analysis of a process recording, but that involves review of one transcript of an interaction by a group, with discussion of content, techniques, observations, and interpretations (Shattell, Hogan, & Hernandez, 2006). These are all important tools that can help the nurse gain insight into the meaning and interpretation of his or her own, as well as the patient's, communication.

Process Recording

The **process recording** is a written record of an interaction between two or more individuals (Table 8-7). It has been used for many years as a reflective process in programs in which students are learning to interact with patients using therapeutic communication techniques, including social work, psychotherapy, and nursing education programs (Bodley, 1992; Hudson, 1955; Peplau, 1960; Shattell, Hogan, & Hernandez, 2006; Smith, 1986). Although it is typically used to record interactions between two people, it may involve recording of the content and process of both family and group meetings. The process recording offers one way for feedback to be provided on communication skills and dynamics in the therapeutic relationship when direct observation is not an option. Both student accounts (Turzynski & Morgan, 2001) and study of the use of process recordings identify that 90% of students who used process recordings felt they had benefited from use, identifying their usefulness as a tool for reflection and developing greater self-awareness of communication skills (Clarke, 1998). The purpose of the process recording is to reflect on and evaluate the dynamics of a specific interaction and to provide a sample of interaction for consideration in supervision or consultation with others. The record can offer insight on many levels, depending on how it is structured, including information about both nonverbal communication and the thoughts and feelings of the

Sample Process Recording

table 8-7

Introduction: [Identifies situation, setting, purpose of interaction, information about other events, or information important to interaction]

Situation and Setting: The patient is Amber, a 32-year-old, single African American female who was admitted to an inpatient psychiatric unit 3 days ago after making a suicide attempt. After her boyfriend left for work one night, she ingested a bottle of sleeping pills and expected to die in her sleep. Amber recently lost her job as a nurse's aide and has been in an emotionally and physi-

cally abusive relationship with her boyfriend of 3 years. After she lost her job, Amber's boyfriend threatened to throw her out on the street if she couldn't keep up her part of the expenses for the household.

The conversation was held in a small private interview room on the inpatient psychiatric unit.

Purpose of Interaction: The nurse asked to meet with Amber to determine her plans for after her discharge from the inpatient setting.

Nonverbal Communication	Dialogue	Nurse's Feelings and Thoughts	Analysis
Animated expression describing situation, restless, moving in chair.	AMBER: "I can't believe it! He's throwing me out like I'm trash. At my worst moment. Now where will I go?" NURSE: "Throwing you out of your apartment?"	• I'm fearful Amber might get more agitated. • I'm surprised that her boyfriend would do this during this crisis. • I think moving might be safer given history of abuse in the relationship.	Amber is very angry; I restated what she said to encourage her to share more information about it. Therapeutic technique: Restating
A little calmer, sitting quietly. Speaks with a resigned quality.	AMBER: "My sister called me and said he dropped off bags of my stuff at her apartment." NURSE: "Did you know that this might happen?"	• I feel sad that she had this unsupportive relationship. • He really is throwing her out. • I wonder where she will live?	Therapeutic technique: Seeking information
As Amber describes the situation she gets a little louder and sounds more upset. She begins tapping her leg and motioning as she speaks. I begin to lean forward.	AMBER: "He's threatened to throw me out before. That's how this whole mess started. After I lost my job I got behind on the bills and he was really mad about that. Then he said if I wasn't working by the end of the month, I could find another place to live. That was a couple of weeks ago." NURSE: "So then what happened?"	How committed is he to this relationship if he would do this?	She is accepting poor treatment in this relationship, and this may reflect her own low self-esteem. Therapeutic technique: Exploring
Amber is motioning as she speaks; her voice gets quieter as she talks about taking the pills. She sounds choked up as she says this and looks like she may cry.	AMBER: "Last week, when the end of the month came I knew I would be out on the street and I couldn't handle that. We had a big fight before I took those pills, and I knew things were headed in a bad direction. Usually we fight a lot before he ends up getting really nasty. I figured if he was going to hurt me again, I might as well beat him to it. I was done with it and just couldn't face the mess my life is in now." NURSE: "When you say he gets 'really nasty,' what do you mean?"	I'm concerned that now that he has thrown her out, she will be more in crisis and may feel hopeless and suicidal again.	Cyclical or wave pattern of violence is common, with calm periods and peaks of violence. Therapeutic technique: Seeking clarification
Has an angry tone as she talks about the abuse. Speaks more quietly about her own temper.	AMBER: "He gets physical, he hits me. He broke my nose once. He pushed me down the stairs. Sometimes he throws things, that's not so bad. Once someone in the building called the police. He has a really bad temper. But I do too, my sister says if I kept my mouth shut he wouldn't hurt me." NURSE: "What do you think about that?"	• I was disturbed to hear how abusive he has been toward her. • She talks about this without feeling, like she's talking about what she bought at the grocery store. • I'm surprised that she or her sister would think that this behavior is her fault.	Often victims take responsibility for the abuse. Therapeutic technique: Reflection

Sample Process Recording (continued)   table 8-7

Nonverbal Communication	Dialogue	Nurse's Feelings and Thoughts	Analysis
Sounds a little angry. Hitting her leg with her fist as she discusses him. Chokes up and nearly cries as she talks about his caring behavior. Shakes her head back and forth sadly.	AMBER: "I don't know, I try to calm him down sometimes but it doesn't always work. I'm just so tired of having to be careful about every little thing I say. I know he loves me. After he hurts me, he is really sorry. He always takes good care of me and brings me things. Then he's usually good for a while. Those are good times together." NURSE: "So some of the time, he is loving and does things for you and at other times he threatens to throw you out and hurts you."	• Based on what she says I am glad she may be out of the relationship, even if it's due to his ending it. • I am feeling a little angry and frustrated, because she doesn't see how this keeps her in the relationship, and how trapped she is.	• It is common for victims to forgive the abuser and it allows the cycle to begin again. • I summarized back what she told me. Therapeutic technique: Summarization
Voice sounds lighter, brighter, tries to smile.	AMBER: "Yes, but my mom always says you have to take the good with the bad. No one is perfect."	I can't believe she is willing to accept this.	She is rationalizing about his abusive behavior.

This segment of the interaction provided background information that will be important to plans for Amber's discharge. Her ambivalence about the relationship is clear and her acceptance of being physically abused is disturbing.

clinician. This information offers a way to gain insight about both the patient and the clinician's own reactions and experiences during an interaction. Typically, a process recording involves identification of the individuals involved and the context or situation and setting of the interaction, which allows the reader to more accurately interpret the interaction. The actual words spoken or dialogue of both (or all) parties are recorded as close to verbatim as possible. The nonverbal aspects of the communication—including tone, gestures, facial expression, use of space, and activity/behavior—are specifically recorded for each part of the interaction. Thoughts and feelings of the nurse are identified for each segment of the interaction. Finally, there is an area for interpretation of each segment of the interaction, which is completed after recording all the remembered details of the interaction. If the process recording is being done to learn or improve communication skills, the therapeutic techniques used are also identified in each segment. After the record of the interaction, there is typically a summary of impressions from the interview, identification of any hypotheses made, and analysis of the overall interaction with plans for future directions for work with that patient. Writing down exactly what happened in a difficult interaction can allow the writer to better understand aspects of the interaction, providing a way to abstract from the interaction and gain insight into otherwise unexamined aspects of the experience.

Taping

Taping may be used to help the nurse reflect on an interaction, providing an actual record of what was said in real time. Interactions may be taped using audio or video recording; this type of recording is done only with written consent of all parties involved in the interaction. This tool allows the nurse to actually hear what the patient heard in the interaction. Often communication habits and mannerisms can be identified using this method, offering the nurse greater awareness of both verbal and nonverbal communication skills. Taping is also useful in the supervision process, in which the nurse seeks guidance

from a mentor on therapeutic techniques. The supervisor can review tapes and offer the nurse feedback on particular aspects of an interaction, using the actual tape to provide examples. In the process of obtaining consent, the nurse must be explicit about how the tapes will be protected and when and how the tapes will be destroyed. Most settings have specific procedures that must be followed to obtain informed consent.

Clinical Supervision

Clinical supervision is one of the most important tools for reflective practice used by students and clinicians in the psychiatric setting. Peplau (1962) identified the importance of students learning psychiatric–mental health nursing to review their nurse–patient interactions with an expert psychiatric nurse. Echternacht & Youngs (2008) identify the importance of reflection on experiential learning by use of clinical supervision for development and integration of skills in psychiatric nursing. Clinical supervision offers important feedback and insight into how the nurse provides care to patients in the therapeutic nurse–patient relationship. Expert supervision provides insights into the care of patients that the nurses may not have identified on their own. It also promotes the growth of the nurses professionally and can improve the relationships of team members when supervision occurs in a group setting. Typically, clinical supervision of practice in the psychiatric–mental health setting involves review of patient care provided and interactions with individuals, families, or groups by the clinician. In both educational and clinical settings, supervision by a more experienced clinician or teacher is often scheduled on a regular basis and may also be available on an as-needed consultation basis. Many psychiatric nursing clinical experiences include a clinical supervision seminar in which groups of students review cases, discuss issues and concerns that have arisen in treatment, and practice applying principles learned in the classroom setting.

Clinical supervision, whether in individual or group settings, is a forum for the nurse to discuss new skill acquisition, application of theory, and the often emotion-laden experiences from the psychiatric setting and obtain support and feedback related to planning for future intervention. It is easy to underestimate the toll that providing psychosocial care takes on the nurse. Regular supervision is one tool that the nurse can use to maintain balance and objectivity in providing care to patients.

SUMMARY

Therapeutic communication within the context of a therapeutic nurse–patient relationship is the primary tool psychiatric–mental health nurses use to assist their patients in making progress toward their treatment goals. To be able to develop a therapeutic relationship and communicate effectively with patients, there are fundamental philosophic issues and principles that assist the nurse to develop a frame of mind or world view that supports the patient's individuality, dignity, and per-

sonal growth. These principles relate to the nurse's perspective on what it means to be mentally healthy and to how the nurse approaches the patient as a human being and assists the patient with the needs presented. Viewing patients with unconditional positive regard is an important requisite to working therapeutically and partnering with the patient so that care is truly patient centered. The nurse uses self as a tool and masters the art of being fully present with the patient within a frame of therapeutic neutrality and uses active listening and empathy in interactions. The nurse develops a therapeutic alliance that follows phases of development and is a goal-directed therapeutic nurse–patient relationship. The nurse maintains boundaries in the therapeutic relationship and is aware of communication skills and techniques used. The nurse also takes responsibility for understanding the dynamics of interactions and uses a variety of tools to increase his or her own awareness of the strengths and areas for growth that require attention over time.

Chapter Highlights

1. Global principles important to caring for individuals include unconditional positive regard and considering the patient an equal partner in care.

2. To be helpful to patients, nurses must be able to set aside their own personal opinions and biases to help others. Centering is one way that can help the nurse be more aware of thoughts and feelings and offer the ability to be available to patients.

3. Empathy is an important skill used in therapeutic relationships and may be one of the most effective healing skills offered by the nurse.

4. The nurse develops a therapeutic relationship with a patient; this relationship progresses through expected phases and assists patients to progress and meet their goals in treatment.

5. Nurses maintain professional boundaries related to the type of relationship they develop with patients and are careful to avoid interactions with patients that focus on the nurse's personal feelings, thoughts, opinions, or experiences.

6. Communication is a complex process that is composed of verbal, nonverbal, and meta-communication.

7. Communication is enhanced when attention is paid to the context of communication, including the setting, space, and time.

8. Active listening indicates the nurse's interest and concern for the patient; promotes sharing of thoughts, feelings, and concerns; and leads to better outcomes in interactions.

9. Therapeutic communication techniques encourage or promote patient interaction and patient healing through a trusting nurse–patient relationship. Nontherapeutic communication often raises barriers or misunderstandings in relationships and is detrimental to patient outcomes.

10. Reflection on the relationship with patients and specific interactions and communication are important to positive patient outcomes. Many tools are available to use to offer reflection and greater understanding of dynamics in relationships, including journaling, process recordings, taping, and supervision.

NCLEX®-RN Questions

1. The nurse is assigned to the care of a patient admitted to the mental health unit. Which behaviors by the nurse reflect the essential principles of therapeutic relationship? Select all that apply.
   a. Empowering the patient to make decisions regarding care
   b. Looking beyond the illness when interacting with the patient
   c. Trying to see things from the unique perspective of the patient
   d. Sharing personal insights that are relevant to the patient's problems
   e. Ensuring that all physical and emotional needs are met by the nurse

2. The nurse is working with a patient who is struggling to overcome a serious mental illness. The patient begins crying after learning that her family will no longer be visiting. Which response by the nurse demonstrates empathy?
   a. "I am not sure what I would do if I were in your shoes."
   b. "You must be wondering why they are acting this way."
   c. "My sense is that this experience has been very painful for you."
   d. "I understand because I went through something similar one time."

3. The nurse is acting as a preceptor to a recent nurse graduate who wants to obtain a job on the mental health unit. The new nurse has been struggling to differentiate between social and therapeutic interactions because so many of the patients are around his own age. Which evaluation finding indicates that nurse is acting in accordance with appropriate professional boundaries? Select all that apply.
   a. The nurse sets limits on inappropriate behaviors.
   b. The nurse uses colloquial language to foster trust.
   c. The nurse brings in clothing for a homeless patient.
   d. The nurse offers a video collection for a group movie night.
   e. The nurse lets a patient know when their time together will end.

4. The nurse is working with a patient who presents in the outpatient setting for the treatment of situational depression. The patient has begun to try out new coping strategies and has taken advantage of a support group the nurse recommended. The nurse recognizes that the patient has entered which phase of therapeutic nurse–patient relationship?
   a. Orientation
   b. Working
   c. Exploitation
   d. Resolution

5. The nurse is working with the patient admitted to the mental health unit. The nurse learns that the patient has a history of exposure to trauma that that the nurse can relate to on a personal level. Which rationale best supports nondisclosure on the part of the nurse?
   a. The patient may use the disclosure against the nurse.
   b. The nurse may be assuming that the experiences are similar.
   c. There is a risk of distortion or shifting of caregiver boundaries.
   d. The patient will not have the same resources to cope as the nurse.

6. The nurse is working in an outpatient mental health clinic. The clinic is implementing an initiative to use telecommunication to deliver care to patients living in remote areas. The nurse understands that this change will be most likely to affect which aspects of communication?
   a. Nonverbal communication only
   b. Nonverbal and meta-communication
   c. Verbal and nonverbal communication
   d. Meta-, nonverbal, and verbal communication

7. The nurse is working with a patient in the context of the therapeutic relationship. Which evaluation finding supports the effectiveness of active listening techniques?
   a. The patient remains focused on the purpose of the interaction.
   b. The patient takes advantage of opportunities to verbalize concerns.
   c. The patient affirms the nurse's interpretation of what was communicated.
   d. The patient provides sufficient information for the nurse to make care decisions.

8. The nurse is caring for a patient who has been in an abusive relationship. The patient relates being concerned that leaving the relationship will result in judgment by family and friends. How should the nurse respond?
   a. Acknowledge that the decision may not be accepted by others.
   b. Ask the patient why she cares so much about what others think.
   c. Remind the patient that everyone has difficult decisions to make.
   d. Advise the patient to share details of the abuse with family and friends.

9. The nurse manager is employing tools to assist staff to maintain a sense of objectivity and balance in the context of the therapeutic inpatient psychiatric milieu. Which intervention is most likely to be effective for new nurses?
   a. Formal education
   b. Journaling exercises
   c. Individual supervision
   d. Peer-led support groups

Answers may be found on the Pearson student resource site: nursing. pearsonhighered.com

Pearson Nursing Student Resources Find additional review materials at **nursing.pearsonhighered.com**

References

American Nurses Association. (2010). Code of Ethics for Nurses with Interpretive Statements. Available at http://nursingworld.org/MainMenu Categories/EthicsStandards/CodeofEthicsforNurses.aspx and http://nursingworld.org/MainMenuCategories/EthicsStandards/Codeof EthicsforNurses/Code-of-Ethics.pdf

Argyle, M. (1988). *Bodily Communication* (2nd ed.) Madison, CT: International Universities Press.

Argyle, M., Salter, V., Nicholson, H., Williams, M., & Burgess P. (1970). The communication of inferior and superior attitudes by verbal and non-verbal signals. *British Journal of Social and Clinical Psychology, 9*, 222–231.

Bachelor, A. (1995). Clients' perception of the therapeutic alliance: A qualitative analysis. *Journal of Counseling Psychology, 42*(3), 323–337.

Barrett-Lennard, G. T. (1962). Dimensions of therapist responses as causal factors in therapeutic change. *Psychological Monographs, 76*, 43, #562.

Beck, A. T. (1976). *Cognitive Therapy and the Emotional Disorders.* Madison, CT: International Universities Press.

Berry, K., Gregg, L., Vasconcelos e Sa, D., Haddock, G., & Barrowclough, C. (2012). Staff-patient relationships and outcomes in schizophrenia: Role of staff attributions. *Behaviour Research and Therapy, 50*(3), 210–214.

Blakemore, S.-J., Bristow, D., Bird, G., Frith, C., & Ward, J. (2005). Somatosensory activations during the observation of touch and a case of vision-touch synaesthesia. *Brain, 128*(7), 1571–1583.

Bodley, D. E. (1992). Clinical supervision in psychiatric nursing: Using the process record. *Nurse Education Today, 12*, 148–155.

Bressington, D., Stewart, B., Beer, D., & MacInnes, D. (2011). Levels of service user satisfaction in secure settings: A survey of the association between perceived social climate, perceived therapeutic relationship and satisfaction with forensic services. *International Journal of Nursing Studies, 48*(11), 1349–1356.

Clarke, D. J. (1998). Process recording: Of what value is examining nursing interaction through assignment work? *Nursing Education Today, 18*, 138–143.

College of Registered Nurses of Manitoba. (2011). Professional boundaries for therapeutic relationships. Available at http://cms.tng-secure.com/file_download.php?fFile_id=144

Cox, R. P. (1998). IPRs revisited: Using process recordings to develop nursing students' critical thinking skills. *Journal of Nursing Education, 37*(1), 37–41.

Darwin, C. (1872). *The Expression of the Emotions in Man and Animals.* London, UK: John Murray.

Dziopa, F., & Ahern, K. (2009a). Three different ways mental health nurses develop quality therapeutic relationships. *Issues in Mental Health Nursing, 30*(1), 14–22.

Dziopa, F., & Ahern, K. (2009b). What makes a quality therapeutic relationship in psychiatric–mental health nursing: A review of the research literature. *Internet Journal of Advanced Nursing Practice, 10*(1), 1–19.

Echternacht, M., & Youngs, R. (2008). Clinical supervision: Instructional strategy in the development of psychiatric nursing skills. *Teaching and Learning in Nursing, 3*, 76–80.

Fluckiger, C., Del Re, A. C., Wamport, B. E., Symonds, D., & Horvath, A. O. (2012). How central is the alliance in psychotherapy? A multilevel longitudinal meta-analysis. *Journal of Counseling Psychology, 59*(1), 10–17. doi: 10.1037/a0025749

Forchuk, C. (1994). The orientation phase of the nurse client relationship: Testing Peplau's theory. *Journal of Advanced Nursing, 20*, 532–537.

Forchuk, C., & Reynolds, W. (2001). Clients' reflections on relationships with nurses: Comparisons from Canada and Scotland. *Journal of Psychiatric-Mental Health Nursing, 8*, 45–51.

Forchuk, C., Westwell, J., Martin, M-L., Bamber-Azzapardi, W., Kosterewa-Tolman, D., & Hux, M. (1998). Factors influencing movement of chronic psychiatric patients from the orientation to the working phase of the nurse-client relationship on an inpatient unit. *Perspectives in Psychiatric Care, 34*(1), 36–44.

Forchuk, C., Westwell, J., Martin, M-L., Bamber-Azzapardi, W., Kosterewa-Tolman, D., & Hux, M. (2000). The developing nurse–client relationship. *Journal of American Psychiatric Nurses Association, 6*(1), 3–10.

Freud, S. (1915). Observations on transference love. In J. Strachey, (Ed. & Trans.). *The Standard Edition of the Complete Psychological Works of Sigmund Freud* (vol. 12). London, UK: Hogarth Press, pp. 157–171.

Gilburt, H., Rose, D., & Slade, M. (2008). The importance of relationships in mental health care: A qualitative study of service users' experiences of pscyhiatric hospital admission in the UK. *BMC Health Services Research, 8*, 92.

Gurman, A. S. (1972). Therapists' mood patterns and therapeutic facilitativeness. *Journal of Counseling Psychology, 19*(2), 169–170.

Haase, R. F., & Tepper, D. T. (1972). Nonverbal components of empathic communication. *Journal of Counseling Psychology, 19*(5), 417–424.

Hart, V. (2010a). *Patient-Provider Communications: Caring to Listen.* Boston, MA: Jones & Bartlett.

Hart, V. (2010b). Text messaging: The antithesis of interpersonal relating; Guest editorial. *Journal of Psychosocial Nursing and Mental Health Services, 48*(12), 5–6.

Hectornelj-Taylor, C. A., & Yonge, O. (2003). Exploring boundaries in the nurse-client relationship: Professional roles and responsibilities. *Perspectives in Psychiatric Care, 39*(2), 55–66.

Holder, K. V., & Schenthal, S. J. (2007). Watch your step: Nursing and professional boundaries. *Nursing Management, 38*(2), 24–29.

Huckshorn, K. A. (2007). Building a better mental health workforce: 8 core elements. *Journal of Psychosocial Nursing, 45*(3), 24–34.

Hudson, B. C. (1955). The nursing process record. *Nursing Outlook, 3*, 224–226.

Humphries, R. H. (1982). Therapeutic neutrality reconsidered. *Journal of Religion and Health, 21*(2), 124–131.

Kaplan, S. H., Greenfield, S., & Ware, J. E. (1989). Assessing the effects of physician-patient interactions on the outcomes of chronic disease. *Medical Care, 27*(3), S110–S127.

Katz, J. S. (2010). Reconsidering therapeutic neutrality. *Clinical Social Work Journal, 38*(3), 306–315. doi: 10.1007/s10615-010-0272-7

King, F. B., & LaRocco, D. J. (2006). E-Journaling: A strategy to support student reflection and understanding. *Current Issues in Education* [On-line], *9*(4). Available at http://cie.ed.asu.edu/volume9/number4

Killian, J. (1999). Journaling. National Staff Development Council. *Journal of Staff Development*, Summer, 36–37.

La Monica, E. (1981). Construct validity of an empathy instrument. *Research in Nursing and Health, 4*, 389–400.

Larson, J. (2011). New principles guide nurses in using social media. Available at http://www.nursezone.com/Nursing-News-Events/more-news/New-Principles-Guide-Nurses-in-Using-Social-Media_38004.aspx

Layton, J. M., & Wykle, M. H. (1990). A validity study of four empathy instruments. *Research in Nursing and Health, 13*(5), 319–325.

Luft, J. (1969). *Of Human Interaction.* Palo Alto, CA: National Press.

Luft, J., & Ingham, H. (1955). The Johari window, a graphic model of interpersonal awareness. *Proceedings of the Western Training Laboratory in Group Development.* Los Angeles, CA: UCLA.

Mehrabian, A. (1969). Significance of posture and position in the communication of attitude and status relationships. *Psychological Bulletin, 71*, 359–372.

Mehrabian, A. (1970). A semantic space for nonverbal behavior. *Journal of Consulting and Clinical Psychology, 35*, 248–257.

Mok, E., & Chiu, P. C. (2004). Nurse–patient relationships in palliative care. *Journal of Advanced Nursing, 48*(5), 475–483.

National Council of State Boards of Nursing. (n.d.). Professional boundaries: A nurse's guide to the importance of appropriate professional boundaries.

Chicago: NCSBN. Available at https://www.ncsbn.org/ProfessionalBoundariesbrochure.pdf

Neuman, B. (1997). The Neuman systems model: Reflections and projections. *Nursing Science Quarterly, 10*, 18–21.

Neuman, B., & Young, R. J. (1972). A model for teaching total person approach to patient problems. *Nursing Research, 21*, 264–269.

Orlando, I. J. (1972). *The Discipline and Teaching of Nursing Process: An Evaluative Study.* New York: G. P. Putnam's Sons.

Peplau, H. E. (1952). *Interpersonal Relations in Nursing: A Conceptual Frame of Reference for Psychodynamic Nursing.* New York, NY: Putnam.

Peplau, H. (1960). Talking with patients. *American Journal of Nursing, 7*, 964–966.

Peplau, H. (1962). Interpersonal techniques: The crux of psychiatric nursing. *American Journal of Nursing, 62*(6), 50–54.

Peplau, H. E. (1991). *Interpersonal Relations in Nursing: A Conceptual Frame of Reference for Psychodynamic Nursing.* New York, NY: Springer Publishing Company.

Peplau, H. E. (1992). Interpersonal relations: A theoretical framework for application in nursing practice. *Nursing Science Quarterly, 5(1),* 13–18.

Peplau, H. E. (1997). Peplau's theory of interpersonal relations. *Nursing Science Quarterly, 10*(4), 162–167.

Pilette, P. C., Berck, C. B., & Achber, L. C. (1995). Therapeutic management of helping boundaries. *Journal of Psychosocial Nursing and Mental Health Services, 33*(1), 40–47.

Pounds, K. G. (2010). Client-nurse interaction with individuals with schizophrenia: A descriptive pilot study. *Issues in Mental Health Nursing, 31*(12), 770– 774. doi: 10.3109/01612840.2010

Prochaska, J. O., DiClemente, C. C., & Norcross, J. C. (1992). In search of how people change: Applications to addictive behaviors. *American Psychologist. 47*(9), 1102–1114.

Reade, M. N., & Smouse, A. D. (1980). Effect of inconsistent verbal-nonverbal communication and counselor response mode on client estimate of counselor regard and effectiveness. *Journal of Counseling Psychology, 27*(6), 546–553.

Registered Nurses' Association of Ontario. (2006). *Establishing Therapeutic Relationships* (rev. suppl.). Toronto, ON: Registered Nurses' Association of Ontario.

Rogers, C. (1951). *Client-Centered Therapy: Its Current Practice Implications and Theory.* Cambridge, MA: Riverside Press.

Rogers, C. (1957). The necessary and sufficient conditions of therapeutic personality change. *Journal of Consulting Psychology, 21*, 95–103.

Rogers, C. (1959). A theory of therapy, personality and interpersonal relationships as developed in the client-centered Framework. In S. Koch, (Ed.). *Psychology: A Study of a Science. Vol. 3: Formulations of the Person and the Social Context.* New York, NY: McGraw Hill.

Rogers, C. (1961). *On Becoming a Person.* Boston, MA: Houghton Mifflin.

Rogers, C. R. (1975). Empathic: An unappreciated way of being. *The Counseling Psychologist, 5*(2), 2–10.

Rogers, C. R. (1980). *A Way of Being.* New York, NY: Houghton Mifflin.

Rollnick, S., & Miller, W.R. (1995). What is motivational interviewing? *Behavioural and Cognitive Psychotherapy, 23*, 325–334.

Rosen, D. C., Miller, A. B., Nakash, O., Halpern, L., & Alegría, M. (2012). Interpersonal complementarity in the mental health intake: A mixed-methods study. *Journal of Counseling Psychology, 59*(2), 185–196.

Roter, D. (1989). Which facets of communication have strong effects on outcome: A meta-analysis. In M. Stewart & D. Roter, (Eds.). *Communicating with Medical Patients.* Newbury Park, CA: Sage Publications.

Roter, D. L., Hall, J. A., Kern, D. E., Barker, L. R., Cole, K. A., & Roca, R. P. (1995). Improving physicians' interviewing skills and reducing patients' emotional distress: A randomized clinical trial. *Archives of Internal Medicine, 155*, 1877–1884.

Roter, D. L., Stewart, M., Putnam, S. M., Lipkin, M., Stiles, W., & Inui, T. S. (1997). Communication patterns of primary care physicians. *JAMA, 277*(4), 350–356.

Sabo, D. (2006). Compassion fatigue and nursing work: Can we accurately capture the consequences of caring work? *International Journal of Nursing Practice, 12*(3), 136–142.

Satir, V. (1995). *Making Contact.* Berkeley, CA: Celestial Arts.

Schafer, P. (1997). When a client develops an attraction: Successful resolution versus boundary violation. *Journal of Psychiatric and Mental Health Nursing, 4*(3), 203–211.

Shattell, M. M., Hogan, B., & Hernandez, A. R. (2006). The interpretive research group as an alternative to the interpersonal process recording. *Nurse Educator, 31*(4), 178–182.

Smith, D., & Fitzpatrick, M. (1995). Patient-therapist boundary issues: An integrative review of theory and research. *Professional Psychology: Research and Practice, 26*(5), 499–506.

Smith, L. (1977). Communication skills. *Nursing Times, 2,* 926–929.

Smith, L. (1986). Talking it out. *Nursing Times, 26,* 38–39.

Sommer, R. (1959). Studies in personal space. *Sociometry,* 247–260.

Stern, W. (1938). *General Psychology* (H. D. Spoerl, Trans.). New York, NY: Macmillan.

Sullivan, H. S. (1953). *The Interpersonal Theory of Psychiatry.* New York, NY: W.W. Norton & Co.

Truax, C. B. (1963). Effective ingredients in psychotherapy: An approach to unraveling the patient-therapist interaction. *Journal of Counseling Psychology, 10,* 256–263.

Turzynski, K., & Morgan, D. (2001). Process recording: a student's perspective. *Journal of Child Health Care, 5*(1), 30–34.

von Uexküll, J. (1957). A stroll through the worlds of animals and men: A picture book of invisible worlds. In C. H. Schiller, (Ed. and Trans.). *Instinctive Behavior: The Development of a Modern Concept.* New York, NY: International Universities Press, Inc., pp. 5–80.

Walker, R., & Clark, J. J. (1999). Heading off boundary problems: Clinical supervision as risk management. *Psychiatric Services, 50*(11), 1435–1439.

Watzlawick, P. (1978). *The Language of Change: Elements of Therapeutic Communication.* New York, NY: W.W. Norton & Co.

Weissman, G. V. (2011). Evaluating associate degree nursing students' self-efficacy in communication skills and attitudes in caring for the dying patient. *Teaching and Learning in Nursing, 6*(2), 64–72.

Weissman, M. M., Markowitz, J. C., & Klerman, G. L. (2000). *Comprehensive Guide to Interpersonal Psychotherapy.* New York, NY: Basic Books.

Weissman, M. M., Markowitz, J. C., & Klerman, G. L. (2007). *Clinician's Quick Guide to Interpersonal Psychotherapy.* New York, NY: Oxford University Press.

Wright, L. D. (2006). Violating professional boundaries. *Nursing, 36*(3), 52–54.

Yalom, I. D. (1995). *The Theory and Practice of Group Psychotherapy.* New York, NY: Basic Books.

Yu, J., & Kirk, M. (2009). Evaluation of empathy measurement tools in nursing: Systematic review. *Journal of Advanced Nursing, 65*(9), 1790–1806.

The Nursing Process in Psychiatric–Mental Health Nursing

9

Joanne DeSanto Iennaco

Learning Outcomes

1. Describe the purpose and phases of the nursing process.

2. Explain the role of assessment in the nursing process.

3. Perform a holistic assessment that incorporates the biological, psychological, sociological, spiritual, and cultural domains for individuals with psychiatric–mental health needs.

4. Demonstrate the ability to perform a mental status exam.

5. Define the components of a nursing diagnosis.

6. Formulate nursing diagnoses based on information gathered during assessment.

7. Identify the components of the planning phase of the nursing process.

8. Describe the role of outcome evaluation in the nursing process.

9. Discuss types of nursing interventions used to support goals and outcomes identified for patients with psychiatric-mental health disorders.

Key Terms

critical thinking

Claudine Initial Onset

Claudine Norvell presents to the emergency department (ED) after having a panic attack while driving to work. She pulled over and called 911 because she was hyperventilating and having pains in her jaw and shoulders; she feared she was having a heart attack and would die. The ED medical evaluation ruled out a heart attack and other physiologic reasons for her symptoms, and referred Claudine to you for a psychiatric evaluation to rule out anxiety-related panic attacks. Precipitants include difficulty in her marriage and fear of a job change or layoff in her school district. Claudine reluctantly agreed to the referral, although she remains concerned about her physical health.

Claudine sought help independently from the health care system. She is hesitant to engage in psychiatric treatment, but on some level sees a need to obtain help, which indicates some insight about her problems.

During the intake interview with Claudine, she says, "Sometimes I have chest pain and trouble breathing and feel like I'm going to die." Claudine describes episodes of difficulty breathing with hyperventilation, rapid pulse, and chest, shoulder, and jaw pain, which start "out of the blue." She has had these episodes with increasing frequency over the past month; this episode is the second one this week. During these episodes, she fears that she will die. Claudine reports that she has been under a lot of pressure at work and home recently, and she fears that if she is laid off at work that will make her marriage problems worse. She complains of fatigue and irritability, trouble sleeping, and difficulty concentrating at work. Claudine tells you that it is hard to get her mind off her financial concerns, especially since her husband Joe was laid off last year and had to take a job at another company with a much lower salary. Claudine says that her mind constantly goes over and over these worries.

You conduct a mental status exam of Claudine to elicit more information. Your findings include the following:

1. Claudine is neatly dressed and groomed and appears to be her stated age of 43 years old. She makes good eye contact and freely shares her history. She appears tense, restless (foot tapping, frequent position changes), and hyper-alert to her surroundings.

2. Her speech is rapid but understandable and circumstantial.

3. Claudine's mood is anxious, and she has a full range of affect, tearing up slightly when discussing her father, smiling with discussion of children. She describes a "tense feeling inside" that at times "feels like every nerve is jumping." She easily describes a range of emotions, although she identifies feeling "detached," as though she isn't real or a part of things when her anxiety increases or during episodes of hyperventilation. Although she describes feeling sad at times, she denies a depressed mood. She reports increased irritability lately, and denies mood swings or episodes of euphoria or elated mood. She denies thoughts about taking her own life, stating that she would never do anything to harm herself due to responsibilities to her children and her religious beliefs. She denies ever having been suicidal in the past and has never made a suicide attempt. She denies homicidal thought or intent and denies history of violent or aggressive behavior.

4. Her thought is logical and goal directed, and, although her thought is also circumstantial, she returns to the focus with cues. She describes ambivalence and difficulty with decision making at work and home related to finances. She identifies difficulty concentrating and inability to read due to rumination about her job and marriage, resulting in distraction at work and difficulty completing tasks.

5. Claudine is alert and responsive to questions; she is oriented to person, place, time, and situation. She has normal recall of recent and remote experiences and is able to identify three of three words. She is able to repeat six digits forward and five backward, and completes serial sevens without difficulty. She possesses a good fund of information and is able to perform simple calculations. She is able to abstract with interpretation of a proverb (A rolling stone gathers no moss: "If you don't stick with things, success is unlikely."). She has good judgment, and some insight of connection of stressors to anxiety symptoms, but less of a relation to panic symptoms.

Claudine identifies this as the first time she has ever had a mental health problem requiring intervention.

APPLICATION

1. Based on these findings, what additional assessment data should you collect?

2. What is/are Claudine's chief complaint(s) and presenting problem(s)? What other symptoms or issues do you think require nursing intervention?

The Nursing Process in Psychiatric–Mental Health Nursing

The nursing profession has a unique perspective that is reflected in the way that nurses think about and care for individuals, families, and groups. This perspective is a humanistic one, focusing on individual patients, the difficulties with which they present, and the context contributing to their experiences. Knowledge of the presenting symptoms is very important, but it offers only a microscopic view and understanding of the problem. To fully understand an individual, the nurse must consider many aspects of that person's life in assessing and comprehensively planning to deliver holistic care. The same is true when a family or group is the focus of care. The nursing process is the framework nurses use to think about the problems for which individuals seek care. This process provides structure to the assessment of the patient and to the way in which nurses identify or clarify problems using nursing diagnosis. The process also guides nurses in planning for care in a cyclical way. This involves review of the process, and builds on itself as the nurse and patient identify progress being made and refine or redefine goals over time. Important to this process is a frame that places the individual(s) seeking care at the core or center of the process.

The goal of patient-centeredness is to customize care to the specific needs and circumstances of each individual; that is, to modify the care to respond to the person, not the person to the care (Institute of Medicine, 2001). All care should be tailored to meet the needs and preferences of individual patients. The critical elements of patient-centered care include (1) respect for patients' values, preferences, and expressed needs; (2) coordination and integration of care; (3) information, communication, and education; (4) physical comfort; (5) emotional support—relieving fear and anxiety; and (6) involvement of family and friends (Institute of Medicine, 2001). A formal definition of patient-centered care is "care that informs and involves patients in medical decision-making and self-management; coordinates and integrates medical care; provides physical comfort and emotional support; understands the patients' concept of illness and their cultural beliefs; and understands and applies principles of disease prevention and behavioral change appropriate to diverse populations" (Maizes, Rakel, & Niemiec, 2009, p. 3).

Patient as the Center of the Process

Perhaps the most important question involved in the assessment of a patient is, "What would you like help with?" or "What goals would you like to accomplish in treatment?" In any setting, joining with patients to help them meet their goals is a core value and is of primary importance. If the nurse pursues goals that the patient does not embrace, the patient is less likely to make progress than if the patient were actively involved in goal setting. Nurses often need to provide care for urgent, even life-threatening, needs when patients are unable to voice their goals. Nurses do so to protect and preserve function and life so the patient can later identify and jointly pursue goals with the health care team. In the psychiatric setting, nurses are sometimes faced with situations in which the patient is attempting to harm himself or herself, or someone else. In these circumstances, the priority is to work with the patient to identify goals that can be pursued without putting the patient or others at risk. Typically, there are many areas for collaborative care planning that involve shared decision making, even with high-risk patients who require more directive care.

Overview of the Nursing Process

The **nursing process** refers to the steps nurses use to identify needs for care; analyze, prioritize and plan for intervention; and evaluate the nursing care that is delivered to patients. This is a process of assessment and problem solving that occurs jointly with patients. Central to the process is the development of a therapeutic relationship and identification of needs that will benefit from attention in the current episode of care. Every interaction nurses have with a patient is an opportunity to engage in the nursing process, and to thoughtfully use the time with the patient to assess the process of caregiving and its effectiveness at meeting patient needs.

The first step of the nursing process is assessment, which may begin prior to the first face-to-face meeting with the patient and continues until the patient leaves the setting. **Assessment** involves the collection of information about the patient across the wellness domains and may include, but is not limited to, data gained through observation, patient interviews, and assessment tools such as vital signs measurements and mental status examinations. **Nursing diagnosis** follows the assessment phase; in this step, the nurse synthesizes the information gathered and identifies and categorizes the presenting needs of the patient in a salient way, following both nursing diagnosis and psychiatric diagnostic criteria. Once problems that will be the focus of care have been jointly identified, planning for care begins. In the **planning** phase, the nurse and patient identify **outcomes** and goals that the patient is interested in achieving, as well as activities required by the nurse to maintain health, safety, and daily function. When the goals and outcomes are defined, interventions to support their achievement are identified. **Interventions** (the activities that nurses employ to achieve the goals established in the planning phase) are carried out in the *implementation* phase of the nursing process and may be affected by a variety of factors. Critically important to the success of the nursing process is **evaluation**, the process by which the nurse determines what progress has been made relevant to the plan of care. The result of this evaluation may include renegotiating needs to be addressed; identifying new, different, or additional goals and outcomes; and redefining the role of the patient and nurse in achieving outcomes. At all times, the nursing process is collaborative, involving the nurse and patient in partnership, and dynamic, responding to changes in the patient's care needs as they occur.

Advances in the Nursing Process

As nursing developed as a profession, the nursing process was first identified by Ida Jean Orlando in the 1950s (Orlando, 1961). Orlando described this process as a systematic one that involved assessment, diagnosis, planning, intervention, and evaluation. The process is cyclical, with the evaluation providing important information to update the assessment of needs. From Orlando's starting point, nurse theorists began developing models that defined nursing and the way nurses cared for their patients. In these models, aspects of how nurses conducted assessments of patients and how they assisted patients to achieve their optimal level of health were identified. Many nursing models offer a philosophical orientation or framework for the assessment of individuals in need of nursing care.

In the 1970s, initial efforts were made to more systematically define the problems or needs that nurses addressed in care. One of the first efforts to define nursing diagnosis occurred in Marjory Gordon's book, *Nursing Diagnosis*, published in 1982. Gordon was the first leader of a task force identified in 1973 to classify nursing diagnoses. Her most recent book, *The Manual of Nursing Diagnosis*, was published in 2010. From Gordon's early work, the **North American Nursing Diagnosis Association** (NANDA) was founded in 1982 and is now an international group (NANDA-I). In addition to the standardization of nursing diagnoses, the group has developed classifications of outcomes (**Nursing Outcomes Classification**, NOC) and nursing interventions (**Nursing Interventions Classification**, NIC). These groups have contributed to the development of standardized diagnosis, outcome, and intervention use in nursing.

Assessment

Assessment begins with the first information the nurse receives about the patient or situation. For example, as the nurse listens to a report about a patient or reviews a file, the nurse begins to collect important information that will help the nurse understand the patient and his or her needs. At this early stage, it is important to consider the information offered but to refrain from making assumptions or judgments about the patient based on this initial information. *By suspending expectations about the patient, the nurse allows the patient an opportunity for a fresh start with the initial patient–nurse interaction.*

Nurses typically begin the assessment by asking the patient what brought him or her to the treatment setting that day. It is important to hear this in the patient's own words, because the patient provides information about how he or she perceives the current situation. The nurse proceeds in collecting information about the current problem that brought the patient in for care, and the associated symptoms and effects on the patient's daily life and functioning. In addition, the nurse asks the patient about any previous history of similar difficulties and obtains a history of prior symptoms and treatment. Critically important is identification of the patient's current and prior approach to coping with difficulties, and the success or limitations of these methods. In addition, the nurse asks permission to obtain information from prior treatment providers that will offer further perspective on caring for the patient and for permission to contact significant others or family members to obtain collateral information about the problems and how they affect the patient's functioning.

With direct assessment of the current problem and past history, the nurse also obtains important information about the patient's family, relationships, occupation, living situation, and supports, and how the current problem has affected these dimensions of the patient's life; these areas constitute the environment within which the patient's symptoms developed. Additional information for assessment includes the following:

- How the patient has attempted to manage the problem, including any remedies or techniques he or she has tried to manage symptoms
- The patient's development and educational background
- A review of the patient's general and physical well-being
- Prescription and over-the-counter medications taken regularly or intermittently
- Use of complementary and alternative medical therapies, including folk remedies, vitamins, and nutritional supplements (see Chapter 22)
- Any history of substance use and abuse
- Cultural background and spiritual beliefs and practices

Framework of Assessment

In the psychiatric setting, nurses use a holistic model to collect information across the domains of wellness that informs care and forms the basis of the care planning process. This model means that the nurse identifies physiological, psychological, social, spiritual, and cultural aspects of the person's life and carefully examines how the current reason for presenting to treatment relates to and influences the patient's life. Nurses working in psychiatric settings think of not only the patient, but also the patient's relationships with family or significant others, and the systems in which the patient plays a role, including extended family, occupation, neighborhood, and other important connections. In this way, nurses collect a holistic view of the patient and how the patient is functioning in life.

The nursing process structures how nurses assess, interpret findings, and plan for and deliver nursing care. It helps nurses identify problems that require intervention as well as rule out possibilities based on patient history and assessment data. The nursing process represents a way to organize signs and related symptoms into patterns requiring intervention. In psychiatric nursing, the nursing process is informed by the system for classification and diagnosis of psychiatric disorders, the *Diagnostic and Statistical Manual of Mental Disorders*, 5th edition (DSM-5) (American Psychiatric Association, 2013). Nurses are expected to be familiar with this manual, which is a vital resource for the field of psychiatric–mental health nursing and informs the collaborative care of patients with mental illnesses. The DSM-5 provides a system to organize psychiatric symptoms, and offers explicit criteria for when a diagnosis can be made for particular disorders.

A complete assessment in psychiatric–mental health settings involves a range of present and historical information that is collected from the patient. Information about the following areas are collected: demographics, mode of presentation, chief complaint, present history of illness, mental status exam and review of psychiatric symptoms, past history of psychiatric illness and treatment history, physical health history, family history of psychiatric illness, family history, developmental history, social history, occupational history, leisure interests, substance use history, legal history, strengths and areas for growth, and patient goals and aspirations. For each area, a rationale for why that information is collected, what the parts of that assessment entail and how they are collected, and information about how data from this section are interpreted and used to plan care will be summarized. The assessment information concludes with the formulation of the problem, which is a concise summary of the patient's presentation and need for treatment.

The assessment interview may be structured by the clinician or it may follow an intuitive flow as the patient relates his or her difficulties and the clinician guides the direction based on the information presented. Typically, the interview, documentation of the interview, and presentation of the results of the assessment to members of the clinical team follow general topic areas that are standard in most settings. Beginners may find a greater need to structure the interview as they learn to guide patients in sharing information needed to complete a comprehensive assessment. Most settings have forms and instructions for collection of assessment information that can help guide the interview. Depending on the setting, the patient, and the time frame for meeting with and interviewing the patient, the assessment may be completed in single or multiple sessions. If multiple sessions are needed, typically the current problem and treatment history are the main focus initially, with further historical and background history collected in future sessions.

Mode of Patient Presentation to Clinical Setting

The *pre-setting* background refers to the information about the patient's situation immediately preceding or precipitating the patient's admission. This would include any information about events occurring prior to treatment, as well as the kind of setting that either referred or planned the admission for the patient. This information is helpful in understanding the context in which the decision to seek treatment was made. In addition, information about the nature of assistance that is being sought by the patient or referring agency is identified. This includes information about whether the patient is seeking treatment voluntarily or the patient was required to enter treatment and is being admitted involuntarily. The circumstances related to how an individual presents to treatment help to determine his or her interest, motivation, and goals for treatment—for example, if the patient is being forced to attend or complete treatment, there may be an unwillingness to change that affects clinical intervention efforts.

Presenting Concerns

Patients generally come to treatment with presenting concerns—symptoms, frustrations, goals, and aspirations that are critically important to them. The patient's concerns help inform the plan of care related to priority diagnoses (for instance, which symptoms most impair the patient's functioning) and in terms of identifying strategies for motivating patient participation in the care plan.

Chief Complaint

The chief complaint, or presenting problem, is usually a direct quote from the patient that identifies the reason for seeking care at this time, such as Claudine's statement, "Sometimes I have chest pain and trouble breathing and feel like I'm going to die." The chief complaint gives the nurse a starting point from which to obtain background information on the problems and immediate symptoms experienced by the patient, and factors that precipitated the current episode of illness. This part of the assessment both provides a concise overview of how the patient perceives the symptoms, and reviews the symptoms and precipitants of the problem.

Goals and Aspirations

The process of planning and providing care in mental health settings must be collaborative, as much of the work and progress that must occur requires individuals to reflect on and be motivated to change. The best way to approach change is to work collaboratively to help the patient to move toward the goals he or she is interested in accomplishing. In addition, the process of identifying goals and aspirations is a positive, hopeful one that can provide motivation to the patient and may be a good note on which to close the assessment process.

History of Present Illness

The history of present illness provides the background information essential to understand what brought the patient to seek treatment now. Present history may include information provided by the patient, as well as collateral information provided by family members, friends, or co-workers. This part of the interview involves asking the patient to describe how he or she decided to seek help; identify symptoms and the time frame of symptom development; describe precipitants of symptoms or behaviors, with pattern of emergence; and discuss previous responses to intervention, periods of remission (if any), and effects of the symptoms on daily life, work, and relationships (Box 9-1).

Other symptoms that should be evaluated in terms of how they relate to the presenting problem include changes in feelings (such as elevated or depressed mood), anxiety, fear, and changes in perception, such as hallucinations, illusions, or experiences of depersonalization or dissociation. Neurovegetative changes are common and should be routinely evaluated; these include the patient's sleep pattern, appetite, and libido. As with other symptoms, it is useful to know what "normal" is or has been for the patient, and when and how symptoms have changed (Box 9-2). In addition, it is important to ask the patient what stressors or precipitants have occurred in the past few months or year(s), including any recent losses. Cognitive changes should be assessed, including whether the patient is oriented and whether there is any impairment in memory, attention, or concentration. Other cognitive symptoms should be identified, including the following:

- Delusions
- Obsessions
- Ideas of reference
- Suspiciousness
- Grandiosity
- Phobias
- Changes in judgment or abstraction

Behavior changes should also be noted, including hyperactivity or slowed behavior, impulsivity, compulsive behavior, substance use or withdrawal symptoms, safety issues, and problems with role performance and interpersonal relationships that are pertinent to the presenting problem. The patient should also be asked to identify his or her goals or expectations of treatment.

Assessment of History of Present Illness   box 9-1

Assessment of the patient's history of present illness includes eliciting data on the following:

- Current symptoms: specific experiences, details of symptoms, timing of development, effect on daily function, relationships, work
- Detail on what brought patient to treatment at this time:
  - Precipitants of symptoms, behaviors, losses, changes
  - When did symptoms first emerge, what decreases or promotes remission
- Symptom areas (in this section, identify how the symptoms contribute/pertain to this episode of illness):
  - Neurovegetative changes (sleep, appetite, libido)

- Feeling changes (mood, anxiety, fear)
- Cognitive changes (orientation, memory, concentration, attention, delusions, phobia, obsessions, ideas of reference, suspiciousness, grandiosity, judgment, abstraction)
- Behavior changes (hyperactive, slowed, impulsive, compulsive), safety (suicidal/homicidal ideation/intent), substance use, substance withdrawal, role performance, interpersonal relationships
- Perceptual changes (hallucinations, depersonalization, derealization, illusions)
- Expectations of treatment
- Treatment goals

Reflection and Clarification

box 9-2

Patients will often report a symptom or behavior and not fully describe it, preventing full understanding of the symptom or patterns of behaviors related to a symptom. It is a common oversight, particularly for new clinicians, to accept a broad statement identifying a symptom without attempting to get further detailed information that helps to clarify the experience.

Patient symptom identification	Nurse Clarification	Patient Response	Information Identified
"I just can't sleep."	"You have trouble sleeping?" "So tell me what happens each night when you try to sleep, the time, the routines, exactly what happens. . ."	"Yes, some nights I don't sleep at all." "I try to get to bed at 11 or so, sometimes I have a drink before bed to help me relax, then I put on the TV and watch until I drift off, it can take up to an hour or two. But lately it seems I am awake later and later. If I do fall asleep, I often wake up by 1 or so and have to go to the bathroom. Then I have to try to sleep again, sometimes I am up all night. Usually once it is light outside, I am up, as early as 5 or 6 a.m."	Sleep problem No sleep at times Sleeps approx. 3–4 hours/night TV watching; alcohol use Difficulty falling asleep (DFA) Middle-night awakening (MNA)
	"What goes through your mind when you are lying there trying to sleep?"	"That's why I watch TV. Everything. I can't stop my brain. I review everything I did that day, mostly what I talked about with my co-workers or husband."	Rumination about interactions, anxiety
"I'm just so nervous all the time! It's horrible." (Patient taps foot repeatedly.)	"You feel nervous a lot? What is that like for you?" "Please describe what that restlessness feels like to you."	"I don't know, I feel on edge a lot. Like I am just so restless." "Yes, sometimes it's so bad that I feel like I am going to jump out of my skin, I just have to move. I never really considered myself a nervous person until now. I just can't believe all of this has happened to me."	Anxiety? Restlessness: (consider anxiety vs. akathisia vs. restless leg syndrome)
	"So you experience a feeling like you physically need to move? Are there times when this is better or worse for you?"	"Well it seems worse when I'm just sitting and trying to relax – it's so frustrating."	This sounds like akathisia, which is a medication reaction.

In this scenario, if the nurse had recorded only the initial statement, or the response to the follow-up question, the nurse would have learned little about the patient's difficulty sleeping or anxiety. Asking for clarification gains much more information that will aid in accurate assessment and planning intervention. In the first example, general principles of sleep hygiene suggest that alcohol be avoided before bedtime, and that the bedroom be reserved only for sleep and sexual activity, not work, TV, or other activities. In the second example, the nurse is able to make an important distinction between the experience of anxiety or nervousness, and the side effect of akathisia.

Biological Domain

Patients presenting with symptoms of mental illness require a thorough assessment that includes their demographic information, physical and developmental health histories, and history of any substance use or abuse (Table 9-1). Careful assessment in the biological domain is necessary given the high occurrence of co-morbid medical and mental health disorders experienced by patients with mental illness.

Demographic Information

It is also important to include demographic information that includes brief identifying information such as gender, age and ethnicity, and marital and socioeconomic status. Awareness of a patient's socioeconomic status is important in care planning, as it helps the nurse understand the patient's situation in life, availability of or need for resources, and areas of support or conflict (Box 9-3).

Socioeconomic status is a broad term that refers to a person's position within society and is often defined by several different kinds of information, including education, income or wealth, occupation, and location of residence. For example, Susan, a 35-year-old single, White female with a high school education who is chronically unemployed, is homeless, and relies on food stamps and government assistance. She has distinctly different needs and resources when compared to Sarah, a 35-year-old single, White female with a master's degree who is employed full-time as an accountant and lives in an apartment in the city. The delineation of these aspects of a patient's background help nurses to best understand the kind of

Assessment Considerations: Biological Domain

table 9-1

Demographic information	Gender Age Ethnicity Marital status Socioeconomic status
Physical health history	*History of medical conditions or diagnoses:* surgical procedures; infectious disease Treatments or therapies: prescribed medications (past and current); over-the-counter medications; vitamins, minerals, or herbal preparations; complementary or alternative therapies *Preventive and health promotion activities:* physical exercise and strength training; smoking history; diet and nutrition status; stress management activities; coping strategies; values, beliefs, and cultural practices related to health; vital signs; height, weight, and BMI *Review of systems:* • Skin/dermatologic • Head, eyes, ears, nose, throat (HEENT); sensory and cranial nerves • Lymphatic, hematologic, and immune • Cardiovascular and peripheral vascular • Respiratory • Gastrointestinal • Endocrine • Genitourinary and reproductive • Musculoskeletal and neurologic
Developmental history	*Developmental history* (for each stage: developmental milestones, significant events, significant relationships, family relationships and changes, achievements and losses): • Birth and early childhood • Childhood and early school years • Adolescence and middle, high school years • Young adulthood and vocational or college years • Adulthood, family development, and career path • Middle adulthood • Older adulthood
History of substance use/abuse	*Assess history of substance use or abuse:* alcohol, tobacco, marijuana, opiates, amphetamines, narcotics *For each substance:* first use, amount used and frequency, how substance is used, tolerance, withdrawal symptoms, date of last use *Substance abuse treatment history:* dates, substances, type of treatment

help and support that would be beneficial to the patient's care. For example, without any added information, the nurse can identify potential needs of each of these two patients: Susan's needs might include assistance to find stable shelter initially and eventually permanent housing, and vocational assistance to find stable employment; Sarah's needs might include how to cope with her symptoms when

returning to work and her apartment and increasing her social support systems.

Physical Health History

Physical health assessment is particularly important in the psychiatric–mental health setting, as the nurse is one of only a few professionals

Demographic Information

box 9-3

Referring to the case study featuring Claudine

Assessment Data
Claudine is a 43-year-old, White, married female. She is the mother of three school-age children. She lives in a house in a nearby suburb and works as a middle-school teacher.

Application
Claudine's demographic information can be used to identify how her symptoms have affected her ability to work and parent.

Critical Thinking Questions
Carl is a 26-year-old single African American male who completed 10th grade, is currently unemployed, and living in an urban homeless shelter after being thrown out of his brother's house.

1. How do Carl's demographics compare to Claudine's?
2. What kinds of needs might Carl have compared to Claudine?
3. What community resources would help Carl now? What resources are available to patients in your community?

with a background in general health and physical assessment. A priority for the nurse is to rule out whether any physical health conditions are causing or contributing to the mental health problems requiring treatment. It is useful to ask initial questions related to any history of medical conditions or disorders, surgical procedures, and medications, vitamins, complementary, or other therapies the patient has experienced or is currently being treated with. A review of systems should be completed, along with a physical assessment related to findings from inquiry about all aspects of physical health. This may mean hands-on assessment techniques, although clinicians are wise to be aware of agency philosophy about "hands-on" skill use and should follow their agency's policies related to both assessment and referral to appropriate providers, should this be needed.

The review of systems is pursued in one of two ways: a comprehensive review of systems to identify overall health status and provide data to support identification of current health problems and related complications, or specific to a particular problem identified by an already established patient. Initially, nurses review the patient's general symptoms and ask about any particular health problems or concerns the patient is experiencing. Then the nurse assesses for symptoms and signs across all systems: skin/dermatologic; eyes, ears, nose, mouth/throat, head and neck; cardiovascular, including peripheral vascular; respiratory; gastrointestinal; genitourinary; musculoskeletal; neurologic; endocrine; and hematologic/lymphatic/immunologic. Each system should be considered and may be assessed following a "head to toe" progression. Excellent resources are available for review of techniques (Bickley, 2012; Seidel et al., 2011); interpretation of findings should be integrated with the psychiatric assessment, formulation, identification of nursing diagnoses, differential diagnoses (for the APRN), and intervention planning.

Developmental History

The patient's developmental history provides a great deal of background information important to understanding who the patient is and the factors that resulted in the ways in which the patient has adjusted to life. Each phase of development can be reviewed, including birth, developmental tasks and milestones, significant events and relationships, family relationships and changes, and achievements as well as losses. It is common to find similar patterns and themes emerging across an individual's development. These offer important clues to difficulties the patient experiences and beliefs the patient holds about self and others.

One way to involve the patient actively in providing historical information such as the developmental history is to start a timeline with the patient (Box 9-4). Using either a regular sheet of paper or a large poster-sized sheet of paper, a draw a line across the paper that starts with the patient's birth. As the patient relays historical information about his or her life, dates and information are added to the timeline. Timelines can be a useful homework assignment for a patient to complete during the course of treatment. As patients reflect on important events and experiences, they gain perspective on difficulties and problems that have not been resolved. This process may lead to important insights that can be discussed in treatment. In addition, a timeline in the patient's record can also offer important background information to the clinician. The timeline can be used with several aspects of the assessment process, including the developmental history, family history, social history, leisure/recreational activities, and occupational or vocational history.

Substance Use History

A complete history of substances the patient uses—including alcohol, tobacco, and drugs—should be identified. Generally, it is helpful to ask an open-ended question about drug use or abuse and then follow with an overview of each substance that might be used. For each substance identified, the nurse identifies and records the start of use, frequency and amount used, how the substance is used (for example, smoked or snorted), and most recent use/last use. It is helpful to ask about substance use in terms of the frequency or amount used, as opposed to asking in a yes-or-no format whether the patient uses a substance. Nurses may also use screening tools to aid in the

Using Timelines to Inform Assessment box 9-4

A timeline can be used to denote significant events across the life span. The nurse might start a timeline with a patient at the initial assessment and add to it in subsequent interviews. Patients often enjoy reflecting back on their experiences, or may need assistance to gain insight and integrate difficult experiences. The activity not only serves an assessment function, but it may also serve as an intervention. As treatment progresses, the timeline may be revisited to add important events, or consider how various aspects of the patient's life were affected by events.

Following is a timeline for April, a 37-year-old married White female patient who presented with recurrent depression and a potential rule-out diagnosis of posttraumatic stress disorder (Chapter 13) after a major car accident and traumatic brain injury (TBI) 4 years ago. At a glance, the timeline provides information about many experiences in the patient's life (Figure 9-1).

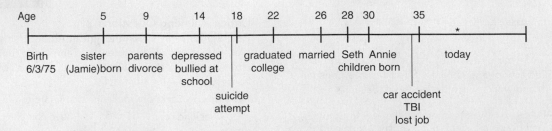

9-1

Claudine Part 2

<table>
<tr><td>

APPLICATION

1. What additional information do you need to get a full picture of Claudine's physical health? Why is this important?

2. Based on the information provided here, what additional concerns do you have about Claudine? How would or should these inform her care plan?

3. What information related to family medical history would be pertinent?

</td><td>

Claudine reports that she has been taking over-the-counter diphenhydramine 25 mg PO QHS prn or Tylenol PM (acetaminophen 500 mg and diphenhydramine 25 mg) two tablets PO QHS prn for sleep, with some relief. She states that her primary care physician prescribed Ambien (zolpidem) 5 mg PO QHS prn approximately 12 months ago after the death of her father, and again 6 months ago with job stressors, but gave her only 10 tablets each time. The Ambien helped her get to sleep at night, but she fears she will "become addicted" to sleep medication.

Claudine reports that she does not have any major health problems. Other than giving birth naturally to her children, she has never been hospitalized nor has she had any major medical or surgical procedures. She has a primary care physician whom she sees for an annual physical. She reports a history of gastroesophageal reflux disease and states that this has been treated in the past with Prilosec (omeprazole). She is visibly overweight and says she has attempted to diet in the past, but in the past year has not felt able to work on losing weight because of other stressors. Her only physical exercise is that associated with work (she stands a lot while teaching), and household chores. She denies smoking. She drinks up to three or four glasses of wine daily and denies history of other substance use.

She has increasingly disturbed sleep, including difficulty falling asleep (DFA) and middle-of-night awakening (MNA), resulting in approximately 4 to 5 hours of sleep per night; she denies snoring or other sleep disturbances. She has a history of "tension headaches," which have increased recently to one or two per month and are successfully treated with extra-strength Tylenol (acetaminophen two 500 mg tabs PO Q 4–6 hours prn); there is no associated aura or nausea with the headaches. She has normal vision and hearing; her teeth are well cared for and she has dental cleanings and exams regularly. Testing of cranial nerves I–XII yields results within normal limits.

Her respiratory rate is 20 and regular and there is no history of wheezing or asthma. She has seasonal allergies but denies food or drug allergies. She reports recent awareness of her heart pounding and reports that she can feel it most at night in bed. She also notices palpitations several times daily and fears there is something wrong with her heart. Her pulse is 76 and regular and her blood pressure is 134/88 mmHg. She denies shortness of breath on exertion and denies dyspnea, with the exception of the panic episodes.

</td></tr>
</table>

identification of substance use disorders (see Chapter 20). Additional assessment of substance use includes history of tolerance to or withdrawal from each substance and dates of substance abuse treatment, as well as how substance use has affected different areas of the patient's life, including significant relationships, responsibilities, and work.

Psychological Domain

The assessment of an individual suspected of having mental illness or of a patient with a confirmed diagnosis will include an assessment related to mental status, cognitive functioning, and psychiatric symptoms (Box 9-5). Although it may seem redundant for particular symptoms that have already been identified, the formal mental status exam provides an overview of all spheres of function important for consideration in understanding a patient's impairment and needs. The major sections of the mental status exam are appearance, attitude, and behavior; speech; emotional status; thought processes; and mental status.

Observations about the patient can be very informative and often may change the interpretation of verbally disclosed information. Nurses can learn a great deal from simply observing the patient's appearance, including his or her dress, hygiene, expression, motor activity, behaviors and mannerisms, and physical features. Changes in expression, mannerisms, behavior, and motor activity often provide important clues to understanding the presenting problem and the difficulties the patient is currently experiencing. How the patient interacts with the clinician is important, as are the patient's ability to establish rapport and the attitude the patient presents regarding both

the interview and treatment. Mental status assessment also examines nonverbal communication along with information about how cooperative or reliable the patient is, whether the patient is able to engage and make good eye contact with the clinician, and whether the patient is motivated for treatment and has insight into the current situation.

An important part of assessment is the patient's past history of psychiatric illness and history of any treatment for symptoms up to the present time. The clinician attempts to understand when the symptoms or problems the patient is experiencing first began and to review precipitants of both initial and intermittent episodes of illness. The duration of symptoms and the effect they have on the patient's role performance at home, work, and in significant relationships are also identified. The nurse inquires about each treatment contact the patient has had, including when it occurred, where treatment was provided, the name and credentials of the provider, precipitants of each episode, the diagnosis and type of treatment, how symptoms changed in response to treatment, and status and stability between treatment episodes. Treatment information includes history of pharmacologic therapy, including specific medications, dosages, start and end dates of treatment, purpose and length of treatment, information about any beneficial effects and adverse effects, and reasons for discontinuation.

Sociological Domain

Assessment of the patient's family, work, and social history can provide information essential to developing the plan of care. Whether or

Assessment of Mental Status and Psychiatric Symptoms
box 9-5

1. **Appearance, Attitude, and Behavior**
   Appearance: dress, posture, expression, motor activity, behavior, mannerisms, physical features
   Rapport and attitude with interviewer/clinician: cooperation, reliability, motivation, insight, engagement, eye contact
   Nonverbal communication
2. **Speech**
   Quantity (freely spoken, mutism)
   Quality (pace [rapid/slow], pressured, clear or mumbled, pitch, volume, vocabulary, word use/misuse, pronunciation, continuity, blocking, responsiveness/reaction time)
   Organization (coherent, logical, circumstantial, tangential, word salad, rhyming, flight of ideas)
3. **Emotional status**
   Mood: as described, depth, intensity, duration, fluctuations
   Affect: observed state, relationship to topic, experiences, content
   Anxiety: objective and subjective levels
   Self-esteem: view of self, ability to accept self
   Connection with feelings: depersonalization, derealization, detachment, dreamlike
   Suicidal ideation/intent
   Homicidal ideation/intent
4. **Thought processes**
   Content of thought: preoccupations, repetitive thoughts, obsessions, rumination, doubting, phobia, theme
   Thought disturbance: delusions (type), ideas of reference, ideas of influence
   Perceptual state: illusions (misinterpretations)

   Hallucinations: details, circumstances, frequency, reaction to; auditory (note if command hallucinations), visual, gustatory, olfactory, tactile
   Dreams and fantasies: dreams (note nightmares, prominent dreams), fantasies (recurrent)
   Coping strategies: response to stressors; strategies used to mitigate stressors and resolve problems; how symptoms are managed and response
5. **Cognitive functioning**
   State of consciousness: alert, responsive, able to understand
   Cognitive functioning: orientation (person, place, time, situation)
   Memory: recent, remote: recent experiences (can retell events of past day); remote experiences (able to identify dates of child's birth, anniversary, jobs, place of birth, schools attended); can recall three unrelated words (ex: 25, green, Alaska) immediately and after 3 to 5 minutes
   General fund of information: names current and past presidents; identifies state capital and governor, distance to California
   Attention and concentration: can repeat at least five or more digits forward and four or more digits backward; can subtract 7 from 100 and continue (average time approximately 60 seconds, with minimal mistakes); can spell the word "world" forward and backward.
   Abstraction capacity: provide a proverb and ask the patient to interpret it, noting the nature of the interpretation (literal, concrete, abstract, incoherent)
   Judgment/insight: social, personal (for example, what to do if there is smoke in a movie theater)

not family members and friends are supportive of the patient or contribute to the patient's symptomatology, as well as the patient's ability to be successful in a vocational setting, can affect the patient's motivation to succeed in treatment as well as the ability to adhere to treatment.

Family History

Assessment of family history includes a review of the patient's family members and the presence of any psychiatric disorders. This can be assessed in a variety of ways. It may be useful to ask specifically about the presence of the most common disorders, including depression, anxiety, bipolar disorder, or alcohol or drug abuse, in addition to whether any family member ever had a psychotic illness, such as schizophrenia. A different way to approach this assessment is to ask whether any family members have ever heard voices or made a suicide attempt or died due to suicide. Depending on the region and cultural background of the patient, the patient may use terms commonly used to identify mental illness that are not part of Western professional terminology. For example, *amok* in the Malaysian culture or *nervios* in Latino cultures will identify the presence of syndromes not otherwise mentioned.

At times, patients will deny any history of mental illness in their family, but may indicate that a family member is currently taking an antidepressant or other psychotropic medication. If a family member is noted to have a history of a psychiatric disorder, it is useful to identify information about the onset of first illness and how the problem has been treated. A family member's successful treatment with a particular antidepressant, for example, may indicate good potential for remission of symptoms in a family member with a similar disorder.

Obtaining a complete family history provides insight into relationships, situational and environmental context, and health risks that are important to consider in planning for care. It is useful to draw a genogram with the help of the patient during a session as you inquire about family relationships and history (Chapter 24). A genogram, with its visual orientation, may help the patient gain insight into family dynamics, health issues, and relationships.

Social History

The social history provides an overview of the most significant relationships and support systems for the patient. In addition, the nurse assesses the connections the patient has in the community and any involvement in community groups or organizations, and also identifies social relationships, including information about the nature of the relationship or membership in community groups. This information is important in understanding how the patient finds support in daily life, and offers resources to use in planning care and suggesting behavioral alternatives and coping strategies.

Occupational/Vocational History

Psychiatric symptoms can be exacerbated by work or can interfere with an individual's ability to work. Occupational and vocational history are important factors for consideration, given that work is an important activity in our lives. It is important to understand what the patient's career goals and aspirations are and how they have changed over time. Identifying vocational training, education history, and work history provides important information about the role of work in the patient's life, significant exposures at work to chemicals or other toxins, any history of injury or disability at work, and adjustment to work life. For patients who are currently working, it is important to get an understanding of the culture and climate in their workplace as well as the demands of the job and the relationship between the patients' psychiatric symptoms and their work. The workplace can be a significant stressor as well as a positive force in a person's life, but can easily be overlooked or forgotten.

Legal History

Information about an individual's involvement with the legal system is needed to understand whether treatment is required due to some legal involvement, as well as whether the patient may be a crime victim or party to a legal suit that is related in some way to the patient's health. If a patient has been arrested, been charged or convicted, and served time in local, state, or federal jail or prison, the information should be recorded in the history. In addition, information about the patient's release or parole, including terms of release and parole, should be identified. For example, some patients may be required to be involved in psychiatric treatment as part of their parole. Past problems with domestic violence or stalking should be identified, including whether restraining orders are in place. If the patient is involved in legal proceedings, information about the situation and the patient's role in the case are important to understanding current stressors and past difficulties that may have led to the legal action.

Recreational Interests and Activities

Leisure and recreational interests and activities are important to quality of life, finding pleasure and enjoyment, and relieving stress. Understanding how individuals spend their free or leisure time and activities that they enjoy will offer information about influences in their lives and assist the nurse to help patients better structure their free time, which is often difficult. Being actively involved in activities that are enjoyable can relieve stress and enhance pleasurable feelings.

Cultural and Spiritual Domains

Assessment of patients' cultural and spiritual practices, values, and beliefs can provide insight into a variety of areas that may affect the treatment plan. For example, if a patient is from a culture or belief system that does not value traditional Western medicine, it may be challenging to gain the patient's cooperation in a treatment plan that involves prescription medications. As another example, therapy sessions may need to be scheduled around times during which a Muslim patient observes prayer. Cultural and spiritual considerations and assessment are discussed in detail in Chapters 5 and 6, respectively.

Strengths and Areas for Growth

Patients have many strengths and resources that offer a foundation for successful coping and can be used to affirm abilities and encourage further growth and hope for the future. After obtaining a comprehensive history with a patient, the clinician usually can easily identify several strengths or assets to help the patient cope with difficulties in his or her life. These may include personal assets such as intelligence, education, physical health or strength, personality style, and communication skills. Other assets may include support systems, vocational skills, financial resources, family supports, or relationships. Jointly identifying strengths and assets both provides the clinician with a perspective of how the patient perceives himself or herself, and affirms important skills, assets, and capacities. Areas for growth may be identified during history taking, through the goals the patient identifies for himself or herself, or framed as changes or areas the patient would like to work on in treatment; or they may relate to stressors and problems that the patient perceives as barriers to health. The ability to name goals and areas for growth are important so that work in treatment is directed to the areas most in need.

Claudine Part 3

critical thinking

APPLICATION

1. What are Claudine's strengths at this time? How might these inform her plan of care? How might they affect her participation in treatment?

2. What areas for growth can you identify?

Claudine has worked as a teacher in the same city since her graduation from college. Prior to the birth of her children, she was active in groups at the school and in the community. Although she was raised in the Episcopal church, she reports attending only occasionally as an adult, finding it helpful when she is struggling. She has not attended recently, reporting, "I just don't feel up to it." Claudine describes herself as extroverted and social, although she tends to keep most difficult problems private. Although she reports having two very close friends and being close to her sisters, whom she sees regularly, Claudine says she has not shared anything about how she is feeling with either her siblings or her close friends. Her most significant relationship is with her husband, whom she describes as her "best friend." When she began dating him, she focused more of her activity on their relationship and less on her other friendships, interests, and activities. In the past they argued infrequently, but lately they argue nearly weekly. The conflicts have never become physical in nature. Most often they focus on finances and the children. She feels hurt that her husband is "taking out his frustration with work on me," which has led to her further disengagement in the relationship. Her three children are ages 6 to 10 and are healthy and doing well in school. She has good relationships with her children, who seek advice from her and tell her their problems.

Claudine played soccer in high school and enjoyed the physical activity; after high school her activities have included hiking and biking. She enjoys sewing and craft projects, although she rarely does one for her own enjoyment, more frequently getting her children started with their own activities and projects. She spends most of her free time making sure her three children are involved in activities they enjoy and transporting them to and from activities and sports. She and her husband are enthusiastic football fans and regularly watch or attend games. She is an avid reader and is a member of a local reading group, although she has felt too busy to attend regularly during the past year.

Formulating a Diagnosis

The formulation of a comprehensive diagnosis is a synthesis, or summary, of the assessment process. It typically is completed at the initial interview and serves as the clinician's initial interpretation of data collected, including the identification of problems, patterns, and themes that inform the initial treatment plan. This summary of information is specific to the current need for treatment. It typically includes a concise description of the patient, the patient's presentation, significant symptoms, mental status findings, prior psychiatric problems, and history of trauma or abuse. The significance of symptoms is determined using the WHODAS Disability Scale, which assists the clinician in assessing the extent to which symptoms impair daily functioning (Chapter 5). It should also identify the presence of any safety concerns (suicide, homicide, inability to care for self), and identify current medication or other treatment. Indication of pertinent social or occupational issues or needs, and legal status (for example, homelessness, unemployed, voluntary or required admission) are included. The formulation also includes an immediate or initial plan for treatment. In the formulation, all pertinent issues are presented concisely, making every word count. In most settings, the formulation will be one or two paragraphs in length; thus, information must be synthesized to convey the needed information as clearly as possible. See Box 9-6 for a sample formulation based on Claudine's scenario.

Diagnosis

Once a comprehensive assessment has been made, the nurse uses clinical judgment to identify problems requiring intervention. This process involves naming the problem(s) using nursing diagnosis, which focuses on how individuals respond to health problems or threats to their health. Integral to the nursing process, nursing

diagnosis is a comprehensive and holistic approach to identifying needs of individuals. Rather than focusing on only the disease or medical condition, the lens includes how that condition affects the patient in life, and the patient's adaptation. The first step in this process is to use nursing diagnoses to name the problems that will be a focus of care. These diagnoses can be about an actual health problem or can relate to a health promotion need or risk factor that has been identified. Identifying the nursing diagnosis can be approached as identifying a single problem with related signs or symptoms, or it can be approached as identifying a cluster of related signs, symptoms, or behaviors that together represent a syndrome or pattern that can be addressed with nursing intervention.

The nursing diagnosis includes three elements:

- Naming of the problem
- Etiology of the problem
- Data that provide evidence of the problem or the signs and symptoms present in the patient

For example, a patient who is experiencing psychosis and has looseness of associations, paranoia, racing thoughts, and auditory hallucinations after using PCP might have the following nursing diagnosis: "Alteration in thinking due to PCP intoxication as evidenced by loose associations, paranoia, racing thoughts, and auditory hallucinations." Identifying these specific elements of the problem helps the nurse to begin to formulate a plan of care because this comprehensive overview of the problem offers identification of symptoms and behaviors that lead to further assessment, monitoring, and intervention.

In addition to identifying the nursing diagnosis, the nurse will also begin to evaluate symptoms presented that are indicative of

---

Formulating a Comprehensive Diagnosis—Sample box 9-6

Claudine is a 43-year-old, married Caucasian mother of three children who presents to the ED after calling 911 from her car due to a panic attack. Anxiety-related symptoms have increased over the past 3–6 months. She is fearful that the symptoms may be due to an undiagnosed heart or physical health problem. Panic attacks have increased in frequency to 3–4 times per week lasting 10–15 minutes, starting without precipitant. Symptoms include chest, shoulder, and jaw pain, palpitations, "pounding chest," hyperventilation, fear that she is dying, and derealization. Reports decreased concentration, restlessness, anhedonia, rumination about finances/marital conflict, ambivalence with decision making, social isolation, and poor sleep (DFA, MNA, 4–5 hrs/night). Speech is rapid, pressured and circumstantial, reports irritability, mood is euthymic with normal range of affect, no evidence of mania. Has occasional passive suicidal thought ("if my life ended, these problems would too"), no current or history of active suicidal ideation or intent, no evidence of homicidal ideation or intent. Thinking is logical and goal-directed without evidence of psychosis. Increased alcohol use from 1–2 glasses of wine/day to 3–4 glasses/day "to relax," denies withdrawal symptoms, denies other substance use. Precipitants include potential job loss, financial strain, marital conflict (finances, child rearing), and father's

death (1 year ago). History of anxiety symptoms since adolescence, binge drinking as young adult, and depressive symptoms with death of grandmother and father. No prior history of psychiatric treatment or physical, sexual or domestic abuse. She is in good physical health. She is one of 4 children, a college graduate, and works as a teacher. Has adequate supports, although does not enlist help for self and has disengaged from community support systems. To begin individual cognitive behavioral therapy 1–2/week to manage anxiety and panic-related symptoms and escitalopram (Lexapro) 10 mg QD.

Diagnostic Formulation
Diagnoses:

- Panic Disorder—Diagnostic severity = severe; symptom severity = severe; psychosocial: potential job loss, death of father
- Differential: Generalized Anxiety Disorder—requires further evaluation
- Differential: Alcohol dependence—requires further evaluation; history of gastroesophageal reflux disorder
- WHODAS-2: disability score = mild disability in daily activities (Chapter 5).

Development of the Nursing Diagnosis

table 9-2

Problem statement	"Due to"	Etiology or related reason	"As evidenced by"	Signs, symptoms, or evidence of problem
Depression	due to	Death of spouse, onset of diabetes	as evidenced by	Depressed mood, poor concentration and attention, poor sleep (DFA, MNA), passive suicidal thought, social isolation, pessimism, low energy, staying in bed all day, anhedonia, irritability, tearfulness, loneliness
Alteration in mood, depressed	due to	Death of spouse, onset of diabetes	as evidenced by	Depressed mood, poor concentration and attention, poor sleep (DFA, MNA), passive suicidal thought, social isolation, pessimism, low energy, staying in bed all day, anhedonia, irritability, tearfulness, loneliness
Risk for metabolic syndrome and cardiovascular disease	due to	Familial risk factors, medication side effects, high-fat diet	as evidenced by	Family history of early cardiac death, quetiapine treatment of psychosis, and dietary excess of red meat and junk/snack foods

particular psychiatric diagnoses. In the preceding example, the nurse would assess the patient's use of substances and attempt to understand whether a DSM diagnosis of substance abuse or dependence is more appropriate. Although nurses do not make clinical diagnostic decisions unless they are at the advanced practice level, nurses are important contributors to the clinical team in understanding and accurately diagnosing the conditions that patients present with. *It is often the information, input, and insight of the clinical nursing staff that provides the evidence that enables advanced practice nurses or physicians to determine particular diagnoses.*

Nursing diagnoses are formulated in a specific manner, and they are identified in the same format as other areas of nursing. A strength of nursing diagnosis as compared to assignment of a DSM diagnosis (which is the same statement for most patients) is that the nursing diagnosis is specific to each particular patient, and reflects the holistic understanding of that person's difficulty. A well-specified nursing diagnosis should convey the most pertinent aspects of a patient's problems, symptoms, and need for care. A difference in diagnoses of psychiatric–mental health problems is that they may involve much more detail regarding the symptoms, precipitants, and patterns of behavior that commonly occur (Table 9-2).

The first part of the nursing diagnosis statement identifies the focal pattern, problem, or behavior that is observed. The focal point or problem is either named outright (e.g., depression), or termed as an alteration or impairment in normal function (e.g., alteration in mood, depressed). The second part of the nursing diagnosis identifies the nurse's assessment of the cause of the problem. It is often introduced in the statement with "due to" (e.g., alteration in mood, depressed, due to death of spouse and onset of chronic illness). If a physiologic cause is suspected, that is also identified. The third segment of the nursing diagnosis is the evidence or data that indicate or support the problem statement. Typically this segment is introduced with the statement "as evidenced by." The nurse then identifies the specific signs, symptoms, or behaviors associated with the problem. From this listing, the nurse is then able to design a care plan specific to the symptoms experienced by the patient. In this way, the well-formulated nursing

diagnosis drives the development of goals and interventions specific to the patient's needs. It should be noted that in some electronic health record systems, only the initial label or problem statement is identified. In cases such as this, the nurse communicates the assessment data supporting the diagnosis to provide background to others providing care for the patient.

Planning and Goal Setting

Once all nursing diagnoses are identified, the nurse identifies problems and their priority in care. This prioritization aids in identifying interventions that will be carried out immediately, compared with those that will be done sequentially after the more immediate priorities for care have been addressed. The planning phase involves identifying the outcomes and goals that the patient wants to achieve in care, and interventions that will support the patient in achieving each goal.

It is important to engage the patient as much as possible in identifying outcomes and setting goals of care (Figure 9-2). The *goal* is a

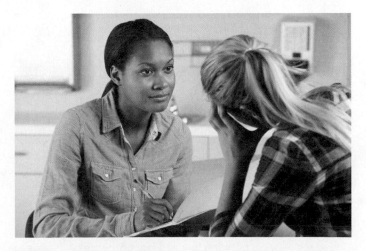

9-2 It is important to engage the patient as much as possible in developing the plan of care.

Source: Monkey Business/Fotolia

statement of what the nurse will assist the patient to achieve. The *outcome* is the description of the step toward change that the patient would like to accomplish; it includes specific measures indicating progress toward the goal. Goals are naturally related to outcomes. Both should be concrete and measurable so it is clear when the outcome and goal have been reached. For example, the following could be the nursing diagnosis, goals, and outcomes in a patient who is alcohol dependent and undergoing detoxification:

- *Nursing diagnosis:* Risk for seizure due to alcohol withdrawal evidenced by elevated blood pressure (BP), pulse (P), temperature (T), and anxiety.
- *Goal:* The patient and nurse will identify signs and symptoms of autonomic hyperactivity, delirium tremens, and alcohol hallucinosis.
- *Outcomes:* Vital signs will remain within normal limits (BP > 90/60, < 140/90; P 60–100 bpm; T 98–99.5°F). Patient will remain calm, oriented, and without hallucinations. No seizure activity.

Indicators of each outcome would be the actual assessment of the outcome: BP 130/70; P 80 bpm; T 99°F; mental status: calm;

oriented to person, place, date, and situation; and presence or absence of hallucinations. Note that indicators that offer the ability to identify the degree that each indicator is met as a way to review progress may also be used.

Pause and Reflect

Reflect on the case study featuring Claudine.

1. *What might be an appropriate nursing diagnosis for Claudine that focuses on a single health promotion need or risk factor?*
2. *What might be an appropriate nursing diagnosis that focuses on a cluster of related signs, symptoms, or behaviors?*
3. *Choose the diagnosis that you believe takes higher priority, and write it fully as depicted in Table 9-2. Then identify possible goals and outcomes. Include indicators for your outcomes.*

Implementation

Interventions are identified to support each goal or outcome. These interventions relate to several kinds of activities carried out by the nurse and patient. They may involve assessments made by the nurse or signs and symptoms as reported by the patient, or they may involve

Adjusting Nursing Care Over the Course of Treatment | table 9-3

	Crisis Stage	Acute Stage	Recovery Stage
Stage characteristics	• Symptoms are emergent and require intervention to prevent harm to patient or others; patient requires daily or inpatient level of care.	• Symptoms are acute, interfere with daily function, quality of life (QOL). Patient requires more frequent appointments, depending on symptom acuity and safety concerns.	• Residual symptoms remain. Patient is able to integrate self-care with role responsibilities. • Referrals are necessary to garner resources to support patient's independent function in the community. Appointments are less frequent.
Assessment	• Focus on safety and stabilization • How symptoms impair QOL	• Focus: What is the problem that brought patient to this setting? • What are associated symptoms? How do they impair QOL? • Consider safety to self and others.	• Focus on management of residual symptoms. What goals will enable patient to achieve full recovery and return to function? • Interpersonal, social, family, vocational, recreational, and spiritual needs are identified.
Diagnosis	• Address priority needs: safety and security first.	• Identify problems and disorders that require a focus in treatment.	• Address return to independent function, symptom management, support systems, and vocational needs.
Planning/ goals	• Maintain safety; stabilize symptoms and identify focus for future intervention.	• Identify priority issues and goals; focus on alleviating symptoms.	• Monitor and manage symptoms and behavior to prevent relapse; focus on independence and interpersonal and community function.
Intervention	• What level of care is required? How frequently does safety (e.g., suicidal or homicidal ideation; ability to care for own needs) require reassessment?	• Monitor safety (suicidal or homicidal ideation; self-care); assess and monitor symptoms; address priorities and goals.	• Monitor symptoms; identify resources and support to improve function, QOL; engage patient in problem solving and coping strategies; provide education to enable early identification of symptom recurrence.
Evaluation	• How stable are symptoms? Is planning for handling recurrence of symptoms in place? What safety needs still need to be met?	• Evaluate level of symptom interference with daily function and QOL. Ensure progress toward meeting goals, identify goals to further improve function.	• Evaluate coping, problem solving, and symptom recurrence. Evaluate progress toward interpersonal, social, familial, vocational, and spiritual goals.

activities to support meeting patient goals such as group or individual areas of counseling. They may also involve educational activities that help the patient to learn more about the health problem and how to prevent complications and manage his or her own care. Interventions are developed in a comprehensive manner to systematically manage the problems, needs, signs, and symptoms identified by the patient. Interventions should support the goals and outcomes collaboratively identified by both the nurse and patient. They should also designate activities the patient will follow through on as well as those for the nurse and other members of the team and the patient's support system.

A number of common nursing interventions are frequently used in psychiatric–mental health nursing practice. The most common problems encountered in psychiatric patients include depression, anxiety, sleep disorder, substance dependence and withdrawal, and psychosis. In some care plans, interventions are organized according to the "type" of intervention: diagnostic, therapeutic, or educational. These categories can be helpful when the nurse is planning care to include interventions of each type to address the problem. Diagnostic interventions involve assessment and evaluative actions by the nurse. Educational interventions provide patients with information to better understand their health and care and to learn ways to better maintain and promote their own health. Therapeutic interventions involve a wide variety of actions that are designed to move patients forward on their therapeutic goals. (See the Nursing Care Plan later in this chapter for examples of goals and interventions for a patient with anxiety.)

Evaluation

Goals and outcomes are evaluated regularly in the treatment process. Goals are specified for defined time periods, and outcomes allow the nurse to quantify the amount of progress the patient has made over that time period. When evaluating a goal, nurses tend to end up with a met versus not-met frame of reference, which is less effective at specifying the progress made toward meeting the goal. Use of outcomes allows the nurse to define the particular steps made toward improved health. It is expected that individuals will make gradual progress over time and that outcomes and goals will change. In some situations, the nurse recognizes that a goal or outcome may not be realistic or the focus of treatment changes such that a new goal with appropriate outcome measures must be defined.

The nursing process is a dynamic process, one in which assessment is continual, goals are renegotiated, and interventions adjusted to support the patient in meeting the mutually agreed-upon goals. If progress is not being made on a goal or outcome, then the nurse reassesses with the patient to determine whether changes can be made in the plan of care to better support patient needs. Table 9-3 illustrates how nurses adjust the care plan during the course of treatment.

SUMMARY

The nursing process is a foundation for nursing practice in all clinical settings. In the psychiatric mental health setting, the nurse assesses patient needs across the domains of wellness to determine

---

Claudine—A Patient With Anxiety   NURSING CARE PLAN

Nursing Diagnosis: Anxiety *related to* occupational, financial, and marital stressors *as evidenced by* anxiety (currently 7 of 10), muscle tension, restlessness, panic attacks (chest, shoulder and jaw pain, palpitations, tachycardia, hyperventilation, fear of dying, derealization), rumination (finances, marriage), decreased concentration, rapid speech, ambivalence, fatigue.

Goals

Within 4 weeks, patient will report:
- Decrease in anxiety level from 7 to 3
- Decrease in panic attack frequency from 2 times per week to 0 to 1 times per week
- Decrease in muscle tension, restlessness, rumination
- Improved concentration and decision making

Interventions

- Assess and have patient rate anxiety severity (0 = none, 10 = worst/most severe), including frequency of symptoms and panic attacks to monitor change and progress.
- Assess precipitants to increased anxiety symptoms; encourage patient to identify precipitants to anxiety and record in journal, with severity.
- Teach patient deep breathing and relaxation techniques, encourage daily use and practice, encourage use when anxiety symptoms and muscle tension increase.
- Assist patient to identify her own symptoms of increased anxiety and recognize them as target symptoms in need of active coping intervention.
- Assist patient to problem-solve related to financial, work, and marital stressors.
- Have patient develop a list of activities that are relaxing and enjoyable to aid in increasing her activity level; have patient integrate one activity into her schedule daily.
- Encourage patient to add 15- to 30-minute intervals of physical exercise (walking, biking, stretching) daily.
- Develop a list of coping strategies that help to reduce anxiety-related symptoms, encourage use of strategies daily with emergence of symptoms.
- Encourage patient to engage in journal writing to monitor symptoms, free mind of worries, and evaluate use of coping strategies.
- Evaluate use of medication(s) prescribed, assess for beneficial effects, side effects of treatment, and educate patient about use, action, and side effects of medication.

signs and symptoms, as well as behavior patterns and coping styles, to better understand the difficulties with which the patient presents. The nurse identifies problems using nursing diagnosis to provide a comprehensive summary of patient needs for intervention that drives the process of collaborative goal setting and identification of outcomes. Interventions are directly related to presenting problems and behavioral concerns, and promote progress toward meeting patient goals. The evaluation phase of the process allows for a reassessment of needs and continues planning with the patient to attain his or her goals.

This chapter also provides a fundamental overview of the psychosocial history and mental status exam completed by the nurse during the assessment phase. Subsequent chapters will review assessment pertinent to specific disorders and problems. In addition, each chapter presents sample plans of care to provide templates for planning and intervention.

Chapter Highlights

1. Elements of patient-centered care include respect for patients' values, preferences, and expressed needs; coordination and integration of care; information, communication, and education; physical comfort; emotional support; and involvement of family and friends.

2. The nursing process refers to the steps nurses use to identify needs for care; analyze, prioritize, and plan for intervention; and evaluate the nursing care that is delivered to patients.

3. The steps of the nursing process are assessment, diagnosis, planning, implementation, and evaluation.

4. Assessment informs the nursing process through the gathering of data, such as patient presenting concerns, demographic information, physical health history, and sociological considerations.

5. How the patient presents to the clinical setting—voluntarily or involuntarily—informs the nursing process.

6. The components of a mental status examination include appearance, attitude, and behavior; speech; emotional status; thought process; and cognitive functioning. These areas provide important information to the nurse regarding the patient's current levels of functioning.

7. The nursing diagnosis involves three components: identifying or naming the problem; the etiology of the problem; and the data that provide evidence of the problem or the signs and symptoms of the patient.

8. Developing the plan of care includes identifying goals and outcomes through a process of shared decision making with the patient.

9. Nursing interventions are activities carried out by the nurse and patient according to the plan of care.

10. Nurses must evaluate patient care according to the established outcomes, adjusting the plan as necessary during the course of treatment.

NCLEX®-RN Questions

1. The nurse educator is orienting a group of new nurses to the mental health unit. Which statement by the educator best represents the essential purpose of the nursing process in providing nursing care to patients experiencing mental illness?
   a. "The nursing process is what differentiates mental health nursing care from that of other professions."
   b. "The nursing process is a framework for planning and delivering holistic patient- and family-centered care."
   c. "The nursing process provides a structure for applying knowledge of mental illnesses and their management."
   d. "The nursing process provides a model for carrying out linear tasks that are intended to lead to a fixed patient outcome."

2. The nurse is carrying out an assessment of a patient presenting with a sudden onset of psychiatric symptoms. Which describes the best approach for the nurse to determine the priority concern for the patient?
   a. The nurse asks the patient directly why he or she is seeking treatment at this time.
   b. The nurse analyzes the patient's pre-setting background for evidence of a precipitating event.
   c. The nurse defers to the diagnosis made after all members of the team have interviewed the patient.
   d. The nurse refers to the primary symptoms identified in the *Diagnostic and Statistical Manual of Mental Disorders*, 5th edition (DSM-5).

3. The nurse is performing an assessment of a patient being admitted to the inpatient psychiatric unit. Which aspect of the pre-setting background would best assist the nurse to determine the patient's current interest and motivation in treatment?
   a. The patient's socioeconomic status and living situation
   b. The patient's and family's understanding of mental illness
   c. The patient's previous history of treatment for mental illness
   d. The patient's circumstances that led to the decision to seek treatment

4. The nurse is performing a mental status exam. Which technique would be best to determine the patient's affect?
   a. Having the patient complete a feelings rating scale
   b. Observing the patient's current behavioral presentation
   c. Asking the patient to describe his or her current emotional state
   d. Having the patient respond to a series of cognitive exercises

5. The nurse has completed an assessment of a patient presenting with acute mental health concerns. The nurse concludes that patient has an alteration in mood characterized by mania. Which component of the diagnostic statement will this finding comprise?
   a. The focal pattern
   b. The assessment of cause
   c. The supporting evidence
   d. The associated symptoms

6. The nurse is caring for a patient presenting with symptoms of anxiety that are interfering with the patient's ability to function at work. The patient states that the anxiety began soon after a traumatic event and is severely impacting the patient's functioning. Which issue will be the focal point for making a nursing diagnosis?
   a. Patient's anxiety due to exposure to a traumatic event
   b. Patient's difficulty coping
   c. Patient's inability to function at work due to underlying anxiety and stress
   d. Making a diagnosis of posttraumatic stress disorder

7. The nurse is carrying out the components of the planning phase for a patient experiencing a mood disorder. Which step will the nurse take first?
   a. Determine which problem will be addressed as the priority
   b. Determine which interventions will support the patient's goals
   c. Differentiate between collaborative and nursing interventions
   d. Identify what the nurse wants to achieve as a result of interventions

8. The nurse is evaluating the outcomes of interventions for a patient who is in the recovery phase of depression. Which finding best indicates that treatment goals have been met?
   a. The patient agrees to report suicidal thoughts.
   b. The patient has resumed occupational functioning.
   c. The patient manages increased interaction with peers.
   d. The patient identifies goals to improve further function.

9. The nurse is developing a plan of care for a patient experiencing an acute mental health crisis. Which action would be most likely to be carried out during the intervention phase of the illness?
   a. Ensuring the safety of the physical environment
   b. Performing vital signs and a mental status exam
   c. Determining what factors precipitated the crisis
   d. Identifying which problem the patient wants to focus on

Answers may be found on the Pearson student resource site: nursing.pearsonhighered.com

---

Pearson Nursing Student Resources Find additional review materials at **nursing.pearsonhighered.com**

References

American Psychiatric Association. (2013). *Diagnostic and Statistical Manual of Mental Disorders* (5th ed.). Washington, DC: American Psychiatric Publishers.

Bickley, L. S. (2012). *Bates' Guide to Physical Examination and History Taking* (11th ed.). Philadelphia, PA: WoltersKluwer Health | Lippincott Williams & Wilkins.

Brokel, J. & Heath, C. (2009). The value of nursing diagnoses in electronic health records. In T. H. Herdman, (Ed.). *Nursing Diagnoses: Definitions and Classification 2009–2011*. Singapore: Wiley-Blackwell.

Bulechek, G., Butcher, H., & Dochterman, J., (Eds.). (2008). *Nursing Interventions Classification (NIC)* (5th ed.). St. Louis, MO: Mosby Elsevier.

Carpenito-Moyet, L. J. (2009). *Nursing Care Plans and Documentation: Nursing Diagnoses and Collaborative Problems*. Philadelphia, PA: Lippincott Williams & Wilkins.

Gordon, M. (1982a). *Manual of Nursing Diagnosis*. New York, NY: McGraw-Hill.

Gordon, M. (1982b). *Nursing Diagnosis: Process and Application*. New York, NY: McGraw-Hill.

Gordon, M. (1998). Nursing nomenclature and classification system development. *Online Journal of Issues in Nursing*, www.nursingworld.org/oljin/tpc7/tpc7_1.htm

Herdman, T. H. (Ed.). (2012). *NANDA International Nursing Diagnoses: Definitions and Classification 20122014*. Oxford, England: Wiley-Blackwell.

Iowa Intervention Project. (1995). Validation and coding of the NIC taxonomy structure. *IMAGE: Journal of Nursing Scholarship, 27*(1), 43–49.

Institute of Medicine. (2001). *Crossing the Quality Chasm: A New Health System for the 21st Century*. Washington, DC: National Academy Press.

Johnson, M., Moorhead, S., Bulechek, G., Butcher, H., Maas, M., & Swanson, E. (2012). *NOC and NIC Linkages to NANDA-I and Clinical Conditions: Supporting Critical Reasoning and Quality Care* (3rd ed.). Maryland Heights, MO: Elsevier Mosby.

Kessler, R. C., Chiu, W. T., Demler, O., & Walters, E. E. (2005). Prevalence, severity, and comorbidity of 12-month DSM-IV disorders in the national comorbidity survey replication. *Archives of General Psychiatry, 62*(6), 617–627.

Lunney, M. (2014). Assessment, clinical judgment, and nursing diagnoses: How to determine accurate diagnoses. In T. H. Herdman, (Ed.). *Nursing Diagnoses: Definitions and Classification 2012–2014*. Oxford, England: Wiley, pp 71–89.

Maizes, V., Rakel, D., & Niemiec, C. (2009). Integrative medicine and patient-centered care. Commissioned for the IOM Summit on Integrative Medicine and the Health of the Public. Available at http://www.iom.edu/~/media/Files/Activity%20Files/Quality/IntegrativeMed/Integrative%20Medicine%20and%20Patient%20Centered%20Care.pdf

Moorhead, S., Johnson, M., Maas, M., & Swanson, E. (Eds.). (2008). *Nursing Outcomes Classification (NOC)* (4th ed.). St. Louis, MO: Mosby Elsevier.

North American Nursing Diagnosis Association. Website link: http://www.nanda.org/

Nursing Interventions Classification (NIC). Website link: http://www.nursing.uiowa.edu/cncce/nursing-interventions-classification-overview

Nursing Outcome Classification (NOC). Website link: http://www.nursing.uiowa.edu/cncce/nursing-outcomes-classification-overview

Orlando, I. J. (1961). *Dynamic Nurse Patient Relationship: Function, Process, and Principles*. New York, NY: Putnam.

Ormel, J., Petukhova, M., Chatterji, S., Aguilar-Gaxiola, S., Alonso, J., Angermeyer, M. C. et al. (2008). Disability and treatment of specific mental and physical disorders across the world. *British Journal of Psychiatry, 192*, 368–375.

Seidel, H. M., Ball, J. W., Dains, J. E., Flynn, J. A., Solomon, B. S., & Stewart, R. W. (2011). *Mosby's Guide to Physical Examination* (7th ed.). St. Louis, MO: Mosby Elsevier.

World Health Organization. (2004). Global burden of disease 2004. Available at http://www.who.int/healthinfo/global_burden_disease/GBD_report_2004update_AnnexA.pdf

10 Ethical and Legal Concepts

Natasha Maynard Thomas

Key Terms

Learning Outcomes

1. Discuss the importance of the American Nurses Association's Code of Ethics for Nurses.

2. Contrast the ethical principles of autonomy, beneficence, nonmaleficence, justice, and veracity.

3. Summarize each of the major ethical theories applicable to nursing.

4. Identify major steps in ethical decision making.

5. Discuss important state and federal laws relevant to patients with mental illness.

6. Distinguish between privacy and confidentiality.

7. Compare and contrast the different types of psychiatric hospital admissions.

8. Examine major legal and ethical dilemmas in psychiatric–mental health nursing practice.

Jason Relapse Phase

APPLICATION

1. What potential legal and ethical concerns do you identify in Jason's case?

2. What other concerns do you have at this time?

You are assigned to a clinical rotation in an urban emergency department (ED). Your first patient, Jason Crander, is a 23-year-old Caucasian male with a history of paranoid schizophrenia and self-mutilating behaviors. He is not compliant with his medication regimen and consistently refuses voluntary psychiatric hospitalization. According to the chart, the local police brought Jason to the hospital after he resisted arrest for disturbing the peace. Jason was yelling obscenities at passersby on a busy street corner while wielding a broken bottle. Upon admission to the ED, Jason resisted medical evaluation and repeatedly attempted to kick and bite staff. He was restrained and received 10 mg of haloperidol (Haldol).

Now much calmer, Jason asks that you remove his wrist restraints: "They're hurting me." He does not appear dangerous at this time. You ask a veteran nurse about the restraints, and she instructs you to leave the restraints in place: "We're short-staffed tonight—and don't be fooled, Jason will swing at you in a minute."

You inform Jason that you are unable to remove the restraints. He responds, "If you don't take these things off of me, I'm suing you and everybody in this place." The tenor in his voice frightens you. A seasoned nurse hears the commotion and, with the help of security, administers another 5 mg of haloperidol (Haldol) as Jason kicks and screams, "No! No! No!" As you exit the room to look for your preceptor, Jason's parents enter the ED, demanding to know their son's condition and insisting that he be committed.

Introduction

Nurses outrank all other professionals—including other health care providers—with respect to the public's perception of their honesty and ethical conduct (Newport, 2012) (Figure 10-1). This profound trust results, in part, from the nurse's obligation to provide clinically competent, patient-centered care in accordance with ethical and legal principles. Sound clinical care is consistent with established nursing standards and evidence-based practice. The American Nurses Association's (ANA's) **Code of Ethics for Nurses** with Interpretive Statements mandates every professional nurse's obligations and commitment to society (ANA, 2001). To comply with legal and regulatory requirements, nurses must possess an understanding of the decisions and guidelines that shape nursing practice from various governmental, quasi-governmental, funding, and accrediting agencies.

In clinical practice, ethical and legal standards are intertwined, yet distinct. In general, ethics dictate what nurses "should" do, whereas laws mandate what nurses "must" do. The term *ethics* derives from the Greek term *ethos*, which refers to character. In practice, *ethics* refers to moral tenets that characterize conduct as right or wrong and reflects individual or societal values. As an area of study, ethics is a branch of philosophy that examines the moral standards or principles

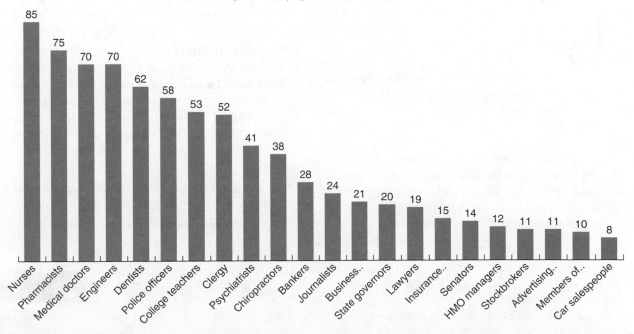

Honesty and Ethics
Percent of respondent saying "very high" or "high" in Gallup Poll

Nurses	85
Pharmacists	75
Medical doctors	70
Engineers	70
Dentists	62
Police officers	58
College teachers	53
Clergy	52
Psychiatrists	41
Chiropractors	38
Bankers	28
Journalists	24
Business..	21
State governors	20
Lawyers	19
Insurance..	15
Senators	14
HMO managers	12
Stockbrokers	11
Advertising..	11
Members of..	10
Car salespeople	8

10-1 Nurses outrank all other professionals in public perception of honesty and ethics.

Data from Newport, F. (2012). Nurses have the highest honesty rating. Retrieved from http://www.gallup.com/poll/159035/congress-retains-low-honesty-rating.aspx and http://www.gallup.com/file/poll/159041/Honesty_Ethics_121203.pdf

that shape decisions. *Nursing ethics* address how nurses determine the appropriate course of action in day-to-day clinical practice.

Laws are rules that organize society and regulate behavior. At their core, they specify minimum standards of conduct. Laws are enforceable in court, and, if necessary, by police power. Ethical standards, in contrast, are more ambitious and aspirational. Nurses study ethics to become better providers in the face of routinely difficult professional and personal choices. Ethics violations are policed by professional organizations or state nursing boards, but are legally enforceable only to the degree that they are incorporated into laws.

In practice, laws and ethics typically reflect and reinforce each other. A nurse's duty to maintain patient confidentiality is consistent with standard clinical, legal, and ethical practice. Often, however, ethical and legal mandates do not neatly align—for example, when a nurse feels compelled to provide care that may be inconsistent with a patient's expressed wishes or when a nurse is prevented from providing needed care. In these circumstances, nurses ask, "What should I do?"

In practice, many nurses find ethical and legal quandaries challenging, if not distressing. This is especially true in psychiatric–mental health nursing. Why? Because psychiatric care is unique. It is one of very few areas of health care in which potentially coercive interventions—such as forced hospitalization or medication administration—are, in certain circumstances, ethically and legally permissible, if not required, to protect patients or others from harm (Sheehan & Burns, 2011). Consequently, perhaps more than any other nursing specialty, psychiatric nurses must regularly weigh the obligation to protect the rights of vulnerable patients against potentially competing obligations to uphold personal, professional, and societal interests. In striking this balance, nurses must know "the Code of Ethics, standards of practice of the profession, relevant federal, state and local laws and regulations, and the employing organization's policies and procedures" (ANA, 2001, p. 14). Acquiring such knowledge is a process that—in keeping with the public's trust in the nursing profession—requires every psychiatric nurse's ongoing commitment to learn the unique ethical and legal particulars of the clinical environment.

To that end, this chapter reviews the most frequent and distressing ethical challenges of psychiatric nursing care, nursing values, and the ethical principles of autonomy, beneficence, nonmaleficence, justice, and veracity in the context of ethical decision making. In addition, it provides an overview of mental health patients' legal rights, including the issues of informed consent, privacy, involuntary hospitalization, and the limited right of patients to refuse treatment, as well as affirmative nursing duties and liabilities. The ultimate goal is to orient the aspiring nurse to the basic ethical and legal issues in day-to-day care and provide the groundwork for navigating such issues in clinical practice.

Ethical Frameworks

Psychiatric–mental health nurses confront a host of ethical issues in daily practice. Beauchamp and Childress define a moral or ethical dilemma as "circumstances in which moral obligations demand or appear to demand that a person adopt each of two (or more) alternative but incompatible actions, such that the person cannot perform all the required actions" (2009, pp. 10–11). Ethical dilemmas present both challenges and opportunities to exercise personal and professional integrity. Common examples of ethical issues in psychiatric nursing include the following:

- Hospitalizing, restraining, or medicating patients against their will
- Telling "white lies" to patients in an effort to "protect" their feelings
- Confronting constraints to delivering care believed to be in the patients' best interests
- Reporting the misconduct of a provider colleague

Resolving ethical conflicts requires nurses understand and be able to apply basic bioethical principles and theories. Nurses must also become aware of their values while adhering to applicable ethical nursing standards.

Ethical Standards

The Florence Nightingale Pledge (Box 10-1) was considered the first ethical standard for nurses. Composed in 1893 by a committee headed by Lystra Gretter of the Farrand Training School for Nurses in Detroit, the vow was reportedly derived from the Hippocratic Oath, the ethical pledge taken by physicians.

At one time, it was common for nurses to state such a pledge upon entry into the profession. Although dated, the pledge speaks to nursing's rich ethical tradition. It addresses many of the fundamental ethical principles, including fidelity, confidence, and competence relevant to modern practice (Miracle, 2009). Other concepts—most notably, subservience to physicians—have been expressly recanted.

ANA Code of Ethics

In 1926, the ANA provisionally adopted and published a "Suggested Code" in the *American Journal of Nursing*. Since then, nursing ethical guidelines have been revised and amended numerous times. In 2001, the ANA adopted the most recent guidelines for nursing practice in the Code for Ethics for Nurses with Interpretive Statements. It serves as a guide for all nurses, regardless of level or setting, and includes the following:

- A succinct statement of the ethical obligations and duties of every individual who enters the nursing profession
- The profession's nonnegotiable ethical standard

The Florence Nightingale Pledge   box 10-1

"I solemnly pledge myself before God and in the presence of this assembly, to pass my life in purity and to practice my profession faithfully. I will abstain from whatever is deleterious and mischievous, and will not take or knowingly administer any harmful drug. I will do all in my power to maintain and elevate the standard of my profession, and will hold in confidence all personal matters committed to my keeping and all family affairs coming to my knowledge in the practice of my calling. With loyalty will I endeavor to aid the physician in his work, and devote myself to the welfare of those committed to my care."

- An expression of nursing's own understanding of its commitment to society (ANA, 2001)

The Code of Ethics does not provide nurses with the "right" answers to the ethical challenges faced in practice. Rather, it is intended to provide a framework to guide nurses in solving ethical conflicts. The Code of Ethics is a dynamic text. The nine stated ethical provisions are relatively fixed, but the interpretive statements are subject to more frequent revision. In an effort to address current challenges faced by nurses, for instance, interpretive statements discuss nurses' efforts to preserve personal and professional integrity via conscientious objection and whistle blowing, as well as collective action as a means to improving working conditions.

ANA Scope and Standards

The ANA requires specific competencies for psychiatric–mental health nurses outlined in *Psychiatric–Mental Health Nursing: Scope and Standards of Practice* (ANA, APNA, ISPN, 2014). Standard 12 identifies ethics competencies for both the psychiatric–mental health registered nurse and the advanced practice nurse. The ethical competencies outlined by the ANA address the nature of the therapeutic relationship, including maintenance of confidentiality; the role of the nurse as an advocate; and the nurse's responsibility for reporting illegal or impaired practice, as well as other standards of professional performance (ANA, APNA, ISPN, 2014).

Other Ethical Obligations

In addition to the ANA Code of Ethics, nurses should be familiar with the International Council of Nurses' (ICN's) ethical guidance. The ICN Code of Ethics for Nurses identifies four principal elements that outline the standards of ethical conduct: Nurses have fundamental responsibilities to promote health, prevent illness, restore health, and alleviate suffering (ICN, 2012).

In addition to specific nursing ethics articulated by the ANA and ICN, nurses are also obligated to comply with ethical mandates of the organizations or agencies in which they practice. Governmental and quasi-governmental agencies, as well as professional, consumer, and accrediting organizations, have ethical codes to which nurses must adhere in the course of practice with such organizations. Examples include the variety of patients' rights conferred by the Joint Commission, the Centers for Medicare and Medicaid Services, and the American Hospital Association.

Authority of Ethical Codes

Nurses are professionally obligated to comply with ethical standards to uphold nursing's commitment to society, as well as the integrity of the individual nurse and the profession. Lachman reports that the Code of Ethics for Nurses is "grossly underutilized in everyday nursing practice" because nurses fail to recognize their professional obligations (2007, p. 132). "Individuals who become nurses are expected not only to adhere to the ideals and moral norms of the profession but also to embrace them as part of what it means to be a nurse" (ANA, 2001, p. 5).

Although not all ethical violations may be enforceable by courts of law, as a practical matter many ethical violations have corresponding legal liability. Regardless of legal liability, nurses who violate ethical standards may be subject to disciplinary action by state licensing boards, as well as employing or professional organizations. Equally important, nurses who engage in unethical practice may experience career-jeopardizing distress as a result of sacrificing their personal and professional integrity.

Pause and Reflect

1. *What do you think of the Nightingale Pledge?*
2. *What would you include in a modern-day pledge?*
3. *What conflicts between ethical and legal mandates have you already encountered or observed?*

Ethical Principles

The ethical principles of autonomy, beneficence, nonmaleficence, justice, veracity, and fidelity are used to guide nurses' preferred conduct (Figure 10-2). These principles reflect the inherent dignity of all persons; nurses may use these concepts to clarify what should be done in a particular situation. These principles provide basic tools to approaching nursing ethical dilemmas.

The ethical principle of **autonomy** refers to an individual's right to self-determination with freedom over oneself and one's affairs. From patients' perspectives, autonomy is the right to direct their own care and make independent decisions consistent with their personal values. Providers exercise the greatest respect for a patient's autonomy when they honor a patient's choice with which they (the providers) disagree. Nurses advance patient autonomy when they facilitate informed decision making. Nurses also maintain their own autonomy when they provide care consistent with their own professional judgment (Box 10-2).

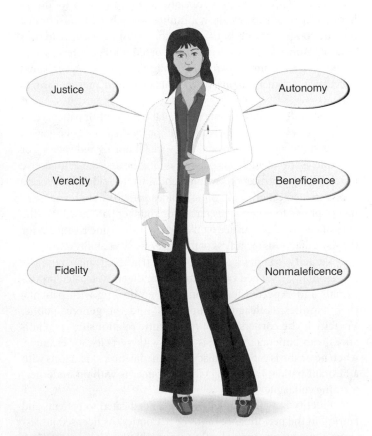

10-2 The ethical principles of autonomy, beneficence, nonmaleficence, justice, veracity, and fidelity guide nurses' conduct.

Nursing Autonomy

box 10-2

Nursing autonomy refers to a nurse's ability to provide care consistent with the nurse's professional judgment and with professional practice standards and state and federal laws. As members of interprofessional teams, nurses may work alongside other providers who may not understand or appreciate the independent contribution of nursing professionals. Nurses who are unable to maintain their professional and personal integrity are more vulnerable to dissatisfaction, stress, and burnout.

Beneficence refers to the nurse's moral obligation to "do good." Promoting "good" is typically defined as advancing the autonomous interests of the patient. A nurse demonstrates beneficence when advocating on behalf of a patient. For example, if a patient complains of excess sedation after taking a particular medication, beneficence requires the nurse to confer with the treatment team regarding less-sedating alternatives.

Paternalism is a concept similar to beneficence, under which providers also intend to "do good." Beauchamp and Childress define paternalism as "the intentional overriding of one person's preferences or actions by another person, where the person who overrides justifies this action by appeal to the goal of benefiting or of preventing or mitigating the harm to the person whose preferences or actions are overridden" (2009, p. 208). Paternalism is typically justified as being in the patients' or society's best interests. It frequently occurs when patients are considered incapable of making decisions, such as when psychiatric symptoms impair decision making. The risk of paternalism, however, is that the nurse or health care team may inappropriately negate the decision-making ability of those whom society seeks to protect.

Nonmaleficence refers to a provider's obligation to "do no harm." It is an affirmative duty, meaning not only that nurses must provide competent care, but also that they must be attentive to risks of harm. Adherence to evidence-based practice reflects the desire to protect patients from harm. A nurse's obligation to report an impaired colleague is another example of how nurses actively prevent harm to patients.

Justice mandates the fair and equal treatment of patients and others. Determinations of what is "just" or "fair" can be quite gray, as they are influenced by personal and societal norms and values. For example, is it preferable for patients on public assistance to receive less-expensive medications with potentially more side effects, or no access to medication at all? Should older patients have fewer treatment options to preserve resources for younger patients? From the patient's perspective, justice would demand the same treatment for the same diagnosis regardless of the patient's age or ability to pay.

Veracity is a nurse's obligation to be truthful, transparent, and forthcoming. As stated earlier, nurses are the most trusted professionals and expected to be honest when dealing with patients, their families, colleagues, employers, and the general public. Veracity is the cornerstone of therapeutic relationships and alliances with patients. A nurse is acting with veracity, for example, when he or she is candid in discussing medication side effects with a hesitant patient or sharing clinical concerns with an underperforming colleague.

Fidelity is a nurse's obligation to be dedicated to patients and faithful in the performance of his or her duties. As licensed professionals, nurses are individually accountable for their practice. A nurse demonstrates loyalty by practicing evidence-based, patient-centered care. Together, veracity and fidelity are essential to developing trusting, therapeutic relationships with patients.

Pause and Reflect

1. *Thinking back to the opening case study, what ethical standards apply to nurses caring for Jason?*
2. *Which ethical principles have implications for the nurses caring for Jason? Why?*
3. *Why are veracity and fidelity so important to developing trusting, therapeutic relationships with patients?*

Ethical Theories

Ethical theories are sets of moral concepts or belief systems that provide a framework or structure for prioritizing one ethical principle over another. There are various ethical theories, and no one theory explains all behavior. Instead, clinicians are challenged to balance the diversity of values in various theories. Theories particularly applicable to nursing include deontology, utilitarianism, the ethics of care, and virtue ethics.

Deontology is derived from the Greek word *deon* for duty. Under this theory, ethical behavior is characterized by adherence to unchanging, self-evident moral duty. For this reason, deontology is also referred to as *rule-based ethics*. Motive, such as fulfillment of the duty to be honest, rather than consequence, determines the moral "rightness" of a particular course of action. Nurses operate in this framework when they make a decision because "it's the right (moral) thing to do." Aiken (2004, p. 117) notes examples of deontological standards encountered in nursing ethics:

- "Humans should always be treated as ends and never as means."
- "Human life has value."
- "One is always to tell the truth."
- "Above all in health care, do no harm."
- "The human person has a right to self-determination."
- "All persons are of equal value."

Utilitarianism, in contrast, focuses on the consequences of an action, with good or pleasure as the ethical imperative. Utilitarianism is associated with the concepts of "the greatest good for the greatest number" and "the end justifies the means." Under this theory, morality is a function of benefit or outcome: morally right approaches promote happiness; morally wrong actions diminish happiness. Utilitarian principles often guide health care decision-making situations that focus on the distribution of finite resources. Triage, for example, involves the prioritization of care based on assessments of patients' survivability. Managed care, in theory, similarly aims to allocate resources efficiently to increase the potential benefit to the largest group of covered patients in need of care.

Whereas utilitarianism and deontological theories view impartial reasoning and justice as drivers of moral action, the **ethics of care** identifies empathy and emotional connectedness as dictating moral behavior. Morality under this theory is grounded in the context of relationships. Moral choices reflect recognition of our interdependence and the responsibility to accommodate individual care needs.

Virtue ethics dates back to the ancient Greek philosophers Aristotle and Plato. Whereas deontology and utilitarianism are concerned primarily with actions, virtue ethics asks: "What kind of person should I be? Is this action consistent with my being the person I wish to be?" This inquiry will affect how nurses apply their personal and professional values in practice.

Pause and Reflect

1. *Which of these theories have you seen applied in nursing care? How have they been applied in those instances?*
2. *Why are clinicians "challenged to balance the diversity of values in various theories"?*

Ethical Decision Making

Ethical dilemmas occur frequently in health care settings (Box 10-3). Although nursing education highlights essential clinical skills and evidence-based practices, it does not ensure competence with respect to ethical decision making. Finding workable solutions to inevitable ethical conflicts requires the development of a unique skill set. Roberts and Dyer (2004) identify essential ethical skills for clinical practice. A mnemonic to help students remember the ethical skills in clinical practice as established by Roberts and Dyer is PILLAR:

P—the ability to appreciate how one's PERSONAL experiences, knowledge, and values may affect patient care

I—the ability to IDENTIFY ethical issues in patient care

L—the ability to appreciate and work within professional LIMITATIONS

L—the ability to LESSEN the LIKELIHOOD of future ethical dilemmas

A—the ability to ANTICIPATE ethical problems

R—the ability to access needed RESOURCES (information/expertise) to clarify and resolve conflict

Ethical decision making involves a deliberate approach to problem solving, rather than simply revealing the "right" answer. Ethical frameworks will help nurses organize their thought processes and avoid reliance on factors that might jeopardize patient care and nursing integrity. Potentially inappropriate influences on decision making include emotion or deference to other providers.

Numerous decision-making models exist to assist nurses in approaching ethical issues. No model reveals the "right" answer; rather, each serves to remind nurses of salient issues to consider. Prominent themes gleaned from various ethical decision-making models can be found in Table 10-1, which uses a mnemonic for ethical decision making: DILEMMA.

Ethical decision making often involves *compromise*, or a balance between unattractive alternatives. How nurses strike this balance is a function of their values. **Values** are the ideals that assign meaning to our decisions. Our values, in essence, tip the scale in one direction or the other when we are confronted with choices. **Integrity** is the ability to consistently adhere to character-resonating values. Some of the most challenging legal and ethical issues confronted by nurses involve threats to personal and professional integrity. Threats to integrity include requests to deceive patients, withhold information, or falsify records. Verbal abuse and requests that the nurse behave in a way that goes against the Code of Ethics also are considered threats to integrity (ANA, 2001).

In the course of resolving ethical dilemmas, nurses must often identify **integrity-preserving compromises**. These are positions or actions that simultaneously account for potentially conflicting alternatives and assist the nurse in resolving conflicts. Integrity-preserving compromises require that nurses understand their professional and legal obligations and have assessed their own and others' values (Box 10-4). Values are dynamic factors that influence how we make decisions. They are the standards that confront and give meaning to facts and circumstances. They are reflected in our attitudes and beliefs, and they evolve as our knowledge and experience expand.

Examples of Frequent Ethical Dilemmas   box 10-3

- Abigail is a feisty 89-year-old widow. She has been living alone for more than twenty years. A former attorney, Abigail is fiercely independent. Her only adult child is deceased. Abigail is admitted to the emergency department for smoke inhalation after a small kitchen fire. She admits that she forgot to turn off the oven and that her memory "isn't what it used to be." Members of the treatment team express concern about whether Abigail is safe alone at home. She insists on immediate release. *Should the nurse process the discharge?*
- Joseph was diagnosed with bipolar disorder in his early twenties. He resisted treatment until he was placed on probation for stealing a car and engaging in a police chase that injured two pedestrians. He has been stable on lithium for more than 15 years. Recently, however, he has been complaining that he no longer needs the medication. *Should he be forced to continue taking medication?*
- Jim is a nurse on an inpatient psychiatric unit. After three months of "chatting" with Sarah on an online social

networking website, they decide to meet in person. As he approaches their meeting place, he recognizes Sarah as a former patient from the unit. *Does he proceed with the date?*
- Sam is a 78-year-old widower of one year. Last month he fell and broke his hip. He has been increasingly depressed since his admission to the nursing home, refusing physical therapy and meals. He has lost 10% of his body weight in the past month and is increasingly weak. The treatment team recommends an antidepressant. Sam refuses. A staff member suggests placing the pill in Sam's daily applesauce, which Sam happily consumes. *Should the nurse administer the antidepressant to Sam in this manner?*
- A nurse observes a co-worker charting care that was not performed. She had confronted the co-worker regarding similar concerns just last week. At that time, the co-worker responded that inadequate staffing leaves her unable to provide care as ordered. *What should the nurse do next?*

Guidelines for Ethical Decision Making   table 10-1

D	Describe the conflict	What is the dilemma? What is the nature of the ethical conflict? When is the deadline for a decision? Identify any conflict in your personal or professional values with those of the patient, agency, and/or society.
I	Identify stakeholders and their values and obligations	Who is involved? Who is the primary decision maker? Who is affected by the decision? Who is able to consent? What are the rights, values, and obligations of stakeholders? Who might be consulted?
L	Learn background information	What information is known? What information is needed? What are the relevant nursing evidence-based practices? Are there relevant ethical and legal standards? Are there relevant policies or procedures? What available resources exist?
E	Explore options	What are the alternatives? Solicit input from others/colleagues, managers/ethics committee. Adopt a broad perspective and consider creative possibilities. Identify the likely consequences of each option.
M	Moral hierarchy	What is the basis for choosing among alternatives? Evaluate options by applying relevant ethical principles and theories including perceiving options as ones that lead to: • The nurse being the person he or she wishes to be (virtue) • The greatest good for the greatest number (utilitarianism) • Equal treatment for all people (justice) • Fulfillment of duty to stakeholders (deontology) Identify how your values or feelings might be affecting your ethical approach. Identify why each option is more or less acceptable/feasible.
M	Make decision	What action will be taken? While acknowledging legal requirements and social expectations, identify rationale for action to be taken. Maintain accountability: How would you defend your action if required to do so? Anticipate objections and consider your response. Failure to make a decision is, in fact, a decision in itself. Identify and collaborate with others needed to execute the action. Assess personal/professional risks inherent in decision (e.g., potential disciplinary action or threats to integrity)
A	Act and assess	What was the impact? Was the goal achieved? Would you choose another course of action in the future? Identify, if necessary, system measures that should be implemented to address the ethical conflict.

Based on Curtin, L. L. (1978). A proposed critical model for ethical analysis. *Nursing Forum, 17,* 12–17; Chally, P. S., & Loriz, L. (1998). Ethics in the trenches: Decision making in practice. *American Journal of Nursing, 96,* 17–20; Velasquez, M., Moberg, D., Meyer, D., Shanks, T., McLean, M., DeCosse, D., André, C., & Hanson, K. (2009). A framework for thinking ethically. Available at http://www.scu.edu/ethics/practicing/decision/framework.html; Taft, S. H. (2000). An inclusive look at the domain of ethics and its application to administrative behavior. *Online Journal of Issues in Nursing, 6.* Available at http://www.nursingworld.org/MainMenuCategories/ANAMarketplace/ANAPeriodicals/OJIN/TableofContents/Volume62001/No1Jan01/ArticlePreviousTopic/DomainofEthics.html; Gilliland, M. (2010). A systematic approach to ethical decision-making for nurses confronted with ethical problems involving elder abuse. *Health Careers Today,* (August), 16–23.

Patients are entitled to receive care consistent with their own values. Nurses, in turn, must recognize their own value systems to prevent unduly influencing or interfering with patient care or preferences. Similarly, nurses must collaborate with providers who hold potentially unique or competing values. Nurses who understand their personal and professional values will be better positioned to respect patient preferences; anticipate and effectively manage provider conflicts; engage in deliberative assessments when confronted with difficult decisions; and, if necessary, take moral action with full awareness of the potential consequences.

Values Clarification Exercise

box 10-4

Because interpersonal and professional value conflicts are almost inevitable, nurses increase their self-awareness and decision-making preparedness by proactively engaging in *values clarification*, a process that involves identifying and prioritizing the unarticulated beliefs that drive decision making. To start this process, identify which is most important to you between the following options:

Career *or* family

Prestige *or* purpose

Personal freedom *or* respect for authority

Creativity *or* conformity

Self-sufficiency *or* sense of community

Accuracy *or* demonstrated effort

Honesty (veracity) *or* sparing another's feelings (nonmaleficence)

Improving patient care *or* avoiding conflict

Do you see a pattern in the items you identified as important? What implications do these choices have for you as a nurse?

Ethical dilemmas can be stressful. Consequently, it is wise to be familiar with available resources in advance. In addition to the ANA Code of Ethics and related ANA publications, other potential resources for ethical problem solving include colleagues, nursing supervisors and mentors, employer/facility ethical policies and committees, and clergy members or spiritual advisors.

Hospital ethics committees are an important resource for nurses. Initially sparked by end-of-life ethical issues that resulted in significant litigation, ethics committees were eventually included in accreditation requirements aimed at protecting patient rights and ensuring mechanisms for addressing ethical concerns. In practice, these committees are intended to provide a neutral forum for the discussion of ethical issues and resolution of conflicts; develop and monitor policies that impact ethical issues; and educate committee and staff members about ethical concerns. Common topics of discussion include allocation of health care resources, involuntary/futile care, and informed consent.

Committee composition varies by facility but generally includes clinicians (including nurses), administration, community, and patient representation. In addition to or in lieu of an ethics committee, some facilities have a dedicated ethics consultant who provides and coordinates consultations. Most facilities actively inform staff and patients of specific procedures for contacting the committee or initiating an ethics consult. Anonymous hotlines are not uncommon. Nurses who are unaware of these procedures or are interested in participating in their facility's committee should confer with their supervisor or human resources representative.

Pause and Reflect

1. *Why is the ability to anticipate ethical dilemmas important?*
2. *How can nurses lessen the likelihood of future ethical dilemmas?*

Referring to the scenario given at the beginning of the chapter and to the guidelines in Table 10-1:

3. *Who are the stakeholders involved in Jason's care?*
4. *As a nurse assigned to care for Jason, what additional information would you want to know about Jason?*

Legal and Regulatory Frameworks

Psychiatric nurses provide care in a complicated health care system. Much of the complexity is due to the fact that the patchwork of laws and regulations affecting the quality, oversight, and financing of care derives from multiple levels of government—federal, state, and local—each with separate but equal executive, legislative, and judicial branches. This power-sharing system is often referred to as *checks and balances*. Federal and state entities may vest their authority in or partner with quasi-governmental or private entities with subject matter expertise in accomplishing identified mandates. Examples include accrediting organizations and the role of state boards of nursing for local nursing oversight.

Although not laws per se, contractual obligations and requirements mandated by payors and accrediting bodies are key considerations that shape the delivery of care. Accrediting organizations include the Joint Commission and the Commission on Accreditation of Rehabilitation Facilities. These entities evaluate provider compliance with state, federal, and private payor safety and quality mandates.

Accreditation is not a legal requirement. It is often, however, a requirement for provider licensing or reimbursement. Failure to comply with specific guidelines and standards of care may not be a violation of law, but may indicate lapses in quality that create safety concerns and jeopardize reimbursement.

State and Local Laws

The laws affecting mental health care are primarily state laws. State laws vary significantly. Consequently, nurses must be aware of laws in the particular state in which they practice.

Nursing practice is authorized and guided by individual state statutes; each state has its own **Nurse Practice Act** (NPA). Among other important provisions, each state's NPA proscribes licensing requirements, permitted nursing titles, and functions composing the legal scope of practice in that state. State boards of nursing (discussed later) are empowered to regulate nursing practice and may publish guidelines, hold hearings, and issue rulings that impact a nurse's ability to practice.

Provided they are not inconsistent with federal law, other important state laws affecting care of patients with mental illness are listed here and discussed in greater detail later in this chapter:

- Specific procedures requiring and regarding informed consent
- Standards for involuntary commitment
- Patients' right to refuse medication
- Other civil rights of patients
- Insanity defense
- Privacy protections

Federal Laws Affecting Care of Patients with Mental Illness

table 10-2

Health Insurance Portability and Accountability Act (HIPAA) of 1996	Federal law explicitly addressing patient privacy.
Patient Self-Determination Act (PSDA)	Requires providers to give patients written notice of their right to direct and participate in their treatment, including the right to refuse treatment.
Mental Health Bill of Rights	A congressional model that states have adopted to varying degrees.
Mental Health Parity and Addiction Equity Act	Requires health plans to cover mental health and substance abuse treatment on par with the treatment of nonpsychiatric medical conditions.
Protection and Advocacy for Mentally Ill Individuals Act of 1986	Augments state funds with federal funds if states appoint a specific agency with broad authority to advocate on behalf of and investigate suspected or reported abuse and neglect of individuals with mental illness.
Patient Protection and Affordable Care Act	This law does not specifically address mental health. However, when fully implemented, it is expected to increase access to currently uninsured Americans, of which individuals with mental illness are disproportionately represented.

- Psychiatric advanced directives
- Exceptions to confidentiality
  - Duty to warn
  - Mandatory reporting of patient abuse or impaired colleagues
- Existence of any nurse–patient privilege
- The use of restraint/seclusion
- Civil and criminal liability for nursing practice

This is not an exhaustive list. All nurses should become aware of the relevant laws in their state of practice by conferring with a reliable source such as their agency's legal office, a local law librarian, or a health law attorney.

Federal Laws

Despite the predominance of state law governing mental health care, federal laws are supreme. Thus, a federal law will "trump" a conflicting state law. However, federal power also is limited. Provided they do not violate federal law, state laws govern the day-to-day lives of citizens. This structure reflects a fundamental national preference against concentration of power, for checks and balances, as well as for government to reflect the "will of the people." Overarching federal legislation that affects care of mental health patients includes the Health Insurance Portability and Accountability Act of 1996 (HIPAA) and the Patient Self-Determination Act (PSDA) (Table 10-2).

As citizens and providers, nurses must comply simultaneously with federal and state laws. In practice, these laws often work in tandem, with the state law elaborating on the details of a federal law. For example, federal laws require that individuals facing involuntary psychiatric hospitalization receive due process. The specific requirements of due process, however, are a matter of state law. Moreover, state law may preexist a federal law covering the same subject matter. Federal privacy laws, for example, preempt conflicting state privacy laws. State privacy laws that are more protective of patient rights, however, govern privacy practices as long as they do not conflict with the federal law. Whether a state violates federal law is a matter of interpretation that is played out in the courts of the judicial branch.

Types of Laws

In addition to distinguishing between state and federal laws, laws are also broadly categorized by subject matter. *Criminal laws* are enforced by government entities and seek to protect the public from undesirable or dangerous conduct. Actions against nurses that fall into this category include falsification of medical records, diversion (stealing drugs), certain HIPAA violations (such as knowingly acquiring patient health information in violation of law), manslaughter, and negligent homicide. Nurses convicted of criminal charges are subject to punishment up to, and including, loss of license and imprisonment.

Civil laws seek to protect and regulate individual and property rights. Those wronged may attempt to enforce their rights by filing an action in court for money damages. Civil law is further divided into several areas, with tort law most applicable to nursing practice. **Tort law** deals with harmful or wrongful acts resulting in either injury to another person or another person's property. Resulting from carelessness, unintentional tort claims against nurses include negligence and **malpractice** (professional negligence). In contrast, intentional tort liability arises from willful acts. Potential claims against nurses include assault, battery, and false imprisonment.

State Boards of Nursing

Nurse practice acts (NPAs) empower state nursing boards to implement and enforce state nursing regulations. Among their important functions, state boards of nursing investigate allegations of nursing misconduct, incompetence, and negligence, often in tandem with state civil or criminal proceedings (Table 10-3). Allegations most frequently investigated include nursing substance abuse, patient endangerment, and fraudulent documentation (Aiken, 2004).

Pause and Reflect

1. *What are your state's laws regarding the care of patients with mental illness? Which one do you believe to be most important? Why?*
2. *Why do you think state boards of nursing view overstating credentials or experience as fraudulent?*

Examples of Conduct Resulting in Disciplinary Action

table 10-3

Types of Cases	Sample Conduct
Practice-related	• Failure to assess changes of condition • Failure to implement appropriate or ordered interventions • Failure to accurately document assessment information or nursing care provided • Failure to follow drug administration procedures
Drug-related	• Misappropriation of medications intended for patients • Failure to document or falsely documenting that medications were administered to patients • Engagement in intemperate use of medications causing impairment • Attempt to obtain drugs by communicating or presenting unauthorized prescriptions to pharmacies
Boundary violations	• Sharing stories of personal challenges to entice gifts or money from patients • Establishing gratifying personal relationships with current or former patients
Sexual misconduct	• Inappropriate physical or sexual contact, by either the nurse touching a patient sexually or causing a patient to touch the nurse sexually
Abuse	• Hitting • Slapping • Threats • Verbal assaults
Fraud	• Overstatement of credentials or experience • Claiming unworked hours or visits on payroll • Falsely documenting care or procedures when related to payments • Submitting inaccurate billing records to defraud insurance companies

Source: Adapted from National Council of State Boards of Nursing (NCSBN), Discipline: Initial Review of a Complaint. Available at https://www.ncsbn.org/3772.htm#types

Responsibilities of Nurses

Nurses have many legal and ethical obligations to patients. These include providing competent care; acting to reduce the potential for error, injury, and liability; and maintaining professional boundaries. Nurses must know the applicable state and federal laws that address these obligations, as well as the relevant professional guidelines and procedures at their place of employment.

Standard of Care

Among the most basic responsibilities is that nurses provide competent care. Nursing standards are the legal benchmarks for assessing the quality of patient care. They are intended to protect the public from harm by establishing minimum safety requirements. In a lawsuit, a nurse's actions will be judged against the relevant **standard of care**. "It is a nurse's duty to exercise the degree of skill ordinarily employed, under similar circumstances, by the members of the nursing or health care profession in good standing in the same community or locality, and to use reasonable care and diligence, along with his or her best judgment, in the application of his or her skill to the case" (*Reilly v. Spinazze*, 2010). Failure to adhere to standards of care may result in civil or criminal liability, as well as administrative claims that result in the restriction or revocation of the right to practice nursing.

Individual nursing practice must be consistent with the knowledge and ordinary skill of nurses actively practicing in the relevant specialty. Thus, psychiatric–mental health nurses are held to standards of care consistent with "what any ordinary, reasonable, and prudent psychiatric nurse would do, based on what any other reasonable and prudent psychiatric nurse would have done in a similar situation" (Wysoker, 2001, p. 166). Nurses often ask: "Will I get sued?"

The more helpful question is: "What would a reasonable, prudent nurse do under these circumstances?" It is also important to keep in mind that nursing standards are not necessarily standards of excellence. Furthermore, poor patient outcomes do not imply nursing negligence, and nursing actions are not judged in hindsight (*Hinson v. Glen Oak Retirement System*, 2003).

Psychiatric nursing standards are derived from numerous sources to reflect diverse legal, professional, accrediting, and organizational norms, including the following:

1. Relevant state statutes and regulations, including those contained in the applicable NPA

2. State board of nursing guidelines and decisions

3. Relevant civil/criminal laws affecting nursing (e.g., privacy)

4. Relevant guidelines issued by federal or state agencies or other organizations overseeing the quality or funding care, such as the Joint Commission, the Centers for Disease Control and Prevention, or the Centers for Medicare and Medicaid Services

5. The ANA's standards and guidelines, including the Code of Ethics and the Standards of Psychiatric and Mental Health Nursing Practice

6. Employer or agency policies and procedures and nursing job descriptions

7. Instructional manuals for any medical equipment or devices used in practice

8. Standards established by any other professional or specialty organizations in which the nurse is a member (e.g., the American Psychiatric Nurses Association's position statements on various aspects of practice)

9. Current nursing educational materials including textbooks, treatises, and journals (e.g., *Journal of Psychosocial Nursing and Mental Health Services* and the *Journal of the American Psychiatric Nurses Association*).

Nurses are individually responsible for knowing and keeping current with relevant standards. Ignorance is no excuse. To fulfill the duty of care, nurses must adhere to the nursing process and evidence-based practice. Nurses must engage in ongoing education to maintain skills consistent with current practice standards. Nurses risk professional discipline and legal liability if they provide care inconsistent with current standards.

Nursing Liability

Nursing liability refers to legal responsibility for nursing actions or inactions constituting breaches of standard of care and resulting in patient harm. Providers found civilly liable may be required to pay money damages to compensate for or deter wrongdoing; those found criminally liable may face fines or imprisonment. Aiken (2004) identifies potential sources of liability specific to psychiatric–mental health nursing:

- Failure to assess the risk of suicide
- Failure to properly monitor
- Failure to communicate and document observations
- Failure to detect drug toxicity
- Failure to protect the patient from other patients
- Failure to provide a safe environment

As licensed practitioners, nurses are always individually accountable for their actions. This point cannot be overstated. Under limited circumstances, some responsibility for harm caused by nursing actions may be attributed to a nurse's employer via a legal theory called *respondeat superior*. When applicable, this legal theory holds an employer liable for an employee's actions performed in the course and scope of employment. For example, when a patient's family sues a psychiatric hospital for failure to prevent harm (such as preventing a suicide attempt), defense of the nurse is often ancillary to the defense of the hospital. Does this mean that nurses should not be concerned with independent liability? Absolutely not. Nurses must recognize that employers will not always "shield" them from litigation. Specifically,

among other situations, the theory of respondeat superior does not apply if the nurse's actions were not "in the course and scope of employment" and consistent with the employer's policies and procedures. For example, a nurse who fails to follow an employer's policy to assess suicidal patients every 15 minutes will face independent liability for patient harm. The hospital may not only abandon defense of the nurse, but it may also seek damages (indemnity) from the nurse if the hospital is found liable as a result of the nurse's actions. In fact, it is not uncommon for an employer to argue that a nurse was acting outside his or her scope of employment in defense of litigation. For this reason and others, nurses should carry independent malpractice insurance and seek private counsel if they are named in a lawsuit.

Malpractice/Negligence

The primary source of nursing liability is civil malpractice. Malpractice is professional negligence—failure to exercise care—or unintentional carelessness. A nurse is liable for nursing malpractice if he or she does not satisfy the professional nursing standards discussed earlier. As negligence is an unintentional tort, the nurse need not have intended to cause harm to be liable for malpractice.

Nurses may be found guilty of malpractice if a patient–plaintiff is able to establish the following:

1. The nurse owed the patient–plaintiff a duty of care.
2. The nurse breached that duty by failing to meet the standard of care.
3. The patient–plaintiff suffered damages.
4. The nurse's breach caused the patient–plaintiff foreseeable injury.

Croke (2003) identifies the six major categories of negligence that result in malpractice lawsuits against nurses as failure to follow standards of care, failure to use equipment in a responsible manner, failure to communicate, failure to document, failure to assess and monitor, and failure to act as a patient advocate. Certain areas with significant potential for negligence merit more detailed discussion. These include patient safety, suicide, medication error, documentation, boundaries, and self-disclosure (Figure 10-3).

Patient Safety

Nurses have a duty to prevent patient harm. They must continually monitor and intervene to safeguard patient well-being and maintain

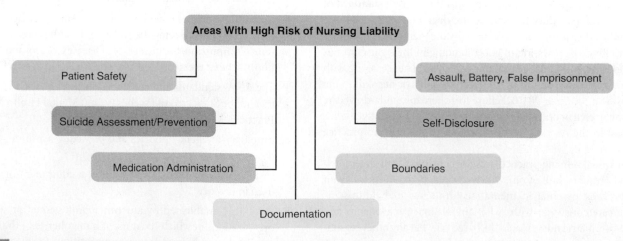

10-3 Areas with high risk of nursing liability.

a safe care environment. Nurses are often the first to observe deterioration in a patient's condition. Failure to monitor, document, and communicate significant changes in a patient's status exposes the nurse to malpractice claims. Satisfying this obligation requires continuous and regular monitoring for a variety of risks to patients' well-being, including harm from restraints, self-harm with items in patients' possession (such as sharp objects), or harm from other patients or providers.

Suicide

Risk of patient suicide is a significant concern, especially for psychiatric–mental health nurses. Whether in the emergency department or inpatient hospitalization, psychiatric–mental health nurses often care for individuals with current or histories of suicidal ideation. Nurses must be vigilant about assessing the risk for suicide and communicating their concerns to other members of the treatment team (Chapter 27). Nurses must be aware of agency policies and procedures concerning suicide prevention.

Medication Errors

Medication errors are another pervasive concern across health care settings. On the front line, nurses must be vigilant about the "six Rs" (the right patient, the right drug, the right dose, the right route, the right time, and the right documentation). They must be knowledgeable about the medications administered, including mechanisms of action, dosage ranges, potential interactions, side effects, and signs of toxicity. Monitoring for adverse drug reactions is especially important, as is following agency policies and procedures for handling medication errors, should they occur.

Documentation

Written documentation is essential to communicating important information among members of the treatment team. Other providers, patients, insurers, and, in the event of a disciplinary action or lawsuit, nursing boards and juries may review nursing documentation. Documentation must be accurate, factual, and objective. Misrepresentation not only jeopardizes patient care, but it can also lead to criminal and/or civil charges of fraud or defamation against the nurse.

Nurses must review and comply with facility policies for documenting, updating, and correcting patient information. In terms of tone, nursing notes should be written as if a patient may read them. For example, rather than document "the patient appeared drunk," note that "the patient's breath smelled of alcohol and his speech was slurred." Sloppy documentation may suggest that a nurse failed to meet the standard of care; strong documentation can reflect, even years later, that nurses performed the required care.

Boundaries

Nurses are responsible for maintaining professional boundaries with patients. "Boundaries are defined as limits that protect the space between the professional's power and the client's vulnerability" (Minnesota Board of Nursing, 2010). Failure to maintain appropriate boundaries jeopardizes patients' recovery and nurses' integrity. Boundary violations range from spending a disproportionate amount of time with a particular patient, to accepting gifts, dating, and sexual relationships (Chapter 8). Boundary issues are ever-present, as nurses provide emotionally intimate care to vulnerable patients.

Self-Disclosure

As discussed in Chapter 8, one potential form of boundary violation is self-disclosure, which occurs when a nurse reveals personal information to a patient. Self-disclosure is controversial. Some disclosures result from patient inquiry; other times, nurses volunteer information. This issue highlights the tension between beneficence (duty to do good) and nonmaleficence (duty to prevent harm). Nurses often self-disclose in an effort to develop trust and therapeutic alliance. A nurse may share his or her history, for instance, to normalize a patient's sense of inadequacy. On the other hand, disclosure can also be very harmful to patients. Lack of professional distance combined with the inherent power of position can result in abuse of an already vulnerable patient.

Whether to self-disclose is a matter of the nurse's clinical judgment. The Code of Ethics allows for rendering an informed opinion on patient request provided that the nurse adheres to professional boundaries (ANA, 2001). The nurse must exercise self-awareness and ask: "Do I have a need to tell, or does the patient have a need to know?" (Moller, 2011, personal communication). If it is the former, the nurse should not disclose. For nurses who decide self-disclosure is appropriate, Deering (1999) offers guidelines for effective therapeutic self-disclosure, including keeping disclosures brief, refraining from implying that the nurse's experience is the same as the patient's, and self-disclosing only situations one has mastered.

Other Forms of Potential Liability

Although less common than negligence-based torts, *intentional torts* are another potential source of psychiatric nursing liability. The most common causes of action are assault, battery, and false imprisonment. Unlike negligent causes of action, to establish an intentional tort the plaintiff must show that the nurse possessed intent to cause the action—not necessarily the harm—that resulted in the injury. For example, consider a nurse's intention to apply physical restraint to confine a patient. A violation of the patient's right to be free from intentional torts is the only damage needed—no other specific injury is required. Defenses to intentional torts include patient consent and legally permissible justifications (such as an emergency to prevent harm to a patient or others).

Assault is the threat of harm from unauthorized touching. Threatening words alone rarely constitute an assault; overt action typically is required. **Battery** is unlawful touching. Unauthorized treatment without informed consent may result in medical battery. These two causes of action, often, but not necessarily, occur simultaneously. A patient may experience reasonable fear (assault) and subsequently be unlawfully touched. In contrast, a patient who is unconscious may not experience fear (therefore no assault), but may claim battery if treated without consent.

False imprisonment is the unlawful confinement of a patient against the patient's will. In addition to physical restrictions, illegal confinement may result from chemical restraint (such as medication) or significant verbal intimidation (threats). Patients may not be detained without their consent, acquiescence, or legal justification. Nurses must know their state law on involuntary hospitalization to avoid liability for false imprisonment.

Psychiatric–mental health nurses also may be liable for intentional infliction of emotional distress if they engage in conduct that is severely distressing to patients. Rude, inconsiderate, or insensitive behavior does not suffice. The conduct in question must be outrageously inappropriate and exceed all possible bounds of decency in a civilized community.

Quasi-intentional torts include a collection of offenses against a patient's dignity. Possible causes of action include defamation and invasion of privacy. *Defamation* is a violation of a patient's right to a positive image. Defamatory statements are derogatory or false statements that harm a patient's reputation or good character. If written, defamation is called *libel*; if oral or verbal, defamation is called *slander*. To minimize liability for defamation, nursing documentation must be opinion free and objective.

Invasion of privacy is a violation of a patient's right to be free from intrusion or the right to be left alone. Nurses are liable for such claims if they release information about a patient without permission. Nurses should be aware that invasion of privacy also occurs with unauthorized disclosure of images. Do not take pictures of patients without prior patient consent and facility authorization.

Pause and Reflect

1. *Which area with the potential for negligence (e.g., patient safety, suicide, medication error, documentation, boundaries, or self-disclosure) concerns you the most? What actions can you take to learn more about this area?*
2. *What do you think Deering means by "self-disclose only situations that you have mastered"?*

Rights of Patients

Americans highly value personal rights and freedoms. As members of organized society, many of our rights reflect well-established ethical and legal norms. Other rights, such as a right to dignity, reflect more generally inferred values but may lack a clear authority or mechanism of enforcement.

Rights vary in the degree to which people define, accept, interpret, or enforce them. Historically, the rights of those with mental illness have not been well delineated or respected. Nurses play an essential role in advocating for the creation and protection of rights that benefit those suffering from mental illness. This advocacy is particularly important, as many individuals suffering from mental illness lack the political, social, or economic power to advocate on their own behalf.

Some individuals with mental illness are uniquely vulnerable in that they may experience symptoms (such as psychosis) that interfere with their ability to know or enforce their rights, or make them less able to conform to societal norms. Consequently, those suffering from mental illness are at high risk for abuse, discrimination, stigma, and marginalization. All patients have a variety of legal rights that nurses are ethically obligated to preserve. Given how broadly we speak of rights, however, discerning among assorted patient rights is not always intuitive. As noted earlier, although federal law confers many essential rights, state law is the primary source of laws governing the rights of mental health patients. Today, patient rights are "almost exclusively the province of individual states" (Talbott, 2011, p. 581). In instances in which federal law does not dictate, it may, however, attempt to guide state policy. The federal Bill of Rights for Mental Health Patients, for instance, is a federal model, rather than a mandate, for states to follow (Box 10-5). States differ widely in their adoption of this model; nurses must become aware of the specific laws in their state. To meet the legal and ethical responsibilities of patient care, nurses are obligated to understand the differences between and the relationship among various rights.

Active Participation in Care

Patients have both an ethical and legal right to active participation in their care. This right is grounded in the principle of autonomy. The ANA Code of Ethics obligates nurses to protect patients' right to self-determination (ANA, 2001). Nurses are also often professionally obligated to uphold patients' rights of self-determination as conferred by government agencies and health care credentialing organizations.

Patients' right to active participation in their care has also been recognized in court decisions and codified in the federal Patient Self-Determination Act (PSDA), enacted in 1991. In 1914, Justice Benjamin Cardozo wrote, "Every human being of adult years and sound mind has a right to determine what shall be done with his own body" (*Schoendorff v. Society of New York Hosp.*). Additionally, the PSDA requires medical providers to give patients written notice of their right to direct and participate in their treatment, including the right to refuse treatment. Most state laws provide similar rights.

Federal Bill of Rights for Mental Health Patients   box 10-5

A person receiving mental health services should be accorded rights including the right to:

(A) Appropriate treatment and related services
(B) An individualized, written, treatment or service plan
(C) Ongoing participation in the planning of care
(D) Refuse treatment in the absence of informed consent (with exceptions for emergency and court ordered treatment)
(E) Refuse participation in experimentation
(F) Freedom from restraint or seclusion (in the absence of treatment, an emergency situation with written order)

(G) Reasonable protection from harm
(H) Appropriate confidentiality of records
(I) Mental health care records (with exceptions)
(J) Converse with others privately, access the telephone and mails, and see visitors
(K) Be informed of his or her rights
(L) Assert grievances with respect to infringement of their rights
(M) Access to rights protection service
(N) Exercise the rights described in this section without reprisal

Source: 42 U.S.C.A. § 9501

The ethical and legal mandates for self-determination are not unlimited. Infringements on autonomy are ethically and legally sanctioned, and in fact are required in certain circumstances. Legal exceptions to a patient's self-determination (discussed later) in large part reflect the ethical concept of paternalism as broad justification for overriding the patient's autonomy.

Psychiatric Advance Directives

Every state allows its citizens to identify certain health care treatment preferences in advance. An **advance directive** is a legal document that specifies health care instructions or identifies a proxy (surrogate decision maker) for making health care decisions. Advance directives often address preferences for end-of-life care, such as cardiopulmonary resuscitation and intubation. A **psychiatric advance directive** (PAD) is a specific type of advance directive that permits individuals to specify treatment options should they become incapacitated due to mental illness (such as psychosis). A PAD may reflect treatment preferences, such as being brought to a specific hospital or receiving a particular antipsychotic medication. In addition to facilitating patient self-determination, PADs are thought to reduce coercive crisis interventions (Swanson et al., 2008), foster therapeutic patient–clinician alliances, and increase patient satisfaction with psychiatric care.

Not all states recognize PADs. Among those that do, state laws vary in terms of when a PAD becomes effective and what treatments it can legally direct or limit. Only certain states, for instance, permit patients to refuse medications in advance. Issues of particular concern include a patient's right to revoke a PAD and clinicians' right to supersede PADs. Most state statutes allow physicians to override PADs when the patient is involuntarily or emergently hospitalized or when the patient's instructions are inconsistent with current standards of care or applicable law.

Informed Consent

Informed consent is the vehicle by which patients exercise their right to self-determination. It is the permission that a patient, or the patient's representative, grants a clinician to provide medical treatment. A provider's responsibilities in obtaining informed consent generally focus on the patient having (1) decision-making capacity and (2) adequate information to make a (3) voluntary choice regarding care.

In theory, providers are ethically and legally obligated to obtain informed consent for all interventions, whether mundane or extraordinary. However, higher thresholds for consent are often required for procedures associated with significant risk, such as electroconvulsive therapy, psychosurgery, or patient participation in research trials or experimental procedures. State law and agency policies may outline specific procedures that require written consent.

With the exception of minors and patients deemed incompetent by a court of law (discussed later), all patients are presumed to be capable and competent to grant informed consent. Unfortunately, patients with mental illness are often assumed to be unable to participate in their care. In fact, no diagnosis or psychiatric symptom automatically negates a patient's capacity or the provider's obligation to obtain informed consent. Patients with psychosis, for instance, do not necessarily lack the ability to give informed consent. Rather, determinations regarding patients' capability to participate in their care should be made on a case-by-case and ongoing basis.

Capacity

The term *capacity* refers to the clinical determination of whether an individual is capable of making health care decisions. Decision-making capacity can be difficult to assess, especially in patients whose illness or treatments may interfere with their insight, judgment, or cognition. State laws specify capacity standards, but generally the term refers to an individual's ability to:

- Communicate a consistent choice
- Understand the relevant information
- Appreciate the situation and its consequences
- Reason about treatment options

Capacity is a fluid concept. It is time and decision specific; a patient may have capacity for certain decisions, such as participation in routine medical procedures, but lack capacity with respect to other decisions, such as whether to consent to psychosurgery. Psychiatric symptoms often pose concerns about capacity assessments. Capacity is a function of the patient's clinical picture at a specific moment in time. It may fluctuate as a result of the exacerbation or treatment of symptoms. Clinicians must consider the degree and temporal nature of various psychiatric illnesses, as well as look for and address reversible causes of incapacity, such as delirium and medication-induced changes in cognition.

The key point is that no psychiatric or cognitive condition automatically eliminates the presumption of capacity. Patients with mild dementia, for instance, may retain significant decision-making capacity. "Despite the presence of bizarre behaviors, inappropriate affects, and disturbances in thought processes or content, such patients may retain the cognitive abilities to understand, recapitulate, and appreciate those factors required to make treatment decisions" (Leo, 1999, p. 137). For example, delusions or hallucinations may impede the decision-making capacity of a patient for a period of time. When the patient is no longer experiencing symptoms (perhaps after administration of medication), the patient may regain capacity. Nurses, therefore, must continually assess for capacity.

Nurses play a critical role in enhancing patient capacity. Nurses are often the first to identify and address factors that may jeopardize capacity, including medication effects, pain, hearing impairments, or language barriers. For a variety of reasons, patients may need to have information repeated and clarified. Additionally, information may need to be reworded and delivered in smaller increments. The use of models, graphs, and other audiovisual tools may also facilitate patient capacity.

There are various assessment tools for assessing capacity. The Mini-Mental State Examination (MMSE) is widely used in clinical practice. Clinicians should note that although it is a significant component of capacity, cognition is not the only criterion for capacity (Sessums, Zembrzuska, & Jackson, 2011). Cognition does not necessarily demonstrate judgment or reasoning abilities relevant to capacity determinations. Other assessment tools include the Aid to Capacity Evaluation (ACE). Developed by the University of Toronto's Joint Centre for Bioethics (n.d.), the ACE uses seven domains to assess the patient's understanding and appreciation of information relevant to the treatment decision confronting the patient.

A mnemonic to assist with evaluating a patient's decision-making capacity is CAPACITY:

C—Communicate consistent choice

A—Appreciate and acknowledge the patient's condition and likely outcomes of treatment options

P—Paraphrase information received (communicate understanding)

A—Ask questions as often as necessary

C—Compare and contrast treatment options

I—Identify rationale for choice among options (reason)

T—Time to consider

Y—Yea or nay the options presented

Competence

A term frequently confused with decision-making capacity is *competence*. Competence is a legal concept and determined by a court of law. Adults are presumed to be competent. Unlike capacity, competence does not fluctuate. Incompetence can be reversed only by court order. An incompetent individual is deprived of the legal right to make decisions. In light of this significant infringement of liberty, a hearing is required to have a patient declared incompetent. In such a proceeding, a judge hears evidence, often with psychiatric testimony, on the following issues:

1. Whether the patient has a mental disease or disorder
2. Whether the patient's judgment is impaired
3. Whether the mental disease or disorder significantly interferes with the patient's ability to reason

If a patient is adjudicated "incompetent," the court will appoint a conservator over the person and/or his or her property. Patients who disagree with the court finding may petition the court for reversal. (Note that competence as it relates to informed consent is distinguished from competence to stand trial in a criminal context, as discussed later.)

Required Disclosures

Consent is "informed" only if a competent patient is provided with sufficient information to make a voluntary and knowledgeable decision. Required disclosures include the risks and benefits of receiving or forgoing treatment, potential complications, and alternatives to a proposed treatment. An ethical dilemma arises when clinicians omit important information—such as medication side effects—for fear that such disclosures will dissuade patients from needed treatments. Moreover, adequately informing patients can be challenging, as every patient has a unique ability to comprehend and appreciate information.

The standard for required disclosures varies by state of practice. Traditionally, disclosure standards had to answer the question: What would a reasonable clinician disclose about the treatment? Currently, the more common standard addresses: What would a reasonable person want to know about the proposed treatment? The latter standard was articulated in a case in which a surgeon performed back surgery on a patient without informing the patient of the small risk of paralysis. Following the surgery, the patient was paralyzed. He then sued, claiming he would not have agreed to the procedure had he been informed of the risk of paralysis (*Canterbury v. Spence*, 1972). The court found that a "reasonable person" would have wanted to know the risk of paralysis.

Voluntary Consent

Patients make a voluntary choice when their preference is free of coercion. **Coercion**, or **undue influence**, refers to the power of one person to affect the decision of another. It includes persuasion and manipulation. Consent based on deceit or deception is not valid.

If a patient is functionally or legally unable to voluntarily consent (for example, an unemancipated minor), clinicians are legally and ethically obliged to identify a surrogate decision maker. State statutes vary, but a surrogate decision maker is generally a person identified as a health care proxy by the patient, or, in the absence of an appointed surrogate, the patient's next of kin. If an incapacitated patient has no identifiable surrogate or a court has deemed a patient incompetent, clinicians must obtain informed consent from the court-appointed surrogate (i.e., conservator or guardian).

Nurses must be aware of the priority of surrogates under applicable state law. In some states, disagreements concerning consent among equal-priority surrogates (such as multiple adult children) are settled by majority rule. Other states require consensus among equal-priority surrogates.

Nurse's Role in Informed Consent

Physicians and other practitioners (such as advanced practice registered nurses) who order procedures or treatments are responsible for obtaining a patient's informed consent (Miller, 2006). Registered nurses, however, play a pivotal role in obtaining, maintaining, and monitoring a patient's informed consent. A nurse's formal role in obtaining informed consent varies by facility. In some cases, depending on provider policy and state law, a primary provider may delegate aspects of the informed consent process to a nurse. In narrow cases, a nurse may act as an agent of the physician in disclosing relevant treatment information (Miller, 2006). More commonly, nurses are tasked with witnessing and obtaining signatures for informed consent. Nurses must be familiar with the specific procedures dictating consent in their state and agency.

The legal and ethical significance of informed consent necessitates that it be well documented. Some employers have specific forms and policies for documenting consent. At other times, day-to-day clinical notes refer to informed consent. It is insufficient for a provider to chart conclusions such as "the patient is unable to give informed consent" or "the patient lacks capacity." Clinicians also must document the basis for such conclusions. For example, with respect to capacity, the patient's medical record should include the assessment questions asked by a clinician and the patient's responses in direct quotes; the consistency with prior decision-making abilities; and the names of any other individuals present for the assessment. If a patient lacks the ability to provide informed consent, nurses should document the same information for surrogate decision makers.

Nurses should confer with the treatment team regarding any concerns about the patient's ability to provide informed consent or whether there is any change in the patient's ability to consent to treatment preferences. The nurse should note any variations in capacity and the existence of factors that may enhance capacity, such as when pain is controlled or family members are present. Capacity is a clinical judgment that demands thorough and ongoing assessment. If the nurse remains concerned about the adequacy of the patient's consent, the nurse should consult with nursing management and, if necessary, elevate his or her concerns to medical administration and the agency's legal counsel.

Exceptions to Informed Consent

There are a limited number of exceptions to the informed consent requirement. They include (1) life-threatening emergencies, (2) patient waiver, (3) prior patient knowledge, and (4) therapeutic privilege. Consent is often implied in emergency situations. Generally, the emergency should involve the patient's inability to participate in an immediate crisis, such as an unconscious patient in need of lifesaving intervention. Additionally, the treatment provided must be consistent with the patient's previously expressed wishes and within well-accepted standards of care.

In the case of waiver, a patient may forgo the right to relevant information by expressly deferring to clinicians. The patient may state: "I leave it up to you [the provider]" or something similar. Courts construe this exception narrowly in part because medical paternalism historically resulted in provider-driven care. Today, in contrast, patients are presumed to be more active health care consumers. Consequently, providers are advised to encourage reluctant patients to become informed (Miller, 2006). Once a patient has consented to a procedure, that prior knowledge constitutes consent for repeated procedures provided there have been no significant changes in risks or benefits.

Therapeutic privilege involves a clinician's withholding information to prevent harm to the patient. The potential detriment (such as anxiety) must be significant and substantiated in the patient's medical record. Clinicians cannot rely on this privilege to prevent a patient's refusing treatment that the provider believes is in the patient's best interest. Some states require that clinicians invoking therapeutic privilege obtain informed consent from the patient's next of kin (Miller, 2006).

Privacy and Confidentiality

Psychiatric–mental health nurses are often entrusted with sensitive and potentially stigmatizing details of patients' lives. **Right to privacy** generally refers to the patient's prerogative to be left alone, free from intrusion, and in command of personal information. Our modern health care system poses challenges to maintaining the privacy of patient's personal information. Clinicians are often required to share information with individuals and entities far from the bedside. Health care administrators, attorneys, law enforcement, and third-party payors may have legitimate needs for patient data. Additionally, the increased use of technology has often compromised the security of patient information.

Despite these challenges, nurses are responsible for safeguarding patient privacy by upholding professional and legal duties to maintain confidentiality. **Confidentiality** is the obligation to not disclose private information. This is an obligation stated in the ANA Code of Ethics, which recognizes confidentiality as essential to the therapeutic relationship and to patient health and privacy. The ANA Code of Ethics also recognizes that there may be legitimate reasons to breach confidentiality; the protection of the patient and public, quality improvement practices, and facilitation of payments may be legitimate exceptions to the obligation of confidentiality (ANA, 2001). In navigating the obligation to maintain patient confidence, nurses must be aware of relevant employer, accrediting agency, and state board of nursing policies with respect to protecting patient privacy. Federal regulations also must be taken into consideration.

The Health Insurance Portability and Accountability Act (HIPAA) of 1996 was the first federal law to explicitly address patient privacy when it implemented its Standards for Privacy of Individually Identifiable Health Information. Effective October 15, 2002 and significantly expanded on April 14, 2003, HIPAA strives to balance the need to protect patient's health information while facilitating the sharing of information among those who legitimately need to know it. "The major purpose of the Privacy Rule is to define and limit the circumstances in which an individual's protected health information

may be used or disclosed by covered entities" (Summary of the HIPAA Privacy Rule, p. 6). "Protected health information" consists of "individually identifiable health information" that is or reasonably can be used to identify an individual. Common identifiers include name, date of birth, Social Security number, address, age, and gender.

HIPAA provides patients with a host of important protections and rights. Significantly, it affords patients the right to limit how their protected information is disclosed. HIPAA also entitles patients to have access to their medical records and the right to request corrections of information therein. It is important to note that HIPAA is a "floor" or minimum level of legal protection; more protective state privacy laws are not preempted by HIPAA.

In addition to protecting privacy, HIPAA facilitates the legitimate sharing of information. HIPAA explicitly permits disclosure of patient health information without authorization in specific circumstances, most significantly for "treatment, payment and health care operations," as well for specifically delineated public interest and safety reasons. Disclosures for any other reason require written patient authorization, also referred to as a "release."

Nurses should be aware that breaches of patient privacy come with significant consequences. Civil penalties may be as high as $25,000 per year and criminal penalties up to $250,000 or 10 years in prison. Nurses also may incur liability under state civil and criminal statutes. Thus, nurses must be clear about when the duty of confidentiality can be breached. Then, even within the realm of permitted disclosures, caution is required. Nurses must disclose only the minimum amount needed for a particular purpose.

A related concept to disclosure is access. Nurses should never access patient information unless they are involved in their care or specifically authorized to receive such information. Unauthorized access to patient information is illegal and is grounds for termination.

Exceptions

There are important exceptions to the patient's right to privacy and the provider's obligation to confidentiality. A clinician's affirmative **duty to warn** potential victims of foreseeable harm was established by the California courts in the case of *Tarasoff v. Regents of the University of California et al.* (1974). In this case, graduate student Prosenjit Poddar told a psychologist of his plan to kill schoolmate Tatiana Tarasoff, in revenge for unrequited love. The clinician notified campus police and attempted to hospitalize Poddar, but he did not warn the potential victim. Ultimately, Poddar killed Tarasoff. Her parents sued the psychologist and the university. In the litigation that followed, the California court concluded that "the public policy favoring protection of the confidential character of patient-psychotherapist communications must yield to the extent to which disclosure is essential to avert danger to others. The protective privilege ends where the public peril begins" (*Tarasoff II*, at 347).

The duty to warn is a matter of state law. Assessing the foreseeability of danger has been a major challenge in clarifying the duty to warn. Consequently, states vary widely as to when and the degree to which clinicians are required to warn. Depending on the state, the duty will reflect the specificity of the threat and the history of the potential assailant. State variations about what constitutes sufficient warning also exist. It is important for nurses to know the law concerning the duty to warn in their state of practice.

In most states, nurses who care for children and older adults are obligated to report suspected patient abuse. The penalty for failure to

Oregon Revised Statutes—Evidence Code	box 10-6

§ 40.240 Rule 504-2.

Nurse-patient privilege

A licensed professional nurse shall not, without the consent of a patient who was cared for by such nurse, be examined in a civil action or proceeding, as to any information acquired in caring for the patient, which was necessary to enable the nurse to care for the patient (1981 c.892 §33b).

Source: https://www.oregonlegislature.gov/bills_laws/Pages/ORS.aspx

report suspected abuse varies by state law. Most states treat failure to report as a criminal misdemeanor, subjecting nonreporters to imprisonment and/or fines; a small number of states classify failure to report as a felony (Child Welfare Information Gateway, 2009).

Privileged Communications

Privilege is a concept related to, but distinct from, confidentiality. Nurses are obligated to keep patient information confidential, meaning they are obligated to refrain from disclosing patient information. **Privileged** is a legal term that pertains to certain confidential communications. Privileged communications often exist between people with special relationships. Generally, conversations between spouses, a minister and a parishioner, an attorney and client, and a health care provider and patient are considered special enough in nature that they deserve these protections.

Whether or not a communication is privileged is a matter of state law. It is typically included in the state rules of evidence. These rules dictate the information that is admissible in court proceedings. Given the special treatment afforded privileged communications, it is a very narrow exception. The privilege may apply only to certain types of discussions at certain times. States vary in the types of professionals involved, the nature of the discussion, and the impact of the presence of third parties.

Most states have a well-established privilege for physician–patient communications. In contrast, nurse–patient communications are privileged in only a small number of states (see Box 10-6 for one example). This creates a dilemma, as nurses are often entrusted with highly sensitive information, but lack the benefit of privilege. Consequently, nurses may be required to reveal information about their patients. Such revelations may cause harm to the patients as well as undermine the trust underlying a therapeutic nurse–patient relationship. Nurses, therefore, must be proactive about addressing this potential dilemma. The first step is for nurses to become knowledgeable about the law in their state of practice. Supervisors, local law librarians, and health care attorneys are sources of this information. Nurses then must educate their patients regarding this potential limitation in confidentiality.

Pause and Reflect

1. *What are the differences between competence and capacity?*
2. *What concerns do you have related to maintaining protected health information confidential? About disclosing it under appropriate circumstances?*

Psychiatric Hospitalization

Patients considering or confronted with psychiatric hospitalization often fear stigma and denial of basic freedoms. The circumstances surrounding a patient's hospitalization (including the patient's involvement in the process, the type of facility, and the participation and/or reaction of family, friends, and facility staff) may contribute to the patient's perception of the experience. In actuality, patients are not summarily stripped of their civil rights on admission to a psychiatric facility. However, patients' rights may be limited, depending on the nature of the admission.

The two main categories of psychiatric hospital admission are voluntary and involuntary. Each state has unique laws outlining the procedures for and rights applicable to various forms of voluntary and involuntary hospitalization. Rights of particular significance to hospitalized patients include the right to discharge, participate in care, refuse treatment and medication, and legal representation. Given the potential for infringement of patient rights and the significant variability in the laws, it is imperative that nurses become familiar with the specific laws of the state in which they practice.

Voluntary Admission

Voluntary admission is the "cornerstone" of inpatient psychiatric treatment (Appelbaum, Appelbaum, & Grisso, 1998). A patient is admitted to a psychiatric hospital "voluntarily" when the patient or someone on the patient's behalf makes a written application for and consents to admission and treatment. (Admission to public or state hospital is sometimes referred to as *commitment*.) Some states have an "informal" voluntary admission process in which the patient's oral request for admission is sufficient consent to admission. Legal guardians and conservators may apply on behalf of minors and individuals who are deemed incompetent. Some individuals may use a psychiatric advance directive to consent to hospital admission in the event they become incapacitated as a result of mental illness.

Admission for voluntary psychiatric treatment largely parallels the admissions process for nonpsychiatric care. In such cases, the patient recognizes the need for treatment, participates in care planning, and submits to agreed-upon treatments. This willingness to partner with the treatment team is thought to expedite recovery.

Providers must understand that voluntary admission to a psychiatric facility, in and of itself, does not overturn the presumption of patients' competence to direct their care. Unless adjudicated otherwise, voluntarily admitted patients are considered competent and retain all of their civil rights, including their right to self-determination. These patients may direct their care, including refusal of treatment and medication, unless they are deemed dangerous to themselves or others. This assessment is based on the "professional judgment" of the patients' providers.

Voluntarily admitted patients may not be forced to remain in or returned to a facility. They may initiate discharge procedures, even against medical advice. Many states require the request for discharge be made in writing. Depending on state law, the patient's release may be delayed for days to weeks. This period is intended to assess the patient's true readiness for discharge and, if necessary, allow time to persuade the patient to remain hospitalized or transition the patient to an involuntary admission. Some advocates believe such provisions violate the patient's right to self-determination.

Involuntary Admission

Some patients in need of hospitalization cannot or will not consent to voluntary treatment. They may be admitted involuntarily if certain commitment standards are satisfied. Involuntary commitment is not uncommon.

The state's authority to compel hospitalization comes from two powers: police power and parens patriae power. Via its *police power,* the state hospitalizes individuals who pose a danger to themselves or to the community. Via its *parens patriae power,* the state hospitalizes citizens who are unable to care for themselves.

Although it is often an act of compassion, **involuntary commitment** is accomplished with coercion. With the exception of confinement for communicable diseases, there is no medical equivalent to psychiatric treatment without a patient's consent. Nurses must assess their beliefs about coercion and the power of the state to override patient autonomy.

Involuntary admission results in substantial infringement of individual freedoms. The Fourteenth Amendment to the U.S. Constitution guarantees citizens due process rights to protect against inappropriate loss of liberty. Due process is the administrative safeguard required for involuntary commitment. In practical terms, "due process" means that the individual in jeopardy of losing his or her liberty is entitled to a meaningful opportunity to object (Box 10-7). The individual must be afforded adequate notice and a hearing of some sort (possibly with legal representation) in which the applicable standard of commitment must be satisfied.

State law determines the due process requirements for involuntary commitment. Despite state-to-state variation, state statutes generally outline a similar process requiring a showing that the individual (1) poses a danger to self or others, (2) suffers from a mental illness and is in need of immediate treatment, and/or (3) is gravely disabled and unable to provide for his or her basic needs. Some states also provide for involuntary commitment for substance abuse. In *O'Connor v. Donaldson* (1975), the U.S. Supreme Court held that the presence of mental illness, in and of itself, does not justify involuntary hospitalization.

Involuntary commitment standards are controversial. Distinguishing between mental illness and eccentricity can be subtle, if not subjective. In particular, the "dangerousness" standard raises ethical and legal concerns. Problems include inability to predict dangerousness, inconsistent state definitions or interpretations of the term of "dangerous," and the potential for reliance on inappropriate social and cultural stereotypes.

Psychiatric–mental health patients are at the unique risk of loss of liberty for what they might do. Mental health advocates argue that the civil commitment standards should be high, given the denial of liberty, and that the threat of danger should be imminent to reflect the extraordinary nature of involuntary commitment. Proponents of lower standards, including the family members of patients who have harmed themselves or others, argue that current standards are too demanding, delay necessary treatment, and require, rather than prevent, harm.

Depending on the specific type of involuntary commitment and relevant state law, different entities are responsible for determining the fulfillment of the commitment criteria. If a judge or jury makes the determination, the admission is referred to as a *judicial commitment.* Medical and administrative commitments are made by health care personnel and hearing officers, respectively.

Each state's standard of proof must be sufficient to prevent unlawful commitment. Until 1979, states differed in the evidentiary standards for commitment. Evidentiary standards establish the state's burden of proof in a commitment hearing. Some states required a showing of the "preponderance of the evidence." This is the lowest standard of proof used in civil cases and minimizes the state's burden for involuntary commitments. Many states required "clear and convincing evidence." This intermediate standard increases the state's burden for involuntary commitments, but not to the highest level. Other states required proof "beyond a reasonable doubt." This highest burden—used in criminal statutes—increased the state's burden for involuntary commitments and potentially results in fewer involuntary commitments.

In 1979, the Supreme Court established a "clear and convincing evidence" standard as the minimum procedural threshold for involuntary commitment proceedings in *Addington v. Texas.* All states and the District of Columbia are required to abide by this minimum standard. A small handful of states have involuntary commitment statutes that require proof beyond a reasonable doubt.

Types of Involuntary Hospitalization

Although state laws vary, there are generally three types of involuntary hospitalization:

1. Emergency involuntary hospitalization

2. Observational or temporary involuntary hospitalization

3. Long-term involuntary admission (commitment)

Nurses must know the types of and requirements for involuntary admission in their state and agencies of practice. Failure

---

Elizabeth Packard, Advocate for Commitment Criteria box 10-7

In 1860, Elizabeth Packard was confined against her will in a state mental hospital for three years pursuant to an Illinois law that allowed a husband to institutionalize his wife without the due process protections in place today. Elizabeth and her husband, a strict Calvinist minister, disagreed on religious matters, among other things. Her husband determined that Elizabeth was "slightly insane" and arranged for a doctor posing as a sewing machine salesman to interview his wife.

Upon her release, Elizabeth's husband locked her in a room in their home. Elizabeth dropped a letter of complaint out of the window. This led to a trial in which the judge ruled that Elizabeth should be free of all restraint. Elizabeth subsequently dedicated her life to changing commitment laws on behalf of those accused of mental illness.

Based on Packard v. Packard, 27 Fam LQ 515 (1864).

to practice within state law exposes a nurse to claims of false imprisonment.

Emergency Admission

Emergency involuntary hospitalizations occur when a patient is imminently dangerous to self or others, and is often undertaken at the behest of family, friends, law enforcement, or health professionals. Nearly every state permits involuntary hospitalization for a short period of time—generally 48 to 72 hours—for psychiatric diagnosis, evaluation, and immediate treatment. The procedural details including the evaluation process and time frame are a matter of state law. At the expiration of the emergency admission, the patient is released, consents to voluntary admission, or is entitled to a hearing in which a court rules on the need for extended involuntary hospitalization.

Observational or Temporary Admission

In contrast to emergency involuntary admissions, temporary involuntary admissions provide for involuntary hospitalization for diagnosis and treatment in nonemergent situations. State laws determine parties eligible to petition, permitted time frame, and other required procedures. Some states require observational hospitalizations as a procedural prerequisite to longer-term involuntary hospitalizations. Generally, as with emergency admissions, on the expiration of the permitted observation period the patient either is released, consents to voluntary admission, or is entitled to a hearing in which a court rules on the need for extended involuntary hospitalization. Similarly, continued involuntary hospitalization triggers due process rights as specified by state statute.

Commitment

In general, longer periods of involuntary hospitalization demand higher procedural safeguards. For example, specific rules regarding eligible petitioners, the contents of the petition, prehearing medical screenings, the requirement for a hearing, or the patient's physical presence at any such hearing vary by state law. Patients committed for longer periods retain rights to due process and opportunities to challenge the basis for ongoing hospitalization. To that end, most states require orders for extended hospitalizations to be reviewed after set periods (such as 90 or 180 days) to ensure that the commitment criteria are still satisfied. Patients discharged after a lengthy hospitalization may be subject to conditional discharge. In such cases, discharge depends on the satisfaction of specific requirements—for instance, the patient's medication adherence. A patient's failure to satisfy requirements of a conditional release may result in his or her rehospitalization.

Patients' Rights

Involuntary psychiatric care, by its very nature, deprives patients of certain fundamental rights and basic freedoms. The significance of the loss of liberty and wrongful commitment has historically dominated the discussion of patients' rights. Over the past 40 years, however, there has been a greater focus on the rights of those committed. Today, loss of freedom via involuntary commitment does not divest patients of all their rights. Which specific rights are retained is typically a matter of state law. See Connecticut's Patient Bill of Rights (Box 10-8) as an example of state-adopted rights.

Among the most significant of rights retained is a patient's general entitlement to autonomy. Unless a court has declared a patient incompetent, the patient retains the right to self-determination and informed consent. As discussed later, a patient may refuse treatment, unless he or she continues to pose a danger to self or others. Treatments should not incapacitate the patient or interfere with his or her ability to participate in commitment hearings. Treatments requiring higher levels of consent (such as electroconvulsive therapy) generally are not permitted without patient consent or court order. If a patient appears to lack decision-making capacity, a surrogate decision maker must be identified. If no surrogate is available, then the court must be petitioned to appoint a guardian. It is important for the nurse to consult state and facility policies regarding appropriate interventions for patients who refuse treatment. Certain important rights merit more detailed discussion.

Pause and Reflect

1. *A patient signs a voluntary admission application. The record includes a note that the patient believed that he was in heaven at the time he was voluntarily admitted. Was his admission "voluntary"? Why or why not?*

2. *Do you think standards for involuntary admission should be lower or higher? Why?*

3. *What are the standards for commitment in your state? How do you think they could be improved? Why?*

Connecticut Patient Bill of Rights   box 10-8

Under the Connecticut Patient Bill of Rights, C.G.S. §§17a-540 et seq., some of your rights include:

- Freedom from physical or mental abuse or harm
- Ability to vote
- Use of personal funds and to manage personal affairs
- Access to individual storage space
- Development of a written, specialized treatment plan that meets your needs
- Participation in developing the treatment plan and to be told of its contents
- Information about a reasonable notice of discharge
- Personalized discharge plan
- Access to medical treatment for illness, injury, or any disability
- Active treatment in combination with medications; medication not to be used as a substitute for treatment Some restrictions apply to the following rights. (Refer to the statute for details.)
- Access to a telephone
- Written correspondence with anyone without interference
- Freedom from restraints and seclusion
- Freedom to attend religious services of personal choice
- Entertain visitors of personal choice
- Wear own clothing
- Keep and use personal possessions
- Ability to request a change of medication as well as the right to refuse medication

Source: Adapted from Connecticut Department of Mental Health and Addiction Services. Your rights as a patient or a client. Available at http://www.ct.gov/dmhas/LIB/dmhas/publications/ptrights.pdf

Right to Treatment

The right to treatment remains a controversial issue as society tries to balance the autonomy and treatment needs of those with mental illness. Discourse regarding the right to treatment dates back to the 1960s and the groundbreaking mental health advocacy of attorney-physician Milton Birnbaum. He argued, against much resistance, that failure to provide adequate care and treatment to involuntarily committed psychiatric patients affords no hope of recovery and amounts to unconstitutional deprivation of liberty (Birnbaum, 2010).

The right to adequate treatment was first recognized by a U.S. court in 1971 (*Wyatt v. Stickney*). The lead plaintiff in the class action lawsuit, Ricky Wyatt, was involuntarily hospitalized at age 14, at the suggestion of his probation officer. A self-admitted "hell raiser," Wyatt was labeled a "juvenile delinquent." Wyatt received no psychiatric diagnosis, yet received antipsychotic medications against his will regularly. In 1971, an Alabama federal circuit court of appeals found:

> To deprive any citizen of his or her liberty upon the altruistic theory that the confinement is for humane therapeutic reasons and then fail to provide adequate treatment violates the very fundamentals of due process.

Most notably, the court outlined three essential conditions for adequate treatment: (1) a humane psychological and physical environment; (2) qualified staff in numbers sufficient to administer adequate treatment; and (3) individualized treatment plans (*Wyatt v. Stickney*, 1971).

The important rights outlined in *Wyatt* have not been expressly affirmed by the U.S. Supreme Court. Consequently, the right to treatment continues to evolve and, as a practical matter, the "right" to treatment does not ensure needed treatment. The high court, however, prohibited purely custodial commitment in *O'Connor v. Donaldson* (1975). Donaldson was diagnosed with paranoid schizophrenia. He had no history of violence or suicidality, but was involuntarily committed to a Florida psychiatric hospital for more than 14 years. He was confined because of concerns that he would fail to achieve a "successful adjustment outside of the institution." The lower courts recognized a right to treatment. The Supreme Court, however, explicitly sidestepped this issue: "There is no reason now to decide whether mentally ill persons dangerous to themselves or to others have a right to treatment . . . this case raises a single, relatively simple, but nonetheless important question concerning every man's constitutional right to liberty" (*O'Connor v. Donaldson*, 1975). The court did, however, recognize that "a state cannot constitutionally confine, without more, a non-dangerous individual who is capable of surviving safely in freedom by himself or with the help of willing and responsible family members or friends." The uncertainty of the phrase "without more" fuels ongoing debate regarding appropriate criteria for involuntary commitment.

Right to Refuse Treatment

A patient's right to refuse treatment is evolving, controversial, and case specific (Cady, 2010). Most patients with mental illness actively participate in their care and treatment planning. Some patients, however, refuse suggested treatments such as hospitalization, medication, or therapy. It is not always clear why patients reject needed treatment. Sometimes, symptoms such as hallucinations or delusions impair the insight needed for informed consent. Other times, patients may be able to withhold consent, despite psychiatric symptoms, for completely "legitimate" reasons, such as fear of side effects. As a practical matter, individuals suffering from severe and persistent mental illness are more likely to refuse treatment. Consequently, patient refusal often leads clinicians to question a patient's ability to make decisions.

The right to refuse treatment gets to the heart of the legal and ethical issues in psychiatric nursing. Forced medication, for example, highlights the struggle between respecting patient autonomy and beneficent intervention for the good of the patient or society. Effective psychopharmacological treatment may reduce or eliminate symptoms that otherwise threaten or limit a patient's quality of life. The concern, however, is that beneficial medications may have a negative impact on cognition and/or volition and dampen patients' ability to resist unwanted treatment.

The right to refuse treatment is controversial because it is so often engulfed by the exceptions. Patients are "often forced or are coerced to comply to take medications" (Lavelle & Tusaie, 2011, p. 275). Involuntary treatment is typically justified on the grounds that patients present a danger to themselves or others, or are incapable of consenting to care. Justifications proffered for coercion and exceptions to a patient's right to refuse treatment include:

- An emergency situation
- Treatment being in the patient's best interest (in a disinterested professional's judgment)
- Judicial determination of incompetence (Hannon-Engel, 2011)

There are arguments both for and against the use of forced medication (Lavalle & Tusaie, 2011). Arguments against the use of forced medications include the following:

- Many people refuse medications because of side effects or other legitimate reasons.
- Forcing someone to do something against his or her will is inherently wrong.
- Coercion creates distrust in the medical community.

Arguments in favor of forced use of medications include:

- The responsibility to care for those who cannot care for themselves
- The responsibility to provide for the safety of others when patients are unable to recognize the risk of harm to others
- Compelling patients may be necessary when they lack insight into their illness

The case law regarding the right to refuse medication is still evolving (Cady, 2010). In the absence of authoritative guidance from the Supreme Court, state and lower federal courts articulate unique standards. Generally, involuntary medication is permitted (1) for a fixed period of time (for example, 72 hours) upon a patient's involuntary hospitalization, (2) upon a patient's judicial commitment, and/or (3) upon a separate judicial or administrative hearing that orders or authorizes involuntary medication (Beinner, 2007). Given the variation in state law, nurses must be very familiar with the requirements surrounding forced medication in the specific jurisdiction in which they practice.

Protecting the patient's autonomy requires the nurse's self-awareness regarding involuntary treatment. Vuckuvich and Artinian found that nurses "justify" coercion by "reconciling themselves to the use of involuntary procedures when the symptoms of psychiatric illness make it impossible to rely on therapeutic alliance" (2005, pp. 378–379). Recall that coercion includes physical force, persuasion, and manipulation. In an examination of how nurses justify coercion, Vuckuvich and Artinian (2005) found that nurses felt that coercive treatment was justified to prevent suffering and if no other alternative were available.

Right to Least Restrictive Setting

Fifty years ago, individuals with severe and persistent mental illness were often institutionalized for most of their lives. With the evolution of patients' rights and social policies such as deinstitutionalization, restrictive settings were increasingly considered dehumanizing. For many years, advocates sought treatment settings and techniques that maximized patient liberty. Today, ANA standards of psychiatric–mental health nursing practice (2014) as well as case law (*Covington v. Harris*, 1969) require that patients receive treatment in the least restrictive environment.

Treatment for psychiatric illness should be individualized to maximize patient autonomy, freedom, and dignity. With respect to treatment setting, for example, a restraint-free environment is less restrictive than a unit where restraints are regularly used; outpatient community or home care is considered less restrictive than inpatient hospitalization. (See discussion of mandatory outpatient programs that follows.) The least restrictive nature and method of treatment might include open, rather than locked, units; unsupervised, rather than supervised, activities of daily living; and greater choice in treatment alternatives.

Restraints and Seclusion

Restraints and seclusion are used to protect patients from harming themselves or others. A **restraint** is a physical, mechanical, or chemical involuntary constraint of a patient's freedom. Physical restraint may involve use of force, such as when used to move a patient. Mechanical restraints are devices, such as ankle or wrist restraints, that limit movement. Seclusion involves involuntary confinement in a room or space. The purpose of seclusion is to decrease stimulation, protect the patient and others, and provide opportunity for self-control.

These high-risk measures raise significant legal and ethical issues. They deprive patients of freedom, jeopardize autonomy, and pose significant risk of injury. Potential harms include skin and nerve damage, respiratory distress, and strangulation and death. Consequently, the use of restraints is highly regulated by state law, governmental agencies such as the Centers for Medicare and Medicaid Services (CMS), and accrediting organizations such as the Joint Commission. In addition, numerous professional organizations, including the ANA and APNA, have issued position statements and standards on the use of restraint and seclusions.

It is imperative that nurses be aware of the specific regulations governing the use of restraints in their state of practice and in their employing facility. Generally however, nurses should know that these interventions are to be used only with a medical order or as a last resort in emergency situations in which there is imminent risk of harm to the patient, staff, or others. When using restraints, nurses must document the specific therapeutic basis for their use. In particular, nurses must provide a thorough assessment of emergent situations requiring the intervention, alternative interventions that failed or were contemplated, ongoing assessment of the patient's condition, and the need for continued restraint or seclusion. When used, restraint and seclusion must be time limited and discontinued when the patient demonstrates control of self-injurious or threatening behavior. In an effort to minimize restrictions, nurses must inform patients of behaviors that would terminate the use of these measures. To avoid repeated use of restraints or seclusion, nurses should debrief with patients and staff to review precipitating factors and potential alternate outcomes.

Nurses must know when restraints are permissible and when they are not (Table 10-4). Restraints or seclusion should never be used for the convenience of staff, to punish a patient, or with patients with impaired cognition (for instance, patients with dementia or who are heavily

Important Considerations for the Use of Restraints   table 10-4

Nurses must understand state, local, and agency policies regarding the use of restraints. The "6 Rs for RESTRAINED patient" is a mnemonic nurses can use to recall important considerations regarding the use of restraints.

R	Restrict freedom/movement as minimally as possible Risk of harm/liability Review and comply with regulations (facility, CMS, state, etc.) Requires medical order Renewal of restraint order requires reassessment Reduce use if possible (goal of being restraint free)
E	Emergency use (limited duration); follow up with medical order for subsequent use
S	Safety monitoring on ongoing basis
T	Time-limited use only (per order); document time applied and removed
R	Reason for use must be specific, based on current behaviors, communicated to patient
A	Assess and continually reassess patient condition/response and need for observation/restraints
I	Indication with medical order
N	Never for staff convenience/patient discipline/vulnerable populations/or PRN (as needed)
E	Educate/debrief patient, staff, and family per episode for future alternatives
D	Document nursing care and compliance with facility policies and procedures

Eligibility for Outpatient Commitment under New York's Kendra's Law box 10-9

No person may be placed under an AOT order unless the court finds, by clear and convincing evidence, that the subject of the petition meets all of the following criteria:

1. be 18 years of age or older; and
2. suffer from a mental illness; and
3. be unlikely to survive safely in the community without supervision, based on a clinical determination; and
4. have a history of non-adherence with treatment that has: a. been a significant factor in his or her being in a hospital, prison or jail at least twice within the last 36 months; or b. resulted in one or more acts, attempts or threats of serious

violent behavior toward self or others within the last 48 months; and

5. be unlikely to voluntarily participate in treatment; and
6. be, in view of his or her treatment history and current behavior, in need of assisted outpatient treatment in order to prevent a relapse or deterioration which would be likely to result in serious harm to the person or others; and
7. be likely to benefit from AOT.

A court may not issue an AOT order unless it finds that assisted outpatient treatment is the least restrictive alternative available for the person.

Source: New York State Department of Mental Health. (2006). An explanation of Kendra's Law. Available at http://www.omh.ny.gov/omhweb/Kendra_web/Ksummary.htm

---

medicated). Providers are strongly encouraged to limit the use of restraint and seclusion. Many facilities strive to be "restraint free." In addition, units are converting seclusion rooms into comfort spaces to allow patients the physical and emotional space to equilibrate voluntarily.

Mandatory Outpatient Commitment

Outpatient treatment is generally thought to be less restrictive than inpatient treatment. Assisted outpatient treatment (AOT) programs, also referred to as mandatory or involuntary outpatient treatment programs, are controversial. They require individuals with mental illness living in the community to comply with treatment plans. AOTs were largely inspired by public outrage following numerous highly publicized incidents in which individuals with insufficiently treated mental illness committed acts of violence.

The New York legislation that serves as a model for many AOT statutes is referred to as **Kendra's Law.** In 1999, Adam Goldstein pushed Kendra Webdale in front of a New York City subway, resulting in her death. He had a long history of uncoordinated mental health care, multiple hospitalizations, and violent assaults. At the time of Kendra's death, he was not taking prescribed medications. Kendra's Law established guidelines for involuntary outpatient commitment in New York (Box 10-9).

Most states have adopted some form of outpatient commitment. Eligibility criteria generally include significant mental illness that interferes with voluntary and effective participation in treatment, history of nonadherence with adverse consequences, and significant risk of future deterioration that would result in harm.

Involuntary outpatient treatment programs raise significant ethical and legal issues. Proponents adopt a paternalistic perspective; they argue that outpatient treatment programs "do good" by facilitating recovery and promoting public safety. AOT programs are needed, advocates claim, to bolster inpatient involuntary commitment laws that require rather than prevent violence. Opponents of AOT programs emphasize the violation of patient autonomy. They argue that the programs deprive patients of liberty and violate the right to self-determination. In short, proponents focus on the benefits; opponents focus on coercive behavior control (Swanson et al., 2009). The effectiveness of AOT programs generally remains debatable, and the efficacy of any AOT program depends on implementation and funding, which are known to vary widely.

Communication Rights

A patient's right to communicate with individuals outside the hospital is particularly significant, given its potential to reveal unlawful deprivations of liberty. Almost all patients have the right to private conversations with attorneys, family, and clergy during scheduled visiting hours. State statutes typically provide access to telephones and mailing materials and permit patients to send and receive communications uncensored. Generally, facilities have significant latitude in limiting communication rights to accommodate facility operations or prevent harm or inappropriate use. Any limitations to otherwise permitted communication should be in writing and part of the patient's clinical record.

Pause and Reflect

1. *Are you personally and professionally comfortable with enforcing a court-mandated treatment?*
2. *What are your thoughts regarding forced medication? How do you think you would feel if you were a patient being forced to accept medication?*
3. *What are your feelings regarding AOT programs in relation to patient autonomy?*

Patients Involved with the Criminal Justice System

Psychiatry and law intersect most publicly in the area of criminal justice. The mental health challenges of those involved in the criminal justice system raise numerous issues. Unfortunately, individuals with mental illness are disproportionately represented in the criminal justice system (Bernstein, 2011). This leads to misconceptions about the relationship between mental illness and crime. In fact, people suffering from mental illness often lack the consistent care and social support that might prevent them from becoming involved with the criminal justice system. As such, it is not uncommon for psychiatric nurses to care for patients accused or convicted of criminal activity. Nurses generally interact with persons involved in the criminal justice system as correctional or forensic nurses.

Correctional Psychiatric Nursing

Correctional psychiatric nurses deliver care to prison inmates, individuals in juvenile detention centers and substance abuse facilities, and individuals found "not guilty by reason of insanity" who have been committed to forensic wards. Many inmates have significant mental health needs. The goal of care in correctional settings is to address patients' current mental health needs in a nontherapeutic environment. Psychiatric nursing care in correctional settings is required to be patient centered, supportive, humane, unbiased, and nonjudgmental. This work can be challenging for many reasons. Nurses must often reconcile their moral objection to acts allegedly perpetrated by their patients. In addition, safety concerns are ever-present and pose significant threats to the nurse–patient therapeutic alliance (Grace, Fry, & Schultz, 2003). The ANA has outlined professional expectations of correctional nurses in *Correctional Nursing: Scope and Standards of Practice* (2013).

Forensic Psychiatric Nursing

In contrast, forensic nurses typically interact with patients from a unique perspective. Rather than concentrate on patients' current mental health needs, forensic nurses work within or in partnership with the legal system. Depending on the nurse's training and experience, a forensic nurse may be involved with a variety of pretrial functions. Forensic nursing includes the collection of evidence, as well as providing assessment, evaluation, and expert testimony regarding a criminal defendant's state of mind at the time of a crime or the ability of the defendant to participate in legal defense proceedings. The goal of the forensic nurse is to provide objective and impartial evaluations. It is important that forensic nurses inform patients of the nature of their relationship and the lack of confidentiality. For example, the nurse must disclose that he or she has been appointed by a court to provide an evaluation to determine competence for ability to stand trial, rather than for patient-centered treatment. The ANA and the International Association of Forensic Nurses have issued joint guidelines for forensic nurses.

Criminal Responsibility

The legal system seeks to hold competent individuals accountable for their actions. Society has long struggled with how mental illness affects treatment of those accused of violent crime. Applicable legal standards have evolved over time, as societal norms have shifted. Generally, to be convicted of a crime, there must be proof of *mens rea*, or, a guilty state of mind; (2) *actus reus*, or, a guilty act; and (3) a connection between the two. The law presumes individuals are competent and that criminal defendants act with intent and volition. Forensic nursing influences how mental illness intersects with these fundamental presumptions.

Competence

Forensic nurses may contribute to competency evaluations. The Fourteenth Amendment to the U.S. Constitution grants defendants the right to due process, which includes competency to stand trial. Competency is a legal concept determined by a court. Distinct from the concept of incompetence discussed with respect to informed consent, forensic evaluations for competency assess the patient's ability to (1) reasonably consult with counsel to participate in the defense proceedings and (2) develop rational and factual understanding of the nature of the proceedings and punishment (*Dusky v. United States*, 1960). Competence is not a function of psychiatric diagnosis or treatment, but rather is an evaluation of an individual's ability to stand trial. Competence is a threshold or pretrial issue: If a defendant

is found incompetent to stand trial due to mental illness, he or she cannot stand trial or be convicted of a crime. Instead, the defendant is remanded to a locked psychiatric facility for treatment (*Jackson v. Indiana*, 1972). The goal of treatment is to restore competency so that the defendant may then stand trial. Incompetent patients cannot be held indefinitely without hearings to reassess the basis for their commitment.

Insanity

The insanity defense is highly controversial and largely misunderstood. Criminal defendants found competent to stand trial may claim insanity to diminish or excuse criminal responsibility. The rationale for the defense comes from society's historical sentiment that only people capable of knowing and controlling their actions should be found culpable for wrongdoing. Defendants found not guilty by reason of insanity (NGRI) are seldom set free. Instead, they are involuntarily committed to state mental hospitals or correctional treatment facilities by the court. Despite public perception to the contrary, the insanity defense is rarely invoked and typically unsuccessful (Knoll & Resnick, 2008).

The criteria and burden required to prove insanity vary by state and change with public opinion. The acquittal of a few high-profile defendants resulted in public outrage and increased scrutiny of the insanity defense. In the past, the prosecution was required to prove that the defendant was sane. Today, the burden is typically on defendants to meet stricter criteria.

The recent trend is that states are narrowing, and in some cases eliminating, the insanity defense. In addition, many jurisdictions have devised an alternate finding—guilty but mentally ill—to emphasize culpability, yet acknowledge mental illness. Advocates for individuals with mental illness argue that this is punitive, perpetuates misunderstanding of the nature of mental illness, and precludes hope of meaningful treatment.

Pause and Reflect

1. *What role should mental illness play in decreasing criminal liability?*
2. *"Should a personality disorder qualify as a mental disease in insanity adjudication?" (Bonnie, 2010)*

Challenges in the Workplace

The ethical and human rights issues most frequently experienced by psychiatric nurses involve protecting patients' rights and human dignity (Grace, Fry, & Schultz, 2003; Ulrich et al., 2010). Patients' rights to autonomy, informed consent, and freedom from coercive interventions (for example, involuntary medication or physical restraints) are at risk in psychiatric care settings. Thus, nurses are both regularly challenged to protect patients' rights and balance the appropriateness of infringements on those rights.

The ethical issue most disturbing or stressful to psychiatric nurses is staffing patterns that adversely affect nursing care (Grace, Fry, & Schultz, 2003; Ulrich et al., 2010; Ohnishi et al., 2010). Other distressing issues for nurses include the following:

- Protecting patients' rights
- Managed care practices that threaten quality of patient care

- Working alongside incompetent/unethical colleagues
- Providing care with health risks to the nurse
- Being required to provide inappropriate care that prolongs living/dying process
- Failure to consider the quality of patients' lives
- Reporting patient abuse or neglect
- Conflicts with other members of the treatment team

When these conflicts occur, nurses may find themselves experiencing moral distress. Wilkinson described moral distress as "psychological disequilibrium and negative feeling state experienced when a person makes a moral decision but does not follow through by performing the moral behavior indicated by that decision" (1987, p. 16). *Moral distress* occurs when there is a disconnect between what the nurse knows ought to be done and what can be done given the multiple constraints in our complex health care system. Lachman (2007) includes lack of familiarity with professional obligations and skills in addition to organizational limitations as constraints that lead to moral distress.

Deady and McCarthy (2010) studied moral distress in Irish psychiatric nurses and found that the interprofessional structure in which nurses work thwarted productive resolution of moral conflict. The nurses identified three situational themes that engendered moral distress: (1) professional and legal conflict, (2) professional autonomy and scope of practice, and (3) standards of care and patient autonomy. Nurses reported feeling disempowered by the hierarchical structure and vulnerable to isolation if they voiced concerns. Most participants relied on less productive coping mechanisms, such as attempting to avoid or normalize the distress. Deady and McCarthy note that moral courage is required for nurses to "act on their convictions" (2010, p. 291). Nurses may reduce risks associated with independent action by initiating and participating in interprofessional dialogue of shared moral conflict.

Working Conditions and Staffing Issues

Psychiatric nurses work in complex and dynamic work environments that have the potential to cause distress and affect patient care. Nurses are continually challenged to work in staff- and resource-constrained environments. Staffing issues have significant ethical and legal consequences. This is especially true in psychiatric–mental health settings, where patients often need direct one-to-one care and unexpected clinical situations can unfold rapidly. In fact, psychiatric nurses report that adverse staffing patterns are a significant cause of ethical distress. (Grace, Fry, & Schultz, 2003; Ulrich et al., 2010; Ohnishi et al., 2010).

Appropriate staffing is essential to protecting the safety of patients and providers. When staffing is inadequate, nurses experience conflict between their primary commitment to the patient and the risks of patient harm and nurse liability. In considering any staffing issues, nurses must be aware of: the applicable provisions or regulations (such as scope of practice) in relevant NPAs; guidance issued by the state board of nursing or other entities (such as accrediting bodies) overseeing safety and quality; and agency, contract, and collective bargaining policies and procedures for accepting, refusing, or delegating nursing assignments.

Accepting or Refusing a Patient Assignment

Accepting or refusing a patient assignment has significant ethical and legal consequences. Nurses have an ethical obligation to accept assignments for patients needing care, as well as an obligation to refuse assignments for which they lack the skills, experience, or physical and emotional stamina necessary to maintain patient and nurse safety (an "inappropriate assignment"). A nurse who accepts an inappropriate assignment risks liability for patient harm. A nurse who refuses an inappropriate assignment risks legal liability and disciplinary action for patient harm, as well as for patient abandonment. Patient abandonment results when a nurse refuses an assignment without transferring care to another qualified clinician. In general, patient abandonment is legally and ethically indefensible.

A nurse confronting an inappropriate assignment must first confer with the assignor and attempt to negotiate a more acceptable assignment. Assignments may become acceptable if, for example, the nurse receives the requisite training, is able to switch assignments with another employee, or is able to limit the scope of the assignment to one that can be accepted. If an appropriate assignment cannot be negotiated, the nurse essentially has three options: (1) accept the assignment, (2) accept the assignment under protest, or (3) refuse the assignment. Questions nurses should ask themselves when considering an assignment include (but are not limited to):

1. Is the assignment permitted by the Nurse Practice Act and Code of Ethics?
2. Are all aspects of the assignment consistent with evidence-based practice, agency policy, and standards of practice?
3. Am I competent in all areas of the assignment?

As noted previously, legal liability or the potential for adverse disciplinary action may arise in all situations, depending on the facts and circumstances of the acceptance or the refusal, as well as the impact on the patient(s) in question. Refusing a patient assignment, however, is very controversial and, given the overwhelming patient safety concerns, almost certainly prompts adverse consequences. State and agency mandatory overtime and float policies are particularly relevant guideposts as nurses navigate this issue (Brooke, 2009). Given the significant risk for adverse consequences of refusal, nurses must understand the intersection of the applicable laws and policies affecting their ability to refuse an assignment, whether they are consistent, and whether they support refusal. In some cases, rather than reject an assignment, nurses might consider accepting an "assignment despite objection" (ADO). Accepting an ADO does not eliminate risk of adverse consequences or shield the nurse from liability in the event of patient harm. It does, however, notify nursing management and any prospective jury regarding the nurse's concerns.

As a practical matter, the objection is a written communication memorializing the nurse's concerns regarding the nature of a specific assignment. At a minimum, communication should address specific grounds for the objection (for instance, lack of experience, training, or staff; patient or nurse safety), factors affecting objection, whom the nurse notified, and alternatives explored. The nurse may prepare the documentation independently; however, many facilities and state nursing associations have communication tools in place.

A position statement published by the American Psychiatric Nurses Association (APNA) notes that "safe staffing is a process that may vary depending upon the multitude of variables that influence staffing decisions" (APNA, 2011). Nurses concerned with the staffing ratios in their practice settings are ethically obligated to take an active role in shaping safe conditions. APNA recommends serving on a committee to evaluate staffing needs and develop and monitor staffing plans. Better staffing and safer working conditions reduce unnecessary legal exposure.

Nurse–Employer Values Conflicts

What recourse does a nurse have if he or she is chronically confronted with unacceptable working conditions? Nurses must be proactive. It bears repeating that nurses are legally and ethically responsible for independent practice. The ANA Code of Ethics and ICN Code address the possibility of conflict between the values of an individual nurse and his or her employer or agency.

The ANA Code of Ethics discusses conscientious objection or the refusal to accept assignments because of a values conflict. It is narrowly construed and cannot be used for personal convenience, preference, or prejudice. Nurses are advised to avoid working in environments where the need for such objection is likely. For example, a nurse who objects to abortions should not work in a clinic that performs abortions. Nurses who conscientiously object are obligated to communicate the refusal in advance to facilitate alternate care for patients. As noted, nurses must know the procedures and the chain of command) for voicing objection.

Ideally, nurses should work individually and collectively to reconcile their employer's policies with their professional and personal values and obligations. If that is not possible, nurses must be aware that actions consistent with personal and professional values, such as conscientious objection, will rarely, if ever, shield them from adverse

employment or legal repercussions. Nurses who are confronted with unacceptable staffing arrangements or circumstances contrary to their personal and professional values but are unable to change the organization should seek alternative employment or risk adverse legal liability or termination.

Pause and Reflect

1. *Kopala and Burkhart (2005) suggest that moral distress and ethical dilemmas should be included in the North American Nursing Diagnosis Association International (NANDA-I) nursing diagnoses. Do you agree? Why or why not?*

2. *You arrive for your scheduled shift and discover there is inadequate staffing to safely care for your assigned patients. What do you do? What do you do if you have previously reported staffing concerns to your supervisor?*

SUMMARY

Nurses are obligated to provide patient-centered care that is consistent with ethical standards and that complies with applicable state and federal laws and regulations. Nurses must be aware of their employer's procedures and resources for reporting ethical and legal concerns and violations. Nurses who provide care at this level help ensure patient safety and improve patient outcomes, actions that prevent further suffering and promote hope among patients and their families.

Chapter Highlights

1. Nurses are obligated to provide clinically competent, patient-centered care consistent with ethical standards and compliant with applicable legal and regulatory requirements.

2. Ethical patient care is consistent with the American Nurses Association's Code of Ethics for Nurses with Interpretive Statements.

3. The ethical principles of autonomy, beneficence, nonmaleficence, justice, veracity, and fidelity reflect the inherent dignity of all persons. Nurses may use these concepts to clarify what should be done in a particular situation.

4. Ethical decision making involves a deliberate approach to problem solving, rather than simply revealing the "right" answer.

5. Federal laws or legislation that affect care of patients with mental illness include the Health Insurance Portability and Accountability Act of 1996 (HIPAA) and the Patient Self-Determination Act (PSDA).

6. Nurse practice acts empower state nursing boards to implement and enforce state nursing regulations, including investigating allegations of nursing misconduct, incompetence, and negligence, often in tandem with state civil or criminal proceedings.

7. The primary source of nursing liability is civil malpractice. Malpractice is professional negligence—failure to exercise care—or unintentional carelessness. A nurse is liable for nursing malpractice if he or she does not satisfy professional nursing standards.

8. The six major categories of negligence that result in malpractice lawsuits against nurses involve failure to follow standards

of care, failure to use equipment in a responsible manner, failure to communicate, failure to document, failure to assess and monitor, and failure to act as a patient advocate.

9. Although less common than negligence-based torts, intentional torts are another potential source of psychiatric nursing liability. The most common are assault, battery, and false imprisonment.

10. Patients have both an ethical and a legal right to active participation in their care.

11. Informed consent is the vehicle by which patients exercise their right to self-determination. Consent is "informed" only if a competent patient is provided with sufficient information to make a voluntary and knowledgeable decision.

12. Capacity is a function of the patient's clinical picture at a specific moment in time. No psychiatric or cognitive condition automatically eliminates the presumption of capacity.

13. A patient is admitted to a psychiatric hospital "voluntarily" when the patient or someone on his or her behalf makes a written application for and consents to admission and treatment.

14. Some patients in need of hospitalization cannot or will not consent to voluntary treatment. They may be admitted involuntarily if certain commitment standards are satisfied. Involuntary commitment carries significant legal and ethical issues and some restriction of patient rights.

15. The ethical and human rights issues most frequently experienced by psychiatric nurses involve protecting patients' rights and human dignity.

16. The ethical issue most disturbing or stressful to psychiatric nurses is staffing patterns that adversely affect nursing care.

17. Accepting or refusing a patient assignment has significant ethical and legal consequences. A nurse confronting an inappropriate assignment must first confer with the assignor and attempt to negotiate a more acceptable assignment.

18. Nurses must be aware of their employer's procedures and resources for reporting ethical and legal concerns and violations.

NCLEX®-RN Questions

1. The nurse is evaluating the implementation of a professional code of ethics on the psychiatric mental health unit. Which outcome best indicates that the model or framework is achieving the intended purpose?
   a. Ethical dilemmas are reduced or eliminated.
   b. Answers to ethical challenges are readily available.
   c. Accountability for resolving issues shifts to the nurse.
   d. Conflicts are addressed through established guidelines.

2. The psychiatric–mental health nurse is performing a quality improvement audit and notices that several weeks earlier she had accidently omitted a dose of a patient's medication. The nurse knows the patient has since stabilized and been discharged to the home setting. Which ethical principle best represents what the nurse is violating when she fails to report the omission?
   a. Veracity
   b. Autonomy
   c. Beneficence
   d. Nonmaleficence

3. The nurse is assigned to a research project and is addressing patients who have agreed to participate. Which action is most consistent with principles of the ethical theory of deontology?
   a. Reinforcing the essential partnership required to meet the project's goals
   b. Determining whether the patients' values really support the completion of the project
   c. Ensuring that the patients understand that consent can be retracted at any time
   d. Reminding the patients that they have committed to do something that will benefit others

4. The mental health nurse is caring for a patient who discloses intent to harm someone else. The nurse refers to the institution's policies to determine whether there are guidelines for dealing with this. Which step in ethical decision making is the nurse carrying out?
   a. Making a decision
   b. Exploring options
   c. Learning background information
   d. Identifying stakeholders' obligations

5. The nurse is conducting a psycho-education group with patients who have histories of mental illness. Which laws would the nurse address when talking about what may differ depending on where in the U.S. patients reside? Select all that apply.
   a. Standards for commitment
   b. Restraint and seclusion laws
   c. Parity in health care coverage
   d. Basic right to informed consent
   e. Confidentiality under the Health Insurance Portability and Accountability Act (HIPAA)

6. The nurse is caring for a young adult in treatment for mental health issues. Which action best represents a violation of the patient's right to confidentiality?
   a. Refusal to honor the patient's request for space
   b. Reading through a patient's journal without permission
   c. Sharing information related to the patient's legal status with the patient's employer without authorization
   d. Imposing consequences if the patient does not provide the information needed for an admission history

7. The nurse is assigned to care for an adult patient suffering from depression. The patient was involuntarily hospitalized after expressing intent to commit suicide. During morning report, the nurse is told that the 72-hour period allowed for emergency admissions will expire. The nurse understands that what is most likely to occur next? Select all that apply.
   a. The patient is discharged to his or her home.
   b. The patient is offered a conditional release.
   c. The patient consents to voluntary treatment.
   d. The patient is provided with due process through a court hearing.
   e. The patient is committed to long-term involuntary hospitalization.

8. The nurse is providing teaching to the family of a patient committed to a locked inpatient unit. The family asks the nurse what it means when members of the health care team state that they strive to provide a restraint-free environment. Which response by the nurse is best?
   a. "We try to maintain very strict rules so patients will not engage in behaviors that result in the need for restraints."
   b. "We don't admit patients who engage in unsafe behavior because we don't have the resources to use restraints."
   c. "Our goal is to provide the least restrictive option for patients with mental illness so we endeavor to eliminate the use of restraints."
   d. "We believe that restraints should be used as a last resort for patients and we incorporate additional measures to avoid their use."

9. A group of mental health nurses is caring for patients with mental illness on a locked inpatient unit. Over the past several months, a patient has assaulted and injured many of the nurses. What should the nurses consider when determining the best course of action?
   a. Nurses' rights may be obscured by policies and laws.
   b. Patients with mental illness are not culpable for their actions.
   c. Workers' compensation covers the emotional impact of violence.
   d. All states have stiff legal penalties against persons who assault nurses.

Answers and rationales may be found on the Pearson student resource site: nursing.pearsonhighered.com

Pearson Nursing Student Resources   Find additional review materials at **nursing.pearsonhighered.com**

References.

Addington v. Texas, 99 S.Ct. 1813, 441 U.S. 418 (1979).

Aiken, T. D. (2004). *Legal, Ethical and Political Issues in Nursing*. Philadelphia, PA: F.A. Davis.

American Association of Colleges of Nursing. (2008). *The Essentials of Baccalaureate Education for Professional Nursing Practice and Tool Kit*. Washington, DC: American Association of Colleges of Nursing.

American Association of Critical Care Nurses. (2004). *The 4 A's to Rise above Moral Distress*. Aliso Viejo, CA: American Association of Critical Care Nurses. Available at http://www.aacn.org/WD/Practice/Docs/4As_to_Rise_Above_Moral_Distress.pdf

American Nurses Association. (n.d.). Short definitions of ethical principles and theories: Familiar words, what do they mean? Washington, DC: American Nurses Association. Available at http://nursingworld.org/MainMenu Categories/EthicsStandards/Resources/Ethics-Definitions.pdf

American Nurses Association. (2001). *Code of Ethics for Nurses with Interpretive Statements*. Silver Spring, MD: American Nurses Publishing.

American Nurses Association (ANA), International Society for Psychiatric Nurses (ISPN), and Association of Psychiatric Nurses (APNA). (2014). *Psychiatric–Mental Health Nursing: Scope and Standards of Practice*. Silver Spring, MD: American Nurses Publishing.

American Nurses Association. (2013). *Correctional Nursing: Scope and Standards of Practice* (2nd ed.). Silver Spring, MD: American Nurses Publishing.

American Psychiatric Nurses Association. (2007). Position statement: Use of seclusion and restraint. Available at www.apna.org

American Psychiatric Nurses Association. (2011). Position statement: Staffing inpatient psychiatric units—A call for new staffing models. Available at http://www.apna.org/i4a/pages/index.cfm?pageid=4662

American Society of Registered Nurses. (2007). Can core nursing values and ethics be taught? Available at http://www.asrn.org/journal-nursing/233-can-core-nursing-values-and-ethics-be-taught.html

Appelbaum, B. C., Appelbaum, P. S., & Grisso, T. (1998). Competence to consent to voluntary psychiatric hospitalization: A test of a standard proposed by APA. *Psychiatric Services, 49*, 1193–1196.

Barrett, M. S. (2012). Ethical decision making: A framework for understanding and resolving mental health dilemmas. In C. Ulrich (Ed.). *Nursing Ethics in Everyday Practice*. Indianapolis, IN: Sigma Theta Tau International, pp. 17–35.

Beauchamp, T. L., & Childress, J. F. (2009). *Principles of Biomedical Ethics* (6th ed.). New York, NY: Oxford University Press.

Beauchamp, T. L., Walters, L., Kahn, J. P., & Mastroianni, A. C. (2007). *Contemporary Issues in Bioethics* (7th ed.). Belmont, CA: Thompson Wadsworth.

Beinner, W. (2007). Non-emergent involuntary medication state-by-state report. National Association of State Mental Health Program Directors (NASMHPD) Legal Division 2007 Annual Meeting, October 22, 2007. Available at http://mentalhealth.vermont.gov/sites/dmh/files/report/DMH-State_by_State_Involuntary_Medication.pdf

Bernstein, R. (2011). White paper: Criminal justice reform: Lessons from the deinstitutionalization movement. Washington, DC: Bazelon Center for Mental Health Law.

Birnbaum, R. (2010). My father's advocacy for a right to treatment. *Journal of the American Academy of Psychiatry and Law, 38*, 115–123.

Bonnie, R. (2010). Should a personality disorder qualify as a mental disease in insanity adjudication? *Journal of Law, Medicine and Ethics, 38*, 760–763.

Brooke, P. S. (2009). Legally speaking…when can you say no? *Nursing, 39*, 42–46.

Burkhardt, M. A., & Nathaniel, A. K. (2007). *Ethics and Issues in Contemporary Nursing* (3rd ed.). Clifton Park, NJ: Delmar Cengage Learning.

Cady, R. (2010). A review of basic patient rights in psychiatric care. *Journal of Nursing Administration's Healthcare Law, Ethics and Regulation, 12*, 117–125.

Canterbury v. Spence, 464 F.2d 772 (1972).

Chally, P. S., & Loriz, L. (1998). Ethics in the trenches: Decision making in practice. *American Journal of Nursing, 96*, 17–20.

Chapman, R., Styles, I., Perry, I., & Combs, S. (2010). Nurses' experience of adjusting to workplace violence: A theory of adaptation. *International Journal of Mental Health Nursing, 19*, 186–194.

Child Welfare Information Gateway. (2009). Penalties for failure to report and false reporting of child abuse and neglect: Summary of state laws. Washington, DC: Child Welfare Information Gateway. Available at www.childwelfare.gov/systemwide/laws_policies/statutes/report.cfm

Connecticut Department of Mental Health and Addiction Services. Your rights as a patient or a client. Available at http://www.ct.gov/dmhas/LIB/dmhas/publications/ptrights.pdf

Corley, M. C. (2002). Nurse moral distress: A proposed theory and research agenda. *Nursing Ethics, 9*, 636–650.

Corley, M. C., & Minick, P. (2002). Moral distress or moral comfort. *Bioethics Forum, 18*, 7–14.

Covington v. Harris, 419 F.2d 617 (1969).

Croke, E. M. (2003). Nurses, negligence, and malpractice, an analysis based on more than 250 cases against nurses. *American Journal of Nursing, 103*, 54–63.

Curtin, L. L. (1978). A proposed critical model for ethical analysis. *Nursing Forum, 17*, 12–17.

De Casterlé, B. D., Izumi, S., Godfrey, N. S., & Denhaerynck, K. (2008). Nurses' responses to ethical dilemmas in nursing practice: Meta-analysis. *Journal of Advanced Nursing, 63*, 540–549.

Deady, R., & McCarthy, J. (2010). A study of the situations, features, and coping mechanisms experienced by Irish psychiatric nurses experiencing moral distress. *Perspectives in Psychiatric Care, 46*, 209–220.

Deering, C. G. (1999). To speak or not to speak?: Self-disclosure with patients. *American Journal of Nursing, 99*, 34–38.

Dock, S. E. (1917). The relation of the nurse to the doctor and the doctor to the nurse. *American Journal of Nursing, 17*, 394–396.

Dusky v. United States, 362 U.S. 402 (1960).

Elliott, A. C. (2001). Cultural relativity of autonomy. *Journal of Transcultural Nursing, 12*, 326–330.

Federal Bill of Rights for Mental Health Patients: 42 U.S.C.A. § 10841.

Fins, J. J., & del Pozo, P. R. (2011, July 18). Too much information: Informed consent in cultural context. Medscape: http://www.medscape.com/viewarticle/746187

Gilbert, A. R., Moser, L. L., Van Dorn, R. A., Swanson, J. W., Wilder, C. M., Robbins, P. S., . . . Swartz, M. S. (2010). Reductions in arrest under assisted outpatient treatment in New York. *Psychiatric Services, 61*, 996–999.

Gilliland, M. (2010). A systematic approach to ethical decision-making for nurses confronted with ethical problems involving elder abuse. *Health Careers Today* (August), 16–23.

Grace, P. J., Fry, S. T., & Schultz, G. S. (2003). Ethics and human rights issues experienced by psychiatric-mental health and substance abuse registered nurses. *Journal of the American Psychiatric Nurses Association, 9*, 17–23.

Guido, G. W. (2010). *Legal and Ethical Issues in Nursing* (5th ed.). Upper Saddle River, NJ: Pearson Education.

Hamilton, P. M. (2009). Pain management: Ethical and legal issues. *Wild Iris Medical Education*. Available at http://www.nursingceu.com/courses/278/index_nceu.html

Hannon-Engel, S. (2011). Regulatory oversight: Do psychiatric patients have the right to refuse treatment? *Archives of Psychiatric Nursing, 25*, 21–23.

Harm. Merriam-Webster http://www.merriam-webster.com/dictionary/harm

Harnett, P. J., & Greaney, A. (2008). Operationalizing autonomy: Solutions for mental health nursing practice. *Journal of Psychiatric and Mental Health Nursing, 15*, 2–9.

Health Insurance Portability and Accountability Act (HIPAA) Final Rule. (2002). 45 C.F.R. Parts 160 and 164.

Helm, A. (2003). *Nursing Malpractice: Sidestepping Legal Minefields*. Philadelphia, PA: Lippincott Williams & Wilkins.

Hinson v. Glen Oak Retirement System, 853 So.2d 726 (2003).

Hoyt, S. (2010). Florence Nightingale's contribution to contemporary nursing ethics. *Journal of Holistic Nursing, 28*, 331–332.

International Council of Nurses (ICN). 2012. *The ICN Code of Ethics for Nurses.* Geneva, Switzerland: ICN.

Jackson v. Indiana, 406 U.S. 715 (1972).

Knoll, J. L., & Resnick, P. J. (2008). Insanity defense evaluations: Toward a model for evidence-based practice. *Brief Treatment and Crisis Intervention, 8*(1), 92–110.

Kohlberg, L. (1973). The claim to moral adequacy of a highest stage of moral judgment. *Journal of Philosophy, 70*, 630–646.

Kopala, B., & Burkhart, L. (2005). Ethical dilemma and moral distress: Proposed new NANDA diagnoses. *International Journal of Nursing Terminologies and Classifications, 16*, 3–13.

Lachman, V. D. (2007). Moral courage: A virtue in need of development? *MedSurg Nursing, 16*, 131–133.

Lachman, V. D. (2008). Whistleblowers: Troublemakers or virtuous nurses? *MedSurg Nursing, 17*, 126–134.

Lavelle, S., & Tusaie, K. R. (2011). Reflecting on forced medication. *Issues in Mental Health Nursing, 32*, 274–278.

Leo, R. J. (1999). Competency and the capacity to make treatment decisions: A primer for primary care physicians. *Journal of Clinical Psychiatry, 1*, 131–141.

Miller, R. D. (2006). *Problems in Health Care Law* (9th ed.). Sudbury, MA: Jones and Bartlett Publishers.

Minnesota Board of Nursing. (2010) Professional boundaries in nursing. Available at http://mn.gov/health-licensing-boards/images/Professional_Boundaries_in_Nursing.pdf

Miracle, V. A. (2009). National nurses week and the nightingale pledge. *Dimensions of Critical Care Nursing, 28*, 145–146.

Moser, J. (2009). Texas nurses under fire for whistleblowing. *American Journal of Nursing, 109*, 19.

National Alliance on Mental Illness (NAMI). (2009). Grading the states: A report on America's health care system for a quality mental health system: A vision of recovery. Available at http://www.nami.org/Content/NavigationMenu/Grading_the_States_2009/Full_Report1/Full_Report.htm

National Council of State Boards of Nursing (n.d.). Discipline: Initial Review of a Complaint. Available at https://www.ncsbn.org/3772.htm#types

Newport, F. (2012, December 3). Congress retains low honesty rating: Nurses have highest honesty rating; car salespeople, lowest. Available at http://www.gallup.com/poll/159035/congress-retains-low-honesty-rating.aspx

New York State Department of Mental Health. (2006). An explanation of Kendra's Law. Available at http://www.omh.ny.gov/omhweb/Kendra_web/Ksummary.htm

O'Connor v. Donaldson, 422 U.S. 563 (1975).

Ohnishi, K., Ohgushi, Y., Nakano, M., Fujii, H., Tanaka, H., Kitaoka, K., Nakahara, J., & Narita, Y. (2010). Moral distress experienced by psychiatric nurses in Japan. *Nursing Ethics, 17*, 726–740.

Packard v. Packard, 27 Fam LQ 515 (1864).

Pavlish, C., Brown-Saltzman, K., Hersh, M., Shirk, M., & Nudelman, O. (2011). Early indicators and risk factors for ethical issues in clinical practice. *Journal of Nursing Scholarship, 43*, 13–21.

Philipsen, N. C., & Soeken, D. (2011). Preparing to blow the whistle: A survival guide for nurses. *Journal for Nurse Practitioners, 7*, 740–746.

Price-Hoskins, P. (2004). Workplace challenges: The right thing—for the right reason. *Journal of Christian Nursing, 21*, 6–12.

Regan, K. (2010). Trauma informed care on an inpatient pediatric psychiatric unit and the emergence of ethical dilemmas as nurses evolved their practice. *Issues in Mental Health Nursing, 31*, 216–222.

Reilly v. Spinazze, 34 So.3d 1069, 2010 La. App. LEXIS 1000 (2010).

Roberts, L. W., & Dyer, A. R. (2004). *Concise Guide to Ethics in Mental Health Care.* Arlington, VA: American Psychiatric Publishing.

Salladay, S. A. (2008). A Christian code of ethics. *Journal of Christian Nursing, 25*, 167.

Schoendorff v. Society of New York Hosp., 105 N.E. 92, 93 (N.Y. 1914).

Sessums, L. L., Zembrzuska, H., & Jackson, J. L. (2011). Does this patient have a medical decision-making capacity? *JAMA, 306*, 420–427.

Sheehan, K. A., & Burns, T. (2011). Perceived coercion and the therapeutic relationship: A neglected association? *Psychiatric Services, 62*, 471–476.

Simon, R., & Shuman, W. (2011). Psychiatry and the law. In R. E. Hales, S. C. Yudofsky, & G. O. Gabbard, (Eds.). *The American Psychiatric Publishing Textbook of Clinical Psychiatry* (5th ed.). Washington, DC: American Psychiatric Publishing. Available at www.Psychiatryonline.com

Slovenko, R. (2009). *Psychiatry in Law/Law in Psychiatry* (2nd ed.). New York, NY: Routledge.

Snow, N., & Austin, W. J. (2009). Community treatment orders: The ethical balancing act in community mental health. *Journal of Psychiatric and Mental Health Nursing, 16*, 177–186.

Swanson, J. W., Swartz, M. S., Elbogen, E. B., Van Dorn, R. A., Wagner, H. R., Moser, L. A., Wilder, C., & Gilbert, A. R. (2008). Psychiatric advance directives and reduction of coercive crisis interventions. *Journal of Mental Health, 17*, 255–267.

Swanson, J., Swartz, M., Van Dorn, R. A., Monahan, J., McGuire, T. G., Steadman, H. J., & Robbins, P. C. (2009). Racial disparities in involuntary outpatient commitment: Are they real? *Health Affairs, 28*(3), 816–826.

Swartz, M. S., Wilder, C. M., Swanson, J. W., Van Dorn, R. A., Robbins, P. C., Steadman, H. J., . . . Monahan, R.. (2010). Assessing outcomes for consumers in New York's assisted outpatient treatment program. *Psychiatric Services, 61*, 976–981.

Taft, S. H. (2000, November 8). An inclusive look at the domain of ethics and its application to administrative behavior. *Online Journal of Issues in Nursing, 6*. Available at http://www.nursingworld.org/MainMenuCategories/ANAMarketplace/ANAPeriodicals/OJIN/TableofContents/Volume62001/No1Jan01/ArticlePreviousTopic/DomainofEthics.html

Talbott, J. A. (2011). The rights of Americans with mental illness. *Journal of Nervous & Mental Disease, 199*, 578–584.

Tarasoff v. Board of Regents of University of California, 592 P.S. 553 (1974); *Tarasoff v. Regents of the University of California* (*Tarasoff II*), 551 P.2d 334 (1976).

Ulrich, C. M., Hamric, A. B., & Grady, C. (2010). Moral distress: A growing problem in the health professions? *Hastings Center Report, 40*, 20–22.

Ulrich, C. M., Taylor, C., Soeken, K., O'Donnell, P., Farrar, A., Danis, M., & Grady, C. (2010). Everyday ethics: Ethical issues and stress in nursing practice. *Journal of Advanced Nursing, 66*, 2510–2519.

University of Toronto Joint Center for Bioethics. (n.d.) Community tools: Aid to capacity evaluation. Available at http://www.jointcentreforbioethics.ca/tools/ace_download.shtml

Velasquez, M., Moberg, D., Meyer, D., Shanks, T., McLean, M., DeCosse, D., André, C., & Hanson, K. (2009). A framework for thinking ethically. Available at http://www.scu.edu/ethics/practicing/decision/framework.html

Vuckovich, P. K., & Artinian, B. M. (2005). Justifying coercion. *Nursing Ethics, 12*, 370–380.

Weston, M. (2010, July 2). Strategies for enhancing autonomy and control over nursing practice. *Online Journal of Issues in Nursing, 15*. Available at http://www.nursingworld.org/MainMenuCategories/ANAMarketplace/ANAPeriodicals/OJIN/TableofContents/Vol152010/No1Jan2010/Enhancing-Autonomy-and-Control-and-Practice.aspx

Westrick, S. J., & Dempski, K. (2009). *Essentials of Nursing Law and Ethics.* Sudbury, MA: Jones and Bartlett.

Wilkinson, J. M. (1987). Moral distress in nursing practice: Experience and effect. *Nursing Forum, 23*, 16–29.

Wocial, L.D. (2012). Finding a voice in ethics: Everyday ethical behavior in nursing. In C. Ulrich (Ed.). *Nursing Ethics in Everyday Practice*. Indianapolis, IN: Sigma Theta Tau International, pp. 37–48.

Wyatt v. Stickney 325 F. Supp. 781 (1971); 1971 U.S. Dist. LEXIS 14217, March 12, 1971; *Wyatt v. Stickney*, 344 F.Supp. 387 (M.D. Ala. 1972).

Wysoker, A. (2001). Standards of care. *Journal of the American Psychiatric Nurses Association, 7*, 166–168.

11

Management and Leadership

Carole Farley-Toombs

Key Terms

Learning Outcomes

1. Examine the unique challenges faced by psychiatric–mental health nurses in creating safe and healing care environments.

2. Describe the potential for burnout due to recurrent stress arousal and how this can have an impact on work satisfaction and patient care.

3. Distinguish between management and leadership skills in creating safe and healing environments for psychiatric–mental health care delivery.

4. Identify examples of management skills that support a healthy, empowering work environment for psychiatric–mental health nurses.

5. Illustrate leadership skills that support the development of empowered psychiatric–mental health nurses at the point of delivery.

6. Summarize the relationship between structural and psychological empowerment and innovative professional nursing practice behaviors in advancing new paradigms of care.

Part 1

You are assigned to a clinical rotation on evening shifts on a 22-bed acute inpatient psychiatric unit in a general hospital. The unit serves patients ages 18 to 60 who are admitted from a psychiatric emergency department for stabilization of acute symptoms of psychiatric disorders.

During report, Nancy, the day charge nurse, remarks that the unit is currently "very acute."

- Paul Croft, a 23-year-old newly admitted male patient, was highly agitated, verbally aggressive, and responding to internal stimuli earlier in the shift. While nursing staff tried to help him to return to his room to decrease stimulation and offer him PRN medications, Mr. Croft struck out at them and hit a nurse in the face. The nurse is being evaluated in the emergency department (ED). It is reported that the staff members were able to avoid use of restraints but that Mr. Croft, while calmer, remains very preoccupied with internal stimuli, is difficult to engage, and remains at risk for more aggressive behaviors.

- The mental health assistant assigned to do checks every 15 minutes found George Blackwell, a 58-year-old patient, trying to tie a pillowcase around his neck. Nursing staff quickly intervened and there was no apparent injury to the patient. The psychiatric nurse practitioner on the unit evaluated Mr. Blackwell and placed him on continual suicide watch with one designated staff member (1:1). Mr. Blackwell's admission earlier this week followed a serious suicide attempt; he continues to report feeling overwhelmed by serious psychosocial stressors and feels hopeless that they can be resolved. Nancy reports that both the event with Mr. Croft and the situation with Mr. Blackwell upset other patients on the unit, requiring increased attention from the nursing staff. As a result, it has been an exhausting day.

- The ED plans to admit Kimberly Turner, a 35-year-old female patient, to the unit on the evening shift. Ms. Turner has had previous admissions for acute symptoms of bipolar disorder with mania. She is being admitted after getting into a physical altercation with her elderly mother, with whom she lives. When police arrived, Ms. Turner's speech was pressured; her thoughts were very tangential and disorganized; and she demanded to be released, as she was needed to save the world. She accepted some medication in the emergency department, but the ED staff reports that she remains activated and intrusive with other patients. Nancy reports that she expects Ms. Turner will be "a handful" when she gets on the unit.

You notice that one of the oncoming staff rolls his eyes and make a comment about "here we go again with her." Another staff member nods and says, "As soon as she leaves here, she's right back at it." The charge nurse acknowledges that it is unfortunate the Ms. Turner requires another admission for the "same old symptoms." The charge nurse adds that the chief social worker will be setting up a meeting early in the admission to explore alternative discharge options for Ms. Turner: Living with her elderly mother is no longer adequate to keep her stable outside the hospital. The staff members agree that such a meeting might help.

The charge nurse continues with report. There are two open beds on the unit, but the psychiatric ED is very busy and it is likely that more patients will need admission. As you listen to report, you learn that another patient is experiencing moderate withdrawal from alcohol use and vital signs are being taken every two hours. In addition, a patient with poorly controlled diabetes has had elevated blood glucose levels all day and her intake is being closely monitored. The medical attending who covers medical issues on the unit has been called and will see the patient with diabetes in the morning.

Nancy also states that a nurse called in sick for the evening shift and that she was able to arrange for one of the nurses on day shift to stay a few hours longer; a night shift nurse will come early to cover the rest of the shift. Another nurse coming onto the evening shift sitting next to you introduces herself. She has been on the unit for 4 weeks and this is her first shift off orientation. She says her preceptor is on the same shift and she is very happy about that.

APPLICATION

1. What is your perception of the change of shift report process as described here?

2. What are your thoughts about the content of what was reported?

3. What potential nursing management and leadership issues can you identify?

4. What are you feeling as you start your shift?

Introduction

Nurses in all care settings benefit from working with nurses and other professionals who possess effective leadership and management skills. This chapter discusses why psychiatric–mental health care settings—in particular, acute care settings—require strong and effective leaders and managers and the qualities that successful leaders and managers possess. Two theories, structural empowerment theory and psychological empowerment theory, emphasize the need for supportive leaders and managers who are able to evaluate both human and material resources and who can help nurses and other staff find congruence between their own beliefs and values and the requirements of their positions and work environments. Nurse leaders and managers who are successful in supporting nurses and other staff promote an environment that encourages innovative practice behaviors as well as partnerships with patients and families, both of which contribute to safe and healing environments (Figure 11-1).

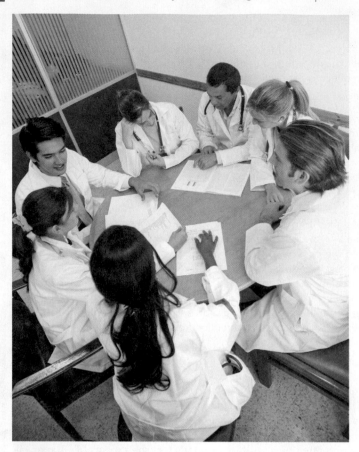

11-1 Nurse leaders and managers who are successful in supporting nurses and other staff promote an environment that encourages innovative practice behaviors as well as partnerships with patients and families, both of which contribute to safe and healing environments.

Source: Andres Rodriguez/Fotolia

Acute Psychiatric Care: Historical Perspective

Prior to the development of effective psychotropic medications, individuals with serious mental illness and psychiatric disorders were often institutionalized in long-term psychiatric care settings. These were typically state hospitals, funded by state budgets. Beginning in the 1970s, the advent of psychopharmacology and an increasing public awareness about some of the dehumanizing aspects of institutionalization led to efforts to move the care and treatment of patients with severe mental illness into community settings. Hospitalization, when needed, changed over time to short-term psychiatric inpatient units in general hospitals.

These settings were designed and staffed primarily to serve patients with less severe symptoms of psychiatric illness. As a result, in these general hospital settings, efforts to maintain the safety of patients with acute psychiatric symptoms who posed an imminent risk of harm to themselves or others often involved the use of controlling interventions, including enforcing rules and expectations; an emphasis on patient "compliance" with treatment; and more restrictive interventions, such as seclusion and restraint.

Psychiatric Care: A Paradigm Shift

In more recent years, the paradigms regarding psychiatric care and treatment have started to shift away from control, consistency, and vigilance to a paradigm of partnership with patients and families, emphasis on individualized care, and the support of hope for recovery. This paradigm shift is shining a light on the **point of service**, meaning the relationship between nurse and patient, as the place where safety and healing can be nurtured. This relationship develops through professional nursing behaviors and interventions to connect and engage in a partnership with patients. These nursing behaviors allow nurses to assist patients to achieve their self-defined goals for the moment, for the day, or for their future wellness (Chapter 8). This therapeutic level of care can be summarized in Hildegard Peplau's statement that "there is a significant difference between taking responsibility for the care of patients and being therapeutically responsive to each patient. Every professional contact with a patient, however brief, is an opportunity to engage" (Peplau, 1994, p. 7).

Today's psychiatric–mental health nurses face many challenges related to the unique needs of the patients they serve, including a regulatory perspective on quality that tends to be reactive instead of proactive, and the allocation of fiscal and human resources for a population that continues to be stigmatized by society (Hanrahan et al., 2010a; Delaney & Johnson, 2008). In many acute psychiatric settings, these challenges have a bearing on the ability to effectively integrate new paradigms of care into daily professional nursing practice. Strong nursing management practices and transformational psychiatric mental health nursing leadership can have a strong positive influence on the clinical work environment to effect evidence-based care, empower psychiatric nursing practice, improve patient outcomes, and improve nurse satisfaction with their work (Blegen & Severinsson, 2011; Smith & Hood, 2005; Tomey, 2009).

Empowering Nurses

Safe and healing psychiatric care environments require frontline nursing leadership and strong collaboration and management skills to assist nurses to integrate varying resources and structures to promote innovative practices consistent with new paradigms of care (Delaney & Johnson, 2008). The **front line** is the environment or space where nurses and patients interact directly on a daily basis. **Frontline nursing leadership** can be defined as the process by which nurses at the unit level motivate themselves and their nursing staff colleagues to engage in professional practice behaviors to accomplish the goal of creating a safe and healing environment (Manojlovich, 2005).

Management skills refer to the ability to mobilize the human and material resources required to meet the organization's goals, which include patient and staff safety and satisfaction and positive care outcomes at the unit level. Strong **collaboration skills** involve the ability to form interpersonal relationships and foster effective communication, using formal and informal power to gain access to information and to support opportunities for professional growth and development (Laschinger, 2009). **Information** includes both formal and informal knowledge needed to be effective in the workplace. **Support** includes regular feedback and guidance to individual nurses to promote optimal nursing professional performance. It also involves valuing the role and contributions of psychiatric–mental health nurses in improving the lives of patients and families struggling with psychiatric disorders and mental health problems.

Strong nursing management and leadership skills support the development of empowered nurses. Spence Laschinger, Finegan, and Wilk (2009) and Knol and van Linge (2009) propose that **empowered nurses:**

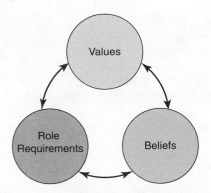

11-2 Congruence among values, beliefs, and role requirements supports the development of empowered nurses.

- Experience congruence between their values and beliefs and the requirements of their role (Figure 11-2).
- Have confidence in their abilities to achieve the goals of optimal patient care.
- Have a sense of being able to influence important patient outcomes.
- Have the potential to engage in innovative practice behaviors essential in implementing new paradigms of care.

This chapter describes how effective leadership and management skills can support nurses working in psychiatric–mental health nursing.

Pause and Reflect

1. *What does it mean to experience congruence between one's values and beliefs and the requirements of a professional role?*
2. *What do you think is the difference between "formal knowledge" and "informal knowledge"?*
3. *What do you need from your work environment to be able to influence patient outcomes?*
4. *What do you need within yourself to be able to influence patient outcomes?*

Environments of Care

More than two-thirds of psychiatric–mental health nurses in the United States work in acute psychiatric care settings, where they comprise the largest proportion of the professional workforce (Hanrahan, Delaney, & Merwin, 2006). Acute psychiatric clinical care settings include inpatient units, psychiatric emergency departments, partial hospital programs, and assertive community treatment teams. These are clinical settings where psychiatric–mental health nurses care for patients experiencing acute or chronically acute symptoms of a mental illness. Psychiatric–mental health nurses focus their work on collaboration with patients, families, and interdisciplinary colleagues to alleviate the intensity of patients' symptoms (such as hallucinations, delusions, severe depression, agitation, and anxiety) and to promote healing.

Violence and aggression are significant issues for patients suffering with acute or chronically acute psychiatric symptoms and for the nurses who care for them (Delaney & Johnson, 2008; Johnson, 2004; Zuzelo, Curran, & Zeserman, 2012). The potential for suicide attempts and/or self-harming behaviors also requires significant attention: Psychiatric nurses continually assess their patients and scan their environment to maintain safety (James, Steward, & Bowers, 2012).

Many patients also present with physical problems related to the following:

- Side effects of medications
- Risk factors such as smoking and substance abuse
- Lack of attention to basic health care needs or access to preventive medical care, including poorly controlled diabetes or hypertension, substance withdrawal symptoms, and chronic respiratory and cardiac conditions that can quickly become acute

In addition, psychotropic medications often are being quickly titrated in these care environments in an effort to improve the acute symptoms of the psychiatric illness. The risk for severe adverse reactions to medications increases in these situations.

As a result of the ever-present patient and staff safety concerns in care environments, an approach to clinical care can develop whereby nurses remain on heightened alert for the potential of an incident. In an attempt to maintain a safe environment, nurses may focus attention on anticipating volatile or violent situations. This can result in a culture in which nurses remain vigilant and on standby for potential difficult situations rather than interacting with patients in a proactive manner (Zuzelo, Curran, & Zeserman, 2012).

The Role of Nurses in Patient Safety

Psychiatric–mental health nurses have a fundamental role in supporting the safety of patients with acute psychiatric symptoms. Delaney and Johnson (2008) assert that patient safety, both physical and psychological, is a central obligation and the key deliverable of acute care psychiatric nursing. This work involves consistently being therapeutically present and engaged with patients whose behaviors, because of the acute symptoms of their illness, may be unpredictable, disruptive, and intrusive and/or pose an imminent danger to themselves or others. Psychiatric nurses face multiple challenges in achieving this mission in acute care settings. Some examples of the clinical and systems challenges are found in Table 11-1.

Emphasis on reduced lengths of stay while maintaining census compresses the amount of time nurses can actually spend with individual patients. The demand for admissions to inpatient psychiatric beds, the variables affecting RN staffing numbers, and the quality of the nursing staff in the short term or the long term may create situations in which staffing expertise no longer matches the acuity needs of the unit (Delaney & Johnson, 2008; Hanrahan et al., 2010b).

Table 11-2 provides examples of variables that can affect the quantity of nursing staffing in the short term and long term. *Short term* is defined has having an impact on unit function from a single shift to up to 6 weeks. *Long term* is defined as greater than 6 weeks and can be a year or more.

Examples of the variables that affect the quality of the psychiatric mental health nursing staff in clinical care settings are provided in Table 11-3.

Challenges Faced by Psychiatric–Mental Health Nurses — table 11-1

Type	Examples
Clinical challenges	• Patients present with a variety of diagnoses and types of symptom acuity in an interactive milieu. • Patients often have co-morbid physiological and medical needs requiring nursing attention and intervention.
Systems challenges	• Reduced numbers of psychiatric inpatient beds contribute to increase in census; at times patient numbers run above census, making it difficult to meet demand. • An emphasis on short-term admissions and reduced lengths of stay means patients are very acute during their admission and there is less time for nurses and staff to get to know them.
Third-party reimbursement	• Health insurance companies often use managed-care models that limit levels of reimbursement for psychiatric–mental health care, affecting the potential revenue for the services. In turn, this can affect how organizations budget for expenses, including staffing models. • Many third-party payors use criteria for approving continuing inpatient care that interprets "active treatment" as frequent changes in medication. This does not take into consideration psychotropic medication half-lives and the complex nature of stabilization of acute symptoms. Premature discharge can result in quick or recurrent readmissions, which can affect psychiatric nurses' sense of efficacy in caring for their patients.
Staffing mix	• Most acute psychiatric clinical care settings include RNs, LPNs, and unlicensed assistive personnel (UAP). The absence of technologically sophisticated medical procedures and equipment in such settings, combined with a lack of understanding on the part of hospital administrations regarding the level of psychiatric nursing expertise and skill required to safely care for persons with acute psychiatric symptoms, can lead to staffing ratios of RN to LPN/UAP that restrict the role of the RN to supervision and delegation rather than direct patient care.

Variables Affecting Quantity of Nursing Staff — table 11-2

Quantity	Short Term	Long Term
Staff member calling in sick; short-term disabilities	x	
Nursing resignations, terminations, retirements, transfers	x	x
Difficulty recruiting to fill vacant positions	x	x
Lack of organizational support for incremental RNs to meet increase in number of patients, patient acuity needs, or higher rate of admissions/discharges	x	x

Variables Affecting Quality of Nursing Staff — table 11-3

Quality Issues	Short Term	Long Term
Institutionally approved ratio of RNs to assistive personnel does not reflect the evolving nursing care needs of the patients; nurses spend more time documenting, administering medications, and putting out fires than in therapeutic interpersonal interactions with patients.	x	x
Service- and unit-based psychiatric–mental health nursing orientation and ongoing professional development are not well developed, of sufficient length, competency-based, or continually reevaluated for consistency with the evidence and new paradigms of care. New nurses remain novice nurses for an extended period of time.	x	x

The use of restraints and seclusion may increase under such circumstances, as nurses revert to attempts to contain and control to maintain safety (Box 11-1). The use of restrictive interventions usually requires hands-on interventions, which increase the risk of psychological and physical injury to patients and staff. Trust among patients and staff may diminish, increasing the level of overall acuity on the unit. Consequently, nurses may find themselves on constant high alert for the potential for danger or adverse events in attempting to fulfill their mission to maintain safety (Zuzelo, Curran, & Zeserman, 2012). The neurobiological processes activated in all human beings by the sense of danger place psychiatric–mental health nurses at the risk of burnout. The symptoms of burnout undermine the fundamental expertise and effectiveness that psychiatric–mental health nurses bring to creating

box 11-1

The Joint Commission

The Joint Commission sets regulatory standards for inpatient settings and accredits more than 19,000 organizations and programs in the United States. It addresses issues related to policies, procedures, and leadership responsibilities to reduce the use of restrictive measures with patients through proactive interdisciplinary treatment planning, nursing staff competency-based training, and continuous performance improvement initiatives.

and sustaining safe and healing environments: the therapeutic use of self.

Burnout as a Management and Leadership Issue

Hanrahan et al. (2010a) conducted a secondary analysis of a large database linking nurse survey data with hospital data to examine the extent to which organizational factors of the psychiatric nurse work environment affect psychiatric nursing report of burnout. Maslach, Jackson, and Leiter (1996) describe **burnout** as consisting of three stages: stress arousal, energy conservation, and exhaustion. Stress arousal involves activation of the neurobiological pathways designed to prepare the body to fight or flee.

Psychiatric–mental health nurses in acute care settings are exposed to actual or potential critical incidents on each shift. A **critical incident** is defined as any sudden, unexpected event that has an emotional impact sufficient to overwhelm the usual effective coping skills of an individual or group. Critical incidents can be events that are perceived to pose a serious threat to safety of patients or staff, including assaults, physical threats, serious suicide attempts, or an acute onset of a serious medical problem. Critical incidents may be experienced as dehumanizing, shocking, or terrifying and may induce feelings of powerlessness, fear, anger, and a constant state of alert (Caine & Ter-Bagdasarian, 2003).

When these events occur, they are initially perceived as a sensation such as a "gut feeling" that precipitates a set of neurobiological reactions (Figure 11-3).

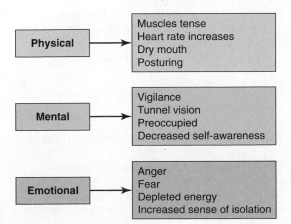

11-3 Neurobiological reactions to stress. Failure to recognize and respond to stress can lead nurses to conserve energy. Increased sick calls, depersonalization, and a reduced sense of accomplishment indicate that the nurse has reached the exhaustion, or burnout, stage.

Physically, muscles tense to prepare the body to fight or flee. The heart rate increases to feed the muscles. The mouth becomes dry to prevent aspiration during fight or flight. The body postures to deflect a potential assault and prepare to defend itself. These physical reactions occur before any cognitive processing of the potential danger actually occurs.

Meanwhile, mental processes go on high alert as the individual becomes vigilant and self-protective, narrowing observations to identify the source of danger. At this stage, there is a preoccupation with protecting self and others and a decreased awareness of how one's body language and appearance are being perceived by others. All these are normal human reactions to the potential for imminent danger.

The potential for imminent danger can be a constant in acute psychiatric clinical care settings; this results in repeated episodes of stress arousal. Repeated episodes of stress arousal deplete energy and lead the nurse to conserve energy by withdrawing physically from the stimulus. This may mean being less present in the milieu, or it could result in increased sick calls. Prolonged stress arousal leads to emotional exhaustion, depersonalization, and reduced sense of personal accomplishment. High levels of emotional exhaustion are related to being emotionally overextended and exhausted by one's work. Depersonalization reflects an unemotional and impersonal response to patients. Low levels of personal achievement reflect feeling detached from potential job rewards (Leiter & Harvie, 1996).

Findings from a large study conducted by Hanrahan et al. (2010b) revealed that manager skill and leadership sustained the highest significance in relation to emotional exhaustion and depersonalization. The findings suggested that skilled managers on psychiatric units are very important to the well-being of the psychiatric nurses. Psychiatric nursing management skills identified as key included the following:

- Supervision
- Organization and direction for the nursing staff
- Negotiating physician–nurse relationships
- Representing the needs of the unit to upper level management to secure adequate resources

The study also found a strong and significant relationship between psychiatric nurses' experience of feeling valued and lower rates of expressed emotional exhaustion and depersonalization. The findings of the study reinforce the premise that psychiatric nurses need to focus on the value of the nurse and support the nursing model of care in their practice settings. Psychiatric nursing management and leadership skills are critical factors in realizing that potential.

Pause and Reflect

1. *Have you ever experienced a setting—at work or somewhere else—where you felt you always had to be on alert for difficult or surprise situations? How did you feel in that setting? How did having to maintain that level of alertness affect your performance? Your attitude toward others in the environment?*

2. *Why do you think there is a relationship between prolonged stress and a reduced sense of accomplishment? How do you think this relationship affects the nursing student? The single, working parent? An older adult caring for a spouse with dementia?*

3. *Why is the ability to negotiate adequate resources a key nursing management skill?*

Management Skills

Nursing management involves the effective mobilization and utilization of human and nonhuman resources to meet the needs of a patient population. Strong nursing management skills involve in-depth knowledge about the organization's budgeting policies and guidelines and the ability to identify and use national benchmarks to advocate for adequate nursing resources to meet patient safety needs. Effective nursing management also involves providing consistent support and supervision to facilitate the development of qualified and satisfied nursing staff. This includes providing education and direction regarding the delegation of tasks to colleagues and unlicensed assistive personnel as a critical element of nursing team function to meet patient care needs (Bittner & Gravlin, 2009; Potter, DeShields, & Kuhrik, 2010). Table 11-4 provides examples of key nursing management functions that support healthy work environments.

Kanter's (1977) theory of structural empowerment provides a useful framework for defining the management skills that create empowering work environments in which nurses use the full extent of their scope of practice to create safe and healing environments. **Structural empowerment theory** asserts that when workplace situations are structured in such a way that employees feel empowered, employees will respond accordingly and rise to the challenges present in their work environment. As a result, the organization is likely to benefit from improved employee attitudes and increased organizational effectiveness (Laschinger, Finegan, Shamian, & Wilk, 2001).

Power, from this perspective, is defined as the ability to mobilize resources, both human and material, to get things done. **Empowerment** refers to individuals' power in relationship to their position in the organization. **Formal power** results from a person's role title and his or her position description that articulates what accountabilities and authority are commensurate with that position (Knol & van Linge, 2009). The position is recognized and relevant within the organization and allows for discretion, flexibility and creativity, and autonomy in decision making (Lethbridge et al., 2011).

A *nurse manager* is an example of a role and position that has formal power in an organization. Nurse managers are accountable for quality of care delivered by nurses in the clinical areas over which they have authority while meeting fiscal expectations. A *charge nurse* is also an example of a role or position with formal power. The charge nurse is accountable for the safety of patients and quality of care delivered by the nursing staff assigned on the shift over which he or she is "in charge."

Informal power emerges from an individual's network of relationships with colleagues within the organization. These relationships provide support for understanding how the organization functions and provide the opportunities to collaborate for achieving

---

Examples of Fiscal and Human Resource Management Functions   table 11-4

Budgeting and fiscal accountability	• Understand the mechanisms by which salary and nonsalary budgets are developed. • Use national benchmarks, when available, for establishing number of nursing staff required to meet patient needs—e.g., RN care hours per patient day for inpatient units. This formula identifies the number of direct care hours each patient on a unit will need from an RN in a 24-hour period (admissions, discharges, medication administration, medication teaching and evaluation of effectiveness, supportive, psychoeducational and psychotherapeutic interventions).
Human resource management	• Fully understand and adhere to all organizational policies related to management of staff, including hiring, orientation, annual mandatory education, time reporting, holiday scheduling and holiday pay, and disciplinary action. • Know how to effectively use the human resources department to support efforts in managing staff to meet performance expectations. • Establish targets for nursing staff retention and collaborate with organizational leaders and interdisciplinary colleagues to develop strategies to meet them. • Have an in-depth understanding of the scope of psychiatric–mental health RN practice and the responsibilities associated with delegating responsibilities and tasks to LPNs and UAP.
Communication	• Use a variety of resources for communicating with staff on a daily basis. • Solicit input from staff regarding new policies, proposed initiatives, environmental redesign, etc. • Keep staff informed of proposed or actual changes and solicit feedback. • Hold regular staff meetings (at least weekly if possible) where information is provided and dialogue is valued. This helps the nurse manager stay informed on what staff perceive as key issues. Ensure that staff from all shifts can participate in staff meetings.

goals in a reciprocal manner. An example is a nurse manager calling a nurse manager on another unit with whom she has developed a collegial relationship to negotiate sharing staff to cover a newly ordered 1:1 for a patient.

Structural empowerment theory states that to create conditions for work effectiveness, managers must ensure that employees have access to four important elements: information, support, resources, and opportunities (Table 11-5).

Leadership Skills

Nursing leadership is the process that supports nurses' intrinsic motivation to meet the care needs of individual patients, the quality and safety goals of the organization, and the professional standards of practice (Table 11-6). **Intrinsic motivation** refers to doing something because it is inherently interesting or enjoyable rather than doing something to attain an unrelated goal such as pay or prestige.

Psychological empowerment, as conceptualized by Spreitzer (1995), informs the discussion on leadership in psychiatric–mental health nursing. **Psychological empowerment** is described as an interpersonal process that is shaped by an individual's personal experiences and belief about the work role (Lethbridge et al., 2011). It is

experienced as an active perspective regarding one's work role and supports an intrinsic motivation to contribute to organizational outcomes. Psychological empowerment consists of four domains: **meaning** (reflecting a congruence between a nurse's beliefs and values and his or her work requirements), competence, self-determination, and **impact** (the nurse's sense that he or she can influence important outcomes) (Table 11-7).

Pause and Reflect

1. *Can you think of a time when rumor or lack of information affected work conditions in a place where you work? How were work conditions affected? What might you have done to improve the situation if you had been one of the managers?*

2. *Think of a situation—paid or volunteer position—in which you or someone you know has informal power. How do you think that informal power developed? What attitudes or behaviors help develop informal power?*

3. *Pretend you are in a position to promote the work of the other student nurses in your class. What unique patient interests do some of your classmates have? What activities might be appropriate to help them develop their interests further?*

Elements of Empowered Workplaces — table 11-5

Information	1. Facts about an alarming situation that occurred on a previous shift.; in the absence of facts, rumors may take hold and undermine a sense of safety or trust.
	2. A strong, evidence-based orientation process for newly hired RNs that defines the competencies the nurses must acquire to meet the role expectations and what will be provided to assist them to achieve the competencies and expectations.
	3. Education about the neurobiological reactions involved in stress arousal, how repeated stress arousal can affect behaviors and emotions, and reinforce healthy coping skills.
	4. Informing nurses about organizational changes that will affect the care environment, such as new admission policies.
Support	1. Ongoing professional development programs to support attainment of new knowledge, skills, and expertise in a rapidly changing health care environment.
	2. Regular feedback and guidance to support achievement of individual professional goals.
	3. Validating that psychiatric nurses routinely deal with difficult—and, at times, frightening—situations and provide opportunities for nursing staff to participate in debriefing sessions when indicated.
	4. Acknowledging the teamwork and individual work that makes a difference on the unit and with individual patients.
Resources	1. Become informed about budget planning process and how decisions are made regarding nursing staffing to develop successful strategies for obtaining the nursing resources needed to meet your patient population needs.
	2. Advocate for the resource needs of the unit. Use data, such as average number of admissions/discharges in a 24-hour period; number of patients with medical co-morbidities that require nursing assessment and intervention; or the number of patients admitted for acute suicidal risk or violence risk that require nursing assessment and psychotherapeutic interventions.
	3. Advocate for resources for patients: educational materials, activities and programs, clean environment, and healthy foods.
Opportunities	1. Encourage nurses' involvement in local, regional and national professional organizations. This broadens the horizon and provides new opportunities for developing networks.
	2. Involve nurses in decisions regarding changes in practice to meet evolving needs of the patient population they serve.
	3. Involve nurses in evaluating outcomes of changes in practice in the spirit of continuous improvement.

Part 2

While the day charge nurse is preparing to give report to the evening shift, the nurse manager goes down to the emergency department to check on Michael Ryan, the nurse who was injured on the day shift. He has a visible bruise on his right cheek and states the he was told that the X-rays revealed no other injury beyond soft tissue. Michael tells the nurse manager he feels like this was his fault: He was standing too close to the patient and should have been more careful.

The nurse manager tells Michael that he was responding in a professional manner to help Mr. Croft, who was frightening other patients with his behaviors, back to his room while also offering him medication to help ameliorate his agitation. She tells Michael that she spoke with other nursing staff that witnessed the incident and they all agreed that Mr. Croft seemed to be cooperating when he turned and struck out suddenly without clear provocation. They believed Mr. Croft was responding to internal stimuli and that his outburst was not directed at Michael. She asks Michael how he is feeling. He tells her he initially felt angry at Mr. Croft and at himself, but that it was helpful to hear the perspective of his colleagues. Michael tells her he is tired now and looking forward to a good night's sleep before returning to his next scheduled shift in two days. The nurse manager tells Michael that Mr. Croft seems to be responding to the medication he did accept and is currently in his room writing in a journal. She also conveys the support and concern of Michael's colleagues and asks Michael to call her if his condition changes or needs to process the event further. Michael thanks the nurse manager for coming to see him.

The nurse manager then goes to the psychiatric emergency department to check in on the possible admissions to the unit on the evening shift. She sees Ms. Turner, who is already planned for admission, and notes that she still appears agitated and intrusive with other patients. She asks the psychiatric nurse if Ms. Turner has been accepting medication to which she responded well on previous admissions. They say she has, and admission orders have been written. The nurse manager reviews these and then asks if the psychiatric nurse can obtain a repeat order for another PRN of her medication prior to sending her to the unit to help her with the transition, as the unit is currently quite stimulating and active. The nurse agrees to the plan and calls the psychiatrist to discuss it and obtain the order. The nurse manager reviews which other patients may need admission on the evening shift and notes that those patients are currently anxious but cooperative, and that they all presented voluntarily for help.

Report is still in progress when the nurse manager returns to the unit. She then goes to her office and calls the service director, explaining the high acuity of the unit and the current staffing situation. The nurse manager obtains permission to call in a per-diem nurse to cover the 1:1. The per-diem nurse is experienced and very familiar with the unit.

The nurse manager also tells the supervisor that she wants to set up a meeting with the finance department in the next two weeks. She has collected data revealing an increase in patient days by 15% over the past year, since the closing of a psychiatric inpatient unit in a local community hospital. The data also reveal a 9% decrease in length of stay on her unit and a 9% increase in number of admissions and discharges. She has also collected data on the increase in the number of patients who have medical needs requiring nursing assessment and intervention such as withdrawal, cardiac and respiratory problems, and diabetes. She plans to present a proposal to increase the authorized number of psychiatric–mental health RNs by 1.5 full-time equivalents to meet the increase in the demand for RN involvement in direct care activities for patient safety and to improve the quality of care. Her supervisor acknowledges her work and agrees to attend the meeting with her to support the proposal.

Application

1. What management skills did the nurse manager demonstrate?

2. What formal power did the nurse manager have, and how did she use it?

3. How did she use informal power?

4. Would you want to work on the unit under the supervision of this nurse manager? Why or why not?

Innovative Practice Behaviors

As discussed earlier in this chapter, frontline nursing leadership is characterized as the process by which nurses at the unit level are motivated to engage in professional practice behaviors to accomplish the goal of a safe and healing environment for their vulnerable patients. This process is enacted within the therapeutic nurse–patient relationship, also called the *point of service*. A review of the nursing literature reveals that there is some consensus that structural empowerment and psychological empowerment are interrelated and that psychological empowerment is the critical variable between structural empowerment and nursing effectiveness and

innovative behaviors (Spence Laschinger, Finegan, & Wilk, 2009; Knol & van Linge, 2009).

Knol and van Linge state that "innovative behaviors of nurses, who are close to the patients, is necessary if they are to be active participants in reaching organizational aims and, in a wider context, the aims of healthcare" (2009, p. 360). The adoption of new paradigms of care and treatment that promote hope and recovery in mental health service delivery requires that psychiatric–mental health nurses engage in innovative practice behaviors, particularly in acute psychiatric settings. Empowered nurses have a level of freedom in deciding how to do their work and a sense of choice or autonomy in initiating

Leadership Activities That Support Intrinsic Motivation in Nurses

table 11-6

Role modeling	One of the most effective strategies for developing an intrinsically motivated staff is to model intrinsically motivated behavior. Examples include the following: • Engage in nursing professional organizations and activities to support professional nursing goals. · • Engage with consumer organizations and facilitate venues for bringing the patients' voices to the table in clinical settings. • Treat the nursing staff as you would have them treat their patients: respectfully, thoughtfully, and supportively. • Engage in continuous learning activities and ongoing professional education. • Present, publish, and teach. • Take care of yourself: Have balance in your life. • Do not have "favorites" among your staff.
Promoting the development of staff leadership skills	• Identify the unique patient-related interests of individual staff and help support their ability to develop these interests. • Provide honest supportive feedback as nurses step up to fulfill leadership responsibilities (e.g., charge nurse). • Provide direction, education and support regarding the use of delegation skills with LPNs and UAP to maximize the contributions of the nursing staff team while retaining a strong direct patient care focus for the psychiatric RNs. • Provide and support engagement in organizational and outside leadership development activities. • Listen to understand.

The Four Domains of Psychological Empowerment

table 11-7

Meaning	1. Reflects that there is congruence between a nurse's beliefs, values, and behaviors and the job requirements. 2. Refers to the level at which people care about their work and feel that it is important.
Competence	Refers to: 1. The confidence in one's abilities to meet role expectations. 2. The perception of self-efficacy to perform their work activities with skill.
Self-determination	Refers to: 1. The feeling that one has control over one's work. 2. The level of freedom that nurses have in deciding how to do their work. 3. A nurse's sense of choice or autonomy in initiating and or continuing work-related behaviors or actions.
Impact	Refers to: 1. The sense that the nurse is able to influence important outcomes in his or her work with patients and colleagues and/or within health care. 2. The level at which a nurse can make a difference in the course of his or her work.

Based on Knol, J., & van Linge, R. (2009). Innovative behavior: The effect of structural and psychological empowerment on nurses. *Journal of Advanced Nursing, 65*(2), 359–370; Laschinger, H. K., Finegan, J., Shamian, J., & Wilk, P. (2001). Impact of structural and psychological empowerment on job strain in nursing work settings. *Journal of Nursing Administration, 31*(5), 260–272; Lethbridge, K., Andrusyszyn, M-A,, Iwasiw, C., Laschinger, H. S., & Fernando, R. (2011). Structural and psychological empowerment and reflective thinking: Is there a link? *Journal of Nursing Education, 50*(11), 636–645.

and/or continuing work-related behaviors. They are intrinsically motivated to improve the quality of care delivered to, and the quality of life experienced by, their patients. They are at the point of service and are uniquely qualified to develop and implement innovative behaviors and interventions that align with new, patient-centered paradigms of psychiatric–mental health care.

Nurse managers and nursing leaders can use the guideposts from structural and psychological empowerment theories to inform the ongoing development of their own management and leadership skills. Through strong, evidence-based, theoretically informed nursing management and leadership skills, they can transform clinical work environments to support the development of empowered nurses who can use innovative behaviors to empower patients to achieve their full potential. This premise is supported through nursing research outcomes, as cited in this chapter, and holds promise for fully realizing the potential of psychiatric–mental health nursing in transforming mental health care delivery.

Part 3

The nurse manager returns to the room prior to the end of report to update everyone on Michael's condition, the plan for admissions, and the additional assistance for the 1:1. She asks the charge nurse to call the attending physician for Mr. Croft to collaborate on adjusting his treatment plan to assist him with his symptoms. She asks that the evening shift staff go out on the unit so the day shift nursing staff can gather briefly prior to their leaving. The day shift staff members come into the conference room a bit warily. The nurse manager then gives them a chance to go over the day's events. This gives them a chance to hear each other's perspectives because, being so busy, each only had one piece of the picture. A psychiatric technician states that the unit can feel "unsafe" when so many issues converge, such as the assault, impending admissions, and sick calls. An experienced nurse begins to talk about the "good old days" when a nurse could stop an admission if he or she thought the unit couldn't handle it. An LPN states that he is concerned about the increased medical acuity of the patients.

The nurse manager acknowledges their concerns. She provides information about the collaboration with the nurses in the emergency department, the service director, and the attending physician to address some of those concerns going into the evening shift. She acknowledges that some things cannot be controlled, such as refusing admissions, but validates how well the nursing staff team work together to meet challenges to promote their safety and the safety of their patients. She updates them on the status of their colleague in the emergency department and that she had conveyed their support to him.

As they talk, she notes that they begin to share positive acknowledgments with each other. The nurse manager reminds them that they did indeed have a very stressful day, much of which they cannot really share with their families, and asks what they will be doing to take care of themselves. Some plan to go for a run or some other physical activity. One is looking forward to her yoga class that evening. They are still talking with each other as they leave.

Later in the shift, you notice the charge nurse sitting with Mr. Croft, who had been violent on the day shift. They are sitting pretty far apart and in an open area at the end of the hall. As you get closer, you can hear the nurse saying to Mr. Croft that it must be very difficult for him to be here on the unit. Slowly Mr. Croft begins to make short responses. Twice he gets up suddenly as if to leave, but then turns and sits back down again. The charge nurse appears calm and attentive.

The two psychiatric technicians on the shift are making rounds on all the patients, making observations and notes on their whereabouts on the unit and their behaviors. They will bring patient concerns that need further assessment to the RN with whom they are co-assigned. The nurse manager leaves for the day, feeling positive about the unit.

APPLICATION

1. What leadership functions did the nurse manager demonstrate?

2. What indications did you see that the nursing staff felt some degree of empowerment?

3. What role did the nurse manager have in supporting the conditions under which these behaviors could occur?

Chapter Highlights

1. In recent years, there has been a shift in the paradigm of care of patients with acute psychiatric symptoms from one of consistency, control, and vigilance to maintain the safety of patients with acute psychiatric symptoms to one of partnership with patients and families, emphasis on individualized care, and the support of hope for recovery.

2. Frontline nursing leadership describes the role of management skills, strong collaboration skills, and leadership skills.

3. Empowered nurses are an outcome of strong nursing management and leadership.

4. Caring for patients whose behaviors may present danger to themselves or others and caring for the co-morbid physiological and medical needs of this patient population in settings that often have some limitations to the amount of medical support available are some of the unique considerations in caring for patients with mental illness.

5. In this context, the physical and psychological safety of persons with acute symptoms of mental illness and psychiatric disorders is identified as the key deliverable of psychiatric–mental health nursing.

6. Challenges posed by systems issues include reduced access to number of inpatient beds, emphasis on shortened lengths of hospital stays, and carve-out behavioral health insurance plans that place limits on reimbursement.

7. Examples of variables that affect the quantity and quality of nursing staff available to meet the acuity needs of a unit include nurses calling in sick, inadequate staffing ratios, and inexperienced staff.

8. Lack of sufficient qualified psychiatric–mental health nurses may result in increased use of seclusion and restraint as an attempt to contain and control the acuity of a unit and maintain safety.

9. Burnout is a nursing management and leadership issue. Nursing research links recurrent stress arousal in nursing staff with behaviors such as energy conservation (e.g., sick calls or reduced presence in the milieu) and exhaustion, leading to burnout.

10. Key management skills that promote safe and healing environments include supervision, organization and direction for the nursing staff, negotiating physician/nurse relationships, and

representing the needs of the unit to upper-level management to secure adequate resources. There is a strong and significant relationship between psychiatric nurses feeling valued and lower rates of emotional exhaustion.

11. Key leadership behaviors that promote safe and healing environments include role modeling and promoting the development of leadership skills in each nurse.

12. The dimensions of psychological empowerment theory support the development of strong nursing leadership skills. The dimensions of this theory are meaning (reflecting a congruence between a nurse's beliefs and values and the nurse's work requirements), competence, self-determination, and impact (the nurse's sense that he or she can influence important outcomes).

13. Frontline nursing leadership is characterized as the process by which nurses at the point of service are intrinsically motivated to engage in professional practice behaviors to accomplish safe and healing environments.

14. Innovative professional practice behaviors and interventions are aligned with new paradigms of psychiatric–mental health care that involve partnership with patients to achieve recovery,

15. Empowered psychiatric–mental health nurses who are intrinsically motivated to engage in innovative professional practice behaviors at the point of service within the therapeutic relationship with the patient are the product of strong nursing management and leadership skills in clinical environments.

NCLEX®-RN Questions

1. The nurse is assigned to care for patients on the psychiatric inpatient unit. Which factor is most likely to be a barrier to developing and maintaining a therapeutic relationship with the patients?
   a. The number of medications the nurse is required to administer
   b. A staffing model that uses high ratios of unlicensed personnel
   c. An absence of technologically sophisticated procedures and equipment
   d. The prevalence of co-morbid medical conditions in the patient population

2. The nurse is managing an acute psychiatric inpatient unit. Over the past few months there have been a number of critical incidents that have affected the staff's morale, and several nurses are expressing the intent to resign. Which elements of leadership skills would be most essential for the manager to self-evaluate?
   a. Capacity to pitch in and provide direct patient care
   b. Expertise in allocating resources and working with less
   c. Competence at managing staff to meet performance expectations
   d. Ability to maintain an environment that supports and values nurses

3. The nurse manager is meeting for an annual performance review. The manager is asked to identify a goal for growth in leadership skills. Which would be most appropriate for the nurse to select?
   a. Reduce annual costs associated with waste
   b. Secure better salaries and benefits for frontline workers
   c. Submit a proposal to increase the number of full-time RNs on the unit
   d. Encourage staff nurse efforts to implement an innovative care model

4. The nurse manger is implementing interventions to maintain a safe and healing work environment. Which strategies are aligned with principles of effective management to achieve this goal? Select all that apply.
   a. Maintaining a quiet, clean area for staff to take uninterrupted breaks
   b. Scheduling routine supervision and group education sessions for all staff
   c. Providing monetary awards to charge nurses who maintain restraint-free shifts
   d. Using data from national sources to determine appropriate nurse-to-patient ratios
   e. Ensuring that new nurse hires have the motivation and energy to put in overtime when acuity is high
   f. Encouraging nurses to delegate most direct patient care activities to unlicensed mental health counselors

5. The nurse preceptor is working with a new nurse who is about to complete an internship in the psychiatric setting. The preceptor highlights the effectiveness of the new nurse participating in quality improvement efforts to effect better outcomes for patients. Which domain of psychological empowerment most closely relates to the nurse preceptor's actions?
   a. Impact
   b. Meaning
   c. Competence
   d. Self-determination

6. The nurse manager has attempted to integrate aspects of both structural and psychological empowerment into leadership practice. Which outcome best demonstrates that the manager has successfully incorporated elements of both?
   a. The nurses are able to discuss principles of evidence-based practice and have taken advantage of opportunities to apply it.
   b. The nurses express the feeling that they are making a difference and convey a sense of confidence when carrying out assigned duties.
   c. The nurses report receiving regular feedback on goals and achievements and share a belief that their work is important and worthwhile.
   d. The nurses demonstrate a working knowledge of the fiscal resources available on the unit and state that they are allowed to have input into the budget.

Answers may be found on the Pearson student resource site: nursing. pearsonhighered.com

Pearson Nursing Student Resources Find additional review materials at **nursing.pearsonhighered.com**

References

Bittner, N. P., & Gravelin, G. (2009). Critical thinking, delegation and missed care in nursing practice. *Journal of Nursing Administration, 39*(3), 142–146.

Blegen, N. E., & Severinsson, E. (2011). Leadership and management in mental health nursing. *Journal of Nursing Management, 19,* 487–497.

Caine, R. M., & Ter-Bagdasarian, L. (2003). Early identification and management of critical incident stress. *Critical Care Nurse, 23*(1), 59–65.

Delaney, K. R., & Johnson, M. E. (2006). Violence on inpatient psychiatric units: State of the science. *Journal of the American Psychiatric Nurses Association, 10*(3), 113–121.

Delaney, K. R., & Johnson, M. E. (2008). Inpatient psychiatric nursing: Why safety must be the key deliverable. *Archives of Psychiatric Nursing, 22*(6), 386–388.

Hanrahan, N. P., Aiken, L., McClaine, L., & Hanlon, A. L. (2010a). Relationship between psychiatric nurse work environments and nurse burnout in acute care general hospitals. *Issues in Mental Health Nursing, 31*(3), 198–207.

Hanrahan, N. P., Delaney, K. R., & Merwin, E. I. (2006). Mental health practitioners and trainees. In R.W. Mandersheid & J. T. Berry, (Eds.). *Mental Health, United States, 2004.* Rockville, MD: DHHS Pub. No. (SMA)-06-4195: Substance Abuse and Mental Health Service Administration, pp. 256–309.

Hanrahan, N. P., Kumar, A., & Aiken, L. H. (2010b). Adverse events associated with organizational factors of general hospital inpatient psychiatric care environments. *Psychiatric Services, 61*(6), 569–574.

Holm, A. L., & Severinsson, E. (2010). The role of mental health nursing leadership. *Journal of Nursing Management, 18,* 463–471.

James, K., Steward, D., & Bowers, L. (2012). Self-harm and attempted suicide within inpatient psychiatric services: A review of the literature. *International Journal of Mental Health Nursing, 21*(4), 301–309.

Johnson, M. (2004). Violence on inpatient psychiatric units: State of the science. *Journal of the American Psychiatric Nurses Association, 10,* 113–121,

Kanter, R. M. (1977). *Men and Women of the Corporation.* New York, NY: Basic Books.

Knol, J., & van Linge, R. (2009). Innovative behavior: The effect of structural and psychological empowerment on nurses. *Journal of Advanced Nursing, 65*(2), 359–370.

Laschinger, H. K., Finegan, J., Shamian, J., & Wilk, P. (2001). Impact of structural and psychological empowerment on job strain in nursing work settings. *Journal of Nursing Administration, 31*(5), 260–272.

Laschinger, H. K., Finegan, J., Shamian, J., & Wilk, P. (2004). A longitudinal analysis of the impact of workplace empowerment on work satisfaction. *Journal of Organizational Behavior, 25,* 527–545.

Laschinger, H. K. S., Leiter, M., Day, A., & Gilin, D. (2009). Workplace empowerment, incivility, and burnout: Impact on staff nurse recruitment and retention outcomes. *Journal of Nursing Management, 17*(3), 302–311.

Leiter, M. P., & Harvie, P. L. (1996). Burnout among mental health workers: A review and research agenda. *International Journal of Social Psychiatry, 42*(90), 90–101.

Lethbridge, K., Andrusyszyn, M-A., Iwasiw, C., Laschinger, H. S., & Fernando, R. (2011). Structural and psychological empowerment and reflective thinking: Is there a link? *Journal of Nursing Education, 50*(11), 636–645.

Manojlovich, M. (2005). The effect of nursing leadership on hospital nurses' professional practice behaviors. *Journal of Nursing Administration, 35*(7/8), 366–374.

Maslach, C., Jackson, S. E., & Leiter, M. P. (1996). *The Maslach Burnout Inventory* (3rd ed.). Palo Alto, CA: Consulting Psychologists Press. (All versions of the MBI, and the manual, are now available at Mind Garden, mindgarden.com)

Peplau, H. E. (1994). Psychiatric mental health nursing: Challenge and change. *Journal of Psychiatric and Mental Health Nursing, 1*(1), 3–7.

Potter, P., DeShields, T., & Kuhrik, M. (2010). Delegation practices between registered nurses and nursing assistive personnel. *Journal of Nursing Management, 18*(2), 157–165.

Smith, H. L., & Hood, J. N. (2005). Creating a favorable practice environment for nurses. *Journal of Nursing Administration, 35*(12), 525–532.

Spence Laschinger, H.K, Finegan, J., & Wilk, P. (2009). Context matters: The impact of unit leadership and empowerment on nurses' organizational commitment. *JONA, 39*(5), 228–235.

Spreitzer, G. Psychological empowerment in the workplace: Dimensions, measurement, and validation. *Academy Management Journal, 38,* 1442–1465.

Tomey, A. M. (2009). Nursing leadership and management effects work environment. *Journal of Nursing Management, 17,* 15–25.

Wagner, J. J., Cummings, G., Smith, D. L., Olsen, J, Anderson, L., & Warren, S. (2010). The relationship between structural empowerment and psychological empowerment for nurses: A systemic review. *Journal of Nursing Management, 18,* 448–462.

Zuzelo, P. R., Curran, S. S., & Zeserman, M. A. (2012). Registered nurses' and behavioral health associates' responses to violent inpatient interactions on behavioral health units. *Journal of the American Psychiatric Nurses Association, 18*(2), 112–126.

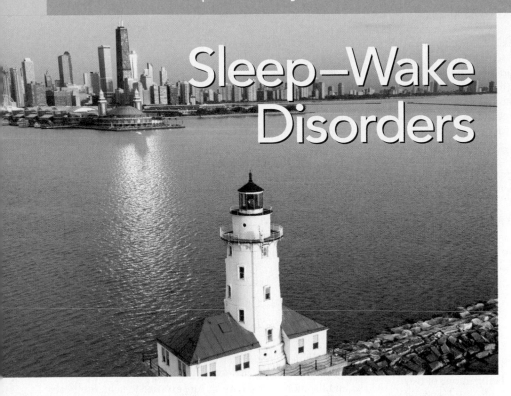

Sleep–Wake Disorders

12

Carla R. Jungquist

Learning Outcomes

1. Examine the etiology, pathophysiology, and impact of sleep–wake disorders.

2. Summarize the impact of biological, psychological, sociological, cultural, and spiritual domains on sleep–wake disorders.

3. Classify treatments for sleep–wake disorders.

4. Contrast different types of sleep–wake disorders and potential interventions.

5. Categorize key symptoms of sleep–wake disorders.

6. Evaluate different pharmacologic and nonpharmacologic therapies used in the treatment of sleep–wake disorders.

7. Plan evidence-based nursing care to promote normal sleep habits for individuals with or without sleep–wake disorders.

Key Terms

central sleep apnea, 227
circadian rhythm, 220
excessive daytime sleepiness, 227
fatigue, 225
insomnia, 225
narcolepsy, 224
obstructive sleep apnea—hypopnea, 227
sleep architecture, 224
sleep continuity, 224
sleep-disordered breathing, 224
sleep latency, 224
sleepiness, 223
sleep-related hypoventilation, 227

Michael Initial Onset

Michael is a 20-year-old male patient who was admitted to the acute psychiatric unit for depression and suicidal thoughts. His vital signs are within normal limits and his affect is flat. He is 5 feet 10 inches tall and weighs 220 pounds. He is a physics student at the local university, in his junior year. He lives on campus. Michael presented to the emergency room with suicidal thoughts, reporting that he is failing his courses; can't function (especially in the mornings); has difficulty getting to sleep, irritability, and difficulty concentrating; generally can't find a reason to live; and feels like a failure. He admits to using marijuana nightly "to help him get to sleep," drinking every weekend with his friends, and smoking approximately one-half pack of cigarettes per day. Michael's family lives out of state, but he has regular contact with them. He is transferred to the unit on the evening shift and requests medication for sleep. He is medicated with diphenhydramine (Benadryl) 25 mg at 10:00 p.m. On hourly rounds, you observe him still awake at 2:00 a.m. You ask him why he is still awake, and he states that he never goes to sleep until 3:00 or 4:00 a.m. You assess Michael for depressive symptoms and suicidal ideations; feeling satisfied that he is sad, but safe, you leave the room. When you return an hour later, you find him sleeping.

After a week on the unit, staff notices that Michael continues to miss breakfast and morning group time, but that by afternoon he is cheerful and attentive.

APPLICATION

1. Address the five domains for Michael:
   a. Biological
   b. Psychological
   c. Sociological
   d. Cultural
   e. Spiritual

2. In what ways do you think Michael may be suffering? Why?

3. How would you prioritize Michael's needs during this encounter, and why?

Introduction

For the most part, patients can be identified as being in one of two states of consciousness: sleep or wake. The sleep–wake pattern is part of a complex biological process that, in part, is driven by the **circadian rhythm** (biochemical, physiological, and behavioral processes that are driven endogenously, spanning a 24-hour cycle). This chapter provides an overview of sleep and sleep disorders, the consequences of sleep loss, and nursing interventions to promote adequate sleep and safe patient care. Nurses, especially when working at the bedside, need to be particularly knowledgeable of the vulnerability of the respiratory system during sleep and states of altered consciousness that are similar to sleep. Several classes of medications have a deleterious effect on sleep and on breathing during sleep. It is imperative that nurses are aware of these medications' effects and are able to promote patient safety through proper nursing assessment and preventive measures, as well as through patient education. The effects of sleep loss are wide-reaching and can have a negative impact on health. Nursing care should always involve awareness of proper sleep-promoting nursing actions and patient behaviors, as well as promotion of patient safety.

Normal Sleep–Wake States

Sleep is a reversible behavioral state of perceptual disengagement and unresponsiveness to environment that is controlled by a complex amalgam of physiological and behavioral processes (American Academy of Sleep Medicine, 2001). The opposing state, wakefulness, involves the same complex physiological and behavioral processes. Having a solid understanding of the mechanisms controlling sleep–wake states will assist nurses in developing appropriate plans of care to prevent the development of and provide treatment for sleep–wake disorders.

Biological Domain

The sleep–wake cycle reflects the changes that occur in the biological rhythm throughout the day–night cycle, the circadian rhythm, as well as the influence of homeostatic drive (Figure 12-1). Homeostatic drive of sleep, sometimes called *sleep pressure*, increases with length of wakefulness, physical exercise, and exposure to light. The longer we are awake, and the more we exercise and are exposed to light, the greater the likelihood of getting to sleep quickly and sleeping in the deeper stages of sleep. In conjunction with the circadian rhythm and homeostatic drive, neurons, neurotransmitters, and hormones in the brain control the sleep–wake cycle. Specific brain regions (and their respective neurotransmitters) are the thalamocortical projection (glutamate), posterior hypothalamus (histamine and orexin), and the basalocortical projections (acetylcholine). Neurons in the ventrolateral preoptic nucleus of the hypothalamus and melatonin produced by the pineal gland promote sleep (Kripke, Youngstedt, Rex, Klauber, & Elliott, 2003; Leger, Laudon, & Zisapel, 2004; Nofzinger, 2008; Olde Rikkert & Rigaud, 2001; Riemann et al., 2002). The wake-promoting mechanisms involve orexinergic, histaminergic, cholinergic, noradrenergic, and serotonergic neurons (Eggermann et al., 2003; Kiyashchenko et al., 2002; Mignot et al., 2002; Nofzinger, 2008; Ohayon, 2009). Wakefulness neurotransmitters also process sensory transmission, promote attention, and regulate motor responses and activity, such as orthosympathetic and neuroendocrine responses.

As mentioned previously, sleep is not just a single behavior. Sleep represents a cycling of brain activity that is closely correlated with cycling of cardiac and respiratory activity. During sleep, brain waves transition from low-frequency, high-amplitude (alpha, beta, and gamma) bands to high-frequency, low-amplitude (theta and delta) bands. The stages of sleep reflect the various frequency bands.

The states of sleep and wake can be identified through observation, but formally require the use of electroencephalography (EEG). *Polysomnography* (a form of EEG procedure performed during sleep) is a sleep study that monitors brain waves along with other physiological measures (see assessment section for full details). Over the normal sleep period, brain waves cycle through two phases and 4 stages. The two phases are rapid eye movement (REM) and non-REM (NREM) sleep. REM sleep is thought to be produced in the brainstem region (pons and adjacent midbrain) and regulated with neurotransmitters. The neurotransmitters responsible for initiating REM sleep are GABA, acetylcholine, glutamate, and glycine (Kilduff

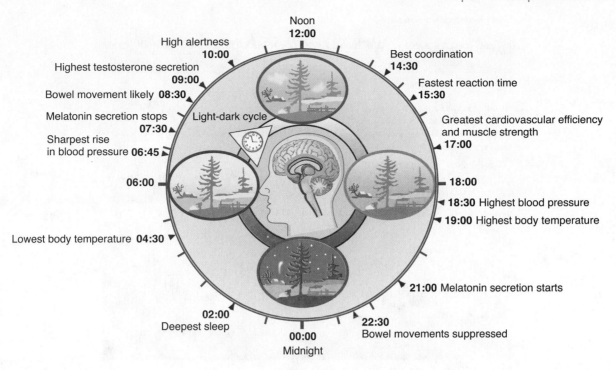

Human biological clock.

& Peyron, 2000; Kiyashchenko et al., 2002; Licata et al., 2009). Neurotransmitters responsible for "turning off" REM sleep are thought to include norepinephrine, epinephrine, serotonin, and histamine. During normal REM sleep, neuroprocessing is active, eyes move rapidly in synchronous movements, and generalized skeletal muscle tone diminishes, resulting in atonia. During NREM sleep, brain waves cycle through four stages, numbered 1 through 4. Stages 3 and 4, in combination, are often referred to as *slow wave sleep* (Figure 12-2). Neurotransmitters and peptides thought to produce slow wave sleep are endogenous opioids (sensory modulation), somatostatin, cortistatin, growth hormone-releasing factor, and adenosine. Although evidence of the function of sleep is underdeveloped, adequate sleep is thought to be necessary for healthy immune function, cognitive performance, mood regulation, restoration of muscles, and neurogenesis (Altena, Van Der Werf, Strijers, & Van Someren, 2008; Backhaus et al., 2006; Daley et al., 2009; Miyata et al., 2010). Hertz (Hz) is a frequency measurement that defines EEG rhythms.

Stage 1 sleep is the transition between wakefulness and sleep. There is low voltage and mixed frequency (2–7 Hz) of EEG activity without any evidence of REM. In adults, the percentage of time spent in stage 1 ranges between 1% and 5% (Mitler, Poceta, & Bigby, 1999). (See Figure 12-3 for examples of sleep stages.) Adults usually spend 15% to 20% of their sleep time in stage 2. This stage is represented on EEG by relatively low voltage and mixed frequency (2–7 Hz) with sleep spindles (12–14 Hz activity for at least 0.5 seconds) and K complexes (triphasic potentials with negative sharp waves followed by positive component lasting more than 0.5 seconds).

Stages 3 and 4 are very similar in character, usually scored together on polysomnography (PSG), and collectively are called slow wave sleep. The normal percentage of slow wave sleep is between 20% and 25% (Carskadon & Dement, 2005). Delta waveforms (2 Hz or slower frequency, with amplitude of 75 μV from peak to peak) are characteristic of this stage of sleep. When delta waveforms occur 20% to 50% of the time, the stage is labeled as stage 3; when they occur more than 50% of the period being examined, the stage is labeled as 4 (Mitler, Poceta, & Bigby, 1999). REM sleep is the period during which most dreaming occurs. The first phase of REM usually occurs after about 80 to 100 minutes of sleep (Carskadon & Dement, 2005). During REM sleep, EEG activity is low voltage and mixed frequency, with characteristic bursts of sawtooth waveforms. Other features unique to REM are that skeletal muscle tone is at a minimum and eye movements are frequent and brisk.

During sleep, the body also goes through physiological changes in the cardiac, respiratory, and endocrine systems that vary according to type and stage of sleep.

Cardiac System

During sleep (especially REM sleep), cardiac rhythm and rate fluctuate due to the result of withdrawal of parasympathetic influence that occurs during REM sleep. During REM sleep, the heart rate increases, then intermittently decelerates due to vagal influence. This alternating pattern of autonomic activation can result in REM sleep-induced cardiac arrhythmias and may contribute to cardiac deaths during sleep (Dergacheva, Wang, Lovett-Barr, Jameson, & Mendelowitz,

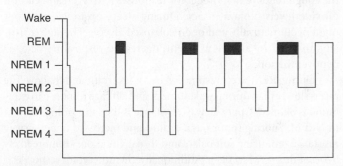

REM and non-REM stages of sleep in an adult.

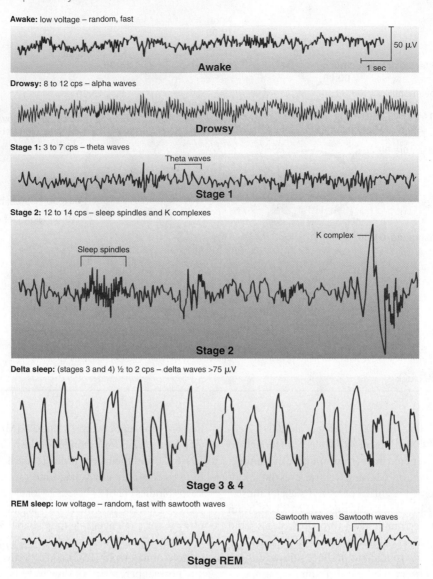

Awake: low voltage – random, fast

50 μV

1 sec

Awake

Drowsy: 8 to 12 cps – alpha waves

Drowsy

Stage 1: 3 to 7 cps – theta waves

Theta waves

Stage 1

Stage 2: 12 to 14 cps – sleep spindles and K complexes

K complex

Sleep spindles

Stage 2

Delta sleep: (stages 3 and 4) ½ to 2 cps – delta waves >75 μV

Stage 3 & 4

REM sleep: low voltage – random, fast with sawtooth waves

Sawtooth waves   Sawtooth waves

Stage REM

12-3   Stages of sleep.

2010). Age, anxiety, and sleep deprivation have been found to result in increased sympathetic tone and blunted parasympathetic antagonism (Nielsen et al., 2010; Schumann, Bartsch, Penzel, Ivanov, & Kantelhardt, 2010; Sgoifo et al., 2006). Specifically, as individuals age, the vagally mediated decelerations diminish (Schumann et al., 2010). Anxiety, panic, and/or posttraumatic stress disorders are associated with sympathetic activation and diminished heart rate variability during sleep (Chung et al., 2009; Nielsen et al., 2010)

Endocrine System

Sleep is regulated in part by the circadian rhythm. The endocrine system is linked directly to the circadian biorhythm. Specifically, the hypothalamo–pituitary–adrenocortical system has a bidirectional relationship with sleep. It is thought that corticotropin-releasing hormone (CRH) impairs sleep, enhances vigilance, and may promote REM sleep (Steiger, 2002).

Respiratory System

During sleep, voluntary control of respiration is absent, and respiratory rate, depth, and rhythm change as the brain moves through

the phases and stages of sleep. During stage 1 and early stage 2 sleep, respiration rate oscillates in response to carbon dioxide and oxygen levels. In late stage 2 and in stages 3 and 4, respiratory rate and volume diminish and rhythm remains regular (Chokroverty, 1999). During all stages of NREM sleep, upper airway resistance increases and motor and neuronal hypotonia occurs, diminishing the cough reflex. Chemoreceptor responses to oxygen and carbon dioxide levels remain intact. During sleep, up to 25 sighs per night occur naturally and open collapsed alveoli. The sigh is usually followed by an apneic event, decreased respiratory rate, or hypoventilation.

During REM sleep, respiration becomes erratic and shallow. The rate is slower than during wakefulness, and rib cage response to expiration is blunted. Upper airway resistance is the same or higher than in NREM. Snoring (poor nasal airflow and increased upper airway resistance producing soft palate and throat vibrations) is more likely to occur during REM sleep. Additionally, chemoreceptor response to oxygen and carbon dioxide levels is blunted. As the result of all the physiological changes that occur during sleep, respiration is most

	Age 13–18	Age 19–29	Age 30–45	Age 46–64
Average Hours Sleep on Weeknights	7h 26m	7h 1m	6h 48m	6h 49m
Rarely/Never Get Good Night's Sleep on Weekdays	46%	51%	43%	38%
Wake Up Feeling Unrefreshed	59%	67%	65%	55%

12-4 Many Americans report insufficient or dissatisfactory sleep during the week.

Data from National Sleep Foundation. (2011). Sleep in America Poll: Communication Technologies in the Bedroom. Retrieved from http://www.sleepfoundation. org/sites/default/files/sleepinamericapoll/SIAP_2011_Summary_of_Findings.pdf

vulnerable during the REM phase of sleep (Hudgel, Martin, Johnson, & Hill, 1984)

Psychological Domain

Sleep and mental health have a reciprocal relationship. When an individual is deprived of adequate sleep, symptoms of depression and anxiety occur. In the presence of depression and anxiety, sleep disruption, either fragmented or prolonged, often occurs. The etiology of the relationship is thought to stem from the sympathetic nervous system and cholinergic neurotransmitters that are shared with symptoms of depression and anxiety and its regulation within REM sleep. There is more recent evidence that melatonin and timing of the circadian rhythm also contribute to mood disorders (Anderson, 2010).

Sociocultural and Spiritual Domains

Although sleep is innate and common to all humans, the timing of sleep differs in cultural regions. It is common in most European and South American regions to have a bedtime of midnight and a rise time after 8 a.m. This is likely related to social influences, such as later evening meal and social gathering times compared with those in the American culture. Ambient temperatures and sunrise and sunset times also influence sleep schedules. Consider tropical regions, where mid-afternoon temperatures are extremely warm, giving rise to the practice of the afternoon siesta.

Societal work ethics and norms also influence opportunity to sleep and timing of sleep. According to the 2011 Sleep in America poll, Americans are chronically sleep deprived due to life and work styles (Figure 12-4). Members of several professions, including firefighters, health care providers, nurses, factory workers, and air traffic controllers are required to stay awake during the period of time when the body has the highest propensity to sleep. Employment in a field requiring shift work often results in sleep deprivation. Among young adults, social networking interferes with sleep: Between 67% and 72% of 13-to-29-year-olds bring their cellphones to bed for use while initiating sleep (National Sleep Foundation, 2011).

Spiritual health, like mental and social health, is enhanced by adequate sleep. The inverse may also be true: Patients with stronger sense of spiritual health have been found to be more likely to experience better quality of sleep (Phillips, Mock, Bopp, Dudgeon, & Hand, 2006).

Sleep Across the Life Span

Timing, duration, and quality of sleep are influenced by age. The ideal duration of sleep decreases over the developmental stages from infancy to young adulthood, then stabilizes through adulthood until death in normal healthy humans. Infants usually require up to 22 hours of sleep in early infancy, and adults usually require 6 to 8 hours of sleep (Figure 12-5). In general, adolescents are more likely to

experience difficulty falling asleep, and older adults are more likely to exhibit fragmented sleep. This is the result of normal fluctuations that occur in circadian rhythm. In other words, it is considered normal for teenagers to exhibit wakefulness until midnight or so and then exhibit **sleepiness** (difficulty maintaining wakefulness) until late morning. This becomes a problem only when societal demands, such as 7 a.m. school start times, go against the normal circadian rhythm. In older adults, fragmented sleep is often due to medical conditions or medications. Early sleep times can occur as the result of boredom, circadian rhythm effects, or poor sleep behaviors. There is sufficient evidence to support the need for adults to attain more than 6 hours and less than 9 hours of sleep, as short sleepers and long sleepers have higher incidence of morbidity and mortality.

Assessing Sleep

As mentioned previously, sleep is a behavioral and physiologic state. During observation of the sleep period, the body is lying

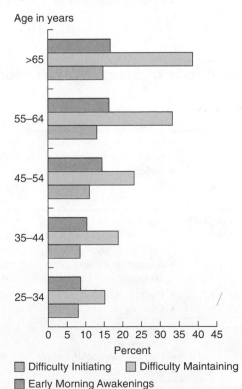

12-5 Sleep complaints over the life span.

Data from Ohayon MM, Reynolds CF (2009). Epidemiological and clinical relevance of insomnia diagnosis algorithms according to the DSM-IV and the International Classification of Sleep Disorders (ICSD). *Sleep Medicine, 10*(9):952-60.

down with limited movement, the eyes are closed, and respiration may be slow and shallow or erratic according to which phase of sleep the person is in. The procedure used to measure sleep objectively is called *polysomnography*. During the PSG procedure, several physiologic variables are measured and recorded during sleep. Physiologic sensors are placed on the head, face, chest, and legs to measure (1) brain electrical activity (electroencephalogram), (2) eye and jaw muscle movement (electrooculogram, electromyogram), (3) leg muscle movement (electromyogram), (4) nasal airflow, (5) respiratory effort (chest belts), (6) cardiac rate and rhythm (electrocardiogram), and (7) vascular oxygenation (peripheral oxygen saturation). The data derived from PSG are collectively used to determine the following:

- **Sleep continuity**, which includes **sleep latency** (minutes to get to sleep), minutes awake during the night, sleep efficiency (total sleep time/minutes in bed × 100), and number of awakenings from sleep)

- **Sleep architecture**, the structure of stages (1, 2, 3, 4) and phases (REM and NREM) of sleep

- **Sleep-disordered breathing**, the presence of partial or complete airway obstruction or dysfunction of the central drive to breath that occurs during sleep (Armon, Johnson, Roy, & Nowick, 2012; Kushida et al., 2005; Stierer & Punjabi, 2005)

Unfortunately, nurses rarely will have access to the results of a sleep study. In the absence of data obtained from a PSG, nurses must be able to use their knowledge and skills to assess sleep subjectively.

Pause and Reflect

1. *How do the circadian rhythm and homeostatic drive work together to control the sleep–wake system?*
2. *How does respiration change during REM sleep?*
3. *How do sociological and cultural factors affect sleep?*

Sleep Disorders

Insomnia, sleep-disordered breathing, and restless legs syndrome are the most common sleep disorders. **Narcolepsy** (a disorder of the wakefulness system) is less common, but can be very disabling. There are also variants of normal sleep, such as REM behavior disorders and parasomnias, that usually do not require treatment unless symptoms interfere with safety. According to the 2005 Sleep in America poll, 21% of the population think they have a sleep disorder (Hiestand, Britz, Goldman, & Phillips, 2006).

A determination of sleep disorder requires significant impairment of functioning. Acute difficulty maintaining daytime wakefulness, issues with safety, difficulty concentrating, and cardiac symptoms represent the range of areas in which impairment in functioning may arise. For many individuals with sleep and wake disorders, manifestations occur across the domains (Table 12-1).

Both the DSM-5 (American Psychiatric Association, 2013) and the International Classification of Sleep Disorders, 2nd edition (ICSD-2) are used to describe the characteristics of sleep–wake disorders given in this chapter. The DSM-5 criteria were designed to facilitate diagnosis of sleep–wake complaints and to help clinicians who are primarily mental health providers clarify whether patient referrals to sleep specialists may be needed (APA, 2013). By contrast,

Manifestations of Sleep–Wake Disorders by Domain table 12-1

Sleep Disorder	Manifestations by Domain			
	Biological	**Psychological**	**Sociocultural**	**Spiritual**
Insomnia	• Decreased immune function • Fatigue	• Depression • Anxiety • Irritability • Decreased cognitive performance	• Social isolation	• Disinterested in attending religious and/or social functions that support spirituality
Breathing-related sleep disorders	• Hypertension • Cardiac disease with left ventricular dysfunction • Altered glucose metabolism • Pedal edema • Obesity	• Anxiety • Depression • Impaired cognitive function	• Isolation • Inability to perform household and work tasks	• Inability to gain pleasure or participate in activities that support spiritual health
Restless legs syndrome	• Uncomfortable, unpleasant leg sensations • Ferritin levels < 45 ng/mL • Fragmented sleep	• Irritability • Inability to concentrate due to discomfort	• Leg movements can disrupt bed partner's sleep	• Inability to attend/enjoy meetings and social functions because of leg sensations
Narcolepsy	• Sleep attacks, sleep paralysis • Hypnogogic/hypnopompic hallucinations • Excessive daytime sleepiness	• Anxiety • Depression	• Potential loss of driving privilege • Inability to maintain employment, family responsibilities	• Loss/impairment of personhood if symptoms are severe • Impaired ability to sustain spiritually supporting activities

the ICSD-2 contains more detailed descriptions of sleep–wake disorders for providers and researchers who specialize in sleep medicine.

In addition to the sleep–wake disorders discussed in this chapter, nurses may encounter patients with less common disorders, including parasomnias, which are characterized by abnormal behaviors, subjective experiences, and/or physiologic events. Parasomnias can occur with sleep, specific sleep stages, and during sleep–wake transitions. The diagnostic criteria for parasomnias include sleepwalking and sleep terrors. There are also diagnostic categories for nightmare disorder (in which dream images that cause anxiety and dysphoria occur) and substance/medication-induced sleep disorder (APA, 2013).

Insomnia

It is estimated that at any one point in time, between 6% and 10% of the population meet the diagnostic criteria for insomnia, although approximately one-third of adults report experiencing symptoms associated with insomnia (APA, 2013). **Insomnia** is the most common sleep disorder in adults and is characterized by repeated difficulty with sleep initiation, duration, consolidation, and/or quality that occurs despite adequate time and opportunity for sleep and results in some form of daytime impairment (APA, 2013). Insomnia can cause real suffering to the individual, as it is associated with high levels of morbidity, injury, poor daytime functioning, and poor quality of life, as well as excessive health care costs. Although insomnia was previously considered to be just a symptom of other medical or psychological disorders, it has become clear that is a multidimensional bio-behavioral disorder with multifactorial etiology. In the past, insomnia occurring in the setting of a medical or psychiatric condition (including other sleep disorders) was considered a symptom and labeled as secondary insomnia. After years of research, it has become apparent that insomnia, in most instances, persists long after the medical or psychiatric condition has resolved. Since the discovery of this phenomenon, coupled with better understanding of the mechanisms of insomnia, insomnia in the setting of other conditions is now labeled *co-morbid insomnia*. Revisions for sleep–wake disorders in the DSM-5 allow the diagnosing clinician to specify etiology of the insomnia disorder as well as co-morbidities. For example, the specifier "non-sleep disorder mental co-morbidity" would be used for a patient with both major depression disorder and an insomnia disorder, because both conditions should be treated. Other specifiers include "with other medical co-morbidities" and "with other sleep disorder" (APA, 2013). Clinicians using the DSM-5 can also describe the duration of the insomnia, using specifiers such as *episodic* (with symptoms lasting at least 1 month but less than 3 months); *persistent* (with symptoms lasting 3 months or longer); and *recurrent* (two or more episodes within a year) (APA, 2013). The ICSD-2 recognizes that patients with insomnia experience varying degrees of severity:

- *Mild insomnia* is characterized by an almost nightly complaint of an insufficient amount of sleep or not feeling rested after the habitual sleep episode. Individuals with mild insomnia experience little or no impairment in social or occupational functioning. Mild insomnia often is associated with feelings of restlessness, irritability, mild anxiety, daytime **fatigue** (a state of physical and/or mental weakness, lethargy), and tiredness.

- *Moderate insomnia* is characterized by a nightly complaint of insufficient sleep or not feeling rested after the habitual sleep

episode. Mild or moderate impairment of social or occupational functioning is seen. Moderate insomnia always is associated with feelings of restlessness, irritability, anxiety, daytime fatigue, and tiredness.

- *Severe insomnia* is indicated by a nightly complaint of an insufficient amount of sleep or not feeling rested after the habitual sleep episode that is accompanied by *severe* impairment of social or occupational functioning. Severe insomnia is associated with feelings of restlessness, irritability, anxiety, daytime fatigue, and tiredness (American Academy of Sleep Medicine, 2001).

Although some individuals have an innate propensity for the development of insomnia, typically an event or stressor precipitates an acute period of poor sleep. The event may emerge from the sociological domain, such as the birth of a child, death of a loved one, loss of a job; or from the biological domain, such as the development of an acute or chronic medical condition. Medications that can interfere with sleep include calcium channel blockers, corticosteroids, beta-blockers, nicotine, xanthenes, dopamine agonists, decongestants, and some antidepressants. Manifestations of insomnia may exhibit across the domains and may include fatigue, anxiety, irritability, and social isolation (see DSM-5 Diagnostic Criteria for Insomnia Disorders).

Poor adaptation to fragmented, nonrestorative sleep can result in the development of chronic insomnia. Examples of poor adaptation are expanding time in bed with the thought that sleep will come; watching television, paying bills, or doing activities other than sleep or sex in bed; taking hot showers at bedtime in the hope of initiating relaxation; and using time in bed to think about stressors or worries. Cognitive and behavioral interventions used to treat insomnia focus on poor adaptation behaviors and the resulting cognitive disconnect of the bed and bedroom with sleep.

Circadian Rhythm Disorders

As mentioned previously, the circadian rhythm consists of oscillations in various hormones and temperature levels in the body. It plays an important role in preparing the body for sleep and wake. The oscillations occur in a 24-hour rhythm and can be influenced by light, physical activity, meal timing, work schedules, and the effects of aging.

The International Classification of Sleep Disorders (American Academy of Sleep Medicine, 2001) recognizes seven circadian-rhythm disorders, whereas the DSM-5 recognizes five subtypes plus an unspecified category (Table 12-2). Common symptoms shared by all circadian rhythm disorders include the following (APA, 2013):

- Ongoing or recurrent sleep disturbance primarily due to an alteration of the circadian system or disalignment between the individual's circadian system and physical environment or work schedule

- Excessive sleepiness and or insomnia

- Significant impairment in functioning

Shift work disorder is prevalent in about 10% of shift workers. Advanced sleep phase disorder (ASPD) is more common in older adults as melatonin levels diminish. Delayed sleep phase disorder (DSPD) is more common in adolescents and young adults and is likely due to genetic predisposition, environmental influences, and physiological changes. The prevalence of DSPD in young adults is 7% to 14% (Ohayon & Bader, 2010; Ohayon & Sagales, 2010). Circadian

Diagnostic Criteria for Insomnia Disorders   DSM-5

A. A predominant complaint of dissatisfaction with sleep quantity or quality, associated with one (or more) of the following symptoms:
   1. Difficulty initiating sleep. (In children, this may manifest as difficulty initiating sleep without caregiver intervention.)
   2. Difficulty maintaining sleep, characterized by frequent awakenings or problems returning to sleep after awakenings. (In children, this may manifest as difficulty returning to sleep without caregiver intervention.)
   3. Early-morning awakening with inability to return to sleep.
B. The sleep disturbance causes clinically significant distress or impairment in social, occupational, educational, academic, behavioral, or other important areas of functioning.

C. The sleep difficulty occurs at least 3 nights per week.
D. The sleep difficulty is present for at least 3 months.
E. The sleep difficulty occurs despite adequate opportunity for sleep.
F. The insomnia is not better explained by and does not occur exclusively during the course of another sleep–wake disorder (e.g., narcolepsy, a breathing-related sleep disorder, a circadian rhythm sleep–wake disorder, or a parasomnia).
G. The insomnia is not attributable to the physiological effects of a substance (e.g., a drug of abuse, a medication).
H. Coexisting mental disorders and medical conditions do not adequately explain the predominant complaint of insomnia.

Source: Reprinted with permission from the *Diagnostic and Statistical Manual of Mental Disorders*, Fifth Edition, (Copyright 2013). American Psychiatric Association.

---

rhythm disorders, if chronic and impairing function, are best treated by sleep specialists. Treatment usually includes supplemental melatonin 3 to 4 hours before the target time of sleep onset and early-morning bright-light therapy.

Approximately 20% of United States employees work shifts other than the traditional 9-to-5 workday (Erren, 2010). As a result, approximately 5 million people nationally suffer from sleep deprivation as the result of shift work: In general, shift workers get about 2 hours less sleep per night than the population at large. This carries a number of potential consequences. About half of shift workers have sleep-related complaints. Shift workers have a higher rate of motor vehicle accidents (Chen et al., 2010; Sandberg et al., 2011). Individuals who work more than 10 years on off-shifts are at higher risk of developing gastrointestinal disorders and cardiac disease (American Sleep Association, 2007). Individuals who develop shift work disorder will report a primary complaint of insomnia or excessive sleepiness and working hours during which they would normally be asleep. To be diagnosed with shift-work disorder, they must not meet the criteria for any other sleep circadian-rhythm or insomnia disorder, and be absent any medical or mental condition accounting for the symptoms.

Both polysomnography and the Multiple Sleep Latency Test (MSLT) confirm the loss of a normal sleep–wake pattern (American Academy of Sleep Medicine, 2001).

Several issues contribute to sleep deprivation secondary to shift work. Two main contributors to inadequate sleep in shift workers are social stressors and biological influences. Social stressors include societal norms to work during the day and socialize at night. As most of society sleeps during the night, shift workers often find their sleep interrupted with environmental noises, telephone calls, medical/dental appointments for themselves or family members, and other family responsibilities and obligations. Biological influences include trying to sleep against the diurnal circadian rhythm that primes the body to sleep best at night.

Nurses are prime candidates for sleep deprivation secondary to shift work, as most nurses are mothers, spouses, and natural caregivers who put others' needs before their own (Box 12-1).

Breathing-Related Sleep Disorders

Breathing-related sleep disorders encompass obstructive sleep apnea–hypopnea, central sleep apnea, and sleep-related hypoventilation. Prevalence of obstructive sleep apnea–hypopnea is estimated to

---

Circadian-Rhythm Disorders   table 12-2

Disorders recognized by the American Academy of Sleep Medicine	• Time Zone Change (Jet Lag) Syndrome • Shift Work Sleep Disorder • Irregular Sleep–Wake Pattern • Delayed Sleep–Phase Syndrome • Advance Sleep–Phase Syndrome • Non-24-Hour Sleep–Wake Disorder • Circadian-Rhythm Sleep Disorder Not Otherwise Specified
Disorders recognized by the American Psychiatric Association	• Delayed Sleep Phase Type • Advanced Sleep Phase Type • Irregular Sleep–Wake Type • Non-24-Hour Sleep–Wake Type • Shift Work Type • Unspecified Type

Data from American Academy of Sleep Medicine. (2001). *The International Classification of Sleep Disorders, Revised.* Available at http://www.esst.org/adds/ICSD.pdf; *Diagnostic and Statistical Manual of Mental Disorders*, Fifth Edition, (Copyright 2013). American Psychiatric Association.

Nurses and Shift Work box 12-1

Nurses in many settings work on shifts that vary in hours required. Many times this is unavoidable, but nurses can advocate for a less disruptive schedule of shift changes that will allow their circadian rhythms to best adapt to sleeping. Tips for nurses related to shift work and reducing the impact of shift work (and thus decreasing the risk for making errors as a result of insufficient or poor sleep) include:

1. Ask yourself if you are suited to shift work:
   a. Do you adjust quickly to jet lag?
   b. Are you a "night owl"?
   c. Can you sleep anywhere?
   d. If you stay up at night, are you able to sleep during the day?
2. Assess yourself for individual factors that predict poor prognosis:
   a. Over 50 years of age
   b. Moonlighting/working more than one job
   c. Heavy domestic workload
   d. Being a morning "lark"
   e. History of sleep disorders, epilepsy, diabetes, heart disease, psychiatric illness, or alcohol or drug abuse
   f. Requiring 9 or more hours of sleep to feel rested
3. Advocate for your schedule to include:
   a. Fewer than four 12-hour shifts in row
   b. Avoidance of excessive overtime
   c. Shift rotation by the week with 2 days off between

4. To address the hazards associated with working off shifts and promote adequate sleep:
   a. Always arrive to work rested.
   b. Avoid complicated and frequently changing schedules, arrange rotating shifts clockwise (new shift starts at time later than previous shift, or at least 2 days between shift changes).
   c. Go to bed and get up at consistent times.
   d. Protect your sleep territory—dark room away from noises, turning off phones and putting signs on the door to prevent interruptions.
   e. Avoid long commute times, and if unavoidable, ask someone to transport you to and from work.
   f. Take breaks during the work shift, and rest if needed.
   g. If work is sedentary, get up and exercise regularly.
   h. Use caffeine judiciously, but no closer than 5 hours before sleep time
   i. Raise light level and decrease environment temperature, as long as this does not interfere with patients' sleep.
   j. Avoid bright light before sleep period.
   k. Allow at least a 5-hour consistent sleep period without interruptions; plan for another 1.5- to 3-hour nap before work.

range between 2% and 15% in adults, with higher rates (more than 20%) seen in older adults (APA, 2013).

Obstructive sleep apnea–hypopnea (also known as OSA) is characterized by recurrent absence of breath for five or more times per hour, accompanied by nocturnal breathing problems such as snoring or breathing pauses and daytime sleepiness or fatigue due to collapse or obstruction of the lower posterior pharynx (APA, 2013). Regardless of symptoms, high numbers of apneic episodes per hour, significant periods of desaturation (less than 90%), and severely fragmented sleep also can indicate obstructive sleep disorders.

Central sleep apnea (CSA) is the repeated absence of breath with five or more central apneas per hour due to the temporary loss of ventilatory effort (White, 2005). Unlike OSA, CSA is characterized by variable respiratory effort without any evidence of airway obstruction (APA, 2013). Some patients with CSA demonstrate a pattern of Cheyne–Stokes breathing. Abusers of opioids may experience central sleep apnea related to a decreased respiratory drive.

Sleep-related hypoventilation is diagnosed when PSG demonstrates episodes of decreased respiration coupled with elevated CO_2 levels (APA, 2013). Sleep-related hypoventilation is graded by severity depending on the degree of hypoxemia and hypercarbia during sleep and end-organ impairment, such as right-side heart failure. It can be idiopathic, congenital, or associated with a co-morbidity such as a pulmonary disorder, neuromuscular disorder, chest wall or spinal cord injury, or use of medications such as benzodiazepines and opiates (APA, 2013).

Sleep–wake disorders often are reported as the average number of apneic–hypopneic events per hour over the night (apnea–hypopnea index [AHI]) (APA, 2013). Severity of breathing-related sleep disorders is graded according to AHI: <15 is mild; 15–30 is moderate;

and an AHI >30 is considered severe. An AHI of ≥15 is highly associated and likely causal for the development of **excessive daytime sleepiness** (inability to maintain wakefulness during the day; a score greater than 10 on the Epworth Sleepiness Scale), systemic hypertension, left ventricular hypertrophy, atrial fibrillation, cerebral vascular accident, diabetes mellitus, depression, and anxiety. Manifestations of breathing-related sleep disorders occur across the domains and can include hypertension, obesity, anxiety, depression, and impaired functioning (see Table 12-1).

The development of OSA is multifactorial and can occur at any point over the life span. Although obesity was originally thought to be the major contributor of the development of OSA, more recent research has shown that may not be the case in all persons. Individuals of normal weight also can develop OSA. OSA results from the collapse of the posterior pharynx during sleep. The cause of the collapse is multifactorial and related to the natural relaxation of airway that occurs at sleep, poor or altered muscle tone of the upper airway/pharynx, and/or, anatomically, a small pharyngeal opening (Abdel-Khalek et al., 2007; Jungquist, Karan, & Perlis, 2011; Tsai et al., 2003). An anatomically crowded airway can be the result of fatty deposits secondary to obesity or the result of congenital jaw structure in which the lower jaw is set back toward the pharynx when compared to the maxilla (retrognathia). Additionally, when an individual is supine, the abdominal weight displaces toward the chest cavity and can collapse the airway.

Although some patients newly diagnosed with OSA initially express fear that they will die in their sleep, this is unlikely to occur. Chemoreceptors in the central nervous system monitor carbon dioxide and oxygen levels and, when changes occur, send an awakening alert. The body's response to the sudden hypoxic awakening includes the activation of the sympathetic nervous system, which increases blood pressure and heart rate. Additionally, intermittent hypoxia can result in endothelial inflammation in the smooth muscles of the vascular system that, in turn, is associated with the development of systemic hypertension, atrial fibrillation, coronary heart disease, and altered glucose metabolism (Alajmi et al., 2007; Budhiraja, Sharief, & Quan, 2005; Hargens, Nickols-Richardson, Gregg, Zedalis, & Herbert, 2006; Ryan et al., 2007; Ryan, Taylor, & McNicholas, 2005).

Risk factors for OSA include obesity, male gender, snoring, witnessed apneas, genetic disorders that reduce airway patency (such as Down syndrome), excessive daytime sleepiness, menopause, and hypertension (APA, 2013; Hirshkowitz, 2008; Young, Peppard, & Gottlieb, 2002). Physical anomalies that increase the likelihood of having OSA include cricomental space of 1.5 cm or less (retrognathia) and the presence of an overbite (Tsai et al., 2003). The diagnosis and treatment of OSA is important to prevent hypertension, cardiovascular morbidity or mortality, sleepiness, impaired cognitive function, decreased quality of life, and motor vehicle accidents (Al Lawati, Patel, & Ayas, 2009; Young, Peppard, & Gottlieb, 2002).

Risk factors for the development of CSA include medical conditions that affect the cardiac and respiratory systems, medications that depress the central nervous system, and age > 65 years. Additionally, central apnea events may occur as the result of hypoxia occurring from OSA and present as either central apneic events or mixed apnea events (APA, 2013; White, 2005).

Treatments for OSA include continuous or bi-level positive airway pressure (CPAP/bi-PAP), oral–pharyngeal surgery, oral appliances affecting tongue placement, or weight loss. Treatment for CSA is usually pointed at the cause of the apnea. For example, treatments may include oxygen therapy for patients with obstructive lung disease, the addition of agents to improve cardiac output in patients with cardiac disease, or weaning from medications that may be inducing the central apneic events. Central apnea events are less likely to be associated with oxygen desaturations, and most times disappear when the obstructive apnea and subsequent intermittent hypoxia is treated. Because of this, CSA is thought to have less clinical relevance as compared with obstructive apneic events.

Restless Legs Syndrome

Restless legs syndrome (RLS) is a neurological disorder characterized by unpleasant sensations in the legs that are characterized by a desire to move the legs or arms (APA, 2013). Other diagnostic criteria include sensations of "creeping" inside the calves that are often associated with general aches and pain in the legs; no evidence of any medical or mental disorders that can account for the movements; and that other sleep disorders may be present but do not account for the symptom (American Academy of Sleep Medicine, 2001). The sensations usually increase as the day goes on and are worse in the evening or at night. To merit diagnosis, RLS must occur at least three times per week for at least 3 months and cause significant distress or impairment in function (APA, 2013). RLS also can negatively affect sleep, mood, energy, and cognition.

Periodic limb movements (PLMs) also characterize RLS during sleep. Some of the uncomfortable sensations reported by patients in addition to the constant desire to move legs or arms are creeping, crawling, tingling, burning, or itching sensations in the limbs. Although not necessary to meet diagnostic criteria, most patients with RLS exhibit PLMs, but the inverse is not always true. Research exploring a genetic component to the development of RLS has resulted in the consideration that RLS and PLMs may not be one disorder, but two separate disorders known as RLS with or without PLMs (Stefansson et al., 2007; Winkelman, 2007). PLMs of sleep in isolation from daytime complaints are associated with aging, depression and antidepressant medications, peripheral neuropathy, spinal cord damage, peripheral vascular disease, mineral and electrolyte imbalance, and iron deficiency (Montplaisir, Allen, Walters, & Ferini-Strambi, 2005). Although the etiology of RLS continues to be investigated, symptoms are known to respond to dopaminergic agents, opioids, anticonvulsants, and benzodiazepines. In addition to the unpleasant leg sensations, manifestations of RLS include fragmented sleep, inability to concentrate, and disruption of partner's sleep (see Table 12-1).

Pause and Reflect

1. How does obstructive sleep apnea differ from central sleep apnea?
2. How can weight loss help improve outcomes for patients with obstructive sleep apnea?
3. In what ways do you think RLS might impair daily functioning?

critical thinking

Michael Recovery Phase

After observing Michael for a week on the unit, it becomes apparent that his function and mood improves as the day progresses. He has been unable to participate in morning group sessions, as he falls asleep if forced to attend. The provider introduces the diagnosis of delayed sleep phase disorder to Michael, questioning whether a reason he was failing school was that he had scheduled all morning classes. Michael agrees with the observation and to adapting his school schedule to afternoon classes, when he is more functional. He also agrees to stop using marijuana and alcohol and to see an outpatient therapist who specializes in adolescent and young adults sleep and mental health disorders. The care plan is initiated while Michael is an inpatient and discharge plans are instituted.

APPLICATION

1. What tools or strategies would you recommend for Michael to use to track his progress toward recovery and rehabilitation? How do you see these as being helpful?

2. What aspects of therapeutic communication do you see as being most helpful when meeting with a patient to evaluate the plan of care?

Disorders of Wakefulness

Disorders of wakefulness include narcolepsy and hypersomnolence disorder. The most common sign of a disorder of wakefulness is excessive daytime sleepiness in absence of a sleep disorder. Inability to maintain wakefulness is a very serious problem that can result in life-threatening motor vehicle and work-related accidents. It is important for nurses to recognize and intervene with patients experiencing these disorders to promote patient as well as community safety.

Narcolepsy

Although originally thought to be a rare form of neurosis, in 2000 narcolepsy was found to be the result of a hypocretin/orexin imbalance. Recent developments from genetic research have found the etiology of narcolepsy likely to be the interaction between genetic susceptibility and environmental factors. Environmental factors include a link to an autoimmune process likely resulting from exposure to infection such as strep throat or influenza. It is theorized that the immune reaction results in destruction of the hypocretin/orexin cells (Sehgal & Mignot, 2011). The key sign of narcolepsy is excessive daytime sleepiness/sleep attacks caused by the intrusion of REM sleep into wakefulness. As mentioned previously, during the phase of REM sleep, brain activity is very high, but muscles are paralyzed with the exception of eye muscles. Thus, the intrusion of REM sleep into wakefulness results in weakness or complete loss of muscle tone. The rarest of sleep disorders, narcolepsy affects 1 in 2000 people in the United States and is gender neutral (Narcolepsy Network, 2010). Symptoms of narcolepsy usually start between puberty and the fifth decade, but peak in the second decade of life (National Institute of Neurological Disorders and Stroke & National Institutes of Health, 2011).

Approximately 10% of people with narcolepsy will also experience cataplexy. Cataplexy is *emotionally triggered* muscle weakness in the presence of excessive daytime sleepiness. Because of the loss of muscle tone, a cataplexic episode can mimic a seizure and is often included in the differential diagnosis during the workup of the etiology of an episode. Narcolepsy with cataplexy can be very disabling and result in loss of driving privileges unless well controlled. Diagnostic criteria for narcolepsy with cataplexy include excessive daytime sleepiness for at least three times per week over the past 3 months, a definite history of cataplexy, and hypersomnia that cannot be attributed to another condition or to medical or substance use (American Academy of Sleep Medicine, 2001). Findings of hypocretin deficiency measured using cerebrospinal fluid and PSG that demonstrate specific abnormalities such as two or more sleep-onset REM periods and rapid sleep latency (length of time required to transition from wakefulness to full sleep) are indicative of narcolepsy (APA, 2013). Other symptoms of narcolepsy with or without cataplexy include sleep paralysis (persistent atonia when awakening from sleep) and hypnogogic/hypnopompic hallucinations (vivid perceptual experiences during transition into or out of sleep).

The diagnosis of narcolepsy is made by sleep specialists and will include a formal in-lab polysomnography study followed by an MSLT. Once it is established that the individual had a good night's sleep, he or she is given the opportunity to nap on four occasions during the following day. To qualify for the diagnosis of narcolepsy on the MSLT, less than 10-minute latency of sleep-onset REM is required in two of the four nap opportunities (American Academy of Sleep Medicine, 2001). Individuals with narcolepsy often report fragmented sleep.

Discovering the biological basis of narcolepsy gives a better understanding of the presence of co-morbid conditions of anxiety, eating disorders, depression, and psychotic symptoms that are known to share hypocretin/orexin in their origin. Co-morbid psychiatric conditions that are commonly seen with narcolepsy may have a common biological link, but also are likely to be associated with stressors and daily coping in the presence of narcolepsy, especially if cataplexy symptoms are present (Droogleever Fortuyn, Mulders, Renier, Buitelaar, & Overeem, 2011).

The treatment for narcolepsy is mainly pharmacologic, although nonpharmacologic treatments such as scheduled naps can decrease the propensity of REM sleep intrusion into wakefulness. Pharmacologic treatment involves medications known to suppress REM sleep, such as antidepressants; medications used to increase wakefulness, such as traditional stimulants (dextroamphetamine and methylphenidate); and nontraditional stimulants (modafinil and armodafinil) and/or a unique medication, sodium oxybate (γ-hydroxybutyrate), which is given at night to consolidate sleep. Sodium oxybate is known to decrease excessive daytime sleepiness and cataplexic events. As modafinil and armodafinil have a high safety profile and low side effect profile, they are commonly used as a first-line treatment for narcolepsy.

Hypersomnolence Disorder

Hypersomnolence disorder (HD) is excessive daytime sleepiness despite a main sleep period of at least 7 hours (APA, 2013). The etiology is thought to be a neurochemical imbalance in the sleep–wake system. Approximately 10% of patients presenting with excessive daytime sleepiness will be diagnosed with HD. Age of onset varies and prevalence is gender neutral. HD is a diagnosis of exclusion—that is, all potential causes of excessive sleepiness should be ruled out before this diagnosis is used. Diagnosis is confirmed with a normal polysomnography and absence of conditions that could present with sleepiness as a symptom. Many individuals with HD present with sleep inertia, also known as sleep drunkenness, in which the patient appears to be awake but displays poor motor dexterity, inappropriate behavior, memory deficiency, time/space disorientation, and grogginess (APA, 2013). Associated symptoms are lack of motivation and energy, decreased attention and cognitive performance, and depressive symptoms (American Academy of Sleep Medicine, 2001). Treatment for HD is primarily stimulant therapy and scheduled brief naps.

Pause and Reflect

1. *What are the main differences between narcolepsy and HD?*
2. *How are medications helpful in the treatment of narcolepsy?*

Collaborative Care

As discussed, treatment for sleep disorders can vary according to the disorder and may require more than one type of therapy. Thorough assessment and determining which symptoms or impairments of functioning are most troublesome to the patient will help identify therapies that are likely to be successful. In some cases, discussion with the patient's sleep partner also may be helpful. The next section focuses on collaborative care of insomnia, the most prevalent sleep disorder.

Psychopharmacology

Several classes of medications are used for insomnia. Unfortunately, most people treat their sleep problems with over-the-counter drugs, such as diphenhydramine, or use alcohol. Because of the adverse effects of these agents, they should not be used to treat sleep disturbance on a long-term basis.

Prescription medications used for treatment of insomnia include benzodiazepines and other CNS depressants (see Medications Commonly Used to Treat Insomnia). Benzodiazepines may be used for short-term treatment related to anxiety; they reduce the length of time it takes to get to sleep, and may decrease frequency of night and early morning awakenings. Estazolam (Prosom), temazepam (Restoril), and triazolam (Halcion) are among the benzodiazepines appropriate for treatment of insomnia. Other drugs that may be used include nonbarbiturate hypnotics such as eszopiclone (Lunesta), zolpidem (Ambien), and zaleplon (Sonata) (Adams, Holland, & Urban, 2013). These medications should be used with caution in patients with depression, history of alcohol or drug use, hepatic or renal impairment, compromised respiratory status, and pregnancy (Wilson, Shannon, & Shields, 2014). Because of research showing decreased clearance in women and increased evidence of next-morning impairment including driving, in 2013 the U.S. Food and Drug Administration (FDA) recommended cutting in half the recommended dosage of zolpidem. Most sleep medications should be administered early enough to allow for at least 6 to 7 hours of sleep prior to awakening to minimize daytime sleepiness.

Insomnia — medications commonly used to treat

Drug	Daily Dose Range	Half-Life	Nursing Considerations
Nonbarbiturate Hypnotics			
zolpidem (Ambien)	5–10 mg	2.5 hours	Newer subclass of hypnotics:
zolpidem CR	6.25–12.5 mg	2.8 hours	• Low adverse effect profiles
zaleplon (Sonata)	5–20 mg	1 hour	• Fewer interactions with other CNS medications
eszopiclone (Lunesta)	2–3 mg adults	6 hours in adults	• Lower lethality risk
	1–2 mg older adults	9 hours in older adults	For all hypnotics, warn patients of potential risk for hazardous activities such as walking, cooking, and eating during sleep. Educate patients to avoid using alcohol while taking these medications. Use with caution in patients with respiratory conditions. Women should receive lower dosages of zolpidem. Monitor for signs/symptoms of depression.
chloral hydrate (Noctec)	500 mg	8–11 hours	CNS depressant: • Potential for tolerance • Withdrawal symptoms can occur if stopped abruptly • Use with caution in patients with history of drug dependency, depression, suicidal tendencies • Monitor for signs/symptoms of allergic skin reaction Instruct patients to avoid driving and potentially hazardous activities.
ramelteon (Rozerem)	8 mg	1–2.5 hours	Melatonin receptor agonist: • May cause disturbances of reproductive hormonal regulation • Of the hypnotics, better choice for sleep phase disorders • Use with caution in patients with depression with suicidal tendencies • Contraindicated in patients with severe sleep apnea or severe COPD Educate patients to avoid taking alcohol while on this medication.
Benzodiazepines			
estazolam (Prosom)	1–2 mg adults 0.5 mg older adults	10–24 hours	Subclass of hypnotics: • Controlled substances with higher lethality and potential for respiratory depression when combined with other CNS depressants

Drug	Daily Dose Range	Half-Life	Nursing Considerations
flurazepam HCl (Dalmane)	15–30 mg adults 15 mg older adults	47–100 hours	• Higher addiction risk • Use with caution in patients with psychosis, history of suicidal ideation, history of addiction, severe depression
triazolam (Halcion)	0.125–0.25 mg adults 0.0625–0.125 mg older adults	2–3 hours	• Assess for safety in older adults because of dizziness and impaired coordination; also acute confusion
temazepam (Restoril)	7.5–30 mg adults 7.5 mg older adults	8–24 hours	

Antidepressants

Drug	Daily Dose Range	Half-Life	Nursing Considerations
trazodone trazodone (Oleptro)	IR (immediate release) 50–200 mg in divided doses ER (extended release) 150–375 mg	5–9 hours	• Commonly used hypnotic at doses less than 100 mg • No significant antidepressant effects at low dose • Instruct male patients on the potential for priapism • Contraindicated in patients with suicidal ideation or undergoing electroshock therapy • Use with caution in patients with bipolar disorder, history of suicidal tendencies • Monitor BP; report tachycardia, bradycardia, palpitations • Monitor for orthostatic hypertension in older adults, patients taking hypertensives
mirtazapine (Remeron)	15–45 mg adults (older adults should receive lower doses)	20–40 hours	• Often used in patients with poor appetite as weight gain is a common side effect • Cautious use required for a number of co-morbid disorders and conditions, including bipolar disorder, mania, depression, and history of suicidal tendencies • Monitor for excessive somnolence or dizziness, which increase injury potential • Should not be administered in conjunction with MAOIs or within 14 days of discontinuation • Monitor for orthostatic hypotension • May lower seizure threshold for patients with history of seizures Educate patients to avoid taking other medications without consulting prescriber and to avoid alcohol while taking this medication.
amitriptyline (Elavil)	25–300 mg adults 10–200 mg in divided doses for older adults/adolescents	10–50 hours	Substantial side effect profile includes potential for: • Excessive dry mouth • Constipation • Orthostatic hypotension • Weight gain • Increased risk of falls in older adults Use with caution in patients with a number of co-morbid conditions including patients with history of alcoholism and in patients with schizophrenia; may turn urine blue-green.
nortriptyline (Aventyl)	25–150 mg adults 10–75 mg older adults	16–90 hours	• Similar effects as amitriptyline, but less carryover sedation the following day • Use with caution in patients with glaucoma, cardiac disease, history of suicidal tendencies, bipolar disorder, asthma. • Contraindicated in patients with suicidal ideation and for patients taking MAO inhibitors

Data from Wilson, B. A., Shannon, M. T., & Shields, K. M. (2014). *Pearson Nurse's Drug Guide 2014.* Upper Saddle River, NJ: Prentice Hall; Adams, M., Holland, N., & Urban, C. (2014). *Pharmacology for Nurses: A Pathophysiologic Approach* (4th ed.) Upper Saddle River, NJ: Prentice Hall.

Over-the-Counter and Complementary Therapies

Over-the-counter (OTC) and complementary therapies for insomnia usually are the first line of treatment used by most patients (Chapter 22). Unfortunately, some of these therapies have significant negative effects and drug interactions that can cause further health problems. The most commonly used sleep aid is diphenhydramine, which is usually found OTC in oral combination tablets containing acetaminophen or ibuprofen. Diphenhydramine is an antihistamine that results in impairment in the normal drive of wakefulness (histamine) that can last for up to 18 hours, especially in older adults. It also has anticholinergic effects that can result in orthostatic hypotension, which increases the risk of falls in older adults. The recommendation of OTC and complementary therapies for sleep disruption should always be accompanied with appropriate assessment and diagnosis of sleep disorders. It is inappropriate to use OTC sleep aids in patients with sleep apnea, as they can result in increased severity of apneic episodes and diminish the propensity to wake in response to an apneic event.

Cognitive–Behavioral Therapy for Insomnia

Cognitive–behavioral therapy for insomnia (CBT-I) directly addresses negative sleep behaviors, beliefs, and cognitions that result in difficulty initiating and maintaining sleep regardless of co-morbid conditions. Therefore, CBT-I may be necessary if sleep disturbance continues after treating the co-morbid sleep disorder. Chronic insomnia is best treated with CBT-I, including the combination of sleep restriction, stimulus control, sleep hygiene, cognitive therapy, and relaxation exercises (Perlis, Jungquist, Smith, & Posner, 2005) (Table 12-3). Insomnia is also treated effectively using medications, although CBT-I offers better long-term gains not seen with medication use (Smith et al., 2002). Although some patients will require a therapist who is especially trained in the delivery of CBT-I, nurses can introduce the concepts in any practice setting. Advanced practice nurses, especially those in the psychiatric setting, are good candidates to learn and deliver the advanced form of CBT-I.

Pause and Reflect

1. *What considerations must nurses keep in mind when working with patients who are prescribed benzodiazepines for insomnia?*
2. *Which cognitive behavioral interventions for insomnia do you think might be most effective for the greatest number of patients? Why?*

Nursing Management

Many Americans experience challenges related to sleep, with between 34% and 45% of adults reporting accidentally falling asleep at least once in the past month (CDC, 2013). Many patients reporting sleep difficulty may not be experiencing an actual disorder. Regardless of the degree of sleep difficulty reported, nurses must complete a thorough assessment to elicit data that will inform the source of the patient's trouble sleeping and, therefore, the care plan. This is particularly important when patients report sleepiness. Sleepiness can be caused by numerous precipitating factors, such as medication side

Cognitive–Behavioral Therapy for Insomnia   table 12-3

Treatment Modality	Description
Stimulus control therapy	A set of instructions designed to re-associate the bed/bedroom with sleep and to re-establish a consistent therapeutic sleep–wake schedule: (1) Go to bed only when sleepy; (2) get out of bed when unable to sleep; (3) use the bed/bedroom for sleep and intimate relations only (e.g., no reading, no watching TV); and (4) arise at the same time every morning; (5) no napping.
Sleep restriction therapy	A method designed to reduce the amount of time spent in bed not sleeping. For example, if a patient reports sleeping an average of 6 hours per night, but spending 8 or 9 hours in bed, the initial recommended time in bed (from lights out to final arising time) would be restricted to 6 hours. Periodic adjustments to this sleep window are made contingent upon sleep efficiency, until optimal sleep duration is reached.
Relaxation training	Clinical procedures aimed at reducing tension (e.g., progressive muscle relaxation) or intrusive thoughts at bedtime (e.g., imagery training, meditation) interfering with sleep.
Cognitive therapy	Therapy aimed at changing misconceptions about sleep and faulty beliefs about insomnia and its perceived daytime consequences. Other cognitive procedures may include paradoxical intention or methods aimed at reducing or preventing excessive worrying about insomnia and its consequences.
Sleep hygiene	General guidelines about health practices (e.g., diet, education exercise, substance use) and environmental factors (e.g., light, noise, temperature) that may promote or interfere with sleep. This may also include some basic information about normal sleep and changes in sleep patterns with aging.
Cognitive–behavioral therapy	A combination of any of the above behavioral (e.g., behavior stimulus control, sleep restriction, relaxation) and therapeutic cognitive procedures.

Based on Morin, C. M., Bootzin, R. R., Buysse, D. J., Edinger, J. D., Espie, C. A., & Lichstein, K. L. (2006). Psychological and behavioral treatment of insomnia: Update of the recent evidence (1998–2004). *Sleep, 29*(11), 1398–1414, table 1, p. 1399; Mayo Clinic. (2011). Insomnia treatment: Cognitive behavioral therapy instead of sleeping pills. Available at http://www.mayoclinic.com/health/insomnia-treatment/SL00013

effects, neurological injury, and certain sleep disorders, such as narcolepsy and sleep apnea. Sleepiness is associated with motor vehicle accidents, and can increase the risk for other types of accidents as well. If a patient complains of inability to stay awake, nursing measures should include reporting the information to the primary care provider, educating on risk of accidents, and advocating for alternative transportation until the cause of sleepiness can be fully diagnosed and treated.

Assessment

When a sleep problem is suspected, full assessment per algorithm is warranted (Figure 12-6). The algorithm assists the nurse in evaluating the patient's symptoms, habits, and environment. Although a sleep study is necessary to diagnose obstructive sleep apnea and narcolepsy, nurses should have the skills to screen for these disorders. Screening tools, such as the Epworth Sleepiness Scale, which measures a patient's report of level of sleepiness, may be used. Nursing assessment questions should target common diagnostic criteria for sleep disorders. Examples of screening questions for sleep-disordered breathing include the following (Jungquist, Karan, & Perlis, 2011):

- Do you wake gasping for breath?
- Has your bed partner witnessed pauses in your breathing while you sleep?
- Do you suffer from excessive daytime sleepiness?
- Do you snore?

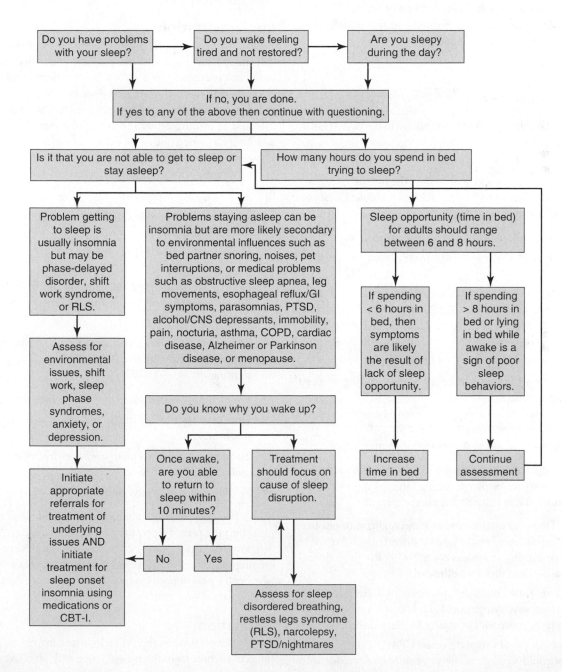

12-6   Algorithm for assessing/screening sleep disorders in adults.

Additional assessment questions related to sleep and wakefulness patterns may include the following:

- What time do you normally go to bed? How long does it take you to fall asleep?
- What do you do to get ready for bed/sleep?
- Do you wake up during the night? If so, how many times per night? What awakens you?
- Do you have difficulty waking up in the morning?
- Do you nap during the day? If so, how do you feel after you nap?
- Do you feel sleepy during the day?
- How do you think your sleep is affecting your daily functioning?

Diagnosis and Planning

It is within the advanced practice nurse's scope of practice to diagnose sleep disorders; generalist nurses should be able to determine the appropriate nursing diagnosis including:

- Sleep Deprivation
- Sleep Pattern, Disturbed
  (NANDA-I © 2014)

All nurses should be able to work with the patient to develop a plan of care that includes patient education in appropriate sleep hygiene.

Plans and Goals

As the nurse develops plans and goals within the nursing care plan, he or she keeps the patient involved as much as possible. Questions the nurse asks include the following:

- Is the patient capable of helping develop a care plan?
- What is the most distressing symptom, from the patient's perspective?
- What specifically does the patient need/want to achieve? How can the patient's needs be articulated and addressed as *specific, realistic,* and *measurable* goals for the patient's care? For example if the patient has difficulty sleeping, the nurse might state the following *specific, measurable,* and *realistic* goals:
  - The patient will demonstrate an understanding of sleep hygiene protocols in one day.
  - The patient will increase sleep time from 5 hours per night to 7 hours per night in 3 days.
  - The patient will report feeling more rested after 3 days.

In developing the plan of care, the nurse will consider with the patient how the five domains are involved. Asking targeted questions may help elicit information that will help inform the care plan.

- *Biological:* Does the patient have any medical conditions that may impede full recovery from sleep disturbance? Are treatments for co-morbid disorders contributing the sleep disturbance? If so, how can these be addressed?
- *Psychological:* How could the diagnosis of a sleep disorder potentiate depressive symptoms? Could depression be contributing to nonadherence with treatment for sleep disorders?
- *Sociological:* Is it possible that the use of CPAP will inhibit sexuality? How could you intervene to promote adherence with treatment due to sexuality concerns?

- *Cultural:* Are there any family traditions or rituals that are impeding or enhancing to the patient's health? Are there cultural obstacles to adherence with treatment for sleep disorders?
- *Spiritual:* Are there any spiritual concerns that could be affecting the patient's motivation to treat the sleep disturbance?

Revising the Care Plan During Recovery and Rehabilitation

As a patient's sleep improves and daytime complaints decrease, the nurse will re-evaluate the plan of care for obstacles to full recovery. If taking hypnotic medications, behavioral therapy can be introduced that may help decrease the patient's need for medications. For patients with sleep apnea, compliance with CPAP use is often challenging, and patients may need re-enforcement of negative health effects of untreated sleep apnea.

Implementation

Appropriate interventions will depend on the individual patient and the specific diagnosis, and may include patient education on use of any prescribed medication, normal sleep requirements, and consequences of insufficient sleep (see the Nursing Care Plan provided in this chapter). For example, interventions for DSPD are directed at forcing advancement of the circadian rhythm and adapting daytime routine to avoid mental activities during the phase of high sleep propensity.

Most patients will require education on one or more of the following:

- Normal sleep requirements, stimulus control, and sleep hygiene (Table 12-4)
- Medications and medical diseases that are known to disrupt sleep
- How to access appropriate referrals and treatment for sleep disorders, including the National Sleep Foundation (www.sleepfoundation.org)

Hospitalized patients require support from the nursing staff to achieve sufficient sleep. Interventions to promote sleep may include the following:

- Ensure uninterrupted sleep time for the patient.
- Offer relaxation using music and/or a warm bath 90 minutes before bedtime.
- Encourage a quiet sleep environment free of staff chatter and unit noise.
- Provide a dark sleep environment.

Patient learning needs and abilities must be addressed and incorporated into the plan. For example, if Disturbed Sleep Pattern is the diagnosis, the patient may need information about sleep hygiene and keeping a sleep log. The nurse will work with the patient to determine whether the patient needs to modify any of the five domains to assist with improved sleep pattern.

Evaluation

The evaluation process should include nursing reassessment of the subjective report from the patient along with objective observation. Assessing for adherence to treatment is of particular importance

Sleep Hygiene Guidelines
table 12-4

Guideline	Rationale
Sleep only as much as you need to feel refreshed during the following day.	Restricting your time in bed helps to consolidate and deepen your sleep. Excessively long times in bed lead to fragmented and shallow sleep.
Get up at the same time each day, 7 days a week.	A regular wake time in the morning leads to regular times of sleep onset, and helps to set your "biological clock."
Exercise regularly.	Exercise makes it easier to initiate sleep and deepen sleep. Schedule exercise times so that they do not occur within 3 hours of when you intend to go to bed.
Make sure your bedroom is comfortable and free from light and noise.	A comfortable, noise-free sleep environment will reduce the likelihood that you will wake up during the night. Even very quiet sounds can lighten your sleep, even though they may not wake you up completely. Carpeting, insulated curtains, and a closed door help.
Make sure that your bedroom is at a comfortable temperature during the night.	Excessively warm or cold sleep environments may disturb sleep.
Eat regular meals and do not go to bed hungry.	Hunger may disturb sleep. A light snack at bedtime (especially carbohydrates) may help sleep, but avoid greasy or "heavy" foods.
Avoid excessive liquids in the evening.	Reducing liquid intake will minimize the need for nighttime trips to the bathroom.
Cut down on all caffeinated products.	Caffeinated beverages and foods (coffee, tea, cola, chocolate) can cause difficulty falling asleep, awakenings during the night, and shallow sleep.
Avoid alcohol, especially in the evening.	Although alcohol helps tense people fall asleep more easily, it causes awakenings later in the night.
Smoking may disturb sleep.	Nicotine is a stimulant.
Don't take your problems to bed.	Plan some time earlier in the evening for working on your problems or planning the next day's activities. Worrying may interfere with initiating sleep and produce shallow sleep.
Do not try to fall asleep.	This only makes the problem worse. Instead, leave the bedroom, and do something quite and nonstimulating like reading a book. Return to bed only when you are sleepy.
Put the clock under the bed or turn it so that you can't see it.	Clock watching may lead to frustration, anger, and worry that interfere with sleep.
Avoid naps.	Staying awake during the day helps you to fall asleep at night.

(see Evidence-Based Practice: Patients Resisting Treatment). Patients should demonstrate knowledge of their disorder, the negative emotional and physical consequences of sleep loss, and the recommended treatment. Patients with DSPD should also be able to demonstrate knowledge of the risks of marijuana and alcohol use and how to access help when or if the depressive symptoms return. The patient's plan of care should be adjusted accordingly; appropriate referrals should be made for post-hospitalization.

Pause and Reflect

1. *In what areas will most patients require patient education related to sleep?*
2. *What sleep hygiene guidelines do you follow? In what areas could you improve?*

From Suffering to Hope

Sleep is innate and necessary to sustain homeostasis, immune function, cognitive performance, mood regulation, and muscle restoration. Sleep disorders are known to impair performance, increase absenteeism from work, decrease quality of life, precipitate depression, and increase the risk of motor vehicle accidents, hypertension, altered glucose metabolism, atrial fibrillation, and stroke. Nurses play a key role in recognizing sleep disorders, initiating referrals to access diagnosis and treatment, and educating patients on the topic of adequate sleep and treatments for sleep disorders. As sleep disorders are all treatable and there are several options for treatment, instilling hope that patients' quality of life can be improved is appropriate and very important.

A Patient with Obstructive Sleep Apnea   NURSING CARE PLAN

Nursing Diagnosis: Disturbed sleep pattern related to obstructed airway during sleep (held breath for >1 minute and O$_2$ saturation dropped to 80%).

Short-Term Goals *Patient will:* *(include date for short-term goal to be met)*	Intervention *Nurse will:*	Rationale
Identify any risk to safety secondary to daytime sleepiness	Assess level of daytime sleepiness. Educate patient about activity risks such as driving and working with machinery. Instruct patient on added risk of unsafe inability to maintain wakefulness if taking sedating medications.	Determine ability to maintain wakefulness during driving or operating heavy equipment.
Identify willingness to undergo sleep study and potential treatment using CPAP.	Instruct patient on signs/symptoms and pathophysiology of sleep apnea, negative health consequences, need for sleep study for diagnosis. Explain a sleep study procedure and how to access a formal sleep evaluation.	Sleep apnea is diagnosed during a sleep study procedure.
Identify risk to safety secondary to inability to maintain patent airway.	Assist patient in maintaining patent airway during conscious sedation by positioning patient in upright position or placing CPAP if ordered and available in facility.	Patients with sleep apnea are at high risk of adverse respiratory event during procedures requiring sedation or when starting medication known to suppress respiratory drive.
Long-Term Goal Adherence with CPAP (wearing more than 4 hours nightly 70% of the time).	Review CPAP use and reinforce importance of adherence.	Research shows that negative health effects and excessive daytime sleepiness resolve once patients adhere to CPAP treatment at a pressure adequate to maintain their AHI < 5.

Clinical Reasoning

1. What other nursing diagnoses might the nurse working with a patient with OSA consider?
2. What are the obstacles to wearing CPAP, and how can the nurse assist the patient with gaining compliance?
3. What could the nurse do for a patient with OSA who does not have the money to afford CPAP treatment?

Patients Resisting Treatment   evidence-based practice

Clinical Problem

A patient is experiencing mood disturbance that is resistant to treatment. On assessing the patient's sleep, it is discovered that the patient is not using the CPAP device as prescribed several months ago.

Evidence

Sawyer, Deatrick, Kuna, and Weaver (2010) reported that an individual's experiences, beliefs, and perceptions are influential in their decision to adhere with CPAP treatment. They found that patients in compliance with CPAP were more likely to:

- Perceive the health and functional risks of untreated OSA.
- Have positive belief in their ability to use CPAP from early in the diagnostic process.

- Have clearly defined outcome expectations.
- Have more facilitators than barriers as they progressed from diagnosis to treatment.
- Identify important social influences and support sources for both pursuing diagnosis and persisting with CPAP use.

Critical Thinking Questions

Identify obstacles to adherence with CPAP using the findings in the Sawyer study. What strategies might you take to address obstacles to adherence in your patients? How do you think these might be helpful?

Chapter Highlights

1. Sleep is innate and necessary for health. It represents a cycling of brain activity that is closely correlated with cycling of cardiac and respiratory activity.

2. Polysomnography (a form of EEG procedure that occurs during sleep) is a sleep study that monitors brain waves along with other physiological measures.

3. Sleep and mental health have a reciprocal relationship. When an individual is deprived of adequate sleep, symptoms of depression and anxiety occur. In the presence of depression and anxiety, sleep disruption, either fragmented or prolonged, often occurs.

4. Timing, duration, and quality of sleep are influenced by age.

5. Insomnia, sleep-disordered breathing, and restless legs syndrome are the most common sleep disorders. Narcolepsy (a disorder of the wakefulness system) is less common, but can be very disabling.

6. Insomnia is characterized by repeated difficulty with sleep initiation, duration, consolidation, and/or quality that occurs despite adequate time and opportunity for sleep and results in some form of daytime impairment.

7. Sleep-disordered breathing has been found to contribute to the development of hypertension, coronary artery disease, altered glucose metabolism, mood dysregulation, and impaired cognitive and immune function.

8. Nurses play a key role in the promotion of adequate sleep, the discovery of sleep disorders, and compliance with treatment.

NCLEX®-RN Questions

1. The nurse is assessing a patient who has been experiencing difficulty falling asleep at night. Which patient factors does the nurse recognize as most likely to interfere with the homeostatic drive of sleep? Select all that apply.
   a. Being 85 years of age
   b. Morbid obesity
   c. Sedentary lifestyle
   d. Frequent daytime napping
   e. Working in a windowless office

2. The nurse is planning care for a group of patients experiencing disturbances in sleep patterns. Which patient does the nurse identify as most at risk for impaired function in the sociocultural domain?
   a. The pediatric patient who is experiencing insomnia related to short-term treatment with steroids
   b. The 40-year-old patient who has been using a CPAP machine for sleep apnea for more than 2 years
   c. The older adult who has been experiencing symptoms of restless legs syndrome three times a week
   d. The 35-year-old patient with narcolepsy with cataplexic episodes occurring most days of the week

3. A patient tells the nurse that her sleeping has improved since she has been getting out of bed when she is not sleepy. The nurse evaluates this is a therapeutic response to which treatment intervention?
   a. Sleep hygiene
   b. Cognitive therapy
   c. Stimulus control therapy
   d. Sleep restriction therapy

4. The nurse is caring for a patient with a shift work sleep disorder. What should the nurse suggest to promote adequate sleep? Select all that apply.
   a. Arrange at least two days off between shift rotations.
   b. Get up and move frequently during the working shift.
   c. Rest or nap whenever there is an opportunity to do so.
   d. Ensure that the sleep area is protected from light and noise.
   e. Try to schedule each shift to start earlier than the previous shift.

5. The nurse is reviewing the records of a patient being admitted to the inpatient mental health unit. It is noted that the patient has been diagnosed with parasomnia disorder. The nurse understands that this type of disorder is likely to be manifested by which of the following?
   a. Persistent early morning awakening
   b. Excessive sleepiness during daytime hours
   c. Intermittent episodes of apnea while asleep
   d. Unusual behaviors demonstrated during sleep

6. The nurse is reviewing the efficacy of pharmacological treatments used for the management of insomnia in older adult patients. Which information should the nurse use to guide practice? Select all that apply.
   a. Melatonin is an endogenous sleep hormone that increases with age.
   b. Diphenhydramine (Benadryl) is a safe, effective over-the-counter medication.
   c. Mirtazapine (Remeron) may be a good choice for the patient who has a poor appetite.
   d. Trazodone (Desyrel) is frequently used for patients undergoing electroconvulsive therapy.
   e. Women may be more susceptible to next-day impairment from agents such as zolipedem (Ambien).

7. The nurse is evaluating the patient who was prescribed a CPAP device several months ago for the management of sleep apnea. Which report by the patient is most likely to indicate that social support influences are a factor in noncompliance?
   a. "I don't want my new partner to know that I use this device."
   b. "A friend gave me an article about other ways to manage apnea."
   c. "I don't think my snoring is that bothersome to my spouse."
   d. "I am not confident about my ability to use the device without help."

Answers may be found on the Pearson student resource site: nursing. pearsonhighered.com

Pearson Nursing Student Resources Find additional review materials at **nursing.pearsonhighered.com**

References

Abdel-Khalek, A. M., Adachi, Y., Yamagami, T., Agargun, M. Y., Kara, H., Ozbek, H., . . . Arnon, Z. (2007). Modafinil: new indication. For a minority of patients with sleep apnoea. *Prescrire International, 16*(89), 102–103.

Adams, M., Holland, N., & Urban, C. (2014). *Pharmacology for Nurses: A Pathophysiologic Approach* (5th ed.). Upper Saddle River, NJ: Prentice Hall.

Al Lawati, N. M., Patel, S. R., & Ayas, N. T. (2009). Epidemiology, risk factors, and consequences of obstructive sleep apnea and short sleep duration. *Progressive Cardiovascular Disease, 51*(4), 285–293.

Alajmi, M., Mulgrew, A., Fox, J., Davidson, W., Schulzer, M., Mak, E., . . . Ayas, N. (2007). Impact of continuous positive airway pressure therapy on blood pressure in patients with obstructive sleep apnea hypopnea: A meta-analysis of randomized controlled trials. *Lung, 185*(2), 67–72.

Altena, E., Van Der Werf, Y. D., Strijers, R. L., & Van Someren, E. J. (2008). Sleep loss affects vigilance: Effects of chronic insomnia and sleep therapy. *Journal of Sleep Research, 17*(3), 335–343.

American Academy of Sleep Medicine. (2001). *International Classification of Sleep Disorders, Revised: Diagnostic and Coding Manual.* West Chester, IL: American Academy of Sleep Medicine.

American Sleep Association. (2007). Shift work disorder. Available at http://www.sleepassociation.org/index.php?p=shiftworkdisorder

American Psychiatric Association. (2013). *Diagnostic and Statistical Manual of Mental Disorders* (5th ed.). Washington, DC: American Psychiatric Publishers.

Anderson, G. (2010). The role of melatonin in post-partum psychosis and depression associated with bipolar disorder. *Journal of Perinatal Medicine, 38*(6), 585–587.

Armon, C., Johnson, K., Roy, A., & Nowack, W. (2012). Polysomnography. *Medscape.* Available at http://emedicine.medscape.com/article/1188764-overview

Backhaus, J., Junghanns, K., Born, J., Hohaus, K., Faasch, F., & Hohagen, F. (2006). Impaired declarative memory consolidation during sleep in patients with primary insomnia: Influence of sleep architecture and nocturnal cortisol release. *Biological Psychiatry, 60*(12), 1324–1330.

Bruls, E., Crasson, M., Van Reeth, O., & Legros, J. J. (2000). Melatonin. II. Physiological and therapeutic effects. *Rev Med Liege, 55*(9), 862–870.

Budhiraja, R., Sharief, I., & Quan, S. F. (2005). Sleep disordered breathing and hypertension. *Journal of Clinical Sleep Medicine, 1*(4), 401–404.

Carskadon, M. A., & Dement, W. (2005). Normal human sleep: An overview. In M. Kryger, T. Roth, & W. Dement (Eds.). *Principles and Practice of Sleep Medicine.* Philadelphia, PA: Elsevier Saunders, pp. 13–23.

Centers for Disease Control and Prevention. (2013). Insufficient sleep is a public health epidemic. Available at http://www.cdc.gov/features/dssleep/

Chen, C. C., Shiu, L. J., Li, Y. L., Tung, K. Y., Chan, K. Y., Yeh, C. J., . . . Wong, R. H. (2010). Shift work and arteriosclerosis risk in professional bus drivers. [Research Support, Non-U.S. Gov't]. *Annals of Epidemiology, 20*(1), 60–66.

Chokroverty, S. (1999). Physiology changes in sleep. In S. Chokroverty (Ed.), *Sleep Disorders Medicine: Basic Science, Technical Considerations, and Clinical Aspects.* Boston: Butterworth Heinemann, pp. 95–120.

Chung, M. H., Kuo, T. B. J., Hsu, N., Chu, H., Chou, K. R., & Yang, C. C. H. (2009). Sleep and autonomic nervous system changes—enhanced cardiac sympathetic modulations during sleep in permanent night shift nurses. *Scandinavian Journal of Work, Environment & Health, 35*(3), 180–187.

Czeisler, C. A., Cajochen, C., & Turek, F. W. (2000). Melatonin in the regulation of sleep and circadian rhythms. In M. Kryger, T. Roth, & W. Dement, (Eds.). *Principles and Practice of Sleep Medicine.* Philadelphia: Saunders, pp. 400– 406.

Daley, M., Morin, C. M., LeBlanc, M., Gregoire, J. P., Savard, J., & Baillargeon, L. (2009). Insomnia and its relationship to health-care utilization, work absenteeism, productivity and accidents. *Sleep Medicine, 10*(4), 427–438.

Dergacheva, O., Wang, X., Lovett-Barr, M. R., Jameson, H., & Mendelowitz, D. (2010). The lateral paragigantocellular nucleus modulates parasympathetic cardiac neurons: A mechanism for rapid eye movement sleep-dependent changes in heart rate. *Journal of Neurophysiology, 104*(2), 685–694.

Droogleever Fortuyn, H. A., Mulders, P. C., Renier, W. O., Buitelaar, J. K., & Overeem, S. (2011). Narcolepsy and psychiatry: An evolving association of increasing interest. *Sleep Medicine, 12*(7), 714–719.

Eggermann, E., Bayer, L., Serafin, M., Saint-Mleux, B., Bernheim, L., Machard, D., . . . Mühlethaler, M. (2003). The wake-promoting hypocretin–orexin neurons are in an intrinsic state of membrane depolarization. *Journal of Neuroscience, 23*(5), 1557–1562.

Erren, T. C. (2010). Shift work, cancer and "white-box" epidemiology: Association and causation. [Editorial]. *Epidemiologic perspectives & innovations: EP+I, 7,* 11.

Hargens, T. A., Nickols-Richardson, S. M., Gregg, J. M., Zedalis, D., & Herbert, W. G. (2006). Hypertension research in sleep apnea. *Journal of Clinical Hypertension 8*(12), 873–878.

Hiestand, D. M., Britz, P., Goldman, M., & Phillips, B. (2006). Prevalence of symptoms and risk of sleep apnea in the US population. *Chest, 130*(3), 780–786.

Hirshkowitz, M. (2008). The clinical consequences of obstructive sleep apnea and associated excessive sleepiness. *Journal of Family Practice. 57*(8), S9–16.

Hudgel, D. W., Martin, R. J., Johnson, B., & Hill, P. (1984). Mechanics of the respiratory system and breathing pattern during sleep in normal humans. *Journal of Applied Physiology, 56*(1), 133–137.

Irwin, M., Clark, C., Kennedy, B., Christian Gillin, J., & Ziegler, M. (2003). Nocturnal catecholamines and immune function in insomniacs, depressed patients, and control subjects. *Brain, Behavior, and Immunity, 17*(5), 365–372.

Johns, M. W. (1991). A new method for measuring daytime sleepiness: The Epworth sleepiness scale. *Sleep, 14*(6), 540–545.

Jungquist, C. R., Karan, S., & Perlis, M. L. (2011). Risk factors for opioid-induced excessive respiratory depression. *Pain Management Nursing, 12*(3), 180–187.

Kilduff, T. S., & Peyron, C. (2000). The hypocretin/orexin ligand–receptor system: Implications for sleep and sleep disorders. *Trends in Neurosciences, 23*(8), 359–365.

Kiyashchenko, L. I., Mileykovskiy, B. Y., Maidment, N., Lam, H. A., Wu, M.-F., John, J., . . . Siegel, J. M. (2002). Release of hypocretin (orexin) during waking and sleep states. *Journal of Neuroscience, 22*(13), 5282–5286.

KräuchI, K., & Wirz-Justice, A. (2001). Circadian clues to sleep onset mechanisms. *Neuropsychopharmacology, 25*(5 suppl), S92–S96.

Kripke, D. F., Youngstedt, S. D., Rex, K. M., Klauber, M. R., & Elliott, J. A. (2003). Melatonin excretion with affect disorders over age 60. *Psychiatry Research, 118*(1), 47–54.

Kushida, C. A., Littner, M. R., Morgenthaler, T., Alessi, C. A., Bailey, D., Coleman, J. J., . . . Wise, M. (2005). Practice parameters for the indications for polysomnography and related procedures: An update for 2005. *Sleep, 28*(4), 499–521.

Leger, D., Laudon, M., & Zisapel, N. (2004). Nocturnal 6-sulfatoxymelatonin excretion in insomnia and its relation to the response to melatonin replacement therapy. *American Journal of Medicine, 116*(2), 91–95.

Licata, S. C., Jensen, J. E., Penetar, D. M., Prescot, A. P., Lukas, S. E., & Renshaw, P. F. (2009). A therapeutic dose of zolpidem reduces thalamic GABA in healthy volunteers: A proton MRS study at 4 T. *Psychopharmacology, 203*(4), 819–829.

Mai, E., & Buysse, D. J. (2008). Insomnia: Prevalence, impact, pathogenesis, differential diagnosis, and evaluation. *Sleep Medicine Clinics, 3*(2), 167–174.

Mayo Clinic. (2011). Insomnia treatment: Cognitive behavioral therapy instead of sleeping pills. Available at http://www.mayoclinic.com/health/insomnia-treatment/SL00013

Mignot, E., Lammers, G. J., Ripley, B., Okun, M., Nevsimalova, S., Overeem, S., . . . Nishino, S. (2002). The role of cerebrospinal fluid hypocretin measurement in the diagnosis of narcolepsy and other hypersomnias. *Archives of Neurology, 59*(10), 1553–1562.

Mitler, M., Poceta, S., & Bigby, B. (1999). Sleep scoring technique. In S. Chokroverty, (Ed.). *Sleep Disorders Medicine: Basic Science, Technical Considerations, and Clinical Aspects.* Boston: Butterworth-Heinemann, pp. 245–262.

Miyata, S., Noda, A., Ozaki, N., Hara, Y., Minoshima, M., Iwamoto, K., . . . Koike, Y. (2010). Insufficient sleep impairs driving performance and cognitive function. *Neuroscience Letters, 469*(2), 229–233.

Montplaisir, J., Allen, R., Walters, A., & Ferini-Strambi, L. (2005). Neurologic disorders. In M. Kryger, T. Roth, & W. Dement, (Eds.). *Principles and Practice of Sleep Medicine.* Philadelphia: Elsevier Saunders, pp. 839–852.

Morin, C. M., Bootzin, R. R., Buysse, D. J., Edinger, J. D., Espie, C. A., & Lichstein, K. L. (2006). Psychological and behavioral treatment of insomnia: Update of the recent evidence (1998–2004). *Sleep, 29*(11), 1398–1414.

Narcolepsy Network. (2010). About Narcolepsy. Available at http://www.narcolepsynetwork.org/about-narcolepsy/about-narcolepsy/

National Institute of Neurological Disorders and Stroke & National Institutes of Health. (2011). Narcolepsy Fact Sheet (NIH Publication No. 03-1637). Available at http://www.ninds.nih.gov/disorders/narcolepsy/detail_narcolepsy.htm#180863201

National Sleep Foundation. (2011). Sleep in America Poll: Communication Technologies in the Bedroom. Available at http://www.sleepfoundation.org/sites/default/files/sleepinamericapoll/SIAP_2011_Summary_of_Findings.pdf

Nielsen, T., Paquette, T., Solomonova, E., Lara-Carrasco, J., Colombo, R., & Lanfranchi, P. (2010). Changes in cardiac variability after REM sleep deprivation in recurrent nightmares. [Research Support, Non-U.S. Gov't]. *Sleep, 33*(1), 113–122.

Nofzinger, E. A. (2008). Functional neuroimaging of sleep disorders. *Current Pharmaceutical Design, 14*(32), 3417–3429.

Oberndorfer, S., Saletu-Zyhlarz, G., & Saletu, B. (2000). Effects of selective serotonin reuptake inhibitors on objective and subjective sleep quality. *Neuropsychobiology, 42*(2), 69–81.

Ohayon, M. M. (2009). Pain sensitivity, depression, and sleep deprivation: Links with serotoninergic dysfunction. *Journal of Psychiatric Research, 43*(16), 1243–1245.

Ohayon, M. M., & Bader, G. (2010). Prevalence and correlates of insomnia in the Swedish population aged 19–75 years. [Research Support, Non-U.S. Gov't]. *Sleep Medicine, 11*(10), 980–986.

Ohayon, M. M., & Sagales, T. (2010). Prevalence of insomnia and sleep characteristics in the general population of Spain. [Research Support, Non-U.S. Gov't]. *Sleep Medicine, 11*(10), 1010–1018.

Olde Rikkert, M. G., & Rigaud, A. S. (2001). Melatonin in elderly patients with insomnia. A systematic review. *Zeitschrift fur Gerontologie und Geriatrie [Journal of Gerontology and Geriatrics], 34*(6), 491–497.

Perlis, M. L., Jungquist, C. R., Smith, M. T., & Posner, D. (2005). *Cognitive Behavioral Treatment of Insomnia: A Session-by-Session Guide.* New York, NY: Springer.

Phillips, K. D., Mock, K. S., Bopp, C. M., Dudgeon, W. A., & Hand, G. A. (2006). Spiritual well-being, sleep disturbance, and mental and physical health status in HIV-infected individuals. [Research Support, N.I.H., Extramural]. *Issues in Mental Health Nursing, 27*(2), 125–139.

Riemann, D., Klein, T., Rodenbeck, A., Feige, B., Horny, A., Hummel, R., . . . Voderholzer, U. (2002). Nocturnal cortisol and melatonin secretion in primary insomnia. *Psychiatry Research, 113*(1–2), 17–27.

Ryan, S., Nolan, G. M., Hannigan, E., Cunningham, S., Taylor, C., & McNicholas, W. T. (2007). Cardiovascular risk markers in obstructive sleep apnoea syndrome and correlation with obesity. *Thorax, 62*(6), 509–514.

Ryan, S., Taylor, C. T., & McNicholas, W. T. (2005). Selective activation of inflammatory pathways by intermittent hypoxia in obstructive sleep apnea syndrome. *Circulation, 112*(17), 2660–2667.

Sandberg, D., Anund, A., Fors, C., Kecklund, G., Karlsson, J. G., Wahde, M., & Åkerstedt, T. (2011). The characteristics of sleepiness during real driving at night—a study of driving performance, physiology and subjective experience. *Sleep, 34*(10), 1317–1325.

Sawyer, A. M., Deatrick, J., Kuna, S. T., & Weaver, T. E. (2010). Differences in perceptions of the diagnosis and treatment of obstructive sleep apnea and continuous positive airway pressure therapy among adherers and nonadherers. *Qualitative Health Research, 20*, 873–892.

Schumann, A. Y., Bartsch, R. P., Penzel, T., Ivanov, P. C., & Kantelhardt, J. W. (2010). Aging effects on cardiac and respiratory dynamics in healthy subjects across sleep stages. *Sleep, 33*(7), 943–955.

Sehgal, A., & Mignot, E. (2011). Genetics of sleep and sleep disorders. *Cell, 146*(2), 194–207.

Sgoifo, A., Buwalda, B., Roos, M., Costoli, T., Merati, G., & Meerlo, P. (2006). Effects of sleep deprivation on cardiac autonomic and pituitary-adrenocortical stress reactivity in rats. *Psychoneuroendocrinology, 31*(2), 197–208.

Smith, M. T., Perlis, M. L., Park, A., Smith, M. S., Pennington, J., Giles, D. E., & Buysse, D. J. (2002). Comparative meta-analysis of pharmacotherapy and behavior therapy for persistent insomnia. [Comparative Study Meta-Analysis]. *American Journal of Psychiatry, 159*(1), 5–11.

Stefansson, H., Rye, D. B., Hicks, A., Petursson, H., Ingason, A., Thorgeirsson, T. E., . . . Stefansson, K. (2007). A genetic risk factor for periodic limb movements in sleep. *New England Journal of Medicine, 357*(7), 639–647.

Steiger, A. (2002). Sleep and the hypothalamo–pituitary–adrenocortical system. *Sleep Medicine Reviews, 6*(2), 125–138.

Stierer, T., & Punjabi, N. M. (2005). Demographics and diagnosis of obstructive sleep apnea. *Anesthesiology Clinics of North America, 23*(3), 405–420.

Tsai, W. H., Remmers, J. E., Brant, R., Flemons, W. W., Davies, J., & Macarthur, C. (2003). A decision rule for diagnostic testing in obstructive sleep apnea. *American Journal of Respiratory and Critical Care Medicine, 167*(10), 1427–1432.

White, D. P. (2005). Central sleep apnea. In M. Kryger, T. Roth, & W. Dement, (Eds.). *Principles and Practice of Sleep Medicine.* Philadelphia: Elsevier Saunders, pp. 969–986.

Wilson, B. A., Shannon, M. T., & Shields, K. M. (2014). *Pearson Nurse's Drug Guide 2014.* Upper Saddle River, NJ: Prentice Hall.

Winkelman, J. W. (2007). Periodic limb movements in sleep — endophenotype for restless legs syndrome? *New England Journal of Medicine, 357*(7), 703–705.

Yee, B., Liu, P., Phillips, C., & Grunstein, R. (2004). Neuroendocrine changes in sleep apnea. *Current Opinion in Pulmonary Medicine, 10*(6), 475–481.

Young, T., Peppard, P. E., & Gottlieb, D. J. (2002). Epidemiology of obstructive sleep apnea: A population health perspective. *American Journal of Respiratory and Critical Care Medicine, 165*(9), 1217–1239.

13

Disorders of Anxiety, Stress, and Trauma

Mertie L. Potter

Key Terms

Learning Outcomes

1. Examine the etiology of anxiety.

2. Summarize the impact of biological, psychological, sociological, cultural, and spiritual domains on anxiety, obsessive–compulsive, and trauma- and stressor-related disorders.

3. Classify defense mechanisms used in anxiety, obsessive–compulsive, and trauma- and stressor-related disorders.

4. Contrast Peplau's four levels of anxiety and potential interventions.

5. Categorize key symptoms of different anxiety, obsessive–compulsive, and trauma- and stressor-related disorders.

6. Evaluate different pharmacologic and nonpharmacologic therapies used in the treatment of anxiety, obsessive–compulsive, and trauma- and stressor-related disorders.

7. Plan evidence-based nursing care for patients diagnosed with anxiety, obsessive–compulsive, and trauma- and stressor-related disorders.

Sondra Initial Onset

Sondra Flores is a 19-year-old Hispanic woman who comes to the local outpatient clinic accompanied by her mother and grandmother. When Carol, a registered nurse working at the clinic, invites Sondra into the examining room, her mother and grandmother accompany her. Sondra is fidgeting and has poor eye contact. Sondra tells Carol that she has a red and itchy rash on both hands. While taking Sondra's health history, Carol learns that Sondra immigrated to the United States from the Dominican Republic at age 16. Sondra lives with her mother, father, brother, and maternal grandmother. She is bilingual in Spanish and English; she speaks both languages well. She is very close to her "Lita" (the Spanish word for grandmother is *abuela*, or the nickname *abuelita*).

Sondra discloses that she has been worried for 3 months about losing her job and that she dreads going to work. She has difficulty getting to work on time and recently received a poor performance evaluation. She reluctantly tells Carol that it bothers her that she takes a lot of time to wash her hands before leaving for work, spending about 5 minutes in the restroom washing her hands upon arrival at work and during her breaks. She also has to wash her hands for 5 minutes once she arrives home and several times before going to bed. Sondra reports washing her hands at least 10 times a day to prevent "getting sick from germs."

Sondra acknowledges a fear of "going crazy" and states she thinks it may be odd that she washes so frequently and for so long. She wonders if the repeated hand washing is causing her rash, but also reports that she cannot keep herself from doing it. Sondra says the rash only is on her hands. She reports getting some temporary relief from her feelings of intense distress and worry when washing her hands during these 5-minute periods.

Carol observes that Sondra's symptoms include the following:

- Dermatitis, possibly related to frequent and excessive compulsory hand washings
- Recurrent and persistent thoughts about germs
- Anxiety that impedes her functioning

Carol brings Sondra to the attention of the clinic's APRN, who orders topical steroids and schedules a follow-up visit in 1 month. The APRN also follows up on Carol's request for a referral to a psychiatric–mental health nurse (APRN-PMH) to help Sondra with issues of stress. Carol encourages Sondra to get some additional support to help her deal with the anxiety associated with her excessive hand washing and offers to arrange an appointment for Sondra. She informs Sondra that the clinic has made referrals to this particular mental health nurse before and that patients have reported being very pleased with her approach and help. Sondra agrees to see the mental health nurse. Carol asks Sondra to sign a release-of-information form that will allow communication between the clinic and the mental health nurse.

APPLICATION

1. Address the five domains for Sondra:
   a. Biological
   b. Psychological
   c. Sociological
   d. Cultural
   e. Spiritual

2. In what ways do you think Sondra may be suffering? Why?

3. How you would prioritize Sondra's needs during this encounter, and why?

4. In what ways does Carol convey hope to Sondra? What might you have done differently to offer hope?

Introduction

Anxiety is a normal, universal, and generally helpful and healthy response to life circumstances that produce stress. For most people, responses associated with anxiety usually subside after the anxiety-producing situation resolves. For others, however, anxiety can be a cause or an outcome of distress within the individual.

Anxiety affects individual functioning; this impact tends to occur on a continuum. At one end of the continuum, positive impact occurs when anxiety promotes healthy responses, such as signaling the body to step away from a moving car. At the other end of the continuum, negative impact occurs when anxiety impedes healthy functioning or prevents a healthy response. The patient who becomes focused on germs to the point of being unable to leave his or her house exemplifies someone experiencing negative impact due to anxiety. When anxiety leads to disruption in normal functioning, it has become problematic. Anxiety that disrupts normal functioning may impair physical health. Quite often, the patient experiencing extreme anxiety seeks help for a medical issue, unaware that the physical symptoms have their origin in or are affected by anxiety. Such is the case of Sondra, a "representative patient" who appears in the critical thinking features presented with this chapter.

Nurses encounter anxiety in patients, family members, staff members, and themselves on a daily basis. It is important for nurses to be aware of their own anxiety and how it may affect others, as well as to know how to help direct their own and others' anxiety constructively when needed. Sometimes, acquiring information about a patient's condition may help alleviate both the nurse's and the patient's anxiety. At other times, the nurse may need additional help from a peer or supervisor to alleviate distress—both for the nurse and the patient. Becoming more comfortable with the experience of anxiety and what it represents for patients and others is key to promoting healing and alleviating suffering.

Theoretical Foundations

Anxiety is a subjective experience that an individual expresses within the biological, psychological, sociological, cultural, and spiritual domains (Table 13-1). An anxiety disorder may develop when anxiety causes an individual significant distress, anxiety is disproportionate to the stressor, and the anxiety is out of the individual's control. Prior to 2013, generalized anxiety disorder, panic disorder, agoraphobia, specific phobia, social phobia, obsessive–compulsive disorder (OCD), posttraumatic stress disorder (PTSD), and acute stress

Anxiety Responses by Domain   table 13-1

Domain	Responses
Biological	• Anorexia, nausea, vomiting • Blurred vision • Chest pain • Diaphoresis • Dilated pupils • Dyspnea or hyperventilation • Elevated pulse, blood pressure, respiration • Fidgeting • Headache • Hypervigilance • Pacing
Psychological	• Confusion • Crying • Decreased interest • Decreased productivity • Depression • Difficulty concentrating • Feelings of apprehension, helplessness, worthlessness • Focusing on past • Forgetfulness • Helplessness • Irritability • Lack of interest or apathy • Persistent worrying • Preoccupation with negatives • Withdrawal
Sociological	• Lacking kinship: feeling alone, without anyone to turn to for help or support • Lack of feeling comfortable and safe in patient's environment, with those around patient • Lacking similar interests or mutual understanding, trust, and agreement with others • Lacking a sense of relation to the whole of society, feelings of loneliness • Challenged in relation to resources
Cultural	• Lack of connectedness or sense of belonging to others from the same race, religion, or culture • Lack of connectedness to those with similar values, shared language or experiences • Lack of access to services due to language or other cultural barriers
Spiritual	• Feeling a lack of connectedness with God or Higher Power and/or with others of like-minded beliefs • Struggling with faith • Struggling with meaning and purpose • Expressing feelings of guilt related to symptoms

disorder were grouped together by symptom similarity—mainly, anxiety—and classified as Anxiety Disorders. Advances in neuroscience, brain imaging, and genetics over the past two decades are reflected in the *Diagnostic and Statistical Manual of Mental Disorders*, 5th edition (DSM-5), in which these disorders are further differentiated into three separate classifications, including Anxiety Disorders, Obsessive–Compulsive and Related Disorders, and Trauma- and Stressor-Related Disorders (American Psychiatric Association, 2013). The scope of this chapter covers the shared theme of anxiety that is observed across these disorders and the ways in which nurses can promote health and healing in individuals who experience them.

Biological Domain

Anxiety and depression (an altered mood state characterized by feelings of sadness and worthlessness, decreased interest in activities,

and diminished concentration) are estimated to have heritability rates between 30% and 40%; they share a common genetic background and tend to include negative emotions of fear, sadness, and anger (Sprangers et al., 2010). Interactions between genes and the environment have been found to play a role in critical developmental phases of neural circuits that regulate emotions and affect the individual's resiliency or propensity toward stress-related illness (Gillespie, Phifer, Bradley, & Ressler, 2009).

Factors affecting mental illnesses are thought to include a combination of genetic, environmental, psychological, and developmental influences. Studies of twins have revealed that there is a genetic role in the development of several disorders presented in this chapter. For example, although trauma clearly is the trigger for the development of PTSD, genetic studies may make clear why some individuals who have been exposed to trauma develop PTSD

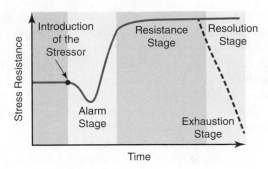

13-1   General Adaptation Syndrome.

symptoms while others do not (National Institute of Mental Health, 2008).

Historical Perspective

Cannon (1939) and Selye (1950) studied responses of animals to stress. Cannon's work involved exploration of the concept of homeostasis, whereas Selye's work resulted in the General Adaptation Syndrome (Figure 13-1). Cannon observed that an animal's sympathetic system combines with the adrenaline hormone to prepare the animal for an emergency response of "fight or flight." The sympathicoadrenal system then changes the blood supply, sugar availability, and the blood's clotting capacity to provide a rush of energy (Cannon, 1915; Brown & Fee, 2002).

Holmes and Rahe (1967) viewed stressors as distinct, measurable events. They developed the Holmes and Rahe Social Readjustment Rating Scale to help predict an individual's risk for becoming ill within 6 months due to an accumulation of positive and/or negative life changes or events. The Holmes and Rahe Scale is discussed in greater detail on page 245.

Lazarus and Folkman (1984) examined how individuals manage an imbalance between demands and resources. They considered stress a transaction through which individuals could manage to cope with stressors.

The normal physiological response of the body to stress and anxiety involves a heightened response in which catecholamine levels become elevated. It is thought that pathologic anxiety results from disturbances in the cerebral cortex, particularly the limbic system (Tefera, Shah, & Hsu, 2012).

Although it was once thought that stress caused only physical and functional damage to an individual, today the more widely held belief is that the impact of stress is mediated by individual perceptions and understanding of what the stress represents; in some cases, the stress response can be beneficial for protection and adaptation (Leonard & Myint, 2009).

General Adaptation Syndrome

Selye (1956) examined an individual's psychophysiological responses to stress with the development of the **General Adaptation Syndrome** (GAS). He described a generalized response with three levels (Table 13-2):

1. *Alarm reaction:* In this acute phase, the body recognizes that there is an internal or external stressor affecting its physiological status. The body reacts the same whether the threat is real or perceived. The sympathetic system becomes aroused, and the body releases cortisol, adrenaline, and other chemicals. These chemicals signal the autonomic nervous system, which releases epinephrine in an attempt to mobilize the body and may decrease the body's immune response.

2. *Stage of resistance:* In this stage, the body continues to defend itself by the fight-or-flight mechanism and tries to repair any damage suffered (for example, in the case of starvation, the body may slow down to conserve energy and use whatever nutrients are available to prevent death) or adapt to the stressor (for instance, a reduced desire for activity). During this stage, the body may function and adapt at lower-than-optimal levels. If the body adapts, anxiety begins to resolve and the individual does not enter the third stage. If the body does not adapt, it enters the third stage.

3. *Stage of exhaustion:* The body experiences a total expenditure of energy at this level. Physical and psychological manifestations may occur at this level (for example, migraine headaches or decompensation resulting in delusions or hallucinations). The body is no longer able to adapt and begins to fail; vital systems become compromised (for example, elevated blood pressure, infection, or stroke). Without relief or resolution of the stressor, death may occur (from, for instance, cardiac arrest or renal failure).

Psychoneuroimmunology

Psychoneuroimmunology (PNI) involves the interaction among the nervous, immune, and endocrine systems and the ways in

General Adaptation Syndrome

table 13-2

Stages	Body's Internal Response	Body's External Response
Alarm reaction	• Sympathetic system aroused. • Release of cortisol, adrenaline, and other chemicals. • Signal to autonomic system. • Release of epinephrine.	• Body mobilized.
Stage of resistance	• Body continues with process in attempt to adapt. • Flight-or-fight mechanisms in action.	• Body adapting and functioning at lower than optimal level. • If body able to adapt, then process resolves at this stage; if not, individual goes to next stage.
Stage of exhaustion	• Body undergoes total expenditure of energy and is no longer able to adapt or function adequately. • Vital systems begin to shut down. • Illness or even death may result.	• Emotional disorders (e.g., migraine headaches, hallucinations) may develop. • Death may occur.

which those systems affect behavior. It is well known that stress increases susceptibility to physical illness. Chronic stress may set off changes within the hypothalamic–pituitary–adrenal (HPA) system and serve as a trigger for anxiety and depression (Leonard & Myint, 2009).

Cytokines are proteins released by immune cells. Cytokines are "signal" molecules that transmit information from the immune system to the endocrine and nervous systems and also within the immune system. Cytokines activate specific receptors on immune, endocrine, or neural cells and directly influence brain function. They can modulate their own function or the function of other types of cells. They influence brain function or "talk" to the brain by activating the hypothalamus and the HPA axis (Leonard & Myint, 2009).

Levels of Anxiety

Even though anxiety is important for survival, it can become so challenging and incapacitating that it can prevent an individual from meeting basic needs. Hildegard Peplau (1963) identified four levels of anxiety: mild, moderate, severe, and panic. Peplau asserted that it is important for nurses to recognize different symptoms within these different levels in order to help patients experiencing anxiety (Figure 13-2). She also examined how anxiety may prevent

the patient from being able to meet basic needs. The levels of anxiety and accompanying symptoms are illustrated in Table 13-3.

In addition to being classified by levels of severity, anxiety may be categorized as normal, acute, or chronic. *Normal anxiety* helps individuals be more alert and think more clearly. Normal anxiety usually occurs during activities such as preparing for an exam or sports event and when handling daily changes and challenges. In these situations, anxiety promotes positive behaviors.

Acute anxiety is a temporary condition in which an individual experiences heightened feelings of apprehension, tension, nervousness, or worry. Acute anxiety also is known as *state anxiety*. State anxiety is a situational anxiety: The individual becomes anxious in response to a particular situation.

Chronic anxiety refers to a more general and long-lasting condition or personality characteristic that has been part of the individual's personality makeup over time. Chronic anxiety also is called *trait anxiety*. Individuals with trait anxiety usually respond to state anxiety situations at a higher level of anxiety and in a more debilitating manner than those without trait anxiety. The patient with chronic anxiety has difficulty performing at work and enjoying relationships. Because trait anxiety can compromise the immune system, physical symptoms may develop. It is important to determine

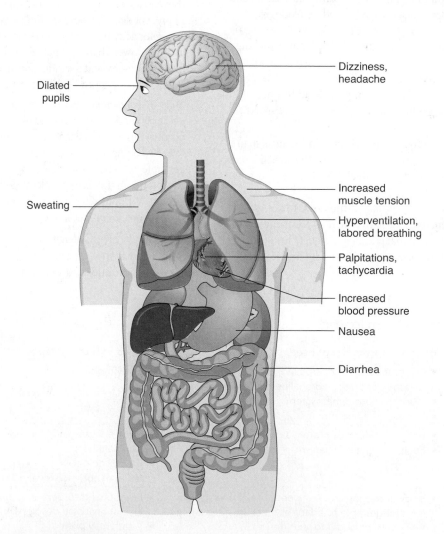

13-2 Selected somatic manifestations of anxiety.

Levels of Anxiety

table 13-3

Anxiety Level	Symptoms
Mild +1	• Restlessness • Irritability • Increased motivation
Moderate +2	Increased • Discomfort • Heart rate • Muscular tension • Perspiration • Respiratory rate • Restlessness • Rate of speech
Severe +3	• Desire to relieve anxiety • Dizziness • Diarrhea • Feelings of dread • Headaches • Hyperventilation • Insomnia • Nausea • Palpitations, tachycardia • Trembling • Urinary frequency • Total focus on self
Panic +4	• Delusions and hallucinations • Diaphoresis • Dilated pupils • Labored breathing • Muscular incoordination, immobility, or purposeless hyperactivity • Palpitations • Sense of impending doom • Sleeplessness • Trembling • Unusual behaviors (shouting, screaming, running about, clinging) • Withdrawal into self

whether anxiety or some other source is the cause for any symptoms that occur. For example, someone experiencing state anxiety may become anxious right before giving a presentation to strangers, but the anxiety will dissipate once the presentation is over. The individual with chronic anxiety, however, may feel anxious most of the time and become ill or incapacitated when it is time to participate in such a presentation.

Psychological Domain

Freud's introduction of the term *anxiety neurosis* dispelled the idea that anxiety was related only to physiological conditions and expanded understanding in this area to include psychological conditions as a basis for anxiety (Freud, 1963). Research later demonstrated a link between emotional factors and physical responses in relation to areas such as the immune and nervous systems, and changed earlier thinking that anxiety originated from either physiological or psychological causes solely (Segerstrom & Miller, 2004). Today, researchers continue to explore the interconnectedness of the spirit with body and mind (Tan, Chen, Wu, & Chen, 2013; Stallwood & Stoll, 1975).

Holmes and Rahe Readjustment Scale

Worry plays a key role in anxiety disorders and their associated psychological distress. There is much debate as to whether normal worry and pathologic worry are distinguishable types of worry or at different ends of a continuum of worry (Olatunji, Broman-Fulks, Bergman, Green, & Zlomke, 2010). Worry and stress may arise from a variety of stressors—positive or negative—as depicted in the Holmes and Rahe Social Readjustment Rating Scale (Holmes & Rahe, 1967) which was developed to help predict potential risk for health changes. The scale is based on the amount of stress experienced by an individual within the previous year. It ranks 43 life change events, including both positive and negative experiences, in descending order. Events that are accompanied by serious changes or consequences, such as death of a close family member or a jail sentence, rank highly, with death of a spouse being identified as the single event with the greatest potential for causing health changes. More benign activities, such as changing recreation activities and vacations, rank lower as they are less likely to result in changes to individual health (Holmes & Rahe, 1967). Scores are tallied and projections given within three categories that indicate an individual's risk for a health change within the near future.

Defense Mechanisms

Anna Freud (1946) explored the idea of **defense mechanisms** as strategies used by the individual when experiencing a threat to the ego that the ego cannot handle through regular problem-solving strategies. Defense mechanisms are listed in Table 13-4. They involve different types of unconscious reactions that the ego uses to protect the conscious mind from threatening feelings and perceptions. Defense mechanisms help an individual cope with reality, maintain

Defense Mechanisms

table 13-4

Defense Mechanism	Definition	Example
Altruism	Emotional conflicts and stressors dealt with by performing helpful service to others that results in satisfaction and pleasure	Serving as a volunteer to a disaster area.
Compensation	Making up for a perceived or real inability by focusing on another area and becoming proficient (may be conscious or unconscious)	A 16-year-old boy is not good at sports. He strives to get the top grades in his class and become a member of his school's honor society.
Conversion	Transfer of a mental conflict into a physical symptom	A concert pianist develops paralysis of his right hand prior to performing his first concert.
Denial	Avoiding, ignoring, or rejecting a real situation and the feelings associated with it	A man tells his wife that he wants a divorce. The wife responds by saying all couples have difficulties and that she is sure he will feel differently tomorrow.
Displacement	Transfer of emotions from one person or object onto another less threatening and more neutral person or object (sometimes called the "scape-goat" defense mechanism)	The staff nurse is yelled at by the unit supervisor at work. When she gets home, the nurse yells at her 12-year-old son for no apparent reason.
Humor	Emphasizing ironic or amusing aspects of a conflict or stressor	A nurse with cold hands comments, "Cold hands but a warm heart" before taking a patient's pulse.
Identification	Process whereby an individual takes on thoughts, mannerisms, or tastes of another individual whom the individual admires	A college student decides to become a physical therapist after spending 3 months in physical therapy due to a knee injury.
Intellectualization	Excessive reasoning or logic to transfer disturbing feelings into the intellectual sphere	A student tells her parents that no one could have done better than she did on the course exam, because the exam material was not covered well enough, and the course instructor is not a very good teacher.
Introjection	Attributing to oneself the qualities of another—intense identification in which the qualities are incorporated into the individual's own ego structure	A patient states he is "General Napoleon" and walks around the unit with his right hand over his heart.
Isolation	Separating ideas, thoughts, and actions from feelings associated with them	A nurse stops on the highway to assist in an accident. The victim's arm has been severed from the body. The nurse does not focus on feelings about the situation but focuses on applying pressure to the wound site, calling for help, and comforting the victim.
Projection	Unconsciously attributing one's thoughts or impulses to another person	Roommate A gets angry at Roommate B for being angry and not listening, when it is actually Roommate A who is angry and has not been listening.
Rationalization	Justifying illogical ideas, actions, or feelings by using acceptable explanations (most common defense mechanism—a form of self-deception)	The college student did not do well on her exam. She calls home and tells her parents that she did not get enough sleep the night before the exam.
Reaction formation	Developing the opposite behavior or emotion to unacceptable feelings or behaviors	A student does not like the teacher or the course being taught by the teacher. The student brings the teacher articles related to the course and comments how much he likes the teacher and her course.

(continued)

Defense Mechanism	Definition	Example
Repression	The *unconscious* exclusion of unwanted experiences, ideas, emotions; repression is a first line of psychological defense against anxiety	A 7-year-old girl displays signs of sexual abuse. Although her family is suspicious of who might have abused her and when, the girl cannot recall anything about the recent visit she had with the potential abuser.
Sublimation	The unconscious substituting of acceptable behaviors for unacceptable behaviors	An 18-year-old male who felt inadequate when compared to his brothers and was bullied in school joins the Marines.
Suppression	The *conscious* denial of a disturbing situation or feeling (Think of the individual as consciously "sitting on" the feelings as compared to repression, in which the individual is not aware.)	One student asks another if he is worried about the exam in their class tomorrow. The student replies, "I'd rather not think about that right now."
Undoing	Making up for an intolerable act or experience to lessen or alleviate feelings of guilt	After being caught by his mother stealing money out of her purse, the 10-year-old boy washes his hands excessively.

self-image, provide protection from anxiety, guard against social sanctions, and provide refuge from a situation with which one cannot cope (Hall, 1954).

Healthy individuals use different defense mechanisms for problem solving. For example, when used temporarily, such as during the grieving process, denial can be a healthy means of protecting an individual who is adapting to a loss. However, when the use of defense mechanisms results in behavior that has a negative impact on physical and/or mental health, those mechanisms are considered unhealthy or pathological. For example, a patient who denies that smoking is harmful and continues to smoke in spite of a positive X-ray for a lung tumor is using denial in a pathological manner.

Sociological Domain

The interplay between genetic and environmental factors is complex. The basis of sociological support lies in one's culture, kinship, and resources. Thus, sociological and cultural domains often overlap. Lack of social connections and a sense of a more threatening environment increases an individual's risk for higher anxiety levels; likewise, disenfranchised populations tend to have higher levels of anxiety (University of Maryland Medical Center, 2013).

For the patient experiencing an anxiety disorder, sociological considerations can affect patient function, hope, and healing. For example, family relationships may play an important role in the patient's ability to participate in and complete treatment. In the case study presented with this chapter, Sondra feels more comfortable disclosing the truth of her anxiety to her mother and grandmother, but decides not to tell her father. Fortunately, Sondra's mother and grandmother support her decision to get help. Nurses working with patients with anxiety disorders must be able to assess the level of family function, the nature of family relationships, and other sociological resources that can have an impact on patient recovery, such as financial resources and access to care. Nurses must also be prepared to help patients with limited resources determine how to make the most of those resources and find new resources and support systems.

Cultural Domain

It is essential to consider cultural issues when assessing a patient experiencing anxiety. Culture plays a key role in how an individual perceives symptoms, prescribes meaning to his or her experience, and shapes the response to treatment, including coping styles and available support systems. The DSM-5 recognizes the diagnostic importance of cultural competence and includes tools for in-depth cultural assessment using cultural formulations (Aggarwal, 2012). Some experts suggest that clinicians use the cultural formulation and sociocultural approach to every diagnostic interview, not only those involving migrants or racial/ethnic minorities (Alarcon et al., 2009). The DSM-5 also includes a detailed discussion of culture-bound syndromes, conditions experienced by specific cultural groups (Chapter 5).

Current understanding of cultural models in relation to somatic syndromes suggests that specific varieties of panic disorder, hypochondriacal worry, and medically unexplained symptoms are related to particular cultures (Kirmayer & Sartorius, 2007).

Culture affects how both families and providers interpret the etiology and origin of anxiety: Some may focus on spiritual, others on physical, and others on social problems (Harmon, Langley, & Ginsburg, 2006). Different beliefs may influence how likely it will be that an individual will adhere to treatment services and how positive treatment outcomes will be (Yeh, Hough, McCabe, Lau, & Garland, 2004). It is critical to treatment that nurses and other clinicians acknowledge and respect client beliefs in the context of symptomatology, as well as being aware of the impact of their own belief systems on the provision of patient care.

Regardless of the patient's cultural background, clarifying the patient's stressors and coping resources is essential. What is stressful in one culture may not be so for another culture. Within a single culture, stressors, coping resources, and perceptions of what is comforting may vary among individual patients. For example, nurses working with patients experiencing anxiety must determine patient history in relation to touch; some patients with histories of physical or sexual abuse may react negatively to touch. By clarifying with patients their level of comfort with touch and by asking permission to touch patients, nurses will avoid inadvertently increasing patient anxiety.

Spiritual Domain

Increasingly, health care providers are recognizing that positive clinical outcomes may not necessarily result in a positive experience for patients. A major academic medical center developed a paradigm of "healing enhancement" within the inpatient setting after recognizing the need to address the patient's total experience related to body, mind, and spirit. The center began offering integrated therapies—such as music therapy, guided imagery, and stress education classes—to reduce patient pain, anxiety, and tension (Curlin et al., 2007). Patients who find comfort in spiritual practices may find that these practices reduce anxiety during times of acute stress. A spiritual assessment, particularly in hospital and inpatient settings, may help nurses facilitate patients' spiritual practices during times of stress and anxiety (Chapter 6).

Pause and Reflect

1. *What implications for nursing are suggested by the role genetics plays in anxiety?*
2. *Referring to Table 13-1, what anxiety responses do you think would have the greatest impact on a patient's ability to function? Why?*
3. *What defense mechanisms do you use when you feel anxious? To what extent are these healthy or unhealthy?*

ANXIETY AND TRAUMA-RELATED DISORDERS

When anxiety rises beyond a mild level, patients often experience distress and suffering. The distress and suffering associated with anxiety can be as painful as physical distress and suffering due to disease or illness. Individuals who are unable to resolve feelings and symptoms of anxiety may develop one of the disorders recognized in the DSM-5 (APA, 2013). This chapter follows the DSM-5 meta-structure with three related but distinct groupings of disorders, including Anxiety Disorders, Obsessive–Compulsive and Related Disorders, and Trauma- and Stressor-Related Disorders (Table 13-5). Although there is overlap among disorders in terms of symptoms, differences regarding core features and underlying vulnerabilities have led to new groupings. **Anxiety disorders** are characterized by psychological (such as fear and anxiety) and somatic (such as nausea or headache) manifestations of anxiety (Stein et al., 2010a). Although anxiety is common in obsessive–compulsive and related disorders, these disorders are more predominantly characterized by "obsessions and compulsive rituals or repetitive, motoric behaviors that resemble compulsions" (Stein et al., 2010a, pp. 496–497). Furthermore, studies using brain imaging have found distinct neurocircuits involved in OCD, including hyperactivity within the orbitofrontal cortex, anterior cingulate cortex, and caudate nucleus. These areas are not implicated in other anxiety disorders (Stein et al., 2010a). Similarly, PTSD, which was previously regarded as an anxiety disorder, now belongs to the cluster of trauma- and stressor-related disorders. This grouping includes disorders precipitated by a traumatic or stressful event (Friedman, Resick, Bryant, & Brewin, 2011).

DSM-5 Overview of Disorders of Anxiety, Stress, and Trauma	table 13-5
Anxiety disorders	• Separation anxiety • Selective mutism • Specific phobia • Social anxiety disorder • Panic disorder • Panic attack • Agoraphobia • Generalized anxiety disorder • Substance-induced anxiety disorder • Anxiety disorder due to medical condition
Obsessive–compulsive and related disorders	• Obsessive–compulsive disorder • Body dysmorphic disorder • Hoarding disorder • Trichotillomania • Excoriation (skin picking disorder) • Substance—medication induced • Obsessive-compulsive disorder due to another medical condition
Trauma-and stressor-related disorders	• Reactive attachment disorder • Disinhibited social engagement disorder • Posttraumatic stress disorder • Acute stress disorder • Adjustment disorder

Data from the Diagnostic and Statistical Manual of Mental Disorders, Fifth Edition, (Copyright 2013). American Psychiatric Association.

Anxiety Disorders

Anxiety disorders are among the most common disorders of mental health; nurses will encounter patients with anxiety disorders in every clinical setting. As stated earlier, patients may initially present with a somatic complaint and be unaware that their discomfort is related to anxiety. Because of these factors, nurses working in all settings must be able to recognize and respond to patient anxiety.

Prevalence

Approximately 15% to 20% of adults within the United States will experience at least one anxiety disorder in their lifetime. With a median age of onset of 11 years, anxiety disorders are one of the earliest-appearing forms of psychopathology (Mohr & Schneider, 2013). Risk factors for anxiety include female gender, problems in school, early separation from a parent, certain perinatal risk factors, parental history of a mental disorder, and poor financial situation and income (Bourne, 2010; Mynatt & Cunningham, 2007). Many individuals diagnosed with an anxiety disorder often have an additional anxiety disorder diagnosis. Anxiety is a clinical feature or co-morbid condition with many psychiatric disorders, especially depression and substance abuse disorders (Kessler, Ruscio, Shear, & Wittchen, 2010). For example, individuals diagnosed with a depressive disorder have a current or lifetime co-morbid anxiety disorder at rates of 67% and 75%, respectively (Lamers et al., 2011).

Separation Anxiety Disorder

Separation anxiety disorder is characterized by excessive fear or anxiety that occurs related to separation from home or from a loved one or caregiver. Individuals with separation anxiety display symptoms and emotions that are developmentally inappropriate and significant, and include a combination of symptoms ranging from somatic symptoms to refusal to participate in normal activities (see DSM-5 Diagnostic Criteria for Separation Anxiety Disorder). As with all psychiatric disorders, the symptoms must persist over time—typically, 4 or more weeks in children and adolescents and at least 6 months for adults (APA, 2013).

Selective Mutism

Selective mutism is characterized by the refusal or withholding of speech in situations in which speech is expected (e.g., school), despite speaking in other situations. The disturbance interferes with educational or occupational achievement or with social communication and is present for at least 1 month (not including the first month of school). The failure to speak is not due to a lack of knowledge or comfort with the spoken language itself (APA, 2013; Scott & Beidel, 2011). Now classified as anxiety disorders, both separation anxiety disorder and selective mutism were previously included among disorders of childhood and adolescents.

Specific Phobia

With specific **phobia**, the individual has a marked fear or anxiety about a specific object or situation; either direct exposure to a stressor or the anticipation of exposure almost always triggers the anxiety response. Degree and context of impairment are relevant: The fear must be excessive in the context of the patient's culture, be out of proportion to the actual danger posed, and cause the patient significant impairment or distress for a period of at least 6 months. Impairment or distress is considered significant in that the individual avoids the object or situation or endures exposure with excessive fear or anxiety. Children may express their distress by crying, throwing tantrums, freezing, or exhibiting clinging behaviors.

Co-morbidity among different types of phobias is common, and 75.8% of individuals with specific phobia are likely to have multiple phobias during their lifetime (LeBeau et al., 2010). Specific phobia co-occurs with other disorders at a rate of approximately 50% to 80%. In general, specific phobia occurs in twice as many women as men, although gender rates differ across phobia specifiers

---

Diagnostic Criteria for Separation Anxiety Disorder   DSM-5

A. Developmentally inappropriate and excessive fear or anxiety concerning separation from those to whom the individual is attached, as evidenced by at least three of the following:
   1. Recurrent excessive distress when anticipating or experiencing separation from home or from major attachment figures.
   2. Persistent and excessive worry about losing major attachment figures or about possible harm to them, such as illness, injury, disasters, or death.
   3. Persistent and excessive worry about experiencing an untoward event (e.g., getting lost, being kidnapped, having an accident, becoming ill) that causes separation from a major attachment figure.
   4. Persistent reluctance or refusal to go out, away from home, to school, to work, or elsewhere because of fear or separation.
   5. Persistent and excessive fear of or reluctance about being alone or without major attachment figures at home or in other settings.
   6. Persistent reluctance or refusal to sleep away from home or to go to sleep without being near a major attachment figure.
   7. Repeated nightmares involving the theme of separation.
   8. Repeated complaints of physical symptoms (e.g., headaches, stomachaches, nausea, vomiting) when separation from major attachment figures occurs or is anticipated.
B. The fear, anxiety, or avoidance is persistent, lasting at least 4 weeks in children and adolescents and typically 6 months or more in adults.
C. The disturbance causes clinically significant distress or impairment in social, academic, occupational, or other important areas of functioning.
D. The disturbance is not better explained by another mental disorder, such as refusing to leave home because of excessive resistance to change in autism spectrum disorder; delusions or hallucinations concerning separation in psychotic disorders; refusal to go outside without a trusted companion in agoraphobia; worries about ill health or other harm befalling significant others in generalized anxiety disorder, or concerns about having an illness in illness anxiety disorder.

Source: Reprinted with permission from the *Diagnostic and Statistical Manual of Mental Disorders,* Fifth Edition, (Copyright 2013). American Psychiatric Association.

Phobia Specifiers

table 13-6

Subtype	Examples
Animal Type	Fear prompted by animal or insects. Usual onset in childhood.
Natural Environment Type	Fear prompted by elements in the environment, such as storms, heights, or water. Usual onset in childhood.
Blood–Injection–Injury Type	Fear prompted by seeing blood or an injury or receiving injection or other invasive procedure. Familial and often results in vasovagal response.
Situational Type	Fear prompted by specific situation including: public transportation, tunnels, bridges, elevators, flying, driving, or enclosed places. Two peaks of onset: childhood and mid-20s.
Other Type	Fear prompted by other stimuli, such as fear of choking vomiting; in children, fear of loud sounds or costumed characters falls within this subtype.

Based on the *Diagnostic and Statistical Manual of Mental Disorders*, Fifth Edition, (Copyright 2013). American Psychiatric Association; LeBeau, R. T., Glenn, D., Liao, B., Wittchen, H.-U., Beesdo-Baum, K., Ollendick, T., & Craske, M. G. (2010). Specific phobia: A review of DSM-IV specific phobia and preliminary recommendations for DSM-V. *Depression and Anxiety, 27*(2), 148–167; Specific Phobias. (2014). Available at http://www.webmd.com/anxiety-panic/specific-phobias

(LeBeau et al., 2010). There is an increased risk in families who have members with specific phobias (APA, 2013; LeBeau, et al., 2010). Phobias usually are classified according to specifiers (Table 13-6).

Social Anxiety Disorder

In social anxiety disorder, formally known as *social phobia*, the patient has marked fear or anxiety about social situations in which there is a potential for embarrassment or scrutiny by others. Types of social situations that trigger the anxiety involve one or more of the following: interaction, observation, or performance (Bogels et al., 2010). In community studies, social phobia is more common in women than in men, but it is equally distributed in clinical studies.

Cultural differences may occur in relation to being concerned about offending others. For example, in Japan and Korea, distress may arise if an individual blushes, makes eye contact, or becomes aware of offending others by having body odor (Lewis-Fernandez et al., 2010). There is a higher rate of social phobia among individuals having relatives with the disorder (Bogels et al., 2010). The onset of social phobia usually is around 13 years of age (Kessler, Berglund, Demler, Jin, & Walters, 2005).

Panic Disorder

Panic disorder generally occurs between adolescence and the mid-30s, although it can begin earlier or later. Panic disorder is characterized by recurrent, unexpected panic attacks (Box 13-1) followed with at least one month of one or both of the following:

- Persistent concern about having additional panic attacks or their consequences
- Significant change in behavior related to the attacks (APA, 2013; Craske et al., 2010)

The course of panic disorder varies with some having intermittent episodes and others experiencing continuous symptoms.

Agoraphobia

Patients with **agoraphobia** have a marked fear or anxiety about situations in which escape could be difficult or help not immediately

Panic Attacks

box 13-1

Panic attacks are not classified as a disorder but may occur with a number of anxiety disorders, other mental disorders (mood and substance-related), and general medical conditions. Panic attacks last for a discrete period of time and involve a period of intense fear or discomfort in which the individual senses impending doom. They typically involve at least four of the following symptoms:

- Palpitations, pounding heart, or accelerated heart rate
- Sweating
- Trembling or shaking
- Shortness of breath
- Feeling of choking

- Chest pain or discomfort
- Feeling dizzy, unsteady, lightheaded, or faint
- Chills or hot flashes
- Nausea or abdominal cramping
- Paresthesia (numbness or tingling)
- Derealization (feelings of unreality) or depersonalization (being detached from oneself)
- Fear of loss of control, going crazy
- Fear of dying

When associated with a psychiatric disorder, panic attacks signal greater symptom severity and risk for suicidality.

Based on Craske, M. G., Kircanski, K., Epstein, A., Wittchen, H.-U., Pine, D. S., Lewis-Fernández, R., & Hinton, D. (2010). Panic disorder: a review of DSM-IV panic disorder and proposals for DSM-V. *Depression and Anxiety, 27*(2), 93–112; Mayo Clinic. (2012). Panic attacks and panic disorder: Symptoms. Available at http://www.mayoclinic.com/health/panic-attacks/DS00338/DSECTION=symptoms; Medline Plus. (2013). Panic disorder with agoraphobia. Available at http://www.nlm.nih.gov/medlineplus/ency/article/000923.htm

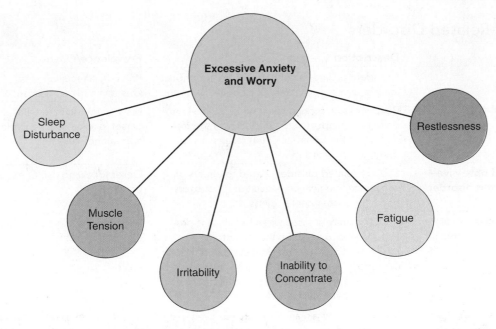

13-3 Key symptoms of generalized anxiety disorder.

accessible, leading to avoidance or enduring with distress. Typically, agoraphobia occurs when an individual experiences difficulty within two or more of these areas (APA, 2013; Wittchen, Gloster, Beesdo-Baum, Fava, & Craske, 2010):

1. Public transportation
2. Open spaces
3. Shops, theaters, or cinemas
4. Standing in line or being in a crowd
5. Being outside the home alone in other situations

The median age of onset for agoraphobia is 20 years of age (Kessler, Berglund, Demler, Jin, & Walters, 2005). Agoraphobia is seen in approximately twice as many females as males, with a 1-year prevalence rate of about 5% (National Institute of Mental Health, 2010).

Generalized Anxiety Disorder

Generalized anxiety disorder (GAD) is characterized by symptoms of excessive anxiety and worry about two or more domains of activities or events (e.g., family, health, finances, school, or work) that occur more days than not during a period of at least 3 months. The anxiety and worry are associated with restlessness, feeling on edge, and/or muscle tension and are not related to another psychiatric disorder (Figure 13-3). Patients with GAD report significant distress or impaired functioning in social, occupational, or other areas. One or more of the following behaviors must be present (Andrews, et al., 2010):

- Marked avoidance of activities or events with possible negative outcomes
- Marked time and effort preparing for activities or events with possible negative outcomes
- Marked procrastination in behavior or decision making due to worries
- Repeatedly seeking reassurance due to worries

Although GAD can occur at any point in the life span, GAD is rarely seen in children and has a median onset of around 30 years of age, with a lifetime risk of 9.0%. The prevalence of GAD among women is almost double compared with that among men (APA, 2013).

Other Types of Anxiety Disorders

With *substance-induced anxiety disorder*, patient history, diagnostic testing, and/or physical assessment indicate that anxiety symptoms result from the physiological effects of a substance, such as medication or an illicit drug, or from toxin exposure (APA, 2013).

Another category, *anxiety disorder due to another medical condition*, may be used when the health care provider determines that another medical condition is directly related to anxiety and distress resulting in significant impairment for the patient. The provider must specify whether the disorder is accompanied by generalized anxiety or panic attacks (APA, 2013). Medical conditions that increase the risk for panic disorder include migraines, obstructive sleep apnea, mitral valve prolapse, irritable bowel syndrome, chronic fatigue syndrome, and premenstrual syndrome (University of Maryland Medical Center, 2013).

Other specified anxiety disorder may be used when symptoms of anxiety impair functioning and cause marked distress but do not meet the criteria for any other specific disorder (APA, 2013).

Obsessive–Compulsive and Related Disorders

This group of disorders is a new category first introduced in the DSM-5 in 2013 (APA, 2013). Prior to the publication of the DSM-5, obsessive–compulsive disorder was included with the anxiety disorders; however, researchers have found distinct neural circuits that differentiate obsessive–compulsive disorder from the other anxiety disorders (Radua, van den Heuvel, Surguladze, & Mataix-Cols, 2010). Obsessive–compulsive disorder, body dysmorphic disorder, and hoarding disorder are described in this section. Other related disorders are outlined in Table 13-7.

Other OCD-Related Disorders

table 13-7

Disorder	Description	Prevalence/Onset
Trichotillomania	Recurrent pulling out of hair, despite attempts to stop or decrease the frequency of the behavior.	Primarily affects females. Onset in early adolescence.
Skin picking disorder (excoriation)	Recurrent skin picking resulting in skin lesions, despite attempts to stop or decrease the frequency of the behavior. Often results in tissue damage and scarring.	More common in females. Onset in adolescence, typically coinciding with appearance of acne.
Substance-induced obsessive–compulsive or related disorder	OCD or related disorder related to effects of substance (medication or illicit drug) or toxin based on assessment findings.	Onset following use or exposure to substance or toxin.
Obsessive–compulsive or related disorder due to other medical condition	Category may be used when health care provider is able to establish that symptoms are attributed to another medical condition. Health care provider must specify which symptoms are present—e.g., appearance preoccupation, hoarding, hair pulling.	Basis for onset in a medical condition, so age of onset varies.
Obsessive–compulsive or related disorder not otherwise specified	May be used when an individual has prominent symptoms characteristic of the category but does not meet the criteria for being diagnosed with a specific disorder.	Onset has not been determined, but given that most of the disorders in this category have an onset in adolescence, symptoms are likely to appear during that time.

Based on the *Diagnostic and Statistical Manual of Mental Disorders,* Fifth Edition, (Copyright 2013). American Psychiatric Association; Mayo Clinic. (2011). Trichotillomania: Symptoms. Available at http://www.mayoclinic.com/health/trichotillomania/DS00895/DSECTION=symptoms; Stein, D. J., Grant, J. E., Franklin, M. E., Keuthen, N., Lochner, C., Singer, H. S., & Woods, D. W. (2010b). Trichotillomania (hair pulling disorder), skin picking disorder, and stereotypic movement disorder: Toward DSM-V. *Depression and Anxiety, 27*(6), 611–626; Trichotillomania Learning Center. (2012). Skin Picking: Signs and Symptoms. Available at http://www.trich.org/about/skin-signs-symptoms.html

Prevalence

The lifetime prevalence of OCD is 2.3% (Ruscio, Stein, Chiu, & Kessler, 2010). The estimated prevalence of hoarding disorder is between 2% and 5% of the population (Mataix-Cols et al., 2010). Statistics on lifetime prevalence of skin picking disorder range from 2% to 5.4% (Grant & Odlaug, 2009).

Obsessive–Compulsive Disorder

The patient with **obsessive–compulsive disorder** (OCD) has recurring obsessions or compulsions that are so persistent that they take up an unreasonable amount of time (for example, more than 1 hour each day) or cause severe distress or impairment (Table 13-8). **Obsessions** are recurrent and persistent thoughts, urges, or images that cause significant anxiety or distress. Themes of obsessions may include contamination, repeated doubts, the need for things to be in a particular order, aggressive or unpleasant impulses, and sexual imagery. In OCD, the individual attempts to ignore or suppress these obsessions or to neutralize them by engaging in a compulsion. **Compulsions** are repetitive behaviors (such as hand washing or ordering) or mental acts (for example, counting or repeating words) that the individual feels driven to perform in response to an obsession or according to rules that must be applied rigidly. Compulsions help lower the individual's anxiety or distress; however, they are either excessive or not connected in a realistic way with the distress and may result in other challenges for the individual, such as interrupting work flow or creating conflict with family members or colleagues. Individuals with OCD have varying levels of insight into their OCD beliefs, ranging from good/fair to poor or absent (APA, 2013; Leckman et al., 2010).

The intrusive nature of obsessions is considered to be **ego dystonic**, because the individual has an uncomfortable sense of self. Individuals who are comfortable with their sense of self in relation to how they perceive their world are referred to as being **ego syntonic**, whether or not they are deemed mentally healthy or mentally unhealthy by society.

OCD usually begins in adolescence or early adulthood with a mean age of onset of 19.5 years, although it may begin in childhood. Although the course of OCD varies over time, stress may exacerbate symptoms. Males and females with adult-onset OCD experience it in equal rates. In childhood onset, males tend to have a higher rate than females (Ruscio et al., 2010).

Body Dysmorphic Disorder

In **body dysmorphic disorder** (BDD), patients engage in repetitive behaviors (for example, mirror checking, excessive grooming, or reassurance seeking) or mental acts (such as comparing their appearance with that of others) in response to preoccupation with perceived deficits or flaws in physical appearance that are not observable or appear slight to others. Diagnostic criteria include muscle dysmorphia, the belief that one's body build is too small or insufficiently muscular (Phillips et al., 2010). As with OCD, individuals with this disorder have varying levels of insight regarding the extent to which they are affected by the disorder.

Hoarding Disorder

Hoarding disorder is characterized by continued difficulty discarding or parting with possessions due to a perceived need to save the items and distress associated with discarding them. The hoarding behavior results in accummulation of possessions that fill active living areas to the point that living spaces may become no longer fit for use; this leads to impairment in social, occupational, or other important areas of functioning (APA, 2013; Mataix-Cols et al.,

Frequent Obsessions and Compulsions

table 13-8

To be considered either an obsession or compulsion, the items below need to occur for more than 1 hour a day or cause significant distress or impairment to the individual.

Obsessions (thoughts, images, or impulses; obsessions may also involve intrusive or distressing sexual or religious imagery)	Recurring fear of: • Causing harm or being harmed • Contamination and illness • Making mistakes • Losing things
Compulsions Repetitive behavioral acts	• Washing (hands) and cleaning • Counting and checking (stove, locks, lights) • Ordering and arranging • Requesting or demanding assurances • Extreme hoarding and saving
Repetitive mental acts	• Praying • Counting • Repeating words silently

Based on Leckman, J. F., Denys, D., Simpson, H. B., Mataix-Cols, D., Hollander, E., Saxena, S.,. . . Stein, D. J. (2010). Obsessive–compulsive disorder: A review of the diagnostic criteria and possible subtypes and dimensional specifiers for DSM-V. *Depression and Anxiety, 27*(6), 507–527; National Alliance on Mental Illness. (2012). Obsessive compulsive disorder. Available at http://www.nami.org/Template.cfm?Section=By_Illness&Template=/TaggedPage/TaggedPage-Display.cfm&TPLID=54&ContentID=23035; National Institute of Mental Health. (2013). What are the signs and symptoms of OCD? Available at http://www.nimh.nih.gov/health/publications/obsessive-compulsive-disorder-when-unwanted-thoughts-take-over/what-are-the-signs-and-symptoms-of-ocd.shtml

2010). The individual's level of insight into the disorder is similar to those with OCD.

Hoarding symptoms typically emerge in childhood or early adolescence; however, research suggests that it is not until the mid-30s that symptoms begin interfering with daily functioning (Mataix-Cols et al. 2010). See other OCD-related disorders in Table 13-8.

Trauma- and Stressor-Related Disorders

With its 2013 publication, the DSM-5 recognized this new category, which includes reactive attachment disorder, disinhibited social engagement disorder, PTSD, acute stress disorder, and adjustment disorder (APA, 2013). For the individual with one of these disorders, onset of symptoms is clearly linked to a traumatic or stressful event, and the symptoms are so great as to result in significant disruption of functioning over a prolonged period of time. Two of the disorders, reactive attachment disorder and disinhibited social engagement disorder, manifest during childhood. The other disorders may manifest at any point in the life span.

Prevalence

Prevalence varies among the trauma- and stressor-related disorders. For example, lifetime prevalence for PTSD is estimated to occur in approximately 7% to 8% of the U.S. population. Although many individuals experience trauma, about 5.2 million adults will be diagnosed with PTSD (U.S. Department of Veterans Affairs, 2012). Reactive attachment disorder and disinhibited social engagement disorder, however, are relatively rare (APA, 2013).

Reactive Attachment Disorder

Children with *reactive attachment disorder* (RAD) typically do not seek comfort when distressed and barely respond to efforts to comfort them. In addition, they often display limited positive affect and experience periods of irritability and sadness even during normal interactions with caregivers. Fearfulness also is seen, despite the absence of apparent stressors. A history of persistent neglect and repeated changes in caregivers are common among children with RAD (APA, 2013; Zeanah & Gleason, 2010).

Disinhibited Social Engagement Disorder

The same characteristics of pathogenic care described in RAD are thought to be responsible for *disinhibited social engagement disorder.* Children with this disorder readily engage with unfamiliar adults, typically using language and behaviors that are outside the cultural norms of familiarity. These children tend to wander from caregivers without seeking permission, even in unfamiliar settings. They often go willingly with strangers (Zeanah & Gleason, 2010). Nurses caring for children with histories of neglect or foster care should be aware that behaviors associated with disinhibited social engagement disorder may persist once the child is placed in an appropriate care setting.

Posttraumatic Stress Disorder

Posttraumatic stress disorder (PTSD) refers to a group of characteristic symptoms that occur following exposure to traumatic events. The exposure may be experienced directly or through witnessing trauma to others. The DSM-5 includes exposure to death, the threat of death, serious injury, and sexual violence as traumatic events that may result in PTSD (APA, 2013). The highest rates of PTSD are seen in individuals who witness someone being badly injured or killed; are involved in fire, flood, or natural disaster; experience a life-threatening accident; experience rape, captivity, or genocide; or experience combat exposure (Figure 13-4) (U.S. Department of Veterans Affairs, 2010). Immigrants from areas of social disturbances and civil conflict may display increased rates of PTSD. In addition, there are some differences and similarities in traumatic events related to males and females:

- *For males:* Rape, combat exposure, childhood neglect, and childhood physical abuse
- *For females:* Rape, sexual molestation, physical attack, being threatened with a weapon, and childhood physical abuse (National Center for PTSD, 2006)

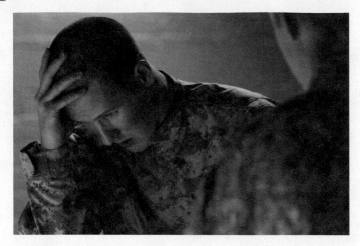

13-4 Survivors of military combat are among those with the highest rates of PTSD.

Source: Burlingham/Fotolia

PTSD is characterized by symptoms of intrusion, including distressing memories of or dreams related to the event and marked distress at occurrences that mimic or are associated with the event—for example, loud noises or sounds that remind the individual of the event. These associations can result in physiologic symptoms of a heightened stress response as well as labile mood states, cognitive disturbances, and hypervigilance. Sleep disturbances, self-destructive behavior, irritability, and aggression are common (APA, 2013; Friedman et al., 2011). *Flashbacks,* dissociative reactions in which the individual feels or acts as if the traumatic event is recurring, are a characteristic symptom. Individuals with PTSD also experience negative alterations in cognition and mood following the event, and as a result may grow increasingly distrustful of others, become persistent in exaggerated negative beliefs and expectations of themselves, and grow increasingly disinterested in activities and disengaged from others (Figure 13-5).

PTSD may occur at any age. The DSM-5 identifies slightly different criteria for PTSD for children ages 6 or younger. Although it acknowledges that children experience many of the same symptoms seen in adults, the DSM-5 recognizes that other symptoms may manifest in children, including physical symptoms such as headache and stomachache. In addition, temper tantrums may be seen, despite the apparent absence of provocation. Children with PTSD may engage in repetitive play that expresses themes or aspects of the event, reenact the event, or have nightmares with unrecognizable content (APA, 2013; Scheeringa, Zeanah, & Cohen, 2011).

Acute Stress Disorder

The key feature of acute stress disorder is the occurrence of symptoms for at least 3 days and up to 1 month after exposure to traumatic event. Significant distress or impairment in social, occupational, or other important areas of functioning occurs. Traumatic events meeting the criteria for acute stress disorder are the same as those for PTSD. Many of the symptoms of acute stress disorder are those of PTSD, including distressing memories of the traumatic event; recurrent, distressing dreams whose content is associated with the event; flashbacks; and efforts to avoid distressing memories or external reminders (such as people, places, or activities) of the event. Additional symptoms include hypervigilance, irritability, aggression, sleep disturbance, and difficulty concentrating (APA, 2013; Bryant et al., 2011). Acute stress disorder is a time-limited condition: If symptoms continue after 4 weeks, the diagnosis of PTSD may be made.

13-5 Patients with PTSD experience a variety of overwhelming symptoms following a traumatic event. These symptoms cause great distress and often result in marked impairment in functioning.

PRACTICE ALERT Patients who are immigrants, especially those from areas with widespread torture and trauma, may be hesitant to share their experiences if they feel their immigrant status is vulnerable (Lindert & Schinina, 2012).

Adjustment Disorder

Similar to the other trauma- and stressor-related disorders, adjustment disorder is a response to a stressful event or events, but in adjustment disorder the response may be out of proportion to the stressor. Symptoms must occur within 3 months of onset of the stressor(s) and not continue for more than 6 months after the termination of stressor (or its consequences) (Strain & Friedman, 2011). In addition, the stressor identified is not an event that rises to the level of severity of those identified under PTSD. When making a diagnosis of adjustment disorder, clinicians should specify a subtype, based on the patient's presentation and history. Subtypes that are recognized in the DSM-5 include adjustment disorder with depressed mood; anxiety; mixed anxiety and depressed mood; disturbance of conduct; mixed disturbance of emotions and conduct; and unspecified (APA, 2013).

Pause and Reflect

1. *How does PTSD differ from generalized anxiety disorder?*
2. *Do you know anyone who has a phobia? How does that person handle his or her anxiety associated with the phobia?*
3. *What concerns do you have about working with military veterans who have PTSD? Where would you go to get more information?*

Collaborative Care

For most patients with anxiety and trauma/stressor disorders, symptoms can be managed and controlled through treatment with medication, different forms of psychotherapy, alternative therapies, or a combination of therapies. Individual style, preferences, and history of success or failure in treatment greatly determine how a patient will or will not pursue treatment. A combination of psychotherapy and medications typically is most effective in treating anxiety disorders, obsessive–compulsive and related disorders, and trauma- and stressor-related disorders. The collaborative process involves development of an interprofessional treatment plan in which members from all the disciplines involved in the patient's care and the patient participate (Ash & Miller, 2013; Craven & Bland, 2006).

Failure of treatment may occur when the patient does not continue treatment for a sufficient period of time. With some antianxiety and antidepressant medications, a number of weeks of treatment may be necessary before the patient experiences satisfactory relief. Patients experiencing high levels of anxiety or other distressing symptoms who want immediate and complete relief will benefit from patient education about the need for continuing psychotherapy and maintaining a course of medication. It may be necessary to try different treatments or different combinations of treatment to find what works best for a specific patient (NIMH, 2008; Stahl, 2011).

Patients experiencing anxiety also benefit from education about anxiety itself. Providing information to patients about their anxiety and diagnoses can be reassuring and promotes collaboration between patients and care providers. A general guideline for initiating treatment with patients experiencing anxiety is to "start low and go slow" (Bandelow et al., 2012; Lieberman & Tasman, 2006, p. 131).

Psychopharmacology

Antianxiety drugs, antidepressants, and beta-blockers are the main categories of medications used to treat anxiety disorders, obsessive–compulsive and related disorders, and trauma- and stressor-related disorders. With symptoms under control, many individuals with anxiety disorders function normally and lead satisfying lives (NIMH, 2008). However, it is important to note that equal efficacy in relation to pharmacotherapy among the different disorders does not exist, nor is the patient's response rate to a medication predictable (Baldwin, 2008). Treatment efficacy and responsiveness to medication vary in relation to the specific disorder (Farach et al., 2012) (see Table 13-9).

An effective working relationship between health care providers and patients is critical for successful treatment. Before initiating medication treatment, the nurse or prescribing provider needs to discuss the following with the patient:

- Indications and side effects of the medication
- Current alternative treatments

table 13-9

Efficacy of Pharmacotherapy in Relation to Specific Disorders

Disorder	Efficacy
Panic disorder	Good
Social anxiety disorder (SAD)	Less efficacious
GAD	Less efficacious
PTSD	Marginal to good
OCD	Marginal to good
Specific phobias	Lack efficacy—medications rarely used

- Other medications (prescription or over-the-counter) that the patient is taking
- How the most effective medication and dose will be determined
- Plan for stopping the medication, as some medications need to be tapered gradually
- Awareness that symptoms may recur if the medication is discontinued
- Family history of success or failure with any medications used to treat anxiety

Antidepressants

In the 1960s, benzodiazepines were the first-line treatment approach for anxiety, primarily because of their rapid onset of action. Problems arose, however, related to craving, dependence, and the withdrawal that follows abrupt discontinuation. Although the benzodiazepines continue to be used for panic and other anxiety disorders, most psychiatric clinicians prefer to use antidepressants as a first-line approach to treatment.

The effectiveness and lack of addictive characteristics of antidepressants, particularly the selective serotonin-reuptake inhibitors (SSRIs) and the serotonin–norepinephrine-reuptake inhibitors (SNRIs) make them useful for treating anxiety (Bandelow et al., 2012; Lieberman & Tasman, 2006). Given that most antidepressants take at least 2 to 4 weeks to become fully effective, patients may become discouraged while waiting for them to begin working. As a result, some patients may even experience a transient period of increased anxiety. Approximately one-third of patients stop taking their antidepressants before completing an initial period of treatment for anxiety (Health Central Network, 2011). Therefore, a benzodiazepine may be prescribed along with an antidepressant to prevent initial anxiety symptoms and to hasten control of panic symptoms. The benzodiazepine often is withdrawn once the antidepressant takes full effect (Bandelow et al., 2012; Farach et al., 2012; Health Central Network, 2011).

Monoamine Oxidase Inhibitors

Monoamine oxidase inhibitors (MAOIs) are used rarely and with caution, because they can cause dangerous increases in blood pressure (hypertensive crisis) if mixed with food or products containing tyramine, which include aged cheese, red wines, some types of birth control pills, some pain relievers, cold and allergy medications, and herbal supplements. MAOIs in combination with SSRIs can produce serotonin syndrome, which can cause a number of troubling symptoms, including confusion, hallucinations, muscle stiffness, and changes in blood pressure or heart rhythm (Farach et al., 2012; Perry, Alexander, Liskow, & DeVane, 2007).

Antianxiety and Sedative–Hypnotic Medications

Antianxiety (anxiolytic) medications reduce anxiety, whereas sedative–hypnotic mediations induce sleep.

Benzodiazepines

Benzodiazepines are effective for anxiety at lower dose levels and for insomnia at higher dose levels (Stahl, 2011). As stated earlier, a major concern with benzodiazepines is their potential for addiction, especially with individuals who already may be abusing drugs and alcohol. Therefore, benzodiazepines generally are prescribed for short periods of time. An exception to this occurs with the diagnosis of panic disorder, in which case individuals may take benzodiazepines

Anxiety   medications commonly used to treat

Anxiolytic Medications
Onset after oral dose:
[1]= Rapid
[2]= Intermediate

[3]= Slow	Usual Adult Daily Dosage (mg)	Nursing Considerations
Benzodiazepines		**For all Anxiolytics**
alprazolam (Xanax)[2]	0.75–4 2–3 × per day	• Avoid heavy machinery and driving. • Avoid alcohol.
chlordiazepoxide(Librium)[2]	15–100 divided in 3–4 doses	• Caution about dependency, confusion, memory loss, drowsiness. • Speak with prescribing provider about taking other medications,
clonazepam (Klonopin)[2]	0.25–4.0	as some can increase the effects of benzodiazepines.
chlorazepate (Tranxene)[1]	7.5–15.0 2–4 × per day	• Instruct patient to speak with prescribing provider about how to discontinue benzodiazepine to prevent withdrawal.
diazepam (Valium)[1]	2–10 2–4 × per day	• Watch for paradoxical reactions in older adults and children. • Caution patient about possibility of impaired mobility related
lorazepam (Ativan)[2]	0.5–6 in 2–3 divided doses	to oversedation. • Inform patient that treatment effects may take several weeks.
midazolam (Versed)[2]	7.5–15	
Other anxiolytic		
buspirone (Buspar)	15–60 in 3 divided doses	

Antidepressant medications	Dosages (mg)	Nursing Considerations
SSRIs		**For all SSRIs**
citalopram (Celexa)	10–40	Provide patient education regarding:
fluvoxamine (Luvox)	50–300 (once greater than 50 mg, divide bid)	• GI distress • Sexual dysfunction
fluoxetine (Prozac)	10–60	• Nausea or diarrhea
paroxetine (Paxil)	20–60	• Tremors
sertraline (Zoloft)	25–200	• Insomnia
escitalopram (Lexapro)	10–20	• Daytime drowsiness • Serotonin syndrome
SNRIs		**For all SNRIs**
duloxetine (Cymbalta)	40–120 in 1–2 doses	In addition to SSRI-like side effects, can cause increased blood
venlafaxine (Effexor)	75–375 (divided into 2–3 doses)	pressure. Provide patient education regarding dry mouth, dizziness, consti-
Tricyclics		pation, weight gain, urinary retention.
clomipramine (Anafranil)	25–250	Inquire about cardiac history. Inform patient that treatment effects may take several weeks.
MAOIs		**For all MAOIs**
isocarboxazid (Marplan)	10 2–3 × per day	• Instruct patient regarding dietary restrictions (foods and products with tyramine).
phenelzine (Nardil)	15–90 After 15, divide into 2–3 doses per day	• Provide education regarding orthostatic hypotension, constipation, nausea. • Determine normal liver functioning prior to administering
tranylcypromine (Parnate)	10–60	medication.
selegiline (Emsam)	4 mg patch	

Antidepressant medications	Dosages (mg)	Nursing Considerations
Other		Instruct patient to change patch daily as ordered.
nefazadone (Serzone)	200–600 in 2 divided doses	Avoid use with MAOIs. Caution about dizziness, drowsiness, GI distress, blurred vision, sexual dysfunction.
mirtazapine (Remeron)	15–45	May cause sedation and weight gain. Sedation does not worsen at higher doses.

Beta-Blockers	Dosage (mg)	Nursing Considerations
propranolol (Inderal)	10–80	Patient should try medication prior to first-time use for performance anxiety.

Calcium Channel Modulators	Dosage (mg)	Nursing Considerations
gabapentin (Neurontin)	900–1800 in 3 divided doses	Educate to avoid mixing with alcohol or other CNS depressants.
pregabalin (Lyrica)	150–600 in 2–3 doses	May cause sedation and dizziness.

Antihistamine	Dosage (mg)	Nursing Considerations
hydroxyzine (Vistaril)	50–100 taken 4 times/day	Can be very sedating and cause excessive dry mouth. May be used as adjunct to SSRIs or SNRIs.

Data from Adams, M., Holland, N., & Urban, C. (2014). Pharmacology for Nurses: A Pathophysiologic Approach (4th ed.). Upper Saddle River, NJ: Prentice Hall; Stahl, S. M. (2011). Essential Pharmacology—The Prescriber's Guide. New York, NY: Cambridge University Press.

for up to a year. Patients may experience withdrawal symptoms if a benzodiazepine medication is discontinued abruptly rather than tapered slowly. Anxiety also may return once the medication is stopped.

Short-acting benzodiazepines generally are used for patients who have sleep-onset insomnia but no daytime anxiety. Benzodiazepines with a longer duration of action are used to treat insomnia in patients with daytime anxiety (Stahl, 2011).

Special consideration should be given when administering benzodiazepines to older adults. Slower rate of clearance due to a slowed metabolism rate, increased problems with accumulation, and greater sensitivity to central nervous system depressants can cause difficulties such as falls. Therefore, shorter-acting benzodiazepines or those without active metabolites, such as oxazepam (Serax) and temazepam (Restoril), should be considered over longer-acting ones and those with active metabolites.

PRACTICE ALERT Older adults often are prescribed one-half the usual adult dose of a benzodiazepine (Bandelow et al., 2012). Older adults also may exhibit a paradoxical reaction, in which the opposite effect of what is expected occurs when a medication is administered. In the case of benzodiazepines, this would mean excitement or agitation.

Nonbenzodiazepines

Buspirone (Buspar), an azapirone, is used to treat GAD. A nonbenzodiazepine, buspirone's anxiolytic effect often takes four weeks to be effective. Possible side effects include dizziness, headaches, and nausea. Buspirone's main advantages are that it does not produce dependence or withdrawal symptoms with long-term use. It is nonsedative and does not exert anticonvulsant or muscle-relaxant effects (Stahl, 2011).

Beta-Blockers

Beta-blockers, such as propranolol (Inderal), can prevent physical symptoms that accompany anxiety disorders such as social phobia.

In the case of a predictable feared situation, such as giving a speech (performance anxiety) or flying in an airplane, a beta-blocker may be prescribed to control physical symptoms of anxiety during the stressful situation only (Stahl, 2011).

Cognitive–Behavioral Therapy

Cognitive–behavioral therapy (CBT) is a main form of treatment for anxiety disorders (Montgomery, Kunik, Wilson, Stanley, & Weiss, 2010). In addition to helping patients change or modify unhealthy thought patterns and change their responses to anxiety-provoking situations, CBT therapists also teach deep breathing and other types of exercises to relieve anxiety and encourage relaxation. CBT can be conducted individually or with a group of patients who exhibit similar symptoms. Group therapy is particularly effective for social phobia. Homework assignments frequently are given between sessions. Medication often is combined with psychotherapy for specific anxiety disorders (Bandelow et al., 2012; NIMH, 2008). Table 13-10 offers several examples of how CBT can be helpful to patients with specific anxiety disorders.

Forms of CBT for PTSD include exposure therapy, eye-movement desensitization and reprocessing (EMDR), stress-inoculation training, cognitive processing therapy (CPT), behavioral activation, and acceptance and commitment therapy (Benedek, Friedman, Zatzick, & Ursano, 2009; Tull, 2008). Research done with 108 female rape survivors found significant improvements in health concerns and sleep impairment when using CPT and prolonged exposure (PE) to trauma triggers (Galovoski, Monson, Bruce, & Resick, 2009). PE typically includes (1) education about trauma and causes of chronic posttrauma challenges; (2) repeated reimagining of the traumatic memory or event; and (3) direct confrontation of triggers (e.g., circumstances, objects) when the individual is safe, which helps gradually reduce the severity of the individual's response to the trigger (Substance Abuse and Mental Health Services Administration, 2014).

Examples of Cognitive–Behavioral Therapy for Disorders of Anxiety, Stress, and Trauma	table 13-10

Disorder	Cognitive–Behavioral Therapy
Social anxiety disorder	Exposure to situations that trigger anxiety. Envisioning situation in advance to discuss social mistakes patient most fears making and how to avoid them.
Specific phobias	Gradual encounters with the object or situation that the patient fears are planned. Encounters may begin through pictures or tapes and progress to "real life" situations.
Obsessive–compulsive disorder	Therapist works with patient to gradually gain control of anxiety. For example, patient may get hands dirty and increase the amount of time before washing. Repeating such exercises generally decreases the patient's anxiety.
Posttraumatic stress disorder	CBT helps desensitize patients to the traumatic event by allowing them to reprocess the event and become better at decreasing the sense of threat. CBT also helps patients restructure or reframe negative thinking related to the event.

Complementary and Alternative Therapies

Many complementary and alternative therapies provide relief from the distress experienced by those suffering with anxiety. Some of the more common ones include exercise, relaxation techniques, breathing techniques, herbs, and vitamins (Rouse, 2010). See Chapter 22 for more information.

Exercise

Many types of exercise are free or relatively inexpensive and accessible to most people. Exercise may be helpful in reducing symptoms of anxiety in patients with anxiety disorders when used as a complementary treatment alongside CBT and/or medication (Jayakody, Gunadasa, & Hosker, 2014). Regular exercise lowers stress levels and can release mood-enhancing endorphins. Exercise has additional psychological and emotional benefits, such as helping patients gain confidence and relieve feelings of worry through reaching exercise goals; providing a distraction from negative thoughts; and increasing social interaction (Mayo Clinic Staff, 2011).

Relaxation Techniques

Similar to exercise, relaxation techniques, including meditation, yoga, t'ai chi, and progressive relaxation, help relieve anxiety by lowering stress levels. Meditation and relaxation techniques such as biofeedback can lessen anxiety, improve mood, and relieve symptoms of distress (Bandelow et al., 2012; Davis, 2006). Slow, gentle yoga practice that focuses on postures that calm the heart and the mind may help individuals balance emotions and release tension, thereby lowering anxiety

Sondra Recovery Phase

critical thinking

Sondra follows through on the referral and sees Marilyn, It should be PMH-APRN. Partway through her initial interview, Sondra shares that she was raped at work one evening 2 months ago. She states that she has difficulty sleeping, because she keeps dreaming about the rape and the man who raped her. She is ashamed and does not want her grandmother, Lita, to know. This is becoming difficult: Lita keeps asking what is wrong, having noticed that Sondra has started jumping every time someone walks into a room and that Sondra is not spending as much time with Lita as she used to.

Marilyn makes a primary diagnosis of Posttraumatic Stress Disorder (PTSD). She sets up a weekly counseling schedule with Sondra and prescribes sertraline (Zoloft) 25 mg daily to be taken by mouth every morning and increased to 50 mg daily after 1 week. Marilyn tells Sondra that if she becomes sleepy, she can take her medication before bedtime the day after her last morning dose.

* * * *

Sondra returns to the outpatient clinic in a month's time for her follow-up appointment there. Her mother and her grandmother, Lita, accompany her into the examining room. Sondra speaks with Carol for the first time about her rape. Lita starts to cry and says, "I had no idea what my little Sondra went through." Carol asks how Sondra is doing now and how the rest of the family is doing. Sondra assures her that she is continuing to attend sessions with Marilyn, and that her mother and grandmother have also participated. They have not yet told Sondra's father.

The rash on Sondra's hands has resolved. Sondra reports that her hand washing has returned to "normal": what it was before the rape. She reports that her medication (sertraline) has been increased to 100 mg daily and that this has helped her sleep better and be less anxious. Carol notes that Sondra is calmer, the rash on her hands has resolved, and that she is making good eye contact during the appointment. Carol and Sondra decide that Sondra should return in 6 months' time.

APPLICATION

1. Address the five domains for Sondra.

2. What are the criteria for PTSD? What symptoms of PTSD does Sondra exhibit?

3. How does Sondra's disclosure change her diagnoses and care plan?

4. Why is sertraline an appropriate recommendation for Sondra?

levels (Harvard Mental Health Letter, 2009). In a systematic review of 40 studies involving 3,817 subjects, t'ai chi was associated with improvements in reduced stress, anxiety, depression, and enhanced mood (Wang et al., 2010).

Breathing Techniques

Controlling one's breathing can be helpful in easing a panic attack (Rouse, 2010) or for helping someone who is very distressed. Nurses can help patients control their breathing by guiding them to do the following:

- Breathe in slowly through the nose in 4 counts.
- Hold breath for 2 counts.
- Blow air out through the mouth as if blowing up a balloon slowly for 4 counts.

Herbs, Vitamins, and Supplements

Herbs, vitamins, and other supplements are used in the treatment of anxiety disorders. Chamomile, ginkgo biloba, and rhodiola may be effective for relieving anxiety and insomnia (Bourne, 2010; LeRoy, 2006). In particular, the *B vitamins*—biotin, niacin, thiamine, pantothenic acid, riboflavin, B6, B12, and folic acid—are all important for the production of neurotransmitters. Thiamine is very important for those prone to panic, anxiety, and depression. Becoming angry, crying, or getting run down expends thiamine. A daily B-complex supplement (50–100 mg per day) is helpful. Other herbs, vitamins, or supplements that may be helpful include *alpha-linolenic acid,* which has been shown to improve anxiety symptoms within 2 to 3 months; magnesium (200 mg 2–3 times per day), which may help improve anxiety and panic symptoms because it assists with muscle relaxation; and vitamin C (250–500 mg per day), which reduces swelling and helps improve immune function (Bourne, 2010; Godlewski, 2006).

Pause and Reflect

1. *What are important nursing considerations associated with selective serotonin-reuptake inhibitors?*
2. *How does exercise help to prevent or relieve anxiety? What factors might inhibit patients with anxiety disorders from engaging in regular exercise?*
3. *What do you do to prevent or relieve your own anxiety?*

Nursing Management

Individuals respond uniquely and subjectively to different anxiety-provoking situations and stressors. Intervening to prevent a patient's level of anxiety from increasing further is essential. Identifying the source of a patient's anxiety may be challenging and may not always be possible. It usually is more realistic to identify what helps a patient relieve distress; this can help prevent patient anxiety from rising to a higher level and may restore the patient to a more functional level of anxiety (Figure 13-6). Learning ways to decrease a patient's distress level and direct the anxiety in a constructive and functional manner is critical to meeting patient needs. These interventions, when validated with the patient as being helpful, result in good nursing care (Kaya, Özcan, & Yilmaz, 2013; Orlando, 1961; Potter & Bockenhauer, 2000).

Anxiety has a "contagious" nature to it. Individuals often sense when someone is anxious and may, in turn, become anxious

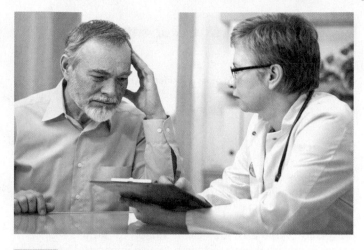

13-6 Nurses help patients with anxiety by acknowledging patients' discomfort, providing a calm presence, and helping patients identify what helps them relieve their anxiety.

Source: Alexander Raths/Shutterstock

themselves. Patients may "spread" anxiety to one another on a unit. Anxiety affects an individual's interpretation of cues, especially in relation to the context of the cues given; interpretations often are more negative when the conditions occurring at the time also are negative (Blanchette, Richards, & Cross, 2007). If anxiety begins to spread, the nurse must intervene to minimize its effects and to direct patient anxiety to the most functional level possible. It also is essential for nurses to sense when their own anxiety is rising, and address their anxiety before it begins to affect others (see Evidence-Based Practice: Anxiety in Nursing Students).

A good strategy for nurses who sense their own anxiety rising is to lower their voice and slow down their rate of speech—in other words, "Speak lowly and slowly." This is a good self-calming strategy that nurses can use themselves and that they can teach to patients who are anxious.

Self-awareness is important when working with patients. Some questions for nurses to explore when working with patients with anxiety include the following:

- Do I get anxious easily?
- What kinds of circumstances make me anxious?
- What do I do to manage my anxiety?
- How do I feel when I am around individuals who are anxious?
- Do I think I can help individuals who are anxious?

As discussed in Chapter 7, Orlando's deliberative nursing process can be helpful in working with individuals who are anxious. By validating the nurse's own perceptions, thoughts, and feelings about an interaction with a patient, the nurse can determine whether he or she is accurately assessing the patient's needs. This may seem difficult when nurses have little time with patients during short interactions or interventions. However, determining with the patient what the immediate needs of the patient are at each interaction can help relieve patient distress (see Perceptions, Thoughts, and Feelings: Validating the Needs of a Patient with Obsessive–Compulsive Symptoms, which appears near the end of this chapter).

Anxiety in Nursing Students   evidence-based practice

Clinical Problem

High levels of anxiety within nursing students working in the clinical environment can affect performance and success. What strategies can nursing faculty incorporate within the learning environment to decrease students' levels of distress?

Evidence

Cheung and Au (2011) reported on their findings from an experimental study of 30 undergraduate nursing students in either their third or fourth year in a 4-year nursing program at a university in Hong Kong. Performance of a newly learned stitch-removal procedure was assessed after participants viewed either an "anxiety-provoking" video clip or a "calm" video clip. Results support a causal relationship between the negative impacts of anxiety on performance.

In a literature review, Moscaritolo (2009) found three strategies that decrease student anxiety and distress in the clinical setting: (1) humor (dependent on cultural sensitivity, circumstances, and context); (2) peer instructors and mentors (peer instructors were perceived as less threatening than faculty and nursing staff mentors being involved as part of a triad with student and instructor was found to be helpful); and (3) mindfulness training (for example, body scanning, meditation, yoga, and guided audiotapes on relaxation practices).

In a qualitative, phenomenological research study, Melincavage (2011) described student nurses' anxiety in the clinical setting. The research was a descriptive report on lived experience and based on interviews with seven student nurses from two baccalaureate nursing programs in the United States. Common themes regarding sources of anxiety included being inexperienced, feeling demeaned, being exposed, being abandoned, competition among peers, and uncertainty about ability. Melincavage (2011) proposes interventions on a larger scale to address group norms and challenges the status quo in terms of how some staff nurses treat nursing students. Interventions include a curriculum in which faculty teach students conflict resolution strategies and coping skills students can use to decrease anxiety both during and outside the clinical day. The author also suggests interventions to target nurses and other hospital staff including role-play presentations in which the students act out scenarios of their experiences. Another intervention is for faculty to share anonymous student evaluations with nursing and hospital staff at the end of each semester.

Implications for Nursing Practice

Nursing students experience increased anxiety in clinical settings related to the following:

- First clinical experience
- Performance of clinical skills
- Assisting dying patients
- Fear of making mistakes
- Evaluation by faculty
- Lack of support by nursing staff
- Feeling demeaned or abandoned
- Gaps between theory and practice

Nursing faculty can use humor, peer instructors and staff mentors, and mindfulness activities to minimize student nurses' anxiety in clinical settings. In addition, nursing faculty may want to consider teaching conflict resolution skills as part of the curriculum and providing additional opportunities for students to practice healthy coping skills.

Critical Thinking Questions

1. Identify strategies that decreased nursing student anxiety in the studies cited. Which of these strategies do you find most helpful when you are anxious?
2. What additional strategies might help you or other students?

Assessment

Keen observation skills help nurses assess and alleviate patient anxiety and its accompanying distress and suffering. By using the senses to attend to a patient's affect, appearance, and behaviors, nurses can gather cues to address the patient's distress and suffering associated with anxiety. In addition, assessing the patient's developmental level according to Erikson's stages of development is helpful when planning nursing care. Determining actual developmental stage in reference to expected developmental stage can promote nursing care that is tailored to the patient's abilities.

Observation and Physical Assessment

When assessing an anxious patient, it will be most helpful if the nurse:

- Remains calm.
- Uses open body language (uncrossed arms, hands at sides or in lap if sitting, staying at eye level with patient if possible—not standing above the patient).
- Keeps voice low and speaks slowly.
- Uses simple and clear phrases.
- Speaks in an assuring and calming manner.
- Provides amount and type of information patient needs to lower anxiety level.

During observation and physical assessment, the nurse notes the following about the patient:

- *Vital signs:* When anxious, patients' vital signs (blood pressure, pulse, and respirations) will be increased.
- *Demeanor:* How does the patient come across in general? Is the patient fidgety, restless, or distracted, or have excessive body movements?
- *Facial expression:* Where are the patient's eyes focused? Is the patient able to maintain eye contact with the nurse? What is the patient doing with his or her mouth (biting lips, making movements with his mouth)? Is the patient grimacing? Are the patient's eyebrows tense, furrowed, or drawn?
- *Body movements:* What is the patient doing with his or her hands and feet? Does the patient exhibit any other body movements, such as twitches or tics (muscle twitch especially in neck, face, or shoulder)?

- *Voice:* What is the patient's voice level (high-pitched, barely audible, soft/loud/normal volume)? What is the pace of speech (pressured and rapid, slow, normal)? What is the tone of speech (mild/agitated/aggressive/normal)? Is the patient's mouth dry when he or she attempts to speak?

- *Behaviors:* Does the patient exhibit any rituals or compulsions?

- *Thoughts:* Is the patient coherent? Is the patient able to grasp what the nurse is saying? Does the patient have repeated and troublesome thoughts or obsessions? Does the patient acknowledge having racing thoughts that he or she cannot stop?

- *Content of conversation:* Does the patient's conversation center on things that are anxiety or fear producing for the patient?

- *Level of anxiety:* Mild, moderate, severe, or panic? (See Table 13-3 Levels of Anxiety.)

Patient Interview

Pertinent questions to ask patients when interviewing and obtaining an assessment of anxiety will address each of the five domains of wellness. For example, assess for somatic complaints, such as headaches, stomachaches, and sleep disturbance. Inquire about psychological symptoms, including worry, irritability, or aggression. Ask how things are going in relation to social and cultural factors, such as difficulty maintaining normal activities or engaging with family members and coworkers. Evaluate whether there are spiritual concerns, such as a change in spiritual practices or evidence of spiritual distress. Also, assess for any recent environmental changes. This latter area can be especially important when assessing children who exhibit symptoms of anxiety.

Rating scales may be helpful to establish mutual understanding between nurse and patient. Questions to ask may include the following:

- How would you rate your anxiety (on a scale of 0, meaning no anxiety, to 10, meaning highly anxious)?

- What is a "normal" level of anxiety for you (on a scale of 0–10)?

- How long have you been experiencing your current level of anxiety?

- Are you aware of anything that may have precipitated or triggered your anxiety?

- What has helped you in the past to deal with your anxiety?

- What would be helpful in lowering your anxiety?

Differences among Initial/Relapse, Recovery, Rehabilitation Phases

Patients in an initial or relapse phase are at a high level of anxiety and need very direct and concrete directions. Typically, patients at this level of anxiety seek help or are directed to help by others. For example, the patient having a panic attack may go the hospital emergency department concerned about having a "heart attack." Nursing staff intervene to assist the patient to rule out heart attack and to decrease the patient's anxiety.

The patient experiencing a relapse may have a better working knowledge of how his or her anxiety manifests and what strategies help lower the anxiety levels. The patient may or may not recognize what happened to exacerbate the relapse. Hopefully, the relapse period will be shorter than the initial episode and the patient will be able to activate strategies to decrease anxiety. For example, the patient may be at work and start to feel chest pain. By employing some of the

approaches the patient learned previously (stress management breathing, for example), the patient will be able to decrease anxiety, with the result that the chest pain ceases.

PRACTICE ALERT Helping the patient recognize that important anniversary dates (e.g., anniversary of the death of a spouse) may activate symptoms is an important educational goal.

The patient in recovery begins to learn more about personal precipitants/triggers for anxiety and may begin apply strategies to avoid relapse. With practice, the patient will be able to employ these strategies more quickly and successfully.

The patient who has reached the rehabilitation phase knows what triggers to avoid and how to cope with them when they arise. The patient actively promotes health by implementing different strategies to prevent relapse and maintain health. For example, the patient may participate in a regular exercise program.

Diagnosis and Planning

Thorough and accurate assessment advances appropriate nursing diagnosis and planning. Working with patients to develop nursing diagnoses and plans can be a rewarding and affirming experience for both the nurse and the patient.

Common Nursing Diagnoses

Nursing diagnoses for patients with disorders of anxiety, stress, and trauma are identified and prioritized based on patient needs. Although a number of nursing diagnoses address various aspects of anxiety, some specific nursing diagnoses are seen more frequently. These include the following:

- Sleep Pattern, Disturbed
- Anxiety
- Fear
- Coping, Ineffective
- Fatigue
- Spiritual Distress, Risk for
- Stress Overload
- Powerlessness
- Rape-Trauma Syndrome

(NANDA-I © 2014)

Disturbed sleep (both initiating and maintaining sleep) is a common problem for patients with these disorders. Patients with disturbed sleep may encounter multiple challenges, such as confusion, appetite disturbances, and interference with reality testing. Often one problem area connects with another. In addition to selecting nursing diagnoses based on what is most problematic or symptomatic for the patient, nurses may also select one or more diagnoses based on patient behaviors that create difficulties for others in the patient's life.

Prioritizing Nursing Diagnoses

Both student and seasoned nurses often wonder what makes a good nursing care plan. The ideal nursing care plan is one in which the nurse involves the patient in its formulation, and together the nurse and patient determine priorities for the patient's care. If that is not possible, the nurse must address the most significant observed needs of the patient and select nursing diagnoses that are realistic in terms of the patient's ability to achieve goals in a reasonable time frame.

Working with the patient will help determine the nursing diagnoses that are most relevant for the patient and will help the patient "buy in" to the care plan. This will increase the likelihood that the patient will adhere to the plan of care.

In Sondra's first visit to the clinic, for example, Carol identifies fear as a priority nursing diagnosis to address with Sondra. Together they develop a nursing care plan to address Sandra's fear (see the Nursing Care Plan). The fear a patient experiences may range from mild to severe. The nurse will need to assist the patient from becoming impaired or immobilized by fear.

Plans and Goals

As the nurse develops plans and goals within the nursing care plan, he or she keeps the patient involved as much as possible. Questions the nurse should consider when developing the plan include the following:

- Is the patient capable of helping develop a care plan?
- What is the most distressing symptom from the patient's perspective?
- What specifically does the patient need/want to achieve? How can patient needs be articulated and addressed as *specific, realistic,* and *measurable* goals for the patient's care? For example if the patient has difficulty sleeping, the nurse might state the following specific, realistic, and measurable goals:
    - The patient will demonstrate an understanding of sleep hygiene protocols in 1 day.
    - The patient will increase sleep time from 4 hours per night to 5 hours per night in 3 days.
    - The patient will report feeling more rested after 3 days.

In developing the plan of care, the nurse will consider with the patient how the five domains are involved. Asking targeted questions may help elicit information that will help inform the care plan.

- *Biological:* Does the patient have any medical conditions that may impede return to health? Does the patient need additional resources to treat these conditions?

- *Psychological:* Are there triggers that make the patient's condition flare or become worse? What might be done to lessen the negative impact of such triggers?
- *Sociological:* Are there relationships that are having a positive or a negative impact on the patient's needs? Is the patient under duress at home, work, or school? Are there other circumstances affecting the patient's environment? Is the environment conducive to sleep or is the environment loud, noisy, chaotic, crowded, distracting, and so on?
- *Cultural:* Are there any family traditions or rituals that are impeding or enhancing to the patient's health? How? For example, what is the patient's cultural background in relation to alcohol and caffeine?
- *Spiritual:* Are there any spiritual concerns (such as guilt, loneliness, or fear) that could be affecting the patient's anxiety level negatively? Are there spiritual supports in the patient's life and, if so, how might they be incorporated to assist the patient?

Patient Education

Patient learning needs and abilities must be addressed and incorporated into the plan. For example, if sleep disturbance is identified as a priority, the patient may need information about sleep hygiene and keeping a sleep log. The nurse will work with the patient to determine whether the patient needs to modify any of the five domains to assist with improved sleep pattern.

Revising the Care Plan During Recovery and Rehabilitation

As patients improve and anxiety levels decrease, the nurse will re-evaluate progress and make necessary adjustments. Patients need support and affirmation that temporarily returning to old patterns does not mean they cannot be restored to better health once again. In fact, being aware that relapses are likely to happen but can be handled better and with less impact on the patient's functioning is a good goal for patients, which may make their expectations of the recovery process more realistic.

During rehabilitation, the patient will be better able to identify triggers and symptoms of relapse and minimize their impact by getting help more quickly.

(See Appendix B for a complete list of NANDA-approved Nursing Diagnoses.)

Sondra—A Patient with Obsessive–Compulsive Disorder		NURSING CARE PLAN

Nursing Diagnosis: Fear related to perceived threat of dirt in environment. Manifested by recurrent and persistent thoughts about germs, frequent and excessive compulsory hand washings (totaling more than 1 hour each day for a duration of 10 minutes each time), and contact dermatitis on both hands.

Short-Term Goals *Patient will:* (include date for short-term goal to be met)	Intervention *Nurse will:*	Rationale
Identify thoughts related to "germs" during first interview.	Ask Sondra to list thoughts that precipitate hand-washing behaviors.	Determine thinking related to need to wash hands
State what hand washing behaviors occur when Sondra is distressed during first interview.	Ask Sondra to list hand-washing rituals.	Clarify what activities actually take place during hand-washing rituals.
During first interview, identify 1–3 stressors that cause Sondra to engage in hand-washing behaviors.	Assist Sondra in identifying stressors that precipitate hand-washing behaviors.	Precipitating stressors trigger certain behaviors.

Short-Term Goals Patient will: (include date for short-term goal to be met)	Intervention Nurse will:	Rationale
During first interview, recognize time frame of relief with hand washing.	Help Sondra estimate how much relief she experiences when beginning hand washing and how long it lasts.	The compulsive behavior being used to manage anxiety may or may not be effective.
Decrease in persistent thoughts about "germs" from constant to 3–4 times a day 1 week after first interview.	Provide patient education in relation to thought stopping: Ask Sondra to say "STOP" in her mind. Assess need for education related to "germs." Replace the thought about "germs" with healthier thoughts.	Thought stopping helps interrupt obsessive thoughts. Education related to "germs" may be helpful. Negative thoughts need to be replaced with positive thoughts.
Adhere to skin care treatment and any medications as ordered by providers (if prescribed).	Provide teaching related to treatments prescribed by care providers.	Patient adherence to treatment often depends on patient understanding of the treatment.
Decrease hand washing to 1 minute and add another constructive activity right after it within 3 days of first interview.	Encourage Sondra to agree to hand-washing schedule that allows her 1 minute to perform her hand-washing ritual. Determine what other activities (including use of therapeutic hand cream) might provide some relief for the Sondra's anxiety and promote healthy skin.	Excessive and prolonged hand washing causes skin breakdown. When an established negative behavior is being decreased, it is important to replace it with a positive behavior.
Resolve contact dermatitis on both hands within 1 week.	Assist Sondra in developing measurement to track healing progress on her hands.	Tracking progress reinforces positive behaviors and boosts self-esteem.
Long-Term Goal Sondra's contact dermatitis will resolve. She will wash her hands for less than 1 minute no more than 10 times a day, and she will report decrease in persistent thoughts about "germs."	Affirm Sondra's progress and check in with her to monitor her anxiety level and if she has been able to redirect her thoughts about "germs" to more positive thoughts.	Acknowledging positive behaviors can be reinforcing. It is important to ensure that the patient's anxiety is decreasing and that the patient is able to redirect negative thinking as a result of interventions.

Clinical Reasoning

1. What other nursing diagnoses might the nurse working with Sondra consider?
2. Do you think the selection of *Fear* as the priority diagnosis is appropriate? Why or why not?
3. In addition to promoting skin integrity, why else might it be helpful to get Sondra to reduce her hand washing to 1 minute?

Implementation

Determining the patient's level of anxiety is important when implementing nursing care. Interventions will depend on the patient's ability to concentrate and listen, learn new information, and make decisions. Where the patient is along the continuum of initial episode/relapse, recovery, or rehabilitation also influences nursing interventions. In addition, patient (and often family) support for the plan of care can influence the success of the interventions. Special circumstances, such as the patient's level of consciousness or whether or not the patient has a guardian, also may affect implementation of nursing care.

In the chapter example, Sondra does not initially disclose the real source of her anxiety. The patient's own behaviors, unforeseen circumstances or triggers, and factors beyond the patient's control can affect patient domain considerations. It is critical to bear in mind that each patient's life story is unique and to plan nursing interventions that treat each patient and circumstance uniquely. For example, a patient may be working 12-hour shifts and not be allowed to bring medications to work, or may travel frequently for work and have difficulty maintaining regular therapy appointments. The nurse will

need to work with other disciplines while ensuring patient confidentiality to help the patient receive treatment. Nurses must consider each patient's circumstances and work with the patient and other individuals and systems to promote continuity of care and minimize increased anxiety in the patient's life.

Interventions for Different Levels of Anxiety

When a patient is experiencing a high level of suffering, it may be difficult for the patient to sense hope. Presence, active listening, and helping the patient meet basic needs are powerful interventions that may be most helpful for the patient with extreme anxiety. The nurse will need to be more directive than usual, because the patient's capacity to hear and receive information may be reduced.

Once the patient becomes less anxious and begins moving toward recovery or rehabilitation, the nurse can offer other strategies to promote hope, such as helping the patient establish goals for the future and promoting social connections and supports.

The four levels of anxiety, their impact on the patient's ability to engage in the teaching process, and basic nursing interventions to help decrease symptoms at each level are described in Table 13-11.

Nursing Interventions for Different Levels of Anxiety   table 13-11

Anxiety Level	Patient Perceptions	Patient Teaching	Nursing Interventions
Mild +1	• Improved learning • Heightened perceptions • Increased awareness and alertness	• Learning abilities are enhanced.	• Encourage patient in information gathering and problem solving. • Explore alternative strategies for coping.
Moderate +2	• Narrowed perceptual field • Selective inattention	• Decreased attention span and ability to concentrate; able to learn with support.	• Remain calm; speak slowly and in a low voice. • Provide support and presence. • Help patient focus. • Assist patient as needed with problem solving. • Encourage activities (such as exercise) to help patient direct feelings of anxiety. • Administer SSRIs and antianxiety medications as prescribed.
Severe +3	• Sensory perceptual fields greatly reduced	• Patient has a very limited attention span. Productive learning cannot occur.	• Provide a calm presence; acknowledge patient's discomfort. • Speak in a low voice. • Use slow, direct, clear, and simple phrases. • Help patient regain a sense of control. • Help patient identify triggers (thoughts and feelings) that increase patient's anxiety. • Determine with patient what has worked in the past to relieve anxiety. • Problem-solve with patient. • Incorporate stress management exercises as tolerated by patient. • Encourage activities to help patient direct feelings of anxiety, such as walking with patient or some other activity as tolerated by patient. • Administer medications as prescribed.
Panic +4	• Unable to focus • Misperceptions common • Behaviors markedly disturbed	• Learning does not occur. • Unable to focus. • Difficulty understanding simple directions.	• Remain calm. • Stay with the patient. • Use simple, clear, and direct communication with patient. • Help patient regain a sense of control. • Ensure safety of patient and others. • Ensure adequate nutritional and fluid intake. • Provide quiet environment for patient. • Respect patient's need for personal space but do not leave patient unattended. • Administer medications as prescribed. • Incorporate stress management techniques as tolerated by patient. • Reinforce reality. • Get assistance as needed.

Primary, Secondary, and Tertiary Interventions

Nursing interventions may be made on the primary, secondary, or tertiary levels in relation to decreasing anxiety and its associated distress. The main focus in primary intervention is to reduce the risk of the occurrence of anxiety or the risk of a normal level of anxiety escalating to an unhealthy level or chronic state. The goal is to channel the anxiety in a positive and constructive manner. This is achieved by lowering the distress associated with the anxiety. Education is aimed at prevention.

Secondary intervention involves early intervention and treatment. A secondary level of intervention would involve managing anxiety that is escalating out of control. Patient education is focused on the elimination of unhealthy response.

Tertiary intervention involves post-intervention with an established unhealthy behavior or risk of recurrence of an unhealthy behavior. The goal is to restore and rehabilitate individuals whose functioning has been impaired by their level of anxiety. Education is directed toward reducing established behavior or the risk of recurrence and promoting restoration and functioning of the individual to a healthier state (Table 13-12).

Patient Education

Before beginning patient education, the nurse needs to assess whether the patient is ready to receive instruction. If the timing is appropriate, the nurse helps the patient understand triggers that set

Primary, Secondary, and Tertiary Levels of Intervention

table 13-12

Level of Intervention	Teaching Opportunity
Primary intervention	Senior-level nursing students provide a class for first and second year students related to understanding suffering prior to the underclass students' affiliation on a psychiatric unit.
Secondary intervention	A nurse works with a patient in the emergency department who is hyperventilating. The nurse instructs the patient to use slow, deep breathing strategies by inhaling slowly and deeply through the nose and exhaling slowly through the mouth as if blowing up a balloon.
Tertiary intervention	The nurse in an outpatient clinic co-leads a support group for PTSD survivors. They share with one another strategies that have helped them cope and return to more normal functioning.

off the anxiety symptoms and strategies that may alleviate the symptoms (Box 13-2). If the patient is highly anxious, instruction efforts may need to be concise and limited or postponed until the patient is ready to accept teaching. For the patient with extreme anxiety, the nurse needs to remain with the patient or delegate another to do so to ensure that the patient will not act impulsively or harm self or others.

As discussed previously, one of the most challenging areas for anxious individuals is getting sufficient rest and sleep. Instructing patients in positive sleep hygiene strategies may be very beneficial, especially for those who are unaware of poor habits and how to break them. (See Chapter 12 for information on sleep hygiene.)

Factors that Influence the Success of Interventions

Nurses plan interventions on the major assumption that patients tell them the truth. However, as mentioned earlier, a patient may fail to disclose important information, such as substance use or abuse, other types of trauma, financial issues, or legal issues. When the nurse suspects that a patient is withholding information, the nurse needs to inquire tactfully without impeding development of trust and rapport with the patient. Some situations may not be evident and may not be disclosed until later in the development of the therapeutic relationship. It is important that the nurse not criticize or judge the patient for not sharing everything initially. Nurses must be ready to adjust interventions based on unfolding information as well as changes in patient circumstances.

Nurses also must engage in self-care to relieve their own anxieties and to ensure that they do not pass their anxieties along to their patients. What constitutes self-care is different for each individual, but exercise; appropriate nutrition; relaxing activities, such as massage and yoga; planning fun times; enjoying hobbies; and appropriate rest, including vacations, all help alleviate anxiety. Humor can be a potent stress reliever as well (Box 13-3).

Minimizing Symptom Recurrence

Patients who recognize symptoms of their anxiety disorder and who have a good working relationship with their care providers may seek help earlier rather than later. Helping patients develop a plan for

Strategies to Alleviate Anxiety

box 13-2

- Talking
- Exercising or some form of physical activity
- Journaling
- Listening to music
- Playing an instrument
- Learning stress management breathing techniques
- Using positive thinking
- Meditating
- Performing yoga
- Using relaxation techniques

- Limiting caffeine, nicotine, and alcohol
- Maintaining good nutrition and fluid intake
- Getting sufficient rest and sleep
- Drinking chamomile tea or warm milk (warm milk releases tryptophan, a natural sleep inducer)
- Getting a massage
- Employing environmental interventions (e.g., being in a quiet area and having someone present)
- Taking prescribed medications

Using Humor to Relieve Anxiety

box 13-3

Nurses use humor in various circumstances and in diverse ways when faced with situations that produce stress in the work environment. Examples of difficult situations that might provoke the use of humor to decrease anxiety include dealing with difficult patients, work relationships, patient and family anxiety, patient care, mistakes, and miscellaneous nursing situations (Bourne, 2010; Wanzer, Booth-Butterfield, & Booth-Butterfield, 2005). The manner in which nurses use humor can be categorized as low humor (acting silly), nonverbal (gestures, making faces), impersonation, language/word play (witty, clever communication), other orientation (including others), expressiveness/general humor (joking), and laughter (Bourne, 2010; Wanzer, Booth-Butterfield, & Booth-Butterfield, 2005). Timing of delivery, individuals involved, and circumstances at hand are critical considerations whenever using humor to ease anxiety.

recurrences is important. Some of the following should be considered when working to minimize relapses:

- What triggers anxiety for the patient?
- What are the symptoms of the patient's anxiety disorder?
- What should the patient do when first noticing reoccurrence of symptoms?
- Who are the patient's supports?
- How does the patient access these supports?

Evaluation

During evaluation, the nurse determines whether the patient's goals and objectives have been met—fully, partially, or not at all—and notes the date the evaluation took place. Improvement is evaluated by seeing whether the specific, realistic, and measurable goals were attained. For example, if the goal indicated that sleep needed to increase by 1 hour within 3 days, and it increased by only half an hour, the patient's goal would be noted as partially met on the day of evaluation. If goals are written *specifically, realistically,* and *measurably,* evaluating their attainment is easier.

How well the patient is adhering to the treatment plan is part of evaluating the success of the treatment plan. Points to consider include whether or not the patient is following the medication regimen, attending counseling, participating in stress reduction activities, sleeping and eating well, and maintaining healthy support systems. In addition, it is important to determine whether the patient has begun using any complementary and alternative medical (CAM) therapies. Evaluating whether or not the CAM interventions are compatible with other treatments for the patient is critical. For example, if the patient were prescribed an SSRI antidepressant for co-morbid anxiety and depression and then began taking St. John's wort, the patient could develop serotonin syndrome, a potentially fatal condition (see Chapter 22).

Once patients begin to feel better, they often need reassurance and a reminder of the importance of continuing on their medications, as symptoms may return with abrupt discontinuation. Treatment with antidepressant medication may be continued 6 months to a year for a first-time episode of anxiety with co-morbid depression and maintained indefinitely with repeated exacerbation (Antai-Otong, 2008; Bandelow et al., 2012).

The frequency and nature of evaluation change as the patient progresses through the phases of healing. Depending on symptom severity, evaluations during the initial or relapse phase should occur more frequently and continue until the patient's anxiety symptoms are improved. During the recovery phase, patient symptoms stabilize. Evaluations can be less frequent with the understanding that any increase of anxiety symptoms or changes in the patient's overall health should be reported. During rehabilitation, the patient should be seen annually and be evaluated for any changes in weight, vital signs, and circumstances. Routine lab work should be performed annually.

A change in any one domain may not necessarily put patients with anxiety disorders at risk for relapse. However, reviewing with patients how they are doing in all domains (biological, psychological, sociological, cultural, and spiritual) may help identify areas that need attention or could increase patients' resilience. For example, if a patient discontinues antidepressant medication to become pregnant,

it would be important for the nurse to evaluate how the patient is doing while pregnant and without the medication. Pregnancy might enhance the patient's psychological, sociological, cultural, and spiritual domains while at the same time compromise the patient's biological domain if she were to experience heavy nausea and lose weight. Similarly, worrying about the health of her baby during pregnancy might compromise the patient's psychological domain.

Examples of other impacts on the domains might include the following:

- *Biological:* Side effects of medications, impact of various medication combinations, use of CAM treatments concomitantly with medications, resistance to treatment, and the need to change medications a number of times.
- *Social and cultural:* Lack of support from family and friends, stigma, finances.
- *Psychological and spiritual:* Self-imposed pressure to "be strong" and not need treatment "because I should be able to do this on my own."

Pause and Reflect

1. *How might patient vital signs inform assessment and care planning for the patient with anxiety?*
2. *How does the nurse prioritize nursing diagnoses for the patient with symptoms of an anxiety, obsessive–compulsive, or trauma- or stressor-related disorder?*
3. *How do severe levels of anxiety affect the patient's ability to learn information and follow a therapeutic regimen?*

From Suffering to Hope

Sometimes nurses have difficulty identifying patient suffering in relation to mental illness symptoms, especially in relation to anxiety symptoms. The nurse may wonder why the patient is reporting such a high level of distress when, in the nurse's mind, the circumstances may not seem to warrant such distress. Acknowledging the pain the patient is experiencing can advance and solidify the nurse–patient relationship. Patients want to feel they are not only being "heard" but also are really being "listened to" when they share their distress and suffering. It is not the nurse's role to judge whether or not the level of distress is warranted, but rather to assist the patient in lowering whatever level of distress is being expressed. The anxiety exhibited by the patient may indicate something more serious is occurring, as demonstrated during Sondra's disclosure to the mental health nurse.

Patients who are suffering as a result of stress, various anxiety disorders, or trauma- or stressor-related disorders often lose hope. They may feel overly burdened and oppressed. This is especially true when patients experience severe anxiety over a long period of time, as with PTSD. Whatever the basis for an individual's experience of anxiety and distress, the nurse has a unique opportunity to "break into" the cycle of intensifying anxiety by helping the patient direct the anxiety constructively and decrease the patient's experience of distress.

Hope will flow from meeting the immediate needs of patients. Working with a patient who feels low self-esteem and helping the patient regain self-worth promotes hope that the patient can return to a more normal level of functioning. The nurse may affirm the

PERCEPTIONS, THOUGHTS, & FEELINGS: Validating the Needs of a Patient with Obsessive–Compulsive Symptoms

Patient's behavior(s)	Nurse's perceptions, thoughts, feelings	Exploration with patient
Sondra is seen in an outpatient clinic. Sondra is seated in a chair in the NP's examining room. Her eyebrows are furrowed slightly, and she is hunched over. When the RN walks into the room, Sondra looks up as if through her eyebrows.	*Perceptions:* Sondra looks worried. *Thoughts:* I wonder what is going on.	*Nurse:* Hello, Sondra. You have a worried look on your face. What brings you here today?

VALIDATION Carol senses Sondra is worried and wants Sondra to state in her own words what she feels her needs are.

Patient's behavior(s)	Nurse's perceptions, thoughts, feelings	Exploration with patient
Sondra: Do you have something you can give me for my hands? They're all red and itchy.	*Perceptions:* Sondra's hands are really red and covered with a rash. *Thoughts:* I believe she has some kind of dermatitis, but I need a little more information. She does seem anxious. I need to know the cause of the dermatitis.	*Nurse:* Have you been exposed to any different irritants or put any new products on your hands lately?

VALIDATION Validating with Sondra whether her hands have come in contact with a potential irritant.

Patient's behavior(s)	Nurse's perceptions, thoughts, feelings	Exploration with patient
Sondra: Not really … ahhh, I have been washing my hands more than usual.	*Thoughts:* I wonder if she has been washing in a compulsive manner.	*Nurse:* What does "more than usual" mean for you, Sondra?

VALIDATION Clarifying exactly what Sondra means by "more than usual."

Patient's behavior(s)	Nurse's perceptions, thoughts, feelings	Exploration with patient
Sondra lifts her chin up and makes direct eye contact. *Sondra:* For the past 3 months I have been washing my hands 10 minutes each morning before I leave for work, when I arrive at work, on all my breaks, when I get home, before I go to bed, and any other time I think I may have been contaminated by something I touched. I'm crazy, aren't I?	*Thoughts:* I'm thinking Sondra needs to hear she isn't "crazy," but I also must address how her behaviors are impairing her functioning. *Feelings:* I hope I can help her.	*Nurse:* No, Sondra. You're not "crazy." That *is* a lot of hand washing, and it may have caused your rash. I hope we can work together so your hands will heal. I will ask the nurse practitioner to come in and see if she can give you something to promote healing. It also will be good for us to work together to help you feel less of a need to wash your hands so often. Does that make sense?

VALIDATION Affirming to Sondra that she is not "crazy" and enlisting her participation in getting help to stop her excessive hand washing.

Patient's behavior(s)	Nurse's perceptions, thoughts, feelings	Exploration with patient
Sondra: Yes, it does. I'm relieved to hear you say you don't think I'm crazy. I don't know how I'm going to stop washing my hands so often, because I am afraid of getting diseases from germs. I'm also afraid I'm going to lose my job, because I recently received a poor performance evaluation because I spend so much time washing my hands.	*Thoughts:* This is sounding like an obsessive–compulsive type of disorder. I think she probably should see someone in psychiatric–mental health for her obsessions and compulsions. I will have to approach this topic gently.	*Nurse:* Sondra, it sounds like you have a lot going on recently. I think you may be feeling pressured to wash your hands due to distress in your life. Does that sound like an accurate assessment of what is going on?

VALIDATION Inviting Sondra to acknowledge or disclaim the assessment.

Patient's behavior(s)	Nurse's perceptions, thoughts, feelings	Exploration with patient
Sondra: Yes. I have been under a great deal of stress. Sondra smiles some.	**Feelings:** I feel sorry for Sondra that she has experienced some difficult times. I want to help her. **Thoughts:** Her smile, even though small, makes me think she is "with me." I need to try to encourage her to see a counselor.	**Nurse:** Sondra, we have a wonderful nurse practitioner colleague who helps individuals who are struggling with issues that lead to heavy emotional distress. Do you think you might be willing to see her if I made a referral?

VALIDATION Continuing to enlist Sondra in the process of getting the help that she needs.

Patient's behavior(s)	Nurse's perceptions, thoughts, feelings	Exploration with patient
Sondra: I'd be willing to go at least once. It's difficult for me to connect with people sometimes.	**Thoughts:** At least she is willing to try. I will reassure her about my NP colleague.	**Nurse:** I'm pleased to hear that. Her name is Marilyn Whittaker and her office is here in town. I've made a number of referrals to her and have only heard good things about her. If you prefer to see someone else, I can give you additional names.

VALIDATION Empowering Sondra by giving her a choice of practitioners.

Patient's behavior(s)	Nurse's perceptions, thoughts, feelings	Exploration with patient
Sondra's eyes brighten slightly. **Sondra:** I'd like to see that Marilyn you mentioned. I know I have to do something. I haven't been getting any better lately. I feel stressed so much of the time.	**Thoughts:** Sondra seems committed to this plan and receptive to meeting with the psychiatric–mental health NP at least once. I want to affirm her health-seeking behaviors.	**Nurse:** I think it is important that you came in today to get started on treating your hands and feeling less stressed. I'd like to see you in a follow-up visit in a week about your hand condition. I believe Marilyn will be able to help you. Please let me know how you do after you see her. Are you ready for me to ask the secretary to make the referral?

VALIDATION Affirming Sondra's healthy choices and reassuring her of continued involvement by this NP in these current needs.

Patient's behavior(s)	Nurse's perceptions, thoughts, feelings	Exploration with patient
Sondra: That sounds okay.	**Thoughts:** This seems to have worked out well. I need to get the ointment samples and explain how she should use them. **Feelings:** I feel good about this interaction.	**Nurse:** I'll get some samples of ointment for the contact dermatitis and explain how to use them.

VALIDATION Tending to Sondra's physical need presented today.

Based on Orlando, I. J. (1972). *The Discipline and Teaching of Nursing Process (An Evaluative Study).* New York, NY: G. P. Putnam's Sons.

patient's self-worth by noting a strength or positive observation or characteristic of the patient. Specific examples might be sharing with the patient observations made about the patient's kindness to another patient; acknowledging patient efforts toward getting healthier; or affirming the patient's effective decision making.

Individuals with anxiety disorders, as well as those with moderate to high levels of anxiety, suffer on many levels. For a patient such as Sondra, decreasing her anxiety level can alleviate some of her suffering, promote healing, and assist her in moving toward recovery.

Sondra Rehabilitation Phase

APPLICATION
1. Address the 5 domains for Sondra:
a. Biological
b. Psychological
c. Sociological
d. Cultural
e. Spiritual
2. What level of anxiety does Sondra exhibit at this time?
3. What steps has Sondra taken to gain control of her anxiety? How or why have these been helpful?
4. How you would prioritize Sondra's needs during this encounter and why?

By the end of six months, Sondra has moved to a day position, socializes with a group of girls her age from work, and is feeling less threatened, although she does have some occasional dreams about the rape. She reports to Marilyn that she feels much less anxious generally, but does not feel ready to date again yet. Sondra has begun to take an assertiveness training class and is thinking about enrolling at the local community college to study early childhood education. Sondra and Marilyn acknowledge that Sondra has returned to a more productive lifestyle and schedule their next appointment in 6 months' time. Sondra asks how long she will need to be on sertraline (Zoloft). Marilyn tells her they can look at how she is doing over the next 6 months and may be able to discontinue it at the end of that time if things continue to progress. She asks Sondra to think about it but assures her that they will work together to determine what is best for Sondra.

Sondra also follows up with Carol for a recheck on her skin. Her mother and grandmother accompany her to the appointment. Sondra updates Carol on her progress and adds that things have been hard for her family since her aunt died. Carol asks Sondra's mother and grandmother how they are doing. They tell Carol that they went to see Marilyn as a family, "because she was really helpful before, and we are glad you gave us her name for Sondra." Carol comforts and acknowledges the family's care for one another. Carol also notes that Sondra's skin continues to look good; determines that Sondra is doing well, in spite of this recent loss; encourages Sondra to call if she has any concerns. Carol also verbalizes support for the family's efforts to get help. Carol and Sondra agree that Sondra will return in a year's time for her annual physical unless she has any concerns before then.

Chapter Highlights

1. Anxiety is a universal and normal experience that may result in feelings of distress and suffering. If anxiety symptoms are not relieved, an individual may develop one or more anxiety disorders.

2. Anxiety has a high rate of co-morbidity with depression and substance disorders.

3. Culture can affect how an individual expresses anxiety, copes with anxiety, and receives help to handle anxiety.

4. Anxiety disorders include separation anxiety disorder, selective mutism, phobias, social anxiety disorder, panic disorder, and generalized anxiety disorder.

5. Obsessive–compulsive and related disorders have been identified with distinct neural circuit involvement that is different from the other anxiety disorders.

6. Obsessive–compulsive and related disorders include body dysmorphic disorder, hoarding disorder, trichotillomania, and skin-picking disorder.

7. Trauma- and stressor-related disorders include reactive attachment disorder, dishinhibited social engagement disorder, posttraumatic stress disorder, acute stress disorder, and adjustment disorder with various specifiers.

8. Cognitive–behavioral therapy (CBT) is one of the most effective treatments for anxiety disorders.

9. Antianxiety (anxiolytic) medications are the most widely prescribed medications in the United States. They are highly addictive and may cause withdrawal symptoms if stopped abruptly.

10. Antidepressant medications are considered the first-line treatment for anxiety.

11. Nurses can promote patient healing through thorough assessment, developing a plan of care in collaboration with the patient and the health care team, and identifying and reducing factors that have a negative impact on the success of interventions.

NCLEX®-RN Questions

1. The nurse is assessing a patient with an anxiety disorder. Which key finding best supports a neurobiological basis for the illness?
   a. The patient has a family history of anxiety.
   b. The patient has a co-morbid medical illness.
   c. The patient has multiple stressors.
   d. The patient has had positive responses to antianxiety medication.

2. The nurse is documenting assessment findings for a patient presenting with symptoms of anxiety. Under which category would the nurse include the observation that the patient is constantly scanning the environment to detect threats?
   a. Spiritual domain
   b. Cultural domain
   c. Biological domain
   d. Psychological domain

3. The nurse is working with a patient who is overcome by feelings of anxiety, each time experiencing thoughts of losing control. The patient states that reorganizing the environment temporarily relieves the anxiety. The nurse correctly interprets this as the use of which defense mechanism?
   a. Denial
   b. Undoing
   c. Projection
   d. Conversion

4. The nurse is using Peplau's four levels of anxiety as a model for assessing a patient who has been experiencing panic attacks. At which stage would the nurse anticipate detecting the onset of tachycardia and tachypnea?
   a. Mild +1
   b. Moderate +2
   c. Severe +3
   d. Panic +4

5. The nurse is caring for a patient presenting with symptoms of anxiety. The patient states that he has started to avoid any situations that induce panic, such as going to the mall or the theater without a family member. The nurse recognizes that the patient's symptoms are most consistent with which type of anxiety disorder?
   a. Agoraphobia
   b. Social anxiety
   c. Panic disorder
   d. Separation anxiety

6. The nurse is evaluating a patient who has been taking fluvoxamine (Luvox) for the management of obsessive–compulsive disorder (OCD) for 1 week. Which statements by the patient would be cause for concern? Select all that apply.
   a. "My thoughts and compulsions are still bothersome sometimes."
   b. "I have needed to drink more because my mouth is frequently dry."
   c. "I take this medication when I experience the compulsion to clean."
   d. "My spouse is concerned that I will become addicted to this medication."
   e. "I have been using Ativan as needed when I have trouble getting to sleep."

7. The nurse is planning care for a patient experiencing an anxiety disorder. Which variable is essential for the nurse to consider first?
   a. The research supporting various treatment modalities
   b. The patient's personal perspective on the anxiety disorder
   c. The behavioral manifestations related to mental health domains
   d. The nurse's previous experience with patients with similar disorders

Answers may be found on the Pearson student resource site: nursing.pearsonhighered.com

Pearson Nursing Student Resources   Find additional review materials at **nursing.pearsonhighered.com**

References

Adams, M., Holland, N., & Urban, C. (2014). *Pharmacology for Nurses: A Pathophysiologic Approach* (4th ed.). Upper Saddle River, NJ: Prentice Hall.

Aggarwal, N. K. (2012). The psychiatric cultural formulation: Translating medical anthropology into clinical practice. *Journal of Psychiatric Practice, 18*(2), 73–85.

Alarcon, R. D., Becker, A. E., Lewis-Fernandez, R. L., Like, R. C., Desai, P., Foulks, E., . . . Primm, A. (2009). Issues for DSM-V: The role of culture in psychiatric diagnosis. *Journal of Nervous and Mental Disease, 197*(8), 559–560.

American Psychiatric Association. (2000). *Diagnostic and Statistical Manual of Mental Disorders*, Fourth Edition, Text Revision. Arlington, VA: American Psychiatric Association.

American Psychiatric Association. (2013). *Diagnostic and Statistical Manual of Mental Disorders* (5th ed.). Washington, DC: American Psychiatric Publishers.

Andrews, G., Hobbs, M. J., Borkovec, T. D., Beesdo, K., Craske, M. G., Heimberg, R. G., . . . Stanley, M. A. (2010). Generalized worry disorder: A review of DSM-IV generalized anxiety disorder and options for DSM-V. *Depression and Anxiety, 27*(2), 134–147.

Antai-Otong, D. (2008). The art of prescribing. *Perspectives in Psychiatric Care, 44*(1), 48–53.

Ash, L. & Miller, C. (2013). Interprofessional collaboration for improving patient and population health. In S. M. Denisco & A. M. Barker (Eds.). *Advanced Practice Nursing: Evolving Roles for the Transformation of the Profession.* Burlington, MA: Jones & Bartlett Learning, pp. 631–653.

Baldwin, D. S. (2008). Room for improvement in the pharmacological treatment of anxiety disorders. *Current Pharmaceutical Design, 14*, 3482–3491.

Bandelow, B., Sher, L., Bunevicius, R., Hollander, E., Kasper, S., Zohar, J., & Möller, H. J. (2012). Guidelines for the pharmacological treatment of anxiety disorders, obsessive-compulsive disorder and posttraumatic stress disorder in primary care. *International Journal of Psychiatry in Clinical Practice, 16*(2), 77–84.

Benedek, D. M., Friedman, M. J., Zatzick, D., & Ursano, R. J. (2009). Guideline watch (March 2009): Practice guideline for the treatment of patients with acute stress disorder and posttraumatic stress disorder. *FOCUS: The Journal of Lifelong Learning in Psychiatry, 7*(2), 204–213.

Blanchette, I., Richards, A., & Cross, A. (2007). Anxiety and the interpretation of ambiguous facial expressions: The influence of contextual cues. *Quarterly Journal of Experimental Psychology, 60*(8), 1101–1115.

Bogels, S. M., Alden, L., Beidel, D. C., Clark, L. A., Pine, D. S., Stein, M. B., & Voncken, M. (2010). Social anxiety disorder: Questions and answers for the DSM-V. *Depression and Anxiety, 27*(2), 168–189.

Bourne, E. J. (2010). *The Anxiety and Phobia Workbook* (5th ed.). Oakland, CA: New Harbinger Publications, Inc.

Brown, T. M., & Fee, E. (2002). Voices from the past. *American Journal of Public Health, 92*(10), 1593–1596.

Bryant, R. A., Friedman, M. J., Spiegel, D., Ursano, R., & Strain, J. (2011). A review of acute stress disorder in DSM-5. *Depression Anxiety, 28*, 802–817.

Cannon, W. B. (1915). *Bodily Changes in Pain, Hunger, Fear and Rage.* New York, NY: D. Appleton & Company.

Cannon, W. (1939). *The Wisdom of the Body* (2nd ed.). New York, NY: Norton Publishers.

Cheung R. Y., & Au, T. K. (2011). Nursing students' anxiety and clinical performance. *Journal of Nursing Education, 50*, 286–289.

Cooper, J., & Barnett, M. (2005). Aspects of caring for dying patients cause anxiety to first year student nurses. *International Journal of Palliative Nursing 11*(8), 423–430.

Craske, M. G., Kircanski, K., Epstein, A., Wittchen, H.-U., Pine, D. S., Lewis-Fernández, R., & Hinton, D. (2010). Panic disorder: a review of DSM-IV panic disorder and proposals for DSM-V. *Depression and Anxiety, 27*(2), 93–112.

Craven, M. A., & Bland, R. (2006). Better practices in collaborative mental health care: An analysis of the evidence base. *Canadian Journal of Psychiatry, 51*(Supplement 1), 1S–72S.

Curlin, F. A., Lawrence, R. E., Odell, S., Chin, M. H., Lantos, J. D., Koenig, H. G., & Meador, K. G. (2007). Religion, spirituality, and medicine: Psychiatrists' and other physicians' differing observations, interpretations, and clinical approaches. *American Journal of Psychiatry, 164*(12), 1825–1831.

Cutshall, S. M., Fenske, L. L., Kelly, R. F., Phillips, B. R., Sundt, T. M., & Bauer, B. A. (2007). Creation of a healing enhancement program at an academic medical center. *Complementary Therapies in Clinical Practice, 13*(4), 217–223.

Davis, J. L. (2006). Best ways to ease anxiety disorders: Meditation and other relaxation techniques work equally well against anxiety. Available at http://www.webmd.com/anxiety-panic/guide/20061101/best-ways-to-ease-anxiety-disorders

Farach, F. J., Pruitt, L. D., Jun, J. J., Jerud, A. B., Zoellner, L. A., & Roy-Byrne, P. P. (2012). Pharmacological treatment of anxiety disorders: Current treatments and future directions. *Journal of Anxiety Disorders, 26*(8), 833–843.

Flaskerud, J. H. (2000). Ethnicity, culture, and neuropsychiatry. *Issues in Mental Health Nursing, 21*, 5–29.

Freud, A. (1946). *The Ego and the Mechanisms of Defence*. New York, NY: International Universities Press, Inc.

Freud, S. (1963). The common neurotic state. In J. Strachey, J. (Ed.). *The Standard Edition of the Complete Psychological Works of Sigmund Freud*, Volume 16, Part III. London, UK: Hogarth, pp. 378–391.

Friedman, M. J., Resick, P. A., Bryant, R. A., & Brewin, C. R. (2011). Considering PTSD for DSM-5. *Depression and Anxiety, 28*(9), 750–769.

Galovski, T. E., Monson, C., Bruce, S. E., & Resick, P. A. (2009). Does cognitive–behavioral therapy for PTSD improve perceived health and sleep impairment? *Journal of Traumatic Stress, 22*(3), 197–204.

Gillespie, C. F., Phifer, J., Bradley, B., & Ressler, K. J. (2009). Risk and resilience: Genetic and environmental influences on development of the stress response. *Depression Anxiety, 26*(11), 984–992.

Godlewski, S. (2006). Vitamins for anxiety and panic disorders. Available at http://ezinearticles.com/?Vitamins-for-Anxiety-and-Panic-Disorders&id=301888

Gorman, J. M. (1992). Anxiety and anxiety disorders. In R. I. Kass, J. M. Oldham, & H. Pardes, (Eds.). *The Columbia University College of Physicians and Surgeons Complete Home Guide to Mental Health*. New York, NY: Henry Holt, pp. 99–107.

Grant, J. E., & Odlaug, B. L. (2009). Update on pathological skin picking. *Current Psychiatry Reports, 11*(4), 283–288.

Griffin, M. T., Salman, A., Lee, Y., Seo, Y., & Fitzpatrick, J. J. (2008). A beginning look at the spiritual practices of older adults. *Journal of Christian Nursing, 25*(2), 100–102.

Hall, C. S. (1954). *A Primer of Freudian Psychology*. New York, NY: The World Publishing Company.

Harmon, H., Langley, A., & Ginsburg, G. S. (2006). The role of gender and culture in treating youth with anxiety disorders. *Journal of Cognitive Psychotherapy, 20*(3), 301–310.

Harvard Mental Health Letter. (2009). Yoga for anxiety and depression. Available at http://www.health.harvard.edu/newsletters/Harvard_Mental_Health_Letter/2009/April/Yoga-for-anxiety-and-depression

Health Central Network. (2011). Medications. Available at http://www.health-central.com/anxiety/introduction-000028_7-145.html

Holmes, T. H., & Rahe, R. H. (1967). The social readjustment rating scale. *Journal of Psychosomatic Research, 11*, 213–218.

Jayakody, K., Gunadasa, S., & Hosker, C. (2014). Exercise for anxiety disorders: A systematic review. *British Journal of Sports Medicine, 48*(3), 187–196.

Kaya, F., Özcan, A., & Yilmaz, M. (2013). Comparing communication and empathic ability levels of nurses with patients' perception of nursing care. *Peak Journal of Public Health and Management, 1*(1), 1–8.

Kessler, R. C., Berglund, P. A, Demler, O., Jin, R., & Walters, E. E. (2005). Lifetime prevalence and age-of-onset distributions of DSM-IV disorders in the National Comorbidity Survey Replication (NCS-R). *Archives of General Psychiatry, 62*(6), 593–602.

Kessler, R. C., Chiu, W. T., Demler, O., & Walters, E. E. (2005). Prevalence, severity, and comorbidity of twelve-month DSM-IV disorders in the National Comorbidity Survey Replication (NCS-R). *Archives of General Psychiatry, 62*(6), 617–627.

Kessler, R. C., Ruscio, A. M., Shear, K., & Wittchen, H. U. (2010). Epidemiology of anxiety disorders. *Current Topics in Behavioral Neuroscience, 2*, 21–35.

Kirmayer, L. J., & Sartorius, N. (2007) Cultural models and somatic syndromes. *Psychosomatic Medicine, 69*, 832–840.

Lamers, F., van Oppen, P., Comijs, H. C., Smit, J. H., Spinhoven, P., van Balkom, A. J.,... Penninx, B. W. (2011). Comorbidity patterns of anxiety and depressive disorders in a large cohort study: The Netherlands Study of Depression and Anxiety (NESDA). *Journal of Clinical Psychiatry, 72*(3), 341–348.

Lazarus, R. S., & Folkman, S. (1984). *Stress, Appraisal, and Coping*. New York, NY: Springer Publishing Company.

LeBeau, R. T., Glenn, D., Liao, B., Wittchen, H.-U., Beesdo-Baum, K., Ollendick, T., & Craske, M. G. (2010). Specific phobia: A review of DSM-IV specific phobia and preliminary recommendations for DSM-V. *Depression and Anxiety, 27*(2), 148–167.

Leckman, J. F., Denys, D., Simpson, H. B., Mataix-Cols, D., Hollander, E., Saxena, S.,... Stein, D. J. (2010). Obsessive–compulsive disorder: A review of the diagnostic criteria and possible subtypes and dimensional specifiers for DSM-V. *Depression and Anxiety, 27*(6), 507–527.

Leonard, B. E., & Myint, A. (2009). The psychoneuroimmunology of depression. *Human Psychopharmacology: Clinical and Experimental, 24*(3), 165–175.

LeRoy, S. (2006). What are the best natural herbs for anxiety? Available at http://ezinearticles.com/?What-Are-The-Best-Natural-Herbs-for-Anxiety?&id=337960

Lewis-Fernández, R., Hinton, D. E., Laria, A. J., Patterson, E. H., Hofmann, S. G., Craske, M. G.,... Liao, B. (2010). Culture and the anxiety disorders: Recommendations for DSM-V. *Depression and Anxiety, 27*(2), 212–229.

Lieberman, J. A., & Tasman, A. (2006). *A Handbook of Psychiatric Drugs*. Hoboken, NJ: John Wiley & Sons, Inc.

Lindert, J., & Schinina, G. (2012). Mental health of refugees and asylum-seekers. In B. Rechel, W. Devillé, P. Mladovsky, B. Rijks, & R. Petrova-Benedict, (Eds.). *Migration and Health in the European Union*. New York, NY: McGraw-Hill Companies, pp. 169–181.

Mataix-Cols, D., Frost, R. O., Pertusa, A., Clark, L. A., Saxena, S., Leckman, J. F.,... Wilhelm, S. (2010). Hoarding disorder: A new diagnosis for DSM-V? *Depression and Anxiety, 27*(6), 556–572.

Mayo Clinic. (2011). Trichotillomania: Symptoms. Available at http://www.mayoclinic.com/health/trichotillomania/DS00895/DSECTION=symptoms

Mayo Clinic Staff. (2011). Depression and anxiety: Exercise eases symptoms. Available at http://www.mayoclinic.com/health/depression-and-exercise/MH00043

Mayo Clinic. (2012). Panic attacks and panic disorder: Symptoms. Available at http://www.mayoclinic.com/health/panic-attacks/DS00338/DSECTION=symptoms

Medline Plus. (2013). Panic disorder with agoraphobia. Available at http://www.nlm.nih.gov/medlineplus/ency/article/000923.htm

Melincavage, S. M. (2011). Student nurses' experiences of anxiety in the clinical setting. *Nurse Education Today, 31*(8), 785–789.

Mohr, C., & Schneider, S. (2013). Anxiety disorders. *European Child and Adolescent Psychiatry, 22*(1), S17–S22.

Montgomery, E. C., Kunik, M. E., Wilson, N., Stanley, M. A., & Weiss, B. (2010). Can paraprofessionals deliver cognitive-behavioral therapy to treat anxiety and depressive symptoms? *Bulletin of the Menninger Clinic, 74*(1), pp. 45-62.

Moscaritolo, J. M. (2009) Interventional strategies to decrease nursing student anxiety in the clinical learning environment. *Journal of Nursing Education, 48*(1), 17–23.

Mynatt, S., & Cunningham, P. (2007). Unraveling anxiety and depression. *The Nurse Practitioner, 32*(8), 28–36.

National Alliance on Mental Illness. (2012). Obsessive compulsive disorder. Available at http://www.nami.org/Template.cfm?Section=By_Illness&Template=/TaggedPage/TaggedPageDisplay.cfm&TPLID=54&ContentID=23035

National Center for PTSD. (2006). Facts about PTSD. Available at http://psychcentral.com/lib/2006/facts-about-ptsd/

National Institute of Mental Health. (2008). Anxiety disorders. Available at http://www.nimh.nih.gov/health/publications/anxiety-disorders/complete-publication.shtml

National Institute of Mental Health. (2010). Mental Health: A Report of the Surgeon General. Available at http://www.surgeongeneral.gov/library/mental-health/chapter4/sec2.html

National Institute of Mental Health. (2013). What are the signs and symptoms of OCD? Available at http://www.nimh.nih.gov/health/publications/obsessive-compulsive-disorder-when-unwanted-thoughts-take-over/what-are-the-signs-and-symptoms-of-ocd.shtml

Olatunji, B. O., Broman-Fulks, J. J., Bergman, S. M., Green, B. A., & Zlomke, K. R. (2010). A taxometric investigation of the latent structure of worry: Dimensionality and associations with depression, anxiety, and stress, *Behavior Therapy, 41*, 212–228.

Orlando, I. J. (1961). *The Dynamic Nurse-Patient Relationship*. New York, NY: G. P. Putnam's Sons.

Orlando, I. J. (1972). *The Discipline and Teaching of Nursing Process (An Evaluative Study)*. New York, NY: G. P. Putnam's Sons.

Peplau, H. (1963). A working definition of anxiety. In S. Burd & M. Marshall, (Eds.). *Some Clinical Approaches to Psychiatric Nursing*. New York, NY: Macmillan, pp. 323–327.

Perry, P. J., Alexander, B., Liskow, B. I., & DeVane, C. L., (2007). *Psychotropic Drug Handbook* (8th ed.). New York, NY: Lippincott Williams & Wilkins.

Phillips, K. A., Wilhelm, S., Koran, L. M., Didie, E. R., Fallon, B. A., Feusner, J., & Stein, D. J. (2010). Body dysmorphic disorder: Some key issues for DSM-V. *Depression and Anxiety, 27*(6), 573–591.

Potter, M. L., & Bockenhauer, B. J. (2000). Implementing Orlando's nursing theory: A pilot study. *Journal of Psychosocial Nursing and Mental Health Services, 38*, 14–21.

Radua, J., van den Heuvel, O. A., Surguladze, S., & Mataix-Cols, D. (2010). Meta-analytical comparison of voxel-based morphometry studies in obsessive-compulsive disorder vs other anxiety disorders. *Archives of General Psychiatry, 67*(7), 701–711.

Rouse, J. (2010). Six alternative treatments for anxiety and panic attacks. Available at http://life.gaiam.com/gaiam/p/AnxietyandPanicAttacksTreatthe-CausesWith.html

Ruscio, A. M., Stein, D. J., Chiu, W. T., & Kessler, R. C. (2010). The epidemiology of obsessive–compulsive disorder in the National Comorbidity Survey Replication. *Molecular Psychiatry, 15*, 55–63.

Scheeringa, M. S., Zeanah, C. H., & Cohen, J. A. (2011). PTSD in children and adolescents: Toward an empirically based algorithm. *Depression and Anxiety, 28*(9), 770–782.

Scott, S., & Beidel, D. C. (2011). Selective mutism: An update and suggestions for future research. *Current Psychiatry Reports, 13*(4), 251–257.

Segerstrom, S. C., & Miller, G. E. (2004). Psychological stress and the human immune system: A meta-analytic study of 30 years of inquiry. *Psychological Bulletin, 130*(4), 601–630.

Selye, H. (1950). Stress and the general adaptation syndrome. *British Medical Journal, 4667*, 1383–1392.

Selye, H. (1956). *The Stress of Life*. New York, NY: McGraw-Hill

Sleep Disorders Center of University of Maryland Medical Center. (2013). Sleep hygiene: Helpful hints to help you sleep. Available at http://www.umm.edu/sleep/sleep_hyg.htm

Specific Phobias. (2014). Available at http://www.webmd.com/anxiety-panic/specific-phobias

Sprangers, M. A. G., Bartels, M., Veenhoven, R., Baas, F., Martin, N. G., Mosing, M., ...The GENEQOL Consortium. (2010). Which patient will feel down, which will be happy? The need to study the genetic disposition of emotional states. *Quality of Life Research, (19)*10, 1429–1437.

Stahl, S. M. (2011). *Essential Pharmacology—The Prescriber's Guide*. New York, NY: Cambridge University Press.

Stallwood, J., & Stoll, R. (1975). Spiritual dimension of nursing practice. In I. L. Beland & J. Y. Passos (Eds.). *Clinical Nursing* (3rd ed.). New York, NY: Macmillan, pp. 1086–1098.

Stein, D. J., Craske, M. G., Friedman, M. J., & Phillips, K. A. (2011). Meta-structure issues for the DSM-5: How do anxiety disorders, obsessive–compulsive and related disorders, post-traumatic disorders, and dissociative disorders fit together? *Current Psychiatry Reports, 13*(4), 248–250.

Stein, D. J., Fineberg, N. A., Bienvenu, O. J., Denys, D., Lochner, C., Nestadt, G., Leckman, J.F., Rauch, S.L., & Phillips, K. A. (2010a). Should OCD be classified as an anxiety disorder in DSM-5? *Depression and Anxiety, 27*(6), 495–506.

Stein, D. J., Grant, J. E., Franklin, M. E., Keuthen, N., Lochner, C., Singer, H. S., & Woods, D. W. (2010b). Trichotillomania (hair pulling disorder), skin picking disorder, and stereotypic movement disorder: Toward DSM-V. *Depression and Anxiety, 27*(6), 611–626.

Stein, D. J., Phillips, K. A., Bolton, D., Fulford, K. W. M., Sadler, J. Z., & Kendler, K. S. (2010c). What is a mental/psychiatric disorder? From DSM-IV to DSM-V. *Psychological Medicine, 40*(11), 1759–1765.

Stephenson, P. L. (2006). Before the teaching begins: Managing patient anxiety prior to providing education. *Clinical Journal of Oncology, 10*(2), 241–245.

Strain, J. J., & Friedman, M. J. (2011). Considering adjustment disorders as stress response syndromes for DSM-5. *Depression and Anxiety, 28*(9), 818–823.

Substance Abuse and Mental Health Services Administration. (2014). National Registry Evidence-Based Programs and Practices. Prolonged exposure therapy for posttraumatic stress disorders. Available at http://www.nrepp.samhsa.gov/ViewIntervention.aspx?id=89.

Szpak, J. L., & Kameg, K. M. (2013). Simulation decreases nursing student anxiety prior to communication with mentally ill patients. *Clinical Simulation in Nursing, 9*(1), e13–e19.

Tan, C., Chen, Y., Wu, Y., & Chen, S. (2013). Chinese medicine for mental disorder and its applications in psychosomatic diseases. *Alternative Therapies in Health & Medicine, 19*(1), 59–69.

Tefera, L., Shah, A. M., & Hsu, K. (2012). Anxiety. Available at http://www.emedicine.com/EMERG/topic35.htm

Tull, M. (2008). How do CBT and psychodynamic treatments differ? Available at http://ptsd.about.com/od/faq/f/CBTPsychodyn.htm

Trichotillomania Learning Center. (2012). Skin Picking: Signs and Symptoms. Available at http://www.trich.org/about/skin-signs-symptoms.html

U.S. Department of Veterans Affairs. (2010). Epidemiological facts about PTSD. Available at http://ncptsd.va.gov/ncmain/ncdocs/fact_shts/fs_epidemiological.html

U.S. Department of Veterans Affairs. (2012). How common is PTSD? Available at http://www.ptsd.va.gov/public/pages/how-common-is-ptsd.asp

U.S. Office of the Surgeon General; U.S. Center for Mental Health Services; National Institute of Mental Health. (2001). Mental Health: Culture, Race, and Ethnicity: A Supplement to Mental Health: A Report of the Surgeon General. Rockville, MD: U.S. Substance Abuse and Mental Health Services Administration. Available at http://www.ncbi.nlm.nih.gov/books/NBK44246/#A1014

University of Maryland Medical Center. (2013). Anxiety Disorders—Risk Factors. Available at http://www.umm.edu/patiented/articles/who_gets_anxiety_disorders_000028_3.htm

Wang, C., Bannuru, B., Ramel, J., Kupelnick, B., Scott, T., & Schmid, C. H. (2010). Tai chi on psychological well-being: Systematic review and meta-analysis. *BMC Complementary and Alternative Medicine*. Available at http://www.biomedcentral.com/1472-6882/10/23

Wanzer, M., Booth-Butterfield, M., & Booth-Butterfield, S. (2005). "If we didn't use humor, we'd cry": Humorous coping communication in health care settings. *Journal of Health Communication, 10*, 105–125.

Wittchen, H.-U., Gloster, A. T., Beesdo-Baum, K., Fava, G. A., & Craske, M. G. (2010). Agoraphobia: A review of the diagnostic classificatory position and criteria. *Depression and Anxiety, 27*(2), 113–133.

Yeh, M., Hough, R., McCabe, K., Lau, A., & Garland, A. (2004.). Parental beliefs about the causes of child problems: Exploring facial/ethnic patterns. *Journal of the American Academy of Child and Adolescent Psychiatry, 43*(5), 605–610.

Zeanah, C. H., & Gleason, M. M. (2010). *Reactive Attachment Disorder: A Review for DSM-V*. Washington, DC: American Psychiatric Association.

Somatic Symptom Disorders and Dissociative Disorders

14

Pamela Marcus

Learning Outcomes

1. Examine the etiology of somatic symptom disorders and dissociative disorders.

2. Summarize the impact of biological, psychological, sociological, cultural, and spiritual domains on somatic symptom disorders and dissociative disorders.

3. Contrast the symptoms of somatic symptom disorders and dissociative disorders.

4. Appraise key symptoms and characteristics of dissociative disorders and how they affect care for patients in medical settings.

5. Differentiate pharmacologic and nonpharmacologic therapies used in the treatment of somatic symptom disorders and dissociative disorders.

6. Plan evidence-based nursing care for patients with somatic symptom disorders and dissociative identity disorders.

Key Terms

alexithymia, 276
amnesia, 282
conversion disorder, 277
depersonalization, 282
derealization, 282
dissociation, 282
dissociative identity disorder, 282
dissociative fugues, 284
factitious disorder, 278
functional neurological symptom disorder, 277
illness anxiety disorder, 277
somatic symptom disorder, 275

Grace Initial Onset

Grace is a 45-year-old married woman who does not have any children. Ten years ago, she sustained a fall at work, which caused a back injury. She was unable to return to work after the fall and received surgery and physical therapy over a period of 3 months. Even though her MRI and physical therapy evaluation showed that the injury was almost healed, Grace experienced a great deal of pain that reminded her of the original injury. She would report the pain as excruciating and rate it as a 10 out of 10, especially when sitting. She was unable to return to work after attempting several times, including using the option of working from home. She was evaluated by a pain specialist, who ordered a trans-cutaneous electric nerve stimulating (TENS) unit, therapeutic massage, trigger point injections, and pain medications. The patient did not experience any relief from the TENS unit or the therapeutic mas-sage. She would increase the pain medications on her own and was seen as "medication seeking" by the urgent clinic staff when she would seek care there for "breakthrough pain." Grace has been unable to function because of the pain that "travels" though several areas in her body. She spends the major-ity of her time in bed, getting up for meals, and taking care of her pets. Her marriage has become strained; her husband will not discuss her physical problems, as he feels she should "push through the pain." They no longer go out together, nor do they sleep together. Her husband is angry that she spends the majority of her time in bed. He feels that he cannot participate in her staying in bed and is staying in the spare bedroom. Her feeling is that "no one has walked in my shoes." She reports pain in her jaw and her back, sometimes radiating down her legs, alternating between legs. Grace has diges-tive problems, including alternating between constipation and diarrhea. She reports difficulty swallow-ing at times and heartburn after meals. Grace reports excruciating menstrual pains, with a heavy flow and pain that she rates as a 9 on a scale from 0 to 10. Her friends are frustrated with her, as she will make plans to meet them for lunch and then will cancel at the last minute, owing to pain or gastric discomfort. Her friends have commented to her that she needs to talk about something other than her medical illnesses.

APPLICATION

1. Assess Grace in the five domains:
   a. Biological
   b. Psychological
   c. Sociological
   d. Cultural
   e. Spiritual

2. In what ways do you think Grace may be suffering? Why?

3. How would you prioritize Grace's needs during this encounter? What is your rationale?

4. What interventions would assist Grace to begin to determine some hope in her situation?

Introduction

This chapter covers two very complex sets of disorders, both of which can cause great disruption in the lives of individual patients and fam-ilies, as well as on the inpatient care unit. The disorders classified in the DSM-5 as somatic symptom and related disorders are discussed first. These include somatic symptom disorder (previously called somatization disorder), functional neurological symptom disorder (previously called conversion disorder), illness anxiety disorder (pre-viously called hypochondriasis), and factitious disorder. Individuals who have these disorders are usually seen by physicians because the presentation of these disorders centers on physical symptoms, although they have a strong psychological component. Individuals who have any one of these disorders experience a great deal of suffer-ing. Often, family members and health care practitioners discount the patient's symptoms. The nurse can act as an advocate for the patient with a somatic symptom disorder by understanding these disorders and assisting the patient to articulate his or her needs.

Next, the chapter focuses on dissociative disorders. Individuals with these disorders also sustain a great deal of suffering. This category includes dissociative identity disorder, dissociative amnesia, and derealization/depersonalization disorder. These disorders are associ-ated with a traumatic experience in which the individual unconsciously dissociates as a coping mechanism to deal with an overwhelming, potentially life-threatening psychological trauma. The individual may not remember the trauma until an environmental cue causes a flash-back. This can happen many years after the original trauma.

Individuals with dissociative disorders often are unable to reach out to others and remain isolated, thinking that other people will not understand what they are experiencing and that others will judge their actions or thoughts. Profound feelings of internal conflict, hopelessness, and worthlessness constrict the individual's thinking and prevent the ability to problem-solve. Nurses can assist patients with dissociative disorders by using the therapeutic relationship to listen to their problems without judging. This is critical, as these patients often are "not believed" and are labeled in a negative manner by the nursing and medical staff. This chapter gives the nurse the opportunity to gain understanding of both somatic symptom disor-ders and dissociative disorders.

SOMATIC SYMPTOM AND RELATED DISORDERS

Theoretical Foundations

Patients with somatic symptom and related disorders complain of somatic, or biological, symptoms. Although there may or may not be a co-occurring medical illness, these patients focus on their somatic complaints to the extent of risking functional impairment in all areas, including the biological domain (Table 14-1). Historically, individu-als who reported multiple body complaints that did not appear to

have "medical cause" were labeled as having "hysteria," which is Latin for "wandering uterus." In 1859, Charles Briquet began to conduct research in France to determine the causal factors for individuals who had these multiple somatic complaints. Briquet believed that the patients were not "hysterical" but that they had real-life stressors, such as abuse, rape, marital problems, and significant losses. He wrote about somatization in *Traité clinique et thérapeutique de*

Symptoms of Somatic Symptom and Related Disorders by Domain

table 14-1

Domain	Responses
Biological	• Anorexia, nausea, vomiting, diarrhea, bloating • Intolerance of certain foods, without an allergy • Apathy toward sexual activity, difficulty sustaining an erection or achieving ejaculation, menstrual irregularity, nausea and vomiting throughout pregnancy • Urinary retention • Blurred vision, double vision, blindness • Impaired coordination or balance, loss of touch • Seizures • Pain • Inability to hear • Difficulty swallowing, reduced speech volume
Psychological	• Dissociation • Hallucinations • Crying • Decreased interest • Decreased productivity • Depressed • Difficulty concentrating • Feelings of apprehension, helplessness, worthlessness • Focusing on past • Forgetfulness • Helplessness • Hypercritical • Irritability • Lack of interest or apathy • Persistent worrying • Preoccupation with negatives • Withdrawal
Sociological	• Feeling alone, believing no one understands the physical symptoms and therefore there is no one to turn to for help or support • Focus on physical feelings, therefore feeling unable to take part with hobbies or interests with others • Lacking a sense of relation to the whole of society, feelings of loneliness, feels judged by others • Challenged in relation to resources
Cultural	• Lack of connectedness to those with similar values or shared language or experiences due to focus on somatic sensations rather than on relating to others • Lack of access to services due to language or other cultural barriers
Spiritual	• Feeling a lack of connectedness with God or higher power and/or with others of like-minded beliefs • Struggling with faith • Struggling with meaning and purpose • Expressing feelings of guilt and stigma related to the physical symptoms

l'hystérie [Treatise on Hysteria] (Briquet, 1859, Dinwiddie, 2013; Loewenstein, 1990). Briquet devised a list of symptoms that he found to constitute this syndrome, later labeled as *Briquet's Syndrome* in DSM-III and reclassified as *somatization disorder* in DSM-IV.

Biological Domain

Patients with **somatic symptom disorder** and its related disorders express symptoms through their body, feeling pain and other somatic sensations that others may not experience (Figure 14-1). These sensations become the individual's focus and concern, often to the exclusion of other areas of life, resulting in functional impairment. Individuals with somatic symptom and related disorders have a more acute and heightened sense of pain and normal body sensations (American Psychiatric Association [APA], 2013). Imagine having a

microphone inside the body that amplifies each body sensation and sometimes distorts the interpretation of the body feeling; this is what occurs in somatic symptom disorders, resulting in the individual believing that he or she is experiencing a medical condition that has not been thoroughly investigated or diagnosed.

Research in the biological domain of somatic symptom and related disorders is minimal. One area to consider is the role Substance P may have on symptoms of pain and nausea. Substance P is a neuropeptide neurotransmitter that is involved in the dopamine reward system due to the activity of the neurokinen-1 receptor, which modulates the rewarding effects of opioids (Robinson et al., 2012). Substance P is involved in the regulation of affective behavior, emesis, and the experience of pain (Chappa, Audus, & Lunte, 2006). Although the current research on Substance P is pharmaceutical in

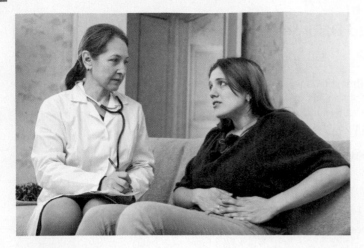

14-1   Patients with somatic symptom disorders often report pain as a predominant symptom.

Source: JackF/Russian Federation/Fotolia

nature, this neurotransmitter may be one of the structures involved in the biological domain of somatic symptom disorder.

Psychological Domain

Individuals with somatic symptom and related disorders are immersed in their bodily sensations, whereas their ability to experience the depth and range of emotions is limited. It is hypothesized that individuals who have somatic symptom disorders have the personality trait of **alexithymia**, which is defined as the inability to label feelings with words. Individuals suffering with alexithymia have difficulty identifying the affective states of self and others, which leads to misunderstanding of the emotional component of relationships. Alexithymia has been linked to early child abuse, posttraumatic stress disorder (PTSD), and early emotional neglect (Aust, Härtwig, Heuser, & Bajbouj, 2013). PTSD and alexithymia also have been linked to chronic pain. Balaban-Murat et al. (2012) studied medical students in Turkey who had migraine headaches. It was reported that the medical students who experienced several migraine headaches also satisfied the diagnostic criteria for PTSD and alexithymia. More research is needed to determine the relationship between alexithymia and somatic symptom disorders.

Another personality trait that is associated with individuals with somatic symptom and related disorders is negative affectivity. The DSM-5 identifies negative affectivity as an independent risk factor for having multiple somatic symptoms (APA, 2013).

Recent research has explored the emotional response individuals experience in relation to their physical state. DeSteno, Gross, and Kubzansky (2013) point out that early childhood distress occurring around ages 7 or 8 is associated with adult obesity, inflammation, and several physical illnesses. These authors suggest that the emotional responses that are experienced at that age can influence the physiologic response toward the events that the individual encounters. This has powerful implications for problem solving when an individual's physiological response is greater than the responses of others to the same stressors. Nurses can capture this information during a thorough assessment. Interventions based on reducing alexithymia and creating new options for problem-solving emotionally laden events, such as mindfulness meditation, can reduce some of the individual's focus on physiological processes (Grepmair et al., 2007).

Sociological Domain

Individuals who have somatic symptom and related disorders generally are female, older, and/or of lower socioeconomic status, with frequent unemployment and fewer years of education. Often there is a history of neglect, physical, and/or sexual abuse during childhood. Chronic physical illness and emotional illness, such as depression or an anxiety disorder, may also be present (APA, 2013).

Because of the extent of focus on their physical symptoms, individuals with somatic symptom disorders may not fully participate in family life or social activities. The individual may perceive the physical symptoms as restricting his or her ability to join in with a physical activity for fear that this participation may make the symptoms worse. The individual often feels alone and misunderstood by others.

Cultural Domain

The DSM-5 (APA, 2013) identifies somatic symptoms as being "culturally bound" syndromes. Worldwide research in primary care facilities and population-based studies demonstrates that there are similar numbers of individuals with somatic concerns and impairments across cultures. Individuals who seek care for multiple somatic concerns are comparable around the world and between ethnic groups in the same country.

Different cultures may describe the somatic changes differently, depending on the meaning of the symptom and the language used to describe the malady. (See Chapter 5 for a discussion and examples of culture-bound syndromes.)

Spiritual Domain

Individuals with somatic symptom and related disorders may seek care from multiple providers, including spiritual resources, as they feel as though other practitioners and family members do not take their symptoms seriously. Individuals may feel spiritually disengaged from others because others have a hard time relating to them. Additionally, patients may experience difficulty in their attempts to find meaning in their symptoms and to seek peace in their lives because of negative thoughts and beliefs.

Pause and Reflect

1. *When assessing the biological domain, what aspects of the patient's presentation may be specific to a somatic symptom disorder?*

2. *How does measuring the patient's experience of pain assist the nurse to understand the patient's suffering?*

3. *What aspects of patient history might be important to the assessment and care of patients with somatic symptom and related disorders?*

Specific Disorders

Individuals with somatic symptom and related disorders present to health care providers with a persistent focus on their physical sensations and with thoughts or behaviors that are negative, fearful, and distressed, along with a concern that the physical symptoms may be related to a life-threatening illness (APA, 2013). Disorders in this category include the following:

- Somatic Symptom Disorder
- Illness Anxiety Disorder

- Conversion Disorder (Functional Neurological Symptom Disorder)
- Psychological Factors Affecting Other Medical Conditions
- Factitious Disorder
- Other Specified Somatic Symptom and Related Disorder
- Unspecified Somatic Symptom and Related Disorder

All the somatic disorders involve symptoms that are physical in nature and cause significant distress and inability to function in daily life. Because individuals with the somatic disorders are commonly seen in primary care and medical offices, it is important for nurses in all settings to be able to recognize when individuals present with these disorders. Often, the patient is labeled as "difficult" or "complex," and sometimes there is a frustration between the clinician and patient that clouds the care delivery. When assessing patients with these diagnoses, it is important to obtain data on the physical manifestations of discomfort as well as the patient's thoughts and feelings about these symptoms and behaviors related to them. Patients with somatic disorders demonstrate maladaptive thoughts, feelings, and behavior patterns in relationship to their physical symptoms. The thoughts about the somatic concern are that the symptoms are due to a very serious illness that has not been discovered by the medical team. Patients with somatic disorders may constantly check their bodies to determine whether there is something wrong. They may become so focused on their condition that they are unable to have a quality relationship with family members, co-workers, and friends (APA, 2013).

Somatic Symptom Disorder

In addition to the symptoms stated earlier, some individuals with somatic symptom disorder report pain as a primary symptom (see DSM-5 Diagnostic Criteria for Somatic Symptom Disorder). Frequently, a diagnosis of the disorder is concurrent with a diagnosis of a medical illness. High levels of worry are common, and the disorder can dominate the individual's life if it becomes severe (APA, 2013).

Currently, it is unknown how many individuals have somatic symptom disorder. It is hypothesized that the prevalence of somatic symptom disorder may be around 5% to 7% of the general adult population. More women report somatic concerns than men; therefore, it is thought that a higher number of women than men will have this disorder (APA, 2013).

Illness Anxiety Disorder

Individuals who have **illness anxiety disorder** experience a preoccupation with having an illness, even though typically there are no physical symptoms of illness. If the individual has an illness, his or her concerns about the illness are excessive and disproportionate for the nature of the condition. Individuals with illness anxiety disorder have a high level of anxiety about health concerns and often obsessively monitor their own health status. Two types of behaviors typically manifest with this disorder. Some people seek care frequently, often checking their bodies for occurrences of illness and seeking tests and procedures to rule out an illness. The second type of symptoms manifest differently as avoidance behaviors, in which individuals do not seek care and avoid seeing practitioners for preventive care or refuse to visit family members or friends who may be in the hospital.

Illness anxiety disorder is a new disorder described in the DSM-5; prevalence statistics are based on estimates of the prior DSM-III and DSM-IV diagnosis of hypochondriasis. Prevalence of this disorder among individuals who have reported symptoms ranges from 1.3% to 10%, based on community surveys and population-based samples. There appears to be no difference in prevalence rates between men and women (APA, 2013).

Conversion Disorder (Functional Neurological Symptom Disorder)

Individuals who have symptoms of **conversion disorder (functional neurological symptom disorder)** experience one or more changes in the performance of a voluntary motor or sensory function; the changes are incompatible with a recognized neurologic or medical condition. Symptoms of abnormal voluntary motor function may

---

Diagnostic Criteria for Somatic Symptom Disorder   DSM-5

A. One or more somatic symptoms that are distressing or result in significant disruption of daily life.

B. Excessive thoughts, feelings, or behaviors related to the somatic symptoms or associated health concerns as manifested by at least one of the following:
   a. Disproportionate and persistent thoughts about the seriousness of one's symptoms.
   b. Persistently high level of anxiety about health or symptoms.
   c. Excessive time and energy devoted to these symptoms or health concerns.

C. Although any one somatic symptom may not be continuously present, the state of being symptomatic is persistent (typically more than 6 months).

Specify if:

With predominant pain (previously pain disorder): This specifier is for individuals whose somatic symptoms predominantly involve pain.

Specify if:

Persistent: A persistent course is characterized by severe symptoms, marked impairment, and long duration (more than 6 months).

Specify current severity:

Mild: Only one of the symptoms specified in Criterion B is fulfilled.

Moderate: Two or more of the symptoms specified in Criterion B are fulfilled.

Severe: Two or more of the symptoms specified in Criterion B are fulfilled, plus there are multiple somatic complaints (or one very severe somatic symptom).

Source: Reprinted with permission from the Diagnostic and Statistical Manual of Mental Disorders, Fifth Edition, (Copyright 2013). American Psychiatric Association.

include weakness or paralysis, abnormal movements, and abnormal extremity functioning or positions, whereas sensory symptoms may present as altered skin sensations or vision or hearing difficulties. Some individuals with conversion disorder may appear to have had an epileptic seizure, with abnormal limb shaking and impaired or loss of consciousness. This is called *psychogenic* or *nonepileptic seizure*. Some individuals experience changes in consciousness, which may appear to be syncope or coma. Other symptoms of conversion disorder include reduced or absent speech volume (dysphonia or aphonia); changes in the ability to articulate words (dysarthria) or a sensation of a lump in the throat (globus), and diplopia (double vision). Some patients with conversion disorder may display a lack of concern about their symptoms (APA, 2013).

PRACTICE ALERT When providing care for an individual with conversion disorder, the diagnosis must be based on all the clinical elements the patient presents, as opposed to one abnormal finding. A thorough assessment and appropriate tests must indicate that the symptoms show clear evidence of incompatibility with other neurologic disorders.

Other Somatic Symptom-Related Disorders

Other disorders in this category relate to psychological factors affecting confirmed medical illnesses; factitious disorder, in which an individual falsifies illnesses; and an "other specified" category.

Psychological Factors Affecting Other Medical Conditions

Individuals who have psychological factors affecting other medical conditions experience psychological or behavioral factors that influence the course of an existing diagnosed medical condition (APA, 2013). For example, a patient with type 1 diabetes mellitus fears becoming obese and takes a higher dose of insulin as a perceived way to prevent weight gain. Taking this dosage of insulin precipitates a hypoglycemic crisis that often results in an evaluation in the emergency department. The patient typically does not reveal the reason for the hypoglycemia and may blame the pharmacy for sending the wrong insulin. This distracts the medical staff from the real cause of the medical problem.

Factitious Disorder

This disorder is characterized by an individual falsifying an illness. A diagnosis of **factitious disorder** requires the practitioner to demonstrate that the individual is taking deceptive steps to fabricate the illness. If the person falsifies an illness of another person, it is called *factitious disorder imposed on another*, formerly called factitious disorder by proxy. The individual who causes the illness in the other person is labeled with the illness.

Other Specified Somatic Symptom and Related Disorders

This classification describes an illness that does not meet the diagnostic criteria for other disorders in the somatic symptom and related disorders category. The disorder must have a presentation that is similar to those described by the other somatic symptom and related disorders and the symptoms must cause the individual significant distress in areas of functioning, such as inability to function at home or at work. An example of this is pseudocyesis, which occurs when a woman believes that she is pregnant and reports symptoms of pregnancy that are not substantiated.

Pause and Reflect

1. *What are the primary differences among the somatic symptom and related disorders?*
2. *What similarities do they share?*
3. *What concerns do you have about working with a patient with somatic symptom disorder? Factitious disorder? How would you go about addressing or resolving your concerns to be more helpful to patients with these disorders?*

Collaborative Care

When working with individuals with somatic symptom and related disorders, a team approach involving clinicians who work in the specialty of the predominant symptom is most effective for both the patient and the practitioners. For example, in addition to consisting of a medical practitioner and the psychological team, the team may include a pain specialist if the disorder involves a pain component, or a gynecologist if the disorder involves a gynecologic symptom. The benefit to the patient is that the team develops a consistent care plan, and the follow-through is smoother and more effective. It is important for the patient to continue regularly scheduled visits with the primary care provider to assist the patient in reducing the focus on the feeling of "not being taken seriously." This also provides an opportunity for the primary care practitioner to monitor the patient's physical presentation on a regularly scheduled appointment, rather than in response to an urgent care or emergency department follow-up. Often, it is difficult for the patient and family members to understand the psychological component of these disorders. Collaboration and follow-up with the psychotherapist assists the patient to develop tools for functioning and redirect attention from the somatic sensation to various aspects of functioning (Dinwiddie, 2013; Kozlowska, Foley, & Savage, 2012; Yates & Dunayevitch, 2012a).

Medications are not advised for individuals with somatic symptom and related disorders. If the patient has a depression or anxiety disorder that is co-occurring with the somatic disorder, then the medication prescribed should focus on decreasing the target symptoms for the depression or anxiety. The most effective way of treating somatic symptom and related disorders is through the use of cognitive–behavioral therapy and collaborative team communication between the medical and psychological practitioners (Yates & Dunayevich, 2012a).

Cognitive–Behavioral Therapy

It is highly recommended that individuals with somatic symptom and related disorders seek psychotherapy. This suggestion often is difficult for the patient and family to hear. From the patient's viewpoint, the symptoms are due to a physical malady and the recommendation to seek psychotherapy must mean that the symptoms are "in my head." Individuals with these disorders are not seeking secondary gain; their symptoms are part of their physical experience and cause great suffering. The best approach is to employ active listening and to restructure thoughts away from the somatic focus toward functioning, activities at the core of cognitive-behavioral therapy. For example, a therapist working with a patient who says she enjoys gardening may suggest that the patient monitor her plants for their needs, both inside the house and outside. During following therapy sessions, the patient is encouraged to briefly share her physical sensations over the week, but also to share the state of her plants. Note that the patient is encouraged to share her own symptoms before discussing her gardening: If the mental health team prohibits discussion of somatic concerns, the patient will feel abandoned and seek care elsewhere. The next practitioner the patient sees may begin another extensive physical systems review and order duplicate tests before making the same conclusion as the previous care team. Spending a short amount of time gathering information on the patient's physical sensations and concerns in the beginning of the session reduces the patient's anxiety and allows for new information to be exchanged (Dinwiddie, 2013; Yates & Dunayevich, 2012a).

Complementary and Alternative Therapies

Individuals with somatic symptom and related disorders often fear that using complementary and alternative therapies reinforces the view that the disorder is "all in your head." Exercise, in particular, is viewed in a negative way, as patients are often afraid they would hurt their bodies by employing exercise. Teaching the patient to gradually observe his or her breathing as an indication of an increase in anxiety is a helpful symptom management strategy. After the patient has learned to monitor his or her breathing, teaching mindfulness meditation will provide a positive influence to experiencing physical sensations. Encouraging the patient to begin exercise at a slow speed and build up to 15 minutes during the day may decrease the perception that exercise will increase negative symptoms. Regular exercise, such as walking and stretching, can be beneficial to individuals with these disorders (APA, 2013; Yates & Dunayevich, 2012a).

Pause and Reflect

1. *Why is psychotherapy important in the treatment of somatic symptom and related disorders?*
2. *Why is collaboration among members of the treatment team important in the care of patients with these disorders?*

Nursing Management

Building the therapeutic relationship is essential in providing quality care to patients with somatic symptom and related disorders. In addition to having a sense of isolation, many patients are distrustful of health care providers because of previous experiences in which they felt criticized or discriminated against. A nonjudgmental attitude and open communication will be especially helpful to nurses working with these patients.

Assessment

Assessment begins by focusing on the problem as defined by the patient. If the nurse dismisses the physical assessment, the patient may feel as though his or her input is not valuable and may withdraw from the process. By evaluating the physical as well as the emotional domains, both the nurse and the patient establish the therapeutic relationship and learn how the other domains can influence the physical domain.

Observation and Physical Assessment

Observation and physical assessment of patients with somatic symptom disorders are comprehensive; the nurse will assess the patient across the domains of wellness, assessing for the presence of underlying medical conditions as well as assessing for symptoms of pain, anxiety, and depression (Box 14-1).

Assessment of Patients with Somatic Symptom Disorders — box 14-1

During observation and physical assessment, the nurse notes the patient's:

- **Vital signs:** When fearful and distrusting or in pain, patients' vital signs (blood pressure, pulse, and respirations) may be increased.
- **Demeanor:** How does the patient come across in general? Are there any movements that appear abnormal?
- **Facial expression:** Is the patient able to maintain eye contact with the nurse? Is the patient grimacing? Is the patient's facial expression flat? Does the facial expression match the content of the patient's discussion?
- **Body movements:** How is the patient moving his or her extremities? Does the patient exhibit any other body movements, such as twitches or tics (muscle twitch, especially in neck, face, or shoulder)? Does the patient present any concerns about abnormal body movements? Does the patient report any seizure activity?
- **Voice:** What is the patient's voice level (high-pitched, barely audible, soft/loud/normal volume)? What is the pace of speech (pressured and rapid, slow, normal)? What is the tone of speech (mild/agitated/aggressive/normal)? Does the patient report any problems with speech? Does the patient report any "lump in the throat" or difficulty swallowing?

- **Pain:** Does the patient report any pain? What is the nature of the pain? What is the sensation of the pain? How often does the pain occur? What is the quality of the pain? Use a predetermined rating scale to assess the patient's pain.
- **Behaviors:** Does the patient exhibit any abnormal behaviors? Are the behaviors geared toward a physical concern?
- **Thoughts:** Is the patient coherent? Is the patient able to grasp what the nurse is saying? Is the patient focused on his or her body sensations? How often does this occur? What helps the patient take the focus off the somatic sensations? Is the patient concerned that he or she may have a severe physical ailment? What is that ailment? Has the patient used the Internet to obtain information? Ask about the content of the information. How has this information helped or caused concern for the patient?
- **Content of conversation:** What does the patient talk about? Is the majority of the discussion focused on the somatic sensations?
- **Patient's level of anxiety:** Mild, moderate, severe, or panic? (See Table 13-3, Levels of Anxiety.) The patient's anxiety level provides context to help the nurse understand how the patient is experiencing his or her physical and emotional feelings.

Patient Interview

When interviewing and obtaining an assessment of the patient, make certain to include all five domains of wellness. Rating scales may be helpful to establish mutual understanding between nurse and patient. Questions to ask may include the following:

- How would you rate your level of concern for the physical symptoms you are experiencing (on a scale of 0, meaning no concern, to 10, highly concerned)? Describe each of the physical symptoms you are experiencing.

- How long have you been experiencing the physical sensation?

- Are you aware of anything that may have caused these sensations?

- What has helped you in the past to deal with these body sensations?

- What would be helpful in refocusing your attention away from the physical sensation to something else? What would be most useful, and the least useful?

- How have these body sensations affected your daily life?

- How has your family responded to your disorder?

- Have you been able to go to work or school? Have you been able to concentrate on completing the work assigned to you?

Diagnosis and Planning

While performing the nursing assessment, the therapeutic relationship develops. This gives the patient and the nurse an opportunity to determine the nursing diagnosis and plan for interventions to relieve the patient's suffering.

Common Nursing Diagnoses

The nursing diagnoses for patients with somatic symptom and related disorders are identified through a thorough assessment and prioritized based on individual patient needs. Appropriate nursing diagnoses may include:

- Pain, Acute

- Pain, Chronic

- Body Image, Disturbed

- Powerlessness, Risk for

- Social Interaction, Impaired

- Hopelessness
  (NANDA-I © 2014)

Determining the optimal care plan is a process between the nurse and the patient. This is especially important for individuals with somatic symptom and related disorders, who are at risk of going from one practitioner to another with increased frustration and hopelessness. The nursing diagnoses and subsequent care should be prioritized with the patient's preference in mind.

Plans and Goals

It is important to collaborate with the patient while determining plans and goals for nursing care. The more the patient is involved in the care, the higher the probability for a reduction in the extent of the focus on the somatic symptoms.

The following questions help the nurse to determine realistic plans and goals related to what is most important to the patient:

1. Is the patient interested in collaborating with the care providers to determine the plan of care?

2. What does the patient identify as the most distressing symptom?

3. What are the patient's goals for care? What contributions is the patient willing to make to participate in the care?

When planning nursing care, determine the patient's needs in each of the five domains. Patients with somatic symptom and related disorders focus on the biological domain, so it is important to continue to provide a periodic assessment as well as assisting the patient to explore alternative ways to deal with the abnormal somatic sensations. This helps reassure the patient that the nurse is taking the patient's concerns seriously, promoting the therapeutic relationship and the patient's continued efforts to engage in treatment. However, the nurse also works to help the patient identify what emotional states may increase the focus on the somatic symptoms. Are there emotional triggers that increase the patient's focus on the somatic symptoms? What types of activities or thoughts might be used to lessen the extent of the somatic symptoms? Within the sociological, cultural, and spiritual domains, the nurse helps the patient determine what affect these domains have related to the somatic concerns, so the nurse and the patient together can identify areas that might need to be incorporated into the plan.

Implementation

Determining the patient's willingness to try a new intervention is an important first step in the implementation aspect of the nursing process. Remember, patients with somatic symptom and related disorders have been obtaining care from many practitioners and may be frustrated with their symptoms and the health care system. A nonjudgmental, therapeutic relationship can assist the patient to begin a new set of interventions.

Promoting Recovery and Restoring Function

The emphasis on implementation of the care plan is to blend biopsychosocial and spiritual domains and to assist the patient to empower himself or herself to increase the ability to function (see the Nursing Care Plan). Nursing interventions to promote return to function may include any of the following:

- Review the patient's daily journal of sleep pattern, appetite, menstrual cycle, mood, and general theme of the day.

- Check the status of the somatic issues, such as pain, nausea, and constipation, in an informational manner, focusing not on the symptom, but rather on what can be done to increase the functioning along with the symptom.

- Monitor the patient's adherence to the treatment plan.

- Encourage use of mindfulness meditation or prayer at least twice a day, when the somatic sensations seem to peak.

- Encourage interactions with family and friends that do not include the discussion of the somatic difficulty.

- Identify an interest or hobby, such as knitting, that the patient can do to shift the focus away from the somatic sensation.

- Discuss activities that the patient can do when the somatic sensation is present to shift the focus away from the sensation. The patient can use tools such as meditation, prayer, music, light chores (sitting at a table, preparing a salad), and playing with children or pets to redirect his or her attention.

The patient should have regular follow-up appointments with the primary practitioner. Ideally, these should be every 3 months to check for physical concerns. Collaboration between the primary practitioner and the psychotherapist should take place on a regular basis.

Patient Education

One of the important aspects of implementing the nursing care plan is to recognize that the patient conceptualizes the symptoms to be physical in nature. Patient education about the integration of biopsychosocial and spiritual aspects of health is an important first step. One basic principle in the patient education is to teach about how stress affects the body. Discussing Hans Selye's theory on the General Adaptation Syndrome will assist the patient to begin to think through what stressors are in his or her life (Chapter 13).

After teaching the patient about the physical effects of stress, discuss how this information applies to the individual. Ask the patient to chart daily activities and note when he or she has been able to function, despite the physical concerns. The journal should note physical and psychological functions, such as sleep pattern, appetite, menstrual cycle, mood, and general theme of the day. This can provide the patient and the nurse with a pattern of the impact the stressors have on the patient's physical sensations and identify activities that help reduce or limit the patient's awareness of physical sensations.

Evaluation

Based on a comprehensive evaluation, the patient and nurse together determine the next set of goals needed to increase the patient's ability to function. The nurse should remember to be objective during evaluation, as achieving the goals and successfully implementing interventions is a long and slow process. Often, the patient has been living with these symptoms for many years and progress will occur with small achievements.

Pause and Reflect

1. *Patients with somatic symptom and related disorders often have been evaluated by numerous providers. How can you make your assessment questions open-ended and nonjudgmental so patients will feel supported and become motivated to explore their symptoms?*

2. *What feedback or response from a patient would indicate that he or she is feeling inundated with questions during the assessment? What would you do if the patient indicated that he or she was feeling overwhelmed?*

Grace—A Patient with Somatic Symptom Disorder	NURSING CARE PLAN

Nursing Diagnosis: Chronic pain related to the patient's current perception of pain originating from a back injury 10 years ago.

Short-Term Goals *Patient will:* (include date for short-term goal to be met)	Intervention *Nurse will:*	Rationale
Describe and rate her pain, when it occurs, and define what steps she can take to reduce the pain and the result. This will take place during the first interview.	Provide a thorough assessment of the presenting physical concerns.	Determine a baseline for Grace's focus on her pain and her psychosocial, spiritual needs
Describe her psychosocial and spiritual circumstances. This will take place during the first interview.	Provide a thorough assessment of the patient's psychosocial and spiritual needs.	Clarify relationships with family members, friends, social and spiritual needs.
During first interview, identify 1 or 2 interventions to try to reduce the focus on her pain.	Through patient education, assist Grace to identify one to two ideas she can use to reduce her focus on her pain.	Encourage a focus on an activity or mindfulness meditation can relieve the extent of the somatic symptom.
Seek psychotherapy after the urgent care visit to assist her to continue to cope with the somatic symptoms within 1 week of the urgent care clinic visit.	Provide a list of three psychotherapists who work with individuals with somatic symptom disorder and coordinate with the primary practitioner and pain specialist.	Cognitive psychotherapy and planned consistent visits with the primary practitioner can reduce the focus on somatic sensations.
Long-Term Goal Grace will seek psychotherapy and will be able to reduce her focus on the pain so she can pursue her gardening for her indoor plants.	She will be able to use mindfulness meditation twice a day when her focus on her somatic symptoms is the highest, prior to going to sleep, and in the morning, upon rising.	Mindfulness meditation may help reduce somatic symptoms and use of analgesics.

Clinical Reasoning

1. What other nursing diagnoses might the nurse working with Grace consider?

2. Do you think the selection of *Chronic Pain* as the priority diagnosis is appropriate? Why or why not?

DISSOCIATIVE DISORDERS

Dissociative disorders are characterized by a combination of fragmented memories (which may result in fragmented personalities), difficulties with memory recall, and dissociative behavior patterns. Often, depersonalization and derealization occur in dissociative disorders. **Dissociation** is defined as a disruption and/or a discontinuity of the individual's normal sense of memory, emotions, perception, motor control, behavior, and sense of identity. Patients have described dissociation as a sense of the body being present with an absent mind. This disruption causes difficulty in daily functioning. The individual usually is embarrassed and attempts to hide the symptoms. Dissociations are unwelcome intrusions that occur with losses of continuity of time, changes in ability to relate to others, and **amnesia**, or the inability to recall what the person was doing during the dissociation. **Depersonalization** is the experience of unreality or detachment from the individual's mind, sense of self, and/or physical body. Patients may describe depersonalization as "I was floating to the ceiling looking down at myself while being beaten." **Derealization**, another symptom, is defined as the experience of unreality or detachment from the person's surroundings. A patient, while describing a severe beating during a domestic argument, stated, "I did not feel a thing; my body felt like jelly being slapped. I smelled the air around me and heard the insects, but I did not know where I was."

Dissociative behavior patterns are labeled as positive and/or negative. *Positive dissociation symptoms* include fragmentation of identity, depersonalization, and derealization and occur to help the person cope with stressors. *Negative dissociative symptoms* include the inability to access information or control mental functions that normally a person can consciously manage, and the primary identity typically has no idea what is happening (APA, 2013).

In addition to **dissociative identity disorder** (DID), the DSM-5 classifies four other types of dissociative disorders:

- *Dissociative amnesia*, which shares the characteristic of amnesia seen in dissociative identity disorder, but not the emergence of multiple personality states

critical thinking

Paula Relapse Phase

Paula Thompson is a 51-year-old woman. Eleven years ago, she discovered that she had several different ego states within her. At that time, she was working with her psychotherapist, an advanced practice clinical specialist, on issues related to a severe rape she experienced when she was 15 years old. At the same time as Paula was discovering that she had several different "people" inside her, Paula's father, George, was placed in a nursing home due to advanced Alzheimer's disease. He was no longer able to care for himself and no longer recognized Paula's mother, Paula's sister, or Paula herself. George experienced a severe alcohol use disorder while Paula was growing up and physically abused both Paula and her sister. Paula and her sister repeatedly witnessed her father beating her mother when he came home drunk after being out all night. When Paula was raped at age 15, she reported the rape to her parents, but they did not take action. After the rape, she turned to alcohol, had difficulty concentrating, and her grades went down. Paula was frequently suicidal and had "a number" of sexual relationships, during which she felt shame and "dirty." Paula married in her early 20s, but divorced her husband, Marc, after only two years of marriage. They both drank alcohol and had physical fights with each other.

After Paula left Marc, she joined Alcoholics Anonymous and has been successful in staying drug and alcohol free since that time. She met her current partner, Abby, in Alcoholic Anonymous. Abby and Paula have been together for 24 years. Paula does not identify herself as a lesbian. She views the several different personalities inside her as having their own relationship with Abby. Some of her personalities call her partner "Abigail" and are very formal with her, sometimes treating Abby in a verbally abusive manner. Abby and Paula have a nonsexual union, due to Paula's decision to work on her abuse and her dissociative identity disorder.

Paula has fragments of memory about her childhood and her abuse. Since she discovered the many "people" inside her, her memories have been fragmented. This is particularly true when she is scared or angry. Paula is frequently suicidal, particularly when there is conflict between personalities inside her.

Paula identifies the ego states in different ways. Some of the personalities have names, hobbies, abilities, and motivations. The more dominant personalities sometimes "punish" the "young ones," to the point at which she physically hurts herself. There is an internal battle about whether to stay alive and work on self or commit suicide with a gun. One dominant male personality, Peter, is obsessed about getting a gun and killing squirrels. He is one of the personalities that beats up the "young ones." Another personality, George, shares many characteristics with Paula's father, often "coming home drunk" and beating on the "young ones."

Paula (presenting as Peter) recently purchased a gun. The dominant male personality, Peter, held the gun to her head, and dared the "younger ones" to defy him. One of her female personalities, Pauline, whom she views as the protector, became frightened and called a woman she knew from the National Alliance on Mental Illness (NAMI) for help. Paula was evaluated in the local emergency department and was hospitalized in the behavioral health (inpatient) unit as a voluntary admission.

APPLICATION

1. How does Paula exhibit behaviors of suffering?

2. Assess Paula in the five domains:
   a. Biological
   b. Psychological
   c. Sociological
   d. Cultural
   e. Spiritual

3. How you would prioritize Paula's needs during this encounter? What is your rationale?

4. What interventions would assist Paula to begin to determine some hope in her situation?

5. What behaviors would help you to measure whether interventions for Paula were effective?

Dissociative Disorder Symptoms by Domain

table 14-2

Domain	Responses
Biological	• During distinct personality states, may experience different sensory or motor functioning; may report that his or her body feels like a child's body or the body of the opposite gender • Alterations in memory • Changes in consciousness • Inability to recall autobiographical information (dissociative amnesia) • Self-mutilation • Flashbacks • Functional neurologic symptoms
Psychological	• Dissociation • Depersonalization • Derealization • Identity disruption • Perceptions of voices: "the little ones are crying" • Sudden strong emotions or behaviors that the individual is unable to control • Difficulty concentrating, due to experiencing multiple, independent thoughts that may belong to different dissociative states • Feelings of apprehension, helplessness, worthlessness • Focusing on past trauma • Forgetfulness • Hopelessness • Spiritual, supernatural being is controlling the individual's behavior in possession form of DID
Sociological	• Patient feels alone, believes no one understands or believes that he or she has DID • Sometimes may take trips in an amnesic state (dissociative fugue) • Different aspects of the personality states vary in their relationships with family members and some friends • Lacking a sense of relation to the whole of society, feelings of loneliness, feels judged by others • Challenged in relation to resources due to inability to read some social cues of others and work effectively, due to shifts in identity • In the possession form of DID, may be "taken over" by a spirit, demon, or deity
Cultural	• Lack of connectedness to those around them, due to changes in behavior patterns, emotional outbursts, amnesia, depersonalization, and derealization experiences • In the possession form of DID, may be rejected due to culturally unaccepted behavior
Spiritual	• Feeling a lack of connectedness with God or higher power and/or with others of like-minded beliefs • Struggling with faith • Struggling with meaning and purpose • Expressing feelings of guilt and stigma related to the symptoms of DID • In the possession form of DID, feels "taken over" by a spirit, demon, or deity, not part of the usual spiritual belief system

• *Depersonalization/derealization disorder*, in which the individual experiences depersonalization, derealization, or both, but in which the individual's reality testing remains intact during episodes

• *Other specified dissociative disorder*, which may be used when symptoms of dissociation are present but do not meet the criteria for the specific disorders; for example, an acute dissociative reaction to stress or trauma for a short duration

• *Unspecified dissociative disorder*, which may be used when dissociative symptoms result in marked distress and impairment, but do not meet the criteria for the other disorders in this category

Symptoms of dissociative disorders by domain are listed in Table 14-2.

Theoretical Foundations

Building on Briquet's research into hysteria as a quantifiable result of trauma, Pierre Janet, a French hypnotist, philosopher, and physician systematically described dissociative states in the late 19th and early 20th centuries (Loewenstein, 1990). Working closely with Jean Charcot, a neurologist at the famous Salpétrière Institute, Janet laid the groundwork for what is known today about dissociation.

Modern researchers such as Bessel van der Kolk, Judith Hermann, and John Briere have made great strides in putting to rest the ideas that dissociation and dissociative disorders are not "real" illnesses. Today, there are established clinical guidelines and professional journals devoted to this important subject. The work continues in the area of understanding how the original identity with which an individual is born fragments into different identity states that emerge at various points in the person's life and various aspects of reintegration into a unified whole. There is controversy as to whether complete reintegration is possible or should even be a goal.

Biological Domain

Because of today's technology, several features of dissociative identity disorders and dissociative amnesia are currently being researched. One area that is being examined is changes in the brain that are implicated with the amnesia aspect of these disorders. Elzinga et al. (2007) studied individuals with a dissociative disorder to determine brain changes related to memory. Using functional magnetic resonance imaging (fMRI) and a verbal working-memory task, they found that the individuals who have a high rate of dissociation have enhanced working-memory capacities. This is in contrast to individuals with posttraumatic stress disorder (PTSD), who have impaired working memory. The individuals with a dissociative disorder in this study demonstrated a higher rate of anxiety and a decrease in concentration during their task performance than the controls. Markowitsch and Staniloiu (2012) explored the current research on amnesic disorders. Brain changes that may occur in episodic autobiographic memory (EAM) loss due to amnesia have been hypothesized to result from hypometabolism in the right temporofrontal regions, particularly the inferolateral prefrontal cortex. The DSM-5 (APA, 2013) lists several brain structures that may be affected with DID: the orbitofrontal cortex, hippocampus, parahippocampal gyrus, and amygdala. Further research will be helpful to determine a possible therapeutic strategy to assist individuals with these disorders.

Psychological Domain

Individuals with dissociative disorders have nearly always sustained severe psychological trauma and abuse incidences during their childhood (APA, 2013; Boysen, 2011; Weber, 2008, 2009). They often experience a discontinuity in their sense of self related to the appearance of the different personalities, the inability to recall events, and/or the experience of detachment from life associated with the disorder. Individuals with DID may be further disoriented or distressed when they experience **dissociative fugues**, episodes of travel with no memory of how the individual reached the location. It is notable that the distance traveled may be as close as the next room or as far as the beach or a place of business (APA, 2013).

With dissociative disorders, strong emotions and impulses may emerge that the individual cannot explain or reports as being beyond his or her control. These also contribute to the discontinuity experienced by the individual.

Sociological Domain

Individuals with dissociative disorders often have chaotic relationships with their family members. There are periods of time when the individual may have amnesia and not recognize his or her children, spouse, and friends. Not surprisingly, family and friends may exhibit skepticism about the disorder. There is, in fact, some skepticism in the professional community about the diagnosis of DID. The question is whether the disorder is due to psychological trauma and attachment difficulties or to a predilection for fantasy, a high suggestibility, and iatrogenic origin—that is, as a result of medical treatment. Reinders et al. (2012) conducted a study in which they tested individuals with DID and controls for high and low fantasy proneness. Both groups were given two autobiographical memory scripts that depicted a neutral and a trauma-related imagery. The control group was asked to enact two DID identity states, while the study group was asked to react to autobiographical memory imagery paradigms that depicted a neutral and a trauma-related imagery. Based on brain imaging and psychophysiological responses (such as heart rate and blood pressure), the researchers determined that the control subjects could not enact DID. This research demonstrates that DID is not due to a sociocultural, fantasy, or iatrogenic origin. Knowing this may help nurses provide information and support to family members and friends of patients with dissociative disorders.

Cultural Domain

Several aspects of DID can be influenced based on cultural practices (APA, 2013). In some cultures, it is common to experience unexplained neurologic changes, such as nonepileptic seizures or sensory loss, as well as possession by unseen spirits, often taking the form of deceased relatives. The difference between the behavior that is part of a cultural norm and DID is that the behavior in individuals with the disorder is involuntary, distressing, and uncontrollable. Often, the possession state of DID involves internal conflict and may occur at times and places that violate the cultural norms.

Xiao et al. (2006) studied individuals in Shanghai, China, to determine the etiology of dissociative disorders. At the time of their study, there was no knowledge of dissociative disorders in China: No information about dissociative disorders was taught in medical school, nor were any depictions of these disorders seen on TV or in the movies. The study participants were selected from inpatients on psychiatric units, outpatient psychiatric patients, and factory workers in Shanghai. The researchers discovered that the individuals who satisfied the diagnosis for dissociative disorders had a previous childhood history of physical and/or sexual abuse. This, again, indicates that dissociative disorders are not due to fantasy or the iatrogenic model.

Spiritual Domain

Individuals with dissociative disorders often experience a religious component to the dissociations and may attribute the dissociation to a religious cause (Dorahy & Lewis, 2001; Rosik & Soria, 2012). When seeking help, they may experience doubt or discrimination from clergy or others who do not understand the true nature of the disorder. Often, individuals with dissociative disorders experience feeling disengaged from others, including their spiritual communities or beliefs. This adds to the isolation these patients often feel. It is important to educate individuals who provide spiritual support to the patient about the biological aspects of dissociative disorders so these people can provide the level of assistance that is desired by the patient.

Pause and Reflect

1. *What implications does the etiology of dissociative disorders have for nursing care and treatment?*
2. *What impact do multiple personality states have on patients?*
3. *How would you deal with a family member who had multiple personality disorders? How do you think this might have an impact on your family?*

Specific Disorders

Individuals with dissociative disorders typically exhibit a disruption or discontinuity of the normal stream of consciousness, memory, identity, emotion, perception, body sensations, and behavior (APA, 2013). These symptoms occur spontaneously, are intrusive, and disrupt the individual's ability to function at work or school or have sustained psychologically healthy relationships with others. Individuals with dissociative disorders who have these symptoms are often embarrassed, question their internal experiences, and try to hide the behaviors that manifest with the dissociations, derealization, and depersonalization. As a result, clinicians who are not experienced in working with these individuals may misdiagnose the patient with another psychiatric disorder (APA, 2013).

Dissociative Identity Disorder

Dissociative identity disorder used to be called *multiple personality disorder*. It occurs in individuals who have sustained horrific physical and psychological abuse over time, usually in early childhood (Brosbe, Faust, & Gold, 2013). During the trauma, the individuals unconsciously dissociated to cope with the trauma. Many years later, an environmental or physical cue may cause the individual to have flashbacks to the early traumatic events. The stress response to the flashback causes the individual to dissociate similarly to when the individual was originally traumatized, and this may result in a fragmented personality. The dissociated fragment of memory may be identified with a personality and may be labeled with a name or act in a different manner than the individual's usual behavior. The dissociated fragment's name and behavior are often based on the original trauma. For example, Paula labeled one of her "people" George; this fragment shares both the name and actions of her father as Paula experienced him. The individual views this part of the individual's sense of self—the alternate identity—as having helped him or her through the original trauma.

Individuals with DID typically have had several life-threatening traumas and therefore may have multiple ego states that helped the individual survive these traumas. The level of personal suffering is so great that the ego states reenact some of the trauma and conflict with one another internally. Suicidal ideation is common among individuals with DID. More than 70% of outpatients with DID have attempted suicide; multiple attempts are common as are self-injurious behaviors (APA, 2013).

The International Society for the Study of Trauma and Dissociation (2011) noted that 1% to 3% of the general population in multiple cities and countries around the world have symptoms of DID. The DSM-5 (APA, 2013) cites a 12-month study in a small community in the United States where 1.5% of the adult population satisfied the criteria for DID, with little difference in prevalence between genders.

It is not uncommon for the symptoms of DID to be observed or reported by family or friends rather than the individual himself or herself (see DSM-5 Diagnostic Criteria for Dissociative Identity Disorder). Despite the level of functional impairment experienced by individuals with the disorder, impairments in memory recall or the appearance of an alternate personality may hamper the individual's ability to remember and report episodes and alterations in function.

The development of DID can occur at any age, but the symptoms may appear differently in children and adolescents. Weber (2008) outlines the following behavior patterns common in children and adolescents:

- *Inconsistent consciousness:* The child manifests changes in attention and may appear to exhibit trance states.
- *Autobiographical forgetfulness:* The child demonstrates episodic autobiographic memory (EAM) loss.
- *Fluctuating mood and behaviors:* The child has periods of rage and mood swings, and has difficulty modulating his or her mood.

Additional symptoms in children and adolescents may include difficulty with concentration, attachment difficulties, and engaging in traumatic play (APA, 2013). Children do not demonstrate identity alterations; they exhibit interference between mental states. Adolescents may experience a change in identity that appears to be part of the adolescent experience of learning about self. Actual changes in identity and dissociative amnesia occur in older individuals. The patient may be diagnosed with mood disorders, OCD, paranoia, psychotic mood disorders, or cognitive disorders rather than DID. Individuals may begin to show signs of changes in identity after events such as leaving a traumatic situation, or when, as a parent, their child reaches the same age that they were when they sustained the initial trauma, or on learning of the terminal illness or death of their abuser (APA, 2013).

Diagnostic Criteria for Dissociative Identity Disorder — DSM-5

A. Disruption of identity characterized by two or more distinct personality states, which may be described in some cultures as an experience of possession. The disruption in identity involves marked discontinuity in sense of self and sense of agency, accompanied by related alterations in affect, behavior, consciousness, memory, perception, cognition, and/or sensory–motor functioning. These signs and symptoms may be observed by others or reported by the individual.

B. Recurrent gaps in the recall of everyday events, important personal information, and/or traumatic events that are inconsistent with ordinary forgetting.

C. The symptoms cause clinically significant distress or impairment in social, occupational, or other important areas of functioning.

D. The disturbance is not a normal part of a broadly accepted cultural or religious practice. *Note:* In children, the symptoms are not better explained by imaginary playmates or other fantasy play.

E. The symptoms are not attributable to the physiological effects of a substance (e.g., blackouts or chaotic behavior during alcohol intoxication) or another medical condition (e.g. complex partial seizures).

Source: Reprinted with permission from the *Diagnostic and Statistical Manual of Mental Disorders*, Fifth Edition, (Copyright 2013). American Psychiatric Association.

Dissociative Amnesia

Individuals with dissociative amnesia have an inability to recall important autobiographical information. This information usually is associated with a traumatic event or something that the individual perceives as stressful. It is information that normally would be stored in the individual's memory and available for recall. *Localized amnesia* occurs when an individual cannot recall specific events, particularly during a precise period of time. Individuals who have suffered child abuse often cannot recall the specifics of the abuse and the memories surrounding it. For example, a patient who was frequently beaten by her father when she did not do household chores to his expectations may not know how to dust or vacuum when she starts her own household.

In *selective amnesia*, the individual can recall some but not all events during a specified period of time. Localized amnesia is the most commonly reported form of dissociative amnesia, but some patients experience both localized and selective amnesia (APA, 2013). *Generalized amnesia* is more rare and represents complete loss of memory of one's life history, including name, place of birth and residence, and parents and siblings. Generalized amnesia occurs rapidly and causes disorientation and wandering. Generalized amnesia may not be discovered until the police are called to perform a welfare check and escort the person to the emergency department for safety.

Individuals with dissociative amnesia may have these symptoms for a long period of time, disrupting their ability to function in an occupation, in a relationship, or as a parent. The individual with dissociative amnesia may become hopeless and attempt suicide. Self-mutilation is common, as well as depersonalization and autohypnotic symptoms, in which the patient appears as if in a hypnotic trance. An individual with dissociative amnesia may have experienced a mild traumatic brain injury prior to the onset of the amnesia.

Depersonalization/Derealization Disorder

Individuals with this disorder experience depersonalization, derealization, or both. The symptoms of depersonalization and derealization are persistent and recur. The individual with depersonalization feels detached from self, experiencing both emotional and physical feelings: "I can't tell where I am, I don't feel anything. I am like a robot walking around, not even feeling my legs." The individual experiencing derealization feels not real and detached from the environment: "I am in a fog, I do not know where I am, it all seems strange." This individual has difficulty keeping a job, as the stimuli related to work tasks and activities become overwhelming, and he or she is unable to perform. Home life becomes chaotic, and the individual loses track of the tasks he or she is doing at home when the surroundings feel unreal.

Pause and Reflect

1. *How does dissociative amnesia differ from dissociative identity disorder?*
2. *Do you know anyone who has experienced amnesia? How has the person dealt with the amnesia?*
3. *What nursing diagnoses might be appropriate for a patient with depersonalization/derealization disorder?*

Collaborative Care

Providing care for an individual with dissociative disorders is very complex, requiring care from a clinician experienced in treating these disorders. For patients who have co-morbid disorders, it is imperative that there is communication among all practitioners who are providing care. Each team member must have a clear role in providing care and consistently communicate that to the patient. This level of collaboration is essential, as the patient with alternate personalities may have relationships that differ with each practitioner, and patients with these disorders may not always remember a discussion they had with a provider. Keeping the lines of communication open between providers assures the patient of comprehensive and safe care (International Society for the Study of Trauma and Dissociation, 2011).

Psychopharmacology

Although research has not focused on the use of medications specifically for dissociative disorders, the clinical guidelines for treating dissociative identity disorder in adults were written by the International Society for the Study of Trauma and Dissociation (2011) and are evidence based. These guidelines suggest that medications are effective on the target symptoms that are disturbing to the patient. For example, selective serotonin-reuptake inhibitors and beta-blockers have been used to treat hyperarousal and intrusive thoughts, depressive symptoms, obsessive–compulsive thoughts and behaviors, and sleep disturbances. At no time should benzodiazepines be used, as they increase the risk of further dissociation (Stahl, 2013). The guidelines also stress the importance of keeping the role of the medicating provider separate from that of the psychotherapist. The individual with a dissociative disorder should have one primary psychotherapist, and the rest of the team should collaborate with that therapist. The medicating provider should see the patient regularly to monitor medications, but should redirect the patient to discuss psychological therapy information with the primary therapist.

Research suggests that alternate identities may respond differently to the medication. For example, the same patient may present with insulin-dependent diabetes and visual impairment requiring glasses with one identity, and require neither insulin nor glasses when in another identity state. It is important to get feedback from the patient over time to determine how the medication is decreasing the target symptoms. Use of medications takes into consideration the whole patient's needs (International Society for the Study of Trauma and Dissociation, 2011). The most effective treatment for individuals with dissociative identity disorder is a combination of affect regulation, grounding, treatment of the PTSD symptoms, and understanding the symptoms of dissociation.

PRACTICE ALERT

- Ask the patient to tell you the medications he or she is currently taking, what symptoms the medications relieve, and any side effects.
- Ask what prompts the patient uses to remember to take medications when he or she is experiencing an increase in symptoms.
- Remember, the patient may experience amnesia when there is an increase in symptoms.
- Some patients have learned ways to work around amnesia in order to take their medications effectively.

Psychotherapy

Individuals with dissociative disorders typically require long-term therapy. The primary psychotherapist conceptualizes the therapy as taking place over years. Most of the therapeutic work is done in an outpatient setting. When the patient is less symptomatic and able to work on issues without safety concerns, psychotherapy once a week may be sufficient. When there are concerns for safety (for instance, the patient is actively suicidal, homicidal, self-mutilating, anorexic, or experiencing an increase in compulsive drives) participating in therapy two or three times a week may prevent a crisis requiring hospitalization. Individual psychotherapy is the best modality for this patient population. Group therapy should be used for building coping skills, not for exploration of psychological dynamics or traumatic material. Community-run groups, such as "Incest Anonymous," are not helpful for this population, as these patients need clear external boundaries and to be able to participate in discussion of psychological trauma in small bursts when the patient is able to process the information. Community groups may not be able to provide that level of boundaries, and psychological flooding may occur as the group members discuss their sexual abuse (International Society for the Study of Trauma and Dissociation, 2011).

There are three phases for providing care for an individual with dissociative disorders:

- Establishing safety, stabilization, and symptom reduction
- Working through and integrating traumatic memories
- Identity integration and rehabilitation

Once the patient's safety and symptoms are stabilized, the therapist begins the work of helping the patient work through and integrate traumatic memories. This may include a number of strategies, depending on the nature of the trauma and the interests and personal preferences of the patient. Art therapy is one strategy that may be used to help patients work through these memories and express their feelings (Figures 14-2 and 14-3).

Complementary and Alternative Therapies

Hypnosis is an effective complementary modality for the individual with DID. Hypnosis is often taught to patients to assist with affective

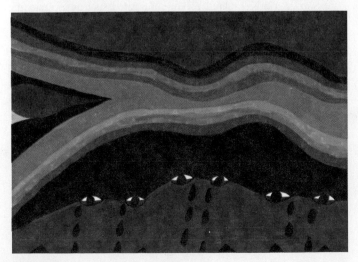

14-2 This drawing by a patient with dissociative identity disorder illustrates the distress the disorder causes in patients' lives.

Source: Pearson Education

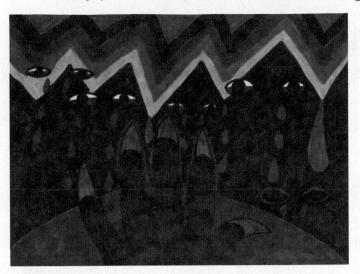

14-3 A patient in therapy drew this picture to illustrate how "the hand of abuse" has affected her life.

Source: Pearson Education

regulation, to assist in modulating anxiety, and to promote self-soothing. This modality needs to be initiated by a practitioner who is knowledgeable about hypnosis and dissociated states. Individuals who have DID are easily hypnotized. Maintaining boundaries and not using hypnosis for psychological explorations are important clinical considerations (International Society for the Study of Trauma and Dissociation, 2011).

Additional modalities, such as art therapy, music therapy, and dance therapy are very helpful for individuals with dissociative disorders. These modalities help the patient to improve concentration, work through affective-laden material, and enhance problem-solving skills (International Society for the Study of Trauma and Dissociation, 2011).

Pause and Reflect

1. *What role does psychotherapy play in the treatment of dissociative disorders?*
2. *Why do you think the ongoing treatment over time is necessary for patients with dissociative disorders?*
3. *Ensuring safety is always the priority for nursing care. Specifically, why do you think is it important when providing care to patients with dissociative disorders?*

Nursing Management

The nursing care of individuals with dissociative disorders is challenging. For many patients, nursing care often takes place in a medical or hospital setting, when the patient is admitted because of either a risk of harming self or others and/or needing further treatment in a structured, safe environment. A particular challenge when working with patients with dissociative disorders is that the patient may have no memory of how he or she came to the hospital (see Perceptions, Thoughts, and Feelings: Validating the Needs of a Patient with Symptoms of Dissociation near the end of this chapter).

Assessment

Individuals with dissociative disorders often have negative views of themselves and feel embarrassed and filled with shame that they experience shifts in alternate identities. The most important questions

Paula Recovery Phase

While in the behavioral health unit, Paula receives psychotherapy from a psychotherapist who is a psychiatric advanced practice clinical nurse specialist. The nurse practitioner on Paula's care team supervises her medications and prescribes prazosin (Minipress) to help alleviate the hyperarousal. While in the hospital, Paula determines that she would like to continue psychotherapy sessions three times a week after discharge, with a medication review every other week. Paula will also e-mail a daily safety check to her psychotherapist. In addition, Paula agrees to short-term, trauma-focused therapy from the local rape crisis center. Prior to Paula's first session, the rape crisis counselor contacts Paula's psychotherapist at the behavioral health unit to ensure that she does not trigger any further flashbacks while exploring the recent memory Paula had experienced immediately prior to her hospitalization. The counselor also wants to work in conjunction with Paula's treating psychotherapist to develop tools that Paula can use if she becomes anxious and experiences emotional flooding.

At each psychotherapy session after discharge, Paula's psychotherapist conducts a safety check. A week after Paula's discharge, Paula reports that Peter is not speaking to her because she sold the gun and that Pauline really likes the counselor at the rape crisis center. The "younger ones" feel calmer now that the gun is gone.

APPLICATION

1. What are Paula's priorities for care at this time?

2. Why do you think Paula was prescribed prazosin? What are some important considerations for patients with dissociative disorders who receive pharmacotherapy?

3. Why was it important for the rape crisis counselor to contact Paula's psychotherapist at the behavioral health unit?

---

relate to safety and the ability to devise a plan for maintaining safety between personality states. Begin the assessment where the patient has defined the problem. It is imperative to understand this disorder and ask questions about dissociative states, using language that the patient has used to describe the alternate identities. If the patient suspects that his or her input is not valuable, he or she may withdraw from the process. By evaluating the patient as the patient describes himself or herself, both the nurse and the patient establish the therapeutic relationship and learn how to meet the needs for safety between alternate identities.

Observation and Physical Assessment

Observation and physical assessment of patients suspected of having dissociative disorders follows the same guidelines for comprehensive assessment as assessment of any patient presenting with impairment in functioning in one or more domains (see Box 14-1).

Patient Interview

For patients with dissociative disorders, it is essential to ask the patient direct questions about the level of risk for suicide (Chapter 27). Approximately 70% of outpatients receiving care for DID have attempted suicide (APA, 2013). Keep in mind that there may be some amnesia for past suicide attempts and that a presenting alternate identity may not feel suicidal, but another personality may be suicidal.

It also is important to assess for the possibility of dissociation and amnesia. An excellent objective tool is the Dissociative Experience Scale (DES) (Bernstein & Putnam, 1986; Wright & Loftus, 1999). This scale assists the clinician to determine whether the individual experiences dissociative and amnesic episodes (Box 14-2).

Difference in Initial/Relapse, Recovery, Rehabilitation Phases

The patient who is in the initial or relapse phase is experiencing a great deal of distress. There is an inability to function, due to a high level of alternating identities or internal conflict among personalities, and an increase in amnesia. The patient seeks help or is directed to receive help by other people in the patient's support network.

Due to the complexity of dissociative disorders, the patient may not be aware of when a relapse is occurring until people who make up the patient's support system request that he or she seek additional care. Some periods of relapse can be anticipated, such as approaching

---

Sample Assessment Questions for Patients with Dissociative Disorders

box 14-2

- Do you have periods of time when you do not remember where you were or what you were doing?
- Have you ever had times when you were dressed in clothes that you did not think you owned or were very different from your usual appearance?
- Did you ever find new things among your belongings that you do not remember obtaining?
- Have you ever had the experience where you feel as though you are not "in your own body," but are looking down at yourself from the ceiling?

- Have you ever had a time in your life when you do not remember important events?
- Have you ever looked in the mirror and did not recognize yourself?
- Have you ever found that you may have done things that you do not remember doing?
- Do you feel sometimes you are looking through a fog and that things feel unclear or removed?

Based on Bernstein, E. M., & Putnam, F. W. (1986). Development, reliability, and validity of a dissociation scale. *Journal of Nervous and Mental Disease, 174,* 727–735; Wright, D. B., & Loftus, E. F. (1999). Measuring dissociation: Comparison of alternative forms of the dissociative experiences scale. *American Journal of Psychology, 112* (4), 497–519.

the anniversary of the abuser's death or of the traumatic event, or when the patient experiences physical illness such as influenza. If the nurse attempts to move the therapeutic interventions faster than the patient can achieve, the patient will react by withdrawing and not disclosing pertinent clinical information.

> **PRACTICE ALERT** Dissociative identity disorder is a chronic illness that may take years of supportive psychotherapy to promote safety and stability. Anticipating when a possible relapse may occur is critical to maintaining safety from suicidal and/or homicidal thoughts and behaviors. It is important to monitor the patient's pace of recovery.

Some individuals with DID have a capacity for higher functioning. These patients have the potential to work with their psychotherapist to understand their trauma and confront the pain and suffering it has caused in their lives. This work is done slowly, as the individual becomes able to integrate new learning styles of coping. Monitor patients for a possible increase in symptoms when working directly on the trauma. It is helpful to empower patients to recognize that the trauma was horrific, but they are now able to make new choices and learn when some of the old abusive behavior is manifested by their own alternate identities.

The rehabilitation phase may be reached by individuals who are high functioning and have minimal dissociation and amnesia. Often, these individuals enjoy "giving back" to people who are experiencing some life challenges. Joining organizations such as NAMI can provide an opportunity for leadership and collaboration with others to help individuals cope with mental illness. The rehabilitation phase for individuals who have DID does not mean that the individuals will not have alternate identities, but that the personalities can work together or coexist without creating conflict or abuse.

Diagnosis and Planning

A thorough assessment helps the nurse and patient to determine the appropriate nursing diagnosis and planning. Collaborating with the patient to develop nursing diagnoses that fit the current circumstance will strengthen the nursing plan and implementation of the interventions.

Common Nursing Diagnoses

The nursing diagnoses selected for the patient with a dissociative disorder are based on the level of safety needed as well as the patient's current intensity of dissociation and amnesia. Appropriate nursing diagnoses may include the following:

- Suicide, Risk for
- Violence: Self-Directed, Risk for
- Self-Mutilation
- Personal Identity: Disturbed
- Parenting, Impaired
- Fear
- Hopelessness
- Powerlessness

(NANDA-I © 2014)

Prioritizing Nursing Diagnoses

The priority for patients with dissociative disorders is to ensure safety. Patients with dissociative disorders may need support for the safety

of others as well as themselves. Patients who are parents may need to determine the level of assistance needed while raising the children to prevent further abuse in the family system. For example, family members need to be aware of the individual's inability to parent when the patient is highly symptomatic. Because of shame and embarrassment, a patient may not disclose periods of possible danger of abuse or harm to children. If the patient has companion pets, monitoring the patient's ability to provide care for these animals can allow the therapist to have insight as to what behaviors may occur in the complexity of a human relationship.

Plans and Goals

As the nurse develops plans and goals within the nursing care plan, the nurse collaborates with the patient as much as possible. While developing the plan of care, the nurse should consider the patient's needs in each of the five domains. Questions the nurse considers when developing the plan of care may include:

- Is the patient capable of helping to develop a care plan and following it?
- What does the patient identify as the most distressing symptom? Is there any memory loss?
- For patients with multiple personalities, how conflicted are the alternate personalities with one another?
- What is the level of danger toward hurting self and/or others?
- What goals does the patient want to achieve?
- What contributions is the patient willing to make to participate in care?

Goals need to be stated in *specific*, *measurable*, and *realistic* terms. For example, if the patient is having obsessive thoughts about hurting the "younger ones," the patient and nurse will develop a safety agreement that the patient can use, both in the hospital and at home to prevent the alternate personalities from harming the "younger ones." The safety agreement will include the following steps:

1. The patient will monitor the internal anxiety level, using the levels of anxiety described in Table 13-3, twice a day.
2. The patient will take medication as needed for panic-level anxiety.
3. The patient will use deep breathing to decrease the anxiety.
4. The patient will divert attention from the dialogue inside to watching TV (no violent programs) or listening to music.

Implementation

Determining the patient's level of safety in the presence of dissociation and amnesia is a priority (see the Nursing Care Plan). Patients who have DID often do not conceptualize the whole person, but become concerned about their own needs depending on the dominant alternate identity. Hospitalization provides a safe stopgap measure to decrease the conflict between the alternate personalities. A safety agreement (Chapter 27) may be developed during hospitalization and implemented and continued after discharge.

Promote Stress Reduction and Healthy Coping

In addition to ensuring safety, nurses help patients with dissociative disorders learn how to recognize triggers and act to reduce the level of their stress response. Nurses do this by providing information about the illness itself, as well as stress reduction techniques. Nurses

Paula—A Patient with Dissociative Identity Disorder   NURSING CARE PLAN

Nursing Diagnosis: Suicide and Risk for Other Directed Violence

Short-Term Goals *Patient will:* (include date for short-term goal to be met)	Intervention *Nurse will:*	Rationale
Be placed on suicidal precautions on the unit, which entails observation to maintain safety.	Provide a thorough assessment. Conduct a thorough search of Paula's belongings to remove any sharp or dangerous items that could be used in a suicidal gesture.	Reduce suicide risk by preventing patient access to sharp or potentially dangerous items while on the hospital unit.
	Place Paula on suicidal precautions, frequent observations to maintain safety.	Provide close observation to reduce isolation and provide therapeutic support to prevent a suicidal gesture.
	Assess level of suicidal thoughts and drive per shift.	Determine level of needed support and observation based on the patient's risk for suicide.
	Monitor patient for changes in mood, affect, thoughts, and ability to control behavior on the milieu to determine if there are any alternate personalities who are feeling angry or wanting to harm self.	Assess patient's level of dissociation and amnesia to promote safety.
Describe her psychosocial and spiritual circumstances. This will take place during the first interview.	Provide a thorough assessment of the patient's psychosocial and spiritual needs.	Clarify relationships with family members and friends, social and spiritual needs.
Seek assistance from staff members if she is experiencing an increase of suicidal thoughts or conflict between Peter and the "younger ones."	The nurse will meet with patient on a one-to-one basis for at least 15 minutes per shift.	Promote a therapeutic relationship with Paula and assess her needs for safety.
	During medication administration and meals, assess Paula for suicidal thoughts.	While giving medications and during meal time, the nurse can facilitate a quick suicide assessment.
	Encourage Paula to seek assistance from staff by being available when she approaches the nursing station.	The patient will be able to disclose suicidal thoughts if she feels that staff members are more open to hearing her needs.
Participate in the structured psychoeducation groups provided in the milieu to promote problem solving and decrease isolation.	Encourage Paula to participate in the psychoeducation groups on the milieu.	Participation in psychoeducation groups will help Paula develop tools she can use to decrease suicidal thoughts when confronted with conflict between alternate personalities.
	Discourage Paula from attending groups that explore emotional issues, as these may increase her symptoms.	Prevent emotional flooding and a potential increase in symptoms.
	Follow up during the one-to-one daily meeting to reinforce information learned during the groups.	Reinforce the information obtained during the group experience.
Develop a safety agreement that can be used as a daily reminder to keep safe. The safety agreement should involve: • Observation of self and behavior • When to take a PRN medication ordered to assist with feeling out of control • Use deep breathing or self-hypnosis • Doing an activity to divert the person's attention away from the negative or upsetting thought pattern and promote self-soothing. • Learning when and how to call for help, both in the hospital and after discharge.	Help the patient to think through and write up a personalized "safety plan" to use during the hospital stay and after discharge. Encourage Paula to review the "safety plan" with the outpatient treatment team of the psychotherapist and NP.	The safety agreement is devised to provide external guidance to Paula when there is conflict between her alternate identities. A safety agreement provides an opportunity to assist Paula to recognize that she may need to use self-hypnosis or a PRN medication to reduce the conflict and tension between alternate personalities. The safety agreement has suggestions on methods to divert attention from internal conflict or upsetting thought patterns to self-soothing. The safety agreement encourages Paula to reach out to ask for help to maintain safety.

Short-Term Goals Patient will: (include date for short-term goal to be met)	Intervention Nurse will:	Rationale
Long-Term Goals Paula will have a reduction in suicidal drive. She will recognize that Peter's desire to kill the "younger ones" will complete suicide for the entire person.	Discuss long-term goals with Paula to confirm that they are consistent with her ultimate goal.	Provides Paula the control to determine her ultimate long-term goal.
Paula will follow up in psychotherapy after discharge from the hospital.	Help Paula determine the safest way to transition from inpatient to outpatient without a loss of progress made during hospitalization.	Supports Paula's transition to outpatient care and promotes her recovery efforts.
Paula will keep a daily journal to determine the needs of the alternate personalities.	Ask Paula if she would like to review any of her journal with the nurse in order to document progress.	Gives Paula ultimate control over her progress. Provides a measure to evaluate Paula's ability to trust the nurse.

Clinical Reasoning

1. What other nursing diagnoses might the nurse working with Paula consider?
2. What interventions may be appropriate for other nursing diagnoses selected?
3. Do you think the selection of *Suicide and Risk for Other Directed Violence* as the priority diagnosis is appropriate? Why or why not?

further act to reduce patient stress by recognizing the significance of the individual's trauma history and incorporating interventions that respect the history and assist the patient in maintaining a measure of control in the clinical setting (see the Nursing Care Plan). Specific nursing interventions that provide support for patients with dissociative disorders include the following:

- Perform safety checks at each health care interaction.
- Due to trauma history, explain all procedures thoroughly; ask for permission to touch patient for any/all interventions (such as taking vital signs).
- Allow patient to determine the extent to which he or she will disrobe for interventions.
- Provide clear information the patient can use to care for self.
- Obtain permission to talk to a family member of the patient's choice to provide education and support.
- Provide information about the illness that is accurate and easy to read; teach the patient how to determine whether Internet sites are peer reviewed, so that the patient knows how to access reliable information.
- Assist the patient and family to make safe provisions for child care, as appropriate.
- Work with the family to ensure monitoring when the patient is overwhelmed.

It is essential that nurses and clinicians caring for patients with dissociative disorders in the medical setting recognize the patient's trauma history. Explaining procedures—even simple ones, such as taking vital signs—and empowering the patient by allowing him or her to determine how much clothing to remove for examinations are essential interventions. Forcing the patient into disrobing or having a procedure that is frightening to the patient can cause increased fear and distrust. In some cases, patients may see the care provider as the abuser and become defensively aggressive (Box 14-3). Patients who understand the procedures can collaborate with the care team to accomplish the goal for the care delivered.

Primary, Secondary, and Tertiary Interventions

Nursing interventions are conceptualized as primary, secondary, or tertiary. Because the etiology of dissociative disorders often arises from severe childhood trauma, primary interventions could be those that help prevent child abuse, sexual molestation, and neglect. The nurse in the community can teach parenting classes. A school nurse can teach 5-to-8-year-old boys and girls about body boundaries, "good" touch, and "don't" touch. Teaching children to report any sexual molestation may reduce long-term effects of the trauma.

Providing secondary intervention involves early detection and treatment. This intervention can be satisfied by assessing all individuals for early trauma and abuse. If a patient states that he or she experienced early childhood abuse, assess for symptoms of dissociation, amnesia, depersonalization, and derealization. Early discovery of symptoms can reduce the severity of the disorder.

Tertiary intervention in the treatment of dissociative disorders assists the individual to improve functioning at home, work, or school; with family members; and within his or her spiritual life. The goal is to decrease the severity of the symptoms to improve the quality of life. Education is directed toward understanding this disorder, maintaining safety, and working through the trauma.

Evaluation

The evaluation phase is a very important part of the nursing process, but one that is not often completed with the patient. Evaluation of care for patients with dissociative disorders should address implications across all the domains of wellness because dissociative episodes and identity fragments may interfere with an individual's physical wellness, either by increasing risk-taking activity or resulting in neglect for another condition (for example, failing to take a medication at a specific time). Evaluation of successful care should show a

Paula's Experience with Nursing Staff in a Medical Setting

box 14-3

Paula agreed to go to the emergency department for an evaluation to facilitate an admission to the behavioral care unit after obsessing about buying a gun. She disclosed to her primary psychotherapist that the obsession was taking over all her thinking and that she was concerned she would purchase a gun and die. Paula and her partner Abby went to the emergency department early in the morning, when there would be less of a wait. After the triage nurse admitted Paula to the emergency department, a male technician requested that Paula change into a patient gown. Paula told him, "I can't." The technician alerted the charge nurse in the ED, and asked the charge nurse to help the patient change into a hospital gown. The security detail was all men; they blocked the entrance to the examining room and demanded that she change into the patient gown. Paula complied. Abby and Paula later told the primary psychotherapist that Paula felt "raped" by the male security guards and the technician. This level of coercion contaminated the hospital stay, as the patient defensively protected herself. She and Abby vowed never to receive care in that facility. The primary psychotherapist brought this incident to the attention of the nursing leadership, the risk management committee, and the physician. Unfortunately, they did not understand why this was a counter-therapeutic intervention. If the staff had allowed Paula to demonstrate that she did not have any contraband or unsafe objects, the admission could have been successful.

Critical Thinking Questions

1. How would you handle a patient who would not disrobe in the emergency department?
2. What is the role of security in the health care setting?
3. What effect does coercing patients to comply with hospital regulations have on the therapeutic relationship?

Unfortunately, this was not the first or only problematic experience Paula had in a medical setting. At the suggestion of her psychotherapist, Paula wrote the following message to nursing staff and other health care providers.

Message from Paula to the Nursing Staff about Her Expectations Based on Her Hospital Experiences

1. Please do not tell me that I don't have dissociative identity disorder; that is not in your role, it damages the possibility of a therapeutic relationship, and I won't trust you.
2. There was only one inpatient nurse during my last hospital stay who sat down and talked to me, listened to what I had to say, and offered suggestions. This is an important part of nursing; the patient needs you to do this.
3. I talked to the nurse about my experience with dissociative identity disorder, I needed to do that, the nurse listened and did not judge me. That was very helpful.
4. Sit down to talk to your patients each shift. Let the person say what they need to say.
5. Educate everyone (nursing staff, case manager, MD, and recreational therapist) about dissociative identity disorder. If the nurse understands what this disorder is, she will be able to determine what her patient needs to do while she is under your care.

   a. It is very hard to explain what DID is to someone who has no idea, and because most nursing staff don't know, it is impossible to trust them.
   b. I certainly did not trust the woman who said, "How do you know you have DID?" That shut me up real fast.
   c. When having to explain DID to someone, mostly you get a blank stare or a question session about it instead of helping the person. Please do your homework before you begin to provide care for a patient. It is hard to trust someone who is questioning you. I question myself enough.

---

decrease in level of frustration with coping with the multiple identities. Other areas to evaluate include increased acceptance by family and friends. Ultimately, individuals should be able to experience improved function at work, maintain housing, and participate in cultural and spiritual activities that provide support or safety.

Pause and Reflect

1. *What do you think might be challenging about providing care for patients with dissociative disorders? How would you address these challenges?*
2. *Why is it so important to offer choices to these patients when they present for treatment?*

From Suffering to Hope

Working with individuals with somatic symptom and related disorders or dissociative disorders is challenging. Imagine what it must feel like to have parts of your personality take over your executive functioning, to have periods of amnesia and not know what happened, or to believe you are dying and have no one believe you. The symptoms are so complex that sometimes staff members are skeptical that patients are telling the truth about how they feel internally.

This doubt can be detected by patients, who are already doubting themselves. Feeling as though one is making up the symptoms is a form of secondary trauma. It is important that the nurse allow himself or herself to become emotionally available to the patient so the patient can sort through the issues.

By taking patients seriously and providing a thorough assessment, nurses can begin to help patients identify the source of their distress. Simply being taken seriously and being treated with respect can help patients begin to hope that they can get the help they need to alleviate distressing symptoms and restore some normalcy to their lives. However, that is just the beginning: Patients with somatic complaints will have difficulty making themselves sufficiently emotionally available to realize that the source of their discomfort is psychological rather than physical, and patients with dissociative disorders will question which memories and behaviors are real and which are from a fragmented personality. Nurses must help these patients identify their strengths and use them as they begin the path to recovery and rehabilitation. By providing nonjudgmental communication, building the therapeutic alliance, providing education to both the patient and family, and helping patients build on their strengths, nurses can help patients find hope and faith in themselves and their ability to return to wellness.

PERCEPTIONS, THOUGHTS, & FEELINGS: Validating the Needs of a Patient with Symptoms of Dissociation

Patient's behavior(s)	Nurse's perceptions, thoughts, feelings	Exploration with patient
Paula is seen in the ED after telling a friend from NAMI that she had put a gun to her head and was feeling scared that she could kill herself. Following evaluation in the ED, Paula is admitted to the behavioral health unit. Paula is in the day room, by herself writing in her journal.	*Perceptions:* Paula's handwriting in her journal looks different from one page to the next. *Thoughts:* This is very unusual. I have never seen anyone write like this in a journal. I heard in report that Paula has DID; I wonder if the different type of writing represents different people inside of her. I have to be careful to ask Paula in a manner that will contribute to her care rather than my curiosity. *Feelings:* I feel uncertain about working with patients with DID, but I know I can't let that stop me from trying to help Paula.	*Nurse:* Hi Paula, how are you doing today? I met you in Community Meeting this morning. My name is Carla, I am your nurse this shift. I usually spend some time with each patient to work on their clinical goals. Is it okay if we spend some time now?

VALIDATION Carla introduces herself and her role, and asks Paula if she is willing to talk, giving Paula the choice to participate in conversation.

Patient's behavior(s)	Nurse's perceptions, thoughts, feelings	Exploration with patient
Paula pulls her knees in closer and continues to write in her journal. Occasionally she looks up at Carla.	*Thoughts:* Paula seems focused on what she is doing. She may not want to share what she is experiencing. It might be best for me to sit near her, and give her time to think and answer.	

VALIDATION By providing patience and presence, Carla extends herself as an empathic listener.

Patient's behavior(s)	Nurse's perceptions, thoughts, feelings	Exploration with patient
Paula continues holding her journal but stops writing and looks up at Carla. *Paula:* Hi, Carla, I remember you from this morning. I am trying to sort out what happened that I ended up here. Can you tell me what happened?	*Perceptions:* Paula seems calm, and appears willing to engage. *Thoughts:* Paula came from the ED after threatening to kill herself. She seems to be asking what happened. I wonder if she is experiencing amnesia. I know that is part of DID.	*Nurse:* I understand that you came to the emergency department early this morning after being suicidal. You had put a gun to your head and told a friend from NAMI that you were scared you would kill yourself with the gun. You gave her the gun. Do you remember doing that?

VALIDATION Validating Paula's need to learn what happened to understand why she is currently on the behavioral health unit. It important to disclose to Paula the facts of her admission so that Carla can assess her current level of safety and determine her needs for care.

Patient's behavior(s)	Nurse's perceptions, thoughts, feelings	Exploration with patient
Paula: I remember now. I just got the gun to kill squirrels. They eat all of the food I put out for the birds. The "younger ones" inside were crying. I can't stand that, I want them to shut up. Paula begins to cry. *Paula:* I hate this illness; it is ridiculous to have all these people inside wanting to tell me what to do all at once. I don't know who to answer first. The journal helps to give everyone a chance to talk, if they want it.	*Perceptions:* Paula seems distressed by her multiple personality states. *Thoughts:* She is beginning to tell me about what is happening in her thoughts. I can see that she has a battle going on inside of her, between her personality states.	*Nurse:* I see that you are using your journal to think things through. Please tell me if you are feeling safe right now. How do you prevent the desire to harm yourself?

VALIDATION Assessing the patient's potential for suicide. Empowering the patient to determine ways she can assist herself to maintain safety.

Patient's behavior(s)	Nurse's perceptions, thoughts, feelings	Exploration with patient
Paula: I don't feel suicidal now. I do feel shaky inside. I am not sure why this happened. My psychotherapist encouraged me to write down my thoughts.	*Thoughts:* I wonder how I determine who is speaking. I wonder if that is something to ask her. Who inside helps her maintain safety? That is really what I need to know.	**Nurse:** Paula, in report they said that you have dissociative identity disorder. What that means to me is that there may be times that you don't remember what happens to you and that you may have shifts between different personalities. Do I understand that correctly?

VALIDATION Carla tries to clarify Paula's understanding of her illness.

Patient's behavior(s)	Nurse's perceptions, thoughts, feelings	Exploration with patient
Paula: Yes. Peter is very strong. I bet he was involved in the gun thing. Everyone is scared now of guns and him; they pushed him down. I don't always know who is talking, who is doing what, but I can help Peter and George not hurt us now. You are listening; that is helpful. It is also important to me that you believe me when I tell you about the others, because it is true.	*Thoughts:* It must be difficult to live with parts of you thinking about and doing things you don't agree with or are dangerous. Keeping that in mind, I want to help her strengthen her position to maintain safety. After discharge, her psychotherapist and NP can work with the day to day issues and the past trauma that may have caused her to dissociate originally.	**Nurse:** Yes, keeping that in mind, can we develop a care plan directed at keeping you safe? This would include tools to use while you are home and no longer have the structure of the unit.

VALIDATION Validating Paula's explanation of her experience of dissociation with other personality states directing the behavior. The priority for care is to work with Paula to reduce her risk for suicide. Involving her and the knowledge of her internal system will be important to sustain safety.

Based on Orlando, I. J. (1972). The Discipline and Teaching of Nursing Process (An Evaluative Study). New York, NY: G. P. Putnam's Sons.

Paula Rehabilitation Phase

Paula is fixing Abby's motorbike and is enjoying this activity. She attends NAMI twice a month to continue to build emotional skills and resources. At times, she finds NAMI difficult, as the meetings are 90 minutes long, and Paula has difficulty sustaining concentration for that period of time. She will continue to challenge herself to go to at least one meeting a month.

During the psychotherapy sessions, her psychotherapist assesses her for safety. The gun has been sold; however, Paula still experiences Peter thinking about getting a gun, especially if there are squirrels in the yard eating the birdseed. Paula communicates about thoughts and feelings about a gun in her daily safety check to her psychotherapist. She assures herself and her treating psychotherapist that she is not going to obtain another gun.

Treating Paula is a commitment—for both the patient and the psychotherapist. Abandonment issues are palpable and easily trigger dissociation to another personality. Daily journaling, celebrating the gains, and encouraging Paula to have a hobby will sustain the recovery phase.

critical thinking

APPLICATION

1. Address the five domains for Paula at this time:
   a. Biological
   b. Psychological
   c. Sociological
   d. Cultural
   e. Spiritual

2. What are Paula's goals at this time? Are these goals realistic? If so, why? If not, why not?

3. What steps does Paula take to prevent her alternative identity from purchasing a gun? Is this realistic? What other interventions can assist with this important safety issue?

4. How you would prioritize Paula's needs during this encounter, and why?

Chapter Highlights

1. Individuals with somatic symptom and related disorders experience symptoms through their body, feeling pain and other somatic sensations that others may not experience. These body sensations become the patient's focus and concern, often to the exclusion of other areas of the patient's life.

2. It is hypothesized that individuals who have somatic symptom disorders have the personality trait of alexithymia—an inability for the individual to label feelings with words.

3. Individuals with somatic symptom disorders often have a history of neglect, physical abuse, and/or sexual abuse during childhood. These individuals may also have chronic physical illness and emotional illness, such as depression or an anxiety disorder.

4. Individuals with a somatic symptom or related disorder may seek care from multiple providers, feeling as though the practitioners and family members do not take their symptoms seriously. They often feel disengaged from others, including spiritual thoughts and beliefs. The person with somatic symptom disorder feels alone and isolated from others.

5. A nurse who takes the time to provide a comprehensive assessment of all aspects of the patient's functioning, body sensations, thoughts, anxiety, and spiritual concerns can plan and deliver interventions that will assist the patient in reducing the symptoms of a somatic disorder.

6. When working with individuals with somatic symptom and related disorders, a team approach is most effective for both the patient and the practitioners. The team must consist of the medical practitioner, a specialty care provider if a predominant symptom warrants a specialist (e.g., a pain specialist), and the psychological team.

7. Individuals experiencing dissociative disorders have sustained horrific physical and psychological abuse that occurred over time, usually in early childhood. During the trauma, the individuals unconsciously dissociate to cope with the trauma. Many years later, an environmental or physical cue may cause the individual to have flashbacks to the early traumatic events.

8. Individuals who experience a dissociated fragment of memory, as is common in dissociative identity disorder, may label the fragment with a name or act in a different manner than their usual behavior. The dissociated fragment's name and behavior are often based on the original trauma.

9. Dissociation is defined as a disruption and/or a discontinuity of the individual's normal sense of memory, emotions, perception, motor control, behavior, and sense of identity. This disruption causes difficulty in day-to-day functioning. The person is usually embarrassed and attempts to hide the symptoms. Dissociations are unwelcome intrusions that occur with losses of continuity of time, changes in ability to relate to others and amnesia, or the inability to recall what the person was doing during the dissociation.

10. Depersonalization is the experience of unreality or detachment from the individual's mind, sense of self and or physical body. Derealization is defined as the experience of unreality or detachment from the person's surroundings.

11. Changes in identity and dissociative amnesia occur in older individuals. The person may be diagnosed with mood disorders, obsessive–compulsive disorder, paranoia, psychotic mood disorders, or cognitive disorders rather than dissociative identity disorder. The individual may begin to show signs of changes in identity after events such as leaving a traumatic situation; having a child reach the same age that they were when they sustained their abuse or trauma; traumatic experiences that occur in adulthood, such as an automobile accident; and the death or terminal illness of the person's abuser.

12. The most effective treatment for individuals with dissociative identity disorder is affect regulation, grounding, treatment of PTSD symptoms, and understanding the symptoms of dissociation.

13. Providing psychotherapy for an individual with dissociative disorders is long term. The primary psychotherapist for this individual conceptualizes the therapy as taking place over years. Most of the therapeutic work is done in an outpatient setting.

14. There are three phases for providing care for an individual with dissociative identity disorder:
    a. Establishing safety, stabilization and symptom reduction
    b. Working through and integrating traumatic memories
    c. Identity integration and rehabilitation

15. Due to the complexity of dissociative disorder, the patient may not be aware of when a relapse is occurring until people who make up the patient's support system request that he or she seek additional care.

16. An individual with a dissociative disorder has many challenges. The first priority is safety—for self and others.

NCLEX®-RN Questions

1. The nurse is planning teaching sessions for patients newly diagnosed with dissociative disorders and for patients who are experiencing somatic symptom disorder. Which statements related to the etiology of the disorders are accurate? Select all that apply.
   a. Both types of disorders have been linked to traumatic experiences.
   b. There is a neurobiological basis for somatic symptom disorders only.
   c. The suffering and pain associated with both types of disorders is overstated.
   d. Research has demonstrated that dissociative disorders cannot be deliberately enacted.
   e. Frequently, a diagnosis of somatic symptom disorder is concurrent with a diagnosis of a medical illness.

2. The nurse is caring for a patient with a somatic symptom disorder. The nurse reflects on her own feelings and beliefs about the disorder in order to provide nonjudgmental care. The rationale for this action relates most closely to which health/wellness domain?
   a. Cultural
   b. Spiritual
   c. Sociological
   d. Psychological

3. The nurse is assessing the patient with a history of severe trauma and abuse. Which finding alerts the nurse to the possibility of a dissociative disorder?
   a. The patient experiences symptoms of abnormal voluntary motor function.
   b. The patient's psychological symptoms affect the course of an associated medical illness.
   c. The patient reports recurrent gaps in the recall of everyday events and important information.
   d. The patient experiences excessive thoughts, feelings, or behaviors related to an associated health concern.

4. The nurse is caring for a patient with a dissociative disorder. The patient reports having been a victim of abuse while in the fourth grade. The patient states she is unable to remember any details of the event or anything else occurring and still cannot apply simple mathematical concepts that may have been introduced at this time. The nurse recognizes that the patient is experiencing which type of amnesia?
   a. Localized
   b. Selective
   c. Generalized
   d. Depersonalized

5. The nurse is caring for a patient experiencing a somatic symptom disorder. The patient's family member asks if there are any medications that can treat the underlying cause of the disorder. How should the nurse respond?
   a. "The treatment of choice is intensive, long-term talk psychotherapy."
   b. "Antidepressants and antianxiety agents are the treatment of choice."
   c. "Somatic symptoms respond to the same medications used to treat a medical condition with the same symptoms."
   d. "Cognitive–behavioral therapy and collaborative health care interventions are used to treat the disorder."

6. The nurse is caring for a patient with a dissociative disorder. Based on an understanding of the nature of the disorder, which of the following nursing diagnoses is priority?
   a. Risk of suicide
   b. Ineffective coping
   c. Posttrauma response
   d. Disturbed body image

Answers may be found on the Pearson student resource site: nursing.pearsonhighered.com

Pearson Nursing Student Resources Find additional review materials at **nursing.pearsonhighered.com**

References

American Psychiatric Association. (2000). *Diagnostic and Statistical Manual of Mental Disorders* (4th Edition, Text Revision). Washington, DC: American Psychiatric Publishing.

American Psychiatric Association. (2013). *Diagnostic and Statistical Manual of Mental Disorders* (5th ed.). Washington, DC: American Psychiatric Publishing.

Aust, S., Härtwig, E. A., Heuser, I., & Bajbouj, M. (2013). The role of early emotional neglect in alexithymia. *Psychological Trauma: Theory, Research, Practice and Policy, 5*(3), 225–232.

Balaban-Murat, H., Serniz, M., Şentürk, İ. A., Kavakçi, Ö., Çinar, Z., Dikici, A., & Topaktaş, S. (2012). Migraine prevalence, alexithymia, and post-traumatic stress disorder among medical students in Turkey. *Journal of Headache Pain, 13*(6), 459–467.

Bernstein, E. M., & Putnam, F. W. (1986). Development, reliability, and validity of a dissociation scale. *Journal of Nervous and Mental Disease, 174*, 727–735.

Boysen, G. A. (2011) The scientific status of childhood dissociative identity disorder: A review of published research. *Psychotherapy and Psychosomatics, 80*(6), 329–334.

Briquet, P. (1859). *Traité clinique et thérapeutique de l'hystérie.* Paris, France: J. Bailliere.

Brosbe, M. S., Faust, J., & Gold, S. N. (2013). Complex traumatic stress in the pediatric medical setting. *Journal of Trauma and Dissociation, 14*(1), 97–112.

Chappa, A. K., Audus, K. L., & Lunte, S. M. (2006) Characteristics of Substance P transport across the blood brain barrier. *Pharmaceutical Research, 23*(6), 1201–1208.

DeSteno, D., Gross, J. J., & Kubzansky, L. (2013). Affective science and health: The importance of emotion and emotion regulation. *Health Psychology, 32*(5), 474–486.

Dinwiddie, S. (2013). Somatization disorder: Past, present, and future. *Psychiatric Annals, 43*(2), 78–83.

Dorahy, M. J., & Lewis, C. A. (2001). The relationship between dissociation and religiosity: An empirical evaluation of Schumaker's theory. *Journal for the Scientific Study of Religion, 40*, 315–322.

Elzinga, B. M., Ardon, A. M., Heijnis, M. K., DeRuiter, M.. et al. (2007). Neural correlates of enhanced working-memory performance in dissociative disorder: A functional MRI study. *Psychological Medicine, 37*(2), 235–246.

Grepmair, L., Mitterlehner, F., Loew, T., Bachler, E., Rother, W., & Nickel, M. (2007). Promoting mindfulness in psychotherapists in training influences the treatment results of their patients: A randomized, double-blind, controlled study. *Psychotherapy and Psychosomics, 76*, 332–338.

Grossman, P., Niemann, L., Schmidt, S., & Walach, H. (2004). Mindfulness-based stress reduction and health benefits: A meta-analysis. *Journal of Psychosomatic Research, 57*, 35–43.

International Society for the Study of Trauma and Dissociation, Chu, J. A., Dell, P. F. Van der Hart, O., Cardeña, E., et al. (2011). Guidelines for treating dissociative identity disorder in adults, 3rd revision. *Journal of Trauma and Dissociation, 12*, 115–187.

Kozlowska, K., Foley, S., & Savage, B. (2012). Fabricated illness: Working within the family system to find a pathway to health. *Family Process, 51*(4), 570–587.

Loewenstein, R. J. (1990). Somatoform disorders in victims of incest and child abuse. In R. P. Kluft (Ed.). *Incest-Related Syndrome of Adult Psychopathy.* Washington, DC: American Psychiatric Press, pp. 75–107.

Markowitsch, H. J., & Staniloiu, A. (2012). Amnesic disorders. *Lancet, 380*(9581), 1429–1440.

Reinders, A. A. T. S., Willemsen, A. T. M., Vos, H. P. J., denBoer, J. A., & Nijenhuis, E. R. S. (2012). Fact or factitious? A psychobiological study of authentic and simulated dissociative identity states. *PloS One, 7*(6), e39279, www.plosone.org

Robinson, J. E., Fish, E. W., Krouse, M. C., Thorsell, A., Heilig, M., & Malanga, C. J. (2012). Potentiation of brain stimulation reward by morphine: Effects of neurokinin-1 receptor antagonism. *Psychopharmacology, 220*(1), 215–224.

Rosik, C. H., & Soria, A. (2012). Spiritual well-being, dissociation, and alexithymia: Examining direct and moderating effects. *Journal of Trauma and Dissociation, 13*(1), 69–87.

Stahl, S. M. (2013). *Stahl's Essential Psychopharmacology: Neuroscientific Basis and Practical Applications* (4th ed.). New York, NY: Cambridge University Press.

Steinberg, M. (2010). *Stranger in the Mirror: The Hidden Epidemic of Dissociation.* New York, NY: Harper Colllins.

Weber, S. (2008). Diagnosis of trauma and abuse-related dissociative symptom disorders in children and adolescents. *Journal of Child and Adolescent Psychiatric Nursing, 21*(4), 205–213.

Weber, S. (2009). Treatment of trauma- and abuse-related dissociative symptom disorders in children and adolescents. *Journal of Child and Adolescent Psychiatric Nursing, 22*(1), 2–7.

Wright, D. B., & Loftus, E. F. (1999). Measuring dissociation: Comparison of alternative forms of the dissociative experiences scale. *American Journal of Psychology, 112*(4), 497–519.

Xiao, Z., Heqin, Y., Wang, Z., Zou, Z., et al. (2006). Trauma and dissociation in China. *American Journal of Psychiatry, 163*, 1388–1391.

Yates, W. R., & Dunayevich, E. (2012a). Somatoform disorders follow-up. *Medscape Reference*, http://emedicine.medscape.com/article/294908-followup

Yates, W. R., & Dunayevich, E. (2012b) Somatoform disorders medication. *Medscape Reference*, http://emedicine.medscape.com/article/294908-medication

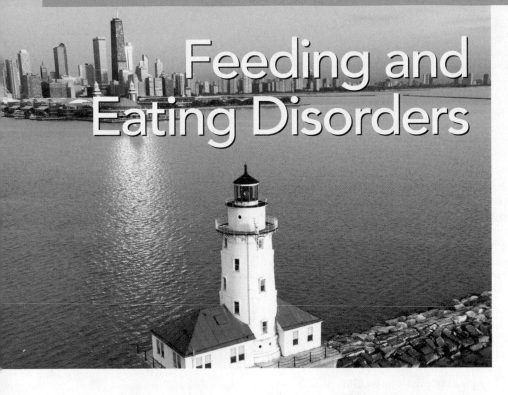

Feeding and Eating Disorders

15

Sandy Hannon-Engel
Elspeth Dwyer

Learning Outcomes

1. Describe core characteristics of feeding and eating disorders.

2. Summarize the impact of biological, psychological, sociological, cultural, and spiritual domains on feeding and eating disorders.

3. Compare and contrast the clinical manifestations of anorexia nervosa, bulimia, and binge-eating disorder.

4. Analyze the importance of nutritional rehabilitation in the treatment of feeding and eating disorders.

5. Evaluate the effectiveness of psychotherapeutic and pharmacologic interventions used in the treatment of feeding and eating disorders.

6. Distinguish characteristics of anorexia nervosa that affect patient suffering and readiness to participate in treatment.

7. Differentiate characteristics of bulimia nervosa that affect patient suffering and readiness to participate in treatment.

8. Plan evidence-based nursing care for patients with feeding and eating disorders.

Key Terms

anorexia nervosa, 298
avoidant/restrictive food intake disorder, 299
binge-eating disorder, 298
bulimia nervosa, 298
cachexia, 310
feeding and eating disorders, 298
night eating syndrome, 299
other specified feeding or eating disorder, 299
pica, 299
purging disorder, 299
refeeding syndrome, 305
rumination disorder, 299
unspecified feeding or eating disorder, 299

Kara Initial Onset

Kara Murphy is a 16-year-old female patient who presents for admission to a psychiatric inpatient unit. She is accompanied by her mother. When Liz, a registered nurse who works on the unit, invites Kara into a room to complete her admission assessment, Kara's mother accompanies her. Kara is casually dressed in baggy clothes, appears to be of average height and weight, and has bloodshot eyes. Her cheeks and neck appear puffy and swollen. During the assessment, Kara appears defensive, slouching in a chair with her arms crossed, and answers questions with one-word answers. Kara's mother gives answers to all questions, even those directed at Kara, while Kara continues to sit with her arms crossed and rolls her eyes and sighs heavily when her mother speaks. Kara's mother reports to the nurse that during a recent argument, Kara "told me she was going to kill herself." Kara's mother adds, "I don't know what to do with her anymore, so I brought her to the hospital."

During the assessment, Liz discovers that Kara had a prior psychiatric hospitalization for the treatment of anorexia nervosa when she was 13, and that Kara has continued to struggle with disordered eating, most recently binging and purging. Kara reports that the argument leading to her hospitalization occurred when her mother woke up late at night to find Kara binging, already having eaten a box of cereal, two large bags of potato chips, two sandwiches, and a large container of pasta salad. Kara reports that when her mother found her binging, she told Kara she was "disgusting" and then tried to physically prevent Kara from entering the bathroom to purge. Kara says at that point she became distraught and reports, "I said I was going to kill myself."

Liz learns that Kara's problems started around age 11, which her mother associates with her having started menarche early and ahead of her friends. Her mother says, "From that point on, she was just really uncomfortable in her own body." Kara's mother also reports that around this time she and Kara's father divorced and she was forced to return to work full time, having been able to stay at home with Kara (who is an only child) until that point. It was around this time that Kara began restricting food and was eventually hospitalized for anorexia at age 13 with a body mass index (BMI) of 14.5. Kara reports that since her hospitalization she has continued to have trouble; most recently, she has had episodes of binging and purging. She says, "I try to restrict what I eat, but I can't. I usually end up totally out of control and binging. Then I feel so bad, I have to try to throw it all up to stop myself from getting fat."

In addition to the ongoing problems with disordered eating, Kara reports that she experiences significant anxiety and depression. She reports she has very poor self-esteem, and constantly has negative self-thoughts about "being fat and ugly." Kara says she feels anxious most days and worries that she is going to have to stay back in school next year because her anxiety has led to her missing school and being unable to attend to her work when she is there. Kara acknowledges that all these problems have left her feeling depressed and that she often contemplates suicide. Her mother reports that Kara has been more irritable at home, and her behavior has been more impulsive, including recently skipping school and sneaking out of the house late at night. Kara and her mother both agree that they feel hospitalization is necessary at this time, and Kara's mother voluntarily signs her into the hospital. Following the assessment, Liz explains the policies of the unit to Kara and her mother and shows Kara to her room.

APPLICATION

1. Address the five domains for Kara:
   a. Biological
   b. Psychological
   c. Sociological
   d. Cultural
   e. Spiritual

2. In what ways do you think Kara may be suffering? Why?

3. How would you prioritize Kara's needs at this time? Why?

4. In what way does Liz convey hope to Kara? What might you have done differently to offer hope?

Introduction

Homeostasis depends on the successful regulation of human eating behavior. **Feeding and eating disorders** are characterized by alterations in normal eating patterns that are marked by distinct and persistent disturbances in eating behaviors, weight regulation, and perceptions toward body weight and shape. Nurses will most commonly encounter three distinct feeding and eating disorders recognized by the DSM-5: anorexia nervosa (AN), bulimia nervosa (BN), and binge-eating disorder (BED). These three eating disorders are discussed fully in this chapter.

Those suffering from **anorexia nervosa** have an unrelenting fear of weight gain in association with extreme distortions of body image, preoccupation with food, and refusal to eat, all in pursuit of thinness. They engage in persistent behaviors that interfere with weight gain, despite markedly low body weight. They can become underweight as a consequence of food restriction, excessive exercise, and other compensatory behaviors (for example, self-induced vomiting and laxative and/or diuretic misuse) (Steinglass et al., 2012).

Bulimia nervosa is characterized by repeated binge-eating episodes and inappropriate compensatory behaviors aimed at controlling weight gain. Individuals affected by this disorder are likely to maintain a normal weight or be overweight despite fluctuations in food intake. Regular attempts at food restriction and dieting are interrupted by repeated binging and purging episodes (Wolfe, Hannon-Engel & Mitchell, 2012).

The criteria for **binge-eating disorder** are recurrent episodes of binge eating in the absence of extreme weight-control behavior, accompanied by a sense of lack of control. As a result, a number of patients with BED are overweight (BMI = 25–30) or meet criteria for obesity (BMI > 30) (Hilbert et al., 2011). However, BED also occurs in individuals of normal weight. BED is distinct from obesity in that most obese individuals do not engage in recurrent binge eating (American Psychiatric Association, 2013).

There are two other related feeding and eating categories. In **other specified feeding or eating disorder**, there are symptoms of a feeding or eating disorder that cause clinically significant impairment or distress but do not meet the full diagnostic criteria. In **unspecified feeding or eating disorder**, symptoms that do not meet the full diagnostic criteria predominate, and the clinician chooses *not* to specify which specific order the presentation resembles. The "specified" category can be used when the clinician can identify the eating disorder, but the duration does not meet full criteria—for instance, a diagnosis of bulimia nervosa "of low frequency" or "of limited duration." Other feeding and eating behaviors that may be specified are **purging disorder**, in which an individual purges to influence weight or shape, and **night eating syndrome**, characterized by excessive eating after the evening meal or after awakening from sleep. Often the "unspecified" category is reserved for a clinician who is having limited contact with the patient, such as in an emergency department setting, and who does not have sufficient information to make an accurate diagnosis (APA, 2013).

Be aware that nurses also may encounter some less familiar feeding and eating disorders: pica, rumination disorder, and avoidant/restrictive food intake disorder (APA, 2013). **Pica** is the persistent eating of substances other than food, such as paper, soap, cloth, hair, paint, gum, and pebbles. Obviously, clinicians will be concerned about the medical complications associated with ingesting foreign substances, such as mechanical intestinal and bowel obstruction and perforation, parasitic infections, and poisoning. **Rumination disorder** is the repeated regurgitation of food. The regurgitated food may be re-chewed, re-swallowed, or spit out. **Avoidant/restrictive food intake disorder** is a lack of interest in food and eating food (when food is available) as supported by weight loss and nutritional deficiencies. These diagnoses all have specific criteria regarding essential characteristics, duration, and exclusions (APA, 2013).

The chronic and debilitating nature of feeding and eating disorders has a significant impact on the psychological and physiological well-being of the individual. Therefore, it is essential that nurses conduct a comprehensive assessment and plan of treatment that promotes opportunities for healing and alleviates the suffering of those with feeding and eating disorders.

Theoretical Foundations

Feeding and eating disorders are multifaceted illnesses that involve the biological, psychological, sociological, cultural, and spiritual domains of wellness (Figure 15-1). Each domain contributes to the overall vulnerability and maintenance factors of these disorders (Table 15-1).

Biological Domain

The biological aspects of eating disorders are complex and not fully understood. During active illness, there are known disturbances in neuroendocrine, neurochemistry, and neurotransmission circuitry and signal pathways (Monteleone & Maj, 2013). Investigators have found disturbances in serotonin and neuropeptide systems that modulate appetite, mood, cognitive function, impulse control, energy metabolism, and hormonal systems (Kaye, 2008). As a result of their malnourished and emaciated state, individuals with AN have alterations of brain structure (Mühlau et al., 2007), metabolism

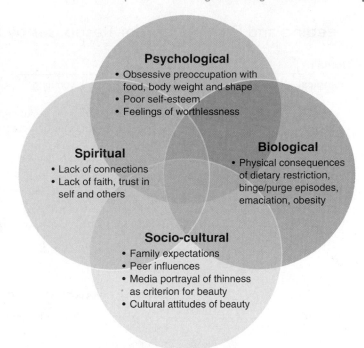

15-1   Domains of wellness and feeding and eating disorders.

(Katzman, 2005), and neurochemistry, whereas those with BN have shown brain atrophy in imaging studies (Kaye et al., 2005).

The genetic heritability of feeding and eating disorders is comparable to other biologically based mental illnesses. Twin studies in AN, BN, and BED estimate that 50% to 83% of the variance is accounted for by genetic factors (Klump & Culbert, 2007). Further, these studies revealed that puberty has a powerful impact in activating the genes of etiological importance in feeding and eating disorders (Klump et al., 2012). Molecular genetic studies are beginning to identify chromosomal genes and regions that may contribute to the etiology of eating disorders (Klump, Bulik, Kaye, Treasure, & Tyson, 2009). Areas on chromosomes 1, 4, and 10 may maintain risk genes for AN and BN (Klump et al., 2009). Additional risk for AN may be in the genes involved in the serotonin and opioid systems and brain-derived neurotrophic factor (BDNF) (Brandys, Kas, van Elburg, Campbell, & Adan, 2011).

Control of Body Weight and Appetite

The regulation of feeding behavior involves a complex integrative central and peripheral signaling network system of positive and negative feedback mechanisms that work to maintain energy homeostasis (Woods & Ramsay, 2011). Positive feedback signals are initiated by feeding behavior. In response, inhibitory or negative feedback signals, requiring greater potency, terminate an episode of eating (Halford & Harrold, 2012). In the case of binge eating, if there is a dysregulation in the relative potency of the negative feedback signaling mechanism, meal size and duration can be increased. Thus, binge eating may reflect a relative dysregulation in the negative feedback system.

During meals, satiety-signaling neuropeptides—cholecystokinin (CCK) and glucagon-like peptide (GLP-1) from the gut (stomach and intestine)—generate sensory nerves impulses to the hindbrain.

Feeding and Eating Disorder Responses by Domain   table 15-1

Domain	Response
Biological	• Anorexia, nausea, vomiting • Headache • Disturbed neuroendocrine function • Physical consequences of dietary restriction, emaciation, binge/purge episodes, and obesity
Psychological	• Poor self-esteem • Poor locus of control • Perfectionism • Anxiety • Tension • Depression • Helplessness • Worthlessness • Self-deprecatory thoughts • Pathological overconcern with body weight and shape • Obsessive preoccupation with food, ruminations, and rituals

Sociological	• Idealization of body image and eating originate from the:
	  • Family
	  • Peers
	  • Media

Cultural	• Culture defines attitudes and beliefs about beauty. • Western industrialized culture values thinness as the ideal. • Feeding and eating disorders are mainly a problem for White women of American or European culture.
Spiritual	• Lack of connectedness to a Higher Power • Lost connection to the universe and all that exists within it • Struggles with loss of faith, hope, forgiveness, and trust in themselves and others

These satiation signals connect with neurons in the brain stem via synapses, where they influence meal size and duration (Woods & D'Alessio, 2008). Ghrelin, a gut peptide that increases appetite, acts on the vagus nerve and stimulates neurons in the hypothalamus. Short-acting satiation signals from the gut to the hindbrain also interact with the long-acting adiposity hormones, leptin and insulin, which are then released and circulated in the blood. These hormones gain access to the hypothalamus in response to the amount of fat stores and energy needs to maintain weight regulation, metabolism, and homeostasis (Figure 15-2). This higher-order integration evaluates inhibitory signals and metabolic state to determine energy storage needs for regulation, whereas the nucleus tractus solitarius in the caudal brainstem primarily controls the amount of food eaten. During food deprivation or restriction, the sensitivity of the short-acting satiation signals decreases. Therefore, it takes larger amounts of food to generate adequate signaling to terminate a meal (Woods & Ramsay, 2011). As seen in Table 15-2, these hormones can affect satiation by either increasing or decreasing the amount of food eaten.

Research has shown that in comparison to individuals without weight issues, those suffering from feeding and eating disorders experience blunted or attenuated functioning in both the short- and long-acting signaling processes responsible for appetite and weight regulation (Table 15-3). When individuals cease eating disordered behaviors, these hormones may return to a normalized state. However, in some individuals these hormones may remain dysfunctional, indicating a *trait*-related phenomenon. Therefore, investigators are

left to determine whether these dysfunctions are a cause, consequence, or maintenance factor in eating disorders.

When individuals who stop engaging in eating disorder behaviors experience normalization of a hormone (such as CCK), this may indicate an adaptive response (Hannon-Engel, Filin, & Wolfe, 2012). Perhaps a recalibration begins to effectively regulate and control the input of neuronal and hormonal signals to the hindbrain. As a result, homeostasis and the stability of the hormone system feedback loops are restored. The resulting responses are the absence of debilitating behaviors (such as binging or vomiting) (Hannon-Engel, 2008). What is unclear is which adaptive mechanism(s) must be present and properly functioning for hormonal response to return to normal and for this behavior to remit. Understanding which biological adaptations must occur before remission and how these can be promoted and maintained is essential to the development of effective treatment strategies and relapse prevention, and merits further investigation.

Psychological Domain

Individuals with eating disorders judge themselves predominately, and often exclusively, on their body shape and ability to control their weight (Murphy, Straebler, Cooper, & Fairburn, 2010). This type of thinking represents distorted cognitive processes. In contrast, those without disordered eating judge themselves on a wide variety of life domains, including relationships, work or academic achievement, public service, and athletic or artistic ability. Therefore, those with eating disorders (who persistently judge themselves on these unobtainable and overvalued beliefs of body shape and weight) feel

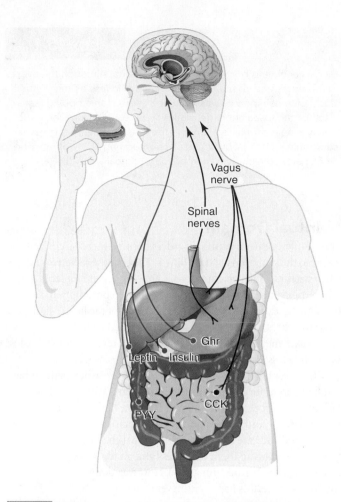

15-2   Hormones acting through the brain help regulate metabolism and short- and long-term appetite.

Select Hormones that Affect Satiation	table 15-2

Hormone	Effect on food intake
Leptin	Decrease
CCK	Decrease
GLP-1	Decrease
Ghrelin	Increase

Changes in Hormones in Active AN and BN	table 15-3

Hormone	AN	BN
Leptin	↓	↓
CCK	↑/↓	↓
GLP-1		↓
Ghrelin	↑	↑

Note: ↑, increase; ↓, decrease; arrows specify that research findings indicate a significant difference in comparison to healthy controls.

immense shame, hopelessness, helplessness, and worthlessness. Furthermore, the severe and disabling cognitive distortions that individuals with eating disorders experience erode their personhood and their abilities to find hope amid their suffering and pain.

Until the 19th century, "anorexia" was characterized as a symptom of several physical and psychological conditions. Previously, forms of long-lasting food refusal, not attributed to a medical condition, would often conjure up rumors about supernatural powers or demonic influences (Fairburn, 2002). Food avoidance and emaciation were common symptoms of "hysteria." At the end of the 17th century, "nervous consumption" was considered a wasting away due to emotional turmoil. It was later dubbed "anorexia hysterica," and, in 1874, Sir William Withey Gull began using the term "anorexia nervosa." From 1945 to 1960, psychiatry was strongly rooted in psychoanalytical views. Thus, AN was viewed as food refusal due to an unconscious fear of oral impregnation. In 1960, American psychiatrist Hilde Brunch focused attention on the lack of self-esteem and body image disturbance (Fairburn, 2002).

The psychopathology of this relentless pursuit of thinness has been labeled as hysteria, a phobia of weight gain, an obsession, and even a delusion. Those with anorexia nervosa will severely restrict dietary intake and protest that they feel and see themselves as fat despite their current state of emaciation. Individuals appear to be genuinely terrified at the prospect of being overweight, and some openly state they would prefer death (Attia, 2010). AN is associated with premorbid perfectionism, introversion, poor peer relations, and low self-esteem. For many, emotional problems arise from separation anxiety, difficulties with identity, and feelings related to lack of control. Other psychological symptoms, many of which can also be contributed to the semi-starvation state, include depressed mood, irritability, social withdrawal, loss of libido, preoccupation with food, obsessional ruminations and rituals, and, eventually, reduced alertness and concentration (Attia & Walsh, 2009).

More than 30 years ago, bulimia nervosa was first described by Russell (1979) as an "ominous variant" of anorexia nervosa. In his initial account, Russell described this "bulimic" group as having core eating-disordered beliefs about weight similar to those of AN. However, unlike those with AN who restrict food consumption, individuals with BN have distinct symptom patterns including an irresistible urge to overeat, followed by self-induced vomiting (Russell, 1979). Pervasive devalued self-worth and loathing of body weight and shape are characteristic of BN. Common premorbid characteristics of impulsivity (Kemps & Wilsdon, 2009), dysregulated emotions, anxiety, depression (Swinbourne et al., 2012), low self-esteem, early menarche, dieting, and critical comments about eating may contribute to the vulnerability and expression of this disorder.

Sociological Domain

The sociological domain includes environmental factors that affect the development and maintenance of an eating disorder. Environmental conditions, such as family and peer relationships and exposure to media images that portray thinness as the ideal, reinforce eating disorder behaviors (Box 15-1) (Wilksch & Wade, 2012). Previous studies have found that age, sex, disparaging remarks about weight, the media, and parental history of an eating disorder can be risk factors in children (Benowitz-Fredericks et al., 2012).

Clustering of individuals with eating disorders has been documented in the literature. Among others, a study by Forman-Huffman

| Influences on Female Body Dissatisfaction | box 15-1 |

Research in the portrayal of women in mass media indicates that the body sizes of women are decreasing steadily. Thinness and beauty are often correlated with success. Consider this: How many thin actresses in television and movies can you name? How many can you name who are overweight?

A recent study surveyed 285 female undergraduates with regard to several criteria, including exposure to mass media, self-esteem, and body dissatisfaction criteria. Although the overwhelming trend of mass media toward thinness as the cultural ideal of female beauty was identified as a factor in body dissatisfaction, the researchers determined that social influences, especially peer influences, and self-esteem were the greatest determinants of body dissatisfaction among the women who took part in the study (van Vonderen & Kinnally, 2012).

and Cunningham (2008) confirmed a clustering by county of high school students exhibiting eating disorders. This supports earlier research on the possibility of a "contagious nature" of eating disorders. Although the reasons for clustering remain unclear, a combination of low self-esteem and peer influences are strongly suspected as two contributing factors.

Disordered eating behaviors also have a direct impact on the individual's ability to function in home, work, school, and other environments. Preoccupations with food and rituals may interrupt or prevent individuals from participating in normal activities (Haines et al., 2011). Decreased energy and associated irritability, related to semi-starvation, can further affect cognitive performance and family and peer relationships (Hatch et al., 2010). This results in increased feelings of alienation and worthlessness.

For the patient experiencing an eating disorder, sociological factors can influence the disease process as well as contribute to hope and healing. For example, in the case study presented in this chapter, Kara identifies that her mother has, in some ways, reinforced her disordered eating through comments about her weight and through her own dieting behavior. The influence of Kara's relationship with her mother also becomes an integral part of her transition from suffering to hope. Comprehensive nursing care will assess the influence of family dynamics on functioning, support, and other sociological dimensions that can affect patient recovery.

Cultural Domain

Implicit in the diagnostic criteria for eating disorders are behaviors and attitudes that carry meaning as symptoms in relationship to core cultural values. For women of Western cultural values who identify appearance as a central component of one's value and for whom thinness is portrayed as the ideal, body dissatisfaction seems almost unavoidable (Mask & Blanchard, 2011). The resulting distorted body image and belief and fear of being fat, which are essentially cultural in origin, are criteria of both AN and BN (George & Franko, 2010).

It has been argued that AN and BN may be culture-bound syndromes (Keel & Klump, 2003). However, recent studies suggest that disordered eating and body image issues are now recognized as affecting all the following racial and ethnic groups in the United States: African Americans, Latino/as, Asians, and Native Americans (George & Franko, 2010). In addition, cross-cultural studies have shown patterns of disordered eating in other cultures; however, these individuals may not meet the full diagnostic criteria of AN or BN. For example, presentations of pathology similar to AN, with the exception of the core diagnostic criterion of fear of being or becoming fat, have been described in populations in Hong Kong, Japan, Singapore, Malaysia, and India (Becker, 2007).

Spiritual Domain

Those suffering from eating disorders become increasingly isolated owing to the symptoms of their illness. They choose secretive and isolative states in which all connections are eclipsed and replaced with a self-perpetuating cycle of food restriction, overconsumption, and loss of control to expelling all nutrients at the cost of the host (Matusek & Knudson, 2009). Loss of connections combined with low self-esteem and an extreme focus on maintaining the disorder can result in a loss of spirit—a loss of faith, hope, and trust in themselves and others.

It is essential that nurses be able to recognize when patients have lost faith, hope, forgiveness, and trust in themselves and others. This lack of spirit affects their connection to their biological and psychological health and their cultural and sociological interests and uniqueness. They are left with the belief that their eating-disordered behaviors will bring them happiness and an ideal body weight and shape (Matusek & Knudson, 2009). However, despite all their suffering and sacrifice, this happiness never arrives.

Spirituality in eating disorders represents a reconnection within the self, reflected in the light of someone or something outside the self. Those struggling with eating disorders have lost their connection to the universe and all that exists within it. Therefore, a reconnection to their spirit allows them to forgive the inadequacies surrounding their weight and shape and embrace their beings without judgment. Connecting to their spirit will hasten the healing and enliven their feelings of hope (Espindola & Blay, 2009).

Nurses can support the individual with an eating disorder by listening, being present, and suggesting a reconnection to past and future strands of hope, spirit, and trust. Assessing which factors or activities brought comfort and happiness prior to the onset of the eating disorder may help identify possibilities for restoring the individual's connections to self and others.

Pause and Reflect

1. *What behaviors does Kara display that you think might be indicative of an eating disorder?*
2. *What other behaviors, apart from those pertaining to eating or weight control, does Kara display that are concerning?*
3. *How would you explain the psychological domain of Kara's suffering?*

Feeding and Eating Disorders

The multifactorial etiology of feeding and eating disorders, combined with their direct and damaging impact on the domains of wellness, make recovering from these disorders especially challenging (Figure 15-3). The dysregulation of hormones can be difficult to overcome, and

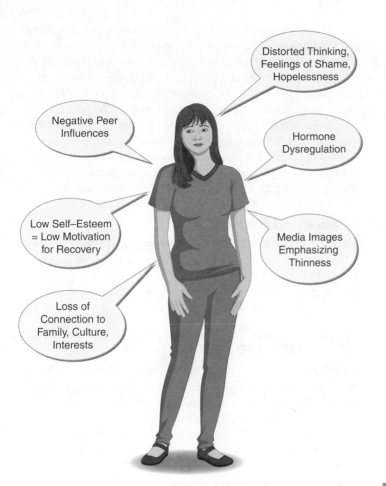

15-3 The multifactorial etiology of feeding and eating disorders makes them particularly challenging to treat.

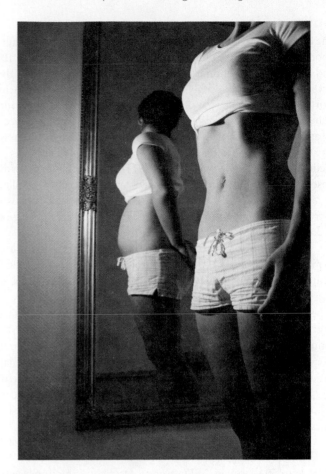

15-4 Individuals with feeding and eating disorders often have a distorted image of their weight and shape.

Source: Xenia-Luise/Fotolia

negative peer influences can create added hostility to the patient's recovery environment. Low self-esteem challenges treatment adherence: Patients who care little for themselves have little motivation for participating in self-care and recovery. A thorough understanding of the symptoms of eating disorders is necessary to promote early identification and treatment of these vulnerable patients.

The average age of onset of AN is 19 years, compared with the average age of onset of 25 years for BN. However, eating disorders are a concern for adolescents, with 2.7% of individuals ages 13 to 18 years diagnosed with an eating disorder (National Institute of Mental Health, n.d.). Lifetime prevalence rates of eating disorders are higher in women (Hudson, Hiripi, Pope, & Kessler, 2007). Longitudinal research indicates that most individuals with eating disorders change in and out of illness states, may vary in diagnosis, display frequent relapses, and show lifetime psychiatric co-morbidity (Eddy et al., 2008; Castellini et al., 2011).

Anorexia Nervosa

Patients suffering with AN persistently restrict energy intake, have an unrelenting fear of weight gain or engage in behavior that interferes with weight gain, and have disturbed self-perceptions regarding weight and shape (APA, 2013). AN is characterized as a refusal to maintain a normal weight for age, sex, developmental trajectory, and physical health and a distorted perception of body weight and shape (Figure 15-4). Some individuals report feeling trapped in and deeply ashamed of their own bodies: "I won't be able to walk through the door because I take up too much

space" (Rørtveit, Åström, & Severinsson, 2009, p. 95). Individuals with AN become underweight largely as a consequence of an unrelenting restriction in the amount and types of food they eat, and they are bound by strict dietary rules. Excessive exercising further contributes to low body weight. Some individuals with AN enjoy the sense of control they gain from depriving their bodies of the essential nutrients to sustain life. In contrast, some individuals experience a loss of control resulting in binge eating followed by self-induced vomiting, laxative and/or diuretic misuse (Matusek & Knudson, 2009). These individuals typically are identified with anorexia nervosa—binging eating/purging type. AN is associated with premorbid perfectionism, introversion, poor peer relations, and low self-esteem. One woman's recollection included, "The false belief of becoming thinner had me believing that happiness was almost within my grasp. It would be mine if I could only lose a few more pounds …then I'd be truly happy" (Matusek & Knudson, 2009, p. 701).

A semi-starvation state can contribute to symptoms of depressed mood, irritability, social withdrawal, excessive preoccupation with food, obsessional ruminations and rituals, and, ultimately, reduced alertness and concentration, and cognitive deficits (Attia & Walsh, 2009). Secondary to being underweight are multiple physiological characteristics, including poor sleep, sensitivity to the cold, heightened fullness, and decreased energy (Murphy, Straebler, Cooper, & Fairburn, 2010). Further physical manifestations of this illness are examined later in this chapter. AN is a serious psychiatric disorder with morbidity and mortality rates that are among the highest of mental disorders (Arcelus, Mitchell, Wales, & Nielsen, 2011).

Bulimia Nervosa

The onset of BN typically starts during adolescence or young adulthood, with an often chronic course of illness (Keel & Brown, 2010) and a substantial economic burden (Stuhldreher et al., 2012). The development of BN generally begins with a pervasive devalued self-worth, loathing of body weight and shape, and depressive mood states (Stice, Marti, & Durant, 2011). Self-worth is unduly influenced by and dependent on the successful attainment of extreme thinness. This quest for perfectionism sets the stage for repeated episodes of dieting and food restriction (Cheney, 2012). A risk factor for the early onset of binge eating is food restriction or fasting (Stice, Davis, Miller, & Marti, 2008). As the individual struggles for control, a compensatory pattern of binging and purging behaviors becomes entrenched (Stice, Rohde, Shaw, & Marti, 2013).

Binging and purging becomes a powerful way for the individual to manage internal emotional states, arbitrate challenges to personal control, and deal with cravings and urges (Stice, Rohde, Shaw, & Marti, 2013). The individual typically engages in binge eating when experiencing negative affect such as interpersonal stressors; dietary restraint; negative feelings related to body weight, body shape, and food; and boredom (see DSM-5 Diagnostic Criteria for Bulimia Nervosa). The inappropriate compensatory purge behaviors may include vomiting (the most common purging method), misuse of laxatives and diuretics, enemas, manipulation of prescription medications such as thyroid hormone and insulin, fasting, and excessive exercise (APA, 2013).

Binge-Eating Disorder

More than 50 years ago, BED was first described as a discrete subgroup of the obese population that displayed recurrent binge-eating behavior without compensatory purging (Stunkard, 1959). Today, the disorder is characterized by recurrent episodes of binge eating accompanied by marked distress about the amount of food consumed and the lack of control associated with the disorder (APA, 2013). Some associated diagnostic criteria regarding the binge-eating episodes include an individual eating more rapidly than normal, eating until feeling uncomfortably full, eating large amounts even when he or she is not hungry, eating alone because of embarrassment over the amount consumed, and feeling disgusted, guilty, or depressed after the episode (APA, 2013). Individual patients may express feelings of hatred and being angry that they cannot resolve their illness; they may despair over their inability to control their binging (McIver, McGartland, & O'Halloran, 2009).

Patients diagnosed with BED also have a higher rate of general psychopathology, lower social adaptation, and greater premorbid exposure to parental mood and substance disorder (Hilbert et al., 2011). Patients who are obese and have BED have shown impaired functioning on psychosocial measures and impairment in physical functioning related to obesity as compared to individuals without eating disorders (Fairburn et al., 2009). Therefore, BED's combination of core eating disorder psychopathology, other co-occurring physical and psychiatric conditions, impaired psychosocial functioning, and overweight state constitute an eating disorder of clinical severity and a significant public health problem (Kessler et al., 2013).

Pause and Reflect

1. *How does bulimia nervosa differ from binge-eating disorder?*
2. *What nursing diagnoses may be appropriate with someone suffering with anorexia nervosa?*
3. *How would the nurse prioritize the plan of care for an individual with anorexia nervosa?*

Collaborative Care

The effective treatment of feeding and eating disorders is a collaborative process among the patient, his or her family members as appropriate, and the members of an interdisciplinary treatment team. Nursing care will include coordination and collaboration with other professionals who are involved in the patient's treatment, such as primary care providers, dentists, registered dieticians, mental health professionals, and school personnel (as applicable). The levels of care begin with the least restrictive outpatient treatment and increase to intensive outpatient, partial hospitalization, residential, and the most restrictive inpatient treatment (APA, 2011). The aims of collaborative treatment include restoring the patient to a healthy weight, treating any physical complications and co-morbid conditions, and reestablishing social engagement (Box 15-2).

Inpatient Treatment

Because of the potentially life-threatening physical and or psychological complications of those with AN, inpatient care may be indicated. Box 15-3 offers general guidance in decision making for those individuals with AN and additional assistance for those with BN and other feeding and eating disorders. These guidelines should not be viewed as standards of medical care. Ultimately, the decision is based on the clinical presentation and the treatment options available.

Diagnostic Criteria for Bulimia Nervosa   DSM-5

A. Recurrent episodes of binge eating. An episode of binge eating is characterized by both of the following:
  1. Eating, in a discrete period of time (e.g., within any 2-hour period), an amount of food that is definitely larger than what most individuals would eat in a similar period of time under similar circumstances.
  2. A sense of lack of control over eating during the episode (e.g., a feeling that one cannot stop eating or control what or how much one is eating).

B. Recurrent inappropriate compensatory behaviors in order to prevent weight gain, such as self-induced vomiting; misuse of laxatives, diuretics, or other medications; fasting; or excessive exercise.
C. The binge eating and inappropriate compensatory behaviors both occur, on average, at least once a week for 3 months.
D. Self-evaluation is unduly influenced by body shape and weight.
E. The disturbance does not occur exclusively during episodes of anorexia nervosa.

Source: Reprinted with permission from the *Diagnostic and Statistical Manual of Mental Disorders*, Fifth Edition, (Copyright 2013). American Psychiatric Association.

Goals of Treatment for Feeding and Eating Disorders   box 15-2

- Restore the patient to a healthy weight.
- Treat physical complications.
- Enhance motivation toward restoration of healthy eating patterns and treatment.
- Provide education (for the patient and family).

- Correct maladaptive thoughts, attitudes, and feelings.
- Treat co-morbid psychiatric conditions.
- Enlist family support.
- Reestablish social engagement.
- Prevent relapse.

Criteria for Hospitalization for Feeding and Eating Disorders   box 15-3

- Weight < 85% of estimated healthy weight
- Heart rate < 40 bpm
- Blood pressure < 90/60 mmHg (< 80/50 mmHg in children/adolescents)
- Electrolyte (e.g., potassium, magnesium, and phosphate) imbalances
- Renal, cardiac, or other organ impairment requiring acute treatment
- Suicidality

- Arrhythmia, hypothermia, hypoglycemia
- Failure to respond to less restrictive treatment

Additional criteria for pediatric patients:

- Orthostatic hypotension (increase in pulse > 20 bpm or decrease in blood pressure of > 10–20 mmHg)
- AN: Body fat < 10%
- BN: Syncope, esophageal tears, inability to control vomiting

Data from American Psychiatric Association. (2012). Guideline Watch: Practice Guidelines for the Treatment of Patients with Eating Disorders. Washington, DC: American Psychiatric Publishers; Halmi, K. A. (2009). Salient components of a comprehensive service for eating disorders. *World Psychiatry, 8*(3), 150–155; Rosen, D. S., & Committee on Adolescence. (2010). Identification and management of eating disorders in children and adolescents. *Pediatrics: Journal of the American Academy of Pediatrics, 126*(6), 1240–1253.

Of note, the DSM-5 uses four stages to denote a patient's severity of anorexia, based on body mass index (BMI). The specifiers are *mild*, with a BMI of 17–18.5 kg/m^2; *moderate*: BMI 16–16.99 kg/m^2; *severe*: BMI 15–15.99 kg/m^2; and *extreme*: BMI ≤ 15 kg/m^2. In contrast, a BMI indicating a normal weight is 18.5–24.9 kg/m^2. In diagnosing children and adolescents with AN, clinicians may determine a BMI-for-age percentage based on developmental trajectories (APA, 2013).

If a patient does require inpatient level of care due to under-weight/malnourished state or associated life-threatening medical conditions, it is essential that the care team develop an understanding and cooperation with the patient regarding nutritional and physical rehabilitation. Weight is restored by first establishing a target weight and rates of weight gain. Generally, intake begins at 30 to 40 kcal/kg per day (approximately 1,000–1,600 kcal/day) and can be increased as appropriate (APA, 2012). Currently, nasogastric feeding is rare and most often reserved for those who are unable or unwilling to ingest essential nutrients to sustain life. Additional interventions include limiting activity and energy expenditure; monitoring vital signs, food and fluid intake/output, and electrolytes; and observing for signs of fluid overload or other evidence of **refeeding syndrome** (O'Connor & Goldin, 2011). Refeeding syndrome is a potentially fatal condition that can occur when severely malnourished patients begin the refeeding process (see Evidence-Based Practice: Refeeding). It is also important to continue to assess/monitor gastrointestinal and cardiac functioning, as necessary. Finally, it is essential to create a milieu that engenders emotional nurturance and genuine opportunities for healing.

PRACTICE ALERT Patients with eating disorders who require hospitalization will need supplementary vitamins and minerals. Administer supplements as necessary for noted deficiencies.

Psychosocial Treatments

Nurses and other professionals establish collaborative goals that aid the patient in understanding and changing maladaptive behaviors and attitudes that reinforce or maintain the eating disorder. Formal psychotherapy typically starts once weight gain begins and the patient is able to cognitively participate in therapy. Although there is a paucity of evidence indicating effective treatment, the APA Practice Guidelines for the Treatment of Patients with Eating Disorders (2012) recommend ongoing individual therapy using cognitive–behavioral, interpersonal, and psychodynamic approaches because of their efficacy when used in adults. Family and couples therapy can be helpful if these relationships are contributing to the maintenance of the disorder. Group psychotherapy can be helpful when using a cognitive–behavioral, interpersonal, and/or psychodynamic focus. However, thoughtful consideration and monitoring of care must be given due to the potential for unhealthy dynamics, such as competition among members to be the thinnest or the sickest of the group.

Family approaches are most effective with children and adolescents, particularly with an illness in duration of less than 3 years. The best-studied approach is the Maudsley model (Stiles-Shields, Hoste, Doyle, & Le Grange, 2012). This approach is operationalized in an outpatient setting and involves 10 to 20 family sessions spaced out over 6 to 12 months. The recommended format is defined as conjoint, meaning that all family members should be seen together. In the initial phase, parental authority is directed and coached on effective means of controlling the child or adolescent's eating and weight. A gradual reduction in parental authority is indicated as the child/adolescent complies with expectations. The adolescent's right to age-appropriate independence is directly related to the resolution of the eating disorder (Lock & Le Grange, 2012).

Clinical Problem

Refeeding, or weight restoration, in severely malnourished individuals with AN is a complex psychological and physiological process that can include overall resistance from the patient and create severe medical complications. Refeeding syndrome (RFS) can cause fluid and electrolyte disorders, including hypophosphatemia, and neurological, pulmonary, cardiac, neuromuscular, and hematologic complications. The traditional and current standard of care advocates a "start low [kcal/kg/day] and go slow" approach. Typically the composition of prescribed meals maintains a high carbohydrate content (30% fat, 15% protein, and 55% carbohydrate) (Mehler, Winkelman, Andersen, & Gaudiani, 2010). However, there is no evidence that suggests that this method is effective in thwarting the occurrence of RFS or the severity of other medical complications. In fact, this approach typically results in a high compensatory insulin response, initial weight loss, extended hospital time, and delayed nutritional recovery (Kohn, Madden, & Clarke, 2011). In severely malnourished patients with AN, how do traditional refeeding practices (low total calories) affect weight restoration during the initial refeeding process compared to observing the dietary composition of macronutrients (avoiding a high proportion of calories from carbohydrates, combined with a higher number of calories)?

Evidence

Current refeeding recommendations for hospitalized patients with AN are conservative due to the belief that this approach will prevent refeeding syndrome. Whitelaw, Gilbertson, Lam, and Sawyer (2010) recently conducted a retrospective study examining their practice of *aggressively* (greater than standard guidelines) refeeding 29 adolescents for the first 2 weeks of their inpatient hospitalization. This practice included meal plans that were 30% fat and 36% to 65% protein for total daily energy. Their findings included a greater-than-average weight gain with no incidents of refeeding

syndrome or medical complications (Garber et al., 2012). To further examine the veracity of the current refeeding protocols, Garber and colleagues (2012) prospectively measured weight change and clinical outcomes in 35 hospitalized adolescents with AN. Initially, 83% of subjects lost weight until day 8, when a mean (SD) of 1,966 (349) kcal/day was reached. When higher calories were prescribed at baseline, there was a significant association with faster weight gain ($p = 0.003$) and a shorter hospital stay ($p = 0.030$). These combined findings suggest the development of more aggressive feeding strategies in adolescents hospitalized with AN. Further research is needed to generalize these findings to an adult population and identify caloric and supplementation regimens that maximize weight gain safely while avoiding refeeding syndrome.

Implications for Nursing Practice

The current refeeding guidelines for malnourished individuals with AN may be conservative and even initially deleterious. Additionally, these "guidelines" are not supported by evidence. Recent research advocates for an increase in kcal/day and a consideration of the dietary composition of macronutrients. For nurses to deliver safe and effective care, it is essential to evaluate the strength or lack of evidence concerning treatment interventions in practice.

Critical Thinking Questions

1. Why might an initial diet that is higher in protein be more beneficial than the high-carbohydrate diet that traditionally has been used with patients with severe anorexia?

2. Given the need for more evidence, what concerns would you have in choosing one diet or another for your patients? Would you feel differently if the patient was your own family member?

All eating disorders share many similar diagnostic features, including the same core pathology. In discerning the core pathology of eating disorders through a cognitive–behavioral framework, it can be understood as the over-evaluation of the importance of body shape and control of body weight (Murphy, Straebler, Cooper, & Fairburn, 2010). Even in the case of binge-eating disorder, for which there is no evidence of extreme weight control behaviors, it is thought that patients have the same process of over-evaluation of weight and body shape, but that they repeatedly fail to adhere to efforts to restrict their eating. This leads to thoughts of incompetence at self-control, deserting struggles with control, and engaging in binge-eating behaviors (Murphy, Straebler, Cooper, & Fairburn, 2010). Given that AN, BN, BED, and related feeding and eating disorders share the same core pathology and that patients diagnosed with an eating disorder often migrate among these diagnoses, it has been suggested that distinguishing between the separate diagnoses has limited value and that treatment approaches should be *transdiagnostic* in nature (Fairburn et al., 2009).

Cognitive–behavioral therapy (CBT) is the most widely studied form of treatment for eating disorders. CBT is strongly supported as the single most effective intervention for the treatment of BN and BED (APA, 2012). Additionally, CBT is associated with a more rapid remission of symptoms and has resulted in better outcomes when compared with other psychotherapies (Wilson, Grilo,

& Vitousek, 2007). Further, the National Institute for Clinical Excellence (NICE) in the UK rates CBT as "grade A" (signifying strong empirical data) and recommends CBT as the first-line treatment in BN, prior to the initiation of medication (Katzman et al., 2010). CBT has resulted in better long-term outcomes than the use of psychiatric medications in BN (APA, 2012). CBT has not shown to be as effective for anorexia, which may be related to a limited motivation for change due to the ego-syntonic nature of the illness. Although most of the research on psychotherapy has focused on BN and BED, there are some promising preliminary data on the use of CBT-E (cognitive–behavioral therapy—enhanced), which incorporates interventions specifically aimed at the core issues of AN, with patients diagnosed with AN (Box 15-4) (Murphy, Straebler, Cooper, & Fairburn, 2010).

In addition to CBT, interpersonal and dialectical behavior therapy (DBT) have shown efficacy in reducing both behavioral and psychological symptoms associated with eating disorders. (See Chapter 24 for a discussion of DBT.)

Psychopharmacology

Pharmacotherapy for patients with eating disorders has met with mixed results. It is generally recommended that pharmacotherapy, when used, be part of an overall plan of care that includes psychotherapy, nutrition counseling, and other interventions. In particular, selective

CBT-E Interventions

box 15-4

- Engaging the patient in treatment and change
- Jointly creating the treatment plan
- Establishing real-time self-monitoring
- Establishing collaborative weekly weighing
- Providing education

- Establishing regular eating
- Involving significant others
- Addressing the overevaluation of shape and weight
- Addressing dietary rules
- Addressing event-related changes in eating

serotonin-reuptake inhibitors (SSRIs) have been shown to have some effectiveness in controlling certain symptoms (see the Medications feature).

PRACTICE ALERT When working with pediatric, adolescent, and young adult patients ages 18 to 24 years, bear in mind that many SSRIs carry an FDA-mandated black-box warning regarding the possibility of increased suicidality in that age bracket; administration of SSRIs may be contraindicated because of this risk. Children and adolescents prescribed SSRIs should also have a safety plan for parents to follow in the event they observe suicidal ideation in their child.

Anorexia Nervosa

Many medications (mainly antidepressants) have been studied in randomized clinical trials, but the majority have failed to show a difference in the treatment of anorexia nervosa in comparison to placebo. However, following weight restoration and depending on remaining symptoms (for example, persistent depression, anxiety, and obsessive–compulsive behaviors), SSRIs have the most evidence for efficacy and the fewest difficulties with adverse effects. Bupropion should be avoided in patients with active eating disorder symptoms (as in AN and BN) due to increased risk of seizures. Tricyclic antidepressants (TCAs) and monoamine oxidase inhibitors (MAOIs) should not be considered in underweight patients, and their overall potential for lethality and toxicity in overdose should be taken into consideration if prescribing for others with disordered eating (APA, 2012).

Evidence from controlled trials is limited; however, for patients with severe symptoms of AN and unremitting resistance to gaining weight, research suggests that second-generation antipsychotic medications (such as olanzapine) may be effective in achieving more rapid weight gain, reducing obsessional thinking, and limiting the denial that can assume delusional proportions (Bissada, Tasca, Barber, & Bradwejn, 2008). No differences in adverse effects were observed; however, the treatment team should monitor for side effects, including laboratory abnormalities and symptoms of metabolic syndrome, if these agents are used.

Bulimia Nervosa

Fluoxetine (Prozac) has an FDA indication for BN. There is strong empirical evidence to support the most effective dose as 60 mg in reducing binging and purging behaviors and eating-disordered attitudes (Powers & Cloak, 2012). Otherwise, other SSRIs have shown some effectiveness in BN with similar dosages used for treatment of depression (Shapiro et al., 2007). Topiramate (Topamax, an anticonvulsant) was studied in controlled trials and found to be statistically superior to placebo in the reduction of binging and purging episodes and weight loss. The current evidence suggests that the SSRI

sertraline and the anticonvulsant topiramate are the most effective at reducing binge eating and weight (Claudino et al., 2007; Aigner, Treasure, Kaye, & Kasper, 2011). Ondansetron (Zofran), a 5HT3 antagonist (antiemetic), has shown significantly greater decreases in binging and vomiting frequencies, time spent engaging in bulimic behaviors, and increase in normal meals (Faris et al., 2006). Initially, treatment with ondansetron was not considered a viable option, in part because of the multiple daily doses of this costly medication and lack of FDA approval for this indication, which resulted in insurance companies' denial to cover the cost (Faris et al., 2008). However, ondansetron is currently available in generic form and may become a feasible treatment option and future line of investigation.

Finally, antidepressant medication combined with CBT was found to be superior to medication alone in reducing binging and vomiting frequency. However, medication alone led to significantly reduced BMI and depression scores compared with CBT alone (Shapiro et al., 2007). In reducing the core symptoms (binging and purging episodes) of BN, the findings to date suggest that the combination of CBT and antidepressants may be the most effective treatment approach (Hay & Claudino, 2012).

Binge-Eating Disorder

Double-blind, placebo-controlled studies suggest that antidepressants are at least as effective in the treatment of BED as in BN. For those who prefer to try medication, topiramate-treated patients displayed reduction of binge eating and weight loss (McElroy et al., 2007). Those in a combined drug and CBT treatment also had a reduction in binge eating, remission rates, and weight loss in comparison to the CBT alone (Claudino et al., 2007).

Orlistat (Xenical) is a medication that produces a dose-dependent reduction in dietary fat absorption. Grilo, Masheb, and Salant (2005) reported better results in the orlistat-plus-CBT guided self-help (CBT-GSH) group for binge remission and significant weight loss. Further, studies using orlistat combined with behavioral weight loss or CBT-GSH showed significantly reduced BED symptoms and greater weight loss. It appears reasonable to augment psychotherapy with an SSRI, topiramate, or orlistat for those suffering from BED.

Pause and Reflect

1. *What are the priority considerations when determining whether hospitalization for eating disorders is necessary?*

2. *In what ways might a patient who requires hospitalization for an eating disorder be suffering? How would you begin to promote hope in patients hospitalized for eating disorders?*

3. *Why do you think a combination of antidepressant medication and cognitive–behavioral therapy has been shown to be effective in treating bulimia nervosa?*

Eating Disorders

medications commonly used to treat

Medication	Dosage	Nursing Considerations
fluoxetine (Prozac) BN: May be helpful in reduction of binge/purge episodes, eating-disordered attitudes	Adult: 20–60 mg PO daily Child ≥ 7 yr: 10–20 mg PO daily in a.m.	• Contraindicated in patients taking MAOIs or thioridazine. • Monitor for worsening depression or suicidal ideation. • Use with caution in patients with AN due to potential presence of hepatic and renal impairment. • Effectiveness may take from several days to 5 weeks to develop fully.
olanzapine (Zyprexa) AN: May help achieve more rapid weight gain, reduce obsessional thinking and denial	Adult: 10–15 mg PO daily; max: 20 mg/day (is available in orally disintegrating tablets for patients prone to cheeking meds as well as an extended-release injectable form) Adolescent: 2.5–5 mg/day (max 10 mg/day)	• Monitor for adverse effects, including extrapyramidal symptoms. • Monitor for laboratory anomalies. • Use with caution in patients with known cardiovascular disease, history of seizures, diabetes mellitus (may cause lack of glycemic control), hepatic or renal impairment. • Should not be used in elderly clients with dementia.
topiramate (Topamax) BN, BED: may be effective in reducing binge-purge or binge episodes, assist in weight loss	Adult: Initiate with 25 mg PO twice a day and titrate to a maximum dose of 200–400 mg daily in two divided doses	• Monitor for and report changes in mental status. • Monitor for laboratory anomalies. • Advise patients not to stop taking this medication abruptly. • Advise patient to drink at least 6 to 8 full glasses of water daily to minimize the risk of kidney stones. • Advise regarding common side effect of sedation, avoiding alcohol and other CNS depressants. • Use with caution in patients with renal and hepatic impairment, pulmonary conditions. • Monitor for cognitive changes.
ondansetron (Zofran) BN: May help reduce binge-purge episodes, increase the frequency of normal meals	Adult: 4–8 mg PO q 8–12 hr (max: 24 mg per dose); also available in IV and orally disintegrating tablets	• Monitor fluid and electrolyte status. • Monitor cardiovascular status. • Use with caution in patients with hepatic disease. • Headaches are a common adverse effect.
orlistat (Xenical) BED: adjunctive therapy that may be helpful in assisting with weight loss	Adult/adolescent: 60–120 mg PO three times a day taken with each meal containing fat	• Monitor weight and BMI, monitor BP. • GI adverse effects such as oily fecal spotting, flatus, and fecal urgency are common; usually resolve within a few weeks; may be minimized by eating low-fat meals. • Monitor for fat-soluble vitamin deficiency (supplements should not be taken within 2 hours before/after taking orlistat).

Nursing considerations based on Wilson, B. A., Shannon, K. T., and Shields, K. M. (2014). *Pearson Nurse's Drug Guide 2014.* Upper Saddle River, NJ: Prentice Hall.

Nursing Management

Unlike most psychiatric disorders, eating disorders can cause severe physiological damage to a patient. Therefore, nursing care focuses on both the physiological and psychological aspects of treatment. Both AN and BN are potentially fatal and, when left untreated, can lead to problems with physical growth and maturation, metabolism, and critical organ functions. In the treatment of eating disorders, physical complications are addressed prior to the psychological aspects of the disease. For patients with AN, the priorities for nursing management typically are managing weight restoration and stabilizing physiological functions.

Assessment

Assessment of patients who present with symptoms of eating disorders includes observation, physical assessment, and a patient interview. Assessment tools have been developed to assist clinicians in the assessment process (Table 15-4). Many of the instruments can be used to assist the nurse in accurately measuring

change in psychopathology over time, allowing for evaluation of treatment strategies, and perhaps identifying those that are effective and those that need modification.

Observation and Physical Assessment

The assessment of patients with feeding and eating disorders requires thorough medical monitoring. This includes frequently assessing vital signs (such as temperature, pulse, and blood pressure), height and weight, urine specific gravity, blood chemistry, and EKG. In addition to monitoring for medical complications, the nurse may assess the content of patients' distorted thinking patterns regarding eating, calories, exercise, and body image. As distorted thinking becomes pervasive and the illness exerts its power and control over the patient's life, the patient is unable to engage in normal activities and maintain productive relationships. A comprehensive nursing assessment also should determine the level of impairment and functioning within the family, relationships with peers, and performance in school or work (Table 15-5).

Kara Recovery Phase

APPLICATION

1. Address the five domains for Kara:
   a. Biological
   b. Psychological
   c. Sociological
   d. Cultural
   e. Spiritual
2. Discuss the DSM-5 criteria for BN. What symptoms of BN does Kara exhibit?
3. Why is medication an appropriate recommendation for Kara?
4. Do you ever experience feelings of worthlessness? How do you handle them?

Kara is admitted to the inpatient psychiatric unit, which specializes in eating disorders, and develops a treatment plan with the psychiatric nurse practitioner, Susan, who works with her while she is hospitalized. As part of this plan, Kara participates in therapeutic groups with other patients from the unit, individual treatment with Susan, and family therapy with her mother and father. Kara also participates in psychopharmacological intervention, including the initiation of 20 mg fluoxetine (Prozac, the only medication approved by the FDA for use in treating depression in children and adolescents) by mouth in the morning to help her with the depression and anxiety that accompany her disordered eating. The focus of the therapeutic groups is helping Kara to understand the process by which distressing events, stress, and resulting moods lead to overevaluation of her weight and shape. During an individual meeting with Susan, Kara is able to identify:

> I'm starting to understand that I feel this pressure to be perfect all the time, and I feel like I don't live up to my parents' expectations most of the time. Especially with my mom: When I was young she would always make comments about my weight and she has always been weird about food and dieting. So that stuck with me, feeling like I was too fat and I didn't have the self-control that she did. Then I start to feel really bad about myself because I've let them down, and I feel like a failure. Plus, I compare myself to the people I see on TV, girls in magazines, and I never look as good or as skinny as they do. Sometimes I think of problems I have and assume it is about my weight. Like my boyfriend broke up with me a while ago, and I think it is because he thought I was too fat. Everything feels so out of my control when I get like this. Then I start focusing on my weight and what I eat because I feel like it is the only thing I can control.

Throughout groups and in individual treatment (while on the unit), Kara is able to further identify how her loss of control around binging reinforced her negative thinking resulting in purging and more dysfunctional thoughts. Her perceived inability to control her weight would start the self-perpetuating pattern over again. During a group session on the unit, she states, "I focus so much of my self-worth on my ability to control what I eat and what I weigh, that when I lose control and binge I feel so bad about myself and start trying to restrict my food again. When I can't binge, then I feel even worse. It is a never-ending cycle."

Therapy with Kara's mother and father focused on how to best support her struggles with disordered eating and often took place during meal times. Kara's mother was able to acknowledge how her own issues with controlling her weight and negative comments she made concerning Kara's weight contributed to her daughter's current problems. The focus became developing a supportive environment for Kara. At the end of her hospital stay there was much less tension at family meals.

Representative Instruments for Assessing Eating Disorders   table 15-4

Instrument	Brief Description
Eating Disorder Examination (EDE)	Used to assess presence and severity of eating disorders
Diagnostic Survey for Eating Disorders (DSED)	Surveys medical history and function in areas such as weight history and body image, eating behaviors and diet, exercise, sexual function, and family history
Bulimia Test Revised (BULIT-R)	Brief instrument that assesses eating behaviors and attitudes related to bulimia
Eating Attitudes Test (EAT)	Self-report screening of symptoms and concerns characteristic of eating disorders
Eating Disorder Examination Questionnaire (EDE-Q)	Self-report version of the EDE
Eating Disorders Inventory–2 (EDI-2)	Standardized measure of traits and symptoms related to eating disorders, including behaviors and attitudes related to food, weight, and body shape
Eating Disorders Questionnaire (EDQ)	Questionnaire that assesses symptoms, course, and treatment
Questionnaire on Eating and Weight Patterns (QEWP)	Questionnaire designed to assess nature of binge-eating episodes

Data from American Psychiatric Association. (2012). Guideline Watch: Practice Guidelines for the Treatment of Patients with Eating Disorders. Washington, DC: American Psychiatric Publishers.

Select Signs and Symptoms of Feeding and Eating Disorders table 15-5

General	• Low body weight • Dehydration • Hypothermia • **Cachexia** (muscle wasting) • Weakness and fatigue with degree of malnutrition
Cardiovascular/Respiratory	• Dizziness, orthostatic hypotension • Shortness of breath, chest pain • Palpitations, arrhythmias, bradycardia • Weak, irregular pulse • Cold extremities • Acrocyanosis • Edema • Cardiac anomalies (tachycardia, prolonged QT and PT intervals, inverted T waves, and decreased cardiac output from use of syrup of ipecac to induce vomiting) (BN)
Neuropsychiatric	• Seizures • Apathy • Poor concentration • Cognitive impairment • Anxious, depressed, irritable mood • Suicidal thinking
Endocrine/Metabolic	• May have amenorrhea or irregular menses, cold intolerance, low body temperature • Electrolyte abnormalities associated with vomiting and laxative abuse (e.g., hypokalemia, hypomagnesemia, and hypophosphatemia) • Dehydration (increased urine specific gravity, osmolality) with purging or diuretic use
Gastroinestinal	• AN: abdominal pain, bloating, constipation, hemorrhoids, abnormal bowel sounds; in vomiters, occasional blood-streaked vomitus, heartburn, gastroesophageal reflux • Increased serum amylase in binging patients • Stool for guaiac: occasionally positive because of purging or laxative abuse
Hematologic	• AN: fatigue • Complete blood count: in AN, anemia (may be normocytic, microcytic, or macrocytic); leukopenia with relative lymphocytosis; low erythrocyte sedimentation rate • Vitamin deficiencies: folate, B12, niacin, and thiamine
Dermatologic	• AN: change in hair, including lanugo (fine, downy body hair); hair loss, dry and brittle hair; self-injury marks; carotenoderma (orange pigmentation); and acne • In vomiters: scarring on dorsum of hand (Russell's sign); conjunctival hemorrhages after vomiting
Reproductive	• AN: may have loss of menses; arrested sexual development or regression of secondary sex characteristics; loss of libido, fertility problems • BN: fertility problems and/or loss of menses • Serum gonadotropins: decreased serum estrogen in female patients with AN or BN; decreased serum testosterone in male patients; prepubertal patterns of luteinizing hormone, follicle-stimulating hormone secretion with amenorrhea
Musculoskeletal	• Muscle cramps and bone pain, short stature, and arrested skeletal growth (more likely in AN than in BN) • Radiography and bone scans: increased rate of pathological stress fractures (more likely in AN than BN); DEXA: osteopenia or osteoporosis, especially in hip and lumbar spine (more likely in AN) • Significant and permanent loss of dental enamel from vomiting (BN)

Based on Academy for Eating Disorders (AED) Medical Care Standards Task Force. (2011). *Eating Disorders: Critical Points of Early Recognition and Medical Risk Management in the Care of Individuals with Eating Disorders* (2nd ed.). Available at http://www.aedweb.org/Medical_Care_Standards; American Psychiatric Association. (2012). Guideline Watch: Practice Guidelines for the Treatment of Patients with Eating Disorders. Washington, DC: American Psychiatric Publishing; the Diagnostic and Statistical Manual of Mental Disorders, Fifth Edition, (Copyright 2013). American Psychiatric Association.

Patient Interview

When conducting an interview with a patient, questions should address each of the previously described five domains. A nursing assessment of a patient with an eating disorder may include asking questions such as:

- On a scale of 0 (none) to 10 (high), how much anxiety does the thought of gaining weight cause you?

- On a scale of 0 to 10, how preoccupied are you with the thought of being overweight?

- Have you ever experienced a person close to you being concerned that you were too thin?

- Do you feel as though food controls your life? In what ways?

- Do you ever make yourself vomit after eating?

- Do you use laxatives or excessive exercise as a means to control your weight?

- Are you aware of anything that precipitates or triggers these behaviors?

- Does your preoccupation with being thin or with food cause problems in relationships with others?

Diagnosis and Planning

Nursing diagnoses are identified and prioritized based on patient needs and include both physiological and psychological components.

Common Nursing Diagnoses

The nursing diagnoses most commonly seen in patients with eating disorders include the following:

- Nutrition, Imbalanced: Less Than Body Requirements
- Body Image, Disturbed
- Fluid Volume: Deficient
- Fatigue
- Cardiac Output, Decreased
- Constipation
- Diarrhea
- Denial, Ineffective
- Coping, Ineffective
- Hopelessness
- Powerlessness
- Self-Esteem, Chronic Low
- Anxiety

(NANDA-I, © 2014)

Given that at the core of most eating disorder pathology is the overevaluation of the importance of body shape and control of body weight, *disturbed body image* is a primary nursing diagnosis for eating disorders. It is imperative for patients to develop a realistic sense of self and body for them to refrain from the compulsive need to control their weight. For patients whose priority in treatment is weight restoration, a primary nursing diagnosis is *imbalanced nutrition: less than body requirements*. When selecting nursing diagnoses, the nurse should assess what symptoms are most life-threatening or problematic for the patient at the time.

Prioritizing Nursing Diagnoses

In creating an effective nursing care plan, the nurse works collaboratively with the patient in determining which nursing diagnoses are priorities for treatment. Collaboration with the patient enhances the development of a therapeutic relationship and increases compliance with the plan of care. Often patients who are diagnosed with an eating disorder are so afraid of gaining weight that they will do almost anything to prevent weight gain. This may make collaboration difficult, if not impossible. When collaboration with the patient on the treatment plan is not possible, the nurse should address the most significant patient need based on observable and measurable symptoms.

For example, in the critical thinking feature Kara identifies many symptoms contributing to her current state. Based on Kara's suicidal ideation and uncontrollable binge and purge cycles, Susan and Kara identify a priority nursing diagnosis of *risk for injury* and work to develop a treatment plan that addresses this priority (see Nursing Care Plan).

Plans and Goals

As the nurse collaboratively creates a treatment plan, the focus should be on creating goals that are *specific, realistic,* and *measurable*. Goals should be focused on patients' needs, capabilities, and desired treatment focus. Further, the five domains should be addressed in the plan of care. For example, in a treatment plan for a patient with an eating disorder, the biological domain should address any potential medical complications; the psychological domain could address underlying negative thought processes that contribute to the maintenance of the disorder; the sociological domain could address family relationships that either hinder or enhance coping; the cultural domain could address how a patient challenges cultural messages of desired thinness; and the spiritual domain addresses any identified spiritual concerns, connections, and/or spiritual supports. Examples of measurable goals include the following:

- Patient will gain ___ ounces per week for 4 weeks.

- Patient will gradually increase caloric intake by ___ calories per week for 4 weeks.

- Patient will actively participate in psychotherapy twice a week for 3 weeks.

Patient Education

It is imperative that the care plan includes an assessment of the patient's learning needs and abilities. For example, a patient with an eating disorder will often benefit from educational counseling by a nutritional expert concerning healthy food choices. To effectively incorporate this information into the treatment plan, the nurse must first assess the patient's knowledge deficits and how the patient can best learn and incorporate this new understanding into lifestyle changes.

Implementation

Determining a patient's willingness to participate in treatment and make changes is especially important when working with eating disorders. Patients with eating disorders, and in particular those with AN, can be disinterested in treatment and resistant to change.

Stress Reduction Interventions

Interventions that focus on reducing stress and not specifically addressing the problematic eating behaviors may help initially to create a therapeutic nurse–patient relationship. In the early stage, patient education about possible stressors that contribute to eating disorder behavior is also appropriate. This approach does not directly

PERCEPTIONS, THOUGHTS, & FEELINGS: Validating the Needs of a Patient with an Eating Disorder

Patient's behavior	Nurse's perceptions, thoughts, and feelings	Exploration with patient
Kara has been sitting in the communal dining area of the unit for 30 minutes. She has moved the food on her plate around with her fork and repeatedly reorganized utensils, condiments, and her drink, but she has not eaten anything. The nurse walks by. *Kara:* I can't eat this.	*Perceptions:* Kara is still eating hardly anything on her tray. *Thoughts:* How can I encourage her to eat? I don't want to put her on the defensive. Maybe I should offer her a meal-replacement shake instead. I know her refusal to eat is part of the core eating disorder pathology. If she continues to refuse food, it will affect her health. *Feelings:* I'm afraid I'm going to say something that will interfere with building a therapeutic relationship, but I am also afraid of what we would have to do if she continues to not eat.	*Nurse:* Kara, I notice you've been reading during your free time. Tell me about the book you're reading.

VALIDATION The nurse chooses a topic of interest to Kara in an attempt to alleviate Kara's anxiety by using distraction.

Patient's behavior	Nurse's perceptions, thoughts, and feelings	Exploration with patient
Kara: Reading is an escape for me. I like reading vampire stuff. It helps me get out of my own head. Kara visibly relaxes as she explains the book she is reading.	*Perceptions:* Kara seems less anxious when she focuses on something other than food. *Thoughts:* How do I help her "get out" of her head more often so that she can feel some relief from her anxieties about eating? *Feelings:* I feel hopeful that Kara wants to make a positive change.	*Nurse:* What else helps you get out of your head? What helps you when you're feeling anxious or stressed out?

VALIDATION The nurse validates Kara's statement by using the same language as Kara, and helps her explore other activities that she enjoys that may help her in her recovery.

Patient's behavior	Nurse's perceptions, thoughts, and feelings	Exploration with patient
Kara: I like to listen to music really loud with my headphones on so I can tune everything out. Also, I like to draw.	*Perceptions:* It may help Kara to offer her some sort of distraction during meals. This might reduce her anxiety. *Thoughts:* I don't know if this will work. Maybe I shouldn't try to force it because she opens up more when I don't talk about food or eating. *Feelings:* I hope I can continue to get her to feel comfortable with me, but I need to encourage her to eat something.	*Nurse:* Would it help if I got your music for you? You could listen with your headphones.

VALIDATION The nurse tries to distract Kara as well as offer a useful coping skill. This strategy keeps the focus on building the therapeutic relationship through offering something that Kara says helps her relax.

Patient's behavior	Nurse's perceptions, thoughts, and feelings	Exploration with patient
Kara: I think that would be helpful. Thank you.	*Perceptions:* I think Kara is open to accepting help. *Thoughts:* I hope this works. I don't know what to try next if it doesn't. *Feelings:* I feel hopeful that this might work, but at the same time I'm a little worried what to do if this does not help Kara eat something.	*Nurse:* Kara, I'll go get your music and headphones. I can see that you get anxious at mealtimes. Maybe listening to your music will help you tune out some of that anxiety so you can eat a little. I understand that it will be hard. I can sit with you while you eat, or I can leave you alone, but I would like you to try.

VALIDATION The nurse acknowledges Kara's feelings and attempts to offer a therapeutic intervention to reduce her anxiety at mealtime. The nurse also offers reassurance while giving Kara control by giving her the choice to eat alone or have the nurse sit with her.

Based on Orlando, I. J. (1972). *The Discipline and Teaching of Nursing Process (An Evaluative Study)*. New York, NY: G. P. Putnam's Sons.

confront the problem behavior, but addresses the stressors that can lead to problem behaviors.

Nursing interventions include decreasing exposure to environmental stress; decreasing anxiety by eliminating caffeine and other stimulants, such as energy drinks; helping patients increase social and familial connectedness through improving communication skills; teaching methods of self-soothing; and encouraging patients to eliminate drugs or alcohol that can increase impulsivity. *If these interventions are framed to patients as a way to reduce stress, rather than directly confronting a behavior they have no desire to change, the interventions will likely be more effective.* (See the Perceptions, Thoughts, and Feelings feature for an example.) Nurses can also begin to offer information concerning the treatment for eating disorders and the pros and cons of treatment choices. Given that there are many risk factors that predict disordered eating behavior, it is also appropriate for the nurse to assess for risk factors that contribute to the problem behaviors, as the patient may be willing to make changes in these areas first. As patients develop a therapeutic relationship and become more open to change, they can be referred to treatment using established methods such as cognitive–behavioral therapy.

Identifying Triggers of the Binge–Purge Process

Patients with BN and a subtype of AN struggle with recurrent episodes and/or urges to binge and purge food. An essential part of treatment is identifying the underlying antecedents, or triggers, to these urges and episodes (see the Nursing Care Plan that follows). It is important that the nurse understands the individual patient's experience, and being aware of others' struggle with this process aids in the development of a comprehensive, evidence-based nursing practice. To implement effective intervention strategies, it is essential that the nurse understand the intricate physical and psychological implications of the binge-and-purge process.

In one study, 39% of participants cited interpersonal relationships as triggers to a binge–purge episode, and 61% noted turbulent internal emotional states as their reason for relapse (Wasson, 2003). The thematic concept of *dealing with interpersonal relationships* represented a compilation of relapse triggers. For example, individuals acknowledged experiencing a trigger to relapse when they found themselves unable to influence or control others' behaviors. Turbulent or negative emotional states that contributed to relapse included "fear, anxiety, depression, loneliness, self-doubt, worry, anger, loss, frustration, guilt, shame and powerlessness" (Wasson, 2003, p. 79). Another study identified that binging and purging provided a measure of relief for patients seeking to divert feelings of shame, guilt, or unpleasant emotional triggers (Rørtveit, Åström, & Severinsson, 2009). Additionally, some individuals reported feeling comforted, soothed, or nurtured, which compensated for emptiness. Therefore, binging and purging served to foster pleasurable emotions while diverting unpleasant ones. Some described a "rush" or "euphoria" or a calmer feeling that they considered more physical than emotional (Jeppson, Richards, Hardman, & Granley, 2003, p. 123).

In contrast, others view purging as a way to exert self-determination and self-control. Purging has been described widely as a feeling of well-being that reaches full potential immediately after completion (Broussard, 2005). Furthermore, purging relieves the discomfort of overeating, such as nausea and severe abdominal pressure (Jeppson, Richards, Hardman, & Granley, 2003). Broussard (2005) noted that her participants reported a strong aversive reaction to the sensation of fullness and that vomiting provided an immediate release. One person described this phenomenon as follows: "That was the one thing I had power over, eat anything desired, and I had the power to get rid of it without gaining weight. It was the only sense of power that I ever had" (Jeppson, Richards, Hardman, & Granley, 2003, p. 119). For many individuals with eating disorders, purging behavior contributes to a marked sense of empowerment, control, and relief from tension.

Nurses can help patients identify triggers by reviewing the events and feelings prior to an episode. This will require some history taking, as a single episode may not identify all key triggers and patterns. Once triggers are identified, nurses and the health care team can collaborate with the patient to identify and practice healthy responses to triggers within a supportive environment. Interventions include providing emotional support at mealtimes, helping patients "reframe" disordered thinking, and monitoring trips to the bathroom and the advent of food hoarding.

Promoting Self-Worth and Positive Regard

Patients with eating disorders often are paralyzed by low self-esteem, but this is particularly true for those with AN, whose self-worth is unduly influenced by and dependent on the successful obtainment of extreme thinness (Broussard, 2005). This quest for perfectionism sets the stage for repeated episodes of dieting and food restriction (D'Abundo & Chally, 2004). As the patient struggles for control, disordered eating patterns become entrenched. One person described this by saying, "I had power over nothing in my life, but I could control that number [my weight]. That's one thing I truly had power over" (D'Abundo & Chally, 2004, p. 1098).

Patients who were overweight during adolescence often were reinforced with increased attention and positive regard following weight loss. Therefore, thinness and personal competence became linked to improved social status and self-regard. Positive reassurance of their weight and shape was the major criterion for truly being accepted by others. One individual believed, "I can be okay, if I'm thin enough" (Matusek & Knudson, 2009).

Nurses can promote self-worth and positive self-regard in patients with eating disorders through a variety of interventions. By providing positive reinforcement when patients adhere to treatment and make efforts to meet goals, patients begin to view their efforts optimistically. Helping patients set short-term, realistic goals that they can easily achieve fosters opportunities for success and allows patients to see and measure their treatment progress. Encouraging patients to reconnect with activities and experiences that they enjoy helps patients begin to regain control over their own behaviors and begin to re-experience positive emotions. These interventions lead to an increase in self-worth and positive self-regard.

Revising the Care Plan During Recovery and Rehabilitation

As treatment progresses, the nurse will evaluate the patient's response to treatment and make modifications to the treatment plan accordingly. The nursing care plan may be adjusted to include support concerning the identification of alternative coping strategies to manage triggers and negative thinking patterns. Additional support and education are needed for times when patients are unable to use alternative skills and may temporarily relapse and re-engage in problem behaviors. The goal in moving from the recovery stage to rehabilitation is to reduce the frequency of problem behaviors and for patients to better understand triggers and ways to cope with them effectively.

Kara—A Patient with Bulimia Nervosa   NURSING CARE PLAN

Nursing Diagnosis: Risk for injury related to suicidal ideation and uncontrollable binge–purge cycles as evidenced by patient self-report of suicidal ideation and binging and purging episodes.

Short-Term Goals *Patient will:* (include date for short-term goal to be met)	Intervention *Nurse will:*	Rationale
Remain free from self-directed harm while on the inpatient unit.	Assess for suicidal thoughts and other self-directed harm and implement suicide precautions as needed.	Priority is given to the continuous monitoring of suicidal thinking and self-directed harm behavior, which is crucial to maintaining safe treatment.
Be able to identify physical complications of binging and purging behaviors by day 3 of her admission.	Teach the patient about harmful effects of binging and purging including dental erosion, cardiac problems, and electrolyte disturbances.	Patient education and health teaching are imperative to treatment and is an integral part of the patient's understanding of the positive outcomes of healthy eating behaviors.
Identify distorted thoughts that precede episodes of binging and purging by day 5 of admission.	Provide emotional support before, during, and after meals and explore dysfunctional thought patterns.	Emotional support by the nurse helps to build therapeutic relationship. Nonjudgmental reframing of distorted thinking engenders improved communication.
Eat a reasonable amount of food without binging or purging 50% of the time by day 7 of admission to the inpatient unit.	Monitor for signs and symptoms of binging and purging behaviors including trips to the bathroom after eating, hoarding food, increased serum amylase, and swollen parotid glands.	Frequent monitoring is essential in the treatment of eating disorders. Patients are often resistant due to intense fears about gaining weight and therefore may not accurately report binging or purging behavior.
Long-Term Goal Kara will abstain from binging and purging and will have identified and used new skills for managing triggers for disordered eating behavior.	Collaborate with Kara to independently implement identified alternative stress-reduction techniques that will prevent disordered eating behavior.	Promoting patient autonomy and independence in managing life stressors is essential in the treatment of eating disorders.

Clinical Reasoning

1. What other nursing diagnoses might be appropriate for Kara?
2. What strategies or techniques might help Kara to process distorted thinking or reduce her stress level?

Evaluation

The evaluation phase focuses on the assessment of whether the goals and objectives are being met, including how well a patient is following the treatment plan. Patients may meet their planned goals and objectives fully; however, it is common for goals and objectives to be met only partially or not at all. The inclusion of specific time frames and measurements in goals and objectives makes evaluating a patient's progress easier. Based on how a patient is progressing and adhering to the nursing care plan, modifications can be made that address current treatment needs. When evaluating and revising nursing care plans, it is helpful to examine (within the context of the five domains) treatment goals that affect the course, severity, and duration of illness.

From Suffering to Hope

For hope and healing to begin, it is essential that nurses fully understand the meaning of the lived experiences of those with eating disorders. Patients with eating disorders suffer with a pervasive devalued self-worth and loathing of body weight and shape and, as a result, avoid intimacy and closeness and continually live in fear. By recognizing and addressing these dynamics, the nurse will help the patient confront and manage these deep and painful feelings.

As previously discussed, the treatment of eating disorders is incredibly complex and poorly understood. D'Abundo and Chally's (2004) model of recovery included data analysis from individuals who were diagnosed with AN and BN. These researchers proposed a model that recovery from an eating disorder can be viewed in a cyclical process. Essential components involve a process of acceptance through spirituality, which fosters the individual's ability to rejoin society, regain control, and think rationally. Within this model, spirituality encourages a connection between mind and body and increases self-worth and hope, not by the status of the patient's body weight and shape, but through other aspects of the patient's being. Through this model, patients can restore healthy eating patterns, maintain homeostasis, gain hope, and establish authentic power and control.

Pause and Reflect

1. *How do power and control affect those with eating disorders?*
2. *What aspects of binging and purging do you think patients find calming? Why?*
3. *What concerns do you have about working with patients with eating disorders?*
4. *How can the nurse help alleviate patient suffering and promote healing for those with eating disorders?*

Kara Rehabilitation Phase

APPLICATION

1. Address the five domains for Kara.

2. How would you prioritize Kara's needs when she is discharged from the hospital? Why?

3. What steps have Kara and her family taken to control her eating disorder? How or why have these been helpful?

By the end of her hospitalization, Kara reports that she is no longer having thoughts of suicide. Furthermore, she reports that her depression, anxiety, and urges to control her weight through binging and purging have decreased. Kara says that she is looking forward to returning to school and "getting back to my life." Kara acknowledges that her recovery is a process that will continue outside of the hospital, and she has agreed to participate in weekly individual therapy. Kara has an appointment with a dietician who can help support and educate her in making healthy choices about food and eating, as well as monitor her height, weight, and BMI. Kara will also begin weekly cognitive–behavioral group therapy for adolescent girls who have eating disorders.

Kara reports that she is feeling more supported by her parents and believes that they will continue to be supportive in the future. Mealtimes, which had been a time of stress for Kara, have become more manageable; her mother and father each plan on spending more time with Kara during meals, rather than arguing over what she is eating. Her parents also agreed to participate in family therapy with Kara to continue learning how to best support her as she progresses.

Chapter Highlights

1. Homeostasis is dependent on the successful regulation of human eating behavior. Alterations in normal eating patterns that are marked by distinct and persistent disturbances in eating behaviors, weight regulation, and perceptions toward body weight and shape are characteristic of eating disorders.

2. Longitudinal research has supported the claim that most individuals with feeding and eating disorders migrate amid the different diagnoses, move in and out of illness states, display frequent relapses, and show lifetime psychiatric co-morbidity.

3. The effective treatment of feeding and eating disorders is a collaborative process between the individual, family members as appropriate, and the members of an interdisciplinary treatment team.

4. Patients will need help in establishing a regular pattern of eating, increasing their variety of foods, correcting nutritional deficiencies, and engaging in healthy but not excessive exercise patterns.

5. It is important to establish collaborative goals that aid patients in understanding and changing core maladaptive beliefs, behaviors, and attitudes that reinforce or maintain their eating disorders.

6. CBT is the most widely studied form of treatment for feeding and eating disorders. CBT is strongly supported as the single most effective intervention for the treatment of BN and BED. Additionally, CBT is associated with a more rapid remission of symptoms and has resulted in better outcomes in comparison to other therapies for BN and BED.

7. Pharmacologic interventions for eating disorders are limited and currently do not have long-term promising results concerning the remission of symptoms. Further investigation is warranted.

8. The nurse can best help the patient with an eating disorder by exhibiting a nonjudgmental, compassionate manner, and listening to the factors that perpetuate this disorder and those that pave the road to recovery.

NCLEX®-RN Questions

1. The nurse is caring for a patient who is demonstrating alterations in eating patterns. Which finding does the nurse recognize as most indicative of an eating disorder?
   a. Anxious appearance
   b. Recent weight changes
   c. Disturbed body image
   d. History of family conflict

2. The nurse is planning a psychoeducation group for individuals at risk for eating disorders that addresses all domains of wellness. Which information is appropriate for the nurse to include? Select all that apply.
   a. Most, if not all, cultures embrace thinness as the ideal for beauty.
   b. Eating disorders are equally prevalent among individuals of both sexes.
   c. Eating disorders have heritability comparable to that of other major mental illnesses.
   d. Distorted cognitive processes have a role in the development of eating disorders.
   e. There may be a "contagious" nature to eating disorders among groups of individuals.

3. The nurse is caring for a patient diagnosed with binge-eating disorder (BED). Which finding does the nurse recognize as distinguishing the patient's condition from other eating disorders?
   a. The patient has experienced severe impairment in psychosocial function.
   b. The patient does not engage in any compensatory measures to control weight.
   c. The patient has demonstrated a variable response to treatment interventions.
   d. The patient experiences feelings of disgust and self-loathing after consuming food.

4. A patient with anorexia nervosa presents for inpatient admission with a body mass index (BMI) of 15.90 kg/m². Which interventions will the nurse carry out as part of evidence-based weight restoration and nutritional rehabilitation? Select all that apply.
   a. Monitor and document food and fluid intake and output.
   b. Consult with a dietician to determine a target weight goal.
   c. Limit excess activity and unnecessary energy expenditure.
   d. Provide a high-fat diet consisting of 1,800 to 2,200 kcal per day.
   e. Supplement oral intake with nasogastric feedings around the clock.

5. The nurse is evaluating outcomes for a patient with anorexia nervosa who has been taking olanzapine (Zyprexa) for the management of the disorder. Which findings indicate that the medication has had the desired effects? Select all that apply.
   a. The patient maintains a BMI of 16.00 kg/m^2.
   b. The patient reports a decreased urge to binge eat.
   c. The patient achieves adequate glycemic control.
   d. The patient reports reduced obsessional thinking.
   e. The patient acknowledges that treatment is needed.

6. The nurse is planning care for a patient with anorexia nervosa. Which aspect of the illness does the nurse recognize as the most significant barrier to recovery?
   a. Impaired social relationships
   b. Patient refusal to acknowledge there is a problem
   c. History of depression and suicidal ideation
   d. Lack of patient interest in pharmacologic interventions

7. The nurse is assessing a patient with bulimia nervosa. The nurse asks the patient to identify feelings and events that typically precede episodes of binging and purging. Which best describes the rationale for this action?
   a. Help the patient recognize that she has a significant problem that requires treatment
   b. Help the nurse to appreciate the extent of the pain and suffering experienced by the patient
   c. Provide the nurse with information necessary to determine the type of eating disorder the patient has
   d. Assist in the design a plan of care that effectively addresses the variables involved in the binge–purge process

8. The nurse is admitting a patient with anorexia nervosa to the inpatient unit. The patient is 30% below her optimal weight for age, sex, and developmental trajectory but believes that it is essential to continue to restrict intake and lose more weight. Which is the priority nursing diagnosis?
   a. Ineffective denial
   b. Imbalanced nutrition
   c. Disturbed body image
   d. Risk for noncompliance

Answers may be found on the Pearson student resource site: nursing.pearsonhighered.com

Pearson Nursing Student Resources Find additional review materials at **nursing.pearsonhighered.com**

References

Academy for Eating Disorders (AED) Medical Care Standards Task Force. (2011). *Eating Disorders: Critical Points of Early Recognition and Medical Risk Management in the Care of Individuals with Eating Disorders* (2nd ed.). Available at http://www.aedweb.org/Medical_Care_Standards

Aigner, M., Treasure, J., Kaye, W., & Kasper, S. (2011). World Federation of Societies of Biological Psychiatry (WFSBP) guidelines for the pharmacological treatment of eating disorders. *World Journal of Biological Psychiatry, 12*(6), 400–443.

Alegria, M., Carson, N. J., Goncalves, M., & Keefe, K. (2011). Disparities in treatment for substance use disorders and co-occurring disorders for ethnic/racial minority youth. *Journal of the American Academy of Child and Adolescent Psychiatry, 50*(1), 22–31.

American Psychiatric Association. (2000). *Diagnostic and Statistical Manual of Mental Disorders* (4th ed. Text Revision). Washington, DC: American Psychiatric Publishing.

American Psychiatric Association. (2011). Practice Guidelines for the Treatment of Patients with Eating Disorders. Rockville MD: Agency for Healthcare Research and Quality (AHRQ).

American Psychiatric Association. (2012). Guideline Watch: Practice Guidelines for the Treatment of Patients with Eating Disorders. Washington, DC: American Psychiatric Publishers.

American Psychiatric Association Work Group on Eating Disorders. (2000). Practice guideline for the treatment of patients with eating disorders (revision). *American Journal of Psychiatry, 157*(1 Suppl), 1–39.

Arcelus, J., Mitchell, J., Wales, J., & Nielsen, S. (2011). Mortality rates in patients with anorexia nervosa and other eating disorders: A meta-analysis of 36 studies. *Archives of General Psychiatry, 68*(7), 724–731.

Attia, E. (2010). Anorexia nervosa: current status and future directions. *Annual Review of Medicine, 61*, 425–435.

Attia, E., & Walsh, B. T. (2009). Behavioral management for anorexia nervosa. *New England Journal of Medicine, 360*(5), 500–506.

Becker, A. E. (2007). Culture and eating disorders classification. *International Journal of Eating Disorders, 40*(S3), S111–S116.

Becker, A. E., Eddy, K. T., & Perloe, A. (2009). Clarifying criteria for cognitive signs and symptoms for eating disorders in DSM-V. *International Journal of Eating Disorders, 42*(7), 611–619.

Benowitz-Fredericks, C. A., Garcia, K., Massey, M., Vasagar, B., & Borzekowski, D. L. G. (2012). Body image, eating disorders, and the relationship to adolescent media use. *Pediatric Clinics of North America, 59*(3), 693–704.

Bissada, H., Tasca, G. A., Barber, A. M., & Bradwejn, J. (2008). Olanzapine in the treatment of low body weight and obsessive thinking in women with anorexia nervosa: A randomized, double-blind, placebo-controlled trial. *American Journal of Psychiatry, 165*(10), 1281–1288.

Brandys, M. K., Kas, J. H., van Elburg, A. A., Campbell, I. C., & Adan, A. H. (2011). A meta-analysis of circulating BDNF concentrations in anorexia nervosa. *World Journal of Biological Psychiatry, 12*(6), 444–454.

Broussard, B. B. (2005). Women's experiences of bulimia nervosa. *Journal of Advanced Nursing, 49*(1), 43–50.

Bulik, C. M., & Reichborn-Kjennerud, T. (2003). Medical morbidity in binge eating disorder. *International Journal of Eating Disorders, 34*, S39–S46.

Castellini, G., Lo Sauro, C., Mannucci, E., Ravaldi, C., Rotella, C. M., Faravelli, C., & Ricca, V. (2011). Diagnostic crossover and outcome predictors in eating disorders according to DSM-IV and DSM-V proposed criteria: A 6-year follow-up study. *Psychosomatic Medicine, 73*(3), 270–279.

Cheney, A. M. (2012). Emotional distress and disordered eating practices among southern Italian women. *Qualitative Health Research, 22*(9), 1247–1259.

Claudino, A. M., de Oliveira, I. R., Appolinario, J. C., Cordás, T. A., Duchesne, M., Sichieri, R., & Bacaltchuk, J. (2007). Double-blind, randomized, placebo-controlled trial of topiramate plus cognitive-behavior therapy in binge-eating disorder. *Journal of Clinical Psychiatry, 68*(9), 1324–1332.

D'Abundo, M., & Chally, P. (2004). Struggling with recovery: Participant perspectives on battling an eating disorder. *Qualitative Health Research, 14*(8), 1094–1106.

Eddy, K. T., Dorer, D. J., Franko, D. L., Tahilani, K., Thompson-Brenner, H., & Herzog, D. B. (2008). Diagnostic crossover in anorexia nervosa and bulimia nervosa: Implications for DSM-V. *American Journal of Psychiatry, 165*(2), 245–250.

Espindola, C. R., & Blay, S. L. (2009). Anorexia nervosa treatment from the patient perspective: A metasynthesis of qualitative studies. *Annals of Clinical Psychiatry, 21*(1), 38–48.

Fairburn, C. G. (2002). Cognitive-behavioral therapy for bulimia nervosa. In C. G. Fairburn & K. D. Brownell (Eds.), *Eating Disorders and Obesity: A Comprehensive Handbook* (2nd ed.). New York, NY: Guilford Press, pp. 303–307.

Fairburn, C. G. (2008). *Cognitive Behavior Therapy and Eating Disorders*. New York, NY: Guilford Press.

Fairburn, C. G., Cooper, Z., Bohn, K., O'Connor, M. E., Doll, H. A., & Palmer, R. L. (2007). The severity and status of eating disorder NOS implications for DSM-V. *Behavioral Research and Therapeutics, 45*(8), 1705–1715.

Fairburn, C. G., Cooper, Z., Doll, H. A., O'Connor, M. E., Bohn, K., Hawker, D. M., Wales, J. A., & Palmer, R. L. (2009).Transdiagnostic cognitive-behavioral therapy for patients with eating disorders: A two-site trial with 60-week follow-up. *American Journal of Psychiatry, 166*(3), 311–319.

Faris, P. L., Eckert, E. D., Kim, S.-W., Meller, W. H., Pardo, J. V., Goodale, R. L., & Hartman, B. K. (2008). Evidence for a vagal pathophysiology for bulimia nervosa and the accompanying depressive symptoms. *Journal of Affective Disorders, 92*(1), 79–90.

Faris, P. L., Hofbauer, R. D., Daughters, R., VandenLangenberg, E., Iversen, L., Goodale, R. L., … Hartman, B. K. (2008). De-stabilization of the positive vago-vagal reflex in bulimia nervosa. *Physiology and Behavior, 94*(1), 136–153.

Forman-Hoffman, V. L., & Cunningham, C. L. (2008). Geographical clustering of eating disordered behaviors in U.S. high school students. *International Journal of Eating Disorders, 41*(3), 209–214.

Garber, A. K., Michihata, N., Hetnal, K., Shafer, M. A., & Moscicki, A. B. (2012). A prospective examination of weight gain in hospitalized adolescents with anorexia nervosa on a recommended refeeding protocol. *Journal of Adolescent Health, 50*(1), 24–29.

George, J. B., & Franko, D. L. (2010). Cultural issues in eating pathology and body image among children and adolescents. *Journal of Pediatric Psychology, 35*(3), 231–242.

Grilo, C. M., Masheb, R. M., & Salant, S. L. (2005). Cognitive behavioral therapy guided self-help and orlistat for the treatment of binge eating disorder: A randomized, double-blind, placebo-controlled trial. *Biological Psychiatry, 57*(10), 1193–1201.

Haines, J., Ziyadeh, N. J., Franko, D. L., McDonald, J., Mond, J. M., & Austin, S. B. (2011). Screening high school students for eating disorders: Validity of brief behavioral and attitudinal measures. *Journal of School Health, 81*(9), 530–535.

Halford, J. C. G., & Harrold, J. A. (2012). Satiety-enhancing products for appetite control: Science and regulation of functional foods for weight management. *Proceedings of the Nutrition Society, 71*(2), 350–362.

Halmi, K. A. (2009). Salient components of a comprehensive service for eating disorders. *World Psychiatry, 8*(3), 150–155.

Hannon-Engel, S. L. (2008). Knowledge development: The Roy Adaptation Model and bulimia nervosa. *Nursing Science Quarterly, 21*(2), 126–132.

Hannon-Engel, S. L., Filin, E. E., & Wolfe, B. E. (2012). Role of altered CCK response in bulimia nervosa. *Physiology & Behavior, 122*, 56–61.

Hatch, A., Madden, S., Kohn, M. R., Clarke, S., Touyz, S., Gordon, E., & Williams, L. M. (2010). In first presentation adolescent anorexia nervosa, do cognitive markers of underweight status change with weight gain following a refeeding intervention? *International Journal of Eating Disorders, 43*(4), 295–306.

Hay, P. J., & Claudino, A. M. (2012). Clinical psychopharmacology of eating disorders: A research update. *International Journal of Neuro-Psychopharmacology, 15*(2), 209.

Hilbert, A., Pike, K. M., Wilfley, D. E., Fairburn, C. G., Dohm, F. A., & Striegel-Moore, R. H. (2011). Clarifying boundaries of binge eating disorder and psychiatric comorbidity: A latent structure analysis. *Behaviour Research and Therapy, 49*(3), 202–211.

Hudson, J. I., Hiripi, E., Pope, H. G., & Kessler, R. C. (2007). The prevalence and correlates of eating disorders in the National Comorbidity Survey replication. *Biological Psychiatry, 61*(3), 348–358.

Jeppson, J. E., Richards, P. S., Hardman, R. K., & Granley, H. M. (2003). Binge and purge processes in bulimia nervosa: A qualitative investigation. *Eating Disorders, 11*(2), 115–128.

Katzman, D. K. (2005). Medical complications in adolescents with anorexia nervosa: A review of the literature. *International Journal of Eating Disorders, 37*, S52–S59.

Katzman, M. A., Bara-Carril, N., Rabe-Hesketh, S., Schmidt, U., Troop, N., & Treasure, J. (2010). A randomized controlled two-stage trial in the treatment of bulimia nervosa, comparing CBT versus motivational enhancement in phase 1 followed by group versus individual CBT in phase 2. *Psychosomatic Medicine, 72*(7), 656–663.

Kaye, W. H. (2008). Neurobiology of anorexia and bulimia nervosa. *Physiology and Behavior, 94*(1), 121–135.

Kaye, W. H., Frank, G. K., Bailer, U. F., Henry, S. E., Meltzer, C. C., Price, J. C., … Wagner, A. (2005). Serotonin alterations in anorexia and bulimia nervosa: New insights from imaging studies. *Physiology and Behavior, 85*(1), 73–81.

Keel, P. K., & Brown, T. A. (2010). Update on course and outcome in eating disorders. *International Journal of Eating Disorders, 43*(3), 195–204.

Keel, P. K., & Klump, P. L. (2003). Are eating disorders culture-bound syndromes? Implications for conceptualizing their etiology. *Psychological Bulletin, 129*, 747–769.

Kemps, E., & Wilsdon, A. (2009). Preliminary evidence for a role for impulsivity in cognitive disinhibition in bulimia nervosa. *Journal of Clinical and Experimental Neuropsychology, 32*(5), 515–521.

Kessler, R. C., Berglund, P. A., Chiu, W. T., Deitz, A. C., Hudson, J. I., Shahly, V., … Xavier, M. (2013). The prevalence and correlates of binge eating disorder in the World Health Organization World Mental Health Surveys. *Biological Psychiatry, 73*, 904–914.

Klump, K. L., Bulik, C. M., Kaye, W. H., Treasure, J., & Tyson, E. (2009). Academy for Eating Disorders position paper: Eating disorders are serious mental illnesses. *International Journal of Eating Disorders, 42*(2), 97–103.

Klump, K. L., & Culbert, K. M. (2007). Molecular genetic studies of eating disorders. *Current Directions in Psychological Science, 16*(1), 37–41.

Klump, K. L., Culbert, K. M., Slane, J. D., Burt, S. A., Sisk, C. L., & Nigg, J. T. (2012). The effects of puberty on genetic risk for disordered eating: evidence for a sex difference. *Psychological Medicine, 42*(3), 627–637.

Kohn, M. R., Madden, S., & Clarke, S. D. (2011). Refeeding in anorexia nervosa: Increased safety and efficiency through understanding the pathophysiology of protein calorie malnutrition. *Current Opinion in Pediatrics, 23*(4), 390–394.

Le Grange, D., & Lock, J. (2007). *Treating Adolescent Bulimia: A Family-Based Approach*. New York, NY: Guilford Press.

Le Grange, D., & Lock, J. (2011). *Eating Disorders in Children and Adolescents: A Clinical Handbook*. New York, NY: Guilford Press.

Linde, J. A., Jeffery, R. W., Levy, R. L., Sherwood, N. E., Utter, J., Pronk, N. P., & Boyle, R. G. (2004). Binge eating disorder, weight control self-efficacy, and depression in overweight men and women. *International Journal of Obesity, 28*(3), 418–425.

Lock, J., & Le Grange, D. (2012). *Treatment Manual for Anorexia Nervosa: A Family-Based Approach*. New York, NY: Guilford Press.

Machado, P. P. P., Gonçalves, S., & Hoek, H. W. (2013). DSM-5 reduces the proportion of ednos cases: Evidence from community samples. *International Journal of Eating Disorders, 46*(1), 60–65. http://dx.doi.org/10.1002/eat.22040

Mask, L., & Blanchard, C. M. (2011). The protective role of general self-determination against "thin ideal" media exposure on women's body image and eating-related concerns. *Journal of Health Psychology, 16*(3), 489–499.

Matusek, J. A., &, Knudson, R. M. (2009). Rethinking recovery from eating disorders: Spiritual and political dimensions. *Qualitative Health Research, 19*, 697–707.

McElroy, S. L., Hudson, J. I., Capece, J. A., Beyers, K., Fisher, A. C., Rosenthal, N. R., & Topiramate Binge Eating Disorder Group. (2007). Topiramate for the treatment of binge eating disorder associated with obesity: A placebo-controlled study. *Biological Psychiatry, 61*(9), 1039–1048.

McIver, S., McGartland, M., & O'Halloran, P. (2009). "Overeating is not about the food": Women describe their experience of a yoga treatment program for binge eating. *Qualitative Health Research, 19*(9), 1234–1245.

Mehler, P. S., Winkelman, A. B., Andersen, D. M., & Gaudiani, J. L. (2010). Nutritional rehabilitation: Practical guidelines for refeeding the anorectic patient. *Journal of Nutritional Metabolism.* http://dx.doi.org/10.1155/2010/625782. Epub February 7, 2010.

Monteleone, P., & Maj, M. (2013). Dysfunctions of leptin, ghrelin, BDNF and endocannabinoids in eating disorders: Beyond the homeostatic control of food intake. *Psychoneuroendocrinology, 38*(3), 312–330.

Mühlau, M., Gaser, C., Ilg, R., Conrad, B., Leibl, C., Cebulla, M., … Nunnemann, S. (2007). Gray matter decrease of the anterior cingulate cortex in anorexia nervosa. *American Journal of Psychiatry, 164*(12), 1850–1857.

Murphy, R., Straebler, S., Cooper, Z., & Fairburn, C. G. (2010). Cognitive behavioral therapy for eating disorders. *Psychiatric Clinics of North America, 33*(3), 611–627.

NANDA International. (2011). *Nursing Diagnoses: Definitions and Classification 2012–2014.* Hoboken, NJ: Wiley-Blackwell.

National Institute of Mental Health. (n.d.) Statistics. Available at http://www.nimh.nih.gov/statistics/index.shtml

O'Connor, G., & Goldin, J. (2011). The refeeding syndrome and glucose load. *International Journal of Eating Disorders, 44*(2), 182–185.

Orlando, I. J. (1972). *The Discipline and Teaching of Nursing Process (An Evaluative Study).* New York, NY: G. P. Putnam's Sons.

Peterson, C. B., Mitchell, J. E., Crow, S. J., Crosby, R. D., & Wonderlich, S. A. (2009). The efficacy of self-help group treatment and therapist-led group treatment for binge eating disorder. *American Journal of Psychiatry, 166*(12), 1347–1354.

Powers, P. S., & Cloak, N. L. (2012). Psychopharmacologic treatment of obesity and eating disorders in children and adolescents. *Child and Adolescent Psychiatric Clinics of North America, 21*(4), 831–859.

Presnell, K., Stice, E., Seidel, A., & Madeley, M. C. (2009). Depression and eating pathology: Prospective reciprocal relations in adolescents. *Clinical Psychology and Psychotherapy, 16*(4), 357–365.

Rørtveit, K., Åström, S., & Severinsson, E. (2009). The feeling of being trapped in and ashamed of one's own body: A qualitative study of women who suffer from eating difficulties. *International Journal of Mental Health Nursing, 18*(2), 91–99.

Rosen, D. S., & Committee on Adolescence. (2010). Identification and management of eating disorders in children and adolescents. *Pediatrics: Journal of the American Academy of Pediatrics, 126*(6), 1240–1253.

Russell, G. (1979). Bulimia nervosa: An ominous variant of anorexia nervosa. *Psychological Medicine, 9,* 429–448.

Shapiro, J. R., Berkman, N. D., Brownley, K. A., Sedway, J. A., Lohr, K. N., & Bulik, C. M. (2007). Bulimia nervosa treatment: A systematic review of randomized controlled trials. *International Journal of Eating Disorders, 40,* 321–336.

Steinglass, J., Albano, A. M., Simpson, H. B., Carpenter, K., Schebendach, J., & Attia, E. (2012). Fear of food as a treatment target: Exposure and response prevention for anorexia nervosa in an open series. *International Journal of Eating Disorders, 45*(4), 615–621.

Stice, E., Davis, K., Miller, N. P., & Marti, C. N. (2008). Fasting increases risk for onset of binge eating and bulimic pathology: A 5-year prospective study. *Journal of Abnormal Psychology, 117*(4), 941–946.

Stice, E., Marti, C. N., & Durant, S. (2011). Risk factors for onset of eating disorders: Evidence of multiple risk pathways from an 8-year prospective study. *Behavioral Research and Therapy, 49*(10), 622–627.

Stice, E., Rohde, P., Shaw, H., & Marti, C. N. (2013). Efficacy trial of a selective prevention program targeting both eating disorders and obesity among female college students: 1- and 2-year follow-up effects. *Journal of Consulting Clinical Psychology, 81*(1), 183–189.

Stiles-Shields, C., Hoste, R. R., Doyle, P. M., & Le Grange, D. (2012). A review of family-based treatment for adolescents with eating disorders. *Review of Recent Clinical Trials, 7*(2), 133–140.

Stuhldreher, N., Konnopka, A., Wild, B., Herzog, W., Zipfel, S., Löwe, B., & König, H. H. (2012). Cost-of-illness studies and cost-effectiveness analyses in eating disorders: A systematic review. *International Journal of Eating Disorders, 45*(4), 476–491.

Stunkard, A. J. (1959). Eating patterns and obesity. *Psychiatric Quarterly, 33*(2), 284–295.

Swinbourne, J., Hunt, C., Abbott, M., Russell, J., St Clare, T., & Touyz, S. (2012). The comorbidity between eating disorders and anxiety disorders: Prevalence in an eating disorder sample and anxiety disorder sample. *Australian and New Zealand Journal of Psychiatry, 46*(2), 118–131.

The Eating Disorders Work Group. (2012). Feeding and Eating Disorders: DSM-V Development. Available at http://www.dsm5.org/ProposedRevision/Pages/FeedingandEatingDisorders.aspx

van Vonderen, K. E., & Kinnally, W. (2012). Media effects on body image: Examining media exposure in the broader context of internal and other social factors. *American Communication Journal,* (14)2, 41–57.

Wasson, D. H. (2003). A qualitative investigation of the relapse experiences of women with bulimia nervosa. *Eating Disorders, 11*(2), 73–88.

Whitelaw, M., Gilbertson, H., Lam, P. Y., & Sawyer, S. M. (2010). Does aggressive refeeding in hospitalized adolescents with anorexia nervosa result in increased hypophosphatemia? *Journal of Adolescent Health, 46*(6), 577–582.

Wilksch, S. M., & Wade, T. D. (2012). Examination of the Sociocultural Attitudes Towards Appearance Questionnaire-3 in a mixed-gender young-adolescent sample. *Psychological Assessment, 24*(2), 352–364.

Wilson, B. A., Shannon, K. T., and Shields, K. M. (2014). *Pearson Nurse's Drug Guide 2014.* Upper Saddle River, NJ: Prentice Hall.

Wilson, G. T., Grilo, C. M., & Vitousek, K. M. (2007). Psychological treatment of eating disorders. *American Psychologist, 62*(3), 199–216.

Wolfe, B. E., Hannon-Engel, S., & Mitchell, J. (2012). Bulimia in DSM-5. *Psychiatric Annals, 42*(11), 406–409.

Woods, S. C., & D'Alessio, D. A. (2008). Central control of body weight and appetite. *Journal of Clinical Endocrinology and Metabolism, 93*(11 Supplement 1), s37–s50.

Woods, S. C., & Ramsay, D. S. (2011). Food intake, metabolism and homeostasis. *Physiology and Behavior, 104*(1), 4–7.

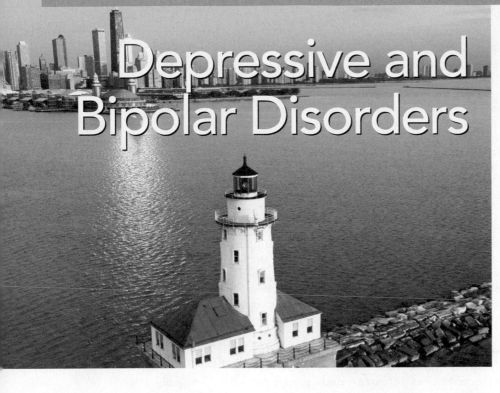

Depressive and Bipolar Disorders

16

Margaret M. McLaughlin

Learning Outcomes

1. Describe the etiology of depressive and bipolar disorders.

2. Summarize the impact of biological, psychological, sociological, cultural, and spiritual domains on depressive and bipolar disorders.

3. Categorize key symptoms associated with depressive and bipolar disorders.

4. Compare pharmacologic therapies used in the treatment of depressive and bipolar disorders.

5. Evaluate pharmacologic and nonpharmacologic therapies used in the treatment of depressive and bipolar disorders.

6. Apply principles of therapeutic communication that demonstrate empathy and instill hope during interactions with patients with depressive and bipolar disorders.

7. Plan evidence-based nursing care for individuals diagnosed with depressive and bipolar disorders.

Key Terms

Vijay Guntupalli Relapse Phase

Vijay Guntupalli is a 21-year-old college senior with a history of bipolar disorder that was first diagnosed at age 16. He is brought to the college health center by his brother Deepak, who is a first-year student at the same college. Deepak's parents implored him to go to the same college as Vijay "to keep an eye on his brother." At first Deepak resisted, but he finally agreed to go to the same college out of respect for his parents. Deepak loves his brother, but has felt burdened by the responsibility, and he feels angry with Vijay and his parents for making him responsible for Vijay's mental illness. Deepak recalls many nights when he was just a kid, listening to his parents argue about what was "wrong" with Vijay. Vijay's behavioral problems were the focus of much of the family's attention while Deepak was growing up. Vijay has been hospitalized a total of six times: four times for manic episodes that have resulted in some significant disruption to social and school functioning and twice for depression. He made a serious suicide attempt at age 19 by trying to hang himself. Vijay has been arrested twice: once for disorderly conduct and public intoxication and another time for driving to endanger when he was clocked going 110 miles per hour.

Vijay and Deepak are seen by the psychiatric nurse practitioner, Michelle Terrien, at the student health center. Vijay is loud and gregarious, laughing inappropriately and making rude comments about the other students in the health center. He is flirtatious with Ms. Terrien, commenting on her hair and figure. Once Deepak begins to voice his worries and discuss Vijay's symptoms, Vijay becomes irritable and agitated, frequently telling Deepak to shut up. Over the past several weeks, Vijay has become increasingly irritable and has not been sleeping well. Deepak reports that Vijay has been up for several nights claiming to be writing a novel that will sell millions. He believes that Vijay stopped taking his medications about three weeks ago.

Ms. Terrien meets with Vijay alone and determines that he is quite delusional, believing that he is on special assignment for the Federal Bureau of Investigation. He denies suicidal ideation, but his judgment is quite impaired, as evidenced by the fact that he believes that he has special powers that will protect him from "any assault or injury." His insight into his illness state is poor. Ms. Terrien inquires as to why he stopped taking his medication and he replies that he has been cured by the creator God, Brahma.

Ms. Terrien calls Vijay's psychiatrist, and the decision for hospitalization is made. Because Vijay is in such an agitated state and demonstrating poor impulse control, campus security is called to escort him to the local emergency department, where a member of the crisis intervention team will evaluate him further and arrange for psychiatric hospitalization. When the security officers arrive in the health center, Vijay attempts to leave and engages in a physical altercation with one of the officers. A scuffle ensues, and Vijay is handcuffed and taken from the health center. After Vijay has left the building, Ms. Terrien finds Deepak alone in the hallway, crying.

APPLICATION

1. Address the five domains for Vijay:
   a. Biological
   b. Psychological
   c. Sociological
   d. Cultural
   e. Spiritual

2. In what ways do you think that Vijay is suffering? How is Deepak suffering?

3. How would you prioritize Vijay's care needs during the initial assessment?

4. How can the nurse convey hope to the family of a person with bipolar disorder during a manic episode?

Introduction

Mood is an internal personal barometer that can be defined as "a pervasive emotional tone that profoundly influences one's outlook and perception of self, others, and the environment" (Kaplan & Sadock, 2005, p. 145). Mood states include **grief** (an individual's unique response to loss), sadness, depression, sorrow, joy, happiness, elation, passion, and pleasure; they are a normal response to the human experience. It is these mood states or emotions that define our existence, give color to our world, and allow us to connect and empathize with others. Normal mood states can vary from hour to hour and day to day and are influenced by biological, psychological, sociological, cultural, and spiritual experiences. Examples of how normal mood states can be influenced by experience include joy at the arrival of a new baby, weariness from caring for an infant, happiness and relief at graduating from college, and grief at the death of a loved one. These are all normal variations of mood that are part of the human experience and are not associated with mental illness.

Although mood states vary according to an individual's biopsychosocial–cultural–spiritual experience, most individuals experience a **euthymic mood** state, or a mood in the "normal" range. Extremes in mood states, such as **depression** (an altered mood state characterized by feelings of sadness and worthlessness accompanied by decreased interest in activities and diminished concentration) or **mania** (an abnormally elevated or irritable mood characterized by high levels of arousal and energy which cause significant social, vocational or academic impairment), are seen in mood disorders. **Mood disorders** refer to sustained emotional states that are a departure from the individual's usual functioning and that cause significant impairment in social or vocational functioning. Mood disorders are outside the boundaries of normal mood states by virtue of their intensity and duration; they tend to have a periodic or cyclical nature.

The DSM-5 describes two broad categories of mood disorders: depressive disorders and bipolar disorders (American Psychiatric Association [APA], 2013). There are a number of subcategories within each classification, detailing related disorders. Regardless of the setting, nurses will regularly encounter individuals with these disorders and need to develop skills in the identification, assessment, and management of the individual experiencing a mood disturbance.

An important consideration for all individuals experiencing a mood disorder is the possibility of suicide. In the United States,

Risk for Suicide in Patients with Depressive and Bipolar Disorders   box 16-1

Patients with depression are at increased risk for suicide and should be assessed for suicidal ideation and potential during initial evaluation and periodically throughout treatment. Recognizing suicidal ideation and risk is essential to determining treatment setting and establishing treatment priorities. Factors that increase patient risk for suicide include history of previous suicide attempt, active substance use disorder, age greater than 65, history of physical or sexual abuse, and access to a firearm (Chapter 27).

The individual with bipolar disorder is at increased risk for suicidal ideation and successful completion of suicide. The following risk factors increase the lifetime risk for suicide for individuals with bipolar disorder (Nabuco de Abreu, Lafer, Baca-Garcia, & Oquendo, 2009):

- Hopelessness regarding the illness state
- Prior suicide attempt

- Early age of onset of bipolar disorder
- Preponderance of depressive episodes and mixed episodes
- Rapid cycling of moods
- Co-morbidity with other psychiatric disorders, especially borderline personality disorder
- Impulsivity, hostility, and aggressiveness
- Childhood history of physical and sexual abuse
- Family history of suicide attempt

38,364 individuals completed suicide in 2010, making suicide the 10th leading cause of death in the United States (American Association of Suicidology, 2013). Not surprisingly, 90% of people who die by suicide have a diagnosable mental health disorder (American Foundation for Suicide Prevention [AFSP], 2011). Between 25% and 50% of people with bipolar disorder will attempt suicide at least once in their lifetime, and as many as 20% will die by suicide (AFSP, 2011). Suicide risk is elevated among individuals with chronic and terminal illness and in those with substance abuse disorders. As suicide is a tragic consequence associated with all depressive and bipolar disorders, assessment for suicidal ideation and intent should be part of the initial and ongoing nursing care of the individual with mood disturbance. All nurses need to develop the necessary skills and comfort level to assess suicide potential and familiarize themselves with risk factors that increase the likelihood of suicide (Box 16-1).

Mood disorders are highly prevalent and exact an enormous burden on individuals, their families, and society. Mood disorders know no age demographic. According to recent statistics from the National Comorbidity Survey-Replication (NCS-R) study, the 12-month prevalence for all mood disorders among U.S. adults ages 18 to 65 is 9.5%, with a lifetime prevalence of 20.8% (National Institute of Mental Health [NIMH], 2011). In older adults, there is wide variability in the estimated frequency of mood disorders due to the significant overlap of mood symptoms with additional medical co-morbidities in this age group. Research indicates that although the incidence of mood disorders is relatively high in the older population, older adults are less likely to seek care for mental disorders, thus further complicating data collection (Hanrahan & Sullivan-Marx, 2005). Regardless, it is clear that mood disorders are underdiagnosed and undertreated in persons over age 65. The most prevalent mood disorder among older adults is major depression; however, persistent depressive disorder (dysthymia), adjustment disorder with depressed mood, depression attributable to medical conditions, and subsyndromal depressive symptoms are also common.

The lifetime prevalence for mood disorders in adolescents ages 13 to 18 is an alarming 14%, with a 4.7% lifetime prevalence of a severe mood disorder that will affect adolescents' quality of life and functioning (NIMH, 2011). Although clear data are lacking on the prevalence of mood disorder in children, information from the National Health and Nutrition Examination Survey (NHANES) estimates the prevalence to be about 3.7% in children 8 to 15 years of age (NIMH, 2011).

As a result of inadequate numbers of trained providers and uneven distribution of services, many people with mood and other mental disorders either go undiagnosed and untreated, or they are identified and treated in primary care and specialty care settings such as emergency rooms or gynecologic settings. For many with complex psychiatric diagnoses or refractory symptoms, long waits for referral to specialty care are the norm (Wang et al., 2005). Of special concern is the fact that of patients with psychiatric disorders who do receive treatment, studies indicate that only a third receive at least minimally adequate treatment. In light of these findings, *nurses across all specialties may be among the first to recognize and evaluate a mood disorder and may be the first step in linking these individuals and their families with other health care professionals and specialty providers.* In addition, nurses can take a role in developing and implementing creative strategies to address the health care disparities in these populations.

In this chapter, the various mood disorders are examined, beginning with the depressive disorders and then bipolar disorder (formerly known as manic–depressive disorder). Although the disorders are discussed separately, it is important to appreciate that there is considerable overlap and range in mood symptoms (Figure 16-1). Although mania and depression may be viewed as being on separate ends of a spectrum, they frequently share similar symptoms, such as sleep and appetite disturbance, cognitive disturbance, and symptoms of restlessness or agitation. Mania and depression both cause significant physical, psychological, social, spiritual, and cultural suffering for the individuals and their families.

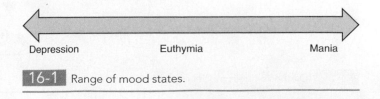

Depression   Euthymia   Mania

16-1   Range of mood states.

DEPRESSIVE DISORDERS

Theoretical Foundations

What causes depression? Why do some individuals develop depression while others do not? Like many disease processes, depression is a multifaceted illness that is most likely due to a complex and dynamic interaction among biological, psychological, sociological, cultural, and spiritual factors. The **diathesis–stress model** postulates that individuals inherit tendencies to express certain traits or behaviors when exposed to the right conditions or stressors (Figure 16-2). Seemingly, psychological events have the ability to initiate or exacerbate a neurochemical imbalance in susceptible individuals. Thus, it would seem that under the right circumstances and given a genetic vulnerability, an individual will develop depression. However, simply having a propensity toward developing depression alone (for example, having a strong family history of depression in one or both parents) is not enough to trigger illness. An individual's diathesis (hereditary predisposition) must interact with life events to set the stage for illness. In addition, it would seem that the greater the inherited vulnerability, the less environmental stress will be needed to trigger depression. Life trauma (such as sexual abuse, physical abuse, political and social violence), especially during the formative years of childhood, may also predispose vulnerable individuals to alterations in brain neurochemistry and set the stage for future mood disorders.

The theoretical foundations of depression will be explored in the following sections (Table 16-1). However, it is important to remember that depression is not linear, and it is impossible to trace its origins to a single cause. This is especially important as nurses teach patients and families about the disorder and employ various treatment modalities. This multidimensional model of causality gives credibility to the effectiveness of the variety of treatments used in the management of depression.

Biological Domain

The biological models of depression have focused on alterations in the neurotransmitters and brain structures responsible for mood regulation, as well as genetic, endocrine, and circadian factors that are responsible for depression (Warren & Lutz, 2009). These models give credence not only to the mood symptoms associated with depression, but also to its physical manifestations.

Neurotransmitters and Brain Structures

The last decade has seen exponential growth in the understanding of the complexities of the brain structures and neurotransmitters that control emotion and regulate mood. Although a full discourse of brain anatomy and physiology is beyond the scope of this chapter, an appreciation of some basic principles is essential.

When studying areas of the brain responsible for emotion and mood regulation, most research focuses on the prefrontal area, the limbic system, and the basal ganglia (Figure 16-3). Extensive functional and neuroanatomic connections exist among these structures. Of these three areas, the limbic system is the area most responsible for mood and emotion. At the base of the forebrain, above the thalamus and hypothalmus, is the limbic system, which includes the hippocampus, cingulated gyrus, septum, and amygdala. This system is responsible for the regulation of emotions and our ability to learn and control our impulses. The basal ganglia has complex fronto-subcortical networks that have an important role in cognition, reward, and mood regulation, whereas the prefrontal area is essential to the creation and expression of emotion. If the pathways to and from the prefrontal area are severed, the person is not able to experience emotions of any kind. All of these structures send signals to one another and the rest of the nervous system via neurotransmitters and their neurotransmitter systems.

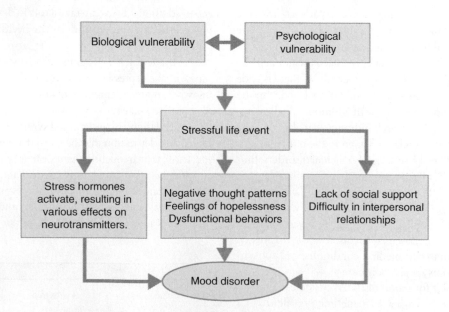

16-2 Diathesis–stress model of depression.

Depressive Responses by Domain
table 16-1

Domain	Responses
Biological	• Changes in weight or appetite • Psychomotor agitation or retardation • Decreased energy/increased fatigue • Somatic complaints of pain or body aches • Lack of sexual interest/sexual dysfunction • Sleep disturbance • Constipation • Decreased self-care • Menstrual changes
Psychological	• Feelings of worthlessness or guilt • Difficulty thinking or concentrating • Suicidal ideation, plans, or attempts • Irritability • Anhedonia • Delusions • Hallucinations • Crying • Ruminations • Anxiety • Anger • Apathy • Despondency
Sociological	• Social withdrawal or isolation • Failure to meet occupational or interpersonal responsibilities • Role strain • Inability to care for oneself or family • Substance use or misuse • Family discord • Economic hardship related to disability; underachievement
Cultural	• Denying, discounting, or explaining away depressive symptoms • Disenfranchisement from cultural group related to stigma • Lack of access to services due to language, cultural barriers or lack of culturally sensitive providers
Spiritual	• Feeling abandoned or punished by God/Higher Power • Loss of hope • Guilt • Loss of purpose or life meaning • View symptoms as punishment for past sins or lifestyle • Belief that his or her faith is not strong enough • Bitterness toward God/higher power

Neurotransmitters are endogenous chemicals that allow the transmission of signals from one neuron to the next across a synapse. Neurotransmitter systems are complex networks or circuits of nerve cells that use the same neurotransmitter to communicate across central nervous system structures. Neurotransmitters bind to multiple receptor subtypes and are responsible for the complexities of human behavior, emotion, and nervous system functioning. For example, at least 18 different subtypes of serotonin receptors have been identified. An appreciation of function of these neurotransmitters is essential to understanding mood disorders and the pharmacotherapies used in their management (Chapter 3).

Dysregulation of the neurotransmitter systems and neurotransmitters has been implicated in mood disorders. The neurotransmitters most commonly linked with mood disorders are known as the *biogenic amines* and include serotonin, norepinephrine, dopamine, histamine, and the inhibitory neurotransmitter gamma-aminobutyric acid (GABA). Recently, the neurotransmitters acetylcholine and glutamate have also been identified as playing an important role in mood regulation. Dysregulation of these neurotransmitters and neurotransmitter systems is responsible for the emotional distress, vegetative symptoms, and physical pain frequently associated with depression. **Vegetative symptoms** are the corporeal manifestations of depression and include sleep and appetite disturbance, decreased energy, psychomotor symptoms (agitation or retardation), sexual dysfunction, and the neurocognitive symptoms of decreased concentration or cognition, lack of pleasure, guilty ruminations, and suicidal ideation.

Recent research points to a complicated interaction among neurotransmitter symptoms as an explanation for mood dysregulation. It would be an oversimplification to say that mood disorders were caused by dysregulation of any one neurotransmitter. In all likelihood, it is almost certain that disturbances are associated with complex and unpredictable interactions among these systems. Dysregulation of one system has profound impacts on the function of other systems. Almost all drug therapies for the management of mood disorders work by either increasing or decreasing the availability of these neurotransmitters.

Further evidence of the role of neurotransmitters in the regulation of mood comes from research that looks at the relationship between pain and depression (Box 16-2). It is widely recognized that a majority of individuals with depression will report a variety of somatic complaints. Indeed, **somatization**, or the process by which psychological distress is expressed in physical symptoms, is common in individuals with major depression. A meta-analysis of 14 studies by Bair et al. (2003) found that, overall, 65% of patients with major depressive disorder reported painful physical symptoms. Data from the Sequenced Treatment Alternatives to Relieve Depression (STAR*D) study, which included both primary care and psychiatric outpatients with nonpsychotic major depression, showed that almost 80% of patients complained about some type of physical pain (Husain et al., 2007).

It is important to recognize the painful symptoms of depression. Some individuals may present with primarily pain or somatic

Pain and Depression
box 16-2

As many as 80% of individuals with depression present with one or more painful symptoms. Stahl (2002) asserts that this may be the result of malfunction in the serotonergic and noradrenergic pathways, causing routine or benign sensory input to be interpreted as discomfort or pain. This may account for the lack of explanation for multiple physical symptoms reported by patients with depression, including headache, abdominal pain, and musculoskeletal pain.

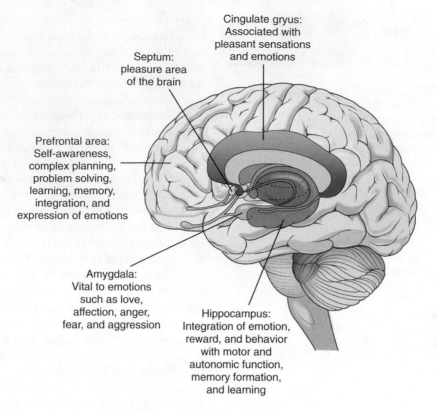

Cingulate gryus:
Associated with pleasant sensations and emotions

Septum:
pleasure area of the brain

Prefrontal area:
Self-awareness, complex planning, problem solving, learning, memory, integration, and expression of emotions

Amygdala:
Vital to emotions such as love, affection, anger, fear, and aggression

Hippocampus:
Integration of emotion, reward, and behavior with motor and autonomic function, memory formation, and learning

16-3 Brain structures responsible for the regulation of mood and emotion.

symptoms and minimize or discount mood symptoms. Often patients say, "If only this pain would go away, my mood would get better" or "Of course I feel depressed—this pain is really getting to me." Pain and depression have a reciprocal relationship in that each heightens the severity of the other. If unrecognized and untreated, painful or somatic symptoms may become a barrier for complete remission of depression (Karp et al., 2005). Several studies have demonstrated that the presence of pain and somatic symptoms may delay remission for as long as 6 weeks (Karp et al., 2005) and may be an indicator of a difficult to treat depression (Kroenke et al., 2008). In addition, individuals with somatic symptoms experience greater social and vocational dysfunction (Demyttenaere et al., 2006).

Genetic and Environmental Models

Depression is believed to be caused by an interaction between genes and environment. Despite clear evidence that depression is transmitted in families, the specific genetic locus for depressive disorders has yet to be discovered. Evidence suggests that it is polygenetic (multiple genes) rather than an isolated gene. In addition, the way in which environmental factors influence this genetic tendency is a matter of much debate. Adverse life advents that occur during early critical phases of brain development are thought to act as the diathesis for the development of depression and other mental health disorders. Current evidence suggests that a combination of genes, environment, and other factors yet to be determined is responsible for expression of disease.

Much of what is known about the genetic and environmental influences of depression comes from twin and adoption studies,

which look at the prevalence of depression in the first-degree relatives of individuals with depression (or the *proband*, the individual who serves as the starting point for a genetic study). A meta-analysis of the genetic epidemiology of major depression conducted by Sullivan, Neale, and Kendler (2000) and a systematic review of the genetic and environmental influences on psychiatric co-morbidity by Cerda, Sagdeo, Johnson, and Galea (2010) highlight several important points:

- There is strong and consistent evidence to support an association between major depression in the proband and major depression in first-degree relatives. The overall heritability of depression is likely to be in the 31% to 42% range. As might be expected, an identical twin is two to three times more likely to present with a depressive disorder than a fraternal twin if the first twin has depression.

- There is little evidence to support that specific environmental influences are important. It seems that individual response, rather than specific behavioral factors (for example, parenting style, socioeconomic status, home environment, or the presence/absence of early life trauma/abuse) is more predictive of mood disturbance. There are "substantial numbers of people with high liability who are not affected with major depression and people with low liability who are affected," making a case for the role of individual intentions, choices, and actions in the development of depression (Sullivan, Neale, & Kendler, 2000, p. 1559). This may point to the concept of resilience as an explanation for why some individuals develop depression and others do not.

- The risk for depression is two times greater in women than in men, indicating a gender-related vulnerability to depression.

- Increased severity and recurrence in the proband was associated with increased incidence of depression in relatives, indicating that the more severe disorders have a stronger concordance than less severe disorders. Specifically, the more profound, recurrent, and impairing a depression is, the more likely there is to be a first-degree relative with depression.

- There is strong evidence to support a shared genetic vulnerability between depression and other psychiatric disorders, particularly anxiety and substance abuse disorders. This link is especially strong between major depressive disorder and generalized anxiety disorder.

These findings have important practice implications for nursing in terms of primary, secondary, and tertiary prevention strategies for depression and other mental disorders. Among the many *Healthy People 2020* topics and objectives are mental health and mental disorders. The overarching goal of these objectives is to improve mental health through prevention and by ensuring access to appropriate, quality mental health services. *Healthy People 2020* offers the following recommendations and suggestions related to mental health and mental disorders:

Primary Prevention

- Strategies aimed at improving family functioning and positive parenting

- School-based preventive interventions aimed at improving social and emotional functioning

- Interventions targeting families dealing with adversities, such as parental depression or divorce, which can be effective in reducing risk for depression among children and adolescents

- Increased attention to at-risk populations (veterans, people in communities with large-scale psychological trauma caused by natural disasters, older adults), thereby facilitating early intervention strategies aimed at eliminating or reducing the risk for depressive disorders

Secondary Prevention

- Screening for major depressive disorder in children, adolescents, and adults when systems are in place to ensure accurate diagnosis, psychotherapy (cognitive–behavioral or interpersonal), and follow-up

- Counseling individuals and families about their relative risks for developing mood disorders

- Measures aimed at reducing harm from traumatic events

Tertiary Prevention

- Collaborative care programs for the management of depressive disorders

- Clinic- and home-based strategies to reduce depression among older adults, especially in those with co-morbid conditions such as cardiovascular disease and diabetes

- Community-based strategies aimed at increasing the amount of mental health services available to homeless adults (U.S. Department of Health and Human Services, 2013)

Neuroendocrine Models

In response to stress, several neuromodulating hormones are released from the hypothalmus thus stimulating the hypothalamic–pituitary–adrenal (HPA) axis. These neuromodulating hormones act very much like neurotransmitters by sending information to other brain structures and the rest of the body, preparing it for real or perceived dangers (fight or flight). Stressful or traumatic experiences during childhood or early adolescence are thought to cause persistent changes to these hypothalamic neuroendocrine circuits, resulting in structural changes within the limbic system, particularly the hippocampus, the source of emotion and mood regulation. These changes are believed to increase the vulnerability to mood and anxiety disorders later in life.

Under normal circumstances following a physical or psychological threat, corticotropin-releasing factor (CRF) is released from the hypothalamus. This, in turn, stimulates the anterior pituitary gland to release adrenocorticotropic hormone (ACTH), which, in turn, stimulates the adrenal gland to increase synthesis and release of cortisol. Through a negative feedback loop to the hypothalmus, hippocampus, and anterior pituitary, cortisol then functions to inhibit further release of ACTH and CRF (Figure 16-4). According to neuroendocrine models of depression, repeated or chronic stress results in over-activity of the HPA axis, ultimately resulting in excessive excretion of stress hormones, particularly cortisol. In essence, the normal feedback loop to suppress cortisol is malfunctioning, causing heightened stress sensitivity. Studies indicate that prolonged elevation of stress hormones can be harmful, especially to developing neurons, and may prevent the development of new neurons (neurogenesis) in the hippocampus resulting in a reduction in hippocampal volume (Nemeroff & Vale, 2005). These findings have important clinical implications in terms of primary prevention of depression and in the development of unique pharmacologic strategies that dampen the HPA axis response to stress.

Circadian Models

Insomnia with early morning awakening is the most common complaint associated with depression; however, hypersomnia is also seen, especially in individuals with atypical depression and those with seasonal affective disorder (SAD). Complaints of poor sleep quality are observed in 50% to 90% of individuals diagnosed with depression. Residual sleep disturbance in an individual recovering from depression is one of the most important predictors of relapse to a new depressive episode. Sleep electroencephalographs (EEGs) are abnormal in up to 90% of individuals with depression. Decreased total sleep time, impaired sleep efficiency, a reduction in slow wave sleep, a shortening of rapid eye movement (REM) sleep latency (a reduction in the time from sleep onset to the beginning of the first REM period), and a reduction and distribution of slow wave sleep characterize the EEG findings in these individuals.

All physiologic and metabolic functions are timed and regulated and occur on a scheduled and periodic basis. These highly regulated processes are known as *circadian rhythms* and are responsible for the 24-hour cycling of numerous physiologic patterns, such as body temperature, blood pressure, digestion, the release of hormones (such as melatonin, cortisol, growth hormone, thyroid hormone), and the timing of sleep and wakefulness (Chapter 12). Disruption to circadian rhythms causes dysregulation of many of these physiologic patterns that results in the

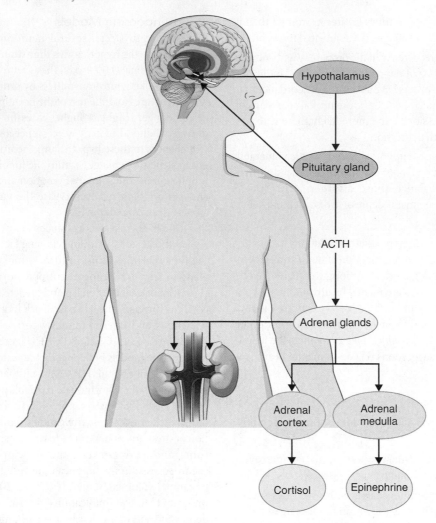

16-4   According to neuroendocrine models of depression, repeated or chronic stress results in overactivity of the HPA axis, ultimately resulting in excessive excretion of stress hormones, particularly cortisol.

symptoms commonly associated with depression, such as appetite disturbance, constipation, fatigue, and sleep disturbance. The high prevalence of sleep complaints in individuals with depression and the response to light therapy in people with clear seasonal patterns to their symptoms provides strong evidence for the circadian models of depression. Research into this relationship has focused on the neuroendocrine abnormalities associated with this sleep disruption, such as elevated cortisol and ACTH levels in depressed individuals throughout the night or 24-hour cycle and alterations in the secretion of hormones that are sleep-stage dependent. For example, slow wave sleep, which occurs predominantly in the first half of the night, is a powerful physiologic stimulus for growth hormone (GH). Polysomnographic abnormalities in individuals with depression are seen regularly in the first half of the night and are associated with blunted GH release. In addition, it has long been recognized that depressive symptoms are acutely alleviated by one night of sleep deprivation in about 60% of individuals with major depressive disorder and that symptoms recur after one night of recovery sleep. Physiologic evidence to support this observation includes a lowering of cortisol levels following sleep deprivation, suggesting that lower HPA activity may be at least partially responsible for the temporary improvement in depressive symptoms (Tsuno, Besset, & Ritchie, 2005).

Circadian models of depression have important implications for nursing practice. Nursing intervention directed at maintaining and supporting regular behavioral and sleep patterns are essential to recovery efforts for individuals with mood disturbance (Chapter 12). A stable sleep–wake schedule and adequate sleep hygiene are crucial in preventing relapse in depressed individuals.

Psychological Domain

As discussed previously, psychosocial stressors often set the stage for the development of future depression by initiating the diathesis-stress cascade responsible for permanent neuronal changes implicated in the development of mood and anxiety disorders. The psychological sequelae of stress and trauma are often unique to the individual (for instance, childhood abuse/trauma, marital discord, parenting stress, vocational failures) and should be viewed within the individual's world view and taken in context. What may be a trigger event for one individual may not be for another. For example, the loss of employment is usually viewed as a severe psychosocial stressor with significant financial and self-esteem ramifications. The individual who was unhappy in his or her job, however, may view this as an opportunity to start anew and perhaps to re-create himself or herself or take time to reappraise life goals. It is not enough to simply identify life events or stressors that may precipitate a depressive episode; it is important to gain an understanding of the relevance the event has for the individual. It is widely recognized that many individuals may experience significant life stressors and traumas and yet not develop depression.

Contemporary research into the psychological domains of depression has focused on the impact of stressful events and the cognitive and behavioral responses to these events that predispose the individual to depression. Learned helplessness and negative cognitive styles result in a cognitive vulnerability to depression, and they are useful theoretical schemas that form the basis of much of our current psychotherapeutic approaches in the management of mood disorders. A fundamental understanding of these models is helpful when planning behavioral strategies for individuals with mood disorders and in employing therapeutic communication aimed at changing negative cognitive and behavioral patterns.

Learned Helplessness

The notion of learned helplessness was first described by Martin Seligman (1975). Seligman observed that dogs that were given repeated electrical shocks without hope of escape became helpless, gave up, and developed an animal equivalent of depression. Seligman later went on to describe depression as a maladaptive cognitive style characterized by the belief that stressful life events are uncontrollable. In short, individuals make an attribution that they are unable to change life events or circumstances and thereafter give up, experiencing a sense of discouragement, hopelessness, and despair. Learned helplessness results from a pessimistic explanatory or attributional cognitive style. The depressive attributional style is (1) *personal*, in that the individual attributes negative events to personal failings; (2) *persistent*, in that even when the event passes, the individual believes that additional bad things will happen; and (3) *pervasive*, in that the attributions extend across a wide variety of issues. Seligman's book, *Learned Optimism* (1998), highlights that one can overcome depression by changing one's explanatory style and developing a more positive outlook.

Negative Cognitive Style

The cognitive model developed by Aaron Beck (1967) hypothesizes that an individual's idiosyncratic responses to life events affect emotions and behavior, and that negative thoughts, attitudes, and behaviors are the hallmarks of depression. Individuals with depression have skewed core beliefs of themselves, their environment, and the future (Beck's cognitive triad for depression) and demonstrate characteristic negative and pessimistic thinking that is responsible for the inability of the individual to change his or her behavior or see the possibility for change or improvement. As a result, individuals with depression develop deep-seated negative life views that are often based on cognitive distortions rather than reality (for example, "I am a bad student because I got a B on my last exam").

Beck observed that individuals with depression often exhibit irrational thinking exemplified by negative automatic thoughts, arbitrary inference, and overgeneralization. *Automatic thoughts* are thoughts and images that go through a person's mind in response to situation-specific events and are based on core beliefs. For example, a pretty, well-educated, professional woman who sees herself as unattractive and uninteresting does not try to meet new men for fear of rejection: "No one would be interested in me anyway; I am not very smart or attractive." *Arbitrary inference* is the tendency to focus on the negative rather than positive aspects of an event or situation.

The same young woman sees it as confirmation of her lack of appeal when a new date fails to call to schedule another meeting. She is not able to think of an alternative explanation, such as his losing her phone number or some type of personal conflict on his part. Explanations tend to focus on the insecurities and perceived faults of the individual. Finally, *overgeneralization* is taking an isolated event and broadly generalizing about it. Again, in the current example, the woman sees it as evidence that no one will want to date her if she is rejected by a single suitor. Negative cognitive styles have important clinical implications with regards to treatment and nursing intervention. Cognitive–behavioral therapy is aimed at restructuring negative thoughts, attitudes, and beliefs. Negative thoughts are challenged in terms of their irrationality and restructured in such a way as to be more adaptive.

Sociological Domain

As discussed earlier, there are probably many pathways that lead to the final endpoint of depressive illness. Recent research into the sociologic conditions and stressors that contribute to depression has focused on the notion of environmental provocation and inclement social events. A number of factors have been implicated, including the current climate of large-scale and long-term unemployment, caregiver burden in the parenting or adult child role, renewed dependency needs of adult children, changing gender roles, marital dissatisfaction, and limited social support.

In a recent poll, 31% of Americans living in poverty reported a diagnosis of depression, as opposed to 15.8% of those living above the poverty line (Brown, 2012). One study demonstrated that job insecurity was strongly associated with feelings of depression even after controlling for age, sex, economic factors, and work characteristics (Meltzer et al., 2010).

Social stressors frequently are viewed as being outside one's personal control and are associated with feelings of entrapment, humiliation, chronic low self-esteem, shame, and personal deprivation. Examples of social stressors include low or threatened socioeconomic status (such as poverty, lack of adequate health insurance, food or housing insecurity), job insecurity or unemployment, single parenthood, legal problems, debt, domestic or community violence, emotionally toxic work environments, and natural or environmental disasters.

Cultural Domain

Culture exerts a powerful influence on the identification, diagnosis, and treatment of mood and mental health disorders. Nurses need to be knowledgeable about the cultural factors that underlie an individual's presentation, perception of depression, and patterns of seeking help in order to effectively assess and provide care. Symptoms are culture and language bound. Some cultures, such as the Hopi Indians of North America, Tahitians, Nigerians, and many Asian cultures, have no word for depression in their language. The lack of appropriate language to describe depression results in alternative cultural labels to describe the mood and physical symptoms we recognize as depression. For example, all people with depression experience a **dysphoric mood**, which is an unpleasant mood state such as sadness, anxiety, or irritability. However, it is the cultural expression of this dysphoric mood that defines the manifestations of symptoms, the clinical course, and treatment outcomes. In

Hispanic people, for example, depressive disorders frequently have a somatic presentation, and individuals tend to have a lower preference for pharmacologic treatments for depression based on less belief in a biomedical explanation for depression (Fernandez y Garcia et al., 2011). This may lead to difficulties in engaging patients fully in care and abandonment of treatment before full recovery. African immigrants have strong family-of-origin connections, and treatment may be influenced by family traditions and customs. Some recent African immigrants believe in magic, sorcery, or witchcraft. This magical belief system may form the basis of an explanation for their physical symptoms and may pose barriers for traditional care and treatment.

Spiritual Domain

Spiritual distress occurs when there is confusion or despair associated with life's meaning or purpose. Spiritual distress is frequently a symptom of depression. The individual who is depressed may question the meaning of life and point to life's vicissitudes as evidence that life is not worth living. Indications of spiritual distress in individuals with depression include searching questions, such as "Why is this happening to me?" or "What have I done to deserve such pain and suffering?" Although rejection of religious beliefs and values may be an obvious indicator of spiritual distress, misplaced anger and hostility, withdrawal, guilt, uncertainty, defensiveness, and a sense of emptiness or aloneness may also indicate spiritual distress (Thompson, 2002).

Depressive symptoms sometimes result from a life crisis that calls into question the purpose and meaning of life. For example, a middle-aged woman who has just lost her 25-year-old son in a motor vehicle accident becomes withdrawn and isolated. She verbalizes anger and inappropriate hostility toward friends and family members who try to provide comfort and support. She asks, "What is the purpose of leading a good life if something terrible like this is going to happen?"

A qualitative study conducted by Greasley, Chiu, and Gartland (2001) looked at how cultural, religious, and spiritual beliefs affected individual response to health and illness in a group of mental health patients and professional caregivers. The study identified the following important themes that nurses should keep in mind when considering the spiritual domain for patients with depression: (1) There is a psychological benefit to the belief in God, an afterlife, and fate, as these beliefs function to give meaning to life events; (2) faith is a source of comfort in times of crisis such as illness; and (3) spiritual guidance and assurance are important during times of crisis.

Pause and Reflect

1. *What physical symptoms are associated with depression? Why? What implications do these have for nursing care?*

2. *Do you know someone who exhibits learned helplessness? How do you feel when you are with that person? What techniques would you use to help a patient exhibiting learned helplessness?*

3. *Ask other students from diverse cultural backgrounds to explain their cultural conception of depression, including asking: "If you are depressed, but your language has no word for depression, how would you describe your depression?"*

Specific Disorders

The DSM-5 (APA, 2013) has identified eight distinct types of depressive disorders. The classic condition in this group is *major depressive disorder* (MDD) or *unipolar depression*, a severe global depressed mood. *Persistent depressive disorder* (PDD, or *dysthymia*) is a chronic depressed mood that frequently has an early onset. MDD and PDD are discussed in detail in this section.

The other depressive disorders included by the DSM-5 in this category are:

- *Disruptive mood dysregulation disorder*, a new diagnosis referring to the presentation of children with persistent irritability and frequent episodes of extreme behavioral dyscontrol. The diagnosis is used for children under 12 years of age.

- *Premenstrual dysphoric disorder*, a treatment-responsive form of depressive disorder that follows ovulation, remits within a few days of menses, and has a marked impact on functioning.

- *Substance/medication-induced depressive disorder*, which is associated with the injection, ingestion, or inhalation of a substance such as a drug of abuse, toxin, psychotropic medication, or other medication.

- *Depressive disorder due to another medical condition*, such as endocrine conditions and other medical conditions.

- *Other specified depressive disorder.*

- *Unspecified depressive disorder.*

Major depressive disorder is characterized according to the presence of anxious distress and severity (mild, moderate, and severe). MDD is also classified by specifiers that describe the current status of the mood episode and its key features, some of which are: anxious distress, atypical, catatonic, melancholic, seasonal, and with peripartum onset (Table 16-2). Although not all mood disorders are accompanied by specifiers, their presence frequently assists in determining the most effective treatment and predicting the future course of the disorder (APA, 2013).

Dysthymic disorder is characterized by a chronically depressed mood for most of the day for more days than not for at least 2 years for adults and 1 year for children and adolescents (APA, 2013). Although dysthymic disorder is clinically viewed as less severe than major depression, individuals with dysthymic disorder experience significant impairment in family, social, and vocational functioning owing to the prolonged nature of symptoms. The other depressive disorders address depressive features that do not necessarily meet full criteria for either a major depressive disorder, dysthymic disorder, or adjustment disorders with associated mood symptoms. However, the other depressive disorders are nonetheless impairing in some way.

Major Depressive Disorder

Major depressive disorder (MDD), sometimes known as *unipolar depression*, is believed to be the most common mood disorder. It may occur in isolation as a single episode, but most people with a clear diagnosis of MDD will experience recurrence at some time during their life. The essential feature of MDD is one or more major depressive episodes without a history of manic or hypomanic episodes.

Clinical Features of Depression

table 16-2

Feature	Characteristics
Anxious distress	Feeling keyed up or tense; feeling unusually restless; difficulty concentrating because of worry; fear that something awful might happen; and fear of loss of control of self.
Atypical features	Overeating, oversleeping, reactive mood, rejection sensitivity.
Catatonia	Total absence of movement; the individual's muscles are waxy and semi-rigid. Mutism, negativism, echolalia, or echopraxia may be present.
Melancholia	Early morning awakening, anhedonia, vegetative symptoms, symptoms worse in morning.
Mixed features	Elevated, expansive mood; inflated self-esteem or grandiosity; more talkative/pressured speech; flight or ideas and subjective feeling of racing thoughts; increase in energy and goal-directed activity; increased involvement in activities that may bring painful consequences; decreased need for sleep.
Peripartum onset	Onset during or following pregnancy.
Psychosis	Presence of hallucinations, delusions, thought disorder.
Seasonal	A pattern of mood disturbance that has a seasonal variation. The most common pattern is a depressive episode that begins in the late fall and terminates in early spring. This condition is known as seasonal affective disorder (SAD). Characterized by increased sleep drive and weight gain.

The DSM-5 indicates two hallmark criteria for a major depressive episode: (1) an extremely depressed mood or (2) loss of interest or pleasure in nearly all activities, known as **anhedonia**, for at least two consecutive weeks. Anhedonia is an extremely important symptom (see DSM-5 Diagnostic Criteria for Depressive Disorders). It implies not only the inability to experience pleasure, but also the inability to experience all positive feelings. Because nothing is capable of making the individual with anhedonia feel better, he or she has little ability or motivation to change behavior. This creates a sense of hopelessness and helplessness for the individual and may cause isolation, alienation, and perpetual despair. The DSM-5 requires individuals to have at least one of these symptoms for diagnosis, but for most people these symptoms co-occur. Many researchers contend that an individual cannot be considered severely

Diagnostic Criteria for Depressive Disorders

Major Depressive Episode

A. Five (or more) of the following symptoms have been present during the same 2-week period and represent a change from previous functioning; at least one of the symptoms is either (1) depressed mood or (2) loss of interest or pleasure. *Note:* Do not include symptoms that are clearly attributable to another medical condition.

1. Depressed mood most of the day, nearly every day, as indicated by either subjective report (e.g., feels sad, empty, hopeless) or observation made by others (e.g., appears tearful). (*Note:* In children and adolescents, can be irritable mood.)

2. Markedly diminished interest or pleasure in all, or almost all, activities most of the day, nearly every day (as indicated by either subjective account or observation).

3. Significant weight loss when not dieting, or weight gain (e.g., a change of more than 5% of body weight in a month), or decrease or increase in appetite nearly every day. (*Note:* In children, consider failure to make expected weight gain.)

4. Insomnia or hypersomnia nearly every day.

5. Psychomotor agitation or retardation nearly every day (observable by others, not merely subjective feelings of restlessness or being slowed down).

6. Fatigue or loss of energy nearly every day.

7. Feelings of worthlessness or excessive or inappropriate guilt (which may be delusional) nearly every day (not merely self-reproach or guilt about being sick).

8. Diminished ability to think or concentrate, or indecisiveness, nearly every day (either by subjective account or as observed by others).

9. Recurrent thoughts of death (not just fear of dying), recurrent suicidal ideation without a specific plan, or a suicide attempt or a specific plan for committing suicide.

B. The symptoms cause clinically significant distress or impairment in social, occupational, or other important areas of functioning.

C. The episode is not attributable to the physiological effects of a substance or to another medical condition.

D. The occurrence of the major depressive episode is not better explained by schizoaffective disorder, schizophrenia, schizophreniform disorder, delusional disorder, or other specified and unspecified schizophrenia spectrum and other psychotic disorders.

E. There has never been a manic episode or a hypomanic episode.

Source: Reprinted with permission from the *Diagnostic and Statistical Manual of Mental Disorders*, Fifth Edition, (Copyright 2013). American Psychiatric Association.

depressed without the presence of anhedonia. Anhedonia is likely to be the cause of many of the other symptoms of depression, such as loss of appetite, impaired libido, and loss of interest, and is believed to have its origins in dysregulation of dopaminergic mesolimbic and mesocortical pathways.

In addition to low mood and anhedonia, a person must have at least four additional symptoms, such as cognitive disturbance (decreased concentration or difficulty making decisions); recurrent thoughts of death or suicide; feelings of worthlessness or guilt; and physical symptoms such as fatigue, sleep disturbance, appetite disturbance, loss of sexual interest, and motor symptoms such as psychomotor retardation or agitation. These additional symptoms are the physical symptoms of depression and are referred to as *vegetative symptoms*. A clever acronym to assist with remembering the diagnostic criteria for major depression is SIG-E-CAPS (suicide, interest, guilt, energy, concentration, appetite, psychomotor, sleep/sex). Symptoms are to such a degree as to cause significant academic, vocational, and social impairment.

Persistent Depressive Disorder (Dysthymia)

Persistent depressive disorder, also known as dysthymia, shares many of the same symptoms as major depressive disorder, but symptoms are often less severe, yet more pervasive. Symptoms are of such duration that the individual frequently does not remember ever feeling any different. Symptoms may be atypical in presentation. Individuals may describe hypersomnia rather than insomnia, or overeating rather than loss of appetite. Low energy, fatigue, low self-esteem, poor concentration, and hopelessness are common. PDD is characterized by a low-grade and protracted depressive state that often has an early onset in childhood, adolescence, or early adulthood. Symptoms are generally milder (but nonetheless disabling) and remain relatively unchanged over a period of years. It is important to recognize that individuals with PDD may also develop more profound symptoms and meet criteria for MDD. This is commonly known as *double depression*.

Other Depressive Disorders

Other depressive disorders include premenstrual dysphoric disorder, minor depressive episodes or episodes that do not meet full criteria, recurrent brief episodes of depression, postpsychotic depressive episodes or depression that is believed to be associated with a psychotic illness, and situations in which the clinician is unable to determine whether the depression is primary, due to a medical condition, or substance induced (APA, 2013).

Premenstrual dysphoric disorder, mentioned previously, was moved from the appendix of the DSM-IV-TR to a full-fledged depressive disorder in the DSM-5 after more than 20 years of confirming research. Another new depressive diagnosis, disruptive mood dysregulation disorder, was also included in the DSM-5. It was developed in response to clinician concerns regarding over diagnosis and treatment of children who displayed persistent irritability and frequent episodes of out-of-control behavior (APA, 2013). This diagnosis reflected the finding that many children displaying this pattern of symptoms frequently develop unipolar depressive disorders or anxiety disorders rather than bipolar disorders as they mature into adolescence and adulthood (APA, 2013).

Pause and Reflect

1. *Why do you think anhedonia is likely to be the cause of other symptoms of depression?*

2. *What are the differences between major depressive disorder and dysthymic disorder?*

3. *Do you know anyone who has been diagnosed with depression? What symptoms did you observe in that person? What treatments has that person found helpful?*

Prevalence and Life Span Considerations

As discussed previously, depression is a multifaceted illness that affects functioning across the domains, and can result in great suffering for individuals and their families.

Prevalence

The World Health Organization (WHO) has ranked depression as the fourth leading cause of disability worldwide and estimates the number of disability-adjusted life years lost to unipolar depression to be 10.3 years (NIMH, 2011). Projections are that by 2020, depression will be second only to heart disease in its contribution to the global burden of disease as measured by disability-adjusted life years (Chapman & Perry, 2008). A study conducted by the Centers for Disease Control and Prevention (CDC) indicated that among 235,067 U.S. adults surveyed between 2006 and 2008, 9.1% met criteria for current depression symptoms (significant symptoms for at least 2 weeks before the survey), including 4.1% who met DSM-IV-TR criteria for major depression disorder (CDC, 2010). This study also confirmed previous findings that individuals who are more likely to meet criteria for major depression include persons 45 to 64 years of age, women, Blacks, Hispanics, non-Hispanic individuals of other races or multiple races, persons with less than a high school education, individuals unable to work or unemployed, and persons without health insurance.

Despite effective detection and treatment, depression continues to be under-recognized and undertreated, with nearly half of all depressions remaining undetected or inadequately controlled. Depressive disorders are a major cause of disability and suffering. Although depression may manifest itself as a single lifetime episode, most individuals experience recurrent episodes with varying degrees of residual symptoms between episodes. The risk for recurrence is higher in younger patients and in individuals with a history of a severe episode (APA, 2013).

Depression and Co-Morbidities

Depression co-occurs with other psychiatric and substance abuse disorders, as well with many medical disorders. There is considerable overlap between depression and anxiety symptoms and disorders. Anxiety symptoms may be a precursor to a depressive episode, may occur during a depressive episode and complicate treatment, or may remain a residual symptom once depression has resolved. Substance misuse/abuse is common in individuals with depression and may represent a first attempt at self-managing depressive symptoms, anxiety, or sleep disturbance.

There is a bidirectional relationship between depression and medical illness, as evidenced by a high incidence of depression among individuals with medical illness and the increased likelihood of developing chronic medical problems in individuals with depression. People with chronic medical illness, such as type 2 diabetes mellitus (DM) and cardiovascular disease (CVD), have been shown to have two- to threefold higher rates of depression compared with age- and gender-matched individuals (Ali et al., 2006; Spijkerman et al., 2005). In addition, depression has been shown to worsen outcomes for medical co-morbidities such as CVD, congestive heart failure (CHF), chronic obstructive pulmonary disease (COPD), and type 2 DM. Depression also increases the risk of rehospitalization for these disorders and compounds the symptom burden and functional impairment associated with these co-morbidities. The co-morbidity of depression and medical illness is a well-recognized marker for severe and treatment-resistant depression.

Of equal importance is the fact that there is evidence to suggest that individuals with depression are at increased risk for CVD, type 2 DM, COPD, and certain cancers as a result of maladaptive health risk behaviors (poor diet, obesity, sedentary lifestyle, and smoking) and the physiologic effects of their psychiatric illness, such as chronic activation of the HPA axis. Increased levels of the stress hormone cortisol and the increase in catecholamine and pro-inflammatory cytokines associated with increased sympathetic activation may be the common pathway that links depression to increased insulin resistance and hypertension, which increases the risk for CVD and type 2 DM (Katon, 2011).

The high rate of co-occurrence of depression and medical illness carries a number of implications for nurses (Katon, 2011): (1) the importance of incorporating depression screening as part of assessment in primary care settings; (2) the need to assess patients with chronic medical illness for depression, as depression may impair a patient's ability to manage chronic medical illness and increase the patient's risk of mortality; and (3) the need to assess patients presenting with pain for depression, as pain is the most common complaint for individuals with depression and medical illness.

Children and Adolescents

Mood disorders occur among children and adolescents with fair regularity. Prevalence rates for depressive disorders based on a recent meta-analysis are 2.8% for children younger than 13 years and 5.6% for 13- to 18-year-olds (Costello, Erkanli, & Angold, 2006; Lack & Green, 2009). Even though the criteria for diagnosing depression are the same for adults and children, many clinicians miss a diagnosis of depression in children, frequently attributing symptoms to the normal variability in mood seen throughout childhood. Symptoms of depression are commonly attributed to "a phase" the child or teenager is currently experiencing. Identification of mood symptoms is especially important, however, in that depression in this age group can be highly debilitating by causing significant disruption in social, academic, family, and interpersonal functioning that may continue to follow the child into young adulthood and beyond. Early age at onset of depression is associated with a high risk of recurrences in adulthood, highlighting the importance of primary prevention strategies aimed at decreasing the risk for depression in children and adolescents and the aggressive identification and treatment of youths with mood symptoms. For more information on the care of children and adolescents with depressive disorders, see Chapter 28.

Women

Female gender itself is a risk factor for depression. Gender-specific differences related to neurobiological, genetic, and psychosocial factors underlie this increased vulnerability. Women are at increased risk for depression at times of hormonal transition, such as during puberty; during premenstruum, perimenopause, and menopause; following miscarriage; and during pregnancy and postpartum (Burt & Quezada, 2009).

As identified earlier, changes in the HPA axis that result in excessive production of the stress hormone cortisol is a likely neuroendocrine explanation for mood disturbance. Estrogen and progesterone have profound and complicated interactions with the HPA axis and may therefore trigger the HPA axis abnormalities in susceptible women (Meltzer-Brody, 2011). Female sex hormones are important modulators of serotonin, norepinephrine, and dopamine transmitter symptoms. As a consequence, fluctuations in estrogen and progesterone levels throughout the menstrual cycle and in the perimenopause can cause changes in these important neurotransmitters that result in changes in emotions, mood, sexual behavior, cognition, and sensory perception.

In addition to these neurobiological factors, women may be more susceptible to the impact of negative life events and a perceived lack of social support than their male counterparts. It seems that the higher rates of child sexual abuse among girls, burdens associated with the caregiving role, and the sociocultural barriers to personal and professional self-fulfillment play a role in the increased risk for depression in women.

The DSM-5 identifies two gender-specific diagnoses: major depressive disorder with the specifier "with peripartum onset" and premenstrual dysphoric disorder (PMDD). MDD with peripartum onset occurs in about 3% to 6% of women during pregnancy or in the weeks to months following delivery. Although the public is most aware of postpartum depression, clinicians now know that 50% of the depressive episodes actually begin prior to delivery. Symptoms can range from the subclinical, such as mild tearfulness and worry about the challenges of caregiving (known as "baby blues"), to severe depression associated with psychotic features (command hallucinations and delusions associated with the infant) and infanticidal/suicidal ideation. Postpartum psychosis is associated with a significant risk of harm to the infant and mother and is considered a psychiatric and obstetric emergency. Postpartum psychosis is more common in primiparous women and women with a history of postpartum psychosis, prior history of depressive or bipolar disease (especially bipolar I), and women with a history of family members with psychotic disorders. The risk of recurrence of postpartum psychosis with each subsequent delivery is between 30% and 50%, highlighting the importance of close follow-up and support for these women in the postpartum period on subsequent pregnancies.

Equally important is *perinatal depression*, which is defined as a depressive episode that occurs during the pregnancy or within the first 6 months postpartum; it has a prevalence of 10% to 15% in women of childbearing age (Meltzer-Brody, 2011). History of prior depression increases the relative risk for prenatal and postpartum depression, making early screening and treatment essential. In women with depression who become pregnant, 70% who discontinue their medication will relapse, with 50% of the relapses occurring within the first trimester and 90% by the end of the second trimester (Meltzer-Brody, 2011).

Perinatal depression has been shown to have significant health consequences for the woman, her infant, and the family, and is associated with poor birth outcomes such as low birth weight, preterm delivery, and poor maternal–infant attachment/bonding. Several studies have demonstrated that children exposed to maternal depression either during pregnancy or in the postpartum period have higher cortisol levels than infants of women who were not depressed. This finding may partially explain the higher rate of psychopathology found in children of depressed women (Diego et al., 2004; Halligan, Herbert, Goodyer, & Murray, 2004). In addition, animal models of maternal deprivation and separation (surrogates for maternal depression and anxiety) have been shown to confer an increased vulnerability for depressive-like behaviors and alterations in response to stressful events (Franklin et al., 2010). Traumatic events occurring at critical times of early brain development may be responsible for the structural and neurobiological manifestations seen with mood disorders; maternal depression indeed may be such an early traumatic event that begins this diathesis—stress cascade. These findings highlight the importance of primary prevention strategies within the obstetric environment. The American Psychiatric Association and the American College of Obstetricians and Gynecologists have co-published guidelines on the management of depression during the perinatal period (Yonkers et al., 2009).

PMDD is associated with a markedly depressed mood occurring during the luteal phase of the menstrual cycle for most months for the previous 12 months. PMDD affects 1.8% to 5.8% of premenopausal women. Symptoms remit within a few days of the onset of the menses and are always minimal or absent in the week following the menstrual flow. Five or more of several key symptoms are required for the diagnosis, including marked mood lability, irritability and increased interpersonal conflict, sadness or hopelessness, sleep disturbance, decreased interest in usual activities, and feeling overwhelmed or out of control (APA, 2013).

As with other psychiatric disorders, symptoms are associated with significant social or vocational disruption. The term *premenstrual syndrome* (PMS) has been commonly used to describe similar symptoms, but these symptoms do not meet the full criteria for PMDD or cause significant social or vocational disruption.

Keep in mind the following implications for nursing practice regarding depression in women (Meltzer-Brody, 2011; Burt & Quezada, 2009):

- Rather than describing sadness or depression, women with peripartum depression may experience and express guilt and confusion. They are unable to understand why they are not experiencing joy at this important life transition and frequently wonder whether there is something wrong with them. They may ruminate about being a "bad mother."

- Screening for suicidal ideation is paramount; maternal suicide accounts for up to 20% of all postpartum deaths.

- Careful follow-up and treatment of depression during the peripartum period may improve maternal and neonatal outcomes that extend into early childhood. Multiple studies have demonstrated that successful treatment of maternal depression has a positive effect on the mental well-being of school-age children and adolescents.

- Pharmacologic treatment of perinatal depression is controversial. There continues to be a lack of well-designed studies because of ethical and practical concerns associated with the treatment of pregnant women and infants. That being said, perinatal depression poses a significant risk to mother and child; the risk–benefit ratio must be assessed with each woman individually.

Specialized assessment tools are available to assist with the screening and diagnosis of depression during the perinatal period. Some examples include the Edinburg Postnatal Depression Scale (EPDS) and the Postpartum Depression Screening Tool (PDSS). The EPDS is available in several languages.

Older Adults

Depression is widely under-recognized and undertreated in the elderly. Both older adults and clinicians tend to focus on physical problems and regularly miss depression. The estimated prevalence of depression in community-dwelling older adults is 1% to 5% in most large-scale epidemiologic investigations in the United States and internationally, whereas rates of depression among older adults living in nursing homes is estimated to be 14% to 42% (Fiske, Loebach-Wetherell, & Gatz, 2009).

Depression is *not* a normal part of aging and should not be viewed as a natural consequence associated with the life changes that accompany aging, such as retirement or the loss of a spouse (Figure 16-5). Risk factors for late-life depression (depression occurring for the first time in advanced age) include female gender, social isolation, lower socioeconomic status, multiple medical co-morbidities (especially pain), cardiovascular and neurologic disorders, past history of depression, and functional impairment. Personal loss (loss of spouse, home, friends, or independence) increases the burden of depressive symptoms and increases the risk for disability, family

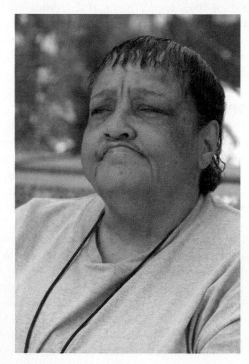

16-5 Depression is not a normal part of aging. Nurses working with older adults should be aware of risk factors for late-life depression, including female gender, social isolation, and multiple co-morbidities.

Source: Greatbass.com/Fotolia

caregiver strain, and successful suicide. Depressive illness in older adults may hasten functional decline, increase the risk for hospitalization and non-adherence to treatment for co-morbidities, and reduce quality of life for individuals and families alike. The additional likelihood of medical co-morbidities (e.g., heart disease, diabetes, stroke, cancer, pain syndromes, and cognitive impairment) compound symptom burden and complicate the assessment, treatment, and ultimate recovery from depressive illness in older adults. Neuropsychiatric disorders such as Parkinson disease and Alzheimer disease increase the risk for depression; conversely, some studies have indicated that depression may be a harbinger of dementia. Depression in older adults frequently is characterized by somatic complaints that may distract clinicians from an accurate diagnosis. Psychotic symptoms can be present in the form of persecutory, guilty, or nihilistic delusions as well as hallucinations. Depression may also present as cognitive impairment in older adults, a condition known as *pseudodementia*.

Although effective treatment is available, several studies indicate that relapse rates are higher in older adults (Mitchell & Subramaniam, 2005) and that fewer than 50% of older adults with major depressive episodes achieve remission with first-line antidepressant pharmacotherapy within the customarily expected response rate of 6 weeks (Mulsant et al., 2006). This highlights the need for longer treatment durations for older patients that include a combined pharmacologic and psychotherapeutic approach, as well as attention to the sociocultural challenges of isolation, **bereavement** (grief associated with the loss of a loved one or object), and social role transition that many older adults face. In addition, older adults are at risk for issues associated with polypharmacy, delayed response time to treatment, and poor tolerability to antidepressants and mood stabilizers.

Keep in mind the following implications for nursing practice regarding depression in older adults (Fiske, Loebach-Wetherell, & Gatz, 2009; APA, 2013):

- Low-grade depressive symptoms, or *subsyndromal depression*, are common in older adults. Even though symptoms may not meet the criteria for a major depressive episode, symptoms are nonetheless impairing and have profound impacts on functioning and quality of life.
- Screening for suicide is paramount; older adults tend to use more immediately lethal means and suicidal behavior is more likely to be successful in older adults compared with other age groups. Of major concern is the observation that older adults are less likely to discuss suicidal ideation or intent.
- Sleep disturbance, fatigue, psychomotor retardation, loss of interest in living, and hopelessness about the future are more prevalent in late-life depression than in younger or middle-age adults. Although some older patients will report dysphoric mood, many do not, a presentation known as "depression without sadness" or "depletion syndrome."
- Depression following certain neurologic disorders, such as stroke, Parkinson disease, or dementia, presents differently than other late-life depressions. Individuals with stroke may present with more vegetative signs, whereas those with Parkinson disease generally do not describe dysphoric mood or anhedonia. Depressive symptoms in those with dementia may be particularly difficult to decipher, but increased agitation, crying, and social withdrawal may point to depression in these individuals.
- Careful assessment is essential to distinguish depressive symptoms from the grief response. The feelings of emptiness and loss as well as preoccupation with thoughts of the deceased that are characteristic of grief typically are not articulated in individuals with depression, and the lack of self-esteem exhibited with depression generally is not associated with grief.
- Interventions aimed at successful aging such as activities that enhance cognitive functioning, promote physical activity, and maintain meaningful social connections are key strategies for wellness and the prevention of depression in this age group.

Specialized assessment tools are available to assist with the screening and diagnosis of depression in the geriatric population. Some examples include the Geriatric Depression Scale—Short Form (GDS-SF) and the Geriatric Depression Scale—Long Form (GDS-LF).

Pause and Reflect

1. *Why do you think individuals with chronic medical illness experience higher rates of depression? What implication does this have for treatment of patients with chronic medical illnesses?*
2. *How may depression present differently in children?*
3. *What symptoms of depression are more prevalent in older adults than in younger or middle-age adults? How does symptom presentation differ in older adults with neurologic disorders?*

BIPOLAR AND RELATED DISORDERS

Theoretical Foundations

Bipolar disorder (formerly known as manic–depressive disorder) is a biological disorder, but its ramifications have wide psychological, social, cultural, and spiritual implications. As with depression, it is probably a complex interaction between biology and environment that is responsible for the manifestations and consequence of the illness. Though treatable, bipolar disorder (BD) is a chronic and frequently disabling illness characterized by significant social and occupational dysfunction and suffering. It is associated with the highest lifetime rate of suicide of all the mental disorders (see Box 16-1). As discussed earlier, between 25% and 50% of people with

BD will attempt suicide at least once in their lifetime; up to 20% will die by suicide (American Foundation for Suicide Prevention, 2011). The following sections will explore the theoretical foundations of bipolar disorders, building on an understanding of depression and gaining an appreciation for the connection between the two disorders (Table 16-3).

Biological Domain

When considering the biological domain of bipolar disorders, it is important to keep in mind what has already been discussed about depression. Mania by itself does occur, but is exceedingly rare.

Bipolar Responses by Domain   table 16-3

Domain	Response
Biological	• Hyperactivity to the point of physical exhaustion • Sleep disturbance • Appetite disturbance • Hypersexuality • Increased distractibility • Altered thought processes • Elation, euphoria
Psychological	• Grandiosity • Pressured speech • Loosening of associations • Paranoia • Psychosis • Suicide • Increased creativity • Impaired judgment and insight • Manipulative behaviors • Exaggerated self-esteem • Lack of insight • Aggressive or argumentative
Sociological	• Interpersonal and occupational difficulties • Substance use/misuse • Increased marital conflict and divorce • Risk taking • Inappropriate intimacy with strangers • Exaggerated sense of importance • Loss of social supports due to behaviors
Cultural	• Rejection by others due to behaviors • Rejection of cultural morals/values
Spiritual	• Rejection of religious beliefs due to manic or hypomanic state • Hyper-religiosity • Delusional religious beliefs • View of symptoms as punishment for past sins or lifestyle • Belief that faith is not strong enough

Large-scale, prospective studies demonstrate that most individuals with bipolar disorder remain symptomatically ill for approximately 50% of their lives, with depression representing the dominant mood state and a reported ratio of depression to mania or hypomania as 3:1 (Kupka et al., 2007). There are convincing data that up to 50% of all depressions may be of the bipolar type, and 75% of all patients with BD present first with depression, reinforcing the need to obtain a careful psychiatric and family history in all individuals presenting with depression. This gives rise to the current concept of bipolar spectrum disorder (Kaplan & Sadock, 2005). Although depression represents the predominant abnormal mood state for treated individuals with BD (Kupka et al., 2007), episodes of mania, **hypomania** (a continuing elevated, expansive, irritable mood state that does not impair functioning), or **mixed episodes** (depression plus mania/hypomania) are the key elements that distinguish BD from MDD

and are frequently related to the psychosocial disruption associated with the disorder.

Just as in depression, there are complex biological interactions involving dysregulation of neuroendocrine systems, biogenic amines and brain structures, intracellular signaling systems, circadian rhythms, and genetic and environmental influences that account for our understanding of BD.

Neurotransmitters and Brain Structures

There is mounting evidence to support neuroanatomic and neurophysiologic abnormalities in individuals with BD. Several investigators have observed structural and functional abnormalities that seem to predate symptom onset and persist during symptom remission and treatment (Bearden, Woogen, & Glahn, 2010). This gives credence to the possibility that changes in brain structure and function are central to the pathophysiology of BD and solidifies the view of BD as a biological illness. The most consistently documented changes are lateral ventricle enlargement, decreased frontal cortical volume, reduced volume of the corpus callosum, and increased rates of deep white matter hyperintensities (Mahon, Burdick, & Szeszko, 2010; Martinowich, Schloesser, & Manji, 2009). These changes result in dysregulation of the neuronal circuits of the prefrontal cortex and limbic system (the sources of mood and emotion regulation, executive function, reasoning, and memory), and may predispose the individual toward the development of bipolar disorder. For example, studies have shown reduced activity in the right prefrontal cortex during an episode of mania, an event that has been associated with poor impulse control, risk taking, distractibility, poor attention, and psychosis, all of which resemble the symptoms of mania (Martinowich, Schloesser, & Manji, 2009). Additional theories as to the biological basis for BD include mitochondrial dysfunction, dysregulation of the monoaminergic neurotransmitter systems (norepinephrine, dopamine, and serotonin) and, most recently, the glutaminergic, cholinergic, and GABAergic systems, abnormalities in signaling pathways, and changes in size and density of neuronal cell types and neuronal cell plasticity.

These changes may be responsible for the observation that many individuals with bipolar disorder do not regain premorbid levels of psychosocial functioning and the consequent high degree of functional impairment observed in the disorder. Even euthymic, asymptomatic patients with BD have been shown to exhibit limitations in several cognitive domains, including executive functioning, memory, and attentional processing; this has been shown to be a reasonable predictor of psychosocial functioning and disability (Bearden, Woogen, & Glahn, 2010). Age at onset of disease, number of depressed and manic episodes, and number and duration of hospitalizations have been associated with degree of functional impairment and degree of structural abnormality noted on imaging studies, which provide evidence that BD may be viewed as a chronic progressive illness. Further research and understanding into the neurobiological basis for BD may improve current treatment options and offer opportunities for primary and secondary prevention strategies.

Genetic and Environmental Models

Family and twin studies suggest a clear genetic predisposition toward the development of BD. If one parent has BD, the risk that a child will have the disorder is about 27%; if both parents have the disorder, that risk increases to 50% to 65% (National Coalition for Health

Professional Education in Genetics [NCHPEG], 2011). Twin studies demonstrate a concordance rate for monozygotic twins of about 77%, versus a 23% rate for dizygotic twins (Goodwin & Jamison, 2007). Equally important is the observation that in families of individuals with bipolar disorder, not only is the risk for BD elevated, but the relative risk for unipolar depression also increases. Interplay between environmental and genetic factors seems a reasonable explanation for the fact that not all individuals with first-degree family members with BD develop the illness, and this interplay may have important implications for primary prevention strategies.

Neuroendocrine Models

As in depression, dysregulation of the HPA axis figures highly in the pathophysiology of bipolar disorder. Mania has been associated with both elevated CSF and urinary-free cortisol concentrations, and depressed patients with bipolar disorder are reported to have significantly greater elevation of cortisol than normal controls or unipolar depressed patients. The mechanism for these alterations in the HPA axis is as yet unknown, but glucocorticoid resistance, similar to the insulin resistance of diabetes, has been suggested (Berns & Nemeroff, 2003).

Circadian Models

Sleep disruption is a key symptom in patients with bipolar disorder; patients suffer profound alterations in their sleep–wake cycles during both the manic and depressive phases of their illness. In contrast to unipolar depression, in which insomnia may be the predominant sleep complaint, the depression of bipolar disorder tends to be atypical; individuals with bipolar depression tend to describe fatigue, hypersomnia, and reverse diurnal mood variability (Berns & Nemeroff, 2003). Patients with bipolar disorder may experience episodes of sleeplessness associated with mania that are described not necessarily as insomnia but rather as a decreased need for sleep.

Changes in sleep patterns or circadian rhythms (timing of work, activity patterns, eating patterns) can have profound effects on mood and may even precede a shift in the mood state in patients with BD. For example, it is well recognized that sleep deprivation or traveling across time zones can trigger a manic episode. Sensitivity to perturbations in circadian rhythm appears to be one characteristic of BD, making an argument for regular sleep–wake and activity patterns.

Psychological and Sociological Domains

The biological basis for bipolar disorder is irrefutable and accounts for the fact that most psychological theories have gone by the wayside. As discussed previously, however, biology alone is an insufficient explanation for the myriad symptoms that constitute the disorder. Even those individuals who adhere to their medication regimens are troubled with symptom recurrence as well as social and vocational disruption. There is good evidence to suggest that psychosocial stressors contribute to symptom burden and that psychological therapies, such as psychoeducation and social rhythm therapy, are effective in reducing symptoms and improving overall functioning. Goodwin and Jamison (2007) proposed three psychosocial factors that interact with biology to create recurrence of bipolar illness: (1) stressful life events; (2) disruption in social rhythms; and (3) medication nonadherence. Additional psychosocial factors for the development of subsequent or persistent mood symptoms have been identified as

lack of social supports, poor family functioning, and functional impairment. Weinstock and Miller (2010) demonstrated that low levels of social support, as measured by material aid, availability of someone to talk with, self-esteem, and meaningful relationships or belonging, predicted an increased risk for subsequent depression but not mania at one year after acute phase treatment of bipolar I disorder.

The sociological consequences of BD are especially troublesome. As many as two-thirds of individuals with BD have some type of inter-episode functional impairment (Tohen et al., 2003); about half are unemployed or have some type of vocational or occupational dysfunction (Altshuler et al., 2007). The source of this persistent distress is likely related to the chronic nature and burden of the disease, the high incidence of psychiatric and medical comorbidities, side effects of medications, and the impact that manic or hypomanic behavior may have on work, family, and community relationships. A study conducted by Jonsson, Skarsater, Wijk, and Danielson (2011) examined the experience of living with a family member having BD and found that family members often feel alone in the experience of dealing with a loved one with BD, are unsure about the future, and struggle with understanding what constitutes normal and abnormal behavior. Family members participating in the study reported feeling stigmatized and experiencing shame, isolation, uncertainty, resentment, hopelessness, and powerlessness. These findings bring into sharp focus the far-reaching burden of BD and demonstrate a need for nursing interventions that provide support and education for families and communities as a standard of care.

PRACTICE ALERT Make sure that family members are also taking care of themselves while caring for a loved one with a psychiatric illness. Assess their nutrition and sleep patterns and coping skills, as well as their community and spiritual supports. Provide education regarding self-care and, when necessary and appropriate, offer referral and respite services through local health care agencies and support groups.

Cultural and Spiritual Domains

Individuals with BD experience significant cultural and spiritual distress; not infrequently, these domains overlap. For example, a young woman with BD is unable to work as a result of fatigue and sleepiness associated with her medication regimen; she feels that she is a burden to her family and is ashamed that she must accept disability in order to live (social domain). Her culture does not recognize her illness and she loses respect and status within her community (cultural domain), which leads to further isolation and feelings of abandonment (spiritual domain). Another example: A well-respected politician loses his standing in the community during a manic episode in which he is hypersexual and exhibits poor judgment managing community finances; his wife leaves him as a result of his sexual indiscretion and he loses his job (social domain). He feels guilty about his extramarital affair and financial recklessness, because he sees himself as a good Christian and family man (spiritual domain). These scenarios highlight the importance of using a holistic cultural perspective to assess the role and influence of culture on the expression of symptoms and management of disease (Jones-Warren, 2007) and the impact that BD has on the individual, the family, and society.

Pause and Reflect

1. *What psychosocial factors can trigger a recurrence of bipolar illness? Why do you think these factors carry such impact for patients with bipolar disorder?*

2. *Why do you think bipolar disorder has such an impact on the family members of patients with bipolar disorder? What implications does this have for nursing care?*

Specific Disorders

DSM-5 has identified three major types of bipolar disorders: bipolar I, bipolar II, and cyclothymic disorder. Bipolar I disorder is characterized by at least one episode of mania and major depression (see DSM-5 Diagnostic Criteria for Bipolar Disorders) (APA, 2013). As previously described, mania in the absence of a history of depression does occur, but is exceedingly rare. In the rare incidences in which this occurs, many of these individuals are found to have alternative medical- or substance-related explanations for the mania. Bipolar II disorder is usually characterized by recurrent episodes of major depression alternating with episodes of hypomania; however, diagnosis can be made when at least one hypomanic and at least one major depressive episode have occurred. Specifiers regarding current severity, presence of psychotic features, course, and so forth are used to further categorize the disorder. For example, a *single manic episode* is used to describe a first manic episode, and a *current episode manic, depressed, or mixed* is used to describe subsequent or recurrent episodes. **Cyclothymic disorder** is a chronic mood disturbance of at least 2 years' duration characterized by numerous episodes of hypomania and depressed mood of insufficient severity to meet the full criteria for bipolar I or bipolar II disorder (APA, 2013).

Bipolar I and Bipolar II Disorders

While it is important to realize that the individual with BD can present with either depression or mania/hypomania, *more than 75% of people with BD will present initially with depression.* As a result, individuals with BD frequently go undiagnosed for many years. Once again, this highlights the importance of a complete and accurate clinical history that includes screening for any episodes of hyperactivity, expansive mood, or marked changes in behavior, as well as a full family history that focuses on screening for bipolarity in any family members.

The predominant mood state for individuals with BD during a manic or hypomanic episode is one of abnormally exaggerated elation, grandiosity, energy, joy, or euphoria. Despite this elation, the mood state is quite unstable and may quickly change to irritability, anger, or even rage. The individual may be belligerent or uncooperative, and frequently lacks insight into the illness and its impact on those around them. During manic or hypomanic episodes, the individual experiences pleasure in every activity. He or she can become extremely hyperactive and may not eat, sleep, or care for basic physical needs such as washing and physical care. Hypersexuality is common and may lead to indiscriminate and unsafe sexual practices. Grandiosity and an inflated self-esteem may cause the individual to make poor choices regarding relationships, work, finances, and personal safety. Pressured speech, loosening of associations, and **flight of ideas** (rapid speech that involves ideas that jump from topic to topic and may be loosely associated) are common language patterns. Psychotic symptoms in the form of paranoia, delusions of grandeur, and hallucinations are possible and indicate a need for immediate hospitalization.

Bipolar I and bipolar II disorder are distinguished from each other by the degree and severity of symptoms that the individual experiences during an "up" period. Thus, mania and hypomania are distinguished from one another by the severity and degree of impairment. The individual who is manic is generally quite impaired and, in most instances, has psychotic symptoms, as we saw in the case of Vijay. In contrast, the individual with hypomania may be capable of a high degree of functioning and indeed may be capable of extraordinary accomplishments. Ludwig von Beethoven, Winston Churchill, Charles Dickens, Ernest Hemingway, and Abraham Lincoln are among some of the many talented and gifted individuals believed to have had BD.

Hypomania is not generally severe enough to cause significant disruption in psychosocial or vocational functioning or require hospitalization, and it is not associated with psychosis. Although hypomania is a less severe version of a manic episode, it is nonetheless dangerous. Whereas the individual with bipolar I disorder who is clearly manic may come into contact with either the police or health care provider fairly quickly, the individual with bipolar II disorder can cause substantial disruption within the family and other relationships during a hypomanic episode, causing significant and often irreparable damage to relationships and reputation.

Diagnosis of bipolar I and II disorders is frequently complicated in that it is not unusual for an individual to present with both depressive symptoms and manic or hypomanic behavior, a condition termed a *mixed episode.* During a mixed episode, a person experiences rapidly alternating moods of sadness, irritability, and euphoria (APA, 2013). A mixed episode is characterized by the presence of both depressed mood and manic or hypomanic symptoms during the majority of the days of the current or most recent episode; the person must meet diagnostic criteria for both disorders simultaneously. Some individuals experience *rapid cycling,* which occurs when mood episodes appear in quick succession (at least four mood episodes within a year) in any combination (depression, mania, or hypomania) and are separated by partial or full remission periods of at least 2 months *or* a switch to the opposing mood episode (e.g., from depression to mania) (APA, 2013).

Cyclothymic Disorder

Cyclothymic disorder is characterized by a biphasic pattern of alternating brief periods of depression and hypomania over a 2-year period (1 year in children and adolescents). There must be no symptom-free periods that last longer than 2 months. The essential feature is a chronic, fluctuating course of mood disturbance involving numerous periods of hypomanic and depressive symptoms (APA, 2013). The symptoms are of insufficient severity to meet full diagnostic criteria for either a major depressive episode or a manic/hypomanic episode, and individuals with this disorder frequently elude evaluation. There is considerable controversy regarding cyclothymic disorder as a distinct condition; probably, this controversy has given rise to the notion of *bipolar spectrum disorder.* Regardless, cyclothymic disorder should not be viewed as "less severe" than bipolar I or bipolar II disorder, as the degree of impairment from the disorder is frequently quite significant and many contend that it may be a precursor of types I and II BD (Baldessarini, Vazquez, & Tondo, 2011). These individuals are frequently misdiagnosed as having atypical depression or personality disorders, especially of the cluster B type (Perugi, Fornaro, & Akiskal, 2011).

Diagnostic Criteria for Bipolar I Disorder

DSM-5

For a diagnosis of bipolar I disorder, it is necessary to meet the following criteria for a manic episode. The manic episode may have been preceded by and may be followed by hypomanic or major depressive episodes.

Manic Episode

A. A distinct period of abnormally and persistently elevated, expansive, or irritable mood, and abnormally and persistently increased goal-directed activity or energy, lasting at least 1 week and present for most of the day, nearly every day (or any duration if hospitalization is necessary).

B. During the period of mood disturbance and increased energy or activity, three (or more) of the following symptoms (four if the mood is only irritable) are present to a significant degree and represent a noticeable change from usual behavior:

1. Inflated self-esteem or grandiosity

2. Decreased need for sleep (e.g., feels rested after only 3 hours of sleep)

3. More talkative than usual or pressure to keep talking

4. Flight of ideas or subjective experience that thoughts are racing

5. Distractibility (i.e., attention too easily drawn to unimportant or irrelevant external stimuli), as reported or observed.

6. Increase in goal-directed activity (either socially, at work or school, or sexually) or psychomotor agitation (i.e., purposeless non–goal-directed activity).

7. Excessive involvement in pleasurable activities that have a high potential for painful consequences (e.g., engaging in unrestrained buying sprees, sexual indiscretions, or foolish business investments)

C. The mood disturbance is sufficiently severe to cause marked impairment in social or occupational functioning or to necessitate hospitalization to prevent harm to self or others, or there are psychotic features.

D. The episode is not attributable to the physiological effects of a substance (e.g., a drug of abuse, a medication, other treatment) or to another medical condition.

Hypomanic Episode

A. A distinct period of abnormally and persistently elevated, expansive, or irritable mood and abnormally and persistently increased activity or energy, lasting at least 4 consecutive days and present most of the day, nearly every day.

B. During the period of mood disturbance and increased energy and activity, three (or more) of the following symptoms (four if the mood is only irritable) have persisted, represent a noticeable change from usual behavior, and have been present to a significant degree:

1. Inflated self-esteem or grandiosity

2. Decreased need for sleep (e.g., feels rested after only 3 hours of sleep)

3. More talkative than usual or feels pressure to keep talking

4. Flight of ideas or subjective experience that thoughts are racing

5. Distractibility (i.e., attention too easily drawn to unimportant or irrelevant external stimuli), as reported or observed

6. Increase in goal-directed activity (either socially, at work or school, or sexually) or psychomotor agitation.

7. Excessive involvement in pleasurable activities that have a high potential for painful consequences (e.g., engaging in unrestrained buying sprees, sexual indiscretions, or foolish business investments).

C. The episode is associated with an unequivocal change in functioning that is uncharacteristic of the individual when not symptomatic.

D. The disturbance in mood and the change in functioning are observable by others.

E. The episode is not severe enough to cause marked impairment in social or occupational functioning or to necessitate hospitalization. If there are psychotic features, the episode is, by definition, manic.

F. The episode is not attributable to physiological effects of a substance (e.g., a drug of abuse, a medication, or other treatment).

Major Depressive Episode

A. Five (or more) of the following symptoms have been present during the same 2-week period and represent a change from previous functioning; at least one of the symptoms is either (1) depressed mood or (2) loss of interest or pleasure.

1. Depressed mood most of the day, nearly every day, as indicated by either subjective report (e.g., feels sad, empty, or hopeless) or observation made by others (e.g., appears tearful). (Note: In children and adolescents, can be irritable mood.)

2. Markedly diminished interest or pleasure in all, or almost all, activities most of the day, nearly every day (as indicated by either subjective account or observation).

3. Significant weight loss when not dieting, or weight gain (e.g., a change of more than 5% of body weight in a month), or decrease or increase in appetite nearly every day. (Note: In children, consider failure to make expected weight gain.)

4. Insomnia or hypersomnia nearly every day.

5. Psychomotor agitation or retardation nearly every day (observable by others; not merely subjective feelings of restlessness or being slowed down).

6. Fatigue or loss of energy nearly every day.

7. Feelings of worthlessness or excessive or inappropriate guilt (which may be delusional) nearly every day (not merely self-reproach or guilt about being sick).

8. Diminished ability to think or concentrate, or indecisiveness, nearly every day (either by subjective account or as observed by others).

9. Recurrent thoughts of death (not just fear of dying), recurrent suicidal ideation without a specific plan, or a suicide attempt or a specific plan for committing suicide.

B. The symptoms cause clinically significant distress or impairment in social, occupational, or other important areas of functioning.

C. The episode is not attributable to the physiological effects of a substance or another medical condition.

BIPOLAR I DISORDER

A. Criteria have been met for at least one manic episode (Criteria A–D under "Manic Episode" above).

B. The occurrence of the manic and major depressive episode(s) is not better explained by schizoaffective disorder, schizophrenia, schizophreniform disorder, delusional disorder, or other specified or unspecified schizophrenia spectrum and other psychotic disorder.

Source: Reprinted with permission from the Diagnostic and Statistical Manual of Mental Disorders, Fifth Edition, (Copyright 2013). American Psychiatric Association.

Other Bipolar and Related Mood Disorders

In addition to the mood disorders discussed previously, bipolar disorders may be associated with a general medical condition or with substance use. Nurses must be aware of medical conditions and substances that can result in mood disorders and help clients manage their care needs.

Bipolar and Related Disorder Due to Another Medical Condition

A bipolar or related disorder due to a another medical condition is the presence of a prominent and persistent period of abnormally elevated, expansive, or irritable mood and abnormally increased activity or energy directly related to the effects of a general medical condition (APA, 2013). To merit this determination, mood symptoms must not have appeared before the initial presentation of the medical condition. Improvement or remission of mood symptoms that are associated with the treatment and/or remission of the medical condition is not uncommon in this diagnostic category. If depressive symptoms are also present but do not predominate, the specifier "with mixed features" is used. Finally, the diagnosis cannot be made during the course of a delirium (APA, 2013).

Medical conditions such as multiple sclerosis, Cushing disease, stroke, and traumatic brain injuries are commonly associated with manic/hypomanic symptoms. Fluid and electrolyte imbalances; endocrine disorders, such as Addison disease and Cushing syndrome; thyroid disorders; parathyroid disorders; and nutritional deficiencies may be associated with either depressive symptoms or mania/hypomania (Hoff & Morgan, 2011). This complex situation highlights the importance of a complete physical evaluation that includes laboratory tests and family history when evaluating individuals with mood symptoms.

Substance/Medication-Induced Bipolar and Related Disorder

In addition to drugs of abuse (e.g., nicotine, caffeine, alcohol, cocaine, amphetamine, marijuana) as possible causes of bipolar disorders and drug withdrawal syndromes, many of the most commonly used medications used to treat hypertension, cardiovascular disease, neurologic disease, and certain dermatologic conditions may also cause bipolar symptoms. Examples of these medications include anxiolytics; antipsychotics; sedative–hypnotics; certain blood pressure medications, such as beta-blockers, hydrochlorthiazide, clonidine, and reserpine; dermatologic agents, such as isotretinoin (Accutane); hormone therapy; steroids; antifungal medications; analgesics; cimetidine and metoclopramide; chemotherapeutics; and antiretroviral therapies (Hoff & Morgan, 2011). This highlights the importance of a complete medication review as part of the assessment for an individual experiencing bipolar symptoms. A clear temporal relationship between the mood symptoms and the use of a medication should prompt discontinuation of the medication and reevaluation.

Of note, a full manic episode that emerges during antidepressant treatment (e.g., medication and/or electroconvulsive therapy) and persists beyond the physiological effects of the treatment is diagnosed as bipolar I; a full hypomanic episode that emerges during antidepressant treatment and persists beyond the physiological effects of the treatment is diagnosed as bipolar II only if preceded by a major depressive episode (APA, 2013).

Pause and Reflect

1. *What symptoms of bipolar disorder do you find most intimidating? How might you address these symptoms in the clinical setting?*
2. *What are the distinguishing features among bipolar I disorders, bipolar II disorder, and cyclothymic disorder?*

Prevalence and Life Span Considerations

As with depression, there are important prevalence and life span considerations related to caring for clients with bipolar disorder.

Prevalence

The lifetime prevalence of bipolar disorder is estimated to be around 3.9%, with 82.9% of these individuals are classified as having severe disease impairing quality of life and overall functioning in some way (NIMH, 2011). Bipolar disorder has been deemed the most expensive behavioral health care diagnosis, costing more than twice as much as unipolar depression per affected individual (CDC, 2011). The cost in terms of years lost to disability, family burden, and impaired health-related quality of life is immeasurable, with fewer than 40% of bipolar individuals maintaining their premorbid levels of functioning (Judd et al., 2002).

Bipolar disorder generally starts in late adolescence or early adulthood, with the average age of onset at 25 years, but many individuals with BD are frequently misdiagnosed or underdiagnosed. This is especially true for individuals with bipolar II disorder and is likely due to the wide variability in clinical presentation for these individuals. Recurrent, brief, episodes of hypomania may occur that elude clinical evaluation, as individuals are not likely to seek treatment or assistance during these times. In addition, individuals with BD may present with psychiatric co-morbidities (for instance, anxiety disorders, substance abuse/use disorders, personality disorders) whose symptoms may overlap with bipolar symptoms, as well as significant psychosocial disruption (such as marital and family discord, legal involvement, gambling) that confounds or distracts from accurate diagnosis and treatment.

Delayed identification and diagnosis of BD is concerning: Evidence suggests that early diagnosis and treatment are critical in preventing illness progression, limiting disability, and preventing social and vocational dysfunction often associated with the illness. Individuals with BD frequently go untreated, with only 48.8% of those with the disorder being treated. Of those individuals, only 18.8% receive minimally adequate treatment (NIMH, 2011).

Co-Morbidities

Patients with bipolar disorder are characterized by high frequencies of co-morbid psychiatric disorders—particularly substance abuse, anxiety, impulse control disorders, eating disorders, attention deficit hyperactivity disorders, and personality disorders (Pompili et al., 2009). These co-morbid psychiatric illnesses frequently delay diagnosis, complicate treatment, and add to the psychosocial burden associated with bipolar disorder. It may be this additional burden that is associated with the relative high risk for suicide in patients with bipolar disorder.

Of special concern is the high association of co-morbid medical illness and increased risk of premature death for individuals with BD.

In addition to the well-recognized increased risk for death associated with unnatural causes such as suicide, homicide, and accident (Angst, Stassen, & Clayton, 2002), a comprehensive review of 17 studies involving more than 331,000 patients demonstrated an increased risk of death from heart disease, respiratory illness, stroke, and diabetes (Roshanaei-Moghaddam & Katon, 2009). Among all causes of death, cardiovascular disease accounted for the majority of premature deaths. Research into the causes of excessive mortality in this population may be associated with risky health behaviors such as unhealthy diet and obesity, physical inactivity, and smoking, and social factors such as homelessness, social isolation, substance abuse, and poor or inadequate access to general health care. Biological explanations, such as stress-related effects on the immune system and HPA axis with resultant increase in cortisol levels, increased activity of the sympathetic nervous system, and the metabolic effects associated with the medications used to treat the illness have also been described (Roshanaei-Moghaddam & Katon, 2009). The widespread use of second-generation antipsychotic medication, with resultant weight gain, has greatly increased the risk and incidence of metabolic syndrome, thereby increasing the overall risk for DM, dyslipidemia, heart disease, and stroke in this population. These findings highlight the need for aggressive co-management of medical disorders and side effects and the need for collaborative health service models that integrate primary care and primary prevention strategies into community mental health services. Unfortunately, there are significant health care disparities for individuals with severe mental illness. Data indicate that they receive lower-quality health care, lack basic primary care, and are regularly not at goal for the management of medical co-morbidities such DM, hypertension, and dyslipidemia (Druss et al., 2002).

Children and Adolescents

Controversy exists regarding the prevalence and diagnostic criteria for BD disorders in pediatric populations. The lifetime prevalence estimates for pediatric bipolar disorder (PBD) range from 1% to 1.6%, but the actual rates are estimated to be much higher due to misdiagnosis and the high incidence of co-morbidities such as ADHD, behavioral and anxiety disorders, and depression that delay recognition and confound diagnosis (McClellan, Kowatch, & Findling, 2007). *Pediatric bipolar disorder differs from adult BD in that it is associated with longer episodes, a higher incidence of mixed episodes and rapid cycling, and prominent irritability* (Carbray & McGuinness, 2009). Children with BD are at increased risk for academic failure, family conflict, substance abuse, accident and injury, unprotected sexual activity, chronic low self-esteem, and suicide and, as such, pose significant treatment challenges. In addition to pharmacotherapy, psychosocial interventions that include family-based psychotherapies are essential for optimal outcomes. The goals of psychotherapeutic interventions include ameliorating mood symptoms, reducing morbidity and mortality, improving family relationships and school functioning, and fostering normal growth and development.

Specialized assessment tools are available to assist with the screening and diagnosis of PBD and are both clinician and parent rated. Some examples include the Young Mania Rating Scale (YMRS), the K-SADS Mania Rating Scale (K-SADS-MRS), and the Child Mania Rating Scale (CMRS). The American Academy of Child and Adolescent Psychiatry has published practice parameters on the assessment and treatment of bipolar disorder in children and adolescent (McClellan, Kowatch, & Findling, 2007). For more information on the care of children and adolescents with mental illness, see Chapter 30.

Women

Even though the incidence and presentation of BD are comparable in men and women, women present unique challenges to its management. Studies have demonstrated that women with BD are more likely to experience rapid cycling, mixed mania, and antidepressant-induced manias compared with men with BD (Marangell, 2008). The normal mood variability seen throughout the menstrual cycle and at times of hormonal change (pregnancy, postpartum, and in menopause), the use of oral contraceptives, and the higher incidence of endocrine disorders (such as thyroid disorders and polycystic ovary syndrome) in women may account for this observation. The peripartum period is a time of particular high risk for mood disturbance for women with BD, with as many as 40% to 67% of women reporting postpartum depression or mania (Freeman et al., 2002). Women with bipolar disorder have a 100-fold higher risk than women without a psychiatric illness history of experiencing postpartum psychosis (Freeman et al., 2002).

Pharmacologic management of BD in women is a challenge, and it can be complicated by hormonal changes, interactions with methods of birth control such as oral contraceptives (OCs), and the desire for pregnancy and breastfeeding. The use of lithium and other mood stabilizers, with their inherent tendency toward weight gain, increases the risk for polycystic ovary and metabolic syndromes. The use of lithium is associated with a greater incidence of hypothyroidism in women as compared to men. The efficacy of many OCs is diminished with the use of certain mood stabilizers, such as carbamazepine and oxcarbazepine, thus necessitating the use of either a barrier method for birth control or an increase in the dose of OCs. The peripartum pharmacologic treatment of BD poses several risks to the woman, her child, and the family. As might be expected, there are no randomized controlled studies that direct care for the treatment of acute BD during pregnancy or postpartum. As a result, it is important that women discuss the timing of a pregnancy with their health care provider, and that clinicians routinely inquire whether a pregnancy is being planned within the next 12 months. Because medications used for the management of BD are teratogenic (causing fetal malformation), prenatal counseling should include a discussion about risks of fetal harm when medication is taken during pregnancy and risks of uncontrolled bipolar symptoms should the mother discontinue medications. Developing a plan to manage symptoms should the woman choose to stop medications is optimal care. Management of sleep disturbances during pregnancy is particularly critical, as sleep disturbance may exacerbate a mood episode (Marangell, 2008).

There are no screening instruments designed specifically for use before or after delivery in women with bipolar disorder. Commonly used screening instruments, such as the Edinburgh Postnatal Depression Scale-23 and the Postpartum Depression Screening Scale-24, have not been validated in women with BD.

Older Adults

Very little is known about BD in older adults. The lack of research in the area creates large gaps in our understanding of the disorder and optimal treatment strategies. Even though BD is much more likely to present in late adolescence or early adulthood, late-onset BD is not unheard of because approximately 10% to 15% experience onset of illness after age 55 (Depp & Jest, 2004). Late-onset illness is much more likely to be associated with structural or metabolic causes. When mania presents as the first affective episode in older adults, as many as 70% have been found to have an underlying neurologic disorder (Luggen, 2005). Thus, the prognosis for late-onset BD is generally poor and is associated with significant morbidity and mortality.

Older adults are at increased risk of adverse medication events. Limited data exist regarding which medications are safest and most effective and which psychosocial interventions provide the greatest benefit. Lithium continues to be the mainstay of treatment but demands aggressive monitoring of cardiovascular, renal, and endocrine function. Medical co-morbidities frequently complicate the diagnosis and management of BD in older adults; careful physical and neurologic examination is indicated. Involvement of family members and significant others in the treatment of older adults has demonstrated efficacy in improving adherence and decreasing the frequency of mood events (Sorrell, 2011).

Pause and Reflect

1. *Why do you think establishing a family pedigree is essential in working with children and adolescents experiencing issues with attention?*
2. *What are some differences nurses should consider when working with women who have bipolar disorder?*

Collaborative Care

Depression and BD are chronic conditions that require management through all stages of the disease (initial onset/relapse, recovery, and rehabilitation). They necessitate a combination of approaches and the expertise of multiple disciplines to meet the recovery needs of patients and their families. Treatments for mood disorders include pharmacotherapy; psychotherapy; neuromodulation therapies, such as electroconvulsive therapy (ECT); and complementary and alternative medical (CAM) therapies, such as massage and acupuncture. Current treatment strategies may employ several modalities together (for example, pharmacotherapy and psychotherapy) to obtain remission and full treatment response. The effectiveness of a multidisciplinary–multimodal treatment approach gives further credence to the heterogeneity and complexities of mood disorders.

In the past, a 50% reduction in depressive symptoms as measured by a clinical evaluation tool measure such as the Hamilton Depression (HAM–D) scale, was deemed an acceptable treatment goal. That being said, the results of the Sequenced Treatment Alternatives to Relieve Depression (STAR*D) study suggested that only about 50% of patients with MDD achieved clinical response, and only one-third achieved remission of their depressive episode following a course of an antidepressant (Trivedi et al., 2006). *The current state of the science is to work toward full remission and wellness.* Remission is viewed as the complete resolution of signs and symptoms of depression. Failure to achieve and sustain full symptomatic relief of depressive symptoms is associated with an increased risk of relapse, more chronic and severe symptoms, progressive functional decline, and increased risk of medical co-morbidities (Trivedi et al., 2006). In addition, several studies have demonstrated that recurrent depressive episodes lead to possible suppression of brain neurogenesis, neuronal atrophy, cell death, hippocampal dysfunction, and

changes visible on magnetic resonance imaging. These changes have been linked to decline in cognitive, executive, and emotional function (Frodl et al., 2008). A 30-year study found that individuals with three or more hospitalizations for a depressive episode had a greater incidence of developing dementia compared with those who had only one or two hospitalizations for depression (Kessing & Andersen, 2004).

Today, nurses and other clinicians strive to go "beyond remission," with the goals of treatment to assist patients to resume premorbid levels of functioning and optimizing quality of life. Complete remission is possible only with the coordinated efforts of patients, families, and providers using a variety of approaches that support all the domains of wellness. Patients who achieve full wellness have a greater likelihood of staying well (Fava, Ruini, & Belaise, 2007).

This notion of treating to remission and optimal wellness extends to BD as well. Many patients with BD experience a suboptimal response to treatment. As a result, they experience frequent impairing mood symptoms, persistent inter-episode symptoms such as insomnia and cognitive impairment, and significant disruption in vocational and psychosocial functioning. Several studies have shown that, on average, individuals with BD suffer from manic, depressive, hypomanic, or mixed symptoms for about half the time despite treatment, and many individuals suffer with a high degree of residual illness-related morbidities (Kupka et al., 2007). Collaborative care models consisting of the patient, family members, the psychiatrist, and a community-based psychiatric nurse or case worker have been shown to be cost effective as well as effective in reducing frequency and severity of manic episodes, improving social and vocational functioning, and improving quality of life in individuals with BD (Bauer et al., 2006a; Bauer et al., 2006b; Simon et al., 2005; Simon et al., 2006). These models are aimed at reducing symptom burden, promoting treatment adherence and self-management, diminishing or eliminating social and vocational disruption, preventing relapse, and providing support to the caregivers.

Nurses play key roles in these collaborative care teams, often functioning as the coordinator or clinical manager. By virtue of their expertise in providing holistic care, nurses are an obvious choice as care coordinators for patients with mood disorders. The American Psychiatric Association's clinical practice guidelines for the treatment of individuals with BD (APA, 2002) state that the major goals of treatment are to maintain adherence with therapy and monitor the patient's psychiatric status, establish and maintain a therapeutic alliance, promote regular patterns of activity and sleep, anticipate stressors, and minimize functional impairment. These goals are consistent with nursing's mission and scope of practice.

Psychopharmacology

Medications used in the treatment of mood disorders include *antidepressants* (selective serotonin-reuptake inhibitors [SSRIs]), atypical antidepressants, dual-action antidepressants (dopaminergic–noradrenergic-reuptake inhibitors [DNRIs] and serotonin–norepinephrine-reuptake inhibitors [SNRIs], monoamine oxidase inhibitors [MAOIs], and tricyclic antidepressants [TCAs]), *mood stabilizers*, and *atypical antipsychotics* (see Medications Commonly Used to Treat Mood Disorders). Antianxiety medications are also used at times for those patients who are experiencing significant anxiety and insomnia symptoms associated with their mood symptoms. Anxiolytics also may be used early in the treatment of mood disorders to decrease possible side effects associated with the other classes of medications.

Key Pharmacological Considerations

box 16-3

Treatment-Induced Manic Switch Once a diagnosis of major depressive disorder has been made, the patient should be evaluated for a personal and family history of mania or hypomania. Initiation of treatment with SSRIs or SNRIs may precipitate a manic or hypomanic episode in a patient with a previously undiagnosed or unrecognized bipolar disorder. Monitor all patients newly started on antidepressants for an unexpected and rapid improvement in mood symptoms.

Antipsychotic FDA Black Box Warning New use of both first-generation and second-generation antipsychotics is associated with increased risk for death in older adult patients with dementia-related psychosis from 30 days to 180 days after initial prescription. Most of these deaths were from cardiovascular causes or pneumonia, making careful nursing assessment of cardiovascular and pulmonary status in this population important.

Antidepressant FDA Black Box Warning Antidepressants of all classes may increase the risk of suicidal thoughts and behaviors in children, adolescents, and young adults ages 18 to 24, usually within the first 2 months. Although these medications may increase risk, they also have demonstrated efficacy in improving depressive symptoms; thus, nursing considerations include careful monitoring of this population during the initial stages of treatment. Family and care providers should be advised of the need for close observation and communication with the prescriber.

Antidepressants

Although there are multiple studies that demonstrate the efficacy and even superiority of MAOIs compared with other classes of antidepressants, MAOIs are rarely used in current clinical practice because of their high side effect and toxicity profile. When combined with food and drinks that contain high levels of tyramine (such as aged cheese, wine, some beers, and organ meats), they may cause hypertensive crisis. In addition, their combination with other antidepressants of other classes and some herbal supplements and over-the-counter medications may potentiate their toxicity profile and increase the risk for serotonin syndrome (Chapter 23 Psychopharmacology). Thus, use of MAOIs is complicated by multiple drug–to–drug interactions and dietary restrictions that many individuals find difficult to follow. The most widely recognized MAOIs include isocarboxazid (Marplan), phenelzine (Nardil), and tranylcypromine (Parnate). More recently, selegiline (Eldapril), a transdermal skin patch that allows for slow continuous absorption, has become available and is associated with a lower side effect profile.

Tricyclic antidepressants (TCAs) work by blocking the presynaptic transporter proteins for the neurotransmitters norepinephrine and serotonin, thereby increasing the amount of norepinephrine and serotonin in the brain. They also block postsynaptic histamine receptors and acetylcholine receptors, mechanisms that are responsible for their high sedation and anticholinergic profiles. In addition to their clear efficacy in relieving depressive symptoms, they have significant anxiolytic and analgesic effects, making them an attractive treatment choice for individuals whose depressive symptoms consist of significant anxiety or painful symptoms. Again, their efficacy is robust, but their use is limited by significant potential for cardiotoxicity and a high anticholinergic side effect profile, as well as their risk of death if taken in overdose. Still, they are used for patients who do not show improvement with newer antidepressants and who are at low risk for side effects and suicide. The most widely recognized TCAs include imipramine (Tofranil), nortriptyline (Pamelor), desipramine (Norpramin), and amitriptyline (Elavil).

Selective serotonin-reuptake inhibitors (SSRIs) are the mainstay for the treatment of unipolar depression, based on their relative safety and overall efficacy. These medications block the function of the presynaptic transporter for serotonin reuptake, resulting in more serotonin being available in the synaptic cleft to activate postsynaptic receptors for serotonin. Increased serotonin is associated with antidepressant and antianxiety effects, but it also is responsible for the common side effects associated with this class of drugs, such as insomnia, agitation, and sexual dysfunction. Even though many individuals may report improvement in depression within several weeks of starting an SSRI, an adequate trial of at least 6 weeks is recommended to determine overall response. The most widely recognized SSRIs include fluoxetine (Prozac), paroxetine (Paxil), sertraline (Zoloft), fluvoxamine (Luvox), citalopram (Celexa), and escitalopram (Lexapro).

Atypical antidepressants also work by altering the neuronal conduction–neurotransmission cascade, but the medications in this class do not necessarily have a common mechanism of action, as is seen with the SSRIs or TCAs. For example, although the exact mechanism is unclear, trazodone (Desyrel) and nefazadone (Serzone) are believed to selectively inhibit neuronal reuptake of serotonin and act as an antagonist at several serotonin receptors subtypes ($5\text{-}HT_2$ and $5\text{-}HT_3$). As a result, they produce beneficial effects on sleep and have fewer sexual side effects than SSRIs, TCAs, or MAOIs. They are known in the literature as serotonin agonist reuptake inhibitors. Mirtazapine (Remeron), another atypical antidepressant, is known as a norepinephrine and serotonin specific agonist. It potentiates noradrenergic and serotoninergic neurotransmission and blocks serotonin $5\text{-}HT_2$ and $5\text{-}HT_3$ receptors, so it does not cause some of the common side effects of other antidepressants, such as agitation, insomnia, and sexual side effects, making it a good choice for individuals who are disturbed by these side effects from other classes of medication.

Dual-action antidepressants act by modulating two different synaptic sites. This dual action is believed to be associated with improved efficacy while limiting side effects. Medications in this family are classified as serotonin–norepinephrine-reuptake inhibitors (SNRIs) and include venlafaxine (Effexor), duloxetine (Cymbalta), and the norepinephrine–dopamine-reuptake inhibitor (NDRI) bupropion (Wellbutrin). Bupropion is currently the only NDRI available in the United States. Bupropion is unique as an antidepressant in that it selectively inhibits dopamine and norepinephrine without affecting serotonin, and has stimulant-like properties. Its effect on dopaminergic transmitters systems also makes it effective in the treatment of nicotine addiction. Venlafaxine (Effexor) and duloxetine (Cymbalta) bind to and block the reuptake transporters for norepinephrine and serotonin, making them excellent choices for individuals with painful symptoms associated with depression as well as individuals with predominantly anxious symptoms.

Mood Stabilizers

Mood stabilizers include lithium and anticonvulsants such as carbamazepine (Tegretol), valproic acid (Depakene), gabapentin (Neurontin), lamotrigine (Lamictal), and topiramate (Topamax). Mood stabilizers are the mainstay for the treatment of acute mania and for maintenance therapy in individuals with BD. These medications also have been used for some people with unipolar depression as an augmentation strategy for individuals with difficult to treat depression or those that do not respond to traditional antidepressants (Bauer et al., 2010).

Lithium continues to be the gold standard for treatment of BD, but it is used less and less in clinical practice because of its narrow therapeutic index and a high and frequently intolerable side-effect profile. Its efficacy in controlling manic symptoms and reducing the rate of reoccurrence is without question, but nonadherence with lithium therapy is high. Despite its clear efficacy and plethora of clinical research, the exact mechanism by which lithium controls mania and BD is yet undetermined. It seem to have wide-reaching biochemical and molecular effects on neurotransmitter/receptor-mediated signaling, hormonal and circadian regulation, ion transport, and gene expression, but how these mechanisms might control mania remains elusive. What does seem clear is that there is strong evidence to support neuronal damage associated with untreated BD, and lithium seems to exert its overall effect by limiting or reversing disease progression directly associated with the activation of neurotrophic effects (Machado-Vieira, Manji, & Zarate, 2009). Thus, it would seem that lithium has some type of neuroprotective properties.

The therapeutic efficacy of lithium is directly related to its level in the blood, with the therapeutic dose established by closely monitoring blood lithium levels. Lithium has a very narrow therapeutic index, meaning that the ratio between the toxic dose and the therapeutic dose of the drug is low, increasing the risk for toxicity and side effects (Box 16-4). Normal blood levels for lithium are 0.5 meq/L to 0.7 meq/L, although some guidelines allow up to 1.2 meq/L. Symptoms of clear toxicity generally are seen with levels greater than 1.5 meq/L and include ataxia, slurred speech, and muscle weakness. The individual who is suffering from lithium toxicity gives the impression of being under the influence of alcohol. Toxicity can progress rapidly, making early detection and treatment essential to prevent untoward complications, including renal failure, cardiac arrhythmias, coma, and death.

Anticonvulsants

Anticonvulsants have gained increased popularity in the treatment of BD as a result of their overall tolerability and efficacy. Once again, as a class of medication, their exact mechanism of action in controlling mania and regulating mood symptoms is unclear but is probably multimodal. The most widely postulated mechanism of action is through modulation of GABA at its pre- and postsynaptic nerve terminals. In addition to their role as anti-mania medications, anticonvulsants are used regularly for the management of multiple additional psychiatric as well as medical illnesses, including migraine, peripheral neuropathies and pain syndromes, substance abuse disorders, pathological gambling, explosive behavioral disorders in adults and children, and sleep disturbance. The term *neuromodulators* has frequently been used to describe this category of medication, owing to their wide range of use and versatility.

All the anticonvulsants are probably equally effective in the management of mania and bipolar disorder, although some individuals will respond to one agent more favorably than to another. It is not unusual to see anticonvulsants combined with lithium. This augmentation strategy can be very effective in lowering the dose of both medications, thereby decreasing the overall side effect burden and toxicity profile of each of the drugs separately. As with lithium, anticonvulsant effectiveness is most likely associated with adequate blood levels, but in clinical practice, blood levels generally do not direct treatment strategies, owing to the relatively lower side effect and toxicity profile of these medications. Of all the anticonvulsants, lamotrigine (Lamictal) is rapidly gaining popularity as an important monotherapy for its effectiveness in the treatment of rapid-cycling bipolar II disorder, prevention of relapse to mania, and reduction of recurrent bipolar depressive episodes.

Some important nursing considerations are related to specific drugs within this category. For example, carbamazepine is associated with myelosuppression (agranulocytosis, aplastic anemia, leukopenia). Individuals should report fever, chills, sore throat, and fatigue. Regular monitoring of complete blood counts is recommended. Carbamazepine may also reduce the efficacy of hormonal contraceptives; thus, alternative or additional forms of birth control may be necessary. Lamotrigine may be associated with the development of serious dermatologic reactions (Stevens-Johnson syndrome, erythema multiforme, or toxic epidermal necrolysis); the development of rash, fever, or flulike symptoms should be reported promptly to the prescriber. The incidence of rash can be reduced by slowly tapering up the dose of medication over a period of several weeks. Strict adherence to the medication regimen is recommended.

Atypical Antipsychotics

Atypical antipsychotics such as olanzapine (Zyprexa), risperidone (Risperdal), quetiapine (Seroquel), ziprasidone (Geodon), and aripiprazole (Abilify) have demonstrated efficacy against acute mania and for psychotic symptoms associated with mania and depression. They are associated with fewer extrapyramidal side effects than traditional antipsychotics, making them an attractive first choice in the early management of acute manic episodes. The exact mechanism of action of the atypical antipsychotics is unknown. They are believed to block

---

Patient and Family Education: Lithium   box 16-4

Lithium has a narrow therapeutic index and levels can quickly become toxic in the setting of dehydration. Instruct patients to avoid dehydration or marked changes in sodium intake. Typical side effects of lithium therapy include thirst, polyuria, weight gain, gastrointestinal disturbance (nausea, vomiting, diarrhea, and abdominal pain), cognitive dulling, and neurologic side effects (slight tremor, lethargy, impaired concentration, dizziness, slurred speech, ataxia, muscle weakness, and nystagmus). Patients should be instructed to have lithium levels drawn at least every 6 months during the maintenance phase of treatment and if symptoms indicating possible toxicity develop. Blood levels should be measured at trough (9 to 13 hours after the last dose). Because long-term lithium use may be associated with renal, hematologic, endocrine, and cardiac effects, routine follow-up with a primary care provider for annual thyroid (TSH) level, renal function (BUN, creatinine), electrolytes, blood count (CBC with differential), and ECG is recommended. Lithium toxicity is also related to diet. Careful monitoring to insure the same amount of sodium daily is ingested either through foods or beverages (tomato juice).

serotonin receptors (specifically $5HT_2$) in the cortex and dopamine D_2 receptors, effects that are responsible for their antipsychotic, anxiolytic, and antidepressant properties. It is not unusual to see atypical antipsychotics combined with either lithium or anticonvulsants for the management of mood symptoms. The most problematic side effects of this category of medication are sedation and weight gain. For some individuals, the weight gain can be in excess of 10 kg (22 lbs) and is the reason most often cited for nonadherence to the treatment regimen. Additional side effects include the development of diabetes, dyslipidemia, QT_c interval prolongation, sexual side effects, and cataracts. This category of medication may also lower the seizure threshold and should be used with caution in patients with known seizure disorders.

Anxiolytics

Benzodiazepines, such as alprazolam (Xanax), lorazepam (Ativan), clonazepam (Klonopin), and diazepam (Valium), are helpful in the management of co-morbid anxiety symptoms in individuals with depressive disorders and in the management of acute manic–hypomanic episodes. They are frequently used as initial management for individuals who experience increased restlessness, agitation, and insomnia when first exposed to antidepressants, especially SSRIs. However, benzodiazepines are not the mainstay of treatment for mood disorders, and because of their abuse potential their use should be limited to initial symptom management and in the management of insomnia associated with the mood disturbance. (See Chapter 13 for a full discussion of benzodiazepine use for the management of anxiety symptoms.)

Psychotherapy

More than 400 different types of psychotherapy have been described; some are more credible than others. Key psychotherapeutic approaches employed in the treatment of mood disorders include dynamic psychotherapy, cognitive–behavioral therapy, interpersonal psychotherapy, family-focused therapy, group therapy, and social rhythm therapy (Table 16-4). Multiple studies have demonstrated the efficacy of these modalities as monotherapies in terms of improved outcomes in individuals with depression and BD (Hollon & Ponniah, 2010). Current research into the mechanisms by which psychotherapeutic approaches reduce and improve mood symptoms include reducing circulating cortisol levels to normal, improving blood flow to brain structures involved with mood regulation (hippocampus and amygdala), increasing prefrontal cortex–limbic connectivity, and increasing the neurotransmitters believed to be responsible for mood regulation (Sharpley, 2010). Thus, psychotherapy is more than "just talk." Evidence suggests that it reverses the structural changes associated with mood disturbance and restores neurotransmitter balance.

Even though most clinicians would agree that some type of psychotherapeutic intervention is an integral part of the overall treatment approach for patients with mood disorders, which therapy to use continues to be the subject of much debate. The comparative effectiveness of various types of psychodynamic therapies have had limited assessment in systematic reviews, and for those reviews available, there is an inability to find a consistent difference in effectiveness across

Psychotherapy for Depressive and Bipolar Disorders   table 16-4

Modality	Description
Interpersonal psychotherapy (IPT)	IPT is a practical, highly structured, time-limited therapy with a focus on the individual's current relationships and interpersonal events (interpersonal disputes, role transitions, grief, interpersonal deficits). The aim is to improve communication, express affect appropriately, and renegotiating the roles in relationships.
Cognitive–behavioral therapy (CBT)	CBT is a structured, goal-oriented, time-limited therapy. Cognitive aspects of the treatment are designed to identify and link maladaptive attitudes and beliefs that contribute to and fuel symptoms. Negative thoughts are challenged in terms of their irrationality and restructured in such a way as to be more adaptive. An increased cognitive awareness is combined with specific behavioral interventions. Behavioral aspects of the treatment involve motivating the individual through activity scheduling and planning and using positive reinforcement of desired behavior.
Dynamic psychotherapy	Emphasizes increasing one's awareness of unconscious thoughts and emotions and developing an understanding of how historical or developmental events influence and control behaviors and feelings. The focus is on gaining greater understanding and self-awareness of one's behavior.
Family-focused therapy	Family-focused therapy evaluates how each person in a system or group functions as a whole. The assumption is that each person is part of a system and changing one person changes the function of the entire system. The focus is on improving family relationships, providing education, building better communication skills, and solving problems together.
Group therapy	Group therapy is led by a trained therapist that is delivered within groups. There is generally a common and specific focus and can include supportive psychotherapy, skills training, problem solving, and psychoeducation. Members provide support and feedback to one another to solve common problems or issues.
Social rhythm therapy	Initially developed for management of BD, social rhythm therapy stresses maintaining a regular schedule of daily activities (work, school, sleep–wake patterns, leisure activities, exercise) and stability in personal relationships. It is based on the notion that disruptions in daily routines and interpersonal relationships can cause recurrence of manic and depressive symptoms.

psychotherapy modalities. A recent systematic review of the effect of interpersonal psychotherapy and other psychodynamic therapies versus treatment as usual in patients with major depression failed to find convincing evidence to support or refute the effect of interpersonal psychotherapy or psychodynamic therapy compared with treatment as usual for patients with MDD (Jakobsen, Hansen, & Simonsen, 2011). Rather, it appears that the nature of the therapeutic alliance and the goals of therapy affect outcomes more than the type of therapy or the therapist's psychodynamic orientation (Martin, Garske, & Davis, 2000). The underlying benefit of the therapeutic alliance may be the soothing effects of receiving compassion and empathy from another individual. These effects have been associated with the release of oxytocin, a neurohormone that engenders emotions of warmth, intimacy, and personal connection with others and reduction in cortisol levels (Sharpley, 2010).

Although each type of therapy is guided by a set of principles and theories that direct the ultimate goal of behavior change, in reality most therapists are versed in many different types of treatment modalities and demonstrate "disciplined flexibility" or the ability to adjust therapeutic strategies to meet the individual needs of the person and family. In clinical practice, the type and duration of therapy depend on individual preference, symptoms and treatment needs, co-morbid psychiatric illness, cognitive ability and personal insight, therapist availability, and, unfortunately, cost.

Neuromodulation Therapies

Most therapeutic strategies used in the treatment of mood disorders are aimed at modulating the neurotransmitters, neuroendocrine hormones, and brain structures responsible for mood regulation. Neuromodulation therapies are no exception; these include ECT,

repetitive transcranial magnetic stimulation (rTMS), vagal nerve stimulation (VNS), light therapy (LT), and deep brain stimulation (DBS) (Table 16-5).

Complementary and Alternative Medicine Therapies

The use of CAM for the management of all disease states is increasing. The 2007 National Health Interview Survey (NHIS), which included a comprehensive survey of CAM use by Americans, showed that approximately 38% of adults use CAM (National Center for Complementary and Alternative Medicine, 2011). Many individuals report using CAM to prevent and treat disease, to restore immune function and spiritual balance, to increase energy and bolster feelings of well-being, and for residual symptom management. There is some evidence to suggest that individuals with mood disorders may be more frequent users of CAM therapies because of the high symptom burden associated with the disorders (Kessler et al., 2001). For many people, the combination of a complementary therapy such as acupuncture, massage, spiritual support, dietary modifications, or megavitamin therapy serves to augment their treatment and provide greater control of the recovery process. Although multiple studies demonstrate the widespread use of CAM therapies for the management of symptoms in individuals with mood disorders (Hsu et al., 2009; Wu, et al., 2007), there is lack of sound scientific evidence surround the quality, safety, and efficacy of many CAM therapies (Chapter 22). The efficacy of CAM largely depends on the user's subjective experience and beliefs in the therapy. Kessler et al. (2001) identified almost 24 different types of CAM therapies used by patients with anxiety and depressive disorders. It is important for nurses to familiarize themselves with these therapies, as many may

Overview of Neuromodulation Therapies	table 16-5

Modality	Biological Basis for Response
Electroconvulsive therapy (ECT)	Although the exact mechanism is unclear, ECT is believed to exert its effect though alteration/modulation of neurotransmitter and hormonal systems responsible for mood and cognition. Given as unilateral or bilateral electrical stimulation under general anesthesia for a total of 6 to12 treatments. Commonly used for individuals with severe mood disorders, including severe mania, for both acute treatment and maintenance treatment.
Repetitive transcranial magnetic stimulation (rTMS)	rTMS uses focused magnet pulses to induce electric currents leading to neuronal depolarization and manipulation of brain structures and neurotransmitters believed to be involved in mood regulation. Approved for treatment of unipolar depression with one failed antidepressant treatment in the current episode.
Vagal nerve stimulation (VNS)	VNS is the surgical implantation of a pulse generator in the chest that delivers intermittent electrical signals to the brain via an electrode wrapped around the left vagus nerve. VNS is thought to alter parasympathetic nervous system activity by affecting acetylcholine receptor function. Commonly used as a long-term maintenance treatment to sustain remission, rather than as an initial treatment for depression.
Light therapy (LT)	LT involves regular daily exposure to ultraviolet-filtered visible light during times of low light exposure. This involves at least 5000 lux-hours per day of exposure, which translates into about 30 minutes per day of light exposure. The therapeutic effect of light is mediated by the eyes and retina, not the skin. Therapy is delivered first thing in the morning for maximal effect. Used in the treatment of seasonal affective disorder (SAD).
Deep brain stimulation (DBS)	DBS uses surgically implanted electrodes into subcortical regions to deliver electrical signals to targeted brain regions. Under clinical investigation for the treatment of severe treatment retfractory depression.

not work synergistically with traditional therapies and, indeed, may cause an exacerbation of symptoms or increase possible toxic effects. Most CAM therapies are self-administered without any professional supervision or guidance, and many individuals do not disclose their use of CAM therapies to providers for fear of disapproval or dismissal (Shelley et al., 2009). This highlights the importance of open dialogue that demonstrates a nonjudgmental acceptance of an individual's choices surrounding CAM and invites communication that allows the nurse to provide direction and education regarding the appropriate application of these therapies. Shelley et al. (2009) demonstrated that patients do not necessarily expect providers to be experts in the CAM they are using. They do, however, want providers to demonstrate openness to these therapies and candor regarding lack of knowledge if that applies.

Although the evidence on CAM is limited, a review of randomized controlled trials of commonly used CAM treatments for major depressive disorder—such as omega-3 fatty acids, St. John's wort, folate, S-adenosyl-ʟ-methionine (SAMe), acupuncture, light therapy, exercise, and mindfulness therapies—showed promising results (Freeman et al., 2010). Based on these recommendations, nurses can feel confident in providing patients with information regarding

these therapies to augment their mood symptoms (see Evidence-Based Practice: Using Omega-3 Fatty Acids: Helping Patients Decide). These researchers point out, however, that none of these therapies is approved as monotherapy for mood disorders, and the greatest risk of pursuing a CAM therapy is the possible delay of well-established therapies. Nurses, therefore, play a key role in assisting patients to integrate CAM into their current treatment regimens and in providing education and guidance regarding the efficacy of these therapies.

Pause and Reflect

1. *For patients with bipolar disorder, what are some of the consequences of inadequate or ineffective treatment?*
2. *How can reducing symptom burden help patients find hope for recovery? How can it help their families?*
3. *What role can antidepressants play in the treatment of patients with mood disorders?*
4. *What are the challenges in using lithium as a treatment for mood disorders?*
5. *What nonpharmacologic therapies exist for the treatment of mood disorders?*

Using Omega-3 Fatty Acids: Helping Patients Decide   evidence-based practice

Clinical Question
Are omega-3 fatty acids helpful in regulating mood symptoms or in the treatment of mood disorders?

Evidence
Omega-3 fatty acids are essential polyunsaturated fatty acids with widely established cardiovascular health benefits. They decrease the risk for arrhythmias and thrombosis, decrease triglycerides, improve endothelial function, and may lower blood pressure. These important nutrients are not manufactured in the body and must come from food sources such as seafood, flaxseed, and some eggs. Most of the health benefits derived from omega-3 fatty acids are specifically associated with eicosapentaenoic acid (EPA) and docosahexaenoic acid (DHA). Because the typical American diet is deficient in these essential nutrients, the American Heart Association recommends that adults eat fish at least twice per week and that individuals with coronary heart disease consume at least 1 gram of omega-3 daily; those with hypertriglyceridemia should have at least 2 grams daily.

Recently, several studies have indicated that these essential fats may play a role in mood regulation and that supplementation for individuals with bipolar disorder and depressive disorders may be a complement to standard care. The exact mechanism of action is unclear, but omega-3 may prove to have a role in neuronal protection and increased serotonergic and dopaminergic neurotransmission, as well as decreasing pro-inflammatory markers associated with depression. It is possible that it promotes mood stabilization by exerting an inhibitory effect on the cell-signaling pathway, a mechanism of action similar to commonly used mood stabilizers such as lithium and valproate (Turnbull, Cullen-Drill, & Smaldone, 2008).

Although studies have varied considerably in terms of specific omega-3 fatty acids used, duration of study, dose, and use of omega-3 as adjunctive or monotherapy, several meta-analyses (Turnbull, Cullen-Drill, & Smaldone, 2008; Lin & Su, 2007; Parker et al., 2006) have demonstrated the benefit of omega-3 over placebo in reducing symptom burden, decreasing subjective measures of

depression, and promoting greater time to relapse of depression or mania/hypomania. Of the studies that have demonstrated a positive effect, most have either used EPA or a combination of EPA and DHA with EPA at a higher dose (Freeman, 2009). However, appropriate dosage levels and ratios of EPA to DHA have yet to be established and are the focus of current research.

Implications for Nursing Practice
Because there are clear general health benefits, modest efficacy data, and low side effect profile associated with the use of omega-3 fatty acids, they are a reasonable augmentation strategy for individuals with mood disorders. In addition, it is widely recognized that individuals with mood disorders are at increased risk for metabolic and cardiovascular consequences associated with their psychiatric disorder, commonly used psychotropic medications, and maladaptive health risk behaviors (poor diet, obesity, sedentary lifestyle, and smoking), making use of omega-3 a complementary health strategy on several levels. The American Psychiatric Association recommends that those with mood disorders, impulse control, or psychotic disorders consume at least 1 gram/day of EPA and DHA; 1 to 3 grams/day appears to be a promising dose for the adjunctive treatment of most mood disorders (Freeman et al., 2010).

Critical Thinking Questions
1. Based on the evidence, would you feel comfortable recommending omega-3 fatty acids as an adjunct to treatment for individuals with mood disorders? Why or why not?
2. What information would you provide to a patient who asks if he could stop his prescription medication and use omega-3 as his only treatment?
3. What side effects (if any) are associated with the use of omega-3 fatty acids?
4. As most supplements are not required to meet standard manufacturing and dosing guidelines, what advice should you give your patients who are using nutraceuticals?

Nursing Management

Nursing considerations of patients with depressive or bipolar disorders focus on safety, reducing symptom burden, and assisting the patient in returning to normal functioning. As with any patient situation, thorough assessment is needed to ensure the plan of care is based on accurate information. Patients with depressive and bipolar disorders often experience prolonged periods of despair. Nursing interventions that promote hope and help patients believe that they can return to normal functioning are essential.

Assessment

All nurses need to be versed in the evaluation and assessment of mood disorders, regardless of practice environment. The U.S. Preventive Services Task Force (2009) recommends screening children, adolescents, and adults for depression in primary care practice. A variety of standardized, easy-to-use, empirically validated assessment tools are available within the public domain and can be used with minimal burden to the patient and clinician (Table 16-6). Many of these tools also are effective measures of clinical improvement and can be used to monitor, modify, and document treatment. Nurses should familiarize themselves with several of these tools and integrate them into the evaluation and treatment of individuals with mood symptoms as part of a strategy to implement measurement-based care (MBC). MBC is enhanced precision and consistency in disease assessment, tracking, and treatment

to achieve optimal outcomes through the use of evidence-based practice and standardized measures (Harding et al., 2011). The use of standardized measures in clinical practice serves to inform the treatment plan, improves communication between providers, and allows for personalized treatment. Once symptoms of depression or other mood disturbance have been identified, a complete evaluation within all the domains of health should be undertaken.

Observation and Physical Assessment

Assessment of patients with depression and bipolar disorders begins with observation. It is through skilled observation that the nurse gains insight into the patient's difficulties and suffering. Observation of the patient's demeanor, facial expressions, body language, behaviors, and communication patterns provides important information that assists the nurse in formulating the nursing diagnosis and plan of care. The nurse should consider the following critical elements in the assessment of patients with depression and bipolar disorders:

Biological Domain

- *Vital signs:* Obtain a complete set of vital signs, including orthostatic vital signs in older adults and those complaining of light-headedness associated with medication.

- *Appearance:* Observe general appearance for hygiene, dress, eye contact, demeanor, overall level of health, and nutrition.

Vijay Recovery Phase

critical thinking

Vijay is admitted to the psychiatric unit in a highly manic state. He is loud and disruptive during the initial intake and is overtly sexual with the nurse, Mary. He is taken to a quiet area, where he is given the choice between taking medication either in injection form or by mouth. After some negotiation, he agrees to take the medication by mouth. He is placed on a one-to-one observation due to his agitation and impulsivity. Labs are drawn to assess for metabolic disturbances and the possibility of substance use; his labs are within normal limits and his toxicology screen is negative. Prior to this hospitalization he was prescribed lithium, but his lithium level on admission was 0.0 meq/L, indicating that he has not been taking his medication as prescribed. He is restarted on lithium (Carbonate) and olanzapine (Zyprexa). He has a difficult few days on the unit, but after 72 hours there is a notable improvement in his thinking and level of agitation. He sleeps for the first time in 3 days and sits down to eat his meals.

Within 1 week of hospitalization, Vijay has improved significantly. His delusions have resolved and he reports being "embarrassed" by his behavior toward Mary. Mary learns that Vijay is quite a talented musician and is working toward a degree in music education. Mary is surprised by how "normal" he actually is. Vijay is quite knowledgeable about BD, and Mary is impressed with his overall understanding, as well as his appreciation for the need for close monitoring and medication adherence. She does not challenge the contradictions in his behavior at this point but makes a note to discuss this with him at some time prior to his discharge. She finds it hard to rectify the incongruence of his current presentation with the young man she met only 1 week earlier and plans to review this with her mentor during their weekly supervision sessions.

Mary has met with Vijay several times during his hospitalization. During these meetings, he frequently talks about how he is a disappointment to his family. Mary senses that there are cultural issues at play that she does not quite understand, and she does some research on the Internet. She learns that in India, disability of any type is viewed as a "tragedy," with a "better dead than disabled" approach. Cultural beliefs about disability include the notion that it is not possible for disabled people to be happy or enjoy a good quality of life. She also learns that people from India tend to accept their own disability as something that has resulted from their past karma and thus show low motivation to overcome the limitation (Gupta & Singhal, 2004). She also learns that social standing is highly valued in Indian communities and illness is frequently associated with loss of status and respect in society. Of special concern for many young Indians is the worry that psychological illness will make them undesirable marriage candidates (Weiss et al., 2001). She wonders whether there are cultural implications associated with Vijay's lack of adherence to his treatment plan and decides to explore this with him further.

APPLICATION

1. How should the nurse respond to Vijay's apology for his manic behavior? How can the nurse use this moment to help the patient to gain insight into his illness?

2. Are you surprised by how rapidly Vijay has responded to treatment? In what ways does this rapid response give credibility to the biological models that explain BD?

3. As Vijay improves, what important teaching points should the nurse stress with regard to recovery and rehabilitation?

4. What family interventions might be appropriate at this time?

Commonly Used Assessment Scales

table 16-6

Scale	Screening Information
PHQ-9 Patient Health Questionnaire-9	Self-rated scale; 9 items. Easy to use and complete in less than 3 minutes.
QIDS$_{16}$-CR Quick Inventory of Depressive Symptomatology—Clinician Rated	Clinician-rated scale; 16 items. Easy to administer and complete in 5–10 minutes.
QIDS$_{16}$-SR Quick Inventory of Depressive Symptomatology—Self- Rated	Self-rated scale; 16 items. Easy to complete in less than 5–10 minutes.
MADRS Montgomery-Asberg Depression Rating Scale	Clinician-rated scale; 10 items. Easy to administer and complete in 10–15 minutes.
IDS$_{30}$-C Inventory of Depressive Symptoms (available in multiple languages)	Clinician-rated scale; 30 items. More difficult to administer and complete in 15–20 minutes.
IDS$_{30}$-SR Inventory of Depressive Symptomatology—Self Report	Self-rated scale; 30 items. More difficulty to complete in 10–15 minutes.
HAM–D 21 Hamilton Rating Scale for Depression (21-item version)	Clinician-rated scale; the HAM-D has several versions, including 17-, 21-, 24-, 28-, and 31-item versions. The 21-item version is most often used in clinical practice. More difficulty to administer and complete in 15–20 minutes.
BDI-21 Beck Depression Inventory (13- and 21-item versions)	Self-rated scale; the BDI has several versions, including a 13- and 21-item versions. The 21-item version is most often used in clinical practice. Easy to use and complete in 5–10 minutes.
Zung Depression Rating Scale	Self-rated scale; 20 items. Easy to use and complete in less than 5 minutes.
CES-D Center for Epidemiologic Studies Depression Scale	Self-rated scale; 20 items. Easy to use and complete in less than 5 minutes.
YMRS Young Manic Rating Scale	Clinician-rated scale; 11 items. Easy to administer and complete in 5–10 minutes.
BMRS Bech-Rafaelsen Mania Rating Scale	Clinician-rated scale; 11 items. Easy to administer and complete in 5–10 minutes.
CARS–M Clinician Administered Rating Scale—Mania	Clinician-rated scale; 15 items. Easy to administer and complete in 10–15 minutes.
ASRM Altman Self-Rating Mania Scale	Self-rated scale; 5 items. Easy to complete in 3–5 minutes.
MDQ Mood Disorders Questionnaire	Self-rated scale to screen for prior manic or hypomanic episodes. Three sections with total of 16 questions. Easy to complete in 5–10 minutes.

- *Activity:* Observe and document activity level, noting psychomotor symptoms of agitation or retardation, anxiety symptoms, and unusual behaviors. Assess for low energy and fatigability in individuals with depression and excessive energy in those individuals with mania or hypomania.

- *Nutrition:* Perform a 24-hour dietary recall, including fluid intake. Obtain a baseline weight. Monitor weight in individuals on SSRIs, SNRIs, and mood stabilizers.

- *Sleep:* Assess sleep patterns, including total sleep time and difficulties with sleep initiation, sleep maintenance, or early morning awakenings. Assess for diurnal variation in activity and mood symptoms.

- *Sexual function:* Inquire about change in libido and menstrual irregularity. Inquire specifically about the occurrence of sexual side effects associated with medication use.

- *Elimination:* Assess bowel and bladder patterns; assess for constipation and urinary retention in elderly individuals on antidepressants.

- *Pain:* Inquire about pain and pain syndromes—in particular, cardiac, gastric, genitourinary, and musculoskeletal disorders. Document level of pain, including measures for pain relief.

Psychological Domain

- *Mood symptoms:* Assess for depression, euphoria, agitation, sadness, and irritability. Use standardized assessment tools to determine severity and monitor treatment response.

- *Affect:* Observe for constricted, tearful, labile, flat, shallow, blunted, hostile, angry, irritable, expansive, or inappropriate affect. Note any incongruence between mood and affect.

- *Communication patterns:* Observe for little or no spontaneous speech, monosyllabic responses, long pauses, and soft or low tone speech in individuals with depression and loud, verbose, pressured, dramatic, exaggerated speech in individuals with mania or hypomania.
- *Thought content:* Note obsessive rumination, pervasive feelings of hopelessness, guilt, worthlessness, somatic preoccupation, decreased concentration and indecisiveness, complaints of memory impairment, disorientation, concrete thinking, poverty of thought, and mood-congruent hallucinations and delusions in individuals with depression. Assess for elevated self-esteem and grandiosity, delusions, inflated self-worth, paranoia, flight of ideas, racing thoughts, circumstantiality, and tangentially in those with mania or hypomania.
- *Insight and judgment:* Assess for impairment in insight and judgment, erratic and disinhibited behavior (such as gambling, excessive spending, impulsive travel, hypersexuality), low frustration tolerance, and difficulty managing anger.

Patient Interview

The patient interview provides an opportunity for the nurse to assess the following:

- History of medical and psychiatric illness; date and results of last physical examination.
- Psychiatric status of each first-degree relative.
- Medications the patient is taking, including over-the-counter medications, herbal remedies, and dietary supplements. Inquire directly about adherence to the medication regimen and barriers to adherence, such as medication cost or side effects.

This is also the opportunity to assess the patient's perception of functioning within the psychological, sociological, cultural, and spiritual domains. Assessment of the psychological domain provides information regarding the patient's mood, affect, thought processes, insight and judgment, and communication patterns. It is also within this domain that the nurse inquires and gains insight into the personal conflicts, troubles, and distress that are responsible for the individual's suffering and formulates assessments about the individual's coping and cognitive behavioral style. As part of the assessment, the nurse inquires about the following:

- Issues that are troubling the patient and family. What problem is the patient currently experiencing that contributes to or exacerbates the mood symptoms? What life events may have precipitated this mood episode? A simple open-ended statement such as "Tell me what is troubling you the most right now" can be effective in helping the patient to articulate concerns.
- Patterns of coping and cognitive style. Does the patient describe helplessness or hopelessness? Does the patient feel that symptoms or troubles are out of his or her control? Does the patient believe that others are responsible for his or her problems or symptoms? How does the patient feel about himself or herself?
- The home environment, including family members and their health status and the patient's safety at home (for instance, screen both genders for interpersonal violence).
- Financial status, including job security and satisfaction and health insurance. What resources does the patient need to meet recovery needs?
- Caregiver strain and burnout.
- Substance use.
- Cultural and spiritual values, beliefs, and practices.

Cultural Context

As previously discussed, culture exerts powerful influences on the expression of disease, especially mental illness. It is essential for nurses to understand these culture influences, but it also is important to be cognizant of ascribing specific behaviors to all individuals of certain cultures, a process known as *stereotyping*. Stereotyping frequently leads to inaccurate assessment. Although it is not possible (or necessary) for the nurse to be an expert with regard to understanding all cultures, the sensitive cultural assessment begins with an appreciation for the uniqueness of each individual and a desire to be open and learn as much as possible. In clinical practice, the nurse will frequently be confronted with cultural issues that will affect care.

Respectfully asking permission to ask questions regarding cultural practices, values, and expectations for health care is generally met with appreciation (Box 16-5). The nurse should consider the following

---

Key Cultural Implications of Mood Disorders   box 16-5

Cultural attitudes and values affect acceptance and adherence to treatment and pharmacologic interventions. Newly arrived immigrants and refugees may be at increased risk for a depressive or bipolar disorder due to social isolation, language barriers, poverty, underemployment, and trauma in their countries of origin.

- There may be a reluctance to disclose emotional problems or mood symptoms outside the family.
- Misdiagnosis and underdiagnosis are common owing to provider–patient language barriers and lack of cultural competence in mental health and primary care providers.
- Lack of culturally responsive treatment options is common.
- Fear of stigmatization or bringing shame to the family are barriers to help-seeking behaviors.

- Many immigrants are highly educated yet underemployed, contributing to decreased self-esteem and depression.
- Financial burdens associated with the cost of care (counseling, medications) complicate care.
- Ethnic differences in drug response related to variability in the rate of biotransformation of medication (pharmacogenetics) may affect drug choice.
- Use of home remedies or complementary therapies is common.
- Consider community resources and religious organizations that engender a sense of support and belonging.

critical elements in the assessment of patients from other cultures, especially patients born in other countries (Kirmayer et al., 2011):

- Adverse experience before resettlement/relocation (trauma, torture, exposure to violence, political involvement)
- Economic, educational, and occupational status in country of origin, including the loss of social status through unemployment or underemployment
- Disruption of social support, roles, and network; separation from family of origin; uncertainty about immigration status; exposure to racism and discrimination
- Difficulties in language proficiency and acculturation
- Taboo subjects, such as sexuality or sexual abuse; fear of disclosure
- Distrust of care providers; use of alternative health care providers

Diagnosis and Planning

The nursing diagnoses for mood disorders are unique to the specific patient; the nurse identifies specific problems and care needs for the individual patient and family and develops plans of care in accordance with patient and family goals and expectations.

Many nursing diagnoses may be applicable to the patient suffering from a mood disorder, including the following:

- Coping, Ineffective
- Self-care Deficit
- Sleep Pattern, Disturbed

- Powerlessness
- Risk for suicide
- Fatigue
- Insomnia

(NANDA-I © 2014)

Nursing care is planned within each of the domains of wellness and is based on symptom management and the relief of biological, psychological, sociological, cultural, and spiritual suffering (see the Nursing Care Plan).

Implementation

Full recovery within each of the domains is possible and is the ultimate goal of care. Recovery is an elusive term but "includes the achievement of personal goals, while having a sense of purpose and hope" (Bond & Campbell, 2008, p. 35). Recovery is a dynamic, nonlinear process that requires active participation of the individual and his or her support systems. There are many pathways to healing and wholeness. The nurse works with individuals to fully engage them in recovery, motivates them to achieve mutually agreed-upon goals, and provides ongoing assessment and support to assist in the recovery process. The nurse functions as a guide in the journey toward recovery, allowing the individual to set the agenda and direct the process. Although ensuring safety and achieving a reduction in symptoms are critical, additional recovery outcomes toward which the nurse and patient work include improvement in social and role functioning,

---

Vijay—A Patient with Bipolar Disorder — NURSING CARE PLAN

Nursing Diagnosis: Alteration in thought process related to illness state (mania, nonadherence to treatment) and as evidenced by agitation and delusions

Short-Term Goals Patient will:	Interventions Nurse will:	Rationale
Begin to develop trust and rapport with the nurse by the end of his first hospital day.	Inform Vijay of the nurse's role and spend short periods of time with him.	Before Vijay can engage in treatment, he needs to be able to have a trusting relationship with those caring for him, especially because he is experiencing delusions.
Agree to develop a safety plan by the second day of hospitalization.	Express concern for Vijay's safety and ask whether he will agree to be safe and tell the nursing staff if he has any thoughts or feelings of hurting himself. Ensure that Vijay's orders for suicidal precautions and safety checks are written and explain to Vijay why he is being placed on suicidal precautions and what that entails.	Empowering the patient by engaging him in decisions related to his care and encouraging him to demonstrate responsibility for part of his care.
Take his medications as prescribed by the second day of his hospitalization.	Provide education regarding Vijay's illness and medications.	Education about bipolar disorder and medications used to treat bipolar disorder may help an individual make informed choices in relation to illness and treatment options.
Long-Term Goal Within 2 weeks, Vijay will exhibit more ordered thought processes, as evidenced by a reduction in agitation and delusions.	Encourage medication adherence and connect Vijay with community supports.	Medication adherence and community supports are critical in the treatment of psychosis.

Clinical Reasoning

1. What additional nursing diagnosis might the nurse working with Vijay want to consider?
2. How might Vijay's impulsivity make him more susceptible to a risk for injury?

increased self-care ability and independent living skills, and improvement in general health and quality of life (Mueser & Drake, 2005).

Promote Communication

The nurse uses therapeutic communication strategies that establish and reinforce the therapeutic relationship. Therapeutic communication is central to all nursing care and is accomplished not just verbally but also through caring touch, empathy, and an understanding of the basic principles of the therapeutic alliance. Thus, the nurse can be said to communicate with the hand, the heart, and the head (see the Perceptions, Thoughts, and Feelings feature later in this chapter). Basic elements of therapeutic communication include establishing trust, establishing understanding, demonstrating respect in all interactions, providing presence, and using empathy and insight (Chapter 8).

In addition, when caring for individuals with mood disorders, nurses should keep these additional principles in mind:

- Patients with depression may have delayed and slowed responses; provide for adequate time to allow patients to respond. Patients in a manic or hypomanic state may have difficulty communicating because of their racing thought processes; keep communication simple by offering limited choices.

- Do not remind patients of inappropriate behavior while they are manic or in an altered state of mental health. Do not remind patients of delusional or psychotic material when symptoms have resolved. Patients may not remember, may feel embarrassed, or may feel frightened by their behavior when in a manic or psychotic state. Reminding patients of their behavior or the things they may have said or did may increase embarrassment, guilt, shame, and fear that they are "crazy." If patients bring up the topic, provide reassurance and seek to clarify and understand the feelings associated with their behaviors. When appropriate, use the interaction as a teachable moment to address relapse prevention strategies.

- Do not challenge or criticize the patient's belief system or values, even if they are in direct conflict with your own.

Promote Physical Wellness

Providing for the physical needs and comfort of the patient and family are an important part of all nursing care regardless of care environment. Nutrition, rest and sleep, activity, and elimination are the building blocks of general health and central to good nursing care. In addition to these basic health needs, key nursing interventions within the biological domain that are essential to the recovery process in individuals with mood disorders include the following:

- Instruction and education regarding attention to a regular daily routine that focuses on promoting self-care activities. A regular daily schedule that includes a regular sleep–wake pattern, regular meals, exercise, work or school obligations, and planned leisure and relaxation activities is an essential component of recovery from mood disorders. Planned activities serve to maintain normal biological rhythms and improve general health. The nurse should encourage the patient to use a log or journal to establish and maintain a schedule.

- Assessment of medication effect, adherence, and side effects. Education for the patient and family regarding the expected effects of medications, side effects, and planned duration of treatment is essential in facilitating adherence. Prompt resolution of bothersome side effects is integral to helping patients adhere to therapy. Rating scales, such as the Frequency Intensity and Burden of Side Effects (FIBSER) scale, may help assess overall burden and function related to side effects of medication. Medication adherence questionnaires may help determine frequency of patient adherence and reasons for lack of adherence to medication regimens.

Promote Psychosocial Supports

An appreciation for the sociological factors influencing depression has important treatment implications. Incorporating psychosocial measures aimed at reducing and eliminating these stressors is a key part of the recovery process and may be influential in instilling the hope that is necessary to begin recovery. Theoretically, contextual interventions aimed at decreasing life stressors should lead to a decreased prevalence of depressive disorders (Gottlieb, Waitzkin, & Miranda, 2011). For example, a 55-year-old woman who is burdened by the care of her frail, elderly mother who has Alzheimer disease may find some symptomatic relief of her depression by obtaining a health aide to provide care for her mother and provide some much-needed respite for her. Psychosocial measures aimed at providing a fresh-start experience may provide the motivation to change behavior and improve symptoms. Gottlieb, Waitzkin, and Miranda (2011) provide an excellent systematic review that presents evidence of the favorable effects of contextual interventions on decreasing depressive symptoms, primarily in low-income, ethnically diverse communities. Key nursing interventions within the social domain include the following:

- Assessing social and community supports (financial, cultural, spiritual)

- Referral for social work services (home safety, meals on wheels, senior center, supported workshop, supported employment)

- Providing education regarding options for self-improvement and improved role functioning

- Empowering patients to embrace and incorporate change

Provide Culturally Competent Care

All nurses need to work toward developing culturally competent strategies to help patients recover from mood disorders. Key interventions to providing culturally competent care include matching ethnic groups of patients and providers, when possible; using compatible languages and professional interpreters, as necessary; and understanding the patient's view of the illness and presenting interventions in a way that fits this view. Additional interventions include reducing stigma and disparities through advocacy and involvement in community and promoting social policies that support patient and family education and support individuals with mood disorders in leading full and productive lives.

Promote Spiritual Well-Being

Spiritual well-being, though a frequently neglected domain in the recovery process, has been associated with improvement in symptoms and quality of life in individuals with mood disorders. Helping individuals to find purpose, acceptance, and a state of inner peace are challenges for nursing and may at times feel like a low priority as nurses plan the complex care their patients require. Sometimes silence and physical presence are the best tools in the nurse's arsenal to help address the spiritual needs of patients. Encouraging and facilitating the use of CAM therapies such as exercise, relaxation, massage, acupuncture, or meditation may be a more tangible path to spiritual well-being. For example, using comfort theory as its theoretical framework, a study done by Alves-Apostolo and Kolcaba (2009) researched the effect of daily guided imagery on the relief of depression, anxiety, stress, and existential suffering in a group of hospitalized depressed patients. The study revealed that the treatment group had significantly improved comfort and decreased depression, anxiety, and stress over time. Simple measures such as these are effective, easy to employ, and are generally met with interest by the patient.

Promote Recovery and Rehabilitation in the Community

Recovery takes place at home and in the community and is measured not only by a reduction or absence of psychiatric symptoms, but also by quality of life measures such as personal contentment. Asking patients whether they are content may provide important insight into a patient's psychological well-being and guide the community treatment plan. For example, a patient whose bipolar disorder is well managed on lithium therapy may describe a poor quality of life associated with medication side effects, unemployment, or social isolation. Full recovery will not be possible until these issues are addressed.

Nurses need to be aware of personal and environmental factors that may be a barrier to rehabilitation or complete recovery and fully assess quality of life issues when planning community-based care. Social isolation, economic hardship, and living in communities with a high prevalence of crime and violence have been shown to predict the onset of major depression and hamper recovery in individuals with serious mental illness. Community resources that include social work services, psychiatric home care, medical care, vocational training, independent living skills and training, safe and affordable housing, and opportunities for rest and leisure activities are essential and should be incorporated into the overall nursing care plan. Key considerations when planning community care strategies include assessing the patient's financial resources and ability to access services; determining whether there is a need for vocational or skills training; assessing the patient's access to transportation; assessing the patient's living environment and self-care ability; and determining the need for additional medical, psychiatric, and social supports.

In addition, nurses identify which family members or caregivers need to be involved in patient and family teaching. Empowering patients and family to become active members of the health care team is essential for full recovery and optimal functioning (Box 16-6). Make sure patients and family members understand the role of each team member and how to contact each team member, as working with multiple providers can confuse and overwhelm.

Evaluation

Nurses play a key role in assessing for residual symptoms and advocating for treating to remission. As stated earlier, working toward a vision of full recovery is now the standard of care. Sleep disturbance, somatic symptoms, poor concentration, and anxiety may all persist even after the individual reports improvement in mood symptoms. Spiritual distress or impairments in social or vocational functioning may linger and increase the risk for relapse. Therefore, assessing patients for improvement in quality of life, overall functioning, productivity, and psychological well-being may be more important than reports of improvement in mood symptoms.

Pause and Reflect

1. *Why are planned leisure and relaxation activities important in the treatment of mood disorders?*
2. *What are some examples of social policies in your state or community that reduce stigma and disparities in care for those with mental illness? Are there any policies that increase stigma or promote or condone disparities? What, if any, responsibilities do nurses have related to these social policies?*
3. *What is a "contextual intervention"? What role do contextual interventions play in helping patients with mood disorders?*

Patient and Family Education: Adhering to the Treatment Plan box 16-6

Recovery from mood disorders and the relief of individual and family suffering are possible only through a coordinated effort among patient, family, and providers. Adherence to a comprehensive treatment plan and early recognition of relapse should therefore be the top priority. Health teaching to assist patients and families includes the following:

- Mood disorders are chronic disorders that are treatable and can be successfully managed though medication and attention to lifestyle. Adherence to the treatment plan is critical.
- Develop a written treatment plan that includes identified goals, a medication schedule, list of providers with contact information, and scheduled follow-up appointments. The treatment plan should be reviewed frequently and modified as necessary.
- Difficulties with adherence to the treatment plan should be reported to the nurse to address issues or advocate for modifications in the treatment plan. This is especially true regarding adherence to the medication regimen. This requires an open relationship between the patient/family and the nurse.
- Identify early indicators of relapse and develop an action plan to prevent relapse.
- Identify and manage stressors that contribute to symptom burden, affect or impede adherence to the treatment plan, or increase the risk for relapse.
- Instruct on self-care strategies such as good nutrition, sleep and rest, physical activity and exercise, avoidance of substance use, and CAM therapies that may augment adherence to the treatment regimen, reduce symptom burden, and prevent relapse.
- Educate the family members regarding their role in facilitating adherence and preventing relapse.

From Suffering to Hope

Mood states vary for individuals in relation to their bio–psycho–socio–cultural–spiritual experiences. Euthymia is the normal and moderate mood state that individuals experience most of the time. Mood disorders are sustained emotional states that depart from an individual's usual state and cause significant disruption in social or vocational functioning. Patients with depressive and bipolar disorders are at increased risk for suicide; ongoing assessment for suicidality is a critical part of nursing care for these patients.

Hopelessness is common among patients experiencing moderate to severe symptoms. Pain, medication side effects, sociological factors, and family relationships can increase patient suffering and complicate treatment. Nurses play a key role in providing hope and care to individuals and their families experiencing such challenges and helping them to minimize disability and distress associated with these mood disorders.

PERCEPTIONS, THOUGHTS, & FEELINGS: Validating Patient Needs

This feature refers to the critical thinking feature in which Vijay Guntupalli suffers from bipolar disorder. Deepak is his brother.

Patient's behavior	Nurse's perceptions, thoughts, feelings	Exploration with patient
Deepak is crying in the hallway after Vijay has been taken from Student Health Services by security. The nurse approaches him. *Deepak:* I can't take this anymore.	*Thoughts:* This is very hard for the family as well as the patient. Deepak has been struggling with managing his brother's illness for some time now. I wonder what supports or help he has available to him. *Feelings:* This situation was disturbing to me; I can't imagine what Deepak must be going through. I am worried about him.	*Nurse:* I can see that you are upset. What can I do for you right now? Would you like to talk about what you have been going through? Let's go into my office for some privacy.

VALIDATION The nurse acknowledges Deepak's distress and offers assistance. She communicates concern through her presence and therapeutic touch. She recognizes the family's need for confidentiality and privacy. These basic strategies work to establish trust quickly.

Patient's behavior	Nurse's perceptions, thoughts, feelings	Exploration with patient
The nurse and Deepak go to her office. The nurse offers tissues. Deepak continues to cry. A couple of times he starts to speak, but cannot complete a sentence.	*Perceptions:* Deepak finds it hard to speak. *Thoughts:* There is a great deal of pain here. It must be hard for this young man to share how he is feeling; I need to give him some space and not probe. There may be some cultural implications here that I am unfamiliar with. Silence may be best right now. *Feelings:* I feel overwhelmed with sadness for this young man; how can I use these feelings therapeutically?	The nurse does not speak, allowing Deepak time to compose himself and to offer information as he is able. She recognizes that there may be cultural implications for care here and remains open to understanding them and learning about them. *Nurse:* This was very hard for you.

VALIDATION The nurse uses nonverbal communication strategies (physical presence, silence, time, and offering tissues) to communicate empathy and validate Deepak's feelings. She validates his suffering and distress through observation.

Patient's behavior	Nurse's perceptions, thoughts, feelings	Exploration with patient
Deepak: I have been dealing with this since I was a kid. My parents don't speak English well, and I have always been the one to deal with the doctors and police. My parents don't believe Vijay has a mental illness.	*Thoughts:* Deepak is burdened by the care of his brother. He feels alone in this. I wonder how he has coped up to this point. I am wondering whether he is safe. I need to gather some more information about his supports and coping. *Feelings:* I am feeling sorry for Deepak. I need to be careful here. Feeling sorry for him may prevent me from being helpful therapeutically.	*Nurse:* Who has helped you deal with all of this? What supports do you have?

VALIDATION The nurse invites Deepak to share some information about his level of coping and tries to identify current supports that would be of help to him at this time.

Patient's behavior	Nurse's perceptions, thoughts, feelings	Exploration with patient
Deepak: I did have a counselor in high school who I talked to a lot but since I've gotten here there really isn't anyone for me to talk to about this. I'm sort of embarrassed by his behavior. I am sorry that he was such a jerk to you. People don't understand that he is ill.	*Thoughts:* Deepak feels alone in this. He is embarrassed by his brother's behavior; he may be feeling shame. It sounds as though Deepak should meet with someone so he can process what has been happening to him. I can offer to see him myself or arrange for a colleague to see him. One of our social workers is Indian; I wonder if he would be more comfortable talking with him.	*Nurse:* Deepak, your brother has bipolar disorder, and I was not offended by his behavior. You are not responsible for Vijay's illness. This is a lot to be going through by yourself right now. How can I be of help to you now?

VALIDATION The nurse recognizes Deepak's conflicts and embarrassment. She exhibits a nonjudgmental attitude towards Vijay's behavior and assures Deepak that he is not responsible for his brother's illness. She attempts to establish a therapeutic alliance with Deepak that will allow him to feel comfortable with asking for help.

Patient's behavior	Nurse's perceptions, thoughts, feelings	Exploration with patient
Deepak: I don't know what would help right now. I'm not thinking straight. I really haven't gotten too much sleep myself the last few nights. I need to call my parents … they are going to freak.	*Thoughts:* Deepak hasn't been taking care of himself. It sounds as though he needs some respite from this situation. He is worried about telling his parents about Vijay's hospitalization.	*Nurse:* What do you think will happen when you call them? Would you like to call your parents now from my phone? I can sit with you if you want while you talk with them.

VALIDATION The nurse seeks to understand what will happen when Deepak calls his parents to help him prepare for the call. She offers assistance in the form of personal support for a difficult task. This helps to establish and build the therapeutic alliance.

Patient's behavior	Nurse's perceptions, thoughts, feelings	Exploration with patient
Deepak: Actually, I would really like that. This is going to be hard. I know that they are going to blame me for not keeping a better eye on Vijay.	*Thoughts:* I know that Deepak is worried about his parents' reaction but I also wonder if he feels responsible for Vijay's need for hospitalization today. This is something that should be explored more once this crisis is over. *Feelings:* I am really worried about Deepak. I'd like to make sure that he is safe before he leaves today and that he has a plan to come back and talk with someone in Student Services tomorrow.	*Nurse:* It might be helpful for us to talk about what you are going to say to your parents before we call them. After we are finished with the call, can we talk about how you can take care of yourself though all of this? I am wondering if you would like to meet with me or one of our social workers tomorrow.

VALIDATION The nurse offers a practical solution to a difficult situation by offering to help Deepak break the news to his parents. Role playing is a key communication strategy that can help patients to process difficult situations. She communicates her concern for him by offering to meet with him again tomorrow. By arranging a meeting for the next day, she is assessing his safety and desire for further assistance.

Based on Orlando, I. J. (1972). *The Discipline and Teaching of Nursing Process (An Evaluative Study).* New York, NY: G. P. Putnam's Sons.

Vijay Recovery Phase (Part 2)

After 10 days, Vijay is well enough for discharge from the hospital but is not fully recovered. His health insurance will allow only a 14-day hospitalization. His thinking is clearer and he is no longer overtly psychotic. He is sleeping better but sleeps only about 5 or 6 hours per night. He has been adherent with medication on the unit, and his lithium level is within an acceptable limit. He reports feeling lethargic on the olanzapine. He is anxious to return to school and is worried that he is falling behind in his studies.

Deepak still has not come to visit, and Vijay is worried that he has damaged their relationship "beyond repair." He tells Mary that he "really blew it this time." His parents have been to visit, but it has been difficult for Mary to assess their level of involvement because they speak limited English. Mary recognizes that the importance of involving Vijay's family in his discharge plan and discusses with the treatment team having a family meeting with a Hindi interpreter.

During the discharge meeting, Vijay's parents are present, but Deepak has not come. This is clearly a source of family tension. The interpreter provides important information regarding the family dynamics and expectations for Vijay's treatment after hospitalization. Vijay's parents demonstrate a poor understanding of Vijay's illness and have continued expectations that Deepak should be "watching his brother" when he returns to school. The treatment team has recommended that Vijay take a leave of absence for the remainder of the school year and attend an outpatient program with community-supported living and medication monitoring. Vijay and his parents reject the treatment team's recommendations and request discharge as soon as possible.

APPLICATION

1. What indications are there that Vijay may be still suffering in one or more domains?

2. How would you prioritize his care needs at this time? How have they changed?

3. What concerns do you have for Vijay as he returns to school? Do you think that he is stable? What indications are there that he may relapse?

4. How can you work with Vijay to negotiate a discharge plan that will support him in his recovery? What suggestion can you make?

5. How will you be able to convey a sense of hope for recovery to Vijay at discharge, especially if you are worried that he is at risk for relapse?

Chapter Highlights

1. Mood is a pervasive emotional tone that affects how an individual perceives self, others, and the environment.

2. Mood states are influenced by biological, psychological, social, cultural, and spiritual experiences.

3. The most likely explanation for depression is the diathesis–stress model, which postulates that individuals inherit tendencies to express certain traits or behaviors when exposed to certain conditions or stressors.

4. Sociological factors contributing to depression include poverty, long-term unemployment, caregiver burden, changing gender roles, marital dissatisfaction, and limited social support.

5. Major depressive disorder is characterized by extremely depressed mood accompanied by a loss of interest or pleasure in activities.

6. Manic episodes characteristic of bipolar disorder feature a persistent elevated, expansive, or irritable mood accompanied by an increase in energy or activity.

7. Cognitive therapies in combination with pharmacotherapy are the most effective treatment for patients with mood disorders.

8. Patients with depressive or bipolar disorder are at increased risk for suicide. Assessment for suicidal ideation and intent should be part of initial and ongoing care of the individual with a mood disorder.

9. Written plans for patients need to include identified goals, medication schedules, list of providers with contact information, and scheduled follow-up appointments.

10. Patients and families need to be empowered to be active members of the health care team for full recovery and optimal functioning.

NCLEX®-RN Questions

1. The nurse is providing teaching to the family of a patient who was recently diagnosed with a mood disorder. The focus of the discussion is on factors contributing to the illness. Which statement by the family indicates the need for further teaching?
   a. "There seems to be an inherited predisposition to these disorders."
   b. "Treatment will depend on determining exactly what triggered this illness."
   c. "Reducing environmental stressors will assist in managing this disease."
   d. "An underlying neurochemical imbalance is one component of mood dysregulation."

2. The nurse is caring for a patient experiencing chronic depression. The patient states that he has lost weight, feels as though he can't move, and is experiencing numerous aches and pains. The nurse understands that what aspects of the illness are likely to be responsible for these findings?
   a. The patient is engaging in negative thinking that distorts the perception of physical well-being.
   b. The patient is experiencing adverse effects from a medication used to treat the mood disturbance.
   c. The patient is experiencing physiological changes related to the same neurobiological factors contributing to depression.
   d. The patient is trying to conceal underlying emotional problems by focusing on physical symptoms.

3. The nurse is planning care for a patient with bipolar I disorder. The patient is currently in the manic phase of the illness. The nurse understands that interventions will be geared toward the management of which manifestations? Select all that apply.
   a. Fatigue
   b. Irritability
   c. Dysphoria
   d. Anhedonia
   e. Impulsivity

4. The nurse is caring for a patient who has been taking lamotrigine (Lamictal) for the management of a mood disorder. The patient is going to be switched to a new medication. Which agents would the nurse anticipate having a comparable therapeutic action to the lamotrigine? Select all that apply.
   a. Sertraline (Zoloft)
   b. Bupropion (Wellbutrin)
   c. Valproic acid (Depakote)
   d. Oxcarbazepine (Trileptal)
   e. Lithium carbonate (Lithobid)

5. A patient asks the nurse whether omega-3 fatty acids are an effective way to manage depression. Which information would be appropriate for the nurse to provide to the patient? Select all that apply.
   a. Omega-3 fatty acids are used only in the treatment of bipolar depression.
   b. Recent studies have shown that omega-3 fatty acids may play a role in mood regulation.
   c. Patients can safely use omega-3 acids as a complement to standard care for mood disorders.
   d. There are research-based guidelines on what dosage of omega-fatty acids is safest and most effective.
   e. It is thought that omega-3 fatty acids may have the potential to exert a mechanism of action similar to prescription mood stabilizers.

6. The nurse is attempting to encourage a patient with depression to participate in activities in the milieu. The patient begins to cry and states, "It won't make any difference, I am always going to feel this way." What should be the nurse's initial response?
   a. "It sounds like you are feeling pretty hopeless."
   b. "Many depressed patients have felt the same way you do."
   c. "Maybe it would help to share those feelings with others."
   d. "It sounds as though participating in groups is hard for you."

7. The nurse is providing disposition teaching to a patient who was hospitalized with a mood disorder. Which aspects of teaching are most essential? Select all that apply.
   a. Determining what the patient's long-term goals are.
   b. Suggesting activities that may keep the patient occupied.
   c. Addressing factors that may affect treatment adherence.
   d. Exploring alternative therapies that may augment treatment.
   e. Ensuring that the patient understands the early signs of relapse.

Answers may be found on the Pearson student resource site: nursing.pearsonhighered.com

Pearson Nursing Student Resources Find additional review materials at **nursing.pearsonhighered.com**

References

Adams, M., Holland, N., & Urban, C. (2014). *Pharmacology for nurses: A Pathophysiologic Approach* (4th ed.). Upper Saddle River, NJ: Prentice Hall.

Ali, S., Stone, M., Peters, J., Davies, M., & Khunti, K. (2006). The prevalence of comorbid depression in adults with Type 2 diabetes: A systematic review and meta-analysis. *Diabetic Medicine, 23*(11), 1165–1173.

Altshuler, L., Tekell, J., Biswas, K., Kilbourne, A., Evans, D., & Bauer, M. (2007). Executive function and employment status among veterans with bipolar disorder. *Psychiatric Services, 58(1),* 1441–1447.

Alves-Apostolo, J., & Kolcaba, K. (2009). The effects of guided imagery on comfort, depression, anxiety, and stress on psychiatric inpatients with depressive disorders. *Archives of Psychiatric Nursing, 23*(6), 403–411.

American Association of Suicidology. (n.d.) National suicide statistics. Available at http://www.suicidology.org/resources/facts-statistics-current-research/suicide-statistics

American Foundation for Suicide Prevention. (2011). Facts and figures. Available at: http://www.afsp.org/understanding-suicide/facts-and-figures

American Psychiatric Association. (2002). Clinical practice guidelines for the treatment of patients with bipolar disorder (revision). *American Journal of Psychiatry, 159*(4 suppl), 1–50.

American Psychiatric Association. (2013). *Diagnostic and Statistical Manual of Mental Disorders* (5th ed.). Washington, DC: American Psychiatric Publishers.

Angst, F., Stassen, H., & Clayton, P. (2002). Mortality of patients of mood disorders: Follow up over 34–38 years. *Journal of Affective Disorders, 68*(2–3), 167–181.

Bair, M. J., Robinson, R. L., Katon, W., & Kroenke, K. (2003). Depression and pain comorbidity: A literature review. *Archives of Internal Medicine, 163*(20), 2433–2445.

Baldessarini, R., Vazquez, G., & Tondo, L. (2011). Treatment of cyclothymic disorder: Commentary. *Psychotherapy and Psychosomatics, 80*(3), 131–135.

Bauer, M., Adli, M., Bschor, T., Pilhatsch, M., Pfennig, A., Sasse, J., Schmid, R., & Lewitzka, U. (2010). Lithium's emerging role in the treatment of refractory major depressive episodes: Augmentation of antidepressants. *Neuropsychobiology, 62*(1), 36–42. doi: 10.1159/000314308

Bauer, M., McBride, L., Williford, W., Glick, H., Kinosian, B., …Sajatovic, M. (2006a). Collaborative care for bipolar disorder: Part I. Intervention and implementation in a randomized effectiveness trial. *Psychiatric Services, 57*(7), 927–936.

Bauer, M., McBride, L., Williford, W., Glick, H., Kinosian, B., …Sajatovic, M. (2006b). Collaborative care for bipolar disorder: Part II. Impact on clinical outcome, function, and cost. *Psychiatric Services, 57*(7), 937–945.

Bearden, C., Woogen, M., & Glahn, D. (2010). Neurocognitive and neuroimaging predictors of clinical outcome in bipolar disorder. *Current Psychiatry Report, 12*(6), 499–504.

Beck, A. (1967). *Depression: Clinical, Experimental and Theoretical Aspects.* New York, NY: Harper & Row.

Berns, G., & Nemeroff, C. (2003). The neurobiology of bipolar disorder. *American Journal of Medical Genetics Part C (Seminars in Medical Genetics), 123C*(1), 76–84.

Bolwig, T. (2011). How does electroconvulsive therapy work? Theories on its mechanism. *Canadian Journal of Psychiatry, 56*(1), 13–18.

Bond, G. R., & Campbell, K. (2008). Evidence-based practices for individuals with severe mental illness. *Journal of Rehabilitation, 74*(2), 33–44.

Brown, A. (2012). With poverty comes depression, more than other illnesses. Gallup. Available at http://www.gallup.com/poll/158417/poverty-comes-depression-illness.aspx

Burt, V., & Quezada, V. (2009). Mood disorders in women: Focus on reproductive psychiatry in the 21st century. *Canadian Journal of Clinical Pharmacology, 16*(1), e6–e14.

Byrne, M., & Deane, F. (2011). Enhancing patient adherence: Outcomes of medication alliance on therapeutic alliance, insight, adherence, and psychopathology with mental health patients. *International Journal of Mental Health Nursing, 20*(4), 284–295. doi: 10.1111/j.1447-0349.2010.00722.x

Carbray, M. J., & McGuinness, T. (2009). Pediatric bipolar disorder. *Journal of Psychosocial Nursing and Mental Health Services, 47*(12), 22–26.

Centers for Disease Control and Prevention (CDC). (2010). Current depression among adults—United States 2006–2008. *Morbidity and Mortality Weekly Report (MMWR), 59*(38), 1229–1235.

Centers for Disease Control and Prevention (CDC). (2011). Burden of mental illness. Available at http://www.cdc.gov/mentalhealth/basics/burden.htm

Cerda, M., Sagdeo, A., Johnson, J., & Galea, S. (2010). Genetic and environmental influences on psychiatric comorbidity: A systematic review. *Journal of Affective Disorders, 126*(1–2), 14–38.

Chapman, D., & Perry, G. (2008). Depression as a major component of public health for older adults. *Preventing Chronic Disease, 5*(1), 1–9.

Chong, W., & Chen, A. (2011). Effectiveness of interventions to improve antidepressant medication adherence: A systematic review. *International Journal of Clinical Practice, 65*(9), 954–975.

Cleary, M., Walter, G., & Matheson, S. (2008). What is the role of e-technology in mental health services and psychiatric research? *Journal of Psychosocial Nursing 46*(4), 42–48.

Compton, W., Conway, K., Stinson, F., & Grant, B. (2006). Changes in the prevalence of major depression and comorbid substance use disorders in the United States between 1991–1992 and 2001–2002. *American Journal of Psychiatry, 163*(12), 2141–2147.

Cooper, L., Gonzales, J., Gallo, J., Rost, K., Meredith, L.,…Ford, D. (2003). The acceptability of treatment for depression among African-American, Hispanic, and white primary care patients. *Medical Care, 41*(4), 479–489.

Costello, E., Erkanli, A., & Angold, A. (2006). Prevalence and development of psychiatric disorders in children and adolescence. *Archives of General Psychiatry, 60*(8), 837–844.

Crowe, M., Whitehead, L., Wilson, L., Caryle, D., O'Brien, A., … Joyce, P. (2010). Disorder-specific psychosocial interventions for bipolar disorder—A systematic review of the evidence for mental health nursing practice. *International Journal of Nursing Studies, 47*(7), 896–908.

Demyttenaere, K., Bonnewyn, A., Bruffaerts, R., Bruqha, T., DeGraaf, R., & Alonso, L. (2006). Comorbid painful physical symptoms and depression: prevalence, work loss, and help seeking. *Journal of Affective Disorders, 92*(2–3), 185–193.

Depp, C., & Jest, D. (2004). Bipolar disorder in older adults: A critical review. *Bipolar Disorders, 6*(5), 343–367.

Dettmore, D., & Gabriele, L. (2011). Don't just do something, stand there: Responding to unrelieved patient suffering. *Journal of Psychosocial Nursing, 49*(4), 35–38.

Diego, M., Field, T., Hernandez-Reif, M., Cullen, C., Schanberg, S., & Kuhn, C. (2004). Prepartum, postpartum, and chronic depression effects on newborns. *Psychiatry, 67*(1), 63–80.

Druss, B., Rosenheck, R., & Desai, M. (2002). Quality of preventive medical care for patients with mental disorders. *Medical Care, 40*(2), 129–136.

Elliot, L., & Masters, H. (2009). Mental health inequalities and mental health nursing. *Journal of Psychiatric and Mental Health Nursing, 16*(8), 762–771.

Fava, G. A., Ruini, C., & Belaise, C. (2007). The concept of recovery in major depression. *Psychological Medicine, 37*(3), 307–317.

Fernandez y Garcia, E., Franks, P., Jerant, A., Bell, R., & Kravitz, R. (2011). Depression treatment preferences of Hispanic individuals: Exploring the influence of ethnicity, language, and explanatory models. *Journal of the American Board of Family Medicine, 24*(1), 39–50.

Fetterman, T., & Ying, P. (2011). Informed consent and electroconvulsive therapy. *Journal of the American Psychiatric Nursing Association, 17*(3), 219–222.

Fiske, A., Loebach-Wetherell, J., & Gatz, M. (2009). Depression in older adults. *Annual Review of Clinical Psychology, 5*, 363–389.

Franklin, T., Russiq, H., Weiss, I., Graff, J., Linder, N., & Mansuy, J. (2010). Epigenetic transmission of the impact of early stress across generations. *Biological Psychiatry, 68*(5), 408–415.

Freeman, M. (2009). Omega-3 fatty acids in major depressive disorder. *Journal of Clinical Psychiatry, 70*(suppl 5), 7–11.

Freeman, M., Fava, M., Lake, J., Trivedi, M., Wisner, K., & Mischoulon, D. (2010). Complementary and alternative medicine in major depressive disorder: The American Psychiatric Association Task Force Report. *Journal of Clinical Psychiatry, 71*(6), 669–681.

Freeman, M., Smith, K., Freeman, S., McElroy, S., Kmetz, G.,…Keck P. (2002). The impact of reproductive events on the course of bipolar disorder in women. *Journal of Clinical Psychiatry, 63*(4), 284–287.

Frodl, T., Koutsouleris, N., Bottlender, R., Born, C., Jaqer, M.,…Meisenzahl, E. (2008). Depression-related variation in brain morphology over 3 years: Effects of stress? *Archives of General Psychiatry, 65*(10), 1156–1165.

Gagne, C., Anthony, W. & White, W. (2011). An analysis of mental health and addiction concepts of recovery. Available at http://www.bbs.ca.gov/pdf/mhsa/resource/recovery/analysis_mental_health_addictions_recovery.pdf

Gigantesco, A., & Giuliani, M. (2011). Quality of life in mental health services with a focus on psychiatric rehabilitation practice. *Annali dell'Instituto di Sanita, 47*(4), 363–372.

Goodwin, F., & Jamison, K. (2007). *Manic-Depressive Illness: Bipolar Disorders and Recurrent Depression* (2nd ed.). New York, NY: Oxford University Press.

Gottlieb, L., Waitzkin, H., & Miranda, J. (2011). Depressive symptoms and their social contexts: A qualitative systematic literature review of contextual interventions. *International Journal of Social Psychiatry, 57*(4), 402–417.

Greasley, P., Chiu, L. F., & Gartland, R. M. (2001). The concept of spiritual care in mental health nursing. *Journal of Advanced Nursing, 33*(5), 629–637.

Gupta, A., & Singhal, N. (2004). Positive perceptions in parents of children with disabilities. *Asia Pacific Disability Rehabilitation Journal, 15*(1), 22–35.

Halligan, S., Herbert, J., Goodyer, I., & Murray, L. (2004). Exposure to postnatal depression predicts elevated cortisol in adolescent offspring. *Biologic Psychiatry, 55*(4), 376–381.

Hanrahan, N., & Sullivan-Max, E. (2005). Practice patterns and potential solutions to the shortage of providers of older adult mental health services. *Policy, Politics & Nursing Practice, 6*(3), 236–245. doi:10.1177/1527154405279195

Harding, K., Rush, A., Arbuckle, M., Trivedi, M., & Pincus, H. (2011). Measurement-based care in psychiatric practice: A policy framework for implementation. *Journal of Clinical Psychiatry, 72*(8), 1136–1143.

Hirshfeld, R., Lewis, L.. & Vornik, L. (2003). Perceptions and impact of bipolar disorder: How far have we really come? Results from the National Depressive and Manic-Depressive Association 2000 survey of individuals with bipolar disorder. *Journal of Clinical Psychiatry, 64*(2), 161–174.

Hoff, L., & Morgan, B. (2011). *Psychiatric and Mental Health Essentials in Primary Care*. New York, NY: Routledge.

Hollon, S., & Ponniah, K. (2010). A review of empirically supported psychological therapies for mood disorders in adults. *Depression and Anxiety, 27*(10), 891–932.

Hsu, M., Moyle, W., Creedy, D., Venturato, L., Ouyang, W., & Tsay, S. (2009). Use of antidepressant and complementary and alternative medicine among outpatients with depression in Taiwan. *Archives of Psychiatric Nursing, 23*(1), 75–85.

Husain, M., Rush, A., Trivedi, M., McClintock, S., Wisniewski, S.,…Zisook, S. (2007). Pain in depression: STAR*D study findings. *Journal of Psychosomatic Research, 63*(2), 113–122.

Jakobsen, J., Hansen, J., & Simonsen, E. (2011). The effect of interpersonal psychotherapy and other psychodynamic therapies versus "treatment as usual" in patients with major depressive disorder. *PloS, 6*(4), e19044.

Jones-Warren, B. (2007). Cultural aspects of bipolar disorder: Interpersonal meaning for clients and nurses. *Journal of Psychosocial Nursing, 45*(7), 32–37.

Jonsson, P., Skarsater, I., Wijk, H., & Danielson, E. (2011). Experience of living with a family member with bipolar disorder. *International Journal of Mental Health Nursing, 20*(1), 29–37.

Judd, L., Akiskal, H., Schettler, P., Endicott, J., Maser, J.,…Keller, B. (2002). The long-term natural history of the weekly symptomatic status of bipolar I disorder. *Archives of General Psychiatry, 59*(6), 530–537.

Kaplan, B., & Sadock, V. (2005). *Pocket Handbook of Clinical Psychiatry*. Philadelphia, PA: Lippincott Williams & Wilkins.

Karp, J., Scott, J., Houck, P., Reynolds, C., Kupfer, D., & Frank, E. (2005). Pain predicts longer time to remission during treatment of recurrent depression. *Journal of Clinical Psychiatry, 66*(5), 591–597.

Katon, W. (2011). Epidemiology and treatment of depression in patients with chronic medical illness. *Dialogues in Clinical Neuroscience, 13*(1), 7–22.

Kessing L., & Andersen, P. (2004). Does the risk of developing dementia increase with the number of episodes in patients with depressive disorder and in patients with bipolar disorder? *Journal of Neurology, Neurosurgery, Psychiatry, 75*(12), 1662–1666.

Kessler, R., Berglund, P., Demler, O., Jin, R., Koretz, D., …Wang, P. (2003). The epidemiology of major depressive disorder: Results from the National Comorbidity Survey Replication (NCS-R). *Journal of the American Medical Association, 289*(23), 3095–3105.

Kessler, R., Soukup, J., Davis, R., Foster, D., Wilkey, S.,…Wang, P. (2001). The use of complementary and alternative therapies to treat anxiety and depression in the United States. *American Journal of Psychiatry, 158*(2), 289–294.

Kirmayer, L., Narasiah, L., Munoz, M., Rashid, M., Ryder, A.,… Pottie, K. (2011). Common mental health problems of immigrants and refugees: General approach in primary care. *Canadian Medical Association Journal, 183*(12), E959–E967.

Klakovich, M. (2009). Interpersonal communication: An essential skill for nursing students. Available at https://www.phoenix.edu/profiles/faculty/marilyn-klakovich/articles/interpersonal-communication-an-essential-skill-for-nursing-students.html

Koenig, H. (2009). Research on religion, spirituality, and mental health: A review. *Canadian Journal of Psychiatry 54*(5), 283–291.

Kroenke, K., Shen, J., Oxman, T., William, J., & Dietrich, A. (2008). Impact of pain on the outcomes of depression treatment: Results from the RESPECT trial. *Pain, 134*(1–2), 209–215.

Kübler-Ross, E. (1967). *On Death and Dying*. New York, NY: Touchstone Publishing.

Kupka, R., Altshuler, L., Nolen, W., Luckenbaugh, D., Leverich, G., … Post, P. (2007). Three times more days depressed than manic or hypomanic in both bipolar I and bipolar II disorder. *Bipolar Disorder, 9*(5), 531–535.

Lack, C., & Green, A. (2009). Mood disorders in children. *Journal of Pediatric Nursing, 24*(1), 13–25.

Lu, P., & Su, K. (2007). A meta-analytic review of double-blind, placebo controlled trials of antidepressant efficacy of omega-3 fatty acids. *Journal of Clinical Psychiatry, 68*(7), 1056–1061.

Luggen, A. (2005). Bipolar disorder: An uncommon illness. Recognizing and caring for the elderly person with bipolar disorder. *Geriatric Nursing, 26*(5), 326–329.

Luoma, J., Martin, C., & Pearson, J. (2002). Contact with mental health and primary care providers before suicide: A review of the evidence. *American Journal of Psychiatry, 159*(6), 909–916.

MacDowell, M., Glasser, M., Fitts, M., Nielsen, K., & Hunsaker, N. (2010). A national view of rural health workforce issue in the USA. *Rural Remote Health, 10*(3), 1531.

Machado-Vieria, R., Manji, H., & Zarate, C. (2009). The role of lithium in the treatment of bipolar disorder: Convergent evidence for neurotrophic effects as a unifying hypothesis. *Bipolar Disorder, 11*(suppl 2), 92–109.

Mahon, K., Burdick, K., & Szeszko, P. (2010). A role for white matter abnormalities in the pathophysiology of bipolar disorder. *Neuroscience and Biobehavioral Reviews, 34*(4), 533–554.

Marangell, L. (2008). Current issues: Women and bipolar disorder. *Dialogues in Clinical Neuroscience, 10*(2), 229–238.

Martin, D., Garske, J., & Davis, K. (2000). Relationship of the therapeutic alliance with outcome and other variables: A meta-analytic review. *Journal of Clinical Consulting and Clinical Psychology, 68*(3), 438–450.

Martinowich, K., Schloesser, R.. & Manji H. (2009). Bipolar disorder: From genes to behavior pathways. *Journal of Clinical Investigation, 119*(4), 726–736.

McClellan, J., Kowatch, R., & Findling, R. (2007). Practice parameter for the assessment and treatment of children and adolescents with bipolar disorder. *Journal of the American Academy of Child and Adolescent Psychiatry, 46*(1), 107–125.

Meltzer, H., Bebbington, P., Brugha, T., Jenkins, R., McManus, S., & Stansfeld, S. (2010). Job insecurity, socio-economic circumstances and depression. *Psychological Medicine, 40*(8),1401–1407.

Meltzer-Brody, S. (2011). New insights into perinatal depression: Pathogenesis and treatment during pregnancy and postpartum. *Dialogues in Clinical Neuroscience, 13*(1), 89–100.

Merikangas, K., He., J., Burstein, M., Swendsen, J., Avenevoli, S., Case, B., … Olfson, M. (2011). Service utilization for lifetime mental disorders in U.S. adolescents: Results from the National Comorbidity Survey Adolescent Supplement (NCS-A). *Journal of the American Academy of Child and Adolescent Psychiatry, 50*(1), 32–45.

Mitchell, A., & Subramaniam, H. (2005). Prognosis of depression in old age compared to middle age: A systematic review of comparative studies. *American Journal of Psychiatry, 162*(9), 1588–1601.

Mueser, K., & Drake, R. (2005). How does a practice become evidenced based? In R. E. Drake, M. R. Merrens, & D. W. Lynde (Eds.). *Evidenced Based Mental Health Practice: A Textbook*. New York, NY: W.W. Norton & Company.

Mulsant, B., Houck, P., Gildengers, A., Andreescu, C., Dew, M., … Miller, M. (2006). What is the optimal duration of a short-term antidepressant trial when treating geriatric depression? *Journal of Clinical Psychopharmacology, 26*(2), 113–120.

Nabuco de Abreu, L., Lafer, B., Baca-Garcia, E., & Oquendo, M. (2009). Suicidal ideation and suicide attempt in bipolar disorder type I: An update for the clinician. *Revista Brasileria de Psiquiatria, 31*(3), 271–280.

Nadeem, E., Lange, J., Edge, D., Fongwa, M., Belin, T., & Miranda, J. (2007). Does stigma keep poor young immigrants and U.S. born black and Latina women from seeking mental health care? *Psychiatric Services, 58*(12), 1547–1554.

Nahas, Z., & Anderson, B. (2011). Brain stimulation therapies for mood disorders: The continued necessity of electroconvulsive therapy. *Journal of the American Psychiatric Nurses Association, 17*(3), 214–216.doi:10.1177/1078390311409037

National Center for Complementary and Alternative Medicine. (2011). 2007 Statistics on CAM use in the United States. Available at http://nccam.nih.gov/news/camstats/2007

National Coalition for Health Professional Education in Genetics (NCHPEG). (2011). Empiric risk data. Available at http://www.nchpeg.org/index.php?option=com_content&view=article&id=120:empiric-risk-data&catid=53:genetics-and-major-psychiatric-disorders-a-program-for-genetic-counselors

National Institute of Mental Health (NIMH). (2011). *Mental Health Statistics*. Available at http://www.nimh.nih.gov/statistics/index.shtml

Nemeroff, C., & Vale, W. (2005). The neurobiology of depression: Inroads to treatment and new drug discovery. *Journal of Clinical Psychiatry, 66*(suppl 7), 5–13.

Nothen, M., Nieratschker, V., Cichon, S., & Rietschel, M. (2010). New findings in the genetics of major psychosis. *Clinical Dialogues in Neuroscience, 21*(1), 85–93.

Orlando, I. J. (1972). *The Discipline and Teaching of Nursing Process (An Evaluative Study)*. New York, NY: G. P. Putnam's Sons.

Parker, G., Gibson, N., Brotchie, H., Heruc, G., Rees, A., & Hadzi-Pavlovic, D. (2006). Omega-3 fatty acids and mood disorders. *American Journal of Psychiatry, 163*(6), 969–978.

Parkes, C., & Bowlby, J. (1972). *Bereavement: Studies of Grief in Adult Life.* New York, NY: Basic Books.

Pelham, B. W. (2009). About one in six Americans report history of depression. *Gallup Wellbeing.* Available at http://www.gallup.com/poll/123821/One-Six-Americans-Report-History-Depression.aspx?CSTS=alert

Perugi, G., Fornaro, M., & Akiskal, H. (2011). Are atypical depression, borderline personality disorder, and bipolar II disorder overlapping manifestations of a common cyclothymic diathesis? *World Psychiatry, 10*(1), 45–51.

Pompili, M., Rihmer, Z., Innamorati, M., Lester, D., Girardi, P., & Tatarelli, R. (2009). Assessment and treatment of suicide risk in bipolar disorders. *Expert Review of Neurotherapeutics, 9*(1), 109–136. doi:10.1586/14737175.9.1.109

Roshanaei-Moghaddam, B., & Katon, W. (2009). Premature mortality from general medical illness among persons with bipolar disorder: A review. *Psychiatric Services, 60*(2), 147–156.

Sajatovic, M., Ignacio, R., West, J., Cassidy, K., Safavi, R.,... Blow, F. (2009). Predictors of nonadherence among individuals with bipolar disorder receiving treatment in a community mental health clinic. *Comprehensive Psychiatry, 50*(2), 100–107.

Seligman, M. (1975). *Helplessness: On Depression, Development and Death.* San Francisco, CA: W. H. Freeman.

Seligman, M. (1998). *Learned Optimism* (2nd ed.). New York, NY: Simon & Schuster.

Sharpley, C. (2010). A review of the neurobiological effects of psychotherapy for depression. *Psychotherapy Theory, Research, Practice, Training, 47*(4), 603–615.

Shelley, B., Sussman, A., Williams, R., Segal, A., & Crabtree, B. (2009). "They don't ask so I don't tell them": Patient-clinician communication about traditional, complementary, and alternative medicine. *Annals of Family Medicine, 7*(2), 139–147.

Simon, G., Ludman, E., Bauer, M., Unutzer, J., & Operskalski, B. (2006). Long-term effectiveness and cost of a systematic care program for bipolar disorder. *Archives of General Psychiatry, 63*(5), 500–508.

Simon, G., Ludman, J., Unutzer, J., Bauer, M., Operskalski, B.. & Rutter, C. (2005). Randomized trial of a population-based care program for people with bipolar disorder. *Psychological Medicine, 35*(1), 13–24.

Sorrell, J. (2011). Caring for older adults with bipolar disorder. *Journal of Psychosocial Nursing, 49*(7), 21–25.

Spijkerman, T., van den Brink, R., Jansen, J., May, J., Crijins, H., & Ormel, J. (2005). Depression following myocardial infarction: First-ever versus ongoing and recurrent episodes. *General Hospital Psychiatry, 27*(6), 411–417.

Stack, J., Mazumdar, S., & Reynolds, C. (2006). What is the optimal duration of a short-term antidepressant trial when treating geriatric depression? *Journal of Clinical Psychopharmacology, 26*(2), 113–120.

Stahl, S. (2002). Does depression hurt? *Journal of Clinical Psychiatry, 63*(4), 273–274.

Stroebe, M., & Schut, H. (1999). The dual process model of coping with bereavement: Rationale and description. *Death Studies, 23*(3), 197–224.

Sullivan, P., Neale, M., & Kendler, K. (2000). Genetic epidemiology of major depression: Review and meta-analysis. *American Journal of Psychiatry, 157*(10), 1552–1562.

Thompson, I. (2002). Mental health and spiritual care. *Nursing Standard, 17*(9), 33–38.

Tohen, M., Zarate, C., Hennen, J., Khalsa, H., Strakowski, S., ... Baldessarini, R. (2003). The McLean-Harvard first-episode mania study: Prediction of recovery and first recurrence. *American Journal of Psychiatry, 160*(12), 2099–2107.

Toperczer, T. (2011). Telepsychiatry in the cloud. *Health Management Technology, 32*(8), 28–29.

Trivedi, M. H. (2006). Major depressive disorder: Remission of associated symptoms. *Journal of Clinical Psychiatry, 67*(suppl 6), 27–32.

Trivedi, M., Lin, E., & Katon, W. (2007). Consensus recommendations for improving adherence, self-management, and outcomes in patients with depression. *CNS Spectrums, 12*(suppl 13), 1–27.

Trivedi, M., Rush, A., Wisniewski, S., Nierenberg, A., Warden, D., ... Fava, M. (2006). Evaluation of outcomes with citalopram for depression using measurement-based care in STAR*D: Implications for clinical practice. *American Journal of Psychiatry, 163*(1), 28–40.

Tsuno, N., Besset, A., & Ritchie, K. (2005). Sleep and depression. *Journal of Clinical Psychiatry, 66*(10), 1254–1269.

Turnbull, T., Cullen-Drill, M., & Smaldone, A. (2008). Efficacy of omega-3 fatty acid supplementation of bipolar symptoms: A systematic review. *Archives of Psychiatric Nursing, 22*(5), 305–311.

Uçok, A., & Gaebel, W. (2008). Side effects of atypical antipsychotics: A brief overview. *World Psychiatry, 7*(1), 58–62.

U.S. Department of Health and Human Services. (2013). *Healthy People 2020*: Mental health and mental disorders. Available at http://www.healthypeople.gov/2020/topicsobjectives2020/overview.aspx?topicid=28

U.S. Preventive Services Task Force. (2009). Screening for depression in adults: U.S. Preventive Services Task Force recommendations statement. *Annals of Internal Medicine, 151*(11), 744–792.

Vallerand, A. H., Sanoski, C. A., & Deglin, J. H. (2013). *Davis's Drug Guide for Nurses* (13th ed.). Philadelphia, PA: F. A. Davis.

Vittengl, J., Clark, L., Dunn, T., & Jarrett, R. (2007). Reducing relapse and recurrence of unipolar depression: A comparative meta-analysis of cognitive-behavioral therapy's effects. *Journal of Consulting and Clinical Psychology, 75*(3), 475–488.

Wang, P., Lane, M., Olfson, M., Pincus, H., Wells, K., & Kessler, R. (2005). Twelve-month use of mental health services in the United States: Results from the National Comorbidity Survey Replication. *Archives of General Psychiatry, 62*(6), 629–640.

Warren, B., & Lutz, W. (2009). The state of nursing science—culture and lifespan issues in depression: Part I: Focus on adults. *Issues in Mental Health Nursing, 28*(7), 707–748.

Weiner, R., & Falcone, G. (2011). Electroconvulsive therapy: How effective is it? *Journal of the American Psychiatric Nurses Association, 17*(3), 217–218.

Weinstock, L., & Miller, I. (2010). Psychosocial predictors of mood 1 year after acute phase treatment of bipolar I disorder. *Comprehensive Psychiatry, 51*(5), 497–503.

Weiss, M., Jadhav, S., Raguram, R., Vounatsou, P., & Littlewood, R. (2001). Psychiatric stigma across cultures: Local validation in Bangalore and London. *Anthropology and Medicine, 8*(1), 71–87.

White, P., & Ferszt, G. (2009). Exploration of nurse practitioner practice with clients who are grieving. *Journal of the American Academy of Nurse Practitioners, 21*(4), 231–240.

Wilson, B. A., Shannon, M. T., & Shields, K. M. (2014). *Pearson Nurse's Drug Guide*. Upper Saddle River, NJ: Prentice Hall.

World Health Organization (WHO). (2001). *Burden of Mental and Behavioral Disorders*. Geneva, Switzerland: World Health Organization, Chapter 2.

Wu P., Fuller C., Liu X., Lee, H., Fan, B.,...Kronenberg, F. (2007). Use of complementary and alternative medicine among women with depression: Results of a national survey. *Psychiatric Services, 58*(3), 349–356.

Yonkers, K. A., Wisner, K. L., Stewart, D. E., Oberlander, T. F., ... Lockwood, C. (2009). The management of depression during pregnancy: A report from the American Psychiatric Association and the American College of Obstetricians and Gynecologists. *General Hospital Psychiatry, 31*(5), 403–413.

Zuckerbrot, R., Cheung, A., Jensen, P., Stein, R., & Laraque, D. (2007). Guidelines for adolescent depression in primary care (GLAD-PC): I. Identification, assessment and initial management. *Pediatrics, 120*(5), e 1299–e1312.

Schizophrenia Spectrum and Other Psychotic Disorders

17

Lora Humphrey Beebe

Learning Outcomes

1. Examine the etiology of schizophrenia spectrum and other psychotic disorders (SSDs).

2. Categorize key symptoms of different SSDs.

3. Summarize the impact of biological, psychological, sociological, cultural, and spiritual domains on SSDs.

4. Evaluate pharmacologic and nonpharmacologic therapies used in the treatment of SSDs.

5. Describe appropriate assessments for patients with SSDs in the initial, relapse, and recovery and rehabilitation phases of illness.

6. Design health promotion activities for patients with SSDs.

7. Plan evidence-based nursing care for patients diagnosed with SSDs.

Key Terms

akathisia, 369
asterognosis, 365
automatic obedience, 365
avolition, 362
body mass index (BMI), 376
delusions, 362
dystonia, 369
echolalia, 365
echopraxia, 365
executive functioning, 363
extrapyramidal side effects, 371
formal thought disorder (FTD), 365
hallucinations, 362
hard signs, 365
negative symptoms, 363
positive symptoms, 362
premorbid, 369
prodrome, 369
psychotomimetic, 364
schizoaffective disorder, 368
schizophrenia, 368
self-efficacy, 380
soft signs, 365
tardive dyskinesia (TD), 369
waxy flexibility, 365

Ming Relapse Phase (Part 1)

Ming is a 21-year-old Asian-American woman who comes to the mental health center for her initial outpatient follow-up after a recent psychiatric hospitalization. Ming was born in the United States and is an only child. Ming's mother immigrated from China at age 15 and met Ming's American father while they were in college. There is no known family history of schizophrenia. Ming lives with her parents, who report that she was a high achiever throughout her elementary and high school years, but that her functioning deteriorated after she left home at age 18 to attend college in another state. Ming became convinced that one of her professors was involved in a plot with the student organizations on campus to discredit and humiliate her. Over the course of 2 months, she refused to attend class or eat, believing the cafeteria food was poisoned. She slept little, being constantly vigilant for attack by "people trying to ruin my life." She did not make friends or attend social functions. She denies alcohol use but reports that during this period she could sleep only after smoking marijuana, which she did approximately 5 nights per week.

Ming eventually left college and returned home, where her symptoms lessened without treatment. During this time, she worked stocking the shelves at her mother's Asian grocery store and spent her free time alone or with her parents. She denies marijuana or other drug use since leaving college. At age 20, Ming again became extremely mistrustful of others—this time, her parents. She withdrew from them, refusing to leave her room for meals or to bathe, accusing her parents of "being in league with the devil" and "spying on me for information." Her parents consulted her primary care physician, who recommended a psychiatrist. The psychiatrist subsequently hospitalized Ming and prescribed olanzapine (Zyprexa). Olanzapine reduced Ming's symptoms, but she gained 15 pounds in the first 3 months and refused to continue the medication. Around this time, Ming took up smoking "to help me slim down" and now smokes one pack of cigarettes per day. She was switched to risperidone (Risperdal) with fair results until recently, when her mother's store underwent remodeling. The stress of the remodeling and the presence of workmen triggered a relapse. Ming became convinced she was involved in a love affair with one of the workmen and pregnant with his child. She feared that her prescribed medication would harm the baby, and discontinued it. When she followed the workman home and threatened suicide if he did not admit his paternity and agree to "help me raise your child," he called the police and she was hospitalized yet again. Records forwarded from the clinic to the hospital indicate that Ming's delusions faded after an increase in her risperidone dosage, but that she refused participation in most unit activities.

APPLICATION

1. Address the five domains for Ming:
   a. Biological
   b. Psychological
   c. Sociological
   d. Cultural
   e. Spiritual
2. In what ways do you think Ming may be suffering, and why?
3. How would you prioritize Ming's needs at this time?
4. How would you offer hope to Ming at this time?

Introduction

Approximately 3 million Americans (1% of the population) suffer from schizophrenia spectrum and other psychotic disorders (SSDs) (National Institute of Mental Health [NIMH], 2008). The major SSDs include schizophrenia, schizoaffective disorder, schizophreniform disorder, delusional disorder, and brief psychotic disorder. These neurobiological illnesses are among the most chronic and disabling of the severe mental disorders, causing psychotic symptoms (hallucinations and delusions), social withdrawal, and bizarre behaviors that are puzzling and sometimes frightening to others. SSD symptoms affect multiple areas of functioning, including language, cognition, perception, attention, emotions, initiative, and social interactions. Some of the features of SSDs—in particular, **avolition**, or lack of motivation—create challenges for clinicians attempting to engage patients in their treatment plan. These same features often prevent the patient from succeeding in accomplishing desired life goals. Therefore it is essential for nurses and other clinicians to understand the commonalities shared by the SSDs, as well as some of the discrete differences.

The symptoms of SSDs have been divided into positive, negative, and cognitive types (Figure 17-1). This makes the diagnostic boundaries with other neurological disorders and within this category challenging (Kirkpatrick, 2014). **Positive symptoms** are symptoms that involve additions (+) to normal experiences and include hallucinations and delusions as well as abnormal movements and problems with speech, referred to as *formal thought disorder*. **Hallucinations** are abnormal perceptual (visual, auditory, olfactory, gustatory, and tactile) experiences that occur without external stimuli. Although hallucinations may involve any of the senses, auditory hallucinations are the most prevalent. Voices conversing or commenting on the individual's behavior occur, but threatening/accusatory voices are more common (Tandon, Nasrallah, & Keshavan, 2009).

Delusions are false beliefs based on incorrect inference or perception. The most common delusions are those of *reference* (the belief that events in life happen just for the benefit of the individual—for instance, a parking space opening up just as one drives in). Other types of delusions include:

- *Nihilistic:* belief that part of the individual is dead or does not exist
- *Religious:* the individual assumes the identity of a religious figure
- *Grandiose:* the individual is the president of the world or, conversely, is so bad that others should not be around him or her
- *Persecutory:* belief that others wish to harm, demean, or belittle the individual

Individuals can also experience bizarre delusions. Bizarre delusions are beliefs that are implausible in a given culture and include

Positive Symptoms	 Negative Symptoms	Cognitive Symptoms
Additions to normal experiences:	Diminished affects and behaviors:	• Memory deficits
• Delusions	• Flat or blunted affect	• Attention deficits
• Hallucinations	• Thought blocking	• Language difficulties
• Abnormal movements	• Avolition	• Loss of executive function
• Formal thought disorder	• Poverty of speech	
	• Social withdrawal	

17-1   The symptoms of SSDs have been categorized as positive, negative, and cognitive.

thought broadcasting (others can hear the person's thoughts), thought withdrawal (others can remove thoughts from the person's mind), thought control (others are controlling the person's thoughts), and thought insertion (others are inserting thoughts or conversations into the person's mind, such as believing that radio or television programs are discussing the individual).

Negative symptoms do not refer to symptoms that are simply bad or challenging, but rather refer to affects and behaviors that are diminished (–) or absent in patients with SSDs. They include having a flat or blunted affect, thought blocking, poverty of speech (alogia), avolition, and social withdrawal. The pathophysiology of negative symptoms is not well understood, however, it is thought to originate in the frontal lobe (Keshavan, Tandon, Boutros, & Nasrallah, 2008). Negative symptoms are difficult to treat, produce significant disability, and are those that most often prevent the individual from fully engaging in society.

Cognitive symptoms include memory and attention deficits, language difficulties, and problems with executive functioning. **Executive functioning** includes the ability to order sequential behaviors, establish goal-directed plans, and monitor personal behavior. Cognitive impairment at some level is nearly universal in patients with SSDs (Harvey & Strassnig, 2013). The cognitive impairments include deficits in episodic memory, verbal fluency, and attention (Costafreda et al., 2011; Leonard et al., 2012; Sanz, Gomez, Vargas, & Marin, 2012). Cognitive deficits are present throughout the disease course, although they may improve somewhat with antipsychotic treatment (Keefe, Bilder, & Davis, 2007; Woodberry, Giuliano, & Seidman, 2008). Cognitive impairment is associated with poorer outcomes, especially socially and vocationally (Bowie, Leung, & Reichenberg, 2008). Other features include disorganized thoughts and or behaviors, motor symptoms, and neurologic signs.

The description, diagnosis, treatment and support of individuals with these illnesses have challenged clinicians and families for hundreds of years. This chapter describes the challenges of patients with SSDs and identifies how nurses can help these patients and their families find hope and recovery.

Pause and Reflect

1. *Which symptoms of schizophrenia would you find most difficult to live with if you were the patient? Why?*
2. *Which symptoms of SSDs do you think would be most challenging for family members? Why?*

Theoretical Foundations

Multiple factors related to etiology and the course of illness affect the illness trajectory and treatment responses across all five of the domains. From genetic indicators to crippling hallucinations and delusions to the impact of SSDs on family members, patients with SSDs face numerous barriers to recovery and rehabilitation. Nurses need a thorough understanding of these factors to help patients find solutions that alleviate the enormous suffering created by the symptoms and promote hope and recovery.

Biological Domain

The complexity of SSDs and the multitude of factors influencing the course of illness and treatment responses have resulted in a variety of biological models that explain various aspects of the etiology and symptom manifestations of these disorders. Biological models of SSDs include genetics, biochemical alterations, neuropathology, neural circuitry deficits, and brain metabolism dysfunction. Additional neurobiological manifestations occur as neurologic signs, motor symptoms, and the form and organization of speech referred to as *formal thought disorder*.

Genetics

The genetic basis of the schizophrenia spectrum disorders has long been documented (Kallman, 1946). SSD risk is higher than in the general population by approximately 12 times if the disease is present in one biological parent and by approximately 40 times if present in both biological parents (Heston, 1966). Concordance among monozygotic twins is more than three times greater than in dizygotic twins (Sullivan, Kendler, & Neale, 2003); however, in monozygotic twins, there is only a 50% likelihood of both twins developing the disorder even though they share 100% of their individual genetics. This implies a relationship between the environment and individual genetic polymorphisms as to which genes are actually expressed. The proportion of SSD risk related to genetic factors is estimated at approximately 80% (Cardno et al., 1999). The Human Genome Project, completed in 2003, has identified that there are approximately 20,500 human genes in our 23 pairs of chromosomes. Linkage studies (which identify regions of the genome where schizophrenia genes might be found) suggest 22 loci associated at genome-wide significance, in particular on chromosomes 1, 2, and 5. Several other regions also receiving strong support include chromosomes 3, 6, 7, 8, 10, 11, 12, 18, and 19 (Ripke et al., 2013).

Biochemical Alterations

A number of neurochemical explanations for SSDs and their associated symptoms have been advanced. The most common is the dopamine hypothesis (Figure 17-2). The most effective medications for managing psychotic symptoms have antagonist action on the dopamine type 2 (D2) receptor; further, drugs that increase dopaminergic activity (e.g., amphetamine and cocaine) are **psychotomimetic**—they produce a condition resembling psychosis (Sadock & Sadock, 2007). Thus, the dopamine hypothesis states that psychotic symptoms result from excess dopaminergic activity in the brain, usually in the mesocortical and mesolimbic tracts. Recent

evidence has confirmed dopamine dysfunction in the striatum affecting reward processing and learning (Sorg et al., 2013).

Neuropathology

Neuropathological processes in SSDs are composed of structural defects in multiple areas. Three-dimensional imaging studies have shown consistent gray-matter reductions in the anterior cingulate, bilateral frontal lobe, hippocampus, and amygdala (Figure 17-3) (Ellison-Wright & Bullmore, 2009; Segall et al., 2009). Many individuals with SSDs also have enlarged third ventricles as compared to persons without these diseases (Wexler et al., 2009). It also is known

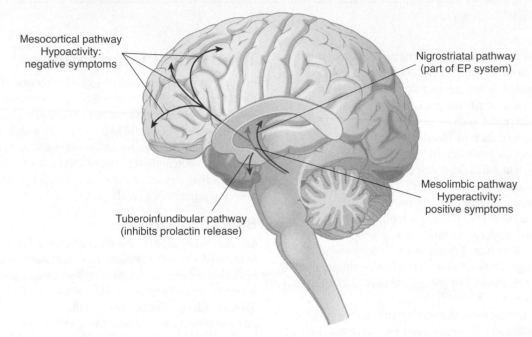

17-2   The dopamine hypothesis states that psychotic symptoms result from excess or deficient dopaminergic activity in the brain, usually in the mesocortical and mesolimbic tracts. Decreased dopaminergic activity in the mesolimbic pathway contributes to the positive symptoms of psychosis; decreased dopaminergic activity in the mesocortical pathway contributes to negative symptoms of mood and psychosis.

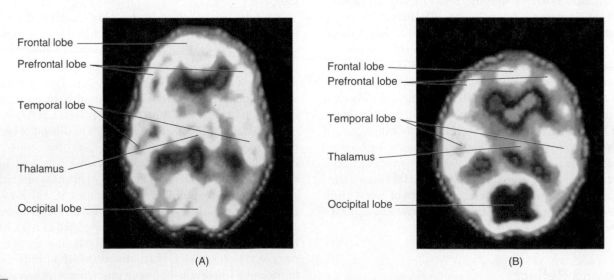

17-3   (A) PET scan of a healthy patient. (B) PET scan of a patient with schizophrenia. This patient will have serious deficits in information processing due to inactivity in the frontal lobe. Red=brain is receiving impulses; Yellow= brain is ready to receive impulses; Green=structures not receiving impulses; Blue=ventricular spaces.

Source: Science Source

that with each psychotic episode, there is atrophy in the neuropil region (synapses) which is visualized as a loss of cortical gray matter (Smiley et al., 2011).

Neural Circuitry Deficits

Neural circuitry deficits may explain the memory alterations observed in patients with SSDs (Citrome, 2011). Two problematic patterns, involving both hypo- and hyper-activation, occur in a variety of cortical and subcortical regions. These alterations cause problems mobilizing neural resources, with the result that individuals with SSDs devote greater cortical resources than the general population to perform similar tasks. In spite of this, patients with SSDs are less accurate and require more time than the general population to complete the same task (Callicott et al., 2000; Vercammen et al., 2012).

Brain Metabolism Dysfunction

Recent studies indicate the presence of mitochondrial dysfunction—including reduced mitochondrial density and volume—as well as defective mitochondrial energy production in patients with schizophrenia (Gubert et al., 2013; Somerville, Conley, & Roberts, 2011). These alterations are associated with oxidative stress, which has been found to induce cell damage (Wang, Shao, Sun, & Young, 2009).

Additional Neurobiological Manifestations

Motor symptoms, neurologic signs, and challenges with speech also plague those who suffer with SSDs. These symptoms can be particularly challenging to family and coworkers.

Motor Symptoms

Motor symptoms are common in individuals with SSDs and range from simple slowing of psychomotor activity, to isolated posturing, to catatonic states (Ungvari, Coggins, Leung, & Gerevich, 2007). Catatonic symptoms are rarely observed today, but when they do occur they involve echolalia, echopraxia, waxy flexibility, and automatic obedience. **Echolalia** is repetition of words spoken by another, whereas **echopraxia** is the compulsive imitation of another's actions. **Waxy flexibility** is a tendency to remain immobile; for instance, if an individual were to move the arm of a patient with waxy flexibility, the arm would remain where it was placed, as though it were made of wax. **Automatic obedience** is an exaggerated, robotic cooperation with requests (Weder, Muralee, Penland, & Tampi, 2008).

Neurologic Signs

Neurologic signs are divided into hard and soft signs. **Hard signs** indicate impaired reflex, sensory, or motor functioning and are localized to a particular brain region. Hard signs include hypoalgesia, impaired olfactory functioning, and oculomotor abnormalities (Tandon, Nasrallah, & Keshavan, 2009). **Soft signs** are deficits that do not implicate a specific brain area. Soft signs include grimacing, increased blink rates, problems sequencing motor tasks, and **asterognosis**—the inability to recognize objects by touch (Sadock & Sadock, 2007).

Form and Organization of Speech

Disruption in the form and organization of speech that can occur in SSDs is referred to as **formal thought disorder** (FTD) because thought process is manifested in speech. FTD is often referred to as symptoms of disorganization. FTD describes a lack of progressive goal-directed thought processes (related to the severity of neurobiological deficits) that manifest in abnormal/odd speech, affecting overall communication. FTD symptoms include loose associations, tangentiality, incoherence/word salad/neologism, illogicality, circumstantiality, pressured/distractible speech, and poverty of speech (Box 17-1).

Behavioral disorganization often accompanies formal thought disorder and ranges from inappropriate affect to attire inappropriate to the season/activity. Symptoms of FTD are more pronounced during illness exacerbations and are associated with poor outcomes (Tandon, Nasrallah, & Keshavan, 2009) due to the overall impairment in the ability to communicate.

Psychological Domain

Only recently has research been published that focuses on the psychological adjustments required to cope with the devastation created by having a psychotic episode and subsequently receiving the diagnosis of schizophrenia (Moller, 2013; Moller & Zauszniewski, 2011). This research outlines a four-phase trajectory from a psychotic episode to return to functioning that takes from 2 to 4 years to achieve and encompasses 50 specific milestones. The phases include cognitive dissonance, insight, cognitive constancy, and ordinariness (Figure 17-4).

A critical feature of psychological adjustment is the courage and ability to re-engage in normal daily interactions. Many patients are afraid to initiate conversation because they associate saying something wrong with being hospitalized. It is important to explain these phases, with the associated milestones, to family members so they can help to monitor and encourage progress. This research is critical, as it identifies significant factors that nurses can address to facilitate patient progress.

Cognitive dissonance describes the time frame of acute psychosis and the initial response to medications (6 months to 1 year) and

---

Symptoms of Formal Thought Disorder
box 17-1

Loose associations: pattern of speech in which a person's ideas slip off track onto another unrelated or obliquely related topic; also known as *derailment*.

Tangentiality: occurs when a person digresses from the topic at hand and goes off on a tangent, starting an entire new train of thought.

Incoherence/word salad/neologism: involves speaking in meaningless phrases with words that are seemingly randomly chosen, often made up, and not connected.

Illogicality: refers to speech in which there is an absence of reason and rationality.

Circumstantiality: occurs when the person goes into excessive detail about an event and has difficulty getting to the point of the conversation.

Pressured/distractible speech: can be identified when the patient is speaking rapidly and there is an extreme sense of urgency or even frenzy, as well as tangentiality. It is nearly impossible to interrupt the person.

Poverty of speech: is the opposite of pressured speech and is identified by the absence of spontaneous speech in an ordinary conversation. The person cannot engage in small talk, and gives brief or empty responses.

Cognitive Dissonance	Insight	Cognitive Constancy	Ordinariness
Period of acute psychosis and initial response to medications. Patients experience: • Loss of self-confidence • Lack of understanding, discrimination by others • Disoriented reality, confusion • Require time to adjust	6–12 months post diagnosis, a period of psychological tasks. Patients: • Learn how to control symptoms, understand limitations • Begin to communicate with others • Experience fatigue	Patients learn how to meet their own needs: • Strengthen support systems • Find purposeful activities • Gain self-confidence • Develop hope for the future • Take care of self	Patients begin to achieve independence: • Secure independent housing • Manage symptoms • Finish education • Become employed

17-4 The Milestones of Adjustment Post-Psychosis model outlines a four-phase trajectory from a psychotic episode to return to functioning that takes from 2 to 4 years to achieve and encompasses 50 specific milestones. The phases include cognitive dissonance, insight, cognitive constancy, and ordinariness.

includes 11 major milestones. During this period, the patient is working through psychological issues related to fear of another episode, loss of self-confidence, embarrassment, loss of friends, and fear of saying something wrong. The individual experiences confusion and frustration in not being able to determine what is reality and what is the illness, and cannot tolerate stress. The role of the nurse in the acute care setting is to reassure the patient that psychosis is temporary and the patient should not lose hope. Upon discharge, patients often spend long periods in isolation, during which they are trying to figure out what happened to their lives. They find it difficult to go out in public and are frequently abandoned by friends and, sadly, by family members. Often, patients are accused of withdrawing from reality and not wanting to engage in normal interactions, but in reality, patients at this stage are engaged in a highly personal time described as "sorting it out." Because of this frustration, patients may use drugs and alcohol as a means to cope and may have no energy for personal hygiene.

Insight describes the time frame (6 months to 1 year) involved in learning how to independently conduct reliable reality checks and five other milestones. The psychological tasks in this phase include learning how to cope with life now, trying to figure out thoughts, getting control of symptoms, getting used to having the diagnosis, and recognizing limitations caused by the SSD. During this period, patients very cautiously try to communicate with others. Fatigue is typical because of the psychological strain of trying to re-enter society and experiencing social setbacks. This is a critical period for family support as well. Patients who are unable to move through the insight phase often do not progress and may end up in a cycle of relapse and rehospitalization.

Cognitive constancy is a 1-to-2-year period in which the patient has the confidence to engage in normal conversation. There are 25 milestones in this period. Eight of these are in the emotional realm and include reflecting on the conditions of the initial hospital experience, the importance of a support system, and the need to have something to do with their time. Other emotional needs include a treatment environment that feels safe, the presence of reassurance and

encouragement, and the need to be around people. Patients reflect that during this phase they should not have too much quiet time, because symptoms seem to escalate when they are left alone. The most important milestone is the ability to have hope that life will get better.

There are six milestones in the cognitive realm. Patients describe the need to be able to distract themselves from the symptoms, accept the need for treatment, get back to what they used to do, and think positively. They also learn they are not the only ones with an SSD and appreciate having choices and control of their treatment.

In the interpersonal realm, seven milestones occur. Patients describe the importance of having others being honest with reality, and having someone to listen to them and understand them as well as talk to about themselves and general things. The importance of having people explain things (psychoeducation) and the need for confidence in the counselor/therapist occur in this phase. Reflection occurs as patients talk about what it was like to try to get help when they first experienced symptoms.

The final set of milestones in this phase are in the physiological realm and include the importance of medication, taking care of the body (exercise and nutrition), and developing a routine.

The final phase, *ordinariness*, lasts at least 2 years and has seven important milestones that reflect that ability to function independently. These milestones include being able to think about the future, accomplish life goals, secure independent housing, manage symptoms, finish education, and become employed. The ultimate milestone is described as being able to do what other people do.

Sociocultural Domain

Cultural factors affect diagnosis, functioning, course, and treatment of SSDs. Culture has an impact on beliefs, opinions, and attitudes that shape not only the individual's help-seeking behavior, but also the mental health system's responses to them. Compared with Caucasians, African Americans (especially men) are more likely to be diagnosed with SSDs and less likely to be diagnosed with an affective disorder (Dealberto, 2010). African Americans with SSDs are less likely to be diagnosed with a co-morbid anxiety or mood disorder

(Barnes, 2008). The source of these differences may include actual variability among cultural groups, but it is also possible that disparities in symptom interpretation, help-seeking behaviors, and treatment referral reflect the cultural bias of clinicians and/or bias in assessment tools. Because of the cultural implications of stigma, lack of public understanding of SSDs, and the use of legal coercion to control behavior, understanding cultural context is especially important for clinicians treating patients with SSDs. Clinicians should also remain mindful of personal, unacknowledged cultural bias.

The SSDs result in severe impairments in the sociocultural domain, including difficulties with maintaining interpersonal relationships. As a result, many individuals with SSDs have problematic family relationships, are socially isolated, and struggle to sustain competitive employment. In addition, a variety of sociocultural factors have been implicated in SSD etiology. Sociocultural conditions include both biological and psychosocial risk factors spanning the period before birth through young adulthood.

A meta-analysis reported significantly higher risk for SSDs in males, those living in urban compared with rural environments, and individuals with a personal or family history of migration (Sutterland et al., 2013). Recent studies have clarified that this association stems from both the tendency of patients with SSDs to congregate in inner cities (Kelly et al., 2010) and an *additional* association between urban birth and childhood (until age 15) with an increased risk for developing SSDs (Kirkbride et al., 2006).

Relative risk of developing SSDs has been documented as 2.7 times greater than the general population for first-generation and 4.5 times greater than the general population for second-generation immigrants. Proposed explanations include the socially isolated status of immigrants, discrimination (Cooper et al., 2008), or biological explanations, such as vitamin D deficiency (Dealberto, 2007); however, a specific factor associated with immigration status remains to be identified. A significantly higher prevalence of SSDs has been observed in more developed as opposed to less developed countries, as well as among individuals of lower as opposed to higher socioeconomic status (Saha, Chant, Welham, & McGrath, 2005).

No single environmental risk factor has thus far been shown sufficient or necessary to cause any SSD. Although biological and environmental influences are clearly important, specific risks and the mechanisms of causation remain a mystery. Associations have been made from the point of conception through pregnancy, birth, childhood, and adolescence to have an association with etiology; these are described in Table 17-1.

Spiritual Domain

Patients with SSDs contend with a chronic illness that affects their reality testing, emotional responses, thinking processes, and communication and judgment. The impact of these symptoms raises multiple questions about life meaning, hope, suffering, coping, and recovery. Although spirituality (which addresses transcendence and life meaning) and religiosity (specific behaviors with social and doctrinal characteristics) are considered by many to provide useful resources in schizophrenia coping and recovery, these aspects of coping have only recently begun to be examined by researchers (Mohr & Huguelet, 2004). Further, many clinicians are reluctant to address religion and spirituality in this group of patients.

Multiple factors may account for a neglect of religious and spiritual themes in psychiatric practice. Mental health professionals receive

Risk Factors Associated with the Development of SSDs　table 17-1

Time Period	Event	Association	Mechanism
Conception	Paternal age greater than 60 years	Doubles the risk of SSDs	Unknown but may be due to impaired spermatogenesis and resultant mutation(s)
First and early second trimester	Maternal influenza, rubella, or toxoplasmosis	Increased risk of developing SSDs	Unknown but may involve suboptimal immune response and/or elevated maternal antibody titers
First trimester	Severe maternal nutritional deficiency, severe maternal stress	Increased risk of developing SSDs	Stress sensitization with resultant hyperdopaminergia
Birthing process	Complicated delivery	Doubles the risk of SSDs	Hypoxia
Birth	During late winter or early spring	5–10% greater likelihood of SSDs	Unknown but may be related to prenatal maternal infection
Childhood	Trauma, head injury, parental separation or death, infection, urban setting, migration	Increased risk of developing SSDs	Unknown
Adolescence	Cannabis use, social adversity, stressful life events	Increased risk of developing SSDs	Unknown

Data from Allardyce, J., & Boydell, J. (2006). Review: The wider social environment and schizophrenia. *Schizophrenia Bulletin, 32*(4), 592–598; Byrne, M., Agerbo, E., & Bennedsen, B. (2007). Obstetric conditions and risk of first admission with schizophrenia: A Danish national register-based study. *Schizophrenia Research, 97*(1–3), 51–59; Cheng, J. Y., Ko, J. S., & Chen, R. Y. (2008). Meta-regression analysis using latitude as moderator of paternal age related schizophrenia risk. *Schizophrenia Research, 99*(1–3), 71–76; Dalman, C., Alleback, P., & Gunnell, D. (2008). Infections in the CNS during childhood and the risk of subsequent psychotic illness: A cohort study of more than one million Swedish subjects. *American Journal of Psychiatry, 165*(1), 59–65; Davies, G., Welham, J., & Chant, D. (2003). A systematic review and meta-analysis of Northern Hemisphere season of birth studies in schizophrenia. *Schizophrenia Bulletin, 29*(3), 587–593; Goldberg, T. E., & Gomar, J. J. (2009). Targeting cognition in schizophrenia research: From etiology to treatment. *American Journal of Psychiatry, 166*(6), 631–644; Khashan, A. S., Abel, K. M., & McNamee, R. (2008). Higher risk of offspring schizophrenia following antenatal exposure to serious adverse life events. *Archives of General Psychiatry, 65*, 146–152.

little training in integration of religion and spirituality into care provision (Borras et al., 2010), and clinicians tend to pathologize the religious dimensions of life (Pesut, 2008). This tendency is reinforced in schizophrenia because, during the course of the illness, religion may be a manifestation of psychosis (delusion) as well as a coping behavior.

Typical religious delusions include persecutory or grandiose themes. Assessment of such themes is a critical safety issue, as these symptoms may lead to violent behavior. In some cases, religiously deluded patients have taken biblical statements literally and attempted to "pluck out" offending eyes or "cut off" offending body parts (Field & Waldfogel, 1995; Waugh, 1986). Religious delusions may affect treatment adherence if patients refuse medication in the hope of supernatural healing. Religious delusions are associated with poorer outcomes and are held more strongly than delusions with nonreligious content (Siddle, Haddock, Tarrier, & Faragher, 2002). Thus, the first step in providing safe care related to the spiritual domain is assessing for delusions with religious content.

Clinicians may differentiate religious delusions from religious beliefs on the basis of three criteria: (1) The patient's self-description of the experience is recognizable as a form of delusion (for example, believing to be God); (2) other symptoms of mental illness are present across multiple domains (for example, cognitive deficits associated with schizophrenia), and (3) behavior following the event is consistent with mental illness rather than a personally enriching life experience—for example, ongoing difficulties in work and/or interpersonal relationships (Sims, 1995).

Although the first responsibility of clinicians is to provide for patient safety, the provision of holistic care dictates that matters concerning the spiritual domain be incorporated into ongoing care when it is safe to do so. The mere presence of religious thought distortions at certain times during the illness trajectory does not negate every religious experience. Individuals with schizophrenia have the same spiritual needs as any other human being. Religion and spirituality are critical to recovery and reconstruction of a functional sense of self. (Leamy et al., 2011).

The first step in successfully addressing patient spiritual/religious needs is the clinician's awareness of his or her own religious or spiritual identity. Patients benefit from open discussion of religious issues, but one study documented that clinicians raise the subject in only 36% of cases (Huguelet et al., 2006). Psychiatric nurses can begin by adding religion and spirituality to every assessment. During such discussions, nurses must cultivate an acceptance of diverse of opinions and practices, respect patient beliefs, and avoid proselytizing (Mohr & Huguelet, 2004). The experience of recovery from schizophrenia has been conceptualized as encompassing several key processes, including finding hope, re-establishing identity, and finding meaning in life (Mohr et al., 2010). Spirituality has a role to play in accomplishing these important recovery-related tasks.

Pause and Reflect

1. *Has anyone you know been diagnosed with an SSD? What are their symptoms? How do their symptoms affect their functioning in the five domains?*

2. *What symptoms or aspects of schizophrenia spectrum disorders do you think that you, as a nurse, would find most challenging, and why? What would you do to make sure that your feelings would not negatively affect the patient?*

Schizophrenia Spectrum Disorders

Schizophrenia is a disturbance lasting at least 6 months (if untreated) that consists of at least two major symptoms from either the list of positive or negative symptoms; one of the cardinal symptoms must be either delusions, hallucinations, or disorganized speech (see DSM-5 Diagnostic Criteria for Schizophrenia). **Schizoaffective disorder** is diagnosed when major mood symptoms (depression,

---

Diagnostic Criteria for Schizophrenia   DSM-5

A. Two (or more) of the following, each present for a significant portion of time during a 1-month period (or less if successfully treated). At least one of these must be (1), (2), or (3):
  1. Delusions.
  2. Hallucinations.
  3. Disorganized speech (e.g., frequent derailment or incoherence).
  4. Grossly disorganized or catatonic behavior.
  5. Negative symptoms (i.e., diminished emotional expression or avolition).
B. For a significant portion of the time since the onset of the disturbance, level of functioning in one or more major areas, such as work, interpersonal relations, or self-care, is markedly below the level achieved prior to the onset (or when the onset is in childhood or adolescence, there is failure to achieve expected level of interpersonal, academic, or occupational functioning).
C. Continuous signs of the disturbance persist for at least 6 months. This 6-month period must include at least 1 month of symptoms (or less if successfully treated) that meet Criterion A (i.e., active-phase symptoms) and may include periods of prodromal or residual symptoms. During these prodromal or residual periods, the

signs of the disturbance may be manifested by only negative symptoms or by two more symptoms listed in Criterion A present in an attenuated form (e.g., odd beliefs, unusual perceptual experiences).
D. Schizoaffective disorder and depressive or bipolar disorder with psychotic features have been ruled out because either (1) no major depressive or manic episodes have occurred concurrently with the active-phase symptoms, or (2) if mood episodes have occurred during active-phase symptoms, they have been present for a minority of the total duration of the active and residual periods of the illness.
E. The disturbance is not attributable to the physiological effects of a substance (e.g., a drug of abuse, a medication) or another medical condition.
F. If there is a history of autism spectrum disorder or a communication disorder of childhood onset, the additional diagnosis of schizophrenia is made only if prominent delusions or hallucinations, in addition to the other required symptoms of schizophrenia, are also present for at least 1 month (or less if successfully treated).

Source: Reprinted with permission from the *Diagnostic and Statistical Manual of Mental Disorders*, Fifth Edition, (Copyright 2013). American Psychiatric Association.

mania, or both) occur during most of the same period of illness as delusions or hallucinations and last at least 2 weeks (American Psychiatric Association [APA], 2013). *Schizophreniform disorder* has the same symptoms as schizophrenia. The only difference in the criteria is that symptoms have lasted between 1 and 6 months, but do not meet the 6-month duration criterion of schizophrenia.

A *brief psychotic episode* consists of one or more of the hallmark symptoms of schizophrenia but lasts from only 1 day to less than 1 month. The patient also returns to the pre-illness level of function.

Delusional disorder is identified by the presence of one or more delusions lasting at least a month or longer. There are several subtypes, which include erotomanic, grandiose, jealous, persecutory, somatic, and mixed. The most frequent type of delusions is persecutory, followed by jealous.

Each of the major disorders has conditions that must be met before the diagnosis can be made, including ruling out medical illnesses and substance use as the primary cause, as well as effect on the ability to function from day to day.

Course of Illness

Seventy-five percent of patients with SSDs are diagnosed in adolescence or early adulthood. Premorbid symptoms occurring in childhood include nonspecific social, cognitive, or motor dysfunctions such as motor delays, social isolation, poor academic performance, or emotional detachment.

Schizophrenia and schizoaffective disorder are often preceded by a prodromal period, which may be more than a year in length. The **prodrome**, or prodromal period, a symptomatic period prior to the diagnosis of SSDs, represents a definite change from premorbid functioning, is clearly identified as problematic, and continues until the emergence of psychotic symptoms. The prodrome may last only weeks but the usual length is between 2 and 5 years (Schultze-Lutter, Schimmelmann, Klosterkotter, & Ruhrman, 2012). The prodrome is associated with severe impairment and nonspecific symptoms such as sleep disturbance, poor concentration, and social withdrawal (Schultze-Lutter, 2009). Later in the prodrome, positive symptoms appear, such as perceptual abnormalities and suspiciousness, and ideas of reference emerge (Woods, Tandy, & McGlashan, 2001). For example, prodromal individuals may believe they have special gifts, such as the ability to communicate with inanimate objects. The first psychotic episode may be insidious or acute and heralds the onset of schizophrenia or schizoaffective disorder, typically occurring between ages 15 and 45 years. The psychotic phase has three distinct phases:

- *Acute:* florid psychosis; for example, delusions, hallucinations, thought disorder.
- *Stabilization:* the 6-to-18-month period following the acute psychosis.
- *Maintenance:* a period when negative and residual symptoms typically remain but are less severe (APA, 2009).

The first 5 years after the first episode are known as the *early course* and may be associated with additional deterioration that tapers off by 5 to 10 years following diagnosis. Long-term outcomes vary between recovery and incapacitation. Some 10% to 15% of those diagnosed with schizophrenia or schizoaffective disorder have no further episodes, but most patients have exacerbations throughout

their lives, and 10% to 15% experience chronic psychosis (Quintero, Barbudo Del Cura, Lopez-Ibor, & Lopez, 2011).

The classic course of both schizophrenia and schizoaffective disorder is one of symptom exacerbations and remissions. Although the positive symptoms appear to plateau within 5 to 10 years of diagnosis, negative symptoms become more pronounced as the disease progresses; as a result, patients become increasingly socially disabled over time. Pronounced negative symptoms, poor social support, and social withdrawal are indicators of a poor outcome, with cognitive deficits being more predictive of poor community functioning than symptom level (Kurtz & Richardson, 2011).

Men with SSDs have a younger age at onset, poorer premorbid history, more negative symptoms, and a poorer course than women with the disease. Women with SSDs have more affective symptoms, more positive symptoms, and a better disease course (defined as fewer hospitalizations and less substance abuse) than men. Women respond more rapidly to medications, showing more symptom improvement regardless of stage of illness and requiring lower medication dosages than men with SSDs. However, women with SSDs experience more **dystonia** (spastic contractions of muscle groups), Parkinsonism, **akathisia** (sensations of restlessness, pacing, and an inability to sit still), and tardive dyskinesia (TD) than men and experience higher medication-related prolactin elevations (Zhang et al., 2009). **Tardive dyskinesia** is a movement disorder characterized by involuntary, repetitive movements often associated with neuroleptic therapy and advanced age.

No single symptom is diagnostic and no laboratory test exists to confirm a diagnosis of an SSD. There is wide variability in symptom expression, affect, and level of functioning both among individuals with SSDs and within the same person over time. Good prognostic indicators include adult onset, the presence of precipitating factor(s), acute onset, high **premorbid** (prior to onset of symptoms) function, mood symptoms, being married rather than single, family history of mood disorders, a good support system, and positive symptoms (e.g., hallucinations). Indicators of a poor prognosis include onset in childhood/adolescence; absence of precipitating factor(s); insidious onset; poor premorbid function; withdrawn/autistic symptoms; being single, divorced, or widowed; family history of SSDs; poor support system; negative/neurologic symptoms; history of prenatal trauma; no remissions in a 3-year period; multiple relapses; and a history of assaultive behavior.

Risk for Co-Morbid Medical Illness

In addition to their chronic psychiatric illness, patients with SSDs are at increased risk for a number of other medical conditions. The rates of obesity, dyslipidemia, glucose dysregulation, and type 2 diabetes are higher in patients with SSDs than in the general population. As a result, the risk for cardiovascular disease among individuals with SSDs is approximately 12 times that of the general population. In addition to taking medications that are associated with weight gain, patients with SSDs have many other risk factors (poor diet, sedentary lifestyle, lack of access to medical care) that lead to increased morbidity and mortality. In addition to type 2 diabetes and dyslipidemias, hypertension is also common in individuals with SSDs (Brunero & Lamont, 2010; DeHert, Schreurs, Vancampfort, & van Winkel, 2009).

The diets of individuals with SSDs are higher in fat and lower in fiber than those of individuals with no mental illness. Studies have documented that patients with SSDs consume more saturated fat and

Comparison of Side Effects of Common Antipsychotic Medications   table 17-2

Medication	Increased Prolactin Level	Hypotension	Sedation	Glucose Abnormalities	Increased QTc Interval
Clozapine	negligible	high	high	high	negligible
Risperidone	high	moderate	low	moderate	low
Olanzapine	low	low	low	high	low
Quetiapine	low	moderate	high	moderate	low
Ziprasidone	low	low	low	low	moderate
Aripiprazole	low	low	moderate	low	low
Iloperidone	negligible	high	low	low	negligible
Asenapine	negligible	low	moderate	low	negligible
Lurasidone	negligible	low	moderate	low	negligible
Thioridizine	moderate	moderate	moderate	low	high
Perphenazine	moderate	low	low	low	negligible
Haloperidol	high	negligible	moderate	negligible	negligible

Medication	Extrapyramidal Symptoms	Lipid Abnormalities	Weight Gain	Anticholinergic Effects
Clozapine	low	high	high	high
Risperidone	moderate	moderate	moderate	negligible
Olanzapine	low	high	high	moderate
Quetiapine	low	moderate	moderate	low
Ziprasidone	low	low	low	low
Aripiprazole	low	low	low	low
Iloperidone	negligible	low	low	negligible
Asenapine	moderate	low	low	negligible
Lurasidone	high	low	low	negligible
Thioridizine	low	low	low	moderate
Perphenazine	moderate	low	low	negligible
Haloperidol	high	negligible	low	negligible

refined sugar than healthy individuals (Bobes, Arango, Garcia-Garcia, & Rejas, 2010; Stokes & Peet, 2003). Poor diet is associated with poverty and unstable living conditions, as well as frequent fast food consumption (Masand, 1999). Further, patients with SSDs may not understand relationships between weight and diet, or how to improve their eating habits (Osborn, Nazareth, & King, 2007).

Individuals with SSDs are less active and less aerobically fit than the general population (Beebe et al., 2010). This is particularly troubling because physical inactivity is one of the most prevalent risk factors for the development of obesity and cardiovascular disease (U.S. Department of Health and Human Services, 2011). Factors contributing to reduced physical activity and exercise in patients with SSDs include negative symptoms such as social withdrawal; lack of access to fitness information, facilities or equipment; and sedative effects of medications.

Collaborative Care

Collaborative care of patients with SSDs requires a multidisciplinary approach that typically includes treatment with antipsychotics and one or more psychosocial treatments. Health promotion and education are critical for patients with SSDs; these are discussed later, in the section on Nursing Management.

Psychopharmacology

The quality of the relationship between the care provider and the patient is critical to treatment success. Initial patient education includes medication indications, expected and adverse effects, when to report adverse effects, alternative treatments available, rationale for dosing decisions, and the likelihood of relapse if medication is discontinued.

Antipsychotics

Antipsychotic medications are the mainstay of SSD treatment. Antipsychotic medications are categorized as either typical or atypical on the basis of similarities in the mechanism of action (Chapter 23). The older, typical, or first-generation antipsychotic (FGA) medications act primarily to reduce positive symptoms by blocking dopamine receptors and increasing dopamine destruction.

Second-generation antipsychotics (SGAs) have an antagonist function against serotonin, as well as dopamine (Citrome, 2012; Stahl, 2013.). Although FGAs are still prescribed, SGAs generally are the treatment of choice based on side-effect profile and improvements in negative symptoms. In 2002, aripiprazole (Abilify), a third-generation antipsychotic, was made available. This medication has a partial agonist function for dopamine rather than an antagonist function. The medications feature provides dosage information, side effects, and nursing interventions for common SGAs and aripiprazole.

A meta-analysis of 150 double-blind studies including 21,533 individuals with SSDs compared FGAs and SGAs. For overall efficacy, the SGAs clozapine, olanzapine, and risperidone were significantly better than the FGAs. The other SGAs were no more efficacious than the FGAs (Leucht, Corves, & Arbter, 2009). See Table 17-2 for a comparison of common side effects of the antipsychotic medications.

Clozapine

Clozapine, the first of the SGAs, was initially pulled from the market as a result of deaths from agranulocytosis. However, because of its efficacy, it was again made available with several strict guidelines related to WBC monitoring. The APA (2004) recommends that patients with SSDs receive a trial of clozapine in the following situations: (1) no response to a 6-week trial of two other antipsychotic medications; and/or (2) persistent suicidal ideation or hostility/aggression. The clozapine trial should be at least 3 months long.

APA (2004) guidelines further specify that clozapine should be stopped immediately when the WBC drops below 2000 or the absolute neutrophil count (ANC) is <1000. When this happens, the WBC with differential should be drawn daily and bone marrow aspiration should be considered. The patient may need to be placed in protective isolation. Clozapine should not be resumed.

If the WBC is between 2000 and 3000 or the ANC is between 1000 and 1500, clozapine should be stopped immediately and the WBC with differential drawn daily. Symptoms of infection must be monitored. Clozapine can be resumed if there is infection as long as the WBC > 3000 and ANC > 1500.

If the WBC is initially between 3000 and 3500 but falls to 3000 in 3 weeks or less and the ANC is >1500 mm^3, the WBC with differential should be repeated twice a week until WBC > 3500.

Extrapyramidal Symptoms

Extrapyramidal side effects (EPSs) are common in patients treated with antipsychotic medications (Veselinović et al., 2011) and involve an imbalance between dopamine and acetylcholine in the extrapyramidal system of the basal ganglia. As such, the symptoms involve the systemic motor system. Side effects may be acute or chronic. Acute EPSs include medication-induced Parkinsonism (e.g., muscle rigidity, tremors, problems with gait), dystonia (acute muscle spasms, often in the extremities), akathisia (intolerable restlessness and inability to sit still), opisthotonus (severe arching of the back), and oculogyric crisis (eyeballs rolling back into the socket). These acute side effects cause extreme distress and pain. They usually occur within the first hours, days, or weeks of treatment, are dose dependent, and are reversible if medication is reduced or discontinued. They are most common with the first generation antipsychotics that are primarily dopamine 2 receptor blockers, many of the antidepressants that effect the norepinephrine/dopamine systems, and antihistamines.

The primary chronic EPS is tardive dyskinesia (TD), which occurs after months or years of medication exposure and typically involve the oral/facial/maxillary muscles, causing uncontrollable twitching of the eyes and neck, tongue thrusting, and eye blinking. Early identification and a withdrawal or reduction of medication may be sufficient to reverse the side effects, but otherwise EPSs—in particular, TD—may be irreversible even if medication is discontinued (Adams, Holland, & Urban, 2014). In the case of acute EPS, anticholinergic/antihistamine medications can be helpful, except in akathisia, in which the treatment of choice is norepinephrine beta-blockers (Aia, Ravuelta, Cloud, & Factor, 2011).

Neuroleptic Malignant Syndrome

Neuroleptic malignant syndrome (NMS) is a rare, life-threatening, and often fatal side effect of antipsychotic medications in which the body temperature can increase to over 105°F quickly. Other symptoms include muscle rigidity and two or more of the following: excessive sweating, difficulty swallowing, tremor, incontinence, changes in the level of consciousness, inability to speak, autonomic dysfunction, leukocytosis, and elevated creatine kinase. Complications include

Schizophrenic Spectrum Disorders

Medication	Usual Adult Dosage Range	Side Effect Profile	Nursing Considerations/Monitoring
clozapine (Clozaril)	12.5 mg/day PO (orally) to start; titrate slowly up to maintenance dose of 350–450 mg/day in divided doses; do not exceed 900 mg/day.	• Sedation • Weight gain • Agranulocytosis • Drooling	• Check WBC prior to starting. Weekly WBC counts for first 6 months and monthly for duration of treatment. Resume weekly WBC for one month after discontinuation. • Report symptoms of infection. • Report tachycardia and sedation during titration. • Teach patients to avoid drugs and foods that may affect clozapine levels or result in interactions, including carbamazepine, phenytoin (Dilantin), St. John's wort, grapefruit juice, fluvoxamine, and erythromycin.
risperidone (Risperdal) risperidone IM (Consta)	2–16 mg/day PO either once a day or in divided doses 25–50 mg IM (intramuscularly) every 2 weeks	All side effects increase above 6 mg daily intake. • Weight gain • Sedation • Orthostatic hypertension • Glucose dysregulation • Hyperprolactinemia	• Monitor fasting blood sugar and lipids. • Provide nutrition and exercise counseling. • Teach patients that fluoxetine and paroxetine may increase risperidone to toxic levels.
paliperidone (Invega) paliperidone palmitate (IM) (Invega Sustenna)	3–9 mg PO 154–256 mg every 4 weeks after loading dose	• Same as risperidone	• Same as risperidone
olanzapine (Zyprexa) olanzapine pamoate (Zyprexa Relprevv) (Zyprexa Zydis)	5–20 mg/day PO 150–300 mg every 2 weeks or 405 mg every 4 weeks IM Sublingual Women have higher olanzapine levels than men at equivalent doses.	• Weight gain • Glucose dysregulation • Metabolic syndrome • Dose-related extrapyramidal symptoms • After IM must stay in the clinic for 3 hours for observation and not allowed to drive because of sedation	• Monitor fasting blood sugar. • Provide nutrition and exercise counseling. • Teach patients to avoid drugs and foods that may affect levels of olanzapine, including phenytoin (Dilantin), St. John's wort, cruciferous vegetables, and smoking. • Use with caution in patients who require insulin, which reduces levels of olanzapine.
quetiapine IR (Seroquel) quetiapine XR (Seroquel XR) (dosing same except take entire dose at HS)	25–800 mg PO daily in divided doses 100–300 mg for depression 300–600 mg for mania 600–800 mg for psychosis	• Sedation • Weight gain • Glucose dysregulation • Metabolic syndrome	• Monitor fasting blood sugar. • Provide nutrition and exercise counseling. • Must take XR no later than 7 pm to avoid daytime sedation. • Teach patients that paroxetine, fluoxetine, tricyclics increase levels; dexamethasone decreases levels.
ziprasidone (Geodon) (Geodon IM)	40–200 mg/day PO in divided doses or 10–20 mg IM for acute agitation	• Sedation • Rhinitis • Muscle weakness • May prolong QT interval	• Use with caution in patients with obesity, diabetes, history of myocardial infarction, or congestive heart failure. • Report syncope, dizziness, palpitations. • Monitor electrolytes and EKG. • Must be taken with food to avoid loss of 40% of absorption. • Caution patients to avoid diuretics, calcium channel blockers, beta-blockers, digoxin. • Dilantin (phenytoin), St. John's wort, cruciferous vegetables, carbamazepine, and phenobarbital decrease ziprasidone levels. • Astemizole (Hismanal), erythromycin (E-mycin), fluvoxamine (Luvox), fluoxetine (Prozac), grapefruit juice, starfruit increase levels.
aripiprazole (Abilify) aripiprazole (IM depot) (Abilify Maintena)	10–30 mg/day PO 400 mg once a month IM	• Agitation • Gastrointestinal distress	• Monitor and report suicidal ideation, tardive dyskinesia, symptoms of neuroleptic malignant syndrome. • Teach patients to avoid drugs and foods that can influence levels of aripiprazole (see ziprasidone).

Medication	Usual Adult Dosage Range	Side Effect Profile	Nursing Considerations/Monitoring
iloperidone (Fanapt)	PO 12–24 mg/day	• Sedation • Dizziness, lightheadedness • Tachycardia • Nausea, vomiting • Anxiety, nervousness • Orthostatic hypotension	• Low incidence of extrapyramidal side effects. • Patient should get up slowly from a lying position. • Teach patients to avoid drugs and foods that can influence levels of aripiprazole (see ziprasidone).
asenapine (Saphris)	5–10mg SL	• Weight gain, but less than others in the class • Sedation • EPS • No reports of hyperprolactinemia	• Monitor cardiovascular system, including signs of orthostatic hypotension, syncope. • Stop dosage and report on signs of neuroleptic malignant syndrome. • Available in cherry and orange flavors. • Avoid food or milk for 10 minutes after taking. • Teach patient to avoid phenytoin (Dilantin), St. John's wort, cruciferous vegetables; use with caution in patients with insulin, which reduces asenapine levels.
lurasidone (Latuda)	40–80 mg PO	• Sedation • EPS • Minimal weight gain or sexual dysfunction	• Must take with food to avoid loss of 40% of absorption • Astemizole, erythromycin, fluvoxamine, fluoxetine, grapefruit juice, starfruit increase levels. • St. John's wort, phenobarbital, carbamazepine decrease levels.

Based on Adams, Holland, & Urban (2014). *Pharmacology for Nurses: A Pathophysiologic Approach* (4th ed.). Upper Saddle River, NJ: Prentice Hall; Wilson, B. A., Shannon, M. T., & Shields, K. (2014). *Pearson Nurse's Drug Guide.* Upper Saddle River, NJ: Prentice Hall; Citrome, L. (2012). A systematic review of meta-analyses of the efficacy of oral atypical antipsychotics for the treatment of adult patients with schizophrenia. *Expert Opinion on Pharmacotherapy, 13*(11), 1545–1573; Stahl, S. (2013). *Essential Psychopharmacology* (4th ed.) New York, NY: Cambridge University Press.

rhabdomyolysis (breakdown of muscle tissue), renal failure, and death. NMS develops within days and can sometimes be hard to diagnose. Treatment involves aggressive supportive measures that include circulatory and ventilatory support as needed; cooling blankets and antipyretics to control temperature; aggressive fluid resuscitation; and alkalization of urine to help prevent acute renal failure and enhance excretion of muscle breakdown products. Typically, all symptoms resolve within 7 to 14 days after antipsychotics are discontinued unless the patient is on long-acting injectable medications, in which symptoms can last up to 30 days.

Treatment Response

Ten to 30 percent of patients with SSDs have little or no response to medications and another 30% have a partial response, defined as ongoing positive symptoms. Partial response may be due to a variety of factors, including suboptimal dosing or nonadherence. Nurses should first assess whether medication was continued for at least 2 to 4 weeks, and that the patient was at least 80% adherent to the medication during that time period. After several such trials with different medications, prescribers may consider augmentation with a second antipsychotic, such as aripiprazole; a mood stabilizer, such as lithium; or a benzodiazepine, such as lorazepam (Stahl, 2009).

Psychotherapy and Social Supports

Because medications alone do not completely address many of the deficits of the SSDs, limiting the focus of treatment to medication alone is a disservice to patients. Although the SGAs have provided a step forward in control of positive symptoms and enhancement of cognitive functions, up to 60% of patients with SSDs who adhere to

pharmacologic therapy continue to experience ongoing positive or negative symptoms (Kaiser, Heekeren, & Simon, 2011). Even among those who respond well to medication, many struggle with impairment in social functioning, have difficulty with activities of daily living, lack productivity, and suffer reduced quality of life. Because of the far-reaching deficits and multifactorial complexity associated with SSDs, myriad psychosocial treatments have been proposed. The Schizophrenia Patient Outcomes Research Team (PORT) recommends the following psychosocial treatments: family therapy, social skills training (SST), vocational rehabilitation, cognitive–behavioral therapy (CBT), and the services of an assertive community treatment (ACT) team (Kreyenbuhl, 2010; Kreyenbuhl, Buchanan, Dickerson, & Dixon, 2010).

Family Psychoeducation

Family psychoeducation is one of the longest standing, best researched, and most successful treatments for SSDs. Studies of family interventions have shown reduced hospitalizations, improved patient–family relationships, improved medication adherence, and improved social functioning. In addition, family psychoeducation provides an opportunity to assess and work toward change at the system level, enabling families to provide optimal support and assistance to their loved ones (Pilling et al., 2002).

Social Skills Training

Social skills training for individuals with SSDs targets a variety of skills, including social, financial, communication, and problem-solving skills. Patients typically require assistance with the acquisition of skills such as conversation, food preparation, shopping, and using public transportation. Although the content and duration of social skills training programs vary, all the programs break target behaviors into smaller tasks. For example, a complex skill such as making friends is divided into manageable steps. The first step teaches the use of introductory remarks, followed by more specific questions (Box 17-2), and, finally, sharing personal information. Nonverbal behaviors, gestures, tone of voice, and mannerisms are likewise broken down, and reminders such as "make eye contact" and "nod your head" are used. Other social skills training techniques include modeling, behavioral rehearsal, corrective feedback, positive reinforcement, and homework assignments. Frequent repetition and handouts are used to cope with the attention and executive functioning deficits that are common in patients with SSDs. Most social skills training is done in small groups in six to eight sessions, meeting two or three times a week for 6 months to 2 years, depending on the program type and the number of skills addressed.

Vocational Rehabilitation

Vocational rehabilitation provides a variety of support services on a continuum from cognitive and skills assessments to supported employment to education and training on how to obtain and maintain competitive employment. Among a wide variety of programs that have been developed are vocational skills training, job placement, transitional employment, supported employment, vocational counseling, and vocational education.

For individuals with SSDs, employment has been associated with increased social contact, reduced severity of positive and negative symptoms, reduced hospitalizations, higher self-esteem, reduced health care costs, better clinician assessments of functioning, and improved quality of life in individuals with SSDs (Uçok, Gorwood, & Karadayi on behalf of the EGOFORS, 2011). Factors associated with improved vocational outcomes include an emphasis on patient preferences, rapid job placement, ongoing support, a focus on problem solving, and support and education for employers and coworkers.

When assisting patients who are receiving vocational rehabilitation services, nurses take a primarily collaborative role, working with other health team members to move the patient toward identified vocational goals. In addition, nurses may play adjunct roles, including the assessment of medication response, coping skills interventions, and/or crisis intervention, all of which may assist patients in meeting vocational goals. Nurses may make referrals and should contact their local mental health center for program and referral information.

Social Skills Therapy for Schizophrenia   box 17-2

Example: Conversation Skills

SKILL: Maintaining conversations

RATIONALE: Asking questions is one way to keep a conversation going. Another way is to give factual information to the other person. This allows people to learn more about each other and identify things they might have in common. Factual information tells who, what, where, when, and how.

Steps of the Skill

1. Greet the person.
2. Give the other person some information.
3. See if the other person is listening and wants to continue the conversation.

Scenes to use in Role Plays

1. Telling someone at the community residence about an outing planned for the weekend.
2. Telling a friend about a movie or TV show that you saw recently.
3. Telling someone at your day program about a current event that interests you.

Special Considerations

Use role-play scenes to help patients identify appropriate information for each situation used. Be sure to discuss which type of information is appropriate in a given situation. For example, personal information that would be appropriate during a therapy session might not be appropriate in a social setting.

I. PRINCIPLES, FORMAT, AND TECHNIQUES
   1. Assess social skills/goal setting via interviewing and behavioral observation of role-plays.
   2. Introduce social skills and steps of social skills training.
   3. Techniques for consolidating social skills include repetition, role play, and homework assignments.

4. Starting a skills group may be considered when at least six patients are in need of social skills training. Consider practical considerations for planning a group, selecting group leaders, selecting patients, preparing patients for participation.
5. Tailor skills for individual needs. Use patient goals to design social skills training groups. Manage the range of skill levels, keep all members involved, and conduct ongoing assessment of progress made in group.
6. Troubleshooting: Anticipate common problems and problems with highly symptomatic patients and those with dual diagnoses.
7. Creating a supportive environment: Develop a social learning milieu, educate family members to support social skills goal attainment.

II. TEACHING SPECIFIC SOCIAL SKILLS

- **Conversation skills:** Listening to others, starting conversations, maintaining conversations by asking questions, maintaining conversations by giving factual information, maintaining conversations by expressing feelings, ending conversations, staying on the topic set by another person, what to do when someone goes off the topic, getting your point across
- **Conflict management skills:** Compromise and negotiation, disagreeing with another's opinion without arguing, responding to untrue accusations, leaving stressful situations
- **Friendship and dating skills:** Expressing positive feelings, giving compliments, accepting compliments, finding common interests, asking someone for a date, ending a date, expressing affection, refusing unwanted sexual advances, requesting that one's partner use a condom, refusing pressure to engage in high-risk sexual behavior

Cognitive–Behavioral Therapy

Research has examined cognitive–behavioral therapy (CBT) as a psychosocial treatment for patients with SSDs to enhance coping and reduce symptoms that do not respond to medications. During CBT interventions, patients with SSDs are encouraged to reframe psychotic symptoms as coping attempts, rather than as signs that the individual is crazy or weak. The problem-solving process is used to identify new coping strategies and reinforce their use. Coping strategies may involve cognitive processes such as distraction, positive self-talk, or behavioral processes such as exercising or taking a walk. Homework consists of practicing techniques and reporting on results. CBT is typically provided in outpatient settings on an individual or group basis and varies from six sessions to more than 20 (Wykes, Steel, Everitt, & Tarrier, 2008). Psychiatric nurses may use CBT principles in interactions to assist patients with SSDs to begin to identify and change cognitive distortions (Box 17-3). The following interaction illustrates how a nurse might use CBT concepts to guide a one-to-one intervention with a patient who is anxious about an interview for a volunteer position.

PATIENT: I don't think I can do that interview.

NURSE: What seems to be the trouble?

PATIENT: I'm nervous; I'll get confused and forget what to say.

NURSE: It's OK to be nervous at first. Let's talk about things that might help. What things have you done that has helped when you've been nervous in the past?

PATIENT: I know how to do deep breathing.

NURSE: That's an important skill. Deep breathing is a good way to cope with nervousness. Can you think of other things that help if you have trouble remembering what you want to say?

PATIENT: Not really.

NURSE: Practicing in advance or writing down a list helps some people remember. Which of these things would you like to try?

PATIENT: I think a list might help.

NURSE: I would be happy to help you write a reminder list of things you'd like to say during the interview. It's also important to think differently about the interview. Everyone gets nervous when starting something new, but we have made a good plan to help you. What might work to help you remember to do the things we have talked about?

PATIENT: Can I ask my dad to remind me?

NURSE: Yes, your dad knows people need extra help sometimes. I will talk with him about our plan before we go for your volunteer interview.

PATIENT: OK. I think that will work.

Cognitive–Behavioral Therapy for Schizophrenia — box 17-3

Example: CBT Techniques

SKILL: Identifying cognitive distortions

RATIONALE: Asking questions of yourself is one way to identify cognitive distortions. Ask yourself whether your beliefs about the situation might have another explanation. This allows you to think about things in new ways and may reduce your worry and anxiety about things.

Steps of the Skill

1. Identify your thoughts about the situation.
2. Examine whether there is any evidence to support your thoughts about the situation.
3. See whether there are other possible explanations of the situation.

Scenes to use for Discussion

1. Experiencing ideas of reference.
2. Negative self-talk.
3. Thoughts that others are not interested in what patient has to say.

Special Considerations

Use scenes to help patients identify distortions for each situation. Be sure to discuss which information is evidence for or against the distortion in a given situation. For example, a verbal response and eye contact from another person would show that the other person is in fact, interested in talking with the patient.

I. PRINCIPLES, FORMAT, AND TECHNIQUES
1. Assess CBT knowledge and skills via interviewing.
2. Introduce CBT concepts.
3. Techniques for consolidating CBT skills include repetition, role play, and homework assignments.
4. Starting a CBT group may be considered when at least six patients are in need of CBT training. Consider practical considerations for planning a group, selecting group leaders, selecting patients, preparing patients for participation.
5. Tailor skills for individual needs. Use patient goals to design CBT groups, manage the range of skill levels, keep all members involved, conduct ongoing assessment of progress made in group.
6. Troubleshooting: Anticipate common problems and problems with highly symptomatic patients and patients with dual diagnoses.
7. Creating a supportive environment: Develop a CBT supportive milieu; educate family members to support CBT goal attainment

II. TEACHING SPECIFIC CBT SKILLS
- **Identifying thought patterns:** Listening to one's internal self talk (differentiate from auditory hallucinations). Learn the common thought distortions and apply this knowledge to personally identified thought patterns.
- **Examining the evidence:** Involves learning to identify and consider alternate explanations for events, obtaining information and opinions of trusted others may also be useful.
- **Identifying alternative explanations:** Nurse and trusted family members may assist, especially in early stages of learning CBT principles. For example, in response to the cognitive distortion, "I am no good; no one wants to be around me," nurse and family can cite examples when others reached out to patient socially and provide alternative explanations for events perceived as rejecting.

Ming Relapse Phase (Part 2)

On assessment today, Ming is 5'5", 170 pounds, and appears her stated age. Her BP is 128/75 mmHg, pulse 80 and regular, and she has no known allergies. Her cranial nerve tests and extraocular movements are intact, reflexes 2+ bilaterally. Ming correctly identifies a pen and a pair of eyeglasses with her eyes closed. She is dressed in clean but wrinkled clothing appropriate to the season, except for a stocking cap she refuses to remove, stating, "It helps keep my thoughts inside my head where they belong."

Ming appears restless, crossing and uncrossing her legs and picking at her fingernails. Her eye contact is poor. Although she answers all questions, her answers are vague and she does not initiate any verbalizations. She exhibits occasional thought blocking, and denies substance use or suicidal or homicidal ideation at this time. She admits to mild paranoia regarding "people reading my thoughts—that's why I wear this hat," and is alert and oriented to time, place, person, and situation. You estimate her to be of above-average intelligence; her memory appears good, but her insight is limited. She relates the reason for her recent hospitalization as "I had a misunderstanding with one of mom's workmen at the store—it's no big deal." Ming reports being concerned about her weight, but says she is not concerned about her smoking habit. Ming's mother, who accompanies her to the appointment, appears tired but genuinely concerned for her daughter. Ming's mother confirms that, to the best of her knowledge, Ming is taking her risperidone as prescribed. Ming has not yet returned to work at the store, although she often stays there in the back room, where her mother can "keep an eye on her."

APPLICATION

1. How would you prioritize Ming's needs at this time? Why?

2. How do Ming's ongoing delusions and minimization of her reason for hospitalization affect her care plan?

3. Why is risperidone an appropriate recommendation for Ming, and what issues are important to discuss with her regarding this medication?

4. What possible repercussions does Ming's relapse have for her parents? How would you assess their needs at this time?

Assertive Community Treatment (ACT) Teams

ACT programs assign identified high-risk patients to a multidisciplinary team (psychiatrist, master's-prepared mental health clinician, registered nurses, and case managers) that delivers around-the-clock care whenever and wherever the patient experiences a need (Chapter 29). ACT teams have demonstrated success in integrating at-risk individuals with severe mental illnesses into the community (Rice, 2011; Shean, 2009).

Pause and Reflect

1. *What is the nurse's role in medication management of patients with SSDs?*

2. *What medication management issue would most complicate the care plan for a patient with an SSD?*

3. *Family therapy has been shown to have positive effects on patient outcomes. Why do you think this is the case? What benefits do you think this type of therapy brings to family members other than the patient?*

Nursing Management

Nursing management of patients with SSDs can challenge even the most experienced nurse. As with all patients, nurses assess for and ensure patient safety and then work to prioritize patient care based on both physiological and psychological indicators.

Assessment

The first step in treatment is a thorough assessment, which includes both psychiatric and medical history, symptom description, precipitating factors (if any), and a suicide/violence assessment. Because of the effects of SSDs on cognition, it is helpful to use additional information from family, friends, or associates to inform the history. A number of physical assessment and monitoring procedures are recommended.

Baseline Assessments

The American Diabetes Association (ADA), in collaboration with the American Psychiatric Association (APA), the American Association of Clinical Endocrinologists (AACE), and the North American Association for the Study of Obesity (NAASO), recommend the following baseline assessments for individuals with SSDs (ADA/APA/AACE/NAASO, 2004):

- Family history, including history of cardiovascular disease, hypertension, diabetes, obesity, and dyslipidemias
- **Body mass index** (BMI) (measurement of body fat based on comparison of weight to height)
- Waist circumference

Measurements should be taken with patients in light clothing and stocking feet, using the same scale each time. The Centers for Disease Control and Prevention (CDC, 2010) guidelines define those with a BMI between 25 and 29.9 as overweight, and those with a BMI ≥ 30 as obese.

Waist circumference is the primary assessment for abdominal obesity. The National Cholesterol Education Panel III (2002) defines abdominal obesity as a waist circumference greater than 40 inches in men and greater than 35 inches in women.

Additional recommended baseline assessments include blood pressure, fasting blood glucose (FBG), and fasting lipid panels. High-risk patients requiring referral include those with blood pressures above 130/85 mmHg, FBS >110 mg/dL, triglycerides > 150 mg/dL, or high-density lipoprotein (HDL) < 40 mg/dL in men, and HDL < 50 mg/dL in women (NCEP, 2002). Recommended assessments for patients with SSDs may be found in Table 17-3.

Ongoing Assessment and Monitoring

Frequency of monitoring is influenced by history, preexisting conditions, and other medications and may be clinically indicated on a more frequent basis than indicated here. Except for patients with BMI below 18.5, an increase of 1 BMI point requires intervention.

Recommended Assessments for Patients with SSDs

table 17-3

Assessment	Baseline	Follow-Up
Vital signs	Pulse, blood pressure, and temperature	At each visit, when clinically indicated, and during medication dosage titration
Height, weight	BMI and waist circumference	At each visit for 6 months and at least quarterly thereafter
Diabetes screening	Family history, sedentary lifestyle, ethnicity, vascular disease, fasting glucose, hemoglobin A1C	Fasting glucose or hemoglobin A1C at baseline, 4 months after initiating new treatment, and at least annually thereafter
Extrapyramidal symptoms	Clinical assessment	Weekly during acute treatment, at each visit during stable phase
Tardive dyskinesia	Abnormal Involuntary Movement Scale (AIMS)	Every 6 months for first-generation and every year for second-generation antipsychotics; high-risk patients: every 3 months for first-generation and every 6 months for second-generation antipsychotics

Ethnicities at risk for diabetes include African Americans, Hispanics, Native Americans, Asians, and Pacific Islanders. Any of these ethnicities, combined with hypertension; high-density lipoprotein (HDL) level < 40 mg/dL in men or < 50 mg/dL in women; triglycerides > 150 mg/dL; and/or fasting glucose >110 mg/dL require medical consultation (NCEP, 2002).

Recommended ongoing monitoring includes monthly weights for the first three months and quarterly thereafter. Blood pressure, fasting glucose, and lipid measurements are recommended at baseline, 3 months, and annually thereafter (ADA/APA/AACE/NAASO, 2004). Clinical status may necessitate more frequent monitoring for some patients (for example, more frequent weighing for patients prescribed olanzapine or clozapine, because weight gain from these medications may continue for up to 1 year). In addition, those with extensive family history of risk or who fail to adhere to dietary/activity recommendations may need more frequent monitoring or a referral for specialty management of medical conditions. Patients at high risk for tardive dyskinesia include older adults, those with a history of acute dystonia, and those with clinically significant extrapyramidal symptoms or akathisia (APA, 2004). These patients may also require more frequent monitoring.

Patient Interview

A thorough patient interview will include questions that address each of the five wellness domains, including symptom history and chief concerns at the time of the interview. During the patient interview, the nurse will observe for the presence of symptoms (positive, negative, or cognitive) as well as for hard and soft neurological signs.

Difference in Initial/Relapse, Recovery, and Rehabilitation Phases

The patient in an initial or relapse phase is often not in touch with reality and is in need of direct, concrete interventions. Nurses working with patients at this stage will need to be very aware of the patient's verbal and nonverbal responses as they assess the patient. Nurses also must be aware of their own feelings and responses when working with the patient (see the Perceptions, Thoughts, Feelings section near the end of the chapter). The patient may be unaware of the need for help and may be brought for treatment by concerned others.

Patients experiencing a relapse may or may not understand their illness and its manifestations. In the case example, although risperidone has diminished Ming's delusions, she is still symptomatic and lacks insight into the severity and nature of her symptoms. Hopefully, over time, patients will learn strategies for understanding their illness, managing their symptoms, and getting along socially. Thorough assessment and planning for a multidisciplinary approach to treatment that includes measurable goals will increase the chances for the patient's recovery.

Diagnosis and Planning

Appropriate nursing diagnosis and planning depends on a thorough and accurate assessment. Nursing diagnoses and care plans are more meaningful and engaging if developed in collaboration with the patient.

Common Nursing Diagnoses

Nursing diagnoses for patients with SSDs are prioritized by patient need. Although many diagnoses might apply to a given patient with an SSD during a specific time in the illness trajectory, some are more common. They include the following:

- Coping, Ineffective
- Injury, Risk for
- Social Isolation
- Social Interaction, Impaired
- Knowledge, Deficient
- Spiritual Distress
- Sleep Pattern, Disturbed
- Anxiety
- Overweight/Obesity
- Fear

(NANDA-I © 2014)

Besides diagnoses based on patient concerns and safety, nurses may also choose diagnoses that address symptoms or behaviors that create problems for those who live or work with the patient.

Prioritizing Nursing Diagnoses

When nurses and patients work together to determine care priorities, patients are more likely to adhere to the care plan, thus increasing the likelihood for success. However, at times, the severity of a patient's symptoms make this type of interaction impractical. At these times, the nurse addresses the most significant patient needs and selects nursing diagnoses based on the patient's ability to participate in goal attainment.

For example, during Ming's clinic visit, the nurse identifies altered thought processes as a nursing diagnosis to address. Together, the nurse and Ming develop a plan to address Ming's delusions of thought broadcasting (see Nursing Care Plan).

Plans and Goals

As the plan develops, the nurse makes every effort to involve the patient when appropriate. Questions the nurse considers when developing the plan of care include the following:

- Does the patient's level of symptoms make it reasonable to expect the patient can be involved in developing the plan of care?
- What does the patient relate as the most distressing symptom?
- What are the patient's goals for treatment? For example, if the patient is distressed by ideas of thought broadcasting, like Ming, the nurse might state the following goals:

  1. The patient will take at least 80% of antipsychotic medication dosages.
  2. The patient will verbalize techniques for distraction from distressing symptoms, such as interacting with others, taking a walk, or reading.
  3. The patient will report a decrease in frequency or distress from ideas of thought broadcasting within 1 week.

In developing the nursing care plan, the nurse should consider, along with the patient, how each of the five domains is affected. Asking the following targeted questions may be helpful in identifying which domains are most affected:

- *Biological:* Does the patient have any medical conditions that may impair overall health? Does the patient need additional care for these conditions? Are there any symptoms affecting the patient's self-care abilities?
- *Psychological:* Are there triggers that increase patient symptoms? What could be done to reduce triggers or enhance patient coping efforts?
- *Social:* Are there relationships or living situations that have an impact on the patient's environment, either positively or negatively? To what extent are the patient's symptoms affecting relationships with family and others?
- *Cultural:* Do cultural beliefs or rituals have impeding or enhancing effects on patient health? For example, what are the patient's cultural beliefs relative to psychiatric symptoms?
- *Spiritual:* Are there any spiritual concerns or religious symptoms that may negatively affect the patient? Does the patient desire spiritual support? If so, how can this be incorporated?

Patient Education

Psychoeducation constitutes a large portion of quality care for patients with SSDs and their families, and therefore must be incorporated into the plan of care. Patients and families have indicated the following areas of need: general information about the disease, symptom coping strategies, and communication and social relationships (Gumus, 2008). Specific information on medication side effects, monitoring, and health promotion activities should be individualized. Patients and families may benefit from referrals for a variety of activities designed to provide support, education, and resources.

To ensure an optimal response to patient education, nurses must first assess the patient's readiness to learn. If the timing is appropriate, the nurse helps the patient understand relapse and symptoms triggers and interventions that alleviate suffering. If the patient's reality testing is impaired, education may need to be concrete and brief or postponed until the patient has gained stability. For the patient with extreme psychotic symptoms, the nurse should remain with the patient or delegate another to ensure safety.

Revising the Care Plan During Recovery and Rehabilitation

As patients improve and symptoms subside, nurses evaluate progress and adjust the care plan as needed. For example, in the recovery phase patients often develop greater awareness of idiosyncratic symptom triggers. Patients need support and affirmation that reaching out for help at such times is not a sign of weakness or that they are "crazy." Rather, being aware of relapse triggers means that treatment can be sought earlier, before symptoms become incapacitating and patients experience loss of function.

Due to the ongoing necessity of medication for most patients with schizophrenia, they remain at risk for chronic EPSs. Individuals receiving antipsychotic medication on an ongoing basis should be assessed using the AIMS (Table 17-4) (Guy, 1976).

Implementation

Nursing interventions depend, in part, on the patient's ability to concentrate and listen, retain new information, and make decisions. Health promotion for patients with SSDs includes psychosocial treatments to prevent relapse (such as education on the importance of treatment adherence) and promote recovery (for instance, involving family members in treatment when possible). In the chapter example, Ming gives vague answers to assessment questions and does not initiate verbalizations. The patient's nonverbal behaviors, as well as circumstances and biological factors, can affect domain considerations. Nurses will do well to remember that each patient's experiences are unique and will plan nursing interventions that honor this uniqueness.

For example, a patient may be cognitively impaired and have trouble remembering to take prescribed medications. The nurse will need to collaborate with other members of the health care team to ensure simplicity of the drug regimen while offering creative suggestions for memory prompts. Memory prompts might include reminder systems in the form of alarms, family caregivers, or signs placed in the environment. Other barriers to medication adherence include lack of transportation and inadequate finances (such as household income or health insurance) to pay for prescribed medications. Nurses must consider each patient's unique circumstances and work with the patients and their support persons to promote quality care and minimize symptom triggers.

Lifestyle Interventions

Commonly recommended lifestyle interventions include dietary changes, physical exercise, and smoking cessation. Dietary changes

The Abnormal Involuntary Movement Scale (AIMS)

table 17-4

Location	Description	Rating (0–4)
Facial and oral	Muscles of facial expression (forehead, eyebrows, periorbital area, and cheeks, including frowning, blinking, smiling, grimacing)	
	Lips and perioral area (puckering, pouting, smacking)	
	Jaw (biting, clenching, chewing, mouth opening, lateral movement)	
	Tongue (rate only increases in movement both in and out of mouth, not inability to sustain movement; darting in and out of mouth)	
Extremities	Upper (arms, wrists, hands, fingers): Include choreic movements, (i.e., rapid, objectively purposeless, irregular, spontaneous) athetoid movements (i.e., slow, irregular, complex, serpentine). DO NOT INCLUDE tremor (repetitive, regular, rhythmic)	
	Lower (legs, knees, ankles, toes): e.g., lateral knee movement, foot tapping, heel dropping, foot squirming, inversion and eversion of foot	
Trunk	Neck, shoulders, hips (e.g., rocking, twisting, squirming, pelvic gyrations)	
Global judgments	Severity of abnormal movements overall	
	Incapacitation due to abnormal movements	
	Patient's awareness of abnormal movements. Rate only patient's report	
	No awareness = 0	
	Aware, no distress = 1	
	Aware, mild distress = 2	
	Aware, moderate distress = 3	
	Aware, severe distress = 4	
Dental status	Current problems with teeth and/or dentures	Yes/no
	Are dentures usually worn?	Yes/no
	Edentia?	Yes/no
	Do movements disappear in sleep?	Yes/no

Note: 0 = none, 1 = minimal (may be extreme normal), 2 = mild, 3 = moderate, 4 = severe

Source: Guy, W. (1976). *Assessment Manual for Psychopharmacology—Revised* (DHEW Publication No. ADM 76-338). Rockville, MD: U.S. Department of Health, Education, and Welfare, Public Health Service, Alcohol, Drug Abuse, and Mental Health Administration, NIMH Psychopharmacology Research Branch, Division of Extramural Research Programs, pp. 534–537. Available at http://imaging.ubmmedica.com/all/editorial/psychiatrictimes/pdfs/clinical-scales-aims-form.pdf

Ming Recovery Phase

Three months later, Ming has been working with a counselor to learn to use cognitive techniques in response to delusions that are not completely controlled with medication; as a result, she has been able to return to church with her parents and has resumed working part-time at her mother's store. After gaining medical clearance for exercise, Ming worked with the nurse at the mental health clinic to increase her physical activity while reducing calorie intake. Ming has lost 5 pounds so far and is pleased with her results. She continues to have occasional thoughts that medications are unnecessary, so the nurse and therapist help her examine the evidence of past events when she discontinued her medications (for instance, increase in symptoms and hospitalization). Ming's parents have been attending a support group through NAMI and find this to be a good source of information and support in dealing with Ming's illness.

APPLICATION

1. Address the five domains for Ming:
   a. Biological
   b. Psychological
   c. Sociological
   d. Cultural
   e. Spiritual
2. How would you prioritize Ming's needs at this time?
3. How would you foster Ming's hope at this time?

critical thinking

and physical exercise are necessary to help patients maintain weight control and reduce their risk for obesity and type 2 diabetes (see Evidence-Based Practice: Nutrition and SSDs). Nurses should plan simple diet teaching, taking into account the memory and attention deficits of patients with SSDs. The use of concrete examples, repetition, reminders, and positive reinforcement helps offset these difficulties. Patients should be frequently reminded to strive for a goal of consuming five servings of fruits and vegetables per day; reducing fat and salt intake by limiting fast food and salty snacks; and limiting foods containing refined sugar, such as baked goods and sweets. In addition, patients with SSDs have been shown to benefit from education regarding proper portion control (Littrell, 2004). For some patients, the use of decaffeinated, unsweetened iced tea to replace high-calorie soda or juice and reminders to drink at least six to eight glasses of water daily would also be helpful in managing intake and satiety.

After medical clearance for exercise is obtained, psychiatric nurses should first focus on motivation. One aspect of motivation is the concept of **self-efficacy**, which includes confidence in one's ability to perform the behavior, along with expectation of benefits from the behavior (Bandura, 1995). Nurses assess patients' confidence in their ability to perform the exercises. Interventions to increase confidence include education, appropriate equipment (for example, verify that the patient has adequate footwear if walking is recommended), memory prompts of earlier physical competence, and discussion of other activities in which the patient is proficient (Beebe, 2006). Walking is the most popular form of exercise for individuals with SSDs. For maximum health benefit, patients need 30 minutes of moderate exercise at least five times per week. When possible, either treatment staff or a buddy should participate, as this motivates participation and increases social interaction. Positive reinforcement, problem solving of exercise barriers, and periodic booster sessions enhance

adherence. Patients must also be educated about the strong evidence for physical, mental, and social benefits of exercise. Pointing out observed improvements as the exercise program continues will reinforce patients' awareness of their progress.

Approximately 65% to 85% of all individuals with SSDs smoke; most consume more than 20 cigarettes per day (de Leon et al., 2005). Persons with mental illness smoke 44% of all the cigarettes smoked in the United States; this is two to four times more than those without a mental illness. Smoking reduces plasma levels of medications, including haloperidol, olanzapine, and clozapine, by approximately one-third through enzyme induction of cytochrome P450. Smoking cessation treatments include nicotine replacement, bupropion, and psychosocial approaches. Research has shown that nicotine replacement therapy (with or without additional behavioral interventions) significantly improves the chances of smoking reduction or cessation in patients with SSDs (George et al., 2008). However, rates of relapse are significant, suggesting that clinicians wishing to support these behaviors over time need to provide ongoing proactive psychosocial support (APA, 2009).

Primary, Secondary, and Tertiary Interventions

Nursing interventions are made on the primary, secondary, or tertiary level to reduce SSD symptoms and their associated distress. Primary interventions seek to alleviate anxiety that may exacerbate psychotic symptoms. Education is aimed at prevention. Secondary intervention involves early intervention and treatment. An example of secondary intervention is patient education about early symptoms of relapse and seeking treatment in a timely manner. Patient education is focused on increasing healthy coping. Tertiary intervention involves post-intervention with an established unhealthy behavior or risk factor. The goal is to restore function in all the domains of wellness. Education is directed toward reducing recurrence and enhancing health functioning.

Nutrition and SSDs   evidence-based practice

Clinical Question
What are effective nutritional interventions for weight loss patients with SSDs?

Evidence
Two studies were located examining nutritional education interventions for patients with SSDs living in the community. Thirty-five outpatients with SSDs participated in a weekly psychoeducational class focused on dietary guidelines, appropriate portion sizes, and the importance of a healthy diet for 4 months, and their weight changes were compared to a control group of 35 outpatients with SSDs receiving standard care (Littrell et al., 2003). At both 4 and 6 months, a statistically significant weight difference was observed between the two groups, with the intervention group exhibiting greater weight loss. Evans, Newton, and Higgins (2005) provided 29 outpatients with SSDs with six 1-hour nutritional education classes over a 6-month period, and compared them with 22 controls receiving standard care. All subjects entered the study upon commencement of treatment with olanzapine. The experimental group had significantly less weight gain than controls at both 3 and 6 months; however, 13% of those in the experimental group still gained more than 7% of their baseline weight (compared to 64% of

controls). This study highlights the serious issue of weight gain (especially when medications such as olanzapine are used), and the need for aggressive management of patients for whom this medication is chosen.

Implications for Nursing Practice
Nurses should plan simple diet teaching, taking into account the memory and attention deficits of patients with SSDs. The use of concrete examples, repetition, reminders, and positive reinforcement helps offset these difficulties. Patients should be reminded frequently to strive for a goal of consuming five servings of fruits and vegetables per day, reducing fat and salt intake by limiting fast food and salty snacks, and limiting foods containing refined sugar, such as baked goods and sweets. Of critical importance is elimination of high-calorie soda and juice from the patient's diet.

Critical Thinking Questions
1. What is the strength of the evidence for nutritional interventions to help patients with SSDs manage medication associated weight gain?
2. On the basis of this evidence, what education would you provide to patients prescribed olanzapine?

Promoting Adherence

Nurses plan interventions assuming that patients will adhere to treatment recommendations and that patients are motivated to improve and exhibit healthy coping. However, the needs of patients with SSDs are complex and multifactorial, and lack of motivation is characteristic of SSDs (Figure 17-5). Treatment response and successful plan implementation depend on treatment adherence as well as the presence of other factors and conditions, such as suicidal thoughts, substance abuse, and pregnancy (Table 17-5).

Rates of adherence to antipsychotic medications range from 11% to 80%, with average rates of 50% (Lang et al., 2013; McCabe et al., 2013). Interventions to improve adherence include problem solving, motivation, behavioral strategies, and/or psychoeducation. Motivational interventions are designed to increase adherence behavior by focusing on the role of medications in reducing symptoms and additional hospitalizations. Problem-solving techniques are used to assist patients in overcoming barriers to adherence, such as forgetfulness or disorganization, with concrete suggestions that may include placing medications in a prominent location or tying medication administration to an established routine. Behavioral strategies include positive reinforcement and the provision of cues; for example, using calendars to mark off doses as they are taken.

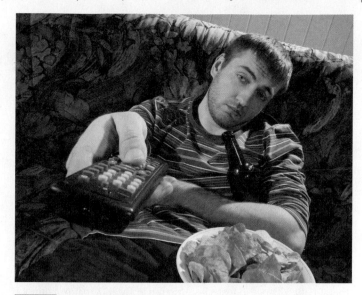

17-5   Patients with schizophrenia experience lack of motivation and difficulty with problem solving. Using motivational interventions and teaching problem-solving techniques helps patients begin to take responsibility for their health and reduce their risk for co-morbid illness.

Source: Nomad_Soul/Fotolia

Interventions for Selected Co-Occurring Conditions   table 17-5

Condition	Risk Factors	Interventions
Suicidal Ideation/Gesture Suicide is the leading cause of premature death in patients with SSDs. Approximately one-third of individuals with SSDs attempt suicide at least once.	• Younger age at onset • High socioeconomic status • High intelligence • Chronic course • Higher premorbid achievement	• Suicide assessment • Mobilization of support team • Antidepressants • Antipsychotic dosage adjustment • Psychotherapy and other supports as indicated
Substance Abuse Co-morbid substance disorders are not uncommon in patients with SSDs.	• Male gender • Single marital status • Lower education level • Early onset of SSD • Increased rates/length of hospitalization • More gray matter volume deficits • Poor treatment adherence • Depression • Legal difficulties • Family burden • HIV/hepatitis C risk	• Regular substance abuse assessments using CAGE questionnaire and collateral information (see Chapter 20) • Toxicology screenings, liver function studies • Careful differentiation of substance-related symptoms from psychotic symptoms • Integrated treatment approach
Pregnancy Women with SSDs who are pregnant require careful attention to both prenatal and psychiatric care. Risks are highest in the first trimester.	• SGAs present relatively low risk of fetal harm. • Mood stabilizers (e.g., lithium) and benzodiazepines carry risk for fetal malformation and behavioral effects.	Assess sexual activity and birth control in women with SSDs of childbearing potential. *If pregnancy occurs:* • Assist patients in obtaining and complying with prenatal care. • Educate women about risks associated with treatment and assist them to make informed decisions. • Encourage smoking cessation, management of co-morbid disorders. • Educate about and encourage exercise and proper nutrition.

Based on Meerwijk, E. L., van Meijel, B., van den Bout, J., Kerkhof, A., de Vogel, W., & Grypdonk, M. (2010). Development and evaluation of a guideline for nursing care of suicidal patients with schizophrenia. *Perspectives in Psychiatric Care, 46*(1), 65–73; Mueser, K. T., & Gingerich, S. (2013). Treatment of co-occurring psychotic and substance use disorders. *Social Work in Public Health, 28*(3–4), 424–439; Tandon, R., Nasrallah, H. A., & Keshavan, M. S. (2009). Schizophrenia: Just the facts. 4. Clinical features and conceptualization. *Schizophrenia Research, 110,* 1–23.

Psychoeducation involves didactic sharing of information about the disease and management of SSDs.

Patients who are defined as partial medication responders (those experiencing ongoing hallucinations and/or delusions) should be assessed for medication adherence. Clinicians should first verify that an adequate trial (taking at least 80% of prescribed doses for 4 to 6 weeks) of antipsychotic medication has taken place. Reasons that patients fail to adhere to medication treatment are variable and include personal factors, system factors, and illness factors. Personal factors include attitudes toward illness, response to medication side effects, and lack of transportation. System factors include the provision of care by multiple practitioners at multiple sites, complex medication regimens, and insurance policies that limit treatment options. Illness factors include psychotic symptoms that inhibit insight into the illness and the need for medication, memory impairments, and dual diagnoses. Clinicians must tailor medication adherence interventions to individual needs, keeping in mind the importance of therapeutic alliance in fostering adherence. By anticipating common problems related to medication adherence, particularly for patients with severe symptoms or dual diagnoses, nurses can promote adherence and provide support as appropriate.

Two prominent reasons patients fail to adhere to medication regimens are failing to remember to take their medications and side effects. Strategies to help patients remember to take their medications include interventions that target memory-related lapses and working with patients and prescribers to simplify the medication regimen, reducing multiple-times-a-day dosing if possible. Encourage patients to tie medication administration to their daily routine, such as at bedtime or during performance of daily hygiene. For issues related to side effects and symptom control, develop strategies for side effects on an individual basis, and provide alternatives to reduce symptoms not completely controlled with medications, such as distraction, physical activity, and socialization.

> **PRACTICE ALERT**   Patients who are actively suicidal, cannot contract for safety, or have few social supports or a history of multiple suicide attempts need inpatient care. Be prepared to discuss inpatient treatment options with the patient and family and to initiate involuntary hospitalization if necessary.

Evaluation

The evaluation process involves determining the extent to which the patient's goals have been met during the specified timeline. For example, if the goal indicated that the patient's delusional verbalizations would decrease from five times a day to once daily within 1 week, and such verbalizations still occur two to three times per day, on evaluation the patient's goal would be noted as being partially met. If goals are *specific*, *measurable*, and *realistic*, their evaluation is less difficult.

The patient's adherence to the treatment plan is one aspect that influences the plan's success. Points to consider include whether the patient is taking at least 80% of prescribed medication doses, appearing for treatment appointments, engaging in satisfying social relationships, and making use of support systems.

Once patients experience relief of positive symptoms, they often need reminders of the importance of continuing prescribed medications, as symptoms often return when medications are discontinued

abruptly. Treatment with antipsychotic medication is lifelong for many patients with SSDs.

The nature and frequency of evaluation is different at each stage of the recovery process. Depending on symptom severity, evaluations will be more frequent during relapse or initial presentation. During the rehabilitation phase, many stable patients with SSDs are seen every 6 months or when symptoms increase or change. See Table 17-3 for recommended assessments for individuals with SSDs during differing phases of illness.

A change in any single domain may or may not put patients with SSDs at risk for relapse depending on other factors, such as medication adherence, coping skills, and environmental supports. A review of all domains (biological, psychological, sociological, cultural, and spiritual) will identify areas needing intervention to increase patient coping. For example, if a patient has co-occurring diabetes mellitus, it would be important for the nurse to evaluate diabetic control and knowledge. Diabetes control in a patient with an SSD would be affected by the psychological domain if the individual were experiencing psychosis or memory deficits. If not well controlled, diabetes could severely compromise the patient's physical health (biological domain).

From Suffering to Hope

Even though it is easy to see that a patient in the grip of a hallucinatory or delusional process is suffering deeply, sometimes nurses have difficulty identifying patient suffering in relation to chronic SSD symptoms, especially in the sociocultural domain. The nurse may wonder why the patient is so reluctant to engage socially when the circumstances do not seem to warrant suspicion and mistrust. Acknowledging the pain the patient is experiencing can foster the therapeutic nurse–patient relationship. Individuals with SSDs desire the same things as everyone else, including a kind word; a hug; encouragement, acceptance, and respect from others; recognition of talents; and to be heard. Patients with SSDs also desire to love, care for, and nurture others. They resist labels and wish to be treated as persons (Beebe et al., 2012).

Nurses can promote hope in patients with SSDs by helping them gain a sense of worth and value. The nurse may affirm a patient's strengths, noting positive characteristics or the strength simply to have held up under such a devastating illness. Specific examples might include observations about patient's talent in art or music, instances of kindness to others, or efforts to abstain from substances or other unhealthy behaviors.

Another way to foster a sense of hope and connectedness is through referrals to self-help activities, such as the National Alliance on Mental Illness (NAMI) and the Schizophrenia and Related Disorders Alliance of America (SARDAA). Participation in such programs has been associated with increased social networks, improved coping, and improved quality of life (Davidson et al., 1999; Raiff, 1984).

> ## Pause and Reflect
> 1. *What common health and recovery issues need to be addressed in patients with SSDs?*
> 2. *How can nurses offer hope to patients with SSDs? To their families?*

Ming—A Patient with Altered Thought Processes   NURSING CARE PLAN

Nursing Diagnosis: Altered thought processes (delusions) related to alteration in structure/function of brain tissue, secondary to schizophrenia evidenced by verbalization that people are trying to read her thoughts.

Short-Term Goals

Patient will: (Include date for short-term goal to be met)	Intervention *Nurse will:*	Rationale
Maintain orientation to time, place, person, and circumstances.	Assess orientation at each encounter and verify information with parents.	Determine presence of delusions.
Identify delusional thoughts during initial interview.	If delusions are expressed, matter-of-factly present reality without arguing. Let Ming know that you do not share the perception.	Reality orientation decreases false perceptions and enhances the patient's sense of self-worth and personal dignity.
Receive feedback about inaccurate reality perception.	Correct Ming's description of inaccurate perception, and describe the situation as it exists in reality.	Explanation of, and participation in, real situations and real activities interferes with the ability to respond to delusions.
Identify stressors contributing to delusions, if any.	Assist Ming to identify stressors that might increase delusional thoughts.	Precipitating stressors can trigger psychiatric symptoms.
Receive reassurance of personal safety.	Provide reassurance of safety if Ming expresses fear due to inaccurate perceptions.	Patient safety is a nursing priority.
Decrease delusional verbalizations to once daily by . . . . [time frame].	Patient education related to thought stopping: Ask Ming to say "STOP" in her mind. Assess need for education related to delusions as illness symptoms. Replace delusional content with healthier thoughts.	Thought stopping helps interrupt nonreality-based cognitions. Education related to illness symptoms may be helpful. Delusional thoughts need to be replaced with positive thoughts.
Adhere to prescribed medication regimen.	Provide teaching related to treatments prescribed and effect on symptoms.	Patient adherence to treatment often depends on patient understanding of treatment.
Long-Term Goal Patient will demonstrate accurate perception of the environment by responding appropriately to stimuli.	Provide periodic "check-in" opportunities for Ming to engage in reality orientation by identifying key triggers that stimulate delusional thoughts.	Allows Ming to control this aspect of her recovery by recognizing that she has the ability to identify delusion triggers and can report her progress in symptom management.

Clinical Reasoning

1. What other nursing diagnoses might the nurse working with Ming consider?
2. Do you think the selection of *Altered Thought Processes* as the priority nursing diagnosis is appropriate? Why or why not?

Ming Rehabilitation Phase

critical thinking

The nurse has been working with Ming for 9 months. Together they have developed a relapse prevention plan, and Ming has become a much more active participant in her ongoing care. She has remained out of the hospital during this time. She is able to tell the nurse about her primary positive symptoms, and together they have developed strategies to help Ming know how to accurately test reality. She is able to describe her delusions and has worked through the embarrassment she felt now that she understands that they were delusions and not reality. She is able to express her frustration at how her life has not turned out as she had originally planned, and she is able to describe other options. Ming is learning how to manage her medications and when to call her provider if symptoms increase, so she can have a temporary increase in medications and avoid another hospitalization. Ming's family has attended the NAMI Family to Family sessions and has learned how to communicate better with Ming. They also are more sensitive to the triggers of her delusions. Ming's parents are able to express the cultural differences in how mental illness is perceived in general in her ethnic group. Ming and her parents both feel that there is hope for her future and she need not be ashamed. Ming has lost 15 pounds and feels better about herself; she is considering going for a job interview.

APPLICATION

1. Why is learning strategies to test reality important for Ming?
2. How does Ming's family play a role in her rehabilitation?

PERCEPTIONS, THOUGHTS, & FEELINGS: A Patient with Disordered Thought Processes

Patient's behavior	Nurse's perceptions, thoughts, feelings	Exploration with patient
Ming appears restless, crossing and uncrossing her legs and picking at her fingernails. Her eye contact is poor. She is dressed in clean but wrinkled clothing appropriate to the season, except for a stocking cap she refuses to remove.	*Perceptions:* Ming is wearing a stocking cap in the summer. *Thoughts:* I wonder what she means by her statement. I think she's still really delusional. *Feelings:* I'm afraid I'm going to say something to interfere with her ability to trust me.	*Nurse:* Thank you for sharing that with me, Ming. I wonder if it would be okay if I asked you a question to help me better understand what you mean.

Ming: It helps keep my thoughts inside my head where they belong.

VALIDATION The nurse acknowledges Ming's statement in a hope to begin to establish trust since this is their first meeting. She honors Ming by asking if it is okay to ask her a question to help her (the nurse) better understand the meaning behind Ming's statement.

Patient's behavior	Nurse's perceptions, thoughts, feelings	Exploration with patient
Ming looks down at the floor.	*Thoughts:* I'm worried I'm going to ask the wrong thing in the wrong way and cause her to feel defensive. *Feelings:* This must be a frightening symptom to have.	*Nurse:* Help me understand what it is like to not have your thoughts stay in your head.

Ming: I suppose so.

VALIDATION The nurse acknowledges Ming's experience of feeling as if her thoughts are escaping from her head. The nurse uses an open-ended question to try to get Ming to share what the experience is like.

Patient's behavior	Nurse's perceptions, thoughts, feelings	Exploration with patient
Ming briefly glances up to give eye contact, but quickly turns her eyes toward the window.	*Thoughts:* What is the best thing to say next? *Feelings:* I'm relieved she answered.	*Nurse:* Thank you, Ming, I appreciate you answering my question. I'm wondering what you remember about it first happening.

Ming: It's been happening for a long time.

VALIDATION Ming was able to answer, but didn't answer the question asked. This gives the nurse permission to continue talking about this symptom.

Patient's behavior	Nurse's perceptions, thoughts, feelings	Exploration with patient
She continues to look down, and her body is still tense.	*Thoughts:* She's talking to me! I think we're going to get somewhere. *Feelings:* I'm so relieved. I hope I can keep the momentum going.	*Nurse:* Oh, Ming, I can't even imagine what that must have been like for you.

Ming: People started reading my thoughts when I was in high school. I tried to ignore it. I didn't know why they wanted my thoughts.

VALIDATION The nurse expresses compassion and empathy for Ming. The nurse waits to ask a second question, realizing that it is difficult for the patient with schizophrenia to process more than one question at a time.

Patient's behavior	Nurse's perceptions, thoughts, feelings	Exploration with patient
Ming raises her eyes and looks briefly at the nurse. She has stopped wringing her hands.	*Perception:* She appears to be relaxing. *Thoughts:* She is still very troubled by her delusions.	*Nurse:* Ming, can you tell me what it is like for you now?

Ming: It's very embarrassing to think that other people can read and take my thoughts.

VALIDATION The nurse needs to clarify what is happening in the here and now.

Patient's behavior	Nurse's perceptions, thoughts, feelings	Exploration with patient
Ming lowers her eyes again and starts fidgeting in the chair.	*Perception:* Ming is showing signs of anxiety. *Thoughts:* She is willing to discuss this further. *Feelings:* I'm worried about pushing her too far in this initial conversation.	*Nurse:* When it happens, what do you do?

Ming: It still happens even with taking the medication.

VALIDATION The nurse continues to validate Ming's symptom experience.

Patient's behavior	Nurse's perceptions, thoughts, feelings	Exploration with patient
Ming looks up at the nurse.	*Thoughts:* I think I should stop now and set up a time to come back and continue the conversation. *Feelings:* I feel more comfortable now that it's okay to talk about her delusions.	*Nurse:* Ming, thank you again for sharing this with me. I would like to discuss this again with you at your next visit and see if we can come up with a plan to help stop this symptom altogether. Would that be okay?

Ming: Wearing this hat helps to keep my thoughts in.

VALIDATION The nurse is establishing credibility with the patient and requesting to discuss her delusions at her next appointment.

Patient's behavior	Nurse's perceptions, thoughts, feelings	Exploration with patient
Ming continues to look at the nurse.	*Thoughts:* We have made progress today for our first meeting. *Feelings:* I'm relieved that we have established a relationship.	*Nurse:* I agree completely and look forward to our next conversation about these symptoms. Let's meet again next week to talk about strategies we can develop so you won't have to keep your hat on all the time.

Ming: Thank you for believing me. I would like these problems to go away.

VALIDATION The nurse verifies that another conversation will occur next week and the nurse "plants the seed" for Ming to think about other ways to manage the symptom.

Based on Orlando, I. J. (1972). *The Discipline and Teaching of Nursing Process (An Evaluative Study).* New York, NY: G. P. Putnam's Sons.

Chapter Highlights

1. SSDs are the most chronic and disabling of the severe mental disorders, affecting multiple areas of functioning, with an exacerbating and remitting course. At present there is no known cure.

2. Theories of SSD etiology include a variety of biological anomalies, environmental conditions, and family interaction patterns.

3. Symptoms are divided into positive, negative, and cognitive types; other characteristics include disorganization, motor symptoms, and neurologic signs.

4. An SSD assessment includes psychiatric and medical history, verification of diagnostic criteria, and a suicide/violence assessment.

5. Antipsychotic medications are the mainstay of SSD treatment.

6. Antipsychotic medications have been divided into the categories of typical and atypical on the basis of similarities in mechanism of action.

7. Antipsychotic medication side effects include both acute and chronic extrapyramidal symptoms.

8. Psychosocial treatments include family therapy, social skills training (SST), vocational rehabilitation, cognitive–behavioral therapy (CBT), and the services of an assertive community treatment (ACT) team.

9. Management issues include physical health promotion, treatment adherence, culture, suicide, substance abuse, smoking cessation education, and self-help referrals.

NCLEX®-RN Questions

1. The nurse is counseling a couple planning to start a family. The couple reveals a family history of schizophrenia and asks about the risks of having a child who develops the illness. Which response by the nurse is accurate?
   a. "Many factors may lead to schizophrenia, but genetics account for the highest proportion of risk."
   b. "Genetic factors are considered significant only when one or both parents have been affected by this mental illness."
   c. "When considering risk factors for this disease, genetic influences are less important than environmental variables."
   d. "Although genetics are a suspected factor in development of schizophrenia, to date there is really limited evidence to support this theory."

2. The nurse is assisting a patient with schizophrenia to complete activities of daily living. Which category of symptoms is being addressed when the nurse lists all the steps that the patient needs to carry out?
   a. Positive symptoms
   b. Negative symptoms
   c. Cognitive symptoms
   d. Prodromal symptoms

3. The nurse is caring for a patient diagnosed with schizophrenia. When reviewing the patient's chart, the nurse recognizes that which sociocultural events are associated with the development of SSDs? Select all that apply.
   a. The patient was raised in a rural area.
   b. The patient's birthday is in the end of February.
   c. The patient's mother did not have access to prenatal care.
   d. The patient's delivery was complicated by a hypoxic episode.
   e. The patient's father was 50 years old when the patient was born.

4. A patient is taking haloperidol (Haldol) for the management of schizophrenia. When evaluating the efficacy of this treatment, the nurse knows this medication is least likely to address which manifestation of the illness?
   a. Avolition
   b. Delusions
   c. Hallucinations
   d. Disorganized speech

5. A patient with a diagnosis of schizophrenia is in the rehabilitation phase of the illness. Which assessments would constitute the focus of nursing care? Select all that apply.
   a. Ensuring the absence of positive, negative, and cognitive symptoms of the illness
   b. Determining whether the patient has resumed functioning consistent with premorbid status
   c. Ascertaining whether family and community supports are available and appropriate to patient needs
   d. Evaluating the patient for extrapyramidal symptoms and other side effects of medication
   e. Appraising the patient's readiness to replace medications with nonpharmacologic treatment interventions

6. The nurse is developing a plan of care for the patient in the rehabilitation phase of treatment of schizophrenia who is struggling to maintain a healthy weight. Which approach is most likely to be effective?
   a. Provide a stimulating multimedia presentation on the deleterious effects of poor lifestyle choices.
   b. Work with the patient to develop simple, manageable goals related to portion control and healthy choices.
   c. Focus efforts on encouraging aerobic exercise for at least 1 hour daily to compensate for increased appetite.
   d. Aim teaching efforts at family members or other support persons who are more capable of influencing the patient's diet.

7. The nurse is providing teaching to the parent of a patient with schizophrenia who has been in remission for 6 months. The parent complains that the patient is no longer ill but sits on the sofa all day watching television instead of looking for work. Which response is most appropriate?
   a. "Your child is lacking any kind of drive to work. It is unrealistic to expect your child to get a job at this time."
   b. "Negative symptoms of schizophrenia include a lack of motivation. Let's discuss practical solutions to address this behavior."
   c. "Social isolation and withdrawal may indicate the recurrence of paranoid delusions. Your child may need an increase in medication."
   d. "Individuals with schizophrenia have difficulty planning and following through with job planning. Your negativity is placing your child at risk of relapse."

Answers may be found on the Pearson student resource site:
nursing.pearsonhighered.com

Pearson Nursing Student Resources Find additional review materials at **nursing.pearsonhighered.com**

References

Acil, A. A., Dogan, S., & Dogan, O. (2008). The effects of physical exercises to mental state and quality of life in patients with Schizophrenia. *Journal of Psychiatric and Mental Health Nursing, 15*(10), 808–815.

Adams, M., Holland, L., & Urban, C. (2014). *Pharmacology for Nurses: A Pathophysiologic Approach* (4th ed.). Upper Saddle River, NJ: Prentice Hall.

Aia, P. G., Revuelta, G. J., Cloud, L. J., & Factor, S. A. (2011). Tardive dyskinesia. *Current Treatment Options in Neurology, 13*(3), 231–241.

American Diabetes Association; American Psychiatric Association, American Association of Clinical Endocrinologists, & the North American Association for the Study of Obesity (2004). Consensus development conference on antipsychotic drugs and obesity and diabetes. *Diabetes Care, 27,* 596–601.

American Psychiatric Association. (2003). *Practice Guidelines for the Assessment and Treatment of Patients with Suicidal Behaviors.* Arlington, VA: American Psychiatric Publishers.

American Psychiatric Association. (2004). *Practice Guidelines for the Treatment of Patients with Schizophrenia* (2nd ed.). Washington, DC: American Psychiatric Publishers.

American Psychiatric Association. (2009) *Guideline Watch: Practice Guideline for the Treatment of Patients with Schizophrenia.* Washington, DC: American Psychiatric Publishers.

American Psychiatric Association. (2013). *Diagnostic and Statistical Manual of Mental Disorders* (5th ed.). Washington, DC: American Psychiatric Publishers.

Andreasen, R., Oades, L., & Caputi, P. (2003). The experience of recovery from schizophrenia: Towards an empirically validated stage model. *Australian and New Zealand Journal of Psychiatry, 37,* 586–594.

Archie, W., Wilson, J. H., Osborne, S., Hobbs, H., & McNiven, J. (2003). Pilot study: Access to fitness facility and exercise levels in olanzapine-treated patients. *Canadian Journal of Psychiatry, 48*(9), 628–632.

Ascher-Svanum H., Zhu, B., Faries, D., Lacro, J. P., & Dolder, C. R. (2006). A prospective study of risk factors for nonadherence with antipsychotic medication in the treatment of schizophrenia. *Journal of Clinical Psychiatry, 67*(7), 1114–1123.

Ball, M. P., Coons, V. B., & Buchanan, R. W. (2001). A program for treating olanzapine related weight gain. *Psychiatric Services, 52*(7), 967–969.

Bandura, A. (1995). *Self-Efficacy in Changing Societies*. New York, NY: Cambridge University Press.

Barnes, A. (2008). Race and hospital diagnoses of schizophrenia and mood disorders. *Social Work, 53*(1), 77–83.

Barnes, T. R. (1989). A rating scale for drug-induced akathisia. *British Journal of Psychiatry, 154*(5), 672–676.

Beebe, L. H. (2006). Walking tall: A person with schizophrenia on a journey to better health. *Journal of Psychosocial Nursing, 44*(6), 53–55.

Beebe, L. H., Smith, K., Burk, R., Dessieux, O. L., Velligan, D., Tavakoli, A., & Tennison, C. (2010). Effect of a motivational group intervention on exercise self efficacy and outcome expectations for exercise in schizophrenia spectrum disorders. *Journal of the American Psychiatric Nurses' Association, 16*(2), 105–113.

Beebe, L. H., Smith, K., Davis, J., Roman, M., & Burk, R. (2012). Meet me at the crossroads: Clinical research engages practitioners, educators, students and patients. *Perspectives in Psychiatric Care, 48*(2), 76–82.

Beebe, L. H., Tian, L., Morris, N., Goodwin, A., Allen, S., & Kuldau, J. (2005). Effects of exercise on mental and physical health parameters of persons with schizophrenia. *Issues in Mental Health Nursing, 26*(6), 661–676.

Bobes, J., Arango, C., Garcia-Garcia, M., & Rejas, J. (2010). Healthy lifestyle habits and 10-year cardiovascular risk in schizophrenia spectrum disorders: an analysis of the impact of smoking tobacco in the CLAMORS schizophrenia cohort. *Schizophrenia Research, 119*(1–3), 101–109.

Borras, L., Mohr, S., Gillieron, C., Brandt, P. Y., Rieben, I., Leclerc, C., & Huguelet, P. (2010). Religion and spirituality: How clinicians in Quebec and Geneva cope with the issue when faced with patients suffering from chronic psychosis. *Community Mental Health Journal, 46*(1), 77–86.

Bowie, C. R., Leung, W. W., & Reichenberg, A. (2008). Predicting schizophrenia patients' real world behavior with specific neuropsychological and functional capacity measures. *Biological Psychiatry, 63*(5), 505–511.

Brunero, S., & Lamont, S. (2010) Health behavior beliefs and physical health risk factors for cardiovascular disease in an outpatient sample of consumers with severe mental illness: A cross sectional survey. *International Journal of Nursing Studies, 47*(6), 753–760.

Byrne, M., Agerbo, E., & Bennedsen, B. (2007). Obstetric conditions and risk of first admission with schizophrenia: A Danish national register-based study. *Schizophrenia Research, 97*(1–3), 51–59.

Callicott, J. H., Bertolino, A., Mattay, V. S., Langheim, F. J., Duyn, J., Coppola, R., Goldberg, T. E., & Weinberger, D. R. (2000). Physiological dysfunction of the dorsolateral prefrontal cortex in schizophrenia revisited. *Cerebral Cortex, 10*(11), 1078–1092.

Cardno, A. G., Marshall, E. J., Coid, B. Macdonald, A. M., Ribchester, T. R., Davies, N. J., … Murray, R. M. (1999). Heritability estimates for psychotic disorders: The Maudsley twin psychosis series. *Archives of General Psychiatry, 56*(2), 162–168.

Centers for Disease Control and Prevention (CDC). (2010). Defining overweight and obesity. Available at http://www.cdc.gov/obesity/defining.html

Centorrino, F., Wurtman, J. J., Duca, K. A., Fellman, V. H., Fogarty, K. V., Berry, J. M., … Baldessarini, R. J. (2006). Weight loss in overweight patients maintained on atypical antipsychotic agents. *International Journal of Obesity, 30*(6), 1011–1016.

Chamove, A. S. (1986). Positive short-term effects of activity on behavior in chronic schizophrenic patients. *British Journal of Clinical Psychology, 25*(2), 125–133.

Chen, C. K., Chen, Y. C., & Huang, Y. S. (2009). Effects of a 10-week weight control program on obese patients with schizophrenia or schizoaffective disorder: A 12- month follow up. *Psychiatry and Clinical Neuroscience, 63*(1), 17–22.

Cheng, J. Y., Ko, J. S., & Chen, R. Y. (2008). Meta-regression analysis using latitude as moderator of paternal age related schizophrenia risk. *Schizophrenia Research, 99*(1–3), 71–76.

Citrome, L. (2011). Neurochemical models of schizophrenia: Transcending dopamine. *Current Psychiatry, 10*(9), S10–S14.

Citrome, L. (2012). A systematic review of meta-analyses of the efficacy of oral atypical antipsychotics for the treatment of adult patients with schizophrenia. *Expert Opinion on Pharmacotherapy, 13*(11), 1545–1573.

Cooper, C., Morgan, C., Byrne, M., Dazzan, P., Morgan, K., Hutchinson, G., … Fearon, P. (2008). Perceptions of disadvantage, ethnicity and psychosis. *British Journal of Psychiatry, 192*(3), 185–190.

Costafreda, S. G., Fu, C. H., Picchioni, M., Touloupoulou, T., McDonald, C., Kravariti, E., … McGuire, P. K. (2011). Pattern of neural responses to verbal fluency shows diagnostic specificity for schizophrenia and bipolar disorder. *BMC Psychiatry, 28*(11), 18.

Dalman, C., Alleback, P., & Gunnell, D. (2008). Infections in the CNS during childhood and the risk of subsequent psychotic illness: A cohort study of more than one million Swedish subjects. *American Journal of Psychiatry, 165*(1), 59–65.

Davidson, L., Chinman, M., Kloos, B., Weingarten, R., Stayner, D., & Tebes, J. (1999). Peer support among individuals with severe mental illness: A review of the evidence. *Clinical Psychology: Science and Practice, 6*(2), 165–187.

Davies, G., Welham, J., & Chant, D. (2003). A systematic review and meta-analysis of Northern Hemisphere season of birth studies in schizophrenia. *Schizophrenia Bulletin, 29*(3), 587–593.

Dealberto, M. J. (2007). Why are immigrants at increased risk for psychosis? Vitamin D insufficiency, epigenetic mechanisms, or both? *Medical Hypotheses, 68*(2), 259–267.

Dealberto, M. J. (2010). Ethnic origin and increased risk for schizophrenia in immigrants to countries of recent and longstanding immigration. *Acta Psychiatrica Scandanavica, 121*(5), 325–339.

DeHert, M., Schreurs, V., Vancampfort, D., & van Winkel, R. (2009). Metabolic syndrome in people with schizophrenia: A review. *World Psychiatry, 8*(1), 15–22.

de Leon, J., Susce, M. T., Diaz, F. J., Rendon, D. M., & Velásquez, D. M. (2005). Variables associated with alcohol, drug, and daily smoking cessation in patients with severe mental illnesses. *Journal of Clinical Psychiatry, 66*(11), 1447–1455.

Ellison-Wright, E., & Bullmore, E. (2009). Anatomy of bipolar disorder and schizophrenia: A meta-analysis. *Schizophrenia Research, 117*(1), 1–12.

Eschweller, G. W., Bartels, M., Langle, G., Wild, B., Gaertner, I., & Nickola, M. (2002). Heart rate variability in the ECG trace of routine EEGs: Fast monitoring for the anticholinergic effects of clozapine and olanzapine? *Pharmacopsychiatry, 35*(3), 96–100.

Evans, S., Newton, R., & Higgins, S. (2005). Nutritional intervention to prevent weight gain in patients commenced on olanzapine: A randomized controlled trial. *Australian and New Zealand Journal of Psychiatry, 39*(6), 479–486.

Ewing, J. A. (1984). Detecting alcoholism: The CAGE questionnaire. *Journal of the American Medical Association, 252*(14): 1905–1907.

Field, H., & Waldfogel, S. (1995). Severe ocular self injury. *General Hospital Psychiatry, 17*(3), 224–227.

Fogarty, M., Happell, B., & Pininkahana, J. (2004). The benefits of an exercise program for people with schizophrenia: A pilot study. *Psychiatric Rehabilitation Journal, 28*(2), 173–176.

Gautam, S., & Meena, P. S. (2011). Drug-emergent metabolic syndrome in patients with schizophrenia receiving atypical (second-generation) antipsychotics. *Indian Journal of Psychiatry, 53*(2), 128–133.

George, T. P., Vessicchio, J. C., Saccok, A., Weinberger, A. H., Dudas, M. M., Allen, T. M., … Jadow, P. I. (2008). A placebo controlled trial of bupropion combined with nicotine patch for smoking cessation in schizophrenia. *Biological Psychiatry, 63*(11), 1092–1096.

Gimino, F. A., & Levin, S. J. (1984). The effects of aerobic exercise on perceived self-image in post-hospitalized schizophrenic patients. *Medicine and Science in Sports and Exercise, 16,* 139.

Goldberg, T. E., & Gomar, J. J. (2009). Targeting cognition in schizophrenia research: From etiology to treatment. *American Journal of Psychiatry, 166*(6), 631–644.

Gubert, C., Stertz, L., Pfaffenseller, B., Rezin, G. T., Massuda, R., Streck, E. L., … Kunz, M. (2013). Mitochondrial activity and oxidative stress markers in peripheral blood mononuclear cells of patients with bipolar disorder, schizophrenia, and healthy subjects. *Journal of Psychiatric Research, 47*(10), 1396–1402.

Gumus, A. B. (2008). Health education needs of patients with schizophrenia and their families. *Archives of Psychiatric Nursing, 22*(3), 156–165

Guy, W. (1976). *Assessment Manual for Psychopharmacology—Revised* (DHEW Publication No. ADM 76-338). Rockville, MD: U.S. Department of Health, Education, and Welfare, Public Health Service, Alcohol, Drug Abuse, and Mental Health Administration, NIMH Psychopharmacology Research Branch, Division of Extramural Research Programs, pp. 534–537. Available at http://imaging.ubmmedica.com/all/editorial/psychiatrictimes/pdfs/clinical-scales-aims-form.pdf

Harvard Mental Health Letter. (2010). Schizophrenia treatment recommendations updated: The new PORT guidelines focus on improving physical as well as mental health. *Harvard Mental Health Letter, 26*(12), 4–5.

Harvey, J. D., & Strassnig, M. (2012). Predicting the severity of everyday functional disability in people with schizophrenia: Cognitive deficits, functional capacity, symptoms and health status. *World Psychiatry, 11*(2), 73–79.

Heston, I. I. (1966). Psychiatric disorders in the foster home reared children of schizophrenic mothers. *British Journal of Psychiatry, 112,* 819–825.

Himelhoch, S., Slade, E., Kreyenbuhl, J., Medoff, D., Brown, C., & Dixon, L. (2012). Antidepressant prescribing patterns among VA patients with schizophrenia. *Schizophrenia Research, 136*(1–3), 32–35.

Huguelet, P., Mohr, S., Borras, L., Gillieron, C., & Brandt, P. Y. (2006). Spirituality and religious practices among outpatients with schizophrenia and their clinicians. *Psychiatric Services, 57*(5), 366–372.

Isaacson, J. H., & Schorling, J. B. (1999). Screening for alcohol problems in primary care. *Medical Clinics of North America, 83*(6), 1547–1563.

Kaiser, S., Heekeren, K., & Simon, J. (2011). The negative symptoms of schizophrenia: Category or continuum? *Psychopathology, 44*(6), 345–353.

Kallman, F. J. (1946). The genetic theory of schizophrenia: An analysis of 691 schizophrenic twin index families. *American Journal of Psychiatry, 103,* 309–322.

Keefe, R. S. E., Bilder, R. M., & Davis, S. M. (2007). Neurocognitive effects of antipsychotic medications in patients with schizophrenia in the CATIE trial. *Archives of General Psychiatry, 64,* 633–647.

Kelly, B. D., O'Callaghan, E., Waddington, J. L., Feeney, L., Browne, S., Scully, P. J., ... Larkin, C. (2010). Schizophrenia and the city: A review of literature and prospective study of psychosis and urbanicity in Ireland. *Schizophrenia Research, 116*(1), 75–89.

Kerfoot, K. E., Rosenheck, R. A., Petrakis, I. L., Swartz, M. S., Keefe, R. S., McEvoy, J. P., Stroup, T. S., & CATIE Investigators. (2011). Substance use and schizophrenia: Adverse correlates in the CATIE study sample. *Schizophrenia Research, 132*(2–3), 177–182.

Keshavan, M. S., Tandon, R., Boutros, N., & Nasrallah, H. A. (2008). Schizophrenia: Just the facts, what we know in 2008: Part 3, Psychophysiology. *Schizophrenia Research, 106,* 89–107.

Khashan, A. S., Abel, K. M., & McNamee, R. (2008). Higher risk of offspring schizophrenia following antenatal exposure to serious adverse life events. *Archives of General Psychiatry, 65,* 146–152.

Kirkbride, J. B., Fearon, P., Morgan, C., Dazzan, P., Morgan, K., Tarrant, J., ... Jones, P. B. (2006). Heterogeneity in incidence rates of schizophrenia and other psychotic syndromes: Findings from the 3-center Aetiology and Ethnicity in Schizophrenia and Related Psychosis (AeSOP) study. *Archives of General Psychiatry, 63,* 250–258.

Kirkpatrick, B. (2014). Developing concepts in negative symptoms: Primary vs. secondary and apathy vs. expression. *Journal of Clinical Psychiatry, 75*(Suppl 1), 3–7.

Knowler, W. C., Barrett-Connor, E., Fowler, S. E., Hamman, R. F., Lachin, J. M., Walker, E. A., & Nathan, D. M. (2002). Reduction in the incidence of Type II diabetes with lifestyle intervention or metformin. *New England Journal of Medicine, 346,* 393–403.

Kopelowicz, A., Ventura, J., Liberman, R. P., & Mintz, J.(2008). Consistency of brief psychiatric rating scale factor structure across a broad spectrum of schizophrenia patients. patients. *Psychopathology, 41*(2):77–84.

Kreyenbuhl, J., Schizophrenia Patient Outcomes Research Team (PORT). (2010). The 2009 Schizophrenia PORT psychosocial treatment recommendations and summary statements. *Schizophrenia Bulletin, 36,* 48–70.

Kreyenbuhl, J., Buchanan, R. W., Dickerson, F. B., & Dixon, L. B.; Schizophrenia Patient Outcomes Research Team (PORT). (2010). The Schizophrenia Patient Outcomes Research Team (PORT): Updated treatment recommendations. *Schizophrenia Bulletin, 36,* 94–103.

Kurtz, M. M., & Mueser, K. T. (2008). A meta analysis of controlled research on social skills training for schizophrenia. *Journal of Consulting and Clinical Psychology, 76,* 491–504.

Kurtz, M. M., & Richardson, C. L. (2011). Social cognitive training for schizophrenia: a meta-analytic investigation of controlled research. *Schizophrenia Bulletin, 38*(5), 1092–1104.

Kwon, J. S., Choi, J. S., Bahk, W. M., Kim, C. Y., Kim, C. H., Shin, Y. C., Park, B. J., & Oh, C. G. (2006). Weight management program for treatment-emergent weight gain in olanzapine-treated patients with schizophrenia or schizoaffective disorder: A 12-week randomized controlled clinical trial. *Journal of Clinical Psychiatry, 67*(4), 547–553.

Lang, K., Federico, V., Muser, E., Menzin, J., & Menzin, J. (2013). Rates and predictors of antipsychotic non-adherence and hospitalization in medicaid and commercially-insured patients with schizophrenia. *Journal of Medical Economics, 16*(8), 997–1006.

Leamy, M., Bird, V., Le Boutillier, C., Williams, J., & Slade, M. (2011). Conceptual framework for personal recovery in mental health: Systematic review and narrative synthesis. *British Journal of Psychiatry, 199*(6), 445–452.

Leucht, S., Corves, C., & Arbter, D. (2009). Second generation versus first generation antipsychotic drugs for schizophrenia: A meta analysis. *Lancet, 373,* 31–41.

Leonard, C. J., Kaiser, S. T., Robinson, B. M., Kappenman, E. S., Hahn, B., Gold, J. M., & Luck, S. J. (2012). Toward the neural mechanisms of reduced working memory capacity in schizophrenia. *Cerebral Cortex, 23*(7), 1582–1592.

Littrell, K. H. (2004). Obesity, diabetes, hyperlipidemia, and antipsychotic medications: Breaking the link. *Advanced Studies in Nursing, 2*(3), 101–109.

Littrell, K. H., Hilligoss, N. M., Kirshner, C. D., Petty, R. G., & Johnson, C. G. (2003). The effects of an educational intervention on antipsychotic induced weight gain. *Journal of Nursing Scholarship, 35*(3), 237–241.

Masand, P. S. (1999). Relative weight gain among antipsychotics. *Journal of Clinical Psychiatry, 60*(10), 706–708.

McCabe, R., Healey, P. G., Priebe, S., Lavelle, M., Dodwell, D, Laugharne, R., Snell, A., & Bremner, S. (2013). Shared understanding in psychiatrist-patient communication: Association with treatment adherence in schizophrenia. *Patient Education and Counseling, 93*(1), 73–79.

McDonagh, M., Peterson, K., Carson, S., Fu, R., & Thakurta, S. (2010). *Drug Class Review: Atypical Antipsychotic Drugs: Final Update 3 Report.* Portland, OR: Oregon Health & Science University.

Meerwijk, E. L., van Meijel, B., van den Bout, J., Kerkhof, A., de Vogel, W., & Grypdonk, M. (2010). Development and evaluation of a guideline for nursing care of suicidal patients with schizophrenia. *Perspectives in Psychiatric Care, 46*(1), 65–73.

Melle, I., Johannson, J. O., & Friis, O. (2006). Early detection of the first episode of schizophrenia and suicidal behavior. *American Journal of Psychiatry, 163,* 800–804.

Menza, M., Vreeland, B., Minsky, S., Gara, M., Radler, D. R., & Sakowitz, M. (2004). Managing atypical antipsychotic associated weight gain: 12-month data on a multimodal weight control program. *Journal of Clinical Psychiatry, 65*(4), 471–477.

Mohr, S., Borras, L., Betrisey, C., Pierre-Yves, B., Gilliéron, C., & Huguelet, P. (2010). Delusions with religious content in patients with psychosis: How they interact with spiritual coping. *Psychiatry, 73*(2), 158–172.

Mohr, S., & Huguelet, P. (2004). The relationship between schizophrenia and religion and its implications for care. *Swiss Medical Weekly, 134*(25–26), 369–376.

Moller, M. D. (2013). Neurobiological responses and schizophrenia and other psychotic disorders. In G. Stuart, (Ed.). *Principles and Practices of Psychiatric Nursing* (10th ed.). St. Louis, MO: C.V. Mosby, pp. 361–362.

Moller, M. D., & Zauszniewsky, J. (2011). Psychophenomenology of the post-psychotic adjustment process. *Archives of Psychiatric Nursing, 25*(4), 253–268.

Mueser, K. T., & Gingerich, S. (2013). Treatment of co-occurring psychotic and substance use disorders. *Social Work in Public Health, 28*(3–4), 424–439.

National Cholesterol Education Panel. (2002). Third report of the National Cholesterol Education Program Expert Panel on Detection, Evaluation and Treatment of High Blood Cholesterol in Adults (Adult Treatment Panel III). Final report. *Circulation, 106,* 3143–3421.

National Heart Lung and Blood Institute. (2010). Assessing your weight and health risk. Available at http://www.nhlbi.nih.gov/health/public/heart/obesity/lose_wt/risk.htm

National Institute of Mental Health. (2008). What is schizophrenia? Available at http://www.nimh.nih.gov/health/publications/schizophrenia/what-is-schizophrenia.shtml

Osborn, D. P., Nazareth, I., & King, M. B.(2007). Physical activity, dietary habits and coronary heart disease risk factor knowledge amongst people with severe mental illness: A cross sectional comparative study in primary care. *Social Work, 42*(10), 787–793.

Pelham, T. W., Campagna, P. D., Ritvo, P. G., & Birnie, W. A. (1993). The effects of exercise therapy on clients in a psychiatric rehabilitation program. *Psychosocial Rehabilitation Journal, 16*, 75–84.

Pendlebury, J., Haddad, P., & Dursun, S. (2005). Evaluation of a behavioral weight management programme for patients with severe mental illness: 3 year results. *Human Psychopharmacology, 20*, 447–448.

Pesut, B. (2008). Spirituality and spiritual care in nursing fundamentals textbooks. *Journal of Nursing Education, 47*(4), 167–173.

Pilling, S., Bebbington, P., Kuipers, E., Garety, P., Geddes, J., Martindale, B., Orback, G., & Morgan, C. (2002). Psychological treatments in schizophrenia: I—Meta analysis of family intervention and cognitive behavior therapy. *Psychological Medicine, 32*, 763–782.

Quintero, J., Barbudo Del Cura, E., Lopez-Ibor, M. I., & Lopez, J. J. (2011). The evolving concept of treatment resistant schizophrenia. *Acta Psychiatrica Espanolas, 39*(4), 236–250.

Raiff, N. (1984). Some health related outcomes of self help participation. Recovery Inc. as a case example of a self help organization in mental health. In A. Gartner & E. Reissman, (Eds.). *The Self Help Revolution*. New York, NY: Human Sciences Press, pp. 183–193.

Remkumar, P., Fannon, D., Kuipers, E., Simmons, A., Frangou, S., & Kumari, V. (2008). Emotional decision making and its dissociable components in schizophrenia and schizoaffective disorder: A behavioural and MRI investigation. *Neuropsychologica, 46*(7), 2002–2012.

Rice, M. J. (2011).Assertive community treatment: Evidence based hope for the seriously mentally ill. *Journal of the American Psychiatric Nurses Association, 17*, 13–15.

Ripke, S., O'Dushlaine, C., Chambert, K., Moran, J. L., Kahler, A. K., Akterin, S., … Sullivan, P.F.. (2013). Genome-wide association analysis identifies 13 new risk loci for schizophrenia. *Nature Genetics, 45*(10), 1150–1159.

Sacchetti, E., Galluzzo, A., Panariello, A., Parrinello, G., & Cappa, S. F. (2008). Self-ordered pointing and visual conditional associative learning tasks in drug-free schizophrenia spectrum disorder patients. *BMC Psychiatry. 8*, 6.

Sadock, B. J., & Sadock, V. A. (2007). *Kaplan and Sadock's Synopsis of Psychiatry* (10th ed.). Philadelphia, PA: Lippincott, Williams and Wilkins.

Saha, S., Chant, D., Welham, J., & McGrath, J. (2005). A systematic review of the prevalence of schizophrenia. *PlosMed, 2*, 413–433.

Sanz, J. C., Gomez, V., Vargas, M. L., & Marin, J. J. (2012). Dimensions of attention impairment and negative symptoms in schizophrenia: A multidimensional approach using the Conners Continuous Performance Test in a Spanish population. *Cognitive Behavioral Neurology, 25*(2), 63–71.

Schultze-Lutter, F. (2009). Subjective symptoms of schizophrenia in research and the clinic: the basic symptom concept. *Schizophrenia Bulletin, 35*, 5–8.

Schultze-Lutter, F., Schimmelmann, B. G., Klosterkotter, J., & Ruhrmann, S. (2012). Comparing the prodrome of schizophrenia-spectrum psychoses and affective disorders with and without psychotic features. *Schizophrenia Research, 138*(2–3), 218–222.

Segall, J. M., Turner, J. A., van Erp, T. G., White, T., Bockholt, H. J., Gollub, R. I., … Calhoun, V. D. (2009). Voxel-based morphometric multisite collaborative study on schizophrenia. *Schizophrenia Bulletin, 35*, 82–95.

Shean, G. D. (2009). Evidence based psychosocial practices and recovery from schizophrenia. *Psychiatry, 72*(4), 307–320.

Siddle, R., Haddock, G., Tarrier, N., & Faragher, E. B. (2002). Religious delusions in patients admitted to the hospital with schizophrenia. *Social Psychiatry and Psychiatric Epidemiology, 37*, 130–138.

Sims, A. (1995). *Symptoms in the Mind: An Introduction to Descriptive Psychopathology*. London, UK: W.B. Saunders.

Smiley, J. F., Rosoklija, G., Mancevski, B., Pergolizzi, D., Figarsky, K., Bleiwas, C., & Dwork, A. J. (2011). Hemispheric comparisons of neuron density in the planum temporale of schizophrenia and nonpsychiatric brains.

Psychiatry Research: Neuroimaging, 192(1), 1–11. doi:10.1016/j.pscychresns.2010.11.007

Somerville, S. M., Conley, R. R., & Roberts, R. C. (2011). Mitochondria in the striatum of subjects with schizophrenia. *World Journal of Biological Psychiatry, 12*(1), 48–56.

Sorg, C., Manoliu, A., Neufang, S., Myers, N., Peters, H., Schwerthöffer, D., & Riedl, V. (2013). Increased intrinsic brain activity in the striatum reflects symptom dimensions in schizophrenia. *Schizophrenia Bulletin 39*, 387–395.

Stahl, S. M. (2009). *The Prescriber's Guide: Stahl's Essential Psychopharmacology*. New York, NY: Cambridge University Press.

Stahl, S. M. (2013). *Stahl's Essential Psychopharmacology. Neuroscientific Basis and Practical Applications* (4th ed.). New York, NY: Cambridge University Press.

Stahl, S. M., & Buckley, P. F. (2007). Negative symptoms of schizophrenia: A problem that will not go away. *Acta Psychiatrica Scandanavica, 115*, 4–11.

Stimmel, G. L., Gutierrez, M. A., & Lee, V. (2002). Ziprasidone: An atypical antipsychotic drug for the treatment of schizophrenia. *Clinical Therapeutics, 24*(1), 21–37.

Stokes, C., and Peet, M. (2003). Dietary sugar and polyunsaturated fatty acidconsumption as predictors of severity of schizophrenia symptoms. *Nutrition and Neuroscience, 7*(4), 247–249.

Sullivan, P. F., Kendler, K. S., & Neale, M. C. (2003). Schizophrenia as a complex trait: Evidence from a meta-analysis of twin studies. *Archives of General Psychiatry, 60*, 1187–1192.

Sutterland, A. L., Dieleman, J., Storosum, J. G., Voordouw, B. A., Kroon, J., Veldhuis, J., Denys, D. A., de Haan, L., & Sturkenboom, M. C. (2013). Annual incidence rate of schizophrenia and schizophrenia spectrum disorders in a longitudinal population-based cohort study. *Social Psychiatry and Psychiatric Epidemiology, 48*(9), 1357–1365.

Swartz, M. S., Wagner, H. R., Swanson, J. W., Stroup, T. S., McEvoy, J. P., Canive, J. M., … Lieberman, J. A. (2006). Substance use in persons with schizophrenia: Baseline prevalence and correlates from the NIMH CATIE study. *Community Mental Health Journal, 194*(3), 164–172.

Swinton, J. (2001). *Spirituality and Mental Health Care*. London, UK: Jessica Kingsley.

Tandon, R., Nasrallah, H. A., & Keshavan, M. S. (2009). Schizophrenia: Just the facts. 4. Clinical features and conceptualization. *Schizophrenia Research, 110*, 1–23.

Turkington, D., Sensky, T., Scott, J., Barnes, T. R., Nur, U., Siddle, R., Hammond, K., Samarasekara, N., & Kingdon, D. (2008). A randomized controlled trial of cognitive behavioral therapy for persistent symptoms in schizophrenia: A 5 year follow up. *Schizophrenia Research, 98*, 1–7.

Uçok, A., Gorwood, P., Karadayi, G., on behalf of the EGOFORS. (2011). Employment and its relationship with functionality and quality of life in patients with schizophrenia: EGOFORS Study. *European Psychiatry, 27*(6), 422–425.

Ungvari, G. S., Coggins, W., Leung, S. K., & Gerevich, J. (2007). Schizophrenia with prominent catatonic features (catatonic Schizophrenia): II. Factor analysis of the catatonic syndrome. *Biological Psychiatry, 31*, 462–468.

U.S. Department of Health and Human Services. (2011). The benefits of physical activity. Available at http://www.cdc.gov/physicalactivity/everyone/health/index.html

Vercammen, A., Morris, R., Green, M. J., Lenroot, R., Kulkarni, J., Carr, V. J., Weickert, C. S., & Weickert, T. W. (2012). Reduced neural activity of the prefrontal cognitive control circuitry during response inhibition to negative words in people with schizophrenia. *Journal of Psychiatry and Neuroscience, 37*(6), 379–388.

Veselinović, T., Schorn, H., Vernaleken, I., Schiffl, K., Hiemke, C., Zernig, G., Gur, R., & Gründer, G.(2011) Effects of antipsychotic treatment on psychopathology and motor symptoms: A placebo-controlled study in healthy volunteers. *Psychopharmacology, 218*(4), 733–748.

Vreeland, B., Minsk, S., Menza, M., Rigussio-Radler, D., Roemheld-Hamm, B., & Stern, R. (2003). A program for managing weight gain associated with atypical antipsychotics. *Psychiatric Services, 54*(8), 1155–1157.

Wang, J. F., Shao, C., Sun, X., & Young, L. T. (2009). Increased oxidative stress in the anterior cingulated cortex of subjects with bipolar disorder and schizophrenia. *Bipolar Disorders, 11*, 523–529.

Waugh, A. (1986). Auto castration and biblical delusions in schizophrenia. *British Journal of Psychiatry, 149*, 656–659.

Weder, N., Muralee, S., Penland, H., & Tampi, R. R. (2008). Catatonia: A review. *Annals of Clinical Psychiatry, 20*, 97–107.

Wexler, B. E., Zhu, H., Bell, M. D., Nicholls, S. S., Fulbright, R. K., Gore, J. C., Colibazzi, T., Amat, J., Bansal, R., & Peterson, B. S. (2009). Neuropsychological near normality and brain structure abnormality in schizophrenia. *American Journal of Psychiatry, 166*(2), 189–195.

Wilson, B. A., Shannon, M. T., & Shields, K. (2014). *Pearson Nurse's Drug Guide.* Upper Saddle River, NJ: Prentice Hall.

Winterer, G. (2010). Why do patients with schizophrenia smoke? *Current Opinion in Psychiatry, 23,* 112–119.

Woodberry, K. A., Guiliano, A. J., & Seidman, I. J. (2008). Premorbid IQ in schizophrenia: A meta analytic review. *American Journal of Psychiatry, 165,* 579–587.

Woods, G., Taggart, C., Boggs, R., & Cadden, I. (2013). Neuroleptic malignant syndrome associated with quetiapine and venlafaxine use: A case report and discussion. *Therapeutic Advances in Psychopharmacology, 3*(1), 53–55.

Woods, S. W., Tandy, M., & McGlashan, T. H. (2001). The "prodromal" patient: Both symptomatic and at-risk. *CNS Spectrums, 6,* 223–232.

World Health Organization. (2011). Metabolic syndrome. Available at http://www.medicinenet.com/metabolic_syndrome/article.htm

Wu, M. K., Wang, C. K., Bai, Y. M., Huang, C. Y., & Lee, S. D. (2007). Outcomes of obese clozapine treated inpatients with schizophrenia placed on a 6 month diet and physical activity program. *Psychiatric Services, 58,* 544–550.

Wu, R. R., Zhao, J. P., Guo, X. F., He, Y. Q., Fang, M. S., Guo, W. B., Chen, J. D., & Li, L. H. (2008). Metformin addition attenuates olanzapine induced weight gain in drug naïve first episode schizophrenia patients, a double blind, placebo controlled study. *American Journal of Psychiatry, 165,* 352–358.

Wykes, T., Steel, C., Everitt, B., & Tarrier, N. (2008). Cognitive behavioral therapy for schizophrenia, effect sizes, clinical models and methodological rigor. *Schizophrenia Bulletin, 34,* 523–537.

Zhang, X. Y., Chen, da C., Qi, L. Y., Wang, F., Xiu, M. H., Chen, S., Wu, G. Y., Kosten, T.A., & Kosten, T R. (2009). Gender differences in the prevalence, risk and clinical correlates of tardive dyskinesia in Chinese schizophrenia. *Psychopharmacology, 205*(4), 647–654

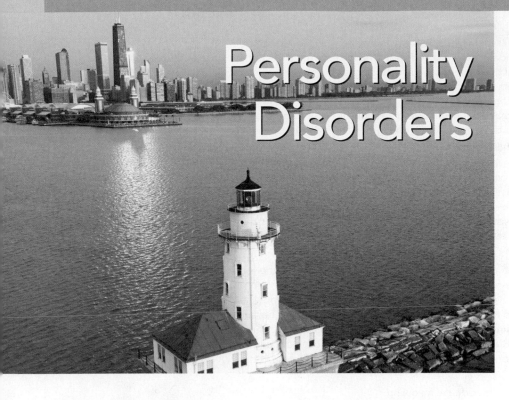

Personality Disorders

18

Kimberley R. Meyer

Learning Outcomes

1. Examine the etiology of personality disorders.

2. Summarize the impact of biological, psychological, sociological, cultural, and spiritual domains on personality disorders.

3. Categorize key symptoms of different personality disorders.

4. Evaluate different pharmacologic and nonpharmacologic therapies used in the treatment of personality disorders.

5. Plan evidence-based nursing care for patients diagnosed with personality disorders.

Key Terms

countertransference, 405
dialectical behavior therapy (DBT), 401
emotional dysregulation, 393
emotional regulation, 392
labile, 397
narcissism, 394
personality, 392
personality disorder, 392
projection, 397
projective identification, 405
reasonable doubt, 406
self-injurious behavior (SIB), 397
splitting, 397
transference, 405
transitional object, 398

critical thinking

Brenda Initial Onset

Brenda Marks is an 18-year-old woman who is being hospitalized following a suspected suicide attempt, in which she cut both her wrists. Brenda is accompanied to the hospital by her stepmother. When Sarah, the admitting nurse on the mental health unit, conducts the admission interview, Brenda tells her that she really did not plan to kill herself, but she just was trying to relieve the incredibly intense feelings of emptiness, pain, and anger she was experiencing. The intake interview and hospital records indicate that Brenda has a history of chaotic and short-lived relationships with others, along with impulsivity, as evidenced by two prior cutting episodes involving her arms and legs. Brenda reports she has a difficult time at school and struggles with academics and relationships.

Although Brenda's family has distanced themselves from her, she lives with her father and stepmother. Her parents divorced when Brenda was 6 years old, and her father is remarried with children. Her step-mother is Nigerian and quite vocal about her belief that Brenda is harassed by evil spirits and may be experiencing punishment because of her promiscuity. Her biological mother, a real estate agent, is very focused on her own career. Brenda's two sisters from her father's first marriage are both married with children. They are busy with their families and have placed limits on Brenda, so their children are not involved with what they term her "chaos."

Brenda complains about her inability to do well at school or keep a job, and the loneliness she feels because of her difficulty with relationships. She recently lent her car to a much older boyfriend, even signing a note granting permission for him to have it. Her boyfriend took the car, and she has not seen it—or him—in 2 months. She is still responsible for the car payments and the insurance, but because she signed a waiver, the police cannot do anything about recovering her car. She misses her boyfriend and really does not want to get him in trouble. Brenda cannot look for a new job without a car, and she is beginning to feel hopeless about her situation. She says she is feeling tempted to resume cutting her wrists.

Sarah determines with Brenda that her symptoms include the following:

- Lacerations with stitches on both her wrists
- Increasing feelings of hopelessness and powerlessness
- Recurrent thoughts of cutting herself
- Difficulty managing the consequences of impulsive decision making

Sarah places Brenda on suicide precautions, under which the staff will check on her every 15 minutes. She establishes a safety agreement, in which Brenda agrees to contact the staff if she is feeling in imminent danger of hurting herself. Sarah contacts the nurse practitioner on the team. The nurse prac-titioner prescribes valproic acid (Depakote) 500 mg twice a day by mouth to help curb Brenda's extreme impulsivity. Sarah suspects that Brenda is suffering with borderline personality disorder (BPD) but further assessment needs to be made to confirm the diagnosis and assess for depression and/or anxiety. Sarah also refers Brenda to the dialectical behavior therapy (DBT) group, which begins in the hospital and follows up in the community. Sarah tells Brenda that from her experience and in the litera-ture, DBT is the most effective therapy to help mitigate her symptoms (see pages 401–402). DBT also will provide Brenda with new skills to help manage the intense pain she is experiencing.

APPLICATION

1. Address the five domains for Brenda:
   a. Biological
   b. Psychological
   c. Sociological
   d. Cultural
   e. Spiritual
2. In what ways do you think Brenda might be suffering? Why?
3. How would you prioritize Brenda's needs at this time, and why?
4. In what ways does Sarah convey hope to Brenda? What might you do differ-ently to offer hope?

Introduction

Personality refers to a distinctive set of traits, behavior styles, and patterns that make up an individual's character. How individuals perceive the world, along with their attitudes, thoughts, and feel-ings, are all part of personality. Personality is developed through a complex combination of genetic and environmental factors (Howland, 2007). Personality characteristics are unique to each individual and influence how individuals think, cope with stress, and relate to others. An individual's affect and **emotional regula-tion,** which includes the ability to control the flux and expression of emotions, are also affected by personality. Those with more adap-tive personalities are able to cope with normal stresses, have very little difficulty managing their emotions, and have no trouble form-ing relationships with family, friends, and co-workers (National Mental Health America, 2013).

For some individuals, certain personality characteristics begin to negatively affect their everyday lives. They find that they are unable to maintain relationships, manage emotions and impulsivity, and generally cope with life's stresses. These individuals experience a fair amount of suffering. They often feel out of control and can feel suspi-cious and mistrustful, as well as powerless and unhappy. They may develop a **personality disorder**—a persistent, maladaptive pattern of thinking, coping, and relating to others. This chapter covers each of the specific personality disorders in turn, but the American Psychiat-ric Association (APA) has identified criteria that are common to all personality disorders (see DSM-5 Diagnostic Criteria for General Personality Disorder).

Personality disorders affect approximately 10% to 13% of people at some point in their lives. Although personality disorders often emerge in childhood, there is some reluctance to diagnose personality

Diagnostic Criteria for General Personality Disorder   DSM-5

A. An enduring pattern of inner experience and behavior that deviates markedly from the expectations of the individual's culture. This pattern is manifested in two (or more) of the following areas:
   1. Cognition (i.e., ways of perceiving and interpreting self, other people, and events).
   2. Affectivity (i.e., the range, intensity, lability, and appropriateness of emotional response).
   3. Interpersonal functioning.
   4. Impulse control.
B. The enduring pattern is inflexible and pervasive across a broad range of personal and social situations.

C. The enduring pattern leads to clinically significant distress or impairment in social, occupational, or other important areas of functioning.
D. The pattern is stable and of long duration, and its onset can be traced back at least to adolescence or early adulthood.
E. The enduring pattern is not better explained as a manifestation or consequence of another mental disorder.
F. The enduring pattern is not attributable to the physiological effects of a substance (e.g., a drug of abuse, a medication) or another medical condition (e.g., head trauma).

Source: Reprinted with permission from the *Diagnostic and Statistical Manual of Mental Disorders*, Fifth Edition, (Copyright 2013). American Psychiatric Association.

disorders in children, because the patterns of behavior and thinking could simply reflect adolescent experimentation or temporary developmental phases (Mayo Clinic, 2012). Diagnosis usually occurs when the individual's symptoms begin to significantly disrupt functioning, or when the individual's behaviors begin to affect others or result in criminal activity. Approximately 20% to 40% of psychiatric outpatients are diagnosed with personality disorders, as are up to 50% of inpatients and up to 66% of the prison population (Winship & Hardy, 2007).

Despite significant interruption to functioning, many people with personality disorders do not seek help from a health care professional. Usually, these patients present with another problem or a co-morbid illness, such as depression or bipolar disorder. In addition, research has demonstrated that inpatients diagnosed with borderline personality disorder scored higher when measured for anger, anxiety, and depression (Sollberg et al., 2012). Not all individuals, however, will experience dysfunction to the extent that hospitalization is required. Individuals with certain disorders (such as borderline and avoidant personality disorders) may experience improvement or remission of symptoms as they grow older, although this may not occur in individuals with other disorders such as obsessive–compulsive and schizotypal personality disorders (APA, 2013). With treatment, individuals can expect to achieve recovery, and even rehabilitation. It has been estimated that individuals who are treated with psychotherapy experience recovery seven times faster compared with those who follow the natural course of the illness (Hadjipavlou & Ogrodniczuk, 2010).

PRACTICE ALERT   Because patients with personality disorders often have identity diffusion, a vague and unsolidified sense of self, it is important that nurses working with these patients have a strong sense of self and identity. It also is important that nurses understand and have the ability to identify and manage their own emotions, because **emotional dysregulation**, in which the experience and expression of emotions feel out of control, is a common characteristic of personality disorders. Maintaining personal and professional boundaries is essential when working with patients with personality disorders.

Personality disorders are often diagnosed in conjunction with another psychiatric disorder. One study found this association most common in individuals with Cluster B personality disorders. Approximately 39% had received treatment for a mental health or substance abuse problem in the past 12 months (Lamont & Brunero, 2009). In a U.S. study of four personality disorder groups (schizotypal,

borderline, avoidant, and obsessive–compulsive), 96% had received psychiatric treatment and 81% had been prescribed some form of psychotropic medication (Lamont & Brunero, 2009). A combination of diagnoses complicates the treatment plan and the prognosis for many patients.

Theoretical Foundations

The etiology of most personality disorders is complex and requires examining the interaction of biopsychosocial models (Figure 18-1). Proposed etiologies can be divided into biological/neurochemical factors, cognitive/behavioral factors, and psychodynamic influences. In addition to these etiologies, various psychological theories inform the treatment of personality disorders. Carl Jung, for example, believed that the unconscious is collective and includes archetypes or inherited predispositions to perceive the world in a certain way (Ewen, 2003). He introduced the characteristics of introversion and extroversion. *Introversion* describes an individual who refuels the self with time alone. Conversely, *extroverted* people are fueled by time with others. From Jung's perspective, pathology occurs when a personality becomes imbalanced. Several theories relevant to caring for individuals with personality disorders, including Maslow's theory of human needs, are discussed in Chapter 4.

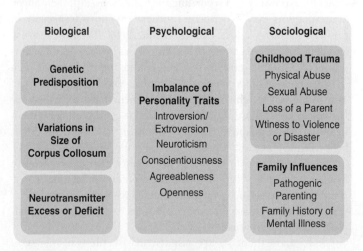

18-1   Selected biological, psychological, and sociological factors in the development of personality disorders.

Biological Domain

From a biological perspective, individuals with personality disorders may have an imbalance in brain chemistry, which may be the result of genetic predisposition, trauma, medical conditions, or a combination of these influences. Most believe the imbalance affects the cerebral cortex, the prefrontal cortex, and parts of the limbic system, especially the amygdala and the hippocampus. For example, individuals diagnosed with borderline personality disorder often are found to have a larger-than-usual amygdala, the primitive part of the brain that focuses on self-protection and anger responses (Shannon, 2011).

Neurotransmitters are an important contributor to the imbalance. Serotonin, dopamine, and norepinephrine excesses or deficits greatly affect mood, behavior, and impulse control. Medication is the treatment of choice for symptoms believed to be caused by neurotransmitter abnormalities. For example, the selective serotonin-reuptake inhibitors (SSRIs) are used to regulate serotonin, which, in turn, maintains normal mood, cognitive acuity and judgment, and impulse control. Treatment options for a neurochemical etiology also include diet and exercise, as well as, to a lesser extent, psychotherapy. As an individual's neurochemistry changes, behavior can begin to change. Conversely, as behavior changes, sometimes neurochemistry will eventually change.

As discussed in Chapter 3, specific neurotransmitters affect certain personality dimensions (Tyrer & Bateman, 2004; O'Donohue, Fowler, Lilienfeld, & Cloninger, 2007):

- *Norepinephrine:* emotional reactivity, arousal, extroversion; reward center
- *Serotonin:* inhibition of impulse/affect, harm avoidance, independence vs. need for reassurance
- *Acetylcholine:* lethargy, exploration, mood/affect
- *Dopamine:* novelty seeking, histrionic traits

Psychological Domain

From a cognitive and behavioral perspective, all behavior is learned and, as such, can be unlearned (Shannon, 2011). For individuals with personality disorders, those learned behaviors have become inflexible and maladaptive. Patients with personality disorders have particular difficulty expressing and regulating their emotions, especially anger. Some patients may experience transient psychosis, especially in response to stress (Sadock, Sadock, & Ruiz, 2009). Paranoia, distrust, and detachment are common. Feelings of inadequacy, fear of abandonment, unstable sense of self, and risk taking may also be seen among a number of the personality disorders. The strong involvement of an individual's psychology supports treatment that involves psychotherapy to target those maladaptive behaviors, substituting for them healthier, more adaptive coping. Cognitive theorists believe that behavior and affect will improve as coping improves (Shannon, 2011).

According to trait theorists, personality disorders can result from an imbalance of certain inherent and predominant traits or personality characteristics. A *trait* is defined as a characteristic that remains relatively stable over time and helps to determine how people act in any given situation (Ewen, 2003).

Two main theorists are associated with the trait theory of personality.

Gordon Allport described three levels of personality traits (Barenbaum & Winter, 2010). *Cardinal traits* are characteristics that dominate a person's entire life, usually developed later in life, and are very rare. These traits are obsessions or passions that drive the person, such as pursuit of fame. *Central traits* are characteristics that form the foundation of a person's personality. Warmth and friendliness are examples of central traits. Finally, *secondary traits* are attitudes and preferences that appear only in certain situations and with specific groups of people. Anxiety when speaking in front of groups is an example of a secondary trait (Ewen, 2003).

Hans Eysenck, a British psychologist, believed that all personality traits could be reduced to three categories: introversion/extroversion, neuroticism/emotional stability, and psychoticism (Barenbaum & Winter, 2010). Currently, five traits emerge as central: introversion/extroversion, neuroticism, conscientiousness, agreeableness, and openness.

When an individual develops an imbalance in any one area, personality can become pathological.

Sociological Domain

Trauma, such as physical or sexual abuse, is often cited as an etiologic force in the development of personality disorders. For example, the percentage of individuals who report experiencing childhood trauma (defined as sexual abuse mostly by a non-caregiver) and are diagnosed with borderline personality disorder is between 40% and 71% (National Institute of Mental Health, 2009). Along with childhood trauma, a co-morbid posttraumatic stress disorder often occurs. In those cases, individuals often experience heightened anxiety, flashbacks, and dissociative episodes that they cannot predict or control.

The focus on family of origin dysfunction and parenting is most prevalent in this etiologic theory. Parenting that is engulfing does not allow a child to separate and individuate. Indifferent parenting may force a child to separate before he or she is ready, and inconsistent parenting (usually involving an overindulging, smothering mother and an indifferent father) also affects the individual's ability to separate and identify as an individual. This is consistent with Carl Rogers's work in humanistic theory. He proposed that pathology occurs with pathogenic parenting, which occurs when parents make their love conditional, demanding that children meet their standards rather than creating standards of their own and moving toward actualization (Baurenbaum & Winter, 2010).

The effects of parenting on personality also appear in the work of Heinz Kohut, who developed a theory in relation to adult narcissistic psychopathology. **Narcissism** is characterized by excessive interest in or preoccupation with the self, which is often illustrated in manipulative or demanding behaviors and a lack of empathy for others. Kohut asserted that such a personality resulted from parental lack of empathy during development. The child then becomes unable to regulate self-esteem and moves between inflated sense of self and feelings of inferiority. The individual ends up looking to others to regulate self-esteem and to receive a sense of self (McLean, 2007).

These factors—childhood trauma and family dysfunction—contribute to an increasing individual risk for developing a personality disorder. Additional risk factors include family history of personality disorder or other mental illness, a diagnosis of childhood conduct disorder, and loss of a parent to death or divorce (Mayo Clinic, 2012). Additionally, research in maternal attachment theory has demonstrated that children who are raised by nurturing caregivers and internalize that support often view themselves positively, whereas children who never experienced approval and encouragement are more apt to develop negative views of themselves (Toth, Cicchetti, Rogosch, & Sturge-Apple, 2009).

Another sociological factor that can affect the diagnosis and treatment of personality disorders is gender. Personality disorders that are characterized by independence and aggression are most often diagnosed in men. Men often enter the system through the courts and legal troubles. However, personality disorders characterized by dependence and emotional dysregulation are most often diagnosed in women. Women are more likely to seek help voluntarily (Bjorklund, 2006).

The same tendency toward emotional dysregulation previously described frequently impairs patient relationships with family, friends, and co-workers. This can present a particular challenge for family members who live in close proximity to the patient. Family-based interventions may be necessary, and patients may need to focus on learning skills that will help them cope in their work environments. Treatment from a psychodynamic perspective historically involved re-parenting, an intensive strategy in which the therapist becomes a surrogate parent and reenacts parenting. Newer approaches involve teaching patients to parent themselves, holding themselves accountable for maladaptive behavior (Shannon, 2011).

Cultural Domain

The diagnosis and treatment of personality disorders vary from culture to culture. This could be due, in part, to differences in diagnostic practices and in help-seeking behaviors. Each culture is unique, yet there are some similarities that are characteristic. Personality characteristics such as passivity, politeness, deferential treatment of others, guardedness, and defensiveness can sometimes be explained culturally (APA, 2013). It is important to note that there is risk for misdiagnosis when differences exist between clinician and patient. Given that some cultural differences exist in all clinician–patient interactions, even between clinicians and patients with somewhat similar cultural backgrounds, all such interactions may be considered transcultural (Tseng & Streltzer, 2006).

There have been several seminal studies of culture and personality disorders. Nukolls (1992) found that clinicians in cultures that suppress affect and discourage individuation are more likely to diagnose schizoid types of personality disorders. Conversely, clinicians in cultures that encourage free expression of affect and individuation are more likely to diagnose borderline and narcissistic personality disorders. In the West, manifestations of personality disorders are more overt. Akhtar (1995) found that in less permissive societies, manifestations are more muted. This could be due, in part, to the fact that in the West, access to alcohol, drugs, firearms, and pornography, which lessen individual inhibition, are more readily available. For example, in Japan, patients diagnosed with borderline personality disorder (BPD) are less often drug and alcohol dependent than in the United States.

BPD is most frequently diagnosed in North America, the United Kingdom, and in Europe. It is less often diagnosed in developing nations. For example, in 1988 Khandelwal and Workneh found that only 1% to 3% of psychiatric outpatients in Ethiopia and India are diagnosed with personality disorders, whereas in Britain the percentage is much larger, at 32% (Bjorklund, 2006). In India, a study was conducted in 2000 by Pinto, Dhavale, Nair, Patil, and Dewan of a population of people who had attempted suicide. They found that 17.3% met the criteria for borderline personality disorder (Bjorklund, 2006).

Even within single cultures there can be wide variance in how individuals and families perceive mental illness and recommended treatments. Individual and family beliefs and preferences will affect different aspects of the treatment plan, and nurses should assess for cultural factors that may need to be considered.

Spiritual Domain

The human need for meaning and purpose, love and belonging, and hope are factors to consider when working with patients with personality disorders. Many of these individuals describe feeling alone, empty, purposeless, and hopeless. Treatment in these cases would include working with patients to find purpose in their lives and establish relationships with support people and hope that the future can be better.

People often use religious and spiritual resources as coping strategies. Religion can help promote a positive world view, help to make sense of difficult situations, give purpose and meaning to life, discourage maladaptive coping, enhance social support, promote other-directedness, help to release the need for control, provide and encourage forgiveness, and provide hope (Koenig, 2005).

There is some evidence that certain personalities are predisposed to religious involvement (Koenig, 2005). As noted earlier, Cloninger (2005) has described personality on three dimensions. An individual who is low in novelty seeking, high in reward dependence, and high in harm avoidance may be able to meet some needs through religious affiliations. Someone who is high in novelty seeking, low in reward dependence, and low harm avoidance may not feel the need for religious affiliation (Koenig, 2005).

Koenig (2005) collated a number of studies about the relationship of personality and religiosity. He stated that religious involvement tends to be associated with "greater cooperativeness, less hostility, lower sense of alienation, more altruism and concern for others, greater capacity to forgive, and a greater sense of internal control" (p. 69). It is also sometimes associated with "greater authoritarianism, guilt, dogmatism and social desirability" (p. 69). Koenig (2005) cited a study of college students conducted by Ramanaiah and colleagues in 1999, in which high and low spiritual well-being were correlated with personality profiles. The investigators administered a personality inventory and the spiritual well-being scale to 319 subjects. They found that students with high spiritual well-being scored lower on neuroticism, and higher on extroversion, agreeableness, and conscientiousness compared with students with low spiritual well-being.

Pause and Reflect

1. *Can you think of any examples of emotional dysregulation that have occurred within your own family? How did this affect your family?*

2. *How is trauma associated with the development of personality disorders? How can knowing this inform assessment and care of patients with personality disorders?*

Personality Disorders

Diagnosis of all mental illness, including personality disorders, is made using the DSM-5, developed by the American Psychiatric Association. In the previous edition, diagnoses were organized on a multiaxial system, using five axes to develop an overall picture of the patient's presentation. Axis I described the main mental illness diagnosis or diagnoses for which the patient is hospitalized and/or treated. Personality disorders were found on Axis II. With the changes in the DSM-5, these axes are no longer recognized, and personality disorders are classified similarly to other psychiatric disorders. The DSM-5 lists 10 personality disorders sorted into three clusters (Figure 18-2). There are also two additional categories. The first is for a personality change related to a medical condition, such as a brain lesion. The second category is for clients who display the criteria for a personality disorder but who do not meet the criteria for a specific disorder, or who have a personality disorder not included in the DSM-5.

Some clinicians may adopt an alternative DSM-5 model for personality disorders, which was aimed at correcting some previous issues with the current method of diagnosis. In the alternative model, personality disorders are characterized by impairments in personality functioning and pathological personality traits. The alternative model recognizes six distinct personality disorders instead of the current 10 disorders (APA, 2013).

Personality disorders are also defined by the International Statistical Classification of Diseases and Related Health Problems (ICD-10), which is published by the World Health Organization (WHO), which also is seeking to develop an international diagnostic system. ICD-10 includes paranoid, schizoid, dissocial, emotionally unstable (impulsive or borderline type), histrionic, anankastic (obsessive–compulsive), anxious (avoidant), and dependent personality disorders (WHO, n.d.).

Cluster A Personality Disorders

The Cluster A disorders, also termed *odd–eccentric*, are marked by atypical behaviors, such as unjustifiable suspicion of others, that greatly impair social functioning.

Paranoid personality disorder is characterized by extreme suspiciousness, mistrust, and guardedness. Patients with this disorder

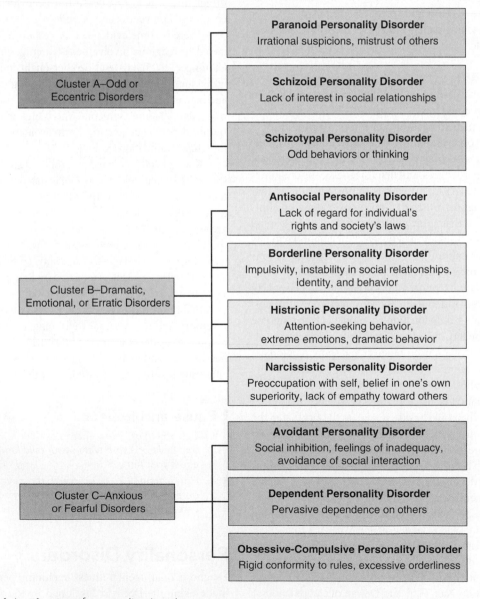

18-2   Overview of classification of personality disorders.

Based on the *Diagnostic and Statistical Manual of Mental Disorders*, Fifth Edition, (Copyright 2013). American Psychiatric Association.

have difficulty confiding in others due to a fear that information they share will be used against them. They have a tendency to view benign comments or situations as insults or threats against them, and are quick to respond with anger or with a counterattack. Brief periods of psychosis, especially in response to stress, are not uncommon. Not surprisingly, the symptoms and behaviors associated with this disorder can result in family conflicts and occupational impairment. Prevalence rates for paranoid personality disorder are estimated between 2.3% and 4.4% (APA, 2013). It is more common in first-degree relatives of people diagnosed with schizophrenia or other psychotic disorders.

Schizoid personality disorder is characterized by a blunted affect, social isolation, and social awkwardness. Reported prevalence rates for schizoid personality disorder vary between 3.1% and 4.9%; it is more often diagnosed in men, who may also experience greater impairment (APA, 2013). The disorder is uncommon in inpatient settings. It is more common in first-degree relatives of individuals diagnosed with schizophrenia or other psychotic disorders. It sometimes appears before the onset of other disorders, particularly schizophrenia or delusional disorder. Rarely, it will precede the development of major depressive disorder (Sadock, Sadock, & Ruiz, 2009). The patient with schizoid personality disorder can experience brief psychosis, especially in response to stress. Difficulty expressing emotions, especially anger, and an inability to relate to others are characteristic of this disorder. As a result, patients with schizoid personality disorder can experience great difficulty at work and in relationships.

Schizotypal personality disorder is characterized by bizarre appearance and behavior, eccentricity, and peculiarity. It is rare, usually diagnosed in less than 3% of the population. Schizotypal personality disorder is rarely found in inpatient settings and is more prevalent in outpatient health care environments (APA, 2013). It is also more prevalent in people with a first-degree relative diagnosed with schizophrenia. Patients with schizotypal personality disorder may experience transient psychosis, including magical thinking, delusions, and hallucinations, especially in response to stress. Some 30% to 50% of these patients experience major depression concurrently (Sadock, Sadock, & Ruiz, 2009). An inability to relate to others creates isolation, although the patient may not be aware that anything is missing. Occupational impairment may also result.

Cluster B Personality Disorders

The cluster B, or *dramatic–emotional*, disorders are marked by impulsivity, lack of regard for others, and exaggerated or extreme emotions and behaviors.

Antisocial personality disorder (APD) has also been called *sociopathic personality*. It is characterized by others feeling manipulated, exploited, and deceived, as well as sensing that the individual is disloyal and lacks remorse for violation of rules and laws. It is found in 3% to 4% of the general population and accounts for 80% of crime in American culture. APD is found more often in men than women; there is a 4:1 gender difference in diagnosis. The greatest percentage of individuals with antisocial personality disorder are men with alcohol use disorder and among those who are incarcerated or in substance abuse treatment facilities (APA, 2013).

The individual diagnosed with APD may use manipulation to manage anxiety and achieve something he or she desires rather than out of a need to control others. When this is the case, the nurse

Impact of Antisocial Personality Disorder on Functioning — table 18-1

Domain	Impact on Functioning
Biological	• Alcohol, drug dependency
Psychological	• Low tolerance for boredom • Impulsive, aggressive behavior that may result in violence toward others • Increased risk for co-morbid disorders, including substance abuse and anxiety disorders
Sociocultural	• Failure to conform to social norms • Uses and manipulates others to meet own needs • Often in trouble with legal authorities • No compassion for others
Spiritual	• Lack of remorse creates inability to process forgiveness

needs to stay objective and try to determine the cause of the patient's distress.

Predictors in childhood of the development of APD include conduct disorder, such as oppositional defiant disorder, or a diagnosis of attention deficit/hyperactivity disorder (ADHD) that is not treated aggressively enough in youth (Shannon, 2011). APD affects functioning in a number of ways (Table 18-1). Patients with this disorder have a low tolerance for boredom and tend to use and manipulate others to meet their own needs. They often exhibit impulsivity, which can lead to using violence in relating to others. They often disregard others' safety and their own, including engaging in high-risk sexual behavior or substance use. Studies indicate that both adopted and biological children of parents with APD are at risk (Sadock, Sadock, & Ruiz, 2009). Individuals with APD are also at increased risk for other mental health disorders (APA, 2013).

Borderline personality disorder was originally named because the symptoms of those diagnosed with BPD were thought to exist on the border between reality and psychosis. Patients with BPD are often emotionally **labile**, exhibiting changeable and unregulated emotions, self-destructive and impulsive behavior, and feelings of emptiness and boredom (Table 18-2). Individuals with BPD often use primitive defense mechanisms such as splitting and projection. **Splitting** is a behavior in which the individual divides and plays one person or group against another. For example, a patient may ask a staff member during one shift if she can have a snack, and be told, "No." The patient may then go to a staff member during another shift, ask the same question, and tell the second staff member that the other shift's staff members always let the patients have snacks, thus causing tension between the two shifts. Nurses can help prevent splitting by using open communication between other staff and shifts and being consistent with unit policies and procedures. **Projection**, the transfer of blame to another person to avoid the feelings that would be experienced by blaming oneself, is common in these patients.

Individuals with borderline personality disorder also tend to use self-injurious behavior as a maladaptive coping mechanism. **Self-injurious behaviors** (SIBs) describe behaviors that individuals

Impact of Borderline Personality Disorder on Functioning
table 18-2

Domain	Impact on Functioning
Biological	• Biologically based emotional vulnerability • Genetic predisposition • Altered HYPAC functioning • Alltered neurotransmitter levels, particularly serotonin
Psychological	• Early trauma (e.g., childhood abuse or sexual abuse) increases risk for developing BPD. • Increased risk for major depression, substance abuse or dependence, eating disorder, PTSD • Difficulty controlling anger • Extreme responses to stress, changes in mood; psychotic-like symptoms may present in response to stress.
Sociocultural	• Splitting in relationships • Sabotage of relationships when rejection and abandonment seem imminent • Impulsivity • Family members and other potentially supportive relationships are easily burned out on the chaos and challenge of relationship.
Spiritual	• Sense of abandonment and emptiness create lack of purpose, love, and relatedness.

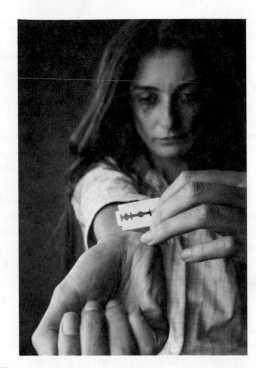

18-3 Patients with borderline disorder may use self-harming behaviors, such as cutting, to help regulate emotions, inflict self-punishment, or express pain. These behaviors do not arise from a desire to die.

Source: Artem Furman/Shutterstock

engage in to cause harm to themselves, and include cutting, abrading, hair pulling, biting, scratching, or burning oneself without the overt purpose of ending life. It is important to note that SIB and suicidal behavior do not necessarily have the same etiology. When patients are self-injurious, they will cut, burn, or harm themselves without intending to end their lives (Figure 18-3). SIB is thought to occur as a self-punishment, as a physical pain that distracts from psychic pain, or as a release of the pain itself. Sometimes patients who dissociate say that self-injury helps to validate reality. Patients often describe feeling relieved after hurting themselves by cutting or burning. It has been postulated that the pain experienced with self-injurious behavior releases endorphins, which provide pain relief and sensations of happiness and contentment (Klonsky, 2007).

Patients who exhibit SIB are at an increased risk for suicide, as are patients who exhibit impulsivity and aggressive behaviors. Nurses working with patients with BPD must be alert to and assess for signs of suicidal ideation. The use of **transitional objects**, such as blankets or stuffed animals, may help provide patients with BPD with a sense of security and comfort.

BPD prevalence rates are estimated to be 1.6%, but they may be higher. BPD is found in about 10% of outpatient psychiatric populations and 20% of inpatient populations. BPD is more common in women than in men, and having a first-degree relative with the disorder increases the risk for developing BPD fivefold (APA, 2013). Nursing considerations for working with patients with BPD are found in Table 18-3.

Histrionic personality disorder is characterized by labile moods, vanity, self-centeredness, and a demand to be the center of attention. People with this disorder have an intense need for constant

reassurance and manipulate others effectively. Their focus on themselves creates difficulty in establishing and maintaining relationships, and family members and caregivers may experience burnout. Histrionic personality disorder is found in less than 2% of the population (APA, 2013). It tends to run in families, and there is a potential genetic link to APD (Sadock, Sadock, & Ruiz, 2009).

Narcissistic personality disorder prevalence rates vary, with samples indicating a range of frequency from 0% to 6.2% of the general population; it is more often diagnosed in men (APA, 2013). It can be divided into two subtypes (Masterson, 1981). The first type is *closeted*, in which the patient exhibits self-absorption, passive–aggressiveness, and hypersensitivity to criticism. Individuals with this type can be superficially nice and function in social situations. The second type is *malignant*, which can be characterized by a firm belief in an innate superiority to others. These individuals are driven by the need for power, wealth, and attention. They have a morbid preoccupation with themselves, and an extreme lack of empathy for others.

Risk factors for narcissistic personality disorder include neglect and emotional abuse in childhood and unreliable or manipulative parenting (Mayo Clinic, 2011). The humiliation and hypercriticism of the self associated with this disorder often are accompanied by social withdrawal and depressed mood, although individuals who experience grandiosity may exhibit hypomanic mood symptoms (APA, 2013)

Cluster C Personality Disorders

Patients with a cluster C, or *dramatic–fearful*, personality disorders engage in pervasive patterns of behavior aimed at trying to reduce a fear (of rejection or abandonment, for example) or maintain control of their environment.

Borderline Personality Disorder Manifestations, Impact on Functioning, and Nursing Considerations

table 18-3

Domain	Manifestations	Impact on Functioning	Nursing Considerations
Biological	• Overactive limbic system • Underactive prefrontal cortex • Decreased amounts of serotonin	• Emotional lability and impulsivity creates a sense of being out of control, decreases ability to focus. • Depression decreases motivation.	*Safety:* • Protect patients from consequences of impulsivity. *Relationship:* • Limit setting for inappropriate displays of emotion. • Remain objective and calm with displays of extreme emotion. • Set daily goals and assist in accomplishing them. Positively reinforce goals that are met. *Teaching:* • Develop written plan to identify adaptive ways to cope with impulsive feelings. • Teach self-management skills for coping with emotions and impulsivity.
Psychological	• Intense and labile moods • Identify diffusion • Maladaptive coping • Suicidal ideation • Self-injurious behavior	• Decreased ability to focus. • Easily takes on characteristics of another, difficulty arises in relationships as patient has no concrete self-image. • Maladaptive coping may work for a time, but eventually has a detrimental effect on health and functioning (for example, use of alcohol or drugs to cope). • Suicidal ideation can decrease anxiety for a time as the patient feels like there is always a way out. Similarly, SIB decreases anxiety for a time but eventually causes harm to the patient.	*Safety:* • Encourage patients to agree to safety, including both SIB and suicidal ideation. • Implement institutional suicide precautions. *Relationship:* • Set limits on inappropriate displays of emotion. • Explore with patients who they are, what they like and don't like, and so on, to begin building a stronger sense of self. *Teaching:* • Adaptive coping strategies, suicide prevention plan.
Sociological	• Chaotic relationships with others • Often crave intimacy but sabotage relationships when they become too intimate or demanding. • Will take on the identity and characteristics of those around them. • Generally find it difficult to stay with a specific job or in a long-term relationship • Impulsivity manifested by substance abuse, sexual promiscuity, spending money. (These symptoms are similar to those of bipolar disorder; it is important for a clinician to make a differential diagnosis.)	• Patient can easily become victimized by others who may take advantage of them. • Relationships usually do not last, as others become burned out or irritated with the emotional lability and lack of boundaries. • Difficulty maintaining employment and an income. • Impulsivity can place a patient at risk physically, psychologically, and financially.	*Safety:* • Discuss with patient limits to relationships and how to stay safe. • Develop a safety plan with coping skills and emergency support people who can be accessed to process interactions, relationships, and impulsive actions. *Relationship:* • The therapeutic relationship will mirror the chaos, splitting, and sabotage of other relationships in the patient's life. Nurses must be objective and maintain awareness to avoid participating in the dysfunction. • Collaborate with colleagues to process interactions with a patient who has BPD. • Provide firm boundaries and consistent enforcement. *Teaching:* • Self-management skills and adaptive coping strategies.

(Continued)

Borderline Personality Disorder Manifestations, Impact on Functioning, and Nursing Considerations (*continued*)

table 18-3

Domain	Manifestations	Impact on Functioning	Nursing Considerations
Cultural	• Differences in the perception of the cause of the patient's distress are culturally based. Punishment? Evil? Victimization? • Characteristics of passivity, deferential treatment of others, politeness, guardedness, and defensiveness can often be culturally explained.	• Relationships can be strained or severed. • Patients can believe they are being punished with their suffering for some real or imagined offense.	*Relationship:* • Explore the patient's cultural context. How is culture influencing their perceptions of themselves, their diagnosis, and relationships?
Spiritual	• Feelings of emptiness • Lack of relatedness to others • Lack of meaning and purpose in life	• Hopelessness can develop, which reinforces maladaptive coping and suicidal ideation.	*Relationship:* • Reinforce the positive and a sense of hope that the future can be better. • Explore with patients what could bring a sense of purpose to their lives. • Explore with patients their relationships. Which have the potential to be supportive? Where could the patient build additional relationships?

Avoidant personality disorder is distinguished by extreme shyness and fear of rejection or disapproval in social situations (Table 18-4). Individuals with this disorder may overreact to slight or perceived criticism. They frequently lack confidence and are reluctant to try new experiences or engage in unfamiliar settings for fear of embarrassment. Avoidant personality disorder is found in approximately 2.4% of the population. There are no gender differences in diagnosis (APA, 2013). Disfiguring illness may play a role in development of avoidant personality disorder in some individuals (MedlinePlus, 2012).

Dependent personality disorder is characterized by low self-esteem and feelings of inadequacy and insecurity. Individuals diagnosed with dependent personality disorder can become extremely dependent on another person, even to the point of relying on that person to define their identity. Dependency may lead to lack of ability to complete certain activities of daily living, ensuring ongoing dependence of those with the disorder. Dependent personality disorder is found in between 0.49% and 0.6% of the general population and is diagnosed more frequently in women (APA, 2013). Chronic physical illness can predispose an individual to dependent personality disorder. Individuals with this disorder may experience mild impairment in occupational and social relationships in which independence is required (Sadock, Sadock, & Ruiz, 2009). They may also be at an increased risk for mood disorders, anxiety disorders, and adjustment disorders (Sadock, Sadock, & Ruiz, 2009).

One of the most common personality disorders, *obsessive–compulsive personality disorder*, is typified by rigidity, perfectionism, and control. It is found in 2.1% to 7.9% of the general population (APA, 2013). It is thought that a serotonin deficiency fuels perfectionism and anxiety in people with obsessive–compulsive personality disorder, and there may be genetic familial connections (Shannon, 2011). Individuals experience difficulty in relationships due to their rigid thinking and issues of control and experience great distress when confronting change or situations that require flexibility (Sadock, Sadock, & Ruiz, 2009).

Impact of Avoidant Personality Disorder on Functioning

table 18-4

Domain	Impact on Functioning
Biological	• No genetic information.
Psychological	• Disfiguring illness may play a role. • Increased risk for mood and anxiety disorders.
Sociocultural	• Social withdrawal; avoidance of occupations that require a great deal of social interaction. • Lack of support systems. • May cancel interviews, appointments out of fear of rejection. • Awkward, fearful behaviors may elicit the very responses from others the individual seeks to avoid.
Spiritual	• Isolation can create a sense of loneliness and lack of connectedness.

Pause and Reflect

1. *Which personality disorders do you find most intimidating? Why? What can you do to gain confidence in working with patients with these disorders?*

2. *Which personality disorder do you think might be the most debilitating for a patient? How would you begin to promote hope and healing for patients with that disorder?*

Collaborative Care

Personality disorders are difficult to treat, as persistence and inflexibility in the individual's thinking and behavior are key elements. Usually, a combination of medication and cognitive–behavioral therapy is used. Treatment protocols are tailored to the patient's level of functioning and symptom presentation. Nurses and other health care providers working with the patient must take into account the patient's priorities regarding treatment (for instance, which symptoms the patient perceives as most troubling). Family members' perspectives regarding which patient behaviors are most difficult to manage also may need to be considered.

Psychopharmacology

Medications are often prescribed for individuals diagnosed with personality disorders; however, they typically are limited to symptom management. For impulse control and aggressive responses, anticonvulsants or mood stabilizers such as valproic acid (Depakote) and carbamazepine (Tegretol) are often used. Clozapine (Clozaril), an antipsychotic medication, has also been effective in controlling aggression in people diagnosed with personality disorders.

In cases of extreme aggression, when a patient is dangerous to self or others, sedation may be used. A common sedation combination is called a "B-52" and includes haloperidol (Haldol) 5 mg, lorazepam (Ativan) 2 mg, and diphenhydramine (Benadryl) 50 mg given intramuscularly (IM) (Lin, 2010). Usually, haloperidol and lorazepam are given in one syringe, and the diphenhydramine is given in another for drug compatibility reasons (the diphenhydramine may crystallize if combined with other drugs). This combination can be used when the patient is in imminent danger and a PRN order (medication order as needed) for another medication is not readily available (B-52, 2011). Other emergency treatments are HAC (Haldol 5 mg, Ativan 2 mg, Cogentin 1 mg IM, all in one syringe); midazolam (Versed), 5 mg IM as a single agent (very short-acting benzodiazepine more consistently absorbed intramuscularly than lorazepam [Ativan]); and haloperidol (Haldol) as a single agent (Lin, 2010). Each institution has standards and policies for the use of psychotropic medications.

For patients with cognitive and perceptual symptoms, such as delusions or hallucinations, antipsychotic medications may be prescribed. For patients with emotional instability, antidepressants, especially the SSRIs, may be effective in regulating emotions. Antianxiety agents may also be used for patients suffering with anxiety (Tyrer & Bateman, 2004).

In Cluster A, the most studied personality disorder is schizotypal personality disorder. It is thought that a dopamine dysregulation is a primary cause of the psychotic symptoms. Many patients diagnosed with schizotypal personality disorder respond well to the typical antipsychotic medications, such as haloperidol (Haldol) and thiothixene (Navane) (Schatzberg & Nemeroff, 2006). Atypical antipsychotics, such as risperidone (Risperdal), may be effective for some patients (Mayo Clinic, 2013).

Cluster B disorders—in particular, BPD—are the most studied personality disorders in terms of medication management. For patients experiencing psychotic symptoms and disinhibition, atypical antipsychotics, particularly olanzapine (Zyprexa) and aripiprazole (Abilify), have been found to have a greater range of efficacy than typical antipsychotics. Dosages of antipsychotics typically are lower for patients with personality disorders than for those suffering from SSDs (Ripoll, 2012).

For patients experiencing emotional dysregulation, the tricyclic antidepressants have shown only modest results and represent an increased risk when used in a suicide attempt because of their cardiotoxicity (Schatzberg & Nemeroff, 2006). They are not recommended as a first line of treatment. Newer-generation antidepressants, including the SSRIs, show some potential in treating mood dysregulation

(Vita, DePeri, & Sachetti, 2011). Mood stabilizers have been shown to help manage impulsivity, especially in terms of aggression. Although lithium is still being used, there is evidence that anticonvulsants, such as carbamazepine (Tegretol) and valproic acid (Depakote), may assist with mood stabilization (Ripoll, 2012; Schatzberg & Nemeroff, 2006).

When treating APD, most health care professionals agree that there is a problem with patient adherence. Some patients with this disorder respond to the mood stabilizers for impulsivity and aggression; however, the evidence is weaker than with the response for BPD (Schatzberg & Nemeroff, 2006).

For Cluster C personality disorders, avoidant personality disorder is the most studied because it appears to be on a continuum with social anxiety disorder (Schatzberg & Nemeroff, 2006). Monoamine oxidase inhibitors (MAOIs) and the SSRIs have been shown to increase patients' comfort levels and confidence in social and occupational situations (Schatzberg & Nemeroff, 2006).

> **PRACTICE ALERT**   Patients may have PRN medications prescribed to help with crisis situations. PRN medications often include low-dose antipsychotic medication and antianxiety medication to be used on a short-term basis. Nurses must assess the need for administration of a PRN medication, and then assess the medication's effectiveness in relieving symptoms as well as its interaction with other prescribed medication.

Psychotherapy

Cognitive–behavioral therapy (CBT) generally is used in the treatment of patients diagnosed with personality disorders. CBT has the greatest efficacy with the Cluster B and C personality disorders; it can reduce self-harm, symptom distress, depression, and interpersonal difficulties (Lamont & Brunero, 2009). CBT focuses on identifying the thoughts and beliefs that underlie maladaptive behavior and changing them to aid in developing more adaptive behavior (see the Perceptions, Thoughts, and Feelings feature near the end of this chapter). Dialectical behavior therapy, group therapy, and music therapy are other forms of therapy that have been found particularly successful with patients suffering from personality disorders.

Dialectical Behavior Therapy

Dialectical behavior therapy (DBT) is a form of CBT introduced by Marsha Linehan (1993a). It employs a unique blend of psychotherapy and skills training that has been shown to be especially effective for patients diagnosed with BPD. Instead of the change focus of CBT, DBT stresses a balance of acceptance and change that is derived from the mindfulness and judgment avoidance of Zen meditation. DBT also emphasizes special focus and treatment of therapy-interfering behaviors, such as splitting and emotional lability; a collaborative therapeutic relationship between patient and therapist; and dialectical processes (Linehan, 1993a). *Dialectics,* in the case of DBT, refers to a principle of interrelatedness and wholeness, the principle of polarity, and the principle of continuous change (Linehan, 1993a). DBT strives to create an accepting environment where patients can grow and change (see Evidence-Based Practice: Dialectical Behavior Therapy).

DBT uses four modes of therapy: individual, group skills training, telephone contact outside usual therapy hours, and a support team for the therapist (Hadjipavlou & Ogrodniczuk, 2010). Skills training modules focus on four areas:

- *Emotion-regulating skills:* DBT teaches patients strategies to reduce negative emotional responses and the impulsive behaviors

Dialectical Behavior Therapy   evidence-based practice

Clinical Question

Is dialectical behavior therapy effective in patients diagnosed with border-line personality disorder?

Evidence

Most research of personality disorders focuses on borderline personality disorder. Marsha Linehan (1993a) began to establish DBT as a modification and alternative to CBT in her seminal two-year study in 1991. Since then, a number of studies have reinforced the belief in mental health circles that DBT is the most effective psychotherapy for BPD. Hadjipavlou & Ogrodniczuk (2010) cited a randomized controlled study published in 2009 by McMain and colleagues with 180 subjects. The subjects showed significant reduction in SIB, reduced patient distress, and improved interpersonal functioning after 1 year of treatment as opposed to a general set of treatment practices based on the guidelines of the American Psychiatric Association (APA) (Hadjipavlou & Ogrodniczuk, 2010). A 2006 study by Linehan and associates showed that the patients receiving DBT as opposed to nonbehavioral therapy were 50% less likely to attempt suicide as those treated by community experts. These patients also had a greatly reduced rate of dropping out of treatment, as well as fewer psychiatric hospitalizations and use of crisis services (Hadjipavlou & Ogrodniczuk, 2010).

Implications for Nursing Practice

DBT is recommended by the APA as the treatment of choice for BPD. DBT has been shown to "reduce depression, anxiety, hopelessness, self-destructive and impulsive episodes, suicidal ideation and hospitalization" (Swift, 2009, p. 31). It is more cost effective and has been shown to improve affect and cognition in patients diagnosed with BPD.

Critical Thinking Questions

1. How might a nurse describe DBT to a patient diagnosed with BPD? What are the benefits? How does it work?
2. If an opportunity does not exist locally to involve a patient in DBT, what principles or strategies might be integrated into a treatment plan? How might you integrate these?

---

that often accompany them. These strategies include identifying and describing emotions, decreasing avoidance of negative emotions, increasing positive emotions, and changing unwanted negative emotions.

- *Distress tolerance training:* Impulse control and self-soothing strategies help patients to survive crises without the use of drugs, SIB, and attempting suicide.
- *Interpersonal effectiveness skills:* DBT teaches assertiveness strategies while maintaining relationships and self-respect.
- *Mindfulness skills:* Patients learn the strategies of focusing attention on the patients' self and immediate context, describing what they see, developing awareness of others' perceptions, and brainstorming what may work in a given situation (Dimeff & Koerner, 2007).

Group Therapy

Group therapy is often helpful in the treatment of personality disorders. Gathering together people diagnosed with similar disorders can help them feel less isolated. Social skills groups can help patients who have difficulty interacting in social situations. Anger management groups can help impulsive patients or any patients who have difficulty controlling and expressing anger appropriately. Groups designed to teach new adaptive coping skills and suicide or self-injury prevention strategies can greatly assist patients who are struggling in those areas. Nurses should note that, especially when dealing with patients diagnosed with APD or BPD whose sense of identity is loosely constructed or not fully developed, issues raised in the group can become "contagious." For example, one patient in the group may bring up an issue in dealing with a mother or other family member. Quickly, each member of the group begins to bring up the same issue for themselves. This unique phenomenon, called *role diffusion*, in which individuals confuse others' attributes or emotions with their own, can complicate the group's goals (Wilkinson-Ryan & Weston, 2000).

Music Therapy

Music therapy is used in mental health settings to help patients better understand their emotions and their responses to the world. Music therapy allows people to explore their feelings more easily, and in many cases can help them begin to turn away from preoccupation with self-harm (Oden-Miller, 2011). Music can also be used as an adaptive coping strategy.

Music therapy is most often accomplished in a group setting. In the past, music via headphones was discouraged, as it seemed to separate and isolate patients from others. More recently, however, music as adaptive coping has been acknowledged as therapeutic. Nurses may need to process the use of headphones, iPods, and MP3 players with patients. When are the times they can be used adaptively? When are the times they may interfere with relationships and create more social isolation?

Pause and Reflect

1. *How might using SSRIs to decrease patient impulsivity be helpful to patients with personality disorders? To their family members or co-workers?*
2. *What is the role of dialectic behavior therapy in treating patients with personality disorders?*
3. *What organizations, therapists, or facilities offer music therapy to patients with mental or physical illness in your area?*

Nursing Management

As with all patients with mental illness, safety is the first priority of care. Beyond that, assessment identifies priorities for care, including patient awareness of the extent of dysfunction, family concerns, and the patient's mental and physical health.

Assessment

Personality disorders involve enduring, inflexible patterns that vary greatly from the individual's culture. Assessment of the patient

Brenda Relapse Phase

APPLICATION

1. What would you include in a safety contract for Brenda?

2. What strategies would you use to get Brenda to "buy in" to the contract?

3. Why do you think a shorter hospitalization period might be in Brenda's best interest?

Brenda called a crisis hotline two weeks after her initial visit, threatening suicide. Her current boyfriend broke up with her and she was so distraught that she did not go in to work and lost her job. The crisis counselor sent an ambulance to her foster home and Brenda was brought back to the hospital. When Sarah meets with her for the first time, Brenda states, "I have nothing to live for . . . it hurts too much." When asked if she has a plan, Brenda confides that she has a bottle of aspirin at home as a fail-safe option for just that purpose. She complains of feeling out of control and empty, and is tempted to cut herself. She is currently unsure about her ability to contract for her safety.

Sarah places Brenda on suicide precautions, which will ensure that staff will check on her every 15 minutes. Her physician decides that the hospitalization should be as short as possible and yet help Brenda to maintain her safety so she can continue to work with her day treatment program on an outpatient basis. She stays in the hospital for 3 days, during which she processes her current situation, and reinforces her suicide prevention plan.

Sarah designs a care plan with Brenda, focusing on safety as her first priority. She includes Brenda in developing realistic goals and interventions (see the Nursing Care Plan).

diagnosed with a personality disorder includes assessing safety and assessing multiple areas of functioning.

Assessing for Safety

Patients with personality disorders are vulnerable and unsafe in a number of different areas. They may be out of touch with reality and may not be aware of how they are coming across in social settings. Impulsivity and self-medication with alcohol and drugs are common. Self-injurious behaviors and suicidality are common: Some 8% to 10% of individuals with BPD complete suicide (APA, 2013). A thorough safety assessment must be done with every patient, especially those diagnosed with personality disorders, as they are correlated with a high incidence of suicidal and self-injurious behavior (Chapter 27).

Assessing Patients Across the Domains

When assessing patients with personality disorders, a holistic focus reveals findings consistent with specific personality disorders across domains. Consequently, it is helpful to organize assessment according to each domain (Table 18-5). For example, during the observation and physical assessment, the nurse will note biological and physical indicators, including vital signs, the patient's appearance, and evidence of SIB. In addition to asking the patient for information regarding family relationships and work situation, the nurse may want to ask family members for their observations to help gain a sense of the patient's awareness of reality, as well as to determine what symptoms family members find most challenging.

Diagnosis and Planning

Nursing diagnoses generally focus on a pattern of symptoms and expressed issues causing the patient distress or interfering with daily functioning. The following is a list of commonly used nursing diagnoses for patients diagnosed with personality disorders:

- Coping, Ineffective
- Social Interaction, Impaired
- Social Isolation
- Violence: Self-Directed, Risk for
- Violence: Other-Directed, Risk for

- Injury, Risk for
- Anxiety
- Personal Identity: Disturbed
- Knowledge, Deficient

(NANDA-I © 2014)

It is important to include the patient in any planning for care. The most important way to enhance patient safety is through the development of a strong nurse–patient relationship. What does the patient see as realistic goals for the issues identified? What would the patient like to see occur in order to mitigate suffering and return to functioning? What interventions would instill hope in the patient?

Goals and outcomes must be measurable and observable. They must also include a target date that is reasonable and realistic. For example, the outcome, "Patient will feel better about herself" is not observable or measurable. Instead, the outcome, "Patient will verbalize that she has accomplished her goal for today (e.g., calling the group home to set up an interview) by 10 p.m." is more specific, concrete, and measurable.

For some patients, the goals of therapy may differ from those of the nurse. For those patients, it might be helpful to ask how their current patterns of functioning are working for them in their present circumstances. Nurses can help patients identify ways in which those patterns are not working well, getting the patient's needs met, and staying out of legal and interpersonal trouble. Understanding the patient's social context and the meaning the patient ascribes to it helps the nurse to facilitate those discussions (Leising, 2008).

Implementation

As with assessment, the priority interventions for patients diagnosed with personality disorders are directed to safety. Once safety is ensured, the nurse turns the focus toward building the therapeutic relationship, which, in turn, supports other nursing interventions in the areas of medication management, facilitating coping skills, strengthening reality orientation, maintaining professional boundaries, and milieu management (Figure 18-4). These interventions help patients begin to feel hopeful that they can progress in their

Assessment by Domain

table 18-5

Domain	Observation and Physical Assessment	Questions for Patient Interview
Biological	**Vital signs (ABC)** **Appearance** • Affect • Dress, hygiene • Speech patterns • Evidence of SIB (e.g., cutting, burns) **Behavior** • Does the patient make eye contact with you? • Does the patient participate in unit activities? • How does the patient act when alone? Around others? **Content of conversation** • What does the patient talk about? • Does the patient talk readily or is the patient reluctant to engage? Is the patient's conversation oriented to reality?	• How have you been feeling physically lately? • How have you been able to function in your everyday life?
Psychological	Does the patient seem depressed? Anxious? Impulsive?	• How have you been feeling emotionally lately? • How do you express your feelings? • What coping strategies do you use? • Are you feeling suicidal? • Do you have a plan to commit suicide? (If patient has a plan, determine level of access to plan requirements.)
Sociocultural	• How does the patient act in response to others? In groups? • Does the patient answer questions readily? • Is there a cultural component to the patient's life that drives relationships and coping mechanisms?	• Explore relationships in the patient's life: What is your relationship like with ___? • What type of work do you do? Are you in school? • What do you do with your leisure time? What do you do for fun? • Who do you have in your life that supports you? • What cultural needs do you have? How can those needs be met?
Spiritual	• Do you notice any jewelry or books in the patient's vicinity that may signal a specific religious affiliation? • Does the patient seem hopeful about the future and empowered to control his or her own life?	• What brings a sense of meaning or purpose to your life? • What close relationships do you enjoy? • What coping strategies do you use when things get tough? • Where do you go for help and strength in tough times?

treatment and improve their ability to function on a daily basis (Table 18-6).

Ensure Safety

After assessing a patient's suicide potential, a nurse establishes an agreement for safety with the patient. Such an agreement usually involves an understanding between the nurse and the patient in which the patient agrees to contact a staff person if feeling imminently self-injurious or suicidal. The nurse and patient can collaborate on a self-harm prevention plan, a written plan that has safety strategies and contact numbers a patient can use when feeling self-injurious or suicidal (Chapter 27).

If a patient does self-injure in some way, it is important for the nurse to remain objective and matter-of-fact. The nurse responds first with the necessary medical attention. Then, when the crisis is over, process the event with the patient. What was the intent of the patient's self-harming episode? What occurred before the incident? How was the patient feeling? What could the patient have done differently? If the patient admits to feeling suicidal, proceed with a suicide assessment. Does the patient have a plan? What is it? Does the patient have access to the planned method? The nurse reinforces safety strategies and alternatives to prevent another incident and promote the patient's ability to make helpful choices under distress.

Specific interventions to ensure safety include frequent assessment for presence of self-injurious or suicidal ideation; frequent observations of patients; following suicide precautions as necessary; ensuring a safe environment; and helping patients find alternative, healthy ways of coping. (See the Nursing Care Plan.)

Establish a Therapeutic Relationship

For patients with personality disorders, there are behaviors inherent to each disorder that can make establishing a therapeutic relationship

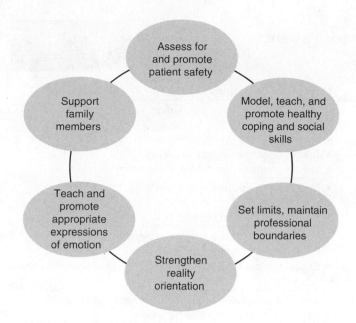

18-4 Essential nursing interventions for patients with personality disorders.

more challenging. Nurses need to be aware of these challenges and strategize to overcome them. Many nurses find themselves increasingly frustrated when working with a patient diagnosed with a personality disorder. Sometimes this frustration may manifest itself in the therapeutic relationship. Individuals diagnosed with personality disorders often describe feeling that their health care providers are negative or unhelpful (Filer, 2005). Many patients are told that they are "attention seeking" and manipulative, which can make them feel dismissed and undeserving of care (Castillo, 2001). Nurses describe feeling helpless, hopeless, angry, and frustrated (Markham, 2003). Sometimes, through a process called **projective identification**, the nurse actually can begin experiencing the emotions of the patient, which can be confusing and even frightening. Those attitudes must be challenged as nurses gain more experience in working with patients who are diagnosed with personality disorders.

Self-awareness is an essential component of the therapeutic relationship, and it is particularly important when working with patients with personality disorders. Nurses must have a strong sense of identity, be willing to set limits and reinforce boundaries, and should have supervision or collaborative relationships with colleagues with whom they can process their relationships with patients. Nurses working with these patients should frequently examine their relationships in order to maintain a consistent and therapeutic effect. Involving a colleague in the process can be helpful: Often, a colleague will see what a nurse misses in interactions with a patient diagnosed with a personality disorder. Nurses must maintain an honest, professional attitude without relating in a manner that is too friendly and warm (Hayward, 2007).

Transference and countertransference often are found in therapeutic relationships between nurses and patients diagnosed with personality disorders. Sometimes, the nurse represents someone else to the patient and the patient responds unconsciously to the nurse accordingly (**transference**). At other times, the patient may represent someone else to the nurse in the nurse's life and evoke unconscious responses (**countertransference**). Help identifying these phenomena usually takes place under supervision; good self-awareness may help the nurse understand and manage these dynamics, should they occur.

Another important feature of the therapeutic relationship is that it provides firm, consistent boundaries. Individuals diagnosed with personality disorders often require limit setting to reinforce those boundaries (Box 18-1). For example, a woman diagnosed with BPD may often attempt to test limits, such as visiting hours. A consistent, firm approach reinforcing those hours is necessary. If reinforcement is inconsistent, a patient with BPD will often engage in splitting by playing one staff person against another, as mentioned earlier. This divisive strategy can be successful in creating strife among nurses and other staff people. Another example may be a patient who manipulates staff by becoming extremely helpful. Then, the patient may begin to ask for and expect special favors and treatment. Nurses may need to enforce boundaries and confront patients who are testing them.

When nurses encounter challenges in establishing a therapeutic relationship, it is important to remember that the main strategy involves "consistency and a willingness to persevere with interventions, despite individuals' behavior" (Wray & Byrt, 2005, p. 42). It is also a good idea to collaborate with others on the health care team, to process and strategize together.

Specific interventions toward developing a therapeutic relationship include maintaining consistent staffing, following through on all agreements and promises, setting limits on inappropriate behavior, maintaining professional boundaries, and processing patient interactions with trusted colleagues.

Facilitate Coping

Nurses can help reconnect patients with coping behaviors they have employed successfully in the past. More often, however, nurses teach patients new coping skills. For example, a patient with avoidant personality disorder might be impulsive and act out aggressively when frustrated. Teaching the patient to count, employ deep breathing exercises, and eventually to express anger verbally can help patients begin to use adaptive coping skills.

Self-management is a process that can help bring a sense of order and empowerment to chronically ill patients' lives (Larsen & Lubkin, 2009). The skills of self-management are similar to coping skills, but they also help patients to live in society as normally as possible. Self-management includes adherence to a treatment plan as well as psychological empowerment and well-being and social skills. Newman, Steed, & Mulligan (2004) call these *self-management interventions*. Nurses help to motivate patients, increase their involvement and control of treatment and symptoms, limit barriers, and teach self-management strategies after assessing the patient's social context. Dialectic behavior therapy dovetails nicely with self-management interventions.

The following are specific interventions related to facilitating adaptive coping and self-management:

- Assess with the patient past coping, both adaptive and maladaptive. Which coping mechanisms work and which do not?

- Teach new coping skills, such as relaxation techniques and anger management strategies. What could the patient try when faced with stressful challenges?

Target Symptoms and Nursing Interventions for Patients with Personality Disorders

table 18-6

	Disorder	Target Symptoms	Nursing Interventions
CLUSTER A	**Paranoid**	• Suspicion and mistrust	• Build trust with consistent staffing, trustworthy and consistent interactions. • Pay special attention to giving patient space. • Teach patient perception checking. • Validate perceptions before acting on them.
	Schizoid	• Blunted affect • Social isolation • Social awkwardness	• Encourage participation in groups; offer to accompany patient if needed. • Teach patient social skills.
	Schizotypal	• Social peculiarity or eccentricity • Bizarre appearance and behavior	• Increase patient's self-awareness by mirroring to patient how he or she comes across to others. • Encourage patient to participate in groups and look for role models.
CLUSTER B	**Borderline**	• Splitting • Emotional acting out • SIB/suicidal ideation and/or actions • Relationship sabotage • Poor impulse control	• Maintain consistency among staff in terms of rules. • Set limits on inappropriate behavior. • Monitor closely for suicidal and self-injurious ideation or actions. • Help patient prepare suicide and self-injury prevention plan. • Teach patient to express emotions adaptively.
	Antisocial	• Manipulation and exploitation of others • Aggressive lack of impulse control	• Assist patient in identifying anxious feelings. • Set limits on inappropriate behavior. • Monitor interactions with others to prevent exploitation. • Teach patient to recognize anxiety and anger and to use other coping skills when responding to others.
	Histrionic	• Emotional dysregulation • Attention-seeking behavior	• Spend time with patient when there is no emotional acting out taking place; reinforce adaptive behavior when patient gets needs met appropriately. • Teach patient adaptive expression of feelings and coping skills.
	Narcissistic	• Self-aggrandizement • Lack of empathy for others	• Encourage other-focused interactions.
CLUSTER C	**Avoidant**	• Social isolation • Inadequacy	• Promote patient's interaction with others. • Promote self-esteem.
	Dependent	• High level of need • Inability to independently achieve normal life goals	• Encourage independence and autonomy. • Include patient in treatment planning and allow for choices.
	Obsessive–compulsive	• Obsessive, recurrent thoughts • Compulsive actions	• Teach anxiety management techniques, such as relaxation strategies.

• Support the patient by being present with the patient and validating the patient's feelings.

• Reinforce the patient's attempts to employ newly learned coping.

• Process with the patient after a challenging event occurs. What coping strategies did the patient use? How did they work? What else could the patient try?

Strengthen Reality Orientation

Some patients with personality disorders experience cognitive distortions bordering on psychosis. It is important to allow patients to talk about their perceptions without reinforcing the ones that are not based in reality. Nurses need to focus on reality in their conversations with these patients, while avoiding arguing with their perceptions. Using the skill of **reasonable doubt**, nurses can question the reality of a perception without arguing. For example, Patient A may tell the nurse that no one likes him. The nurse can respond by saying, "I saw Patient B talking with you earlier today. What did you think about that conversation?" In that way, the nurse has introduced doubt in what the patient has maintained, yet has not argued with the patient's perception. Focusing on the *here and now* is also helpful in keeping patients focused on reality.

Perception checking is a skill that helps patients test reality. Asking questions and checking out a perception of the environment

Limit Setting

box 18-1

The intent of limit setting is to help patients develop more adaptive behaviors and try alternative behaviors to relieve anxiety rather than using acting-out behaviors. Because acceptable behavior varies from culture to culture, it is important for the nurse to first understand the culture in which the patient lives. For example, in some cultures, loud verbal expressions of emotion are considered within normal parameters. Limit setting can help teach patients what is acceptable behavior in a particular context. It also helps patients to interact more effectively with each other and models assertive behavior with others.

Nurses must always remember that limit setting can be considered coercive when used to control the behavior of another (Vatne & Holmes, 2006). Treatment in mental health is predicated on the ethical standard to respect human dignity for both the patient and the nurse. Therefore, if the motivation for limit setting is to control behavior only, it would be considered coercive. If, however, the limit setting is to help the patient by teaching adaptive strategies, it has a therapeutic purpose.

For many patients, entry into the mental health system creates an environment of conflict, as they have never experienced a structured environment in the same way. The structured environment of a mental health care setting generally includes the following specific expectations:

- Staff and patients must respect one another.
- Health care needs of patients will be met.
- The milieu will be structured and orderly.
- Patients will comply with reasonable requests from staff members.
- Patients will observe the usual norms applicable outside the hospital, except when their illness precludes it, and will refrain from behaviors considered inappropriate in a mental health setting (Vatne & Holmes, 2006).

For a patient to understand and respond to limit setting, limits must be enforced consistently by all staff members. This is especially important when working with patients diagnosed with personality disorders, who often use manipulation and defense mechanisms to get their needs met.

Limit setting must never be done out of anger. If the nurse is feeling angry, he or she should deal with that emotion by taking a break or speaking to a colleague about it. Patients with personality disorders will be especially reactive to anger from the nurse or other staff members. This can be challenging, as limit setting should take place as close to the time of the target behavior as possible in order to be effective, and it may not be possible to take time away from the situation before responding. The nurse's understanding of self and management of his or her own emotions are essential.

Make sure expectations are clear. At admission, the nurse can introduce behavioral expectations. A verbal reminder may be necessary as behavior occurs. For example, the nurse could say, "Remember that we talked about acceptable behaviors during your admission interview. Please keep your voice down, as that loud tone is disturbing to others."

Sometimes, limit setting requires removing the patient from the area. In those cases, the patient may be asked to go to his or her room to decrease stimulation and to regain self-control. Offering an ordered PRN medication often is included in the protocol. If the patient declines the medication, the nurse must determine whether or not the patient is in imminent danger of harming self or others. If the answer is "yes," usually the nurse will gather a group of trained staff, as a "show of support." In the presence of the team, the nurse approaches the patient to encourage adherence to the requested limit. Patients often respond positively. Occasions in which they do not respond well may result in imposed limitations, such as medication, seclusion, and/or restraint to protect the patient and others.

---

or another person helps to gather the information needed to respond appropriately (Leising, 2008). For example, a patient may tell her nurse that she believes that the staff is talking about her behind the nursing desk and when they laugh, they are making fun of her. The nurse encourages the patient to check out those perceptions by asking a staff person whether the conversation had anything to do with her. In that way, she can find that the false perception she had of the environment was influencing her thinking negatively.

Specific interventions for reality orientation include avoiding reinforcement of delusions and other cognitive distortions, using reasonable doubt to help strengthen reality orientation, and teaching the patient to check perceptions to test reality.

Patient Education

Patients with personality disorders typically need assistance with developing social skills. Nurses can design groups with role playing and scenario response to help patients learn to respond in certain social situations. Processing social situations with patients is helpful in promoting self-awareness and providing patients with skills to develop healthy relationships. What is the commonly accepted way to behave in this situation? How does the patient's behavior differ

from that? How might others interpret that behavior? These questions are most easily asked in a group setting, where gathering with others can help locate areas of major difference between a patient's perception and the perceptions of those around them (Leising, 2008). Nurses also function as role models as they interact appropriately with patients.

Another area in which nurses can teach patients is the appropriate and adaptive expression of emotion. Many patients are unable to even identify their feelings, much less express them appropriately. Feelings are often experienced viscerally, meaning that people feel them somewhere in their bodies. The ability to connect a body experience to a specific emotion is a beginning for the ability to express emotions. Once feelings are identified, the nurse can teach the patient ways to express them adaptively.

Milieu Management

Creating a safe space for all patients is an essential part of each patient's recovery. Nurses manage the milieu by decreasing stimulation, such as loud noises and conversation, and making sure the milieu is safe and free from dangerous objects and physical and/or emotional abuse. Milieu can function as a "sanctuary for patients, acting as a container for aggressive and self-destructive behaviors,

Brenda—A Patient with Borderline Personality Disorder	NURSING CARE PLAN

Nursing Diagnosis: Risk for self-directed violence related to loss of relationship and lack of adaptive coping strategies as manifested by (1) history of self-injurious behaviors (cutting herself), (2) statement: "I don't know how I'll make it without my boyfriend," and (3) hoarding aspirin for a possible suicide attempt.

Short-Term Goals Patient will: (include date for short-term goal to be met)	Nursing Interventions Nurse will:	Rationale
Patient will not harm herself while she is in the hospital.	Place patient on suicide precautions with 15-minute checks.	When the patient is performing behaviors that may compromise her safety, the need to frequently monitor her for safety increases.
Patient will verbalize options to cutting within 1 day.	Discuss with patient successful past coping strategies.	Sometimes, patients have used adaptive coping in the past but have lost sight of that for various reasons. Reconnecting them with their success in the past plus helping them discover new strategies may create a sense of empowerment.
Patient will engage successfully in alternative strategies to cutting within 1 day.	Teach new alternatives to cutting, such as seeking out staff to talk, using a stress ball, participating in occupational activities offered, and other activities to keep her mind and hands actively engaged in constructive behaviors.	When patients have exhausted their ability to cope, or when a crisis overwhelms their ability to cope, nurses need to teach adaptive coping strategies to create a repertoire from which the patient can choose in order to cope.
Patient will develop a suicide prevention plan outlining adaptive coping strategies and support people/programs within 1 week.	Develop a self-harm prevention plan with patient including adaptive coping strategies and support people/programs and numbers	When a patient begins to feel like self-harming, she can lose sight of potential adaptive coping strategies and support people. Creating a written prevention plan provides the client with a list of strategies and resources when a crisis occurs.
Long-Term Goal Patient will not harm herself and remain safe.	Develop follow-up plans with patient for after discharge: Who is the therapist in the community? Make sure that person or other support persons have sufficient data about work already done in order to continue it. Who are accountability partners?	Continuity of care is essential in the therapeutic relationship. Disruptions in the therapeutic trajectory can create times when the patient feels unsupported and alone. She then may fall back into default habits in order to feel more comfortable.

Clinical Reasoning

1. What other nursing diagnoses might the nurse prioritize with Brenda?
2. What interventions would support these diagnoses?
3. What adaptive coping has Brenda already employed? What other coping skills might the nurse teach Brenda?

which over time lead to substantial clinical improvements" (Winship & Hardy, 2007, p. 150).

Specific interventions to manage milieu environments include removing dangerous objects from the environment, setting limits on behavior that infringes on others or creates confusion, being present in the environment, and modeling a positive perspective and interactions.

Family Considerations

Intervening with families is another important aspect of caring for patients with personality disorders. Family members can feel frustrated, angry, and fearful about the symptoms the patient displays. Sometimes, family members need to disengage from the patient for their own psychological and relational well-being (Stobie & Tromski-Klingshirn, 2009). Family chaos and dysfunction often accompany the patient with a personality disorder.

Teaching family members about the personality disorder is a place to begin. What are the symptoms? What helps? What hinders?

For family members who want to stay connected as a support to the patient, an understanding of boundaries and support to enforce them is crucial. What should the family member do when the patient is actively hurting himself or herself? How should they respond to a midnight phone call for help? What are the limits of their responsibility? Nurses may also encourage counseling for family members to obtain the support and care they need.

Evaluation

In the evaluation phase of the nursing process, nurses must examine the original nursing diagnosis or diagnoses, the goals and desired outcomes, the interventions, and the implementation of the interventions themselves. Modifications can be made in any and all areas of the care plan.

Again, it is important to include the patient in the evaluation of the care plan. From the patient's perspective, have the goals been met? What other areas could be addressed? What other strategies for meeting those goals could be developed?

From Suffering to Hope

Many individuals diagnosed with personality disorders are cared for in community settings such as clinics and outpatient treatment facilities. Follow-up communication between acute care and care in the community is essential for continuity of care to take place. It is often difficult for patients with personalty disorder to transfer learning from the protected environment of the hospital to independent living in the community (Sheldon, Howells, & Patel, 2010). Medication may relieve some symptoms to assist the patient to engage in other therapies that may bring more promising relief. Additionally, patients may feel mistrustful of other patients, group leaders, or therapists and experience a lack of motivation, especially when they are not seeing immediate results. Some patients do not believe they need treatment and drop out of treatment, at least until the next time they experience distress or encounter legal charges.

It is important for nurses to remind patients, as well as themselves, that there is hope for patients with personality disorders living with the pain of feeling alone, empty, purposeless, and hopeless. Treatment can help patients find purpose in their lives, enlist support people, and foster hope that the future can be better. Nurses have a critical role in providing support and hope to patients with personality disorders by setting limits, teaching strategies for self-management, ensuring safety, and teaching patients about their illness and treatment protocols.

PERCEPTIONS, THOUGHTS, & FEELINGS: Validating the Needs of a Patient with Symptoms of Emotional Dysregulation

Brenda has been working with Sarah for 1 week in the hospital. Their focus, besides safety, has been on emotion regulation and identity/self-esteem issues. One day, Brenda is talking to her mother on the phone in the patient lounge. She begins screaming at her and throws the phone down, racing off to her room, where she slams the door. In response, Sarah calms a few of the other patients who are upset by Brenda's outburst, and walks down to Brenda's room to talk with her. Sarah's plan is to interact with Brenda and validate what her specific needs are at this time. When Sarah knocks on the door and announces herself, Brenda calls out, "Come in."

Patient's behavior	Nurse's perceptions, thoughts, and feelings	Exploration with patient
Brenda is on her bed, crying.	**Thoughts:** The outburst really disrupted the milieu. We have talked about this, and I thought this behavior was done. **Feelings:** Anger, frustration, concern.	*Nurse:* Hello, Brenda. That phone conversation seemed to upset you a lot.

VALIDATION Sarah gently validates Brenda's behavior with her.

Patient's behavior	Nurse's perceptions, thoughts, and feelings	Exploration with patient
Brenda: I know. I lost it.	**Thoughts:** Well at least she admits the behavior was a problem. I wonder if she thinks she could have handled it differently.	*Nurse:* Yes, it was pretty disruptive. How else could you have handled it, do you think?

VALIDATION Sarah acknowledges Brenda's behavior as disruptive and inquires how she might have acted differently.

Patient's behavior	Nurse's perceptions, thoughts, and feelings	Exploration with patient
Brenda: Well, I probably could have hung up and found someone to talk to.	**Thoughts:** She is retaining some of what she is learning. Now if only she could do it in the heat of the moment.	*Nurse:* That sounds like a very healthy alternative. So, what happened?

VALIDATION Sarah affirms Brenda's choice and wants Brenda to describe what happened in her own words.

Patient's behavior	Nurse's perceptions, thoughts, and feelings	Exploration with patient
Brenda: Every time I talk to my mom, we end up fighting. She tells me to get it together and to stop wrecking everything. Brenda sits up and wipes her eyes with a tissue.	**Thoughts:** I know it must be hard for Brenda's family to live with the chaos of her life day in and day out. On the other hand, that was a really insensitive thing to say. **Feelings:** Compassion	*Nurse:* I am sorry you are having so much conflict with your mother. You sound like you are feeling really angry and hurt.

VALIDATION Use of reflection helps to validate Brenda's feelings of anger and hurt.

Patient's behavior	Nurse's perceptions, thoughts, and feelings	Exploration with patient
Brenda: I'll say. We can barely speak without accusations. Brenda shakes her head and sighs.	*Thoughts:* It sounds like they ignite each other every time they talk. Anger and guilt seem to emerge and are expressed in yelling and accusations.	**Nurse:** What is your relationship like with your mother?

VALIDATION Further exploration and clarification of relationship that seems to be patient's current focus.

Patient's behavior	Nurse's perceptions, thoughts, and feelings	Exploration with patient
Brenda: Well, when I was little she left me with babysitters a lot. Then, when my parents divorced and I started having trouble in middle school, she just left.	*Thoughts:* Abandonment is a huge issue for patients with BPD, and this sounds like it actually happened. I wonder if she has any supportive people in her life. *Feelings:* Sadness, compassion	**Nurse:** Wow, I am sorry to hear that. It sounds like you feel she abandoned you. Who else do you have in your life that supports you?

VALIDATION Validating feelings of abandonment. Clarifying support system.

Patient's behavior	Nurse's perceptions, thoughts, and feelings	Exploration with patient
Brenda: No one really. Well, my dad calls me once in a while, but his wife doesn't like me. I was dating this new guy, but he drinks a lot and I don't know if I can take that.	*Thoughts:* Brenda does not have much support. It sounds like Brenda's pattern of choosing relationships that are chaotic is continuing.	**Nurse:** It sounds like that is an area we can continue to work. Everyone needs some support in their lives.

VALIDATION Normalizing the need for support and creating goals to work toward.

Patient's behavior	Nurse's perceptions, thoughts, and feelings	Exploration with patient
Brenda: Yeah, you are probably right. I do feel really alone. There are a couple of women in my outpatient support group that have seemed friendly.	*Thoughts:* I hope the women she is referring to are able to be supportive. Having relationships from a therapy group can be great but also can be challenging.	**Nurse:** That sounds like a good beginning. How could you reach out to them?

VALIDATION Exploring this possibility further and empowering Brenda to think of ways she would feel comfortable initiating relationship.

Patient's behavior	Nurse's perceptions, thoughts, and feelings	Exploration with patient
Brenda: Well, maybe after group I could ask them to go out for coffee.	*Thoughts:* Great! She is able to think of ways to connect with the women in her group. *Feelings:* Relief, hopefulness	**Nurse:** Good. Why don't you make it a goal to try that next week?

VALIDATION Affirming her idea. Setting goals with Brenda empowers her and helps increase her self-esteem.

Patient's behavior	Nurse's perceptions, thoughts, and feelings	Exploration with patient
Brenda: OK. I will do that. Brenda sits up and looks at the nurse.	*Perceptions:* Brenda is speaking in a modulated and clear manner. She is sitting up and making eye contact. *Thoughts:* Brenda has a goal and feels empowered to move toward it. *Feelings:* Satisfaction, hope, connectedness	**Nurse:** OK. I will put that on the referral sheet so your therapist can follow up with you after discharge.

VALIDATION Validate with Brenda that she is not alone and even after leaving the hospital she will have professional, continuous support.

Based on Orlando, I. J. (1972). The Discipline and Teaching of Nursing Process (An Evaluative Study). New York, NY: G. P. Putnam's Sons.

Brenda Recovery Phase

APPLICATION
1. How could Sarah reinforce the positive strides Brenda has made?
2. What other areas of Brenda's life could Sarah suggest she focus on in her ongoing therapy?
3. What is necessary for Brenda to continue through recovery to rehabilitation?

Brenda is discharged from the hospital back to her home and the day treatment program. Before discharge, she began to experience some temptation to cut herself because she was feeling anxious about going home. However, she was able to contact nursing staff when she felt she was in imminent danger. She also employed some of her newly acquired techniques for safety. The last time she felt like hurting herself, she called a friend listed on her prevention plan and they went to a movie together. That seemed to distract her from her emotional pain. Sarah shared with Brenda that it is not unusual to feel some anxiety when discharge is looming, which sometimes results in return to previous coping mechanisms, or an earlier stage of functioning (regression). Treatment at this time focused on dealing with anxiety and helping develop plans for her return home.

Brenda feels more confident about her return home. She has a detailed list of coping strategies she has tried and found effective and a list of support people with phone numbers. Her treatment plan has been successful in helping her redirect thoughts related to cutting. However, Brenda is aware that between 40% and 60% of adolescents engage in repeated self-cutting episodes (Puskar et al., 2006).

Chapter Highlights

1. Personality develops from complex biopsychosocial factors.

2. The etiology of personality disorders includes biological, psychological, sociocultural, and spiritual components.

3. Medications used for treatment in personality disorders are indicated to relieve symptoms such as anxiety, depression, impulsivity, aggression, and psychosis.

4. Dialectic behavior therapy (DBT) is shown to be the most effective therapy in treating borderline personality disorder.

5. Nurses can help patients with personality disorders by establishing a therapeutic relationship; managing milieu and medication administration; maintaining patient safety; teaching patients about their illness, medications, social skills and coping mechanisms; and working collaboratively with patients to establish goals for treatment, as well as positive outcomes.

6. Nurses must have a strong sense of identity and the ability to manage emotions in order to work effectively with patients diagnosed with personality disorders, as identity diffusion and emotional dysregulation are common and challenging symptoms.

7. Nurses need to maintain self-awareness and find collegial relationships to offer support and guidance when working with patients diagnosed with personality disorders in order to remain compassionate, yet objective.

NCLEX®-RN Questions

1. The nurse is conducting a psychoeducation group with patients with personality disorders. The discussion has focused on aspects of life experiences that have contributed to maladaptive coping patterns. One patient asks, "How come my adopted sister ended up doing so well, when she has been through the same things as me?" How should the nurse respond?
   a. Suggest the possibility that the sister made better life choices.
   b. Discuss the impact of genetics on resilience and personality.
   c. Remind the patient to stay focused on personal issues and needs.
   d. Explore aspects of the patient's life that may have been more difficult.

2. The nurse is caring for an adult patient diagnosed with borderline personality disorder. The nurse notices that the patient responds automatically to most situations and challenges with destructive, self-defeating thoughts and behaviors. Which interpretation of these behaviors is appropriate at this time?
   a. The patient has learned maladaptive responses over time.
   b. The patient experienced parenting that was often inconsistent and or unavailable.
   c. The patient comes from a culture in which this behavior is acceptable.
   d. The patient is genetically programmed to be defensive and pessimistic.

3. The nurse is planning care for a patient with symptoms of a cluster C personality disorder. The nurse understands that treatment is most likely to be challenged by the need to address which characteristics of behaviors common to this category of disorders?
   a. Odd, eccentric, and/or suspicious
   b. Rigid, dependent, and/or avoidant
   c. Seductive, self-centered, and/or dramatic
   d. Oppositional, impulsive, and/or manipulative

4. The nurse is caring for a patient receiving cognitive–behavioral therapy for the treatment of dependent personality disorder. The family asks what the therapy is supposed to accomplish. Which response is best?
   a. The patient will develop a more appropriate support network.
   b. The patient will gain better insight into factors that led to dependency.
   c. The patient will work to replace dysfunctional behaviors with more adaptive ones.
   d. The patient will learn to break off contact with people on whom the patient has become dependent.

5. The nurse is planning a psychoeducation group for patients diagnosed with borderline personality disorder. The nurse understands that which aspect of group intervention is most essential?
   a. Maintaining consistent limits and boundaries
   b. Providing a relaxed, nonjudgmental atmosphere
   c. Promoting activities that encourage self-reflection
   d. Ensuring opportunities for free expression and disclosure

Answers can be found on the Pearson student resource site: nursing.pearsonhigherred.com

Pearson Nursing Student Resources Find additional review materials at **nursing.pearsonhighered.com**

References

Ado, M. (2006). Culture, spirituality and ethical issues in caring for clients with personality disorder. In National Forensic Nurses Research Group, (Eds.). *Forensic Mental Health Nursing: Intervention for People with Personality Disorders*. London, UK: Quay Books.

Akhtar, S. (1995). *Quest for Answers: A Primer of Understanding and Treating Severe Personality Disorders*. Northvale, NJ: Jason Aronson.

American Psychiatric Association. (2013). *Diagnostic and Statistical Manual of Mental Disorders* (5th ed.). Washington, DC: American Psychiatric Publishers.

B-52. (2011, June 8–11). [Online discussion of the use of the "B-52" cocktail in psychiatric facilities.] Available at http://allnurses.com/psychiatric-nursing/b-52-a-576609.html

Baurenbaum, N., & Winter, D. (2010). History of modern personality theory and research. In O. John, R. Robins, & L. Pervin, (Eds.). *Handbook of Personality*. New York, NY: Guilford Press, pp. 3–23.

Bjorklund, P. (2006). No man's land: Gender bias and social constructivism in the diagnosis of borderline personality disorder. *Issues in Mental Health Nursing, 27*(1), 3–23.

Borderline Personality Disorder support group website: http://www.bpdfamily.com/

Castillo, H. (2001). The hurtfulness of a diagnosis: User research about personality disorder. *Mental Health Care, 4*(2), 53–58.

Chester, R. (2010). Diagnosing personality disorder in people with learning disabilities. *Learning Disability Practice, 13*(8), 14–19.

Cloninger, C. R. (2005). Character strengths and virtues: A handbook and classification. *American Journal of Psychiatry, 162*(3), 802.

Darby, D., & Walsh, K. (2005). *Walsh's Neuropsychology: A Clinical Approach*. New York, NY: Elsevier/Churchill/Livingstone.

Dimeff, L., & Koerner, K. (2007). Overview of dialectical behavior therapy. In L. Dimeff & K. Koerner, (Eds.). *Dialectical Behavior Therapy in Clinical Practice: Applications across Disorders and Settings*. New York, NY: Guilford Press, pp. 1–19.

Erikson Institute. (2012). About Erik Erikson. Available at http://www.erikson.edu/default/aboutei/history/erikerikson.aspx

Ewen, R. (2003). *An Introduction to Theories of Personality*. Mahwah, NJ: Lawrence Erlbaum Associates.

Filer, N. (2005). Borderline personality disorder: Attitudes of mental health nurses. *Mental Health Practice, 9*(2), 34–36.

Hadjipavlou, G., & Ogrodniczuk, J. (2010). Promising psychotherapies for personality disorders. *Canadian Journal of Psychiatry, 55*(4), 202–209.

Hayward, B. (2007). Cluster A personality disorder: Considering the "odd-eccentric" in psychiatric nursing. *International Journal of Mental Health Nursing, 16*, 15–21.

Howland, R. (2007). Pharmacotherapy and personality disorders. *Journal of Psychosocial Nursing, 45*(6), 15–19.

Klonsky, E. D. (2007). The functions of deliberate self-injury: A review of the evidence. *Clinical Psychology Review, 27*(2): 226–239. doi: 10.1016/j.cpr.2006.08.002

Koenig, H. (2005). *Faith and Mental Health: Religious Resources for Healing*. Philadelphia, PA: Templeton Publishing.

Lamont, S., & Brunero, S. (2009). Personality disorder prevalence and treatment outcomes: A literature review. *Issues in Mental Health Nursing, 30*(10), 631–637.

Larsen, P., & Lubkin, I. (2009). *Chronic Illness: Impact and Intervention*. Sudbury, MA: Jones and Bartlett.

Leising, D. (2008). Applying principles of intercultural communication to personality disorder therapy. *Psychology and Psychotherapy: Theory, Research and Practice, 81*(Pt 3), 261–272.

Lin, M. (2010). Tricks of the trade: Chemical sedation options. Available at http://academiclifeinem.com/tricks-of-the-trade-chemical-sedation-options/

Linehan, M. (1993a). *Cognitive-Behavioral Treatment of Borderline Personality Disorder*. New York, NY: Guilford Press.

Linehan, M. (1993b). *Skills Training Manual for Treating Borderline Personality Disorder*. New York, NY: Guilford Press.

Markham, D. (2003). Attitudes towards patients with a diagnosis of borderline personality disorder: Social rejection and dangerousness. *Journal of Mental Health, 12*(6), 595–612.

Masterson, J. (1981). *The Narcissistic and Borderline Disorders*. New York, NY: Bruner/Mazel.

Mayo Clinic. (2011). Narcissistic personality disorder. Available at http://www.mayoclinic.com/health/narcissistic-personality-disorder/DS00652/DSECTION=risk-factors

Mayo Clinic. (2012). Risk factors for personality disorder. Available at http://www.mayoclinic.com/health/personality-disorders/DS00562/DSECTION=risk-factors

Mayo Clinic. (2013). Schizotypal personality disorder. Available at http://www.mayoclinic.com/health/schizotypal-personality-disorder/DS00830/DSECTION=treatments-and-drugs

McLean, J. (2007). Psychotherapy with a narcissistic patient using Kohut's Self Psychology Mode. *Psychiatry, 4*(10), 40–47. Available at http://www.ncbi.nlm.nih.gov/pmc/articles/PMC2860525/

MedlinePlus. (2012). Avoidant personality disorder. Available at http://www.nlm.nih.gov/medlineplus/ency/article/000940.htm

National Institute of Mental Health. (2009). Borderline personality disorder: Raising questions, finding answers. Available at http://www.nimh.nih.gov/index.shtml

National Mental Health America. (2013). Personality Disorders. Available at http://www.nmha.org/index.cfm?objectId=C7DF8E96-1372-4D20-C87D9CD4FB6BE82F

Newman, S., Steed, E., & Mulligan, K. (2004). Self-management interventions for chronic illness. *Lancet, 364*(9444), 1523–1537.

Nukolls, C. (1992). Toward a cultural history of the personality disorders. *Social Science and Medicine, 35*(1), 37–49.

Oden-Miller, H. (2011). Value of music therapy for people with personality disorders. *Mental Health Practice, 14*(10), 34–35.

O'Donohue, W., Fowler, K., Lilienfeld, S., & Cloninger, R. (Eds.). (2007). *Personality Disorders: Toward the DSM V.* Los Angeles, CA: Sage Publications.

Orlando, I. J. (1972). *The Discipline and Teaching of Nursing Process (An Evaluative Study).* New York, NY: G. P. Putnam's Sons.

Potter, M., & Dawson, A. (2001). From safety contract to safety agreement. *Journal of Psychosocial Nursing and Mental Health Services, 39*(8), 38–45.

Puskar, K. R., Bernardo, L., Hatam, M., Geise, S., G., Bendik, J., & Grabiak, B. R. (2006). Self-cutting behaviors in adolescents. *Journal of Emergency Nursing, 32*(5), 444–446.

Ripoll, L. H. (2012). Clinical pharmacology of borderline personality disorder. *Current Opinion on Clinical Psychiatry, 25*(1), 52–58.

Sadock, B., Sadock, V., & Ruiz, P. (2009). *Kaplan and Sadock's Comprehensive Textbook of Psychiatry.* Philadelphia, PA: Lippincott Williams & Wilkins.

Schatzberg, A. & Nemeroff, C. (2006). *Essentials of Clinical Psychopharmacology.* Arlington, VA: American Psychiatric Publishing.

Shannon, J. (2011, May). Understanding and treating personality disorders. In Institute for Brain Potential Conference, *Understanding Personality Disorders*, Minnetonka, MN, http://www.ibpceu.com/

Sheldon, K., Howells, K., & Patel, G. (2010). An empirical evaluation of reasons for non-completion of treatment in a dangerous and severe personality disorder unit. *Criminal Behaviour and Mental Health, 20*(2), 129–143.

Sollberg, D., Gremaud-Heitz, D., Riemenschneider, A., Küchenhoff, J., Dammann, G., & Walter, M. (2012). Associations between identity diffusion, Axis II disorder, and psychopathology in patients with borderline personality disorder. *Psychopathology, 45*(1), 15–21.

Stobie, M., & Tromski-Klingshirn, D. (2009). Borderline personality disorder, divorce and family therapy: The need for family crisis intervention strategies. *American Journal of Family Therapy*, 37, 414–432. doi: 10.1080/01926180902754760

Swift, E. (2009). The efficacy of treatments for borderline personality disorder. *Mental Health Practice, 13*(4), 30–33.

Taylor, E. (2009). *The Mystery of Personality: A History of Psychodynamic Theories.* New York, NY: Springer Science-Business Media.

Toth, S. L., Cicchetti, D., Rogosch, F. A., & Sturge-Apple, M. (2009). Maternal depression, children's attachment security, and representational development: An organizational perspective. *Child Development, 80*(1), 192–208.

Townsend, M. (2011). *Nursing Diagnosis in Psychiatric Nursing.* Philadelphia, PA: F.A. Davis.

Tseng, W-S., & Streltzer, J. (2006). Introduction: Culture and psychiatry. *Focus 4*(1), 81–90. Available at http://focus.psychiatryonline.org/article.aspx?articleID=50459

Tyrer, P., & Bateman, A. (2004). Drug treatment for personality disorders. *Advances in Psychiatric Treatment, 10*, 389–398.

Vatne, S., & Holmes, C. (2006). Limit setting in mental health: Historical factors and suggestions as to its rationale. *Journal of Psychiatric and Mental Health Nursing, 13*(5), 588–597.

Videbeck, S. (2010). *Nursing Practice for Psychiatric Nursing.* Philadelphia, PA: Lippincott Williams & Wilkins.

Vita, A., DePeri, L., & Sacchetti, E. (2011). Antipsychotics, antidepressants, anticonvulsants, and placebo on the symptom dimensions of borderline personality disorder: A meta-analysis of randomized controlled and open-label trials. *Journal of Clinical Psychopharmacology, 31*(5), 613–624.

Wilkinson-Ryan, T., & Weston, D. (2000). Identity disturbance in borderline personality disorder: An empirical investigation. *American Journal of Psychiatry, 157*(4), 528–531.

Winship, G., & Hardy, S. (2007). Perspectives on the prevalence and treatment of personality disorder. *Journal of Psychiatric and Mental Health Nursing, 14*(2), 148–154.

World Health Organization. International Classification of Diseases (ICD 10). Available at http://www.who.int/classifications/icd/en/bluebook.pdf

Wray, C., & Byrt, R. (2005). Towards hope and inclusion: Nursing interventions in a medium secure service for men with "personality disorders." *Mental Health Practice, 8*(8), 38–43.

19

Sexual Dysfunctions, Gender Dysphoria, and Paraphilic Disorders

Barbara Steele

Key Terms

Learning Outcomes

1. Identify the stages of the sexual response cycle.

2. Summarize the impact of biological, psychological, sociological, cultural, and spiritual domains on sexual development and dysfunctions.

3. Compare the differences in sexual dysfunctions experienced by men and women.

4. Categorize key symptoms of sexual dysfunctions.

5. Discuss the possible causes of and treatment options for individuals with gender dysphoria.

6. Describe different types of paraphilic disorders and the role of pharmacotherapy in the treatment of individuals with paraphilic disorders.

7. Plan evidence-based nursing care for patients diagnosed with sexual dysfunctions or gender dysphoria.

Blakeney Carroll Initial Onset

1. Address the five domains for Mr. Carroll:

    a. Biological

    b. Psychological

    c. Sociological

    d. Cultural

    e. Spiritual

2. In what ways do you think Mr. Carroll may be suffering? Why?

3. How you would prioritize his needs during this encounter, and why?

4. If you were the nurse working with Mr. Carroll, what might you do to convey hope to him when he states he never had told any of his counselors about his past sexual abuse? How would you relate that to his current concerns?

Blakeney Carroll is a 33-year-old White male who is seen in the community health care clinic for complaints of delayed or, at times, absent ejaculation in spite of no difficulty with erections. Mr. Carroll has been on numerous antidepressants for major depressive disorder since he was 16 years old. Although some of the past medications did not cause absent or delayed ejaculation, they also did not treat his depression. He has had the most success with the selective serotonin-reuptake inhibitors (SSRIs) and has been on escitalopram (Lexapro) 20 mg PO daily for the past 3 years.

Mr. Carroll has been in a monogamous relationship with a 24-year-old woman named Nancy for the past 6 months. He and Nancy are engaged and hope to start a family. Although he has had some difficulty being able to ejaculate since being on medications from his late teens, he shares that he currently is distressed about this due to the seriousness of his relationship. Mostly he is concerned that his significant other thinks it is her "fault" and that they might not be able to have children.

Melissa, the nurse practitioner seeing Mr. Carroll, inquires about any history of abuse. Mr. Carroll reluctantly shares that he was sexually abused by an older male cousin from ages 6 to 9 years. Melissa asks if he ever addressed that in past counseling sessions. Mr. Carroll acknowledges that he never informed his counselors, because he did not want to get his cousin in trouble and thought he should have prevented it from happening himself.

Melissa also asks Mr. Carroll if he has ever taken bupropion (Wellbutrin). Mr. Carroll recalls that he may have taken it in his early 20s, but he is not sure. Melissa discusses several options with Mr. Carroll. They include (1) add a small amount of bupropion to his current medication regimen, as that sometimes eases sexual side effects; (2) taper off Lexapro and then start bupropion; or (3) lower his dose of Lexapro to 15 mg PO daily, and even 10 mg PO daily if necessary, to see whether that helps his sexual concerns while maintaining his remission from depression.

Additionally, Melissa suggests that Mr. Carroll may want to receive counseling because of the medication adjustment and relationship changes in his life. Mr. Carroll agrees, as long as he can see a female therapist. He states that he would be too embarrassed to discuss these issues with a male therapist.

Introduction

The development of sexuality, sexual identity, gender identity, and related disorders is multifaceted. Clearly there is a biological component, but the way individuals define their own sexuality and what causes them to experience sexual arousal varies, based on a number of factors. When discussing sexual development and sexual identity, the term **sex** generally refers to biological indicators, including sex chromosomes, hormones, and genitalia. The term **gender** is defined by more than simple biology; it is defined as an individual's personal, social, and legal status as a male or female. All the domains—biological, psychological, sociological, cultural, and spiritual—play a role in individual expressions of sexuality and have the potential to affect or be affected by sexual disorders and disorders of gender identity.

Sexuality is the manifestation of several psychosexual factors: sexual identity, gender identity, and sexual orientation. It is a normal and universal part of being human and of relating to another person in the most intimate way possible. In the context of a loving relationship, sexuality can enhance the quality of the relationship as the physical representation of the many dimensions of the relationship. Of course, it is the main means by which children are conceived. It also has the potential for enhancing deeply committed relationships. **Sexual orientation** refers to the object of the individual's sexual attraction. Most individuals begin to identify their sexual orientation in adolescence. *Heterosexuality* refers to attraction to individuals of the opposite gender; **homosexuality** denotes attraction to individuals of the same gender; and *bisexuality* to attraction to individuals of either gender. In the Kinsey reports of 1948 and 1953, 8% of men and 2% to 6% of women in the United States identified themselves as exclusively homosexual. In 2010, 594,000 couples living in same-sex households were identified (U.S. Census Bureau, 2012).

For most human beings, the human sexual response occurs in a predictable cycle. The **sexual response cycle** has four distinct phases: excitement, plateau, orgasm, and resolution. **Sexual dysfunction** refers to interruption or impairment of this cycle or pain associated with intercourse. The term encompasses a number of sexual disorders. Some individuals experience **gender dysphoria**, distress that arises when individuals experience psychosocial incongruence between their assigned gender and the gender with which they more clearly identify.

Paraphilic disorders are a classification of disorders that are characterized by overwhelming sexual arousal and/or behaviors related to unusual objects or activities that result in significant distress and impairment in functioning. Of all the topics discussed in this chapter, paraphilic disorders are often considered to be outside societal norms and carry the greatest risk for legal complications.

Nurses in every area of practice will, at some time, discuss sexuality with their patients. Nurses can play an instrumental role in helping patients understand that aspects of sexuality exist on a continuum of human experience. By addressing patients respectfully and privately, nurses help reduce patient fear and anxiety, making it possible for patients to share their concerns and increasing the likelihood of accurate assessment. In many cases, patients may not ever have discussed sex or issues related to sexuality with another person. Nurses who possess accurate information and have processed their own anxiety about discussing issues related to sex and sexuality will be more comfortable discussing these issues with their patients.

Age-Appropriate Sexual Behaviors   box 19-1

Children are curious by nature, and their curiosity leads them to all kinds of exploration, including wondering about issues related to sex and sexuality. For example, it is common for preschoolers to ask questions about gender and sexuality and to share their knowledge (or their perceptions) with others. The Stop It Now website provides further information on age-appropriate behaviors for the developmental stages of growing children. It also identifies the indicators of unusual sexual behavior by age group which may signify problematic areas, such as possible sexual abuse. The American Academy of Pediatrics offers a toolkit for health care professionals through its website. A number of state agencies and hospitals also provide information about age-appropriate behaviors for both parents and professionals.

Sexual Development

Sexual development begins in early childhood. Appropriate touching and cuddling of the infant, which promotes attachment, lays the groundwork by providing the physical and emotional security necessary to promote the infant's sense of self and self-esteem. In the second year, children begin the normal activity of genital self-stimulation as part of their growing awareness of their bodies. As they become aware of their playmates, they have a natural curiosity about their genitalia (Box 19-1). Genital exhibition and exploration proceed unless excessive shame and punishment intervene. Parents and other adults model appropriate physical affection.

During adolescence, hormones and the development of secondary sexual characteristics produce intensified interest in sexuality. Adolescents need to learn their sexual identity while controlling their sexual impulses. Kissing and caressing help to establish patterns of relating sexually to a potential partner. Manual and oral genital stimulation are a part of the process. Experimentation and sex play with same sex partners are not unusual, even for heterosexual adolescents. In the United States, 17 is the average age at which young people have sex for the first time (Guttmacher Institute, 2013).

Theoretical Foundations

As stated earlier, the individual development of sexuality, sexual identity, and gender identity is influenced by a variety of factors. Hormones, for example, play a critical role in the development of sexuality. Familial, societal, or cultural attitudes may affect an individual's expression of sexuality. Although male erectile dysfunction often results from physiologic changes, the way in which the patient with erectile dysfunction handles it and its impact on his life may vary based on a number of factors. Nurses must be aware of the complex interplay of factors that can affect individual patients.

Biological Domain

The role of biology in gender and sexuality is clear. From determining sex characteristics to influencing the human sexual response, biology carries vast implications for the anatomy and physiology of human gender and sexuality.

Genetic Influence

Genetics certainly plays a role in shaping an individual's gender identity. For example, the sex of a developing embryo is determined at the instant of fertilization as a result of the sex chromosomes. Humans have 23 pairs of chromosomes. The X and Y chromosomes determine an individual's sex. Females carry two X chromosomes and will develop ovaries. Males carry one X and one Y chromosome and will develop testes. Some cultures include greater gender diversity: Sex, gender, and sexual orientation are not always divided along clear lines such as male and female or homosexual and heterosexual.

Occasionally, incorrect combinations of chromosomes occur, leading to abnormalities in sexual development. The most common of these are (World Health Organization, 2013b):

- *In males:* Klinefelter syndrome, which occurs when males have one or more extra X chromosomes (XXY). Males with Klinefelter syndrome typically have small testes that produce lower amounts of testosterone than normal. This can lead to incomplete puberty, reduced amounts of facial and body hair, and sterility.

- *In females:* Turner syndrome, which occurs when the second X chromosome is missing (monosomy). Associated symptoms include short stature, broad chest, low hairline, low-set ears, and a webbed neck. Girls with Turner syndrome typically experience gonadal dysfunction (nonworking ovaries), resulting in amenorrhea and sterility. Secondary sex characteristics are absent or minimal.

Genetics also plays a role in sexual disorders that are not related to chromosomal inheritance. Neurotic personality disorders and submissive personality traits are thought to be associated with erectile issues, as are posttraumatic stress disorder (PTSD), depression, and alexthymia (deficits in cognitive processing of emotions) (American Psychiatric Association [APA], 2013). Likewise, female sexual disorders are thought to have a strong genetic link in relation to vulnerability (APA, 2013)

Hormonal Influence

Hormones play an essential role in the processes of developing sexuality. Fetal hormones affect the development of the genitalia (Box 19-2). Sexual differentiation does not occur until the embryo has developed for more than 6 weeks. Until that point, the embryo is sexually indifferent. As soon as the testes begin to form, at about the 7th week of development, they begin to release testosterone, which causes the development of the penis and scrotum. If testosterone is not present, female genitalia are formed. It sometimes happens that the embryonic testes fail to produce testosterone. The result is a genetic male with female genitalia. In the case of a genetic female, if the mother has a tumor of the adrenal gland that produces testosterone, it will lead to a genetic female with a penis and empty scrotum.

Beginning at puberty, testosterone and estrogen are essential to the development of secondary sexual characteristics. Estrogen is the primary female sex hormone. It stimulates the growth of breasts and causes the mammary glands to prepare for milk production. It stimulates lengthening of the long bones and the female pattern of

Disorders of Sexual Development: An Overview   box 19-2

Disorders of sexual development, sometimes referred to as **intersex** conditions, are a group of conditions resulting from hormonal errors during fetal development in which internal genitalia differ from external genitalia. The nature of the discrepancy determines the type of disorder:

- Individuals with *46, XX intersex* have female chromosomes and ovaries, but their external genitalia appear male.
- Individuals with *46, XY intersex* possess male chromosomes, but their external genitalia appear female or are malformed or ambiguous. Internal testes may be present or absent. If present, they may be normal or malformed.
- Individuals with *true gonadal intersex* have both ovarian and testicular tissue. External genitalia may appear male or female or may be ambiguous.

- A variety of chromosome configurations may result in *complex/undetermined disorders of sexual development.* These may interfere with hormone levels or overall sexual development without resulting in a discrepancy between internal and external genitalia.

Not all intersex conditions are discovered at birth. Some are not discovered until adolescence, when some individuals fail to achieve puberty. Intersex conditions associated with infertility may not be discovered until later in life. Although individuals with hormonal imbalances may require lifelong care, not all will. It is recommended that individuals with disorders of sexual development seek both medical and psychosocial care as necessary, with most health care professionals advocating a collaborative but individually tailored approach.

Based on Medline Plus. (2011). Intersex. Available at http://www.nlm.nih.gov/medlineplus/ency/article/001669.htm; American Psychological Association. (2006). Answers to your questions about individuals with intersex conditions. Available at http://www.apa.org/topics/sexuality/intersex.aspx?item=1; Lee, P. A., Houk, C. P., Faisal Ahmed, S., & Hughes, I. A. (2006). Consensus statement on management of intersex disorders. *Pediatrics, 118,* e488–e501. Available at http://pediatrics.aappublications.org/content/118/2/e488.full.pdf

subcutaneous fat deposits. It also helps to regulate the menstrual cycle by thickening the lining of the uterus, preparing it for ovulation and pregnancy. As estrogen declines in production, the uterine lining no longer thickens and menopause occurs. Testosterone stimulates growth of the external genitalia in males and suppresses mammary gland development. Growth of the larynx and thickening of the vocal cords results from increased production of testosterone, as does growth of pubic, axillary, and facial hair. Bone and muscle mass are increased as well. Testosterone is responsible for the sex drive in both sexes.

Oxytocin is secreted by the posterior pituitary gland. In addition to its role in uterine contractions and lactation, it plays an instrumental role in affiliative behaviors. It promotes grooming, arousal and orgasmic activity, and the maternal activities of breastfeeding and bonding. Research continues to develop an understanding of its role in pair bonding between men and women.

The Sexual Response Cycle

The research team of William H. Masters and Virginia E. Johnson studied the structure, psychology, and physiology of sexual behavior through observing and measuring masturbation and sexual intercourse in the laboratory. In addition to recording some of the first physiological data from the human body and sex organs during sexual excitation, they also framed their findings and conclusions in language that fostered sex as a healthy and natural activity that could be enjoyed as a source of pleasure and intimacy.

One of the most well-known and important aspects of their work was the four-stage model of the human sexual response cycle (Masters & Johnson, 1966). They defined the four stages of this cycle as consisting of the excitement phase (initial arousal), the plateau phase (at full arousal, but not yet at orgasm), the orgasm phase, and the resolution phase (after orgasm) (Figure 19-1). The Masters and Johnson model

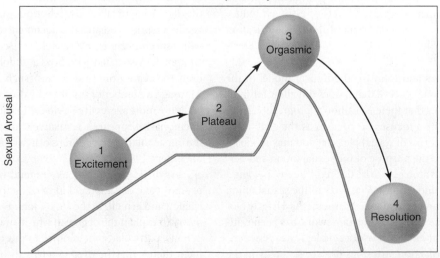

Sexual Response Cycle

Sexual Arousal (vertical axis) — *Time* (horizontal axis)

1 Excitement · 2 Plateau · 3 Orgasmic · 4 Resolution

19-1   The phases of the sexual response cycle may be defined as excitement, plateau, orgasm, and resolution.

proposed that sexual response is linear, such that desire always precedes arousal, and arousal is followed by orgasm and resolution. According to this model, the order of these stages of response does not vary.

Excitement (arousal) is a vascular phenomenon involving the parasympathetic (cholinergic) nervous system. It results in erection, clitoral engorgement, genital and breast swelling, and lubrication caused by the neurotransmitters acetylcholine, dopamine, and nitric oxide. Nitric oxide is synthesized by neurons in the penis. It relaxes smooth muscle in the blood vessels, allowing blood to flow into the penis. In the *plateau* phase, these responses intensify as the result of physical stimulation and extend to the brink of orgasm. *Orgasm* is mediated by norepinephrine, produced by the sympathetic nervous system. Involuntary muscle contractions begin and a sudden, forceful release of sexual tension occurs. For some people, a rash (sex flush) may appear on the chest for a brief period. *Resolution* is defined as the gradual return of the body to its normal state. Erect and engorged body parts return to normal. There is a general feeling of well-being, and often fatigue occurs. A refractory period (during which orgasm is not possible for men) follows resolution. The duration of the refractory period varies with the individual and usually lengthens with age. Women may be able to return to the orgasm phase more quickly (Your Guide to the Sexual Response Cycle, 2012). Note that all phases of the model respond negatively to serotonin. This phenomenon is helpful in deciding which antidepressant to use and under which circumstances. For some individuals (such as those who struggle with hypersexuality or pedophilia), reducing sexual interest is useful. For others, it is problematic.

There are specific changes to the patterns of male and female sexual responses with aging—for example, it takes older men longer to become aroused and they typically require more direct genital stimulation. The speed and amount of vaginal lubrication tends to diminish with age as well. Masters and Johnson noted that many older men and women are capable of excitement and orgasm well into their 70s and even beyond, a finding that has been confirmed in population-based epidemiological research on sexual function in older adults. However, the incidence of sexual disorders also increases with age. Erectile disorders may respond to medication provided there is no underlying medical problem, such as diabetes. For women, decreased levels of estrogen reduce vaginal lubrication, making intercourse painful unless lubrication is augmented with a sterile, water-soluble product such as Sterilube or KY Jelly.

Critics of the Masters and Johnson theoretical model of the human sexual response cycle observe that it does not allow for individual variability. It implies that there is a smooth progression from one stage to the next. It also focuses on orgasm as the goal. In so doing, it overlooks other forms of sexual pleasure and may set up an expectation that orgasm is the purpose of the sexual union and perhaps that multiple orgasms are a goal to be desired. The psychological and relational, cognitive, and emotional aspects of the sexual union are subordinated to the purely physiological aspects. As a largely biological model, the Masters and Johnson framework has been criticized because it does not take into account nonbiological experiences, such as pleasure and satisfaction, nor does it place sexuality in the context of the relationship.

In contrast to the linear model proposed by Masters and Johnson, Basson (2001) proposed a nonlinear model as being representative of a more complex set of response patterns that is a better fit to that of some women. Basson's nonlinear model acknowledges how emotional intimacy, sexual stimuli, and relationship satisfaction affect the female's sexual response. She recognized that many women in long-term relationships do not think of sex or experience spontaneous hunger for sexual activity very often. A desire for emotional closeness and intimacy or the interest expressed by her partner may set the stage for a woman to participate in sexual activity. Beginning from sexual neutrality, where a woman is willing to be sexual but does not initiate sexual activity, her desire for intimacy engenders activities that help her to become sexually aroused. She may engage in conversation, music, reading or viewing erotic materials, or direct stimulation. Once aroused, sexual desire emerges and motivates her to continue the activity. The Basson model clarifies that the goal of sexual activity for women is not always orgasm but may manifest as emotional satisfaction experienced as a feeling of intimacy and connection with a partner.

Psychological Domain

Personality development is deeply affected by sexual development giving rise to the term psychosexual development. *Sexual identity* is the interrelationship of biological factors, including chromosomes, internal and external genitalia, hormones, and secondary sexual characteristics. In most individuals, these factors function in a manner that leaves no doubt about their sexual identity. External manifestations of sexual identity include the secondary sexual characteristics: breast size, muscle mass, hair distribution, subcutaneous fat, and body shape and physical dimensions.

As children grow, they receive many cues to their gender identity. Biological cues are provided by sex hormones. For example, androgens contribute to rough, noisy play in boys. Girls are more likely to engage in more gentle types of play activities. Because of their play style preferences, each is more inclined to seek playmates of the same gender. Environmental factors influencing gender beliefs include the stereotypical modeling activities often provided by adults (for example, mothers cook, fathers fix things) (Putnam, Myers-Walls, & Love, n.d.). These cues have become less prominent as adults in today's society become less inclined to adopt the older, more traditional division of labor. Toy selections may also support or reinforce gender identity. Research has documented that toys can be associated with a specific gender, such as vehicles, science-based toys, and sports equipment associated with boys and dolls and toys that allow children to create domestic scenes (such as dollhouses) with girls. Although a number of studies have documented that boys' toys generally are more aggressive or violent in nature, whereas girls' toys tend to emphasize appearance, relatively little research has documented the impact of toys on children's behavior or development (Blakemore & Centers, 2005).

As discussed in Chapter 4, Freud was one of the first to study psychosexual development, proposing five stages: oral, anal, phallic, latency, and genital. In the 1950s, John Bowlby described *attachment theory* to explain the degree to which an infant can rely on his or her parents, particularly the mother, to meet needs for security. Attachment theory may be used as a lens through which to examine the development of sexual identity and behaviors. Bowlby observed that a distressed infant who is securely attached to the caregiver will turn to the caregiver for solace. If the infant has been deprived in some significant way from developing a secure attachment to the caregiver, however, three other attachment styles may develop. One is a pattern called *preoccupied attachment*, in which the infant has a high desire for intimacy but is fearful of being abandoned. The infant may show clingy behaviors and, if threatened by the potential loss of the caregiver, may react with anger, jealousy, and panic. *Fearful attachment* results in high levels of anxiety and avoidance of dependency on the caregiver. The *dismissive attachment* style results in a child who withdraws from others and relies on himself or herself. The child with dismissive attachment would see intimacy as a sign of weakness.

The patterns of attachment developed in infancy and childhood generally persist into adulthood and may play out in intimate relationships throughout their lives. In the sexual realm, the patterns of attachment manifest in the following ways:

- *Secure attachment:* There is a capacity for high commitment and enjoyment of closeness. The relationship is marked by mutuality, stability, and exploration.

- *Preoccupied attachment:* Commitment and intimacy are low. The relationship is marked by possessiveness, dependency, and idealization.

- *Fearful–avoidant attachment:* Hugging and cuddling are enjoyed more than genital sexuality. The sexual relationship may depend on the partner to initiate a sexual encounter.

- *Dismissive–avoidant attachment:* There is a characteristic "game-playing" in the relationship. Commitment and intimacy are low. Infidelity is routine and may be flagrant.

Individuals who experience what they see as alterations in "normal" related to sexual function or sexual identity may experience symptoms of anxiety or depression. For a sexual dysfunction to be diagnosed, one of the criteria that typically must be met is that the symptoms related to the dysfunction must cause significant distress to the individual (APA, 2013). This distress manifests differently depending on the individual and the disorder. For example, individuals experiencing genitopelvic pain/penetration disorder will experience fear or anxiety associated with vaginal penetration. Men with male hypoactive sexual desire disorder may lose interest in sex altogether, which may result in conflict with the individual's partner, loss of self-esteem, or both. Individuals with gender dysphoria are at high risk for depression related to features associated with their dysphoria, as well as widespread misunderstanding and discrimination of individuals with the condition (Grant, Mottet, & Tanis, 2011).

Sociological Domain

Attitudes and behaviors related to sex, sexuality, and gender are determined largely by society. Many influences within societies change or affect these attitudes and behaviors, including cultural values and practices (Macionis, 2010).

Until the mid-20th century, the predominant view in America was that sex and sexuality occurred within the realm of heterosexual marriage, with an emphasis on sexual expression for reproduction rather than pleasure. Beginning in the 1960s, a trend toward sexual liberation occurred, and more people began to engage in sexual activity before and outside marriage. This change in attitudes and behavior has been attributed (at least in part) to the advent of birth control, legalized abortion, and Alfred Kinsey's publications related to sexuality in the United States (Macionis, 2010). The feminist movement challenged the double standard for acceptable sexual behavior and brought the problems of rape and incest into sharp focus. In the late 1980s, the epidemic nature of HIV/AIDS brought discussions of homosexuality into the mainstream media and resulted in a renewed emphasis on safe sexual practices.

Attitudes toward sexuality are deeply influenced by those held within the family. Parental attitudes play a role in the development of attitudes toward sexuality (Macionis, 2010). Some individuals accept and take on the attitudes of the parents toward sexuality (particularly the attitudes of the same-gender parent), whereas others oppose and reject their parents' values, possibly as a function of the quality of the relationship between parent and offspring. Family attitudes play an instrumental role in the propagation of sexual disorders. For example, in a family in which incest is kept shrouded in secrecy, factors that allow the behavior to persist will likely be carried into the next and subsequent generations. Some 34% of sexual assaults against juveniles are made by family members (Rape, Abuse, and Incest National Network, 2009).

Cultural and Spiritual Domains

For some individuals, cultural and spiritual beliefs and practices influence sexuality. The decision about when to have sex and under what circumstances, for example, may be affected by cultural or religious beliefs. Most cultures agree that incest (sexual relations between certain relatives) is not acceptable on several grounds, including the potential for offspring with mental and/or physical abnormalities (Macionis, 2010).

Sexual freedom and sexual activity may vary by culture. In some cultures, however, sex outside marriage is forbidden and women who engage in extramarital sex may experience shame, torture, or even death. An individual's right or ability to choose when and under what circumstances he or she has sex is at the heart of the issue of consent (Box 19-3). Courtship behaviors—how individuals meet and partner with one another—also vary among cultures. In some cultures, marriages are arranged, with parents and family members choosing partners for their adolescent or grown children. In many Western cultures, courtship begins in social environments or at work.

Female circumcision is one example of a cultural practice related to gender and sexuality. **Female circumcision** (often termed **genital mutilation**) is defined by the World Health Organization (WHO) as "all procedures that involve partial or total removal of the external female genitalia, or other injury to the female genital organs for non-medical reasons" (WHO, 2013a). According to the WHO, female circumcision is practiced in 28 countries (in parts of Africa, Asia, and the Middle East) as well as in some immigrant communities in Europe, North America, and Australia. The WHO estimates that 100 to 140 million women and girls around the world have had the procedure, the majority of them in Africa. The WHO recognizes three different types of female genital mutilation:

- Type I involves the removal of the clitoral hood, usually along with the clitoris itself.

- Type II removes the clitoris and labia minoris.

- Type III (infibulation) removes the labia minoris, the labia majoris, and usually the clitoris.

Following the procedure, the wound edges are sewn together, leaving a small hole for the passage of urine and menstrual blood. The wound is reopened for intercourse and childbirth. In 1996, the

Consent
box 19-3

Sexual activity without consent is considered assault or rape (Chapter 25). Consent given on one occasion does not guarantee consent on any other occasion. To provide consent to have sexual relations with another, an individual must:

- Have the right and ability to say yes or no to sexual contact at any point without the threat of consequences or harm. Individuals with a history of abuse often have an impaired ability to say no. Silence or lack of response does not constitute consent.
- Be of legal age. In the United States and most other countries, children are protected from being permitted to give consent to sexual acts.

- Be in a clear state of mind; in other words, the individual must have the capacity to consent. Impaired states of mind include being under the influence of drugs/alcohol, mental illness or deficiency, developmentally disabled, or unable to speak for oneself (sleeping or injured). Laws regarding capacity vary by state.
- Speak a common language fluently enough to understand fully what is being asked; be able to understand the potential consequences of, and alternatives to, what is being asked.

Based on Rape, Abuse, and Incest National Network. (2013). Was I raped? Available at http://www.rainn.org/get-information/types-of-sexual-assault/was-it-rape; University of North Carolina at Asheville Health and Counseling Center. (2013). What is consent? Available at http://healthandcounseling.unca.edu/what-consent; Northwestern University Women's Center. (n.d.). Defining sexual assault and consent. Available at http://www.northwestern.edu/women-scenter/issues-information/sexual-assault/defining-sexual-assault.html

United States outlawed ritual genital mutilation. It also directed its representatives to deny aid to countries that have not set up educational programs to stop the practice.

Pause and Reflect

1. *What role does genetics play in sexual and gender development?*
2. *What sociological influences affect sexuality or gender identity?*

Sexual Dysfunctions

Both men and women may experience *sexual dysfunctions*, persistent or recurring impairment in achieving sexual arousal or orgasm (APA, 2013). In general, a sexual dysfunction may be diagnosed if it frequently, though not necessarily always: prevents the desired participation in sexual activity; has been present for at least 6 months; and is not caused by some other mental, behavioral, or medical condition. In the DSM-IV-TR, these conditions were called *sexual disorders* and were categorized as they relate to the desire, arousal, and orgasmic phases of the sexual response cycle. The DSM-5 recognizes a slightly different group of sexual dysfunctions and does not categorize them related to the sexual response cycle. The DSM-5 also uses subtypes to designate the onset of sexual dysfunction, as the time of onset may indicate different etiologies and interventions (APA, 2013). These subtypes include the following:

- *Lifelong*: beginning from first sexual experiences
- *Acquired*: developing after normal sexual experiences began
- *Generalized*: occurring regardless of partner, situation, or type of stimulation
- *Situational*: occurring only in specific circumstances or with a specific partner

Clinical judgment and knowledge are required for accurate diagnosis of sexual dysfunction. When making clinical judgments,

providers must consider: *partner factors*, such as a partner's sexual health status; *relationship factors*, such as poor communication and discrepancies in desire for sexual activities; *individual vulnerability*, such as poor body image, history of sexual or emotional abuse, psychiatric co-morbidities, or stressors; *cultural and religious factors*, which may inhibit pleasure in sexual activities; and *medical factors* (APA, 2013). An important diagnostic criterion for all sexual dysfunction and gender dysphoria diagnoses is that the symptoms must cause clinically significant distress in the patient.

Dysfunctions Experienced by Women

Female orgasmic disorder is manifested as difficulty reaching orgasm or decreased intensity of orgasm in almost all or all sexual interactions (APA, 2013; Rellini & Clifton, 2011). It may be acquired after a period of adequate functioning or it may occur as a lifelong inability to achieve orgasm. Reported prevalence for female orgasmic problems varies widely, from 10% to 42% (APA, 2013). The etiology of female orgasmic disorder often is complicated and multifactorial. Psychological elements such as fear of impregnation or vaginal damage and hostility toward a partner may play a role in sexual inhibition. Some women may also experience a fear of losing control or a sense that they are not entitled to gratification. Conversely, some can achieve orgasm through self-stimulation but not with a partner, whereas others are unable to masturbate to orgasm.

Female sexual interest/arousal disorder describes little or no interest or desire in sexual activity. The individual experiences few sexual thoughts or fantasies, has little interest in sexual activity, and is typically unreceptive to a partner's attempts to initiate sexual activity. Psychological and biological factors may both play a role in the development of the disorder. Underlying fears about sex, as well as chronic stress, anxiety, or depression, may be present. In some cases, low serum testosterone and central dopamine blockade have been identified as contributory to low female sexual interest, arousal, and desire. Certain medications (such as oral contraceptives) and relationship problems can affect sexual interest and arousal (Stanford School of Medicine, 2014). Prevalence rates vary and depend on factors including duration of symptoms, age, and cultural setting or expression (APA, 2013).

Genitopelvic pain/penetration disorder, also referred to as *vaginismus*, is manifested as ongoing or recurring difficulty or pain during vaginal intercourse or penetration attempts. Fear or anxiety related to anticipating pain is a common criterion (APA, 2013; Binik, 2010). Lack of lubrication and tense vaginal muscles can contribute to the condition. Physical causes for vaginal pain that must be ruled out prior to confirming a diagnosis of this disorder. Some contributing factors to genitopelvic pain may include vaginal atrophy in postmenopausal women, neurosensory disorders, repeated vaginal infections, long-term use of low-dose contraceptives, sensitivity to spermicide, latex allergy, prolapsed uterus or bladder, ovarian cysts, urinary tract infections, endometriosis, and mittelschmerz (pain associated with ovulation), among others. Other features associated with this disorder may be fear or anxiety in anticipation of pain or marked tensing or tightening of the pelvic floor muscles. For some women, the contractions may be so intense that they may prevent the introduction of a speculum on examination or even prevent the use of tampons. Approximately 15% of women in North America report pain during intercourse (APA, 2013).

Dysfunctions Experienced by Men

Men may experience one of a number of sexual dysfunctions over the course of a lifetime, including erectile disorder and male hypoactive sexual desire disorder. Priapism (a prolonged erection generally lasting more than four hours) is not a disorder, but a medical emergency (Box 19-4).

To be diagnosed, *delayed ejaculation* must be experienced on almost all or all occasions of partnered sexual activity; it is characterized by a marked delay in ejaculation and or marked infrequency or absence of ejaculation despite the presence of adequate sexual stimulation and the desire to ejaculate (APA, 2013; Corona et al., 2011). The man and his partner may report prolonged thrusting to the point of exhaustion or genital discomfort. Although its prevalence is unclear, this is the least common male sexual complaint (APA, 2013). The prevalence of delayed ejaculation disorder appears to remain relatively constant until age 50, when incidence rises significantly.

Age-related loss of peripheral sensory nerves and decreased sex steroid secretion are associated with delayed ejaculation in men older than age 50. Parkinson disease and lumbar and sacral spinal cord lesions are also associated with this disorder. Genitourinary surgery and certain medications, such as antidepressants and antipsychotics, may contribute to this condition. Men who have had transurethral resection of the prostate may be misdiagnosed with delayed ejaculation, when they are actually experiencing retrograde ejaculation, in which seminal fluid passes backward into the bladder (APA, 2013).

Erectile disorder (also called *erectile dysfunction* or *impotence*) may be acquired after a period of adequate functioning (secondary) or it may occur as a lifelong inability (primary) to obtain or maintain an erection firm enough for vaginal penetration. Psychological conflict may contribute to erectile disorder as a manifestation of anger, anxiety, fear, or moral inhibition. For many men, episodic dysfunction may result from stress. Anxiety concerning ability to obtain an erection makes it that much more difficult to do so. In the case of a generalized erectile disorder, the patient is unable to obtain an erection at all, even when masturbating. He also has no early morning or nighttime penile tumescence.

Many diseases and medical conditions can play a role in erectile disorder. Among them are mumps, aortic aneurism, chronic renal failure, cirrhosis, respiratory failure, genetic disorders (such as Klinefelter syndrome), nutritional disorders, endocrine disorders (such as diabetes mellitus), neurological disorders (for example, Parkinson disease), dependence-inducing substances (including alcohol, morphine, and cocaine), and many prescribed drugs (for instance, psychotropics, antihypertensives, and hormones).

Male hypoactive sexual desire disorder is characterized by deficient (or absent) thoughts or fantasies about sex and a decreased or lacking desire for sexual activity occurring on an ongoing or recurring basis. This diagnosis reflects expert clinical judgment regarding factors accounting for sexual functioning, such as age and general and sociocultural contexts in the patient's life. This disorder is sometimes associated with erectile and ejaculatory issues. It is thought that persistent difficulties obtaining an erection may cause a man to lose interest in

---

Priapism

box 19-4

Priapism is the name given to an erection that does not return to its flaccid state following sexual arousal (prolonged erection). Priapism, though relatively uncommon, can be very painful and is considered a medical emergency. A number of factors can lead to priapism. Among them are:

- Prescription medications, including sildenafil (Viagra), tadalafil (Cialis), and vardenafil (Levitra). The SSRIs, several of the antipsychotics, and blood thinners such as warfarin (Coumadin) can also result in priapism.
- Nonpharmacologic drugs, including marijuana, cocaine, and excessive alcohol.
- Medical conditions such as sickle cell anemia, leukemia, spinal cord injury, blood clots, and poisonous venom from scorpions and black widow spiders.

Priapism is considered a urologic emergency because the blood that is trapped in the penis becomes depleted of its oxygen and, over time, becomes toxic to the tissues, ultimately causing damage or destruction. Treatment is aimed at draining the blood from the penis. Needle aspiration can be used to withdraw the blood. Injected sympathomimetic medications such as phenylephrine into the spongy tissue of the penis constrict the incoming blood vessels, allowing the outgoing vessels to drain the blood. Surgical intervention may be necessary if less invasive therapies are not successful.

Based on Mayo Clinic. Priapism: Prolonged erection (2013). Available at http://www.mayoclinic.com/health/priapism/DS00873; Dougherty, C. M., Richard, A. J., & Carey, M. J. Priapism in emergency medicine. (2012). Available at http://emedicine.medscape.com/article/777603-overview; Medline Plus. (2012). Penis pain. Available at http://www.nlm.nih.gov/medlineplus/ency/article/003166.htm

sexual activity. Male patients with hypoactive sexual desire disorder frequently report no longer initiating sexual activity and being minimally receptive to sexual overtures from their partners. Contributing factors to the disorder may include psychiatric illness, use of psychotropic medications (especially antidepressants), low testosterone levels, and certain medical illnesses such as hypothyroidism, coronary artery disease, and diabetes mellitus (Montgomery, 2008). The disorder occurs with greater frequency with age: 41% of men ages 66 to 74 years report problems with sexual desire (APA, 2013).

Premature (early) ejaculation refers to ejaculation that is routinely experienced within 1 minute following penetration and before the man intends it. Approximately 20% to 30% of men ages 18 to 70 report concern about how rapidly they ejaculate (APA, 2013). The disorder may reflect anxiety toward sexual activity, as both anxiety and ejaculation are mediated by the sympathetic nervous system. Other factors include dopamine or serotonin transmitter gene polymorphism, thyroid disease, prostatitis, and drug withdrawal (APA, 2013). The disorder can also develop from conditioning. For example, early sexual experiences in which the man had to hurry to achieve climax to avoid being discovered may establish a pattern that becomes difficult to change later in life.

Dysfunctions Experienced by Women and Men

Substance/medication-induced sexual dysfunction is diagnosed when a patient (male or female) presents with a clinically significant disturbance in sexual function and the patient's history, physical examination, or laboratory findings suggest that the disorder results from recent exposure to a substance or medication. The major diagnostic feature is a disturbance in sexual function that occurs in conjunction with the initiation of medication or substance ingestion, dose increase, or substance/medication discontinuation (APA, 2014; Sachs & Chan, 2013).

Alcohol, opioids, and sedatives are among the many substances that can contribute to sexual dysfunction, either during use or associated with withdrawal from the substance. Medications that can cause sexual dysfunction include antidepressants, antipsychotics, and hormonal contraceptives (Adams, Holland, & Urban, 2014). Many nonpsychiatric medications, such as cardiovascular, cytotoxic, gastrointestinal, and hormonal agents, are associated with sexual dysfunction. Patients using illicit substances also experience sexual dysfunction, especially with chronic drug abuse. The most commonly reported sexual problems are difficulty with orgasm or ejaculation (APA, 2013).

Treatment Considerations

Care of the patient with a sexual dysfunction varies in complexity. Thorough assessment to determine underlying cause of the disorder is essential to developing a plan of care. In some cases, such as male erectile dysfunction, the underlying cause may be medical and pharmacologic therapy may be sufficient to return the patient to more acceptable functioning. Other patients may benefit from nonpharmacologic interventions, including cognitive–behavioral therapy.

Pharmacologic Therapies

Biological treatment is used to address specific problem areas. Erectile function is enhanced by nitric oxide that facilitates the flow of blood to the penis that is needed to obtain an erection. Sildenafil (Viagra) was the first drug to inhibit the enzyme that degrades nitric oxide, thereby permitting the natural process of obtaining and maintaining an erection. It becomes effective about an hour after ingestion and can last for up to 4 hours. Vardenafil (Levitra), with a 36-hour therapeutic window, and tadalafil (Cialis), which has a 4-hour therapeutic window, followed sildenafil. Papaverine is a medication that can be directly injected into the penis and can be used in the treatment of erectile disorder. With these drugs, there have been instances of persistent erections (priapism) lasting more than 3 hours. Such situations constitute a medical emergency that usually responds readily to treatment at a medical facility.

If the cause of sexual problems is related to depression, treatment with antidepressants may be helpful. Conversely, the widespread use of SSRIs has led to some complaints of low libido, impotence, or retarded ejaculation. These are qualities that are helpful in managing premature ejaculation. When this is a problem, switching to bupropion may be helpful. The SSRIs can cause a decrease in dopamine and norepinephrine in an area of the brain, which can have an effect on libido. Bupropion is an antidepressant that works only on dopamine and norepinephrine receptors and can increase libido. Some men have used yohimbine hydrochloride (National Center for Complementary and Alternative Medicine, 2013), which is available only by prescription and is thought to increase production of chemicals that help to produce an erection. Yohimbine is an alpha-2 adrenergic blocker and should not be used with monamine oxidase inhibitors (MAOIs); its use is also contraindicated with serotonergic drugs. The over-the-counter supplement yohimbe is often administered as an aphrodisiac and to aid with sexual function (Wilson, Shannon, & Shields, 2014). It also should not be used with MAOIs and drugs that affect the serotonin system. Other herbal substances that have been tried include dehydroepiandrosterone (DHEA), which seems to increase libido in women and may help erectile dysfunction in men; ginseng, which appears to improve sexual function in men with erectile dysfunction; and ginkgo, which has the potential to increase blood flow to the penis (Wilson, Shannon, & Shields, 2014). Ginseng should not be used with MAOIs and may affect anticoagulants. The nurse should be aware that these products have not been adequately tested and researched for this purpose.

Nonpharmacologic Therapies

Sensate focus exercises consist of a graduated series of exercises (developed originally by Masters and Johnson) that are designed to reduce anxiety and to refocus on erotic pleasure and communication about sexual pleasure. There are four phases to sensate focus exercises. Phase 1 consists of nonsexual touching, in which the couple touch each other but exclude the breasts or genitals. Phase 2 adds genital and breast touching but puts the emphasis on maintaining relaxation while allowing sexual arousal. Phase 3 permits sexual intercourse without thrusting. Relaxation is maintained. Phase 4 resumes thrusting and encourages exploration of different positions.

Cognitive–behavioral sex therapy involves exploring thoughts, feelings, and behaviors for their contribution to tension, anxiety, and pain. It also includes learning relaxation techniques.

Hypnosis focuses on aspects of the sexual relationship that are anxiety producing. In the hands of a qualified practitioner, a careful psychiatric history and mental status examination precede the start of hypnotherapy. Treatment can then focus on changing attitudes and removing symptoms.

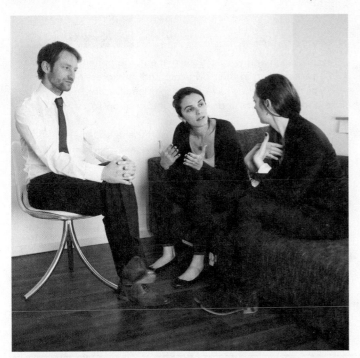

19-2 Therapy offers couples a safe environment in which to talk through problems in the interpersonal relationship that may be affecting sexual dysfunction.

Source: Adam Gregor/Shutterstock

Integrated sex therapy integrates supportive, insight-oriented, and psychodynamic psychotherapies. Problems in the interpersonal relationship and intrapsychic problems can be addressed, as they are frequently found to be underlying the manifestations of a sexual problem (Figure 19-2). Themes that often emerge in integrated sex therapy include fear of intimacy, fear of genital mutilation, difficulties with trust, and fear of punishment.

Mechanical devices such as vacuum pumps can be helpful for men with erectile disorder, provided that they do not have a vascular disease. Male prostheses are available in two varieties for surgical implant. The first is a semi-rigid rod prosthesis that produces a permanent erection. The second is an inflatable type that has its own reservoir and pump for inflation and deflation. Men report greater satisfaction with these approaches than their wives do. Presurgical counseling is essential so expectations are set at a reasonable level (Sadock, 2009).

Pause and Reflect

1. *What are your thoughts about providing nursing care to a female patient with a sexual dysfunction? How comfortable do you think you would be?*

2. *What are your thoughts about providing nursing care to a male patient with a sexual dysfunction? How comfortable do you think you would be?*

3. *Which sexual dysfunctions do you think patients might have the most difficulty discussing? Why?*

Gender Dysphoria

The gender of an individual is usually consistent with chromosomal, or natal, gender. By the age of 2 or 3, most children are very clearly able to say "I am a boy" or "I am a girl." However, young children are not yet clear about what makes a boy or a girl and may think that a change in hair length or clothing will accomplish the change from one to the other. Gender constancy usually is achieved between ages 4 and 6. *Gender identity* is a category of social identity and refers to an individual's identification as male, female, or another category. As stated earlier, gender dysphoria refers to an individual's affective/cognitive discontent with the assigned gender. Gender dysphoria may be said to exist when an individual has a strong and persistent desire to live as a person of the opposite sex. Onset usually occurs between 2 and 4 years of age, and prevalence is relatively low (APA, 2013). Whereas the term *intersex* refers to individuals who possess conflicting or ambiguous biological indicators of sex, the term *transgender* refers to individuals who persistently identify with a gender different from their natal gender. *Transsexual* may be used to refer to an individual who seeks or has undergone a social transition from male to female or female to male. A number of transsexuals undergo physiologic transitions involving cross-sex hormone treatment and genital surgery, known as *sex reassignment surgery.*

Individuals with gender dysphoria feel as though they inhabit the wrong body. With the onset of puberty, boys may shave their legs and bind their genitals in an effort to hide erections. Girls may bind their breasts or wear loose clothing to hide their breasts. They may seek hormone suppressors of gonadal steroids, with or without prescriptions. Older adolescents may not allow partners to see or touch their sexual organs (APA, 2013).

Individual responses to gender dysphoria vary. Some individuals may choose to dress in the gender with which they most closely identify and take on social roles of that gender. Others experience strong, pervasive feelings and sufficient motivation that they seek surgical sexual reassignment. Many will experience some form of discrimination related to their gender identity (Box 19-5).

Sexual reassignment is purposefully a protracted process, by design allowing the patient to make a social transition to the opposite gender, living and working full time in the social role for a period of time, generally 2 or more years, before any hormonal or surgical procedure begins. This social transition usually requires a name change and a change in work status. The rationale is that reversible changes should successfully precede irreversible changes. It is important to note that, according to the World Professional Association for Transgender Health (WPATH), surgical reconstruction is not required for social gender recognition and should not be required for document or record changes (WPATH, 2008).

Treatment Considerations

Individuals seeking to undergo sexual reassignment must undergo several phases, beginning with a diagnostic phase. As a first step, many clinics require that the individual be recommended as a candidate for surgery by at least two mental health providers who are trained and experienced in transgender issues.

The second phase involves hormonal therapy. When cross-sex hormones are started, females are treated with periodic injections of testosterone. The pitch of their voices drops as the vocal cords thicken. The clitoris enlarges to three to four times its original size. Facial hair may grow. Acne may develop. Male pattern hair growth may develop. For males, hormone therapy includes daily estrogen doses. This will result in breast enlargement, testicular atrophy, and decreased libido. The ability to obtain an erection may be diminished. They may also have less dense body hair, and male pattern baldness may be arrested.

Gender Dysphoria and Discrimination   box 19-5

Individuals with gender dysphoria often experience discrimination, especially in institutional settings. In 2013, the family of Coy Mathis, a 6-year-old transgender girl, won a court ruling confirming that Coy's school had discriminated against her by not allowing her to use the bathroom with other girls (Banda & Riccardi, 2013). When Jay Gallo, who transitioned from female to male but decided against sex reassignment surgery, found a lump in his breast, the surgeon was so shocked by his transgender status that the surgeon could not bring himself to inform Gallo that he had breast cancer. Gallo found out by accident when a technician later called to follow up (Donaldson James, 2012).

Nurses are bound by the American Nurses Association (ANA) Code of Ethics to respect each individual patient's dignity and to provide compassionate care regardless of the individual's socioeconomic status, health history, or any other consideration (ANA, 2001). In essence, discriminating against any individual is an ethical violation. Nurses act to reduce and eliminate discrimination when they do the following:

- Approach all patients with an open-minded, nonjudgmental manner.

- Ask open-ended questions that engage patients in actively participating in their own care and in expressing any fears or concerns they have about their health care.
- Provide timely and accurate information to patients and their families.
- Advocate for policies that support the needs of all patients, regardless of ability, social or economic status, or personal attributes.

Critical Thinking Questions

1. What concerns do you have about caring for transgender patients?
2. Do you think the other children at Coy's school need information about transgender individuals? Why or why not? If so, what information should be provided?

Sources: American Nurses Association. (2001). *Code of Ethics for Nurses with Interpretive Statements.* Silver Spring, MD: American Nurses Publishing; Banda, P. S., & Riccardi, N. (2013). Colorado transgender child, 6, wins court ruling, can use girls' bathroom. *Oakland News Press.* Available at http://www.theoakland-press.com/general-news/20130624/colorado-transgender-child-6-wins-court-ruling-can-use-girls-bathroom; Donaldson James, S. (2012). Trans man denied cancer treatment; now feds say it's illegal. *ABCNews.* Available at http://abcnews.go.com/Health/transgender-bias-now-banned-federal-law/story?id=16949817

Before the individual can undergo gender reassignment surgery, the individual must meet any additional surgical requirements. In addition to the recommendation of mental health providers and participation in hormone therapy, requirements may include that the individual be of legal age and in good physical health (Prerequisites, n.d.). The surgery for female-to-male transition usually includes bilateral mastectomy, hysterectomy, and oophorectomy. The patient may have a surgical procedure to free up a portion of the clitoris to create a penis, and the labia may be sutured and prosthetic testicles inserted (phalloplasty). For male-to-female transition, breast augmentation and laser or electrolysis treatment of facial hair may be elected. The surgical procedure of vaginoplasty (to create a vagina) may follow.

A small percentage of those who have undergone surgical sex reassignment have reported some degree of regret over their decision. More often than not, they are those who failed to go through a social transition of living as a member of the opposite gender for a significant period of time (as long as 2 years) prior to undergoing surgery. Many have reported improved social integration and sexual adjustment (Greene, 2009). However, in a Swedish study with 324 sex-reassigned participants, participants were found to have greater risk for mortality, suicidal behaviors, and psychiatric morbidity in spite of some relief with gender dysphoria (Dhejne et al., 2011).

Gender Dysphoria and Suicide

Nurses should keep in mind that adolescents and adults with gender dysphoria are at increased risk for suicidal ideation, suicide attempts, and suicide (APA, 2013). In 2009, 41% of those responding to a survey by the National Center for Transgender Equality (NCTE) reported having attempted suicide in the past, with rates of attempted suicide higher among individuals who transitioned with the help of hormone

therapy or reassignment surgery than among transgender individuals who had not participated in those treatment protocols (NCTE, 2010). The implications for this are clear: Individuals with gender dysphoria are at high risk for depression and suicidal gestures; nurses working with individuals with gender dysphoria of any age, regardless of their gender or treatment status, are well advised to conduct a suicide and safety assessment at each health care interaction. (See Chapter 27 for information on preventing and assessing for suicide risk.)

Pause and Reflect

1. *Why do you think individuals with gender dysphoria have a high rate of suicide?*
2. *What do you think you as a nurse can do to be more supportive of these individuals in the clinical setting?*

Paraphilic Disorders

As stated earlier, *paraphilic disorders* may be defined as a pattern of sexual arousal or behaviors that deviate from the norm and significantly impair relationships and functioning. The word "paraphilia" was created in the early 1900s and refers to forms of sexuality that are not what society defines as normal as determined by cultural and historical standards of behavior. Most paraphilias emerge during adolescence or early adulthood and generally are chronic in nature. "A history of childhood sexual abuse is sometimes seen in individuals with paraphilias" (Sorrentino, 2009, p. 2093).

The DSM-5 defines paraphilias as "any intense and persistent sexual interest other than sexual interest in genital stimulation or preparatory fondling with phenotypically mature, consenting human partners" (APA, 2013, p. 685). Some paraphilias target erotic activities, whereas others target other people. The DSM-5 (APA, 2013) recognizes eight paraphilic disorders:

- Voyeuristic disorder (watching others engaged in private activities)
- Exhibitionistic disorder (exposing the genitals)
- Frotteuristic disorder (touching or rubbing against an individual without consent)
- Sexual masochism (undergoing humiliation, bondage, or suffering)
- Sexual sadism disorder (inflicting humiliation, bondage, or suffering)
- Pedophilic disorder (in which the erotic target is children)
- Fetishistic disorder (in which the erotic target is an object or body part other than the genitals)
- Transvestic disorder (engaging in sexually arousing cross-dressing)

Because of the forensic implications and psychological damage caused to children by pedophilia, pedophilic disorder is covered in this section of the chapter. The paraphilic disorders sexual sadism and sexual masochism are also discussed at more depth later in this chapter.

Pedophilia

Pedophilia is sexual activity with a prepubescent child. Pedophilic disorder involves recurrent, intense sexual thoughts and/or behaviors involving sexual activity with a prepubescent child or children (generally age 13 or under) or recurrent sexual urges or fantasies about children that cause the individual significant psychosocial difficulty or distress (APA, 2013). In addition, for diagnosis, the individual must be at least age 16 and at least 5 years older than the child or children who is/are the focus of the sexual act or fantasy. The individual's awareness or disclosure of sexual urges or activity is not a factor in diagnosis. Extensive use of pornography depicting prepubescent children is a useful diagnostic indicator of pedophilic disorder (APA, 2013). Although pedophilia involves more male offenders than female offenders, research demonstrates females also are involved in pedophilia but may not be detected or reported as frequently (Tewksbury, 2004).

The prevalence of pedophilic disorder among males is estimated at 3% to 5%, whereas the prevalence rate among females is thought to be much lower (APA, 2013). Adult males with pedophilic disorder indicate that they become aware of a preference for children when puberty occurs. Pedophilia appears to be a lifelong condition, and it presents significant treatment challenges (APA, 2013; Sadock & Sadock, 2007).

> **PRACTICE ALERT**   The nurse who has been sexually abused may have great difficulty providing competent nursing care for the patient who has committed sexual abuse. Nurses are called on to have respect for their own boundaries, while at the same time to provide nonjudgmental and competent nursing care to a patient who is, for example, a pedophile. How can this be done if the nurse's own response is one of revulsion and rejection? The answer comes from a process of examining one's own thoughts and feelings at a deep level. Nurses are not required to approve of the behavior of the patient, nor to excuse it in any way, but to work through their own responses so the quality of nursing care provided to a patient whose behavior the nurse finds offensive remains at a professional level and includes an empathic component.

Victims of pedophiles are often relatives (Box 19-6). More than 70% of abusers are known or related to their victims. Over 90% of child sexual abuse is perpetrated by males; and 40% of perpetrators were victims of abuse themselves (Brown, 2012). Some people who have pedophilic inclinations manage to avoid molesting children. Conversely, not all child molesters are pedophiles. Some may be opportunistic sexual offenders for whom children are conveniently available, especially when impulse control is lessened, as when under the influence of mind-altering drugs (Hall & Hall, 2009).

Not infrequently, in the therapeutic setting it is discovered that pedophiles were themselves sexually abused as children (APA, 2013) and became sexually attracted to children who are the age at which they themselves were victimized (Hall & Hall, 2009). This may be viewed as a form of arrested development in the area of sexual interest. Many children who were sexually molested do not become pedophiles as they are somehow sufficiently resilient to resist this phenomenon. However, they may develop other mental or psychosomatic problems, or they may be able to sublimate their pain and, by

---

Protecting Children   box 19-6

Unfortunately, approximately 70% of child sexual abuse victims know their attackers (Brown, 2012). Abuse by a trusted adult, especially when it takes place within the home, is likely to be particularly damaging to the victim. This is sometimes called *sanctuary violation* and refers to the concept that a child ought to be able to count on being safe inside the home, if not outside it. Although even the best-educated child cannot always avoid sexual abuse, children who are well prepared will be more likely to tell someone that abuse has occurred. This is a child's best defense. To protect children, teach them the following:

- To feel good about themselves and how they are loved, valued, and that they deserve to be safe
- The difference between safe, unsafe, and unwanted touches; for example, safety when removing a splinter
- The proper names for all body parts, so they will be able to communicate clearly

- That safety rules apply to all adults, not just strangers
- That their bodies belong to them and nobody has the right to touch them or hurt them
- That they can say "no" to requests that make them feel uncomfortable—even from a close relative or family friend
- To report if any adult asks them to keep a secret
- That some adults have problems, and not all adults are safe to be around
- That there are adults on whom they can rely to believe and protect them if they tell about abuse
- That they are not bad or to blame for sexual abuse

State laws govern the reporting of suspected child abuse and neglect. States generally require a nurse who suspects or knows that a child's physical or mental health or welfare has been or may be adversely affected by abuse or neglect to report the situation to a local or state agency.

"Roy"

box 19-7

My name is Roy. I am a 58-year-old pedophile and child molester. I sexually molested a female from age 13 to 15 by touching her vagina, engaging in oral sex, and mutual masturbation. I groomed her into accepting my abuse by giving her special attention and by my role as a grown-up. I also took pictures of children that I talked into undressing for me. I had an extensive collection of child pornography and was compulsive in my masturbation. I was sentenced to 15 to 30 years in the state prison and served 16 years prior to being granted parole. My other sexual deviance includes massage parlors and peep

shows. My nonsexual deviance includes isolation, secrecy, entitlement, and overwork.

This is a brief statement made by an adult with pedophilic disorder in front of his peers and therapist during the course of treatment and as a component of treatment. Statements like these are given frequently in therapy, particularly during the early phases of treatment, to decrease denial, acknowledge guilt, increase openness, and accept responsibility.

using more advanced coping mechanisms, may enter helping professions such as nursing.

Force is very seldom involved in child molestation. Rather, manipulation and grooming are used to engage the child (Box 19-7). Gifts and special treatment are frequently employed in grooming victims. A pedophile can often tell very quickly which child is most likely to acquiesce to an approach (Hall & Hall, 2009). The victim is likely to be lonely, socially inept, and have few friends. Ongoing research has explored the possibility of structural or functional neurobiological factors that may contribute to the development of pedophilia. Findings of a significant volume reduction in the right amygdala suggest this as a possibility. The reduction in size is not the result of a progressive atrophy or degeneration, nor is it age dependent. This leads to a postulate that it may be a developmental disorder or a preexisting hypoplasia—that is, the amygdala did not develop to its usual size. Head injuries before puberty, but not in adulthood, have been associated with pedophilia (Schiltz et al., 2007).

Women Offenders

It is thought that female pedophilia is under-reported, partly because sex offending has long been viewed as a male-only crime. Gender role stereotypes have portrayed women as nurturing and caregiving, but portrayed men as controlling all sexual encounters and women as passive recipients.

Internet Offending

The Internet has helped to create a new type of sexual offense. Decreased production costs and dramatically increased availability of child pornography, along with a decreased risk of detection, have resulted in an explosion of available sites catering to pedophiles. Even more than the Internet itself, child pornography users are getting images from peer-to-peer file sharing networks, bypassing centralized servers to download files from networks of individual computers. In 2006, there were more than 3500 arrests for crimes involving child pornography. Under the Trafficking Victims Protection Act of 2000, human trafficking has occurred if a person was induced to perform labor or a commercial sex act through force, fraud, or coercion. If the victim is under 18, any commercial sex act is considered human trafficking. The victims of child pornography are mostly female, with 71% between the ages of 13 and 17, and 21% between 6 and 12 years of age. In 26% of victim cases, the offenders who created the pornography were adult family members, and in another 27%, they were acquaintances of the victim. However, 42% of victims met the offender online. Runaway children are at high risk for being sexually exploited via child pornography (Farley et al., 2003).

Internet offending goes beyond child pornography. The National Center for Missing and Exploited Children (NCMEC) reports dramatic increases in online enticement of children and adolescents: At least one in 25 children ages 10 to 17 has received a request to meet in person from someone attempting to solicit them online (Figure 19-3) (NCMEC, 2013).

Masochism and Sadism

Masochism and sadism also fall within the category of paraphilias. Sexual **masochism** is defined as sexual pleasure or arousal derived from receiving physical or mental abuse or humiliation. The main components of sexual masochism are pain, loss of control, and humiliation. One hypothesis as to the origins of sadomasochistic preferences has its roots in the concept that experienced trauma is followed by fantasies related to the trauma and its re-experiencing. The process of fantasizing permits the development of a sense of mastery over the helplessness experienced in the original trauma. The more severe the trauma, the greater is the need to employ fantasy in an effort to "undo" its effects. This then leads to the repetitive behaviors and intrusive imagery that result and are played out in sadomasochistic fantasies (fantasies can be thought of as rehearsals) and behaviors (Grossman, 1991). Another view is that masochism offers a form of *escape* from stress or responsibility; that individuals who are conflicted about domination and submission may defer to submission and eventually come to prefer it; and that the *suppression* of the individual's inappropriate sexual fantasies increases the urge to act on them, and may lead

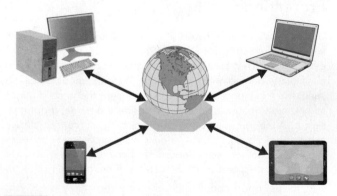

19-3   The Internet plays a role in the increased global trafficking of minors. The National Center for Missing and Exploited Children reports that at least one in 25 children ages 10 to 17 has received a request to meet in person from someone attempting to solicit them online.

to greater confusion regarding sex, pain, and pleasure (Collective Social Services, 2010; Sexual Masochism, n.d.).

A dangerous form of sexual masochism is **hypoxyphilia** (auto-erotic asphyxiation, called *asphyxiophilia* in DSM-5), in which oxygen deprivation enhances sexual arousal and orgasm. This potentially lethal practice produces sexual arousal while restricting the oxygen supply to the brain. Because its proponents seldom present for treatment, there is little evidence related to hypoxyphilia. When a tragic accident occurs and an individual dies while practicing hypoxyphilia, it may come to the attention of the authorities. Many who engage in hypoxyphilia do so alone, using a rope around the neck or a plastic bag over the head. It has been practiced mainly by men under the age of 40 and has often been engaged in by teenage boys. No suggestion of suicidal intent has been found in these cases (Hucker, 2011).

Sexual **sadism** occurs when sexual arousal is associated with causing mental or physical suffering to another person. The sadist's partner may be a masochist who agrees with the practice or may be an unwilling victim. Sexual sadism is most often seen in men but is found in women as well. It can progress to rape, although not all rapists are sadists. As with masochism, theoretical explanations of the causes of sadism include *escape* (feelings of power are gained by people who feel powerless during everyday life), and *suppression* of sexual fantasy (inappropriate sexual fantasies are experienced secretly and bring about confusion and distress, leading to an association between pain and sex). If the desire to dominate accompanies this confusion, sexual sadism may result along with perpetuation of sexual fantasy (milder symptoms progress to more involved behavior). Prevalence rates in the general population are unknown; depending on the criteria, prevalence rates in forensic settings may vary from 2% to 30% (APA, 2013).

Treatment Considerations

Collaborative care is most effective when psychopharmacology and psychotherapy are used in combination. Nurses working with patients experiencing paraphilic disorders promote adherence to the treatment regimen, assess for adverse effects of medication, and continue development of the therapeutic relationship to promote patient confidence in the treatment plan.

Psychopharmacology

Treatment options for paraphilic disorders include a number of pharmacologic agents. SSRIs may be used as a first-line drug because of the underlying depressive state that frequently plays a role in driving the paraphilia. In these cases, sexuality has been used as a coping mechanism to alleviate the depressive experience. In patients for whom paraphilic behavior is more closely related to issues of impulse control, SSRIs may also prove helpful. In some cases, a small dose of an antipsychotic, such as 0.5 to 1 mg of risperidone (Risperdal), may be helpful by lowering aggression (Brannon, 2012). Both mood stabilizers and antipsychotics have been clinically useful in those seeking treatment. These medications should always be used in conjunction with psychotherapy, particularly long-term group psychotherapy, to address their functioning in relational, social, spiritual, and occupational roles at the level that is optimal for that person.

In the most difficult cases, temporary chemical castration with the antiandrogen medroxyprogesterone (Provera or Depo-Provera) reduces the level of testosterone and the associated sex drive in male paraphilics, most particularly in pedophiles. When employed, it is usually for a period of several years in conjunction with cognitive–behavioral therapy,

and is then gradually tapered prior to discontinuation. The clinical marker is to lower the plasma testosterone to a prepubescent level during the early course of treatment. Cyproterone acetate (Cyprostat) is also effective but has not been approved for use in the United States by the FDA. Side effects from the antiandrogens include the risk of weight gain, hyperglycemia, hypertension, muscle cramps, phlebitis, gastrointestinal complaints, and feminization. Generally, the use of an antiandrogen is restricted to the most serious of patients with paraphilic disorders with respect to risk of relapse and committing another act. The benefit for the patients is that their sex drive is totally suppressed for the period of time that they are in treatment, which may permit them to live in the community while they strengthen their ability to avoid relapse through treatment (Codispoti, 2008).

Another approach to reducing plasma testosterone (and thereby reducing sex drive) in men is with the hormonal agents lueprolide (Lupron) or triptorelin (Trelstar), which are long-acting GnRH hormones (Brannon, 2012) that operate by inhibiting the release of luteinizing hormone from the pituitary gland. Side effects with this approach include osteopenia, weight gain, hyperglycemia, hypertension, and insomnia.

Nonpharmacologic Therapies

Psychological and behavioral treatment approaches assist the individual to change the beliefs and attitudes that support paraphilic behaviors. As with any treatment approach, the individual must recognize that there is a problem that needs to be changed. Often this recognition does not emerge until the individual has been arrested and charged. As a result, many states have developed comprehensive treatment programs within their prison systems. Many programs take up to 2 years to complete and are extremely intensive. These programs generally require that the applicant take full responsibility for deviant sexual behaviors prior to the start of treatment. Successful completion of such programs may qualify individuals for earlier parole. Individuals who do not complete treatment will likely be released into the community at the end of their mandatory prison sentence without treatment, and with little likelihood of change in the underlying factors that led to deviant behaviors.

Cognitive–behavioral approaches address cognitive distortions that sustain the continuation of the paraphilic behavior. Defense mechanisms such as rationalization, justification, and minimization are challenged. A relapse prevention model used to assist individuals suffering from paraphilia may be helpful by carefully analyzing and helping the individual understand the pattern of cyclic behaviors. In this way, a stepwise progression from psychological trigger to offending behavior unique to the individual person becomes both predictable and alterable. Occasionally, behavioral techniques are employed to alter sexual fantasies, because the pairing of a deviant fantasy with an orgasm is deeply reinforcing. Breaking this relationship is one of the steps toward rehabilitation. Covert sensitization—the pairing of a harmful fantasy with an unpleasant stimulus—has been found effective in treating pedophilias and sadism (Brannon, 2012).

Group psychotherapy with others suffering from paraphilias is preferable to individual therapy because of the activation of the therapeutic factors inherent in group psychotherapy. In a comprehensive program, psychoeducational elements will address knowledge deficits that may be identified. The objective of group psychotherapy is to heal the character, enhance self-regulation, and increase the capacity for meaningful interpersonal connections.

More advanced concepts of group therapy include the use of psychodynamic psychotherapy, which is the primary treatment for character or personality pathology. Goodman (2009) introduced a type of psychodynamic therapy that integrates three components: understanding, integration, and internalization.

Understanding is described as a cognitive process to learn the meanings of the behaviors individuals have tried in an effort to relieve discomfort. Learning to name what they experience helps to provide perspective. It provides a way to separate thinking from feeling, reduces the likelihood of feeling overwhelmed, and increases the capacity of individuals to learn from their feelings. While it reduces self-blame, it increases responsibility for doing something about it. Participants learn to identify inner processes of which they were previously unaware. They can then begin to see how cognition, affect, and behavior fit together. In the process, participants examine how beliefs, conflicts, and history interrelate. Awareness of this inner landscape leads to the state sometimes called *mindfulness*.

Integration is a mental process linking the subjective experience (needs, fears, wishes, conflicts, and beliefs) with the corresponding verbal description. It is introspective and a conscious awareness of the self-protective process (Goodman, 2009).

Internalization is the gradual acquisition of the self-regulatory function. It helps the individual recognize the need for nurturing, soothing, and holding and provides new opportunities for learning what was inadequately provided during childhood. In addition to the concepts of understanding, integration, and internalization, the relationship to the therapist as both caregiver and authority is essential to the process. The relationship itself provides a means to explore the patient's affects, needs, wishes, fears, inner conflicts, core beliefs, and means of self-protection. The successful therapist is empathic, warm, directive, and encouraging. For better or worse, the characteristics of the therapist account for 40% to 60% of the outcome in this type of therapy, as in other types (Goodman, 2009).

Pause and Reflect

1. *How do you think you would feel if you were asked to provide care to an adult patient recently arrested for sexually abusing a child? What are your obligations in terms of providing care to this patient?*

2. *What concerns would you have about a patient who disclosed masochistic practices? Which of those concerns would be appropriate to communicate to the patient? How would you communicate them?*

Nursing Management

Patients are often uncomfortable discussing problems related to sex and sexuality. This is especially true when the patient feels shame or guilt related to the problem. In many cases, patients with sexual dysfunctions, paraphilias, and gender dysphoria lack information about their condition and may not understand that help is available. Learning ways to approach a patient who may be feeling anxiety, shame, or guilt will allow the nurse to identify and begin to help the patient (see the Perceptions, Thoughts, and Feelings feature later in the chapter).

The key to working effectively with patients who are embarrassed or ashamed to bring up a sexual issue on their own is for nurses themselves to be comfortable discussing these issues. This can be challenging, but practice helps, as does self-awareness. Some questions nurses can use to engage in self-awareness before working with patients on sexual issues include the following:

- Can I use biologically accurate terminology when talking about sex with patients?

- Do I have questions I want to ask but cannot because I am too embarrassed? How can I become comfortable enough to be able to ask these questions?

- How do I feel talking about sexual issues?

- Do I think I can be helpful to patients with sexual problems?

It is also important for nurses to be aware of meaningful differences among patients and to avoid stereotyping. The use of gender-free terminology can be helpful in this regard. For example, nurses should avoid assuming that a male patient's partner is female until the patient confirms the gender of his partner. Using open-ended questions, such as "Tell me about your partner," can help nurses clarify important information without engaging in stereotyping.

Assessment

Some patients will present information in a forthright manner. However, many patients experiencing a sexual dysfunction or disorder may be embarrassed to begin the conversation. Some may wait until their time is almost over—when they have one hand on the doorknob—before they ask the question they would really like to have answered. Patients with gender dysphoria may be reluctant to disclose information if they have not previously received appropriate support in the health care community. Individuals who suffer from paraphilias may be ashamed or fear legal consequences if they

---

critical thinking

Blakeney Carroll Recovery Phase

Mr. Carroll has been meeting with Leslie, the family nurse practitioner, for the past 4 weeks. He tells Leslie that things have been "a little better performance-wise" since he began the low dose of bupropion to counter the sexual side effects of his Lexapro. Mr. Carroll is pleased that his depression has not worsened, and, in fact, he feels a little better overall than he did before he started the bupropion. However, he expresses concern that he does not deserve his fiancée, Nancy. Leslie observes that Mr. Carroll's self-esteem still is low and asks if he would be willing to have Nancy join them for a session or two so they could discuss this concern with Leslie's assistance, if necessary. Mr. Carroll likes that idea and agrees to ask Nancy to join them at his next session.

APPLICATION

1. What is the likely source of Mr. Carroll's low self-esteem? Why might it be helpful for his fiancée to participate in a session to discuss this?

2. How might Mr. Carroll's low self-esteem contribute to his report that things are "a little better performance-wise"?

disclose the nature of their illness. Nurses who sense that a patient is holding something back use open-ended questions and active listening to help patients feel comfortable with disclosure.

In a psychiatric unit, it is understood that the patient's sexual history plays a significant role in his or her psychological, psychiatric, and biological development. This is no less true for patients in other settings. However, the policy of the agency will take precedence in the decision to explore a patient's sexual history.

Obtaining an accurate and thorough assessment requires the nurse to use therapeutic communication and to provide patients with an atmosphere that is free of judgment. Questions nurses can use to help focus their approach include the following:

- Sexually active means different things to different people. What does it mean to you? Do you consider yourself to be sexually active? Do you have any questions you would like to ask me about sexual activity?
- Do you find yourself attracted to men, women, or both?
- On a scale of 0 (not satisfied) to 10 (highly satisfied), how would you describe your satisfaction with your sex life?
- Are you seeing anyone now? How long have you been dating?
- Are there any parts of your sex life or your sexual desires that make you uncomfortable?
- Describe your first important sexual relationship.
- Have you ever or do you currently experience any pain or discomfort with sex? If so, where is it felt and what does it feel like?
- Have ever been asked you to do anything sexually with which you have been uncomfortable?

Before beginning the assessment, nurses must know state and agency policies regarding reportable acts. The nurse's role is to try to help the patient—not to discover criminal behaviors. Nurses must also be familiar with how to refer the patient to social services that can activate access to shelters and services that are available in the community, if necessary.

Diagnosis and Planning

Working with the patient, the nurse develops the nursing diagnoses and plans. Some common nursing diagnoses include the following:

- Sexual Dysfunction
- Sexuality Pattern, Ineffective
- Self-Esteem, Chronic Low
- Coping, Ineffective
- Family Processes, Dysfunctional
- Loneliness, Risk for
- Social Isolation

(NANDA-I, © 2014)

Prioritizing Nursing Diagnoses

Together, the nurse and patient formulate and prioritize the most significant needs of the patient in a manner that is realistic to what the patient can acknowledge and accept as reachable. For example, appropriate nursing diagnoses for Mr. Carroll might include sexual dysfunction and low self-esteem.

Plans and Goals

The nurse continues to work on developing the nursing care plan, working with the patient as much as possible to determine patient education needs. Questions the nurse takes into account include the following:

- Is the patient able to acknowledge that working toward a specific goal would help?
- What difficulty is the patient most in need of addressing?
- What does the patient see as a realistic goal? How can the goal be stated in a way that results in specific, realistic, and measurable goals for the patient's care? As an example, if the diagnosis is related to ineffective sexuality pattern and the patient is a homeless, unemployed woman who trades sex for money or shelter, the nurse might consider the following specific, measurable, and realistic goals:
  ○ The patient will accept and read the information on women's shelters in the area.
  ○ The patient will call two shelters in 5 days and visit one shelter in 1 week.
  ○ The patient will contact her mental health counselor in 1 week to make an appointment for therapy to begin to address breaking the cycle of job insecurity.

The nursing plan of care should incorporate the five domains as much as possible, working with the patient to understand how they affect him or her. This will likely involve speaking with the patient on more than one occasion. The outcome should be a targeted plan that the patient can accept.

- *Biological:* What medical conditions need to be resolved before the patient can move forward with his or her goal?
- *Psychological:* Are there attitudes, behaviors, and thought patterns that will sabotage the patient's efforts toward goal attainment?
- *Sociological:* Is the patient's present living situation dangerous? How does the patient's spouse or partner view the patient's dysfunction or disorder?
- *Cultural:* Can the patient envision living life in a more fulfilled way?
- *Spiritual:* Does the patient participate in any spiritual community that might support his or her efforts?

Implementation

As with all patients, promoting safety and communication are priorities for care. Many patients with sexual dysfunctions or gender dysphoria, as well as patients with paraphilic disorders, may need specific interventions and individualized patient education information to promote healthy sexual behaviors.

Promote Safety

For patients with sexual issues, practicing safe sex may be a priority to achieve wellness. Practicing safe sex is important at any age. Likewise, providing education, information, and, in some cases, resources to prevent risky behaviors will be part of the nurse's role in numerous settings. Being aware of resources and how to refer patients to them is part of promoting safety. In some cases, referring patients to safe houses and helping them find financial resources may be part of promoting safety for patients.

Masturbation

box 19-8

Masturbation plays a role in sexuality. Toddlers explore their genitals and learn that it feels good, even if they are told not to do it. Adolescents masturbate when sexual urges are strong and there is no outlet yet available. The practice usually precedes object-related sexual behavior. Adults may masturbate for pleasure or for more complex reasons. When masturbation becomes a form of escape, becomes compulsive, or begins to impair health, it may be excessive or indicative of the need for psychiatric care. The following guidelines may assist nurses in defining healthy versus unhealthy masturbation for patients:

1. It is done in private—never in a location in which one may be interrupted or seen.

2. When one has an accompanying sexual fantasy, it should not include elements that are illegal or harmful if it were to come true.
3. It is not performed so often that it interferes with any of one's responsibilities or does tissue damage.
4. It is not used as a coping mechanism or an escape from feelings of anxiety or depression.

Promote Communication

Communication in the area of sexuality is sensitive and critical. Developing a therapeutic alliance with the patient helps promote a treatment environment that feels safe and confidential. Using a nonjudgmental approach will enhance that alliance. Additionally, the nurse needs to use communication that is clear and open to questions, and that validates patients' concerns. In the case example of Mr. Carroll, open communication with the nurse allowed Mr. Carroll to share his history of sexual abuse and depression, and the nurse was able to determine factors that may have been affecting his performance during intercourse (see the Nursing Care Plan). It is not as important for the nurse to be an expert in the issue as it is for the nurse to convey acceptance and a willingness to obtain information and to help.

Promote Healthy Behaviors

Patients who seek help related to gender dysphoria and sexual dysfunctions may or may not be actively engaging in unhealthy behaviors. Some may not know that there are behaviors or therapies that may help to relieve the symptoms for which they seek treatment. Others, such as those who are long-term victims of sexual abuse, may need more support. Through careful assessment, the nurse can determine both patient needs and patient readiness to accept help.

Strategies nurses can use to promote healthy behaviors among patients include using charts or models to help clarify anatomical elements of sexual functioning and to support safe sexual practices.

Some patients have difficulty related to excessive masturbation. Occasional masturbation in a private setting can be a healthy, enjoyable behavior for some individuals. For others, it may be a marker of mental illness. Nurses working with patients who admit to excessive masturbation may need to help patients establish healthier behaviors and assess them further for additional physical or psychological symptoms (Box 19-8).

At all times when discussing sexual behaviors, whether healthy or not, the nurse must maintain a nonjudgmental approach to encourage patient trust and disclosure of pertinent health information.

Evaluation

Evaluation of the patient's progress may well occur over a lengthy period of time. As the patient becomes strong enough to tackle the parts of his life that preclude functioning in an optimal manner, support with encouragement and information about options can make a difference in the outcome. To benefit most from improvements, changes must take place at a pace the patient can tolerate. Grief processing for the losses suffered as a consequence of life circumstances, along with acquisition of ego strength to see the possibility of gaining a capacity for increasing self-determination and quality of life, take time. Success in the long term involves learning the potential benefit of delayed gratification and developing a tolerance for it.

From Suffering to Hope

The challenge for the nurse is to see patients as persons of worth with potential, even if the nurse is offended by or uncomfortable with a patient's illness or behaviors. At the same time, patients may rebuff or reject the nurse's efforts to help. Some patients may find the nurse's suggestions to be too challenging or frustrating to implement. Another possibility is that the patient may turn against the nurse's good intentions and view them as interfering or as further proof that the patient is worthless.

Hope for change is the element that is perhaps most needed together with a belief that patients can make changes that will provide an improved quality of life for themselves. Invoking a multidisciplinary approach is likely to improve outcomes. Social work, mental health, community resources, welfare benefits (at least on a temporary basis), and/or vocational training all may need to be activated. It is crucial to note that patients need to participate actively in engaging resources. As each small step is accomplished with active participation by patients, they will increase their belief that they can reach their goals. Patients will probably need much encouragement and inspiration along the way. The nurse's role in this remains instrumental to patients' success in the long term.

Pause and Reflect

1. *What challenges do you think you would face working with a patient with sexual dysfunction? Working with a patient with gender dysphoria?*

2. *How would you go about maintaining a nonjudgmental attitude when working with a patient whose values are in conflict with your own?*

Mr. Carroll—A Patient With Sexual Dysfunction	NURSING CARE PLAN

Nursing Diagnosis: *Sexual dysfunction* related to side effects of SSRIs and depression manifested by lack of ejaculation after erection during sexual activity.

Short-Term Goals *Patient will:*	Intervention *Nurse will:*	Rationale
Participate in therapy to discuss history of child sexual abuse.	Support patient in therapy.	Patient has not previously discussed these experiences with a professional; they are likely the underlying source of his depression and low self-esteem, and may affect his sexual dysfunction.
Participate in a course of bupropion to determine whether it will help lessen the sexual dysfunction that may be occurring related to SSRI use and to see if the additional medication assists in improving his depression.	Monitor patient's adherence to medication therapy and assist him in determining whether it is helpful.	Bupropion has been shown to alleviate sexual dysfunction related to SSRI therapy and to alleviate symptoms of depression.
Explore through therapy the impact of previous sexual experiences on attitudes and behaviors he may be exhibiting in his current relationship.	Assist the patient to explore his attitudes and behaviors in his current relationship.	This may assist the patient in improving his self-esteem.
Long-Term Goal Mr. Carroll's symptoms of depression and sexual dysfunction will improve, and he will articulate being able to discuss these with his fiancée.	Note and affirm progress to patient.	Patient may need help realizing progress is being made in treatment.

Clinical Reasoning

1. What other nursing diagnoses might be useful in working with Mr. Carroll?
2. Do you think the selection of sexual dysfunction as the priority diagnosis is appropriate? Why or why not?

PERCEPTIONS, THOUGHTS, & FEELINGS: Validating the Needs of a Patient with Symptoms of Sexual Dysfunction

Patient's behavior	Nurse's perceptions, thoughts, feelings	Exploration with patient
Mr. Carroll comes in for his appointment following 4 weeks of taking bupropion. Although he shakes hands with Leslie, the nurse practitioner with whom he has been working, he continues to maintain downcast eyes. When he sits down on the sofa, his right hand reaches to play with the fringe on one of the sofa pillows.	*Perceptions:* Mr. Carroll continues to seem depressed, even a little anxious about these appointments. *Thoughts:* Mr. Carroll has continued to participate in therapy, so he must be feeling some benefit. I need to determine how things are going. *Feelings:* I feel sad watching seeing him like this.	*Nurse:* Well, Mr. Carroll, how have things been going since our last appointment?

VALIDATION An open-ended question invites the patient to respond related to his needs or concerns.

Patient's behavior	Nurse's perceptions, thoughts, feelings	Exploration with patient
Mr. Carroll: A little better.	*Thoughts:* That's not much of an answer.	*Nurse:* What is a little better?

VALIDATION The nurse reflects Mr. Carroll's own language back to him in an attempt to get him to open up.

Patient's behavior	Nurse's perceptions, thoughts, feelings	Exploration with patient
Mr. Carroll: Performance-wise, things are a little better.	*Perception:* He seems a little reluctant to get into specifics. *Thoughts:* Maybe I should circle back to that a little later in our session. I think something else must be bothering him.	*Nurse:* I see. What about your depression? Is there any improvement in that since you started the Wellbutrin?

VALIDATION Sensing Mr. Carroll's discomfort, the nurse switches topics.

Patient's behavior	Nurse's perceptions, thoughts, feelings	Exploration with patient
Mr. Carroll: Yes, actually. I feel like I have more energy. Simple tasks don't seem so difficult.	Despite saying this, Mr. Carroll's attitude remains the same, and he continues to play with the fringe on the pillow.	*Perceptions:* His demeanor hasn't changed. *Thoughts:* I wonder what's going on. He is reporting some improvement in both physical function and in his depressive symptoms.	**Nurse:** OK, so the Wellbutrin seems to be helping on all fronts. But you still seem troubled.

VALIDATION The nurse acknowledges Mr. Carroll's progress but continues to try to find the focus of his concerns.

Patient's behavior	Nurse's perceptions, thoughts, feelings	Exploration with patient
Mr. Carroll: It's Nancy. I don't think I'm good enough for her.	Mr. Carroll puts his face in his hands.	*Perceptions:* His lack of sexual performance and depression affect his perspective on their relationship. *Thoughts:* He really seems to love her. I need to try to help him resolve this apparent lack of self-esteem. Nancy may not feel the same way he does. *Feelings:* I hope I can help him.	**Nurse:** I hear what you're saying. You're afraid you're not good enough for her. I'm wondering if Nancy feels that way. What has she said?

VALIDATION The nurse reflects Mr. Carroll's statement back to validate his concerns. She then asks him to try to articulate Nancy's statements regarding their relationship to attempt to help him compare his perceptions to reality.

Based on Orlando, I. J. (1972). *The Discipline and Teaching of Nursing Process (An Evaluative Study).* New York, NY: G. P. Putnam's Sons.

Blakeney Carroll Rehabilitation Phase

After 8 weeks of meeting with Leslie, the nurse practitioner, Mr. Carroll reports feeling more comfortable in his relationship with fiancée, Nancy. They are planning to be married in a few months. Both are excited, as are their families. Mr. Carroll still has some infrequent episodes of delayed ejaculation during orgasm, but he is not as stressed about it as he was before.

Mr. Carroll tells Leslie that he has one major concern at the moment. He is wondering what he will do when his parents make up the wedding invitation list. He does not want to invite the cousin who molested him.

APPLICATION

1. How would you handle Mr. Carroll's concern about his parents likely wanting to invite the cousin who molested him?

2. What concerns do you have about Mr. Carroll's cousin?

3. What follow-up might Mr. Carroll need in the future?

Chapter Highlights

1. The sexual response cycle comprises four stages: excitement, plateau, orgasm, and resolution.

2. Genetic and hormonal influences play a role in the development of sex organs and sexual and gender identity.

3. Gender cues, attachment styles, parental attitudes, and cultural roles and expectations all play a role in the development of gender identity.

4. Sexual dysfunctions involve chronic or recurring impairment in arousal or orgasm.

5. Sexual dysfunctions experienced by women include female orgasmic disorder, female sexual interest/arousal disorder, and genitopelvic pain/penetration disorder.

6. Sexual dysfunctions experienced by men include delayed ejaculation, erectile disorder, male hypoactive sexual desire disorder, and premature ejaculation.

7. Sexual dysfunctions that may be experienced by either men or women can be substance or medication-induced sexual dysfunctions and other (specified or unspecified) sexual dysfunctions.

8. Treatment of sexual dysfunctions may involve pharmacologic or nonpharmacologic therapies appropriate to the nature of the dysfunction.

9. Gender dysphoria occurs when individuals experience marked distress regarding their assigned gender. Individuals who seek to change their gender undergo counseling prior to adopting social roles of the unassigned gender. Some individuals may undergo sexual reassignment surgery.

10. Individuals with paraphilic disorders exhibit sexual arousal or behaviors that are different from the norm and that may be harmful to themselves or others.

11. Nurses working with patients with sexual dysfunctions, gender dysphoria, or paraphilic disorder must maintain a nonjudgmental attitude and promote patient safety, open communication, and healthy sexual behaviors.

NCLEX®-RN Questions

1. The nurse is providing counseling to a female patient who complains that sexual intercourse is sometimes initially painful. The patient relates that it takes time to feel aroused and experience adequate lubrication. The nurse recognizes that the patient is most likely to be experiencing difficulty in which phase of the sexual cycle?
   a. Orgasm
   b. Plateau
   c. Excitement
   d. Resolution

2. The nurse is working with an adolescent struggling with sexual identity. The patient's parents express concern that they have done something to contribute to the patient's problem. Which response by the nurse is most appropriate?
   a. "It is possible that your child was exposed to foods that had hormones in them."
   b. "Your child's sexual identity shouldn't really change your feelings for your child."
   c. "We know now that certain things such as toy selection can support or reinforce sexual identity."
   d. "It is believed that sexual identity relates to the interrelationship of complex biological and environmental factors."

3. The nurse is conducting a psychoeducation group for males experiencing a variety of sexual dysfunctions. The nurse anticipates that participants are likely to have which of the following disorders? Select all that apply.
   a. Impotence
   b. Premature orgasm
   c. Genitopelvic pain disorder
   d. Unspecified sexual dysfunction
   e. Medication-induced sexual dysfunction

4. The nurse is working with a patient with Klinefelter syndrome. The nurse recognizes that this disorder is correctly categorized under which type of disorder?
   a. Genetic
   b. Cultural
   c. Hormonal
   d. Psychological

5. The nurse is caring for a patient with gender dysphoria. Which assessment is priority?
   a. Safety status
   b. Surgical history
   c. Laboratory values
   d. Physical examination

6. The nurse is evaluating a patient diagnosed with a paraphilic disorder. The patient has been prescribed a selective serotonin-reuptake inhibiter (SSRI) as part of the management of the disorder. The nurse understands that the desired effects of the drug have been achieved when what is observed?
   a. Chemical castration of the patient is reported.
   b. The incidence of aggressive behavior is reduced.
   c. The patient reports improved mood and impulse control.
   d. Unnecessary guilt and rumination have been eliminated.

7. The nurse is planning care for the patient experiencing sexual dysfunction that is rooted in fearful–avoidant attachment. Which outcome is most appropriate for the nurse to identify for this patient?
   a. Able to use hugging and cuddling for intimacy
   b. Refrains from game playing and marital infidelity
   c. Initiates sexual activity at least 50 percent of the time
   d. Identifies more realistic expectations for the relationship

Answers may be found on the Pearson student resources site: nursing.pearsonhighered.com

Pearson Nursing Student Resources   Find additional review materials at **nursing.pearsonhighered.com**

References

Adams, M., Holland, N., & Urban, C. (2014). *Pharmacology for Nurses: A Pathophysiologic Approach* (4th ed.). Upper Saddle River, NJ: Prentice Hall.

American Nurses Association. (2001). *Code of Ethics for Nurses with Interpretive Statements.* Silver Spring, MD: American Nurses Publishing.

American Psychiatric Association. (2013). *Diagnostic and Statistical Manual of Mental Disorders* (5th ed.) Washington, DC: American Psychiatric Publishing.

American Psychological Association. (2006). Answers to your questions about individuals with intersex conditions. Available at http://www.apa.org/topics/sexuality/intersex.aspx?item=1

Association of Reproductive Health Professionals. (2008). Female sexual response: Talking to patients about sexuality and sexual health. Available at http://www.arhp.org/publications-and-resources/clinical-fact-sheets/sexuality-and-sexual-health

Baldry, A. C. (2002). From domestic violence to stalking. In J. Boon & L. Sheridan, (Eds.). *Stalking and Psychosocial Obsession*. West Sussex, UK: Wiley & Sons, pp. 83–104.

Banda, P. S., & Riccardi, N. (2013). Colorado transgender child, 6, wins court ruling, can use girls' bathroom. *Oakland News Press*. Available at http://www.theoaklandpress.com/general-news/20130624/colorado-transgender-child-6-wins-court-ruling-can-use-girls-bathroom

Basson, R. (2001). Human sex-response cycles. *Journal of Sex Marital Therapy, 27*, 33–43.

Binik, Y. M. (2010). The DSM diagnostic criteria for vaginismus. *Archives of Sexual Behavior, 39*(2), 278–291.

Black, M. C., Basile, K. C., Breiding, M. J., Smith, S. G., Walters, M. L., Merrick, M. T., Chen, J., & Stevens, M. R. (2011). *The National Intimate Partner Violence and Sexual Violence Survey (NISVS): 2010 Summary Report*. Atlanta, GA: National Center for Injury Prevention and Control, Centers for Disease Control and Prevention.

Blakemore, J. E. O., & Centers, R. E. (2005). Characteristics of boys' and girls' toys. *Sex Roles 53*(9/10), 619–633 doi: 10.1007/s11199-005-7729-0

Brannon, G. E. (2012). Paraphilias. Available at http://emedicine.medscape.com/article/291419-overview

Brown, J. (2012). Child sexual abuse: What we know from practice and research. Available at http://www.nspcc.org.uk/news-and-views/our-news/child-protection-news/12-12-12-child-sexual-abuse/child-sexual-abuse-issue_wda93265.html

Buss, A. H., & Durkee, A. (1957). An inventory for assessing different kinds of hostility. *Journal of Consulting Psychology, 21*(4), 343–348.

Carlat, D. J. (2005). *The Psychiatric Interview* (2nd ed.). Philadelphia, PA: Lippincott Williams & Wilkins.

Center for Sex Offender Management (CSOM). (2007). Female sex offenders. Office of Justice Programs, U.S. Department of Justice. Available at http://www.csom.org/pubs/female_sex_offenders_brief.pdf

Centers for Disease Control and Prevention. (2010). The National Intimate Partner and Sexual Violence Survey. Available at http://www.cdc.gov/violenceprevention/nisvs/

Centers for Disease Control and Prevention. (2012). Sexual violence. Available at http://www.cdc.gov/violenceprevention/sexualviolence

Codispoti, V.L. (2008). Pharmacology of sexually compulsive behavior. *Psychiatric Clinics of North America, 31*(4), 671–679.

Collective Social Services. (2010). Sexual masochism. Available at http://www.regionalcenter.org/mental-health/sexual-masochism

Corona, G., Jannini, E. A., Lotti, F., Boddi, V., De Vita, G. Forti, G., . . . Maggi, M. (2011). Premature and delayed ejaculation: Two ends of a single spectrum. *International Journal of Andrology, 34*, 41–48.

Davin, P. A., Hislop, J. C. R., & Dunbar, T. (1999). *Female Sexual Abusers*. Brandon, VT: Safer Society Press.

Dhejne, C., Lichtenstein, P., Boman, M., Johansson, A. L. V., Langstrom, N., & Landen, M. (2011). Long-term follow-up of transsexual persons undergoing surgery: Cohort study in Sweden. Retrieved from http://www.plosone.org/article/info%3Adoi%2F10.1371%2Fjournal.pone.0016885

Donaldson James, S. (2012). Trans man denied cancer treatment; now feds say it's illegal. *ABCNews*. Available at http://abcnews.go.com/Health/transgender-bias-now-banned-federal-law/story?id=16949817

Dougherty, C. M., Richard, A. J., & Carey, M. J. (2012). Priapism in emergency medicine. Available at http://emedicine.medscape.com/article/777603-overview

Dresher, J. & Byne, W. M. (2009). Homosexuality, gay and lesbian identities, and homosexual behavior. In B. J. Sadock, V. A. Sadock, & P. Ruiz, (Eds.). *Kaplan & Sadock's Comprehensive Textbook of Psychiatry* (9th ed.). Philadelphia, PA: Lippincott, Williams & Wilkins, pp. 2060–2090.

Encyclopedia of Mental Disorders. (n.d.). Sexual masochism. Available at http://www.minddisorders.com/Py-Z/Sexual-masochism.html

Farley, M., Cotton, A., Lynne, J., Zumbeck, S., Spiwak, F., Reyes, M. E., Alvarez, D., & Sezgin, U. (2003). Prostitution and trafficking in nine countries: An update on violence and posttraumatic stress disorder. In M. Farley, (Ed.). *Prostitution, Trafficking and Traumatic Stress*. New York, NY: Routledge, pp. 33–74.

Goodman, A. (2009). Sexual addiction. In B. J. Sadock, V. A. Sadock, & P. Ruiz, (Eds.). *Kaplan & Sadock's Comprehensive Textbook of Psychiatry* (9th ed.). Philadelphia, PA: Lippincott, Williams & Wilkins, pp. 2111–2127.

Grant, J. M., Mottet, L. A., & Tanis, J. (2011). *Injustice at Every Turn: A Report of the National Transgender Discrimination Survey*, Executive Summary. Washington, DC: National Center for Transgender Equality and National Gay and Lesbian Task Force.

Gray, P. B., Kahlenberg, S. M., Barrett, E. S., Lipson, S. F., & Ellison, P. T. (2002). Marriage and fatherhood are associated with lower testosterone in males. *Evolution and Human Behavior, 23*(3), 193–201.

Greene, R. (2009). Gender identity disorders. In B. J. Sadock, V. A. Sadock, & P. Ruiz, (Eds.). *Kaplan & Sadock's Comprehensive Textbook of Psychiatry* (9th ed.). Philadelphia, PA: Lippincott Williams & Wilkins, pp. 2099–2111.

Grossman, W. J. (1991). Pain, aggression, fantasy and concepts of sadomasochism. *Psychoanalytic Quarterly, 60*, 22–51. Available at http://internationalpsychoanalysis.net/wp-content/uploads/2011/02/PainAggressionFantasy.pdf

Groth, A. N. (1979). *Men Who Rape: The Psychology of the Offender*. New York, NY: Plenum Press.

Guess, K. (2008). *Psychiatric-Mental Health Nurse Practitioner*. Silver Spring, MD: American Nurses Credentialing Center, pp. 296–301.

Guttmacher Institute. (2013). Facts on American teens' sexual and reproductive health. Available at http://www.guttmacher.org/pubs/FB-ATSRH.html

Hall, R. C. W., & Hall, R. C. W. (2009). A profile of pedophilia: Definition, characteristics of offenders, recidivism, treatment outcomes, and forensic issues. *Focus, 7*, 522–537.

Hanson, R. K., Bourgon, G., Helmus, L., & Hodgson, S. (2009). A meta analysis of the effectiveness of treatment for sexual offenders: Risk, needs and responsivity. *Public Safety of Canada*. Available at www.publicsafety.gc.ca/res/cor/rep.2009-01-trt-si-eng.aspx

Harrison, P. M., & Beck, A. J. (2005). *Prison and Jail Inmates at Midyear 2004*. Washington, DC: U.S. Department of Justice, Bureau of Justice Statistics.

Hucker, S. J. (2011). Hypoxyphilia/auto-erotic asphyxia. Available at http://www.forensicpsychiatry.ca/paraphilia/aea.htm

Jacklin, C. N., DiPietro, J. A., & Maccoby, E. E. (1984). Sex-typing behavior and sex-typing pressure in child/parent interaction. *Archives of Sexual Behavior, 13*(5), 413–425.

Kafka, M., & Prentky, R., (1998). Attention-deficit/hyperactivity disorder in males with paraphilias and paraphilia-related disorders. *Journal of Clinical Psychiatry, 59*(7), 338–396.

Kinsey, A., & Pomeroy, W. (1948). *Sexual Behavior in the Human Male*. Philadelphia, PA: Saunders.

Kinsey, A., & Pomeroy, W. (1953). *Sexual Behavior in the Human Female*. Philadelphia, PA: Saunders.

Laws, D. R., & O'Donohue, W. T. (2008). *Sexual Deviance, Theory, Assessment and Treatment* (2nd ed.). New York, NY: Guilford Press.

Lee, P. A., Houk, C. P., Faisal Ahmed, S., & Hughes, I. A. (2006). Consensus statement on management of intersex disorders. *Pediatrics, 118*, e488–e501. Available at http://pediatrics.aappublications.org/content/118/2/e488.full.pdf

Macionis, J. J. (2010). *Sociology*. Upper Saddle River, NJ: Pearson Education, Inc.

Masters, W. H., & Johnson, V. E. (1966). *Human Sexual Response*. Toronto, ON and New York, NY: Bantam Books.

Masters, W. H., & Johnson, V. E. (1970). *Human Sexual Inadequacy*. Toronto, ON and New York, NY: Bantam Books.

Mayo Clinic. (2013). Priapism: Prolonged erection. Available at http://www.mayoclinic.com/health/priapism/DS00873

MedlinePlus. (2011). Intersex. Available at http://www.nlm.nih.gov/medlineplus/ency/article/001669.htm

MedlinePlus. (2012). Penis pain. Available at http://www.nlm.nih.gov/medlineplus/ency/article/003166.htm

MedlinePlus. (2013). Turner syndrome. Available at http://www.nlm.nih.gov/medlineplus/turnersyndrome.html

Montgomery, K. A. (2008). Sexual desire disorders. *Psychiatry, 5*(6), 50–55.

National Center for Complementary and Alternative Medicine. (2013). Yohimbe. Available at http://nccam.nih.gov/health/yohimbe

National Center for Missing and Exploited Children. (2013). Key facts. Available at http://www.missingkids.com/KeyFacts

National Center for Transgender Equality (2010). Preventing transgender suicide. Available at http://transequality.org/PDFs/NCTE_Suicide_Prevention.pdf

National Human Genome Research Institute. (2011). Learning about Klinefelter syndrome. Available at http://www.genome.gov/19519068

Northwestern University Women's Center. (n.d.). Defining sexual assault and consent. Available at http://www.northwestern.edu/womenscenter/issues-information/sexual-assault/defining-sexual-assault.html

Orlando, I. J. (1972). *The Discipline and Teaching of Nursing Process (An Evaluative Study)*. New York, NY: G. P. Putnam's Sons.

Polaschek, D. L. L., & Gannon, T. A. (2004). The implicit theories of rapists: What convicted offenders tell us. *Sexual Abuse: A Journal of Research and Treatment, 16*, 299–315.

Prerequisites. (n.d.). The Philadelphia Center for Transgender Surgery. Available at http://www.thetransgendercenter.com/index.php/maletofemale1/pre-requisites.html

Putnam, J., Myers-Walls, J. A., & Love, D. (n.d.). Influences on children's gender development. Available at http://www.extension.purdue.edu/providerparent/child%20growth-development/InfluencesONGender.htm

Rape, Abuse, and Incest National Network. (2009). Who are the victims? Available at http://www.rainn.org/get-information/statistics/sexual-assault-victims

Rape, Abuse, and Incest National Network. (2013). Was I raped? Available at http://www.rainn.org/get-information/types-of-sexual-assault/was-it-rape

Rathus, S. A., Nevid, J. S., & Fichner-Rathus, L. (1998). *Essentials of Human Sexuality*. Needham Heights, MA: Allyn & Bacon.

Rellini, A. H., & Clifton, J. (2011). Sexual dysfunction: Beyond the brain-body connection. *Advanced Psychosomatic Medicine, 31*, 35–56.

Sachs, G. S., & Chan, C. (2013). Medication-induced sexual dysfunction. Available at http://www.medscape.org/viewarticle/420273

Sadock, B., & Sadock, V. (2007). *Kaplan and Sadock's Synopsis of Psychiatry* (10th ed.). Philadelphia, PA: Lippincott Williams, & Wilkins.

Sadock, V. A. (2009). Normal human sexuality and sexual dysfunctions. In B. J. Sadock, V. A. Sadock, & P. Ruiz, (Eds.). *Kaplan & Sadock's Comprehensive Textbook of Psychiatry* (9th ed.). Philadelphia, PA: Lippincott Williams & Wilkins, pp. 2027–2060.

Sands, M., & Fisher, M. A. (2007). Women's endorsement of models of female sexual response: The Nurses' Sexuality Study. *Journal of Sexual Medicine, 4*, 708–719.

Schiltz, K., Witzel, J., Northoff, G., Zierhut, K., Gubka, U., Fellman, H., . . . Bogerts, B. (2007). Brain pathology in pedophilic offenders. *Archives of General Psychiatry, 64*(6), 737–746.

Schwartz, M. F. (2008). Developmental psychopathological perspectives on sexually compulsive behavior. In M. F. Schwartz & F. S. Berlin, (Eds.). *Psychiatric Clinics of North America, Vol. 31 No. 4, Sexually Compulsive Behavior: Hypersexuality*. Philadelphia, PA: W.B. Saunders Company, pp. 567–586.

Shafer, L. (2000). Sexual disorders and sexual dysfunctions. In T. A. Stern & J. B. Herman, (Eds.). *Psychiatry Update and Board Preparation*. New York, NY: McGraw-Hill, Health Professions Division, pp. 157–166.

Smallbone, S. W., & Dadds, M. R. (2000) Attachment and coercive sexual behavior. *Sexual Abuse: A Journal of Research and Treatment, 12*, 3–15.

Sorrentino, R. M. (2009). Paraphilias. In B. J. Sadock, V. A. Sadock, & P. Ruiz, (Eds.). *Kaplan & Sadock's Comprehensive Textbook of Psychiatry* (9th ed.). Philadelphia, PA: Lippincott Williams & Wilkins, pp. 2090–2099.

Stanford School of Medicine. (2014). Female sexual medicine: female sexual arousal disorder. Retrieved from http://obgyn.stanford.edu/fsm/arousal_disorder.html

State of Connecticut, Office of Policy and Management, Criminal Justice Policy and Planning Division. (2012). 2012 recidivism among sex offenders in CT. Available at www.ct.gov.gov/bopp/sex_offender_recidivism_2012_final.pdf

Tewksbury, R. (2004). Experiences and attitudes of registered female sex offenders. *Federal Probation, 68*(3), 30–33.

U.S. Census Bureau. (2012). Households and families: 2010. Available at http://www.census.gov/prod/cen2010/briefs/c2010br-14.pdf

U.S. Department of Justice. (2007). Female sex offenders. Available at http://www.csom.org/pubs/female_sex_offenders_brief.pdf

University of North Carolina at Asheville Health and Counseling Center. (2013). What is consent? Available at http://healthandcounseling.unca.edu/what-consent

Ward, T., & Beech, T. (2006). An integrated theory of sexual offending. *Aggression and Violent Behavior, 11*, 44–63.

Wilson, B., Shannon, M., & Shields, K. (2014). *Pearson Nurse's Drug Guide 2014*. Upper Saddle River, NJ: Pearson.

World Health Organization. (2013a). Female genital mutilation. Available at http://www.who.int/mediacentre/factsheets/fs241/en/

World Health Organization. (2013b). Gender and genetics. Available at http://www.who.int/genomics/gender/en/index1.html

World Professional Association for Transgender Health (WPATH). (2008). WPATH clarification on medical necessity of treatment, sex reassignment, and insurance coverage for transgender and transsexual people worldwide. Available at http://www.wpath.org/site_page.cfm?pk_association_webpage_menu=1352&pk_association_webpage=3947

Your Guide to the Sexual Response Cycle. (2012). Available at http://www.webmd.com/sex-relationships/guide/sexual-health-your-guide-to-sexual-response-cycle

20

Substance-Related and Addictive Disorders

Betty D. Morgan
Donna McCarten White

Key Terms

Learning Outcomes

1. Examine the etiology of addiction.

2. Summarize the impact of the biological, psychological, sociological, cultural, and spiritual domains on substance-related and addictive disorders.

3. Categorize key symptoms of substance-related and addictive disorders.

4. Evaluate different pharmacologic and nonpharmacologic therapies used in the treatment of substance-related and addictive disorders.

5. Compare and contrast the types of care settings and levels of care available to patients diagnosed with substance-related and addictive disorders.

6. Plan evidence-based nursing care for patients diagnosed with substance-related and addictive disorders.

Gerald Kraymore Relapse Phase

APPLICATION

1. Address the five domains for Mr. Kraymore:

   a. Biological

   b. Psychological

   c. Sociological

   d. Cultural

   e. Spiritual

2. What are the priorities of care for Mr. Kraymore?

3. As a nurse, how can you convey or instill hope to patients who feel hopeless about their recovery and dependence on substances?

Gerald Kraymore is a 42-year-old White man who is admitted to the medical unit for treatment of endocarditis and evaluation for depression related to long-term drug use. He states that he first used alcohol at the age of 12. Mr. Kraymore did not realize he had a problem with alcohol until his late 30s. He states he last used alcohol 2 days ago, and before that had been drinking up to 40 ounces of beer every day for approximately 10 days. Mr. Kraymore states that he was recently released from prison and relapsed right away. He reports that his relapses always begin with use of alcohol and progress to use of other substances, notably heroin. When abstinent, Mr. Kraymore craves alcohol more than any other substance. He says he briefly used marijuana when he was 15; he used it "recreationally . . . like other teenagers" but after a "bad experience" he stopped using.

Mr. Kraymore seems sad and is isolating on the unit. He shares very little about his family or having anyone in his life. Mr. Kraymore reports that the longest abstinence he has had lasted for four weeks. Blood cultures now have been positive × 2 for a bacterial infection that led to endocarditis, and his IV antibiotic dosages have been increased. He states he is afraid he will never be able to live a life without drugs. On admission, Mr. Kraymore told the nurse that he no longer feels the high from anything he uses. He states that he worries a lot about "being able to come off drugs and stay off."

Introduction

Substance use often accompanies mental health issues as a dual diagnosis. One in three individuals diagnosed with mental illness has a co-occurring substance use disorder and may be self-medicating with a substance to deal with various symptoms of mental illness (NAMI, 2013). The term **substance** refers to one of several classes of drugs known to act on the brain's reward system. Misuse of these substances may result in a **substance use disorder**, defined as continued use of a substance without regard to negative consequences, including psychological and physiological symptoms (American Psychiatric Association [APA], 2013).

Individuals with a substance use disorder typically display a constellation of symptoms and behaviors: (1) cognitive, behavioral, and physiologic symptoms; (2) desire to reduce use of the substance, but difficulty doing so; (3) need for greater amounts of the substance to achieve the same effect; (4) neglect of normal activities due to focus on obtaining or using more of the substance; and (5) persistent desire, or craving, for the substance (APA, 2013). As with other disorders, symptoms of substance abuse occur across the domains, increasing the likelihood of impairment in multiple areas of functioning, including relationships with others (Table 20-1).

Although *substance use disorder* is sometimes used interchangeably with the term **addiction** or **addictive disorder**, addiction typically refers to the active disease state. The National Institute on Drug Abuse (NIDA) defines addiction as a chronic and relapsing disease depicted by compulsive drug seeking and use in spite of harmful consequences that involve neurochemical and molecular changes in the brain (NIDA, 2012b). Although this term has been used in this chapter to describe extreme presentations and associated patient behavior, it is not applied as a diagnostic term (APA, 2013). Instead, the DSM-5 uses the more neutral term *substance use disorder*.

Historically, society has accepted the use of substances for medical purposes. Heroin was used as a cough suppressant at the turn of the 19th century (Carroll, 1989). Cocaine was given for listlessness in

Impact of Substance Use by Domain	table 20-1

Domain	Responses
Biological	• Dilated or constricted pupils • Tremors (especially notable in eyelids or hands) • Hyperactivity or lethargy • Impaired coordination, unsteady gait • Rapid or slow speech
Psychological	• Emotional lability • Fear, anxiety, panic attacks • Sadness, loneliness • Anger, agitation, irritability • Impulsivity, denial • Easily distracted, disoriented • Impaired concentration or memory • Blackouts
Sociological	• Talking about getting high, using vocabulary typical among drug users • Using despite requests from family, friends to decrease or refrain • Arriving late, leaving early at work or school • Stealing, engaging in risky behaviors • Associating with others who use; withdrawing from those who discourage use
Cultural	• Withdrawal from cultural activities, practices • Use may increase during periods of loss of traditional values
Spiritual	• Withdrawal from spiritual activities, practices • Feelings of helplessness and hopelessness • May question purpose in life

the 1920s and advocated by Freud. Alcohol has been touted for its vasodilative effects, and marijuana is used to countermand the cachexia and anorexia associated with long-term sequelae of cancer. The past few decades have brought new problems and new substances.

Designer drugs are chemical compounds similar to other drugs in effect but slightly different in chemical structure; they are produced illegally and often have more serious and potent effects than the original drug. For example, methylenedioxymethamphetamine (MDMA, or ecstasy) is a designer drug that has gained widespread popularity in the United States. Substances that might once have been considered benign, such as inhalants and substituted cathinones ("bath salts"), are now being used for their euphoric effects, presenting new and different dangers (U.S. Department of Justice, 2013).

Any substance may have deleterious effects on human physiology. Addiction to any substance is a primary disease that implies a comprehensive destruction of individual health and quality of life. It requires daily prioritizing of **abstinence** (refraining from use) if an individual is motivated toward **recovery**, the state in which the individual no longer engages in using the substance or in problem behaviors associated with use. Research continues as to the genetic influence substances have and why some people become dependent and develop addiction disorders while others do not. A complex interplay of factors include the individual, the substance, and the environment. Each factor lends itself to the overall constellation of how a substance use disorder is manifested (Ruiz & Strain, 2011).

Substance use disorders are widespread in the United States, and nurses in all settings will encounter individuals struggling with the effects of substance use (Figure 20-1) (Box 20-1). The goal of this chapter is to examine how addictive substances alter the health and well-being of the individual. The chapter also covers assessment and therapeutic techniques that nurses can use when helping individuals with known or potential substance use disorders.

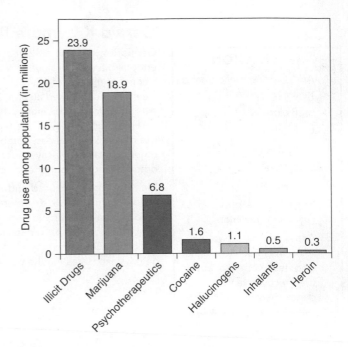

20-1 Past month drug use among persons age 12 and older: 2012. Illicit drugs include marijuana/hashish, cocaine (including crack), heroin, hallucinogens, inhalants, or prescription-type psychotherapeutics used nonmedically.

Data from Substance Abuse and Mental Health Services Administration. (2013). *Results from the 2012 National Survey on Drug Use and Health: Summary of National Findings,* NSDUH Series H-46, HHS Publication No. (SMA) 13-4795. Rockville, MD: Substance Abuse and Mental Health Services Administration.

Pause and Reflect

1. *What is the difference between a substance use disorder and an addiction?*
2. *Why do you think substance use disorders are so prevalent?*

Theoretical Foundations

Initially, use of substances is mostly voluntary. The NIDA (2008) reports that some of these reasons include curiosity, a desire to feel good or feel better (self-medication), and a desire to improve cognitive or physical ability. Which substance an individual uses varies according to demographics, age, drug of choice, and availability. This has implications for prevention and treatment, as individual predispositions, responses, and requirements for treatment vary

greatly. For individuals with a genetic predisposition to addiction, the introduction to addictive substances can create a predictable course of events. Regardless of individual biology and circumstances, addiction has a devastating effect on physiological processes, alters cognitive processes, affects emotional health, and creates social, financial, and spiritual concerns. Additionally, a wide range of dysfunctional behaviors can result from drug abuse. These behaviors interfere with normal functioning in the family, the workplace, and the broader community (NIDA, 2009b). How and why addiction occurs can be best understood from a perspective that includes all the domains—biological, psychological, sociological, cultural, and spiritual.

Prevalence of Substance Use and Addiction in the United States box 20-1

A 2012 survey of Americans ages 12 and older revealed the following:

- 52.1%, or 135.5 million people, reported being current drinkers of alcohol.
- 6.5% (17 million people) reported being heavy drinkers.
- 26.7% of Americans (69.5 million people) used a tobacco product.

- 2.9 million people used an illicit drug for the first time.
- 8.5% (22.2 million people) reported substance dependence or abuse.
- Marijuana, pain relievers, and cocaine (in that order) were the most frequently reported drugs of dependence or abuse.
- Rates of substance dependence or abuse are approximately twice as high among men as women.

Data from Substance Abuse and Mental Health Services Administration. (2013). *Results from the 2012 National Survey on Drug Use and Health: Summary of National Findings,* NSDUH Series H-46, HHS Publication No. (SMA) 13-4795. Rockville, MD: Substance Abuse and Mental Health Services Administration.

Substance Use Terminology

table 20-2

Term	Definition
Compulsivity	Behavior defined as the persistent re-initiation of habitual acts that continue despite the potential for adverse consequences.
Craving	A compelling desire for previously experienced positive or euphoric effects of a psychoactive substance. Cravings can increase in the presence of both internal and external cues (e.g., stressors), particularly with perceived substance availability.
Dependence	The body's physical need for a specific substance. Cessation (abruptly stopping) use of a substance can result in specific withdrawal syndrome.
Detoxification	Process of safely and effectively withdrawing an individual from an addictive substance.
Impulsivity	A predisposition toward rapid, unplanned reactions to internal and external stimuli without regard for negative consequences.
Relapse	The return of symptoms after stabilization. More specifically, the return of drug-seeking behavior in individuals who have been successfully abstaining from use. This can occur both after detoxification and long periods of abstinence. Relapse behavior may be provided by stress, cues, or contexts previously associated with drug use.
Self-medicating	Use of substances to compensate for or improve symptoms resulting from another illness (medical or psychiatric) that has not been treated adequately.
Sobriety	Complete abstinence from alcohol or other drugs of abuse in conjunction with a satisfactory quality of life.
Withdrawal	Onset of signs and symptoms following abrupt discontinuation of or rapid decrease in use of a substance.

Substance use disorders are treatable, but there are divergent opinions in the medical community as to the best approach. When studying the problem of substance abuse, it is important to understand terminology as well as how the use of specific substances create changes in an individual's life (Table 20-2). When an individual's use of psychoactive substances increases, adverse sequelae in all areas of life are predictable. The latest research clearly identifies that addictive processes alter brain functioning (NIDA, 2011). This correlates to an individual's heredity, genetic influence, social surroundings, and emotional health and well-being.

Biological Domain

Prolonged exposure to repeated use of substances precipitates neurological changes in brain circuitry. Learning and memory changes in the brain suggest that a form of neuroadaptation occurs. Some changes occur quickly. Research indicates that some people develop an addictive disorder with only a few exposures to a substance, whereas others may require long-term exposure and others may never develop dependency (Erickson, 2007).

The neural circuits of pleasure (involving the nucleus accumbens, amygdala, and prefrontal cortex) precipitate a cluster of symptoms that emerge when a substance is used. Feelings of euphoria, calm, and well-being often occur with initial and subsequent early use. Continued use may lead to a conditioned response, so the individual will continue to engage in the use of the substance or the behavior in a repeated manner. When this occurs, increasing amounts of the substance are required to achieve the same result, an effect known as **tolerance**. Increasing frequency and amount of use creates *physical dependence*, in which the body becomes so dependent on the substance that, without it, withdrawal symptoms will begin. Continued use leads to a breakdown in patterns of daily living, part of the addictive process. The substance begins to assume an all-important and powerful role in the life of the individual. Daily patterns of existence become consumed with thinking about, obtaining, and using the drug. At this point, the individual becomes incapable of living without the substance and the emotional relief or comfort it provides, a state referred to as *psychological dependence*. This leads to deterioration in other domains.

Medical researchers describe addiction as a "primary chronic disease of brain reward, motivation, memory, and related circuitry" (American Society of Addiction Medicine [ASAM], 2011, para 1). Such a biological view of addiction is a relatively recent development. Until NIDA began in earnest to examine the etiology of brain changes associated with drug use, the disease was considered to be behaviorally based, often with emotional underpinnings. Impaired control was always observed, but research has shown changes in neurochemistry as the basis for the behavior observed in the addictive process. Currently, it is believed that addictive substances act on the mesolimbic system of the brain, where instinctual drives and the pleasure center are located (Brick & Erickson, 2006). The neurotransmitter systems of the brain and related receptors and transporters are being examined for their role in areas of the brain that regulate euphoric effects from drugs and certain behaviors that provide pleasure. Dopamine has been shown to play a key role in the neural pathway that provides activation for the feeling described as *euphoria*. Thus, the brain learns quickly that a drug stimulates a surge of dopamine, activating neural pathways and establishing memory of the pleasurable feeling. Over time, the reward circuits of the individual who is using substances can become low, initiating the individual's requirement for more of the substance to achieve the desired effect. This is the biological basis for tolerance. Individuals who use substances consistently and then suddenly cease using experience *withdrawal*, "a predictable constellation of signs and symptoms following the abrupt discontinuation of, or a rapid decrease in, dosage of a psychoactive substance" (Ries, Miller, Fiellin, & Saitz, 2009, pp. 552–558). Withdrawal may also be referred to as *acute abstinence syndrome*. Withdrawal symptoms vary according to the type of substance or substances used (Table 20-3).

Overview of Commonly Abused Substances

table 20-3

Substance	Clinical Manifestations of Disease	Potential Adverse Effects of Withdrawal	Nursing Considerations
Alcohol (Oral ingestion) A powerful CNS depressant that produces dose-dependent changes in cognitive and motor functioning.	Impaired coordination evidenced by: • Loss of fine and gross motor control (eye–hand coordination, balance) • Impaired reaction time • Changes in speech • Impaired cognition and judgment	Varies—use and tolerance affect timing and extent of withdrawal symptoms, which can include: • Increased cardiac stress with elevated BP and pulse • Diaphoresis • GI distress • Frequent urination • Seizure activity • Difficulty concentrating • Memory loss • Hallucinations • Skin proliferative disorders	• Carefully monitor all body systems. • Assess for last use and monitor for withdrawal. • Assess for signs of recent trauma or head injury. • Assess and monitor existing medical conditions, medications. • Observe for neurological changes, changes in sensorium. • Maintain hydration. • Monitor vital signs and temperature closely. • Observe for possible seizures and hallucinations. • Monitor blood alcohol level. • Monitor for allergic reactions.
Opioids/Opiates (Usual method is oral but may be crushed and snorted or injected) Includes *heroin*, which can be several times stronger than prescription opioids/opiates.	Powerful pain relief that precipitates feelings of euphoria. Manifestations include sluggish demeanor, constricted pupils, delayed reflexes, slowed or slurred speech, and decrease in breathing, BP, and pulse.	Severe craving may facilitate a return to heroin to alleviate symptoms. Refer to clinical indicator of withdrawal (CIWA). • Cardiac palpitations • Poor concentration • Erratic behavior and agitation • Possible tremulousness • Lack of appetite • Poor sleep and wakefulness • Profuse diaphoresis • Lacrimation • Rhinitis • Muscle aches and bone pain • Poor concentration and inability to focus	• Observe for any difficulty breathing. • Monitor O_2 saturation. • Monitor cardiac status. • If cough present, observe sputum. • Observe vital signs closely along with changes in skin color (cyanosis, mottling, etc.). • Observe for any burns on the hands or fingers. Patient may smoke during use of alcohol and depressed CNS effect may intensify drowsiness and result in burns.
Prescription Medications (Injected, crushed and snorted, taken orally) Commonly abused classes of prescription drugs include pain killers, sedatives, and stimulants. Increasing prevalence among teenagers and young adults, many of whom suffer from the misconception that because the drugs are prescription medications, they are safe.	Signs of use and abuse are the same as opioids and heroin. Risk for lethality.	Withdrawal can emerge soon after last dose. Symptoms include: • Clouded perception • Impaired (slowed) memory • Impaired cognitive processes • Impaired coordination • Altered perception of time and disturbance in eye–hand coordination, and impaired reaction time. • Increased appetite during use.	• Monitor all bodily systems. • Observe for dehydration. • Monitor for falls. • Observe cognitive status—monitor for any delirium or changes in sensorium. • Refer to NSG considerations under Alcohol. • Observe for abscesses at the site of injection (IDU/Skin-popping if using injection as route of administration). • Obtain urine drug screen report if available. • Assess the reason for why the prescription was ordered. • Individual may have difficulty separating from the substance. • Offer nonpharmacological interventions for poor sleep.

Substance	Clinical Manifestations of Disease	Potential Adverse Effects of Withdrawal	Nursing Considerations
Cocaine (Smoked, injected, or snorted) A short-acting stimulant, which can lead abusers to "binge" (to take the drug many times in a single session). Quick high (rush) but effects of certain stimulants can be long lasting.	Cocaine abuse can lead to severe medical consequences related to the heart and the respiratory, nervous, and digestive systems.	• Profound loss of weight • Delays fatigue • Individual may eventually present as depressed, violent, anxious, or confused. • Disturbed sleep cycle • Irritability and restlessness	• Monitor for rapid breathing, tremors, loss of coordination. • Monitor for paranoia and aggressiveness. • Maintain a calm atmosphere. • Offer medications as prescribed to ameliorate agitation.
Marijuana, THC (Smoked, inhaled and may be cooked in foods. Medical THC is available in pill form.) Intense ideological debate in the United States as to potential harmful effects. Permanent brain damage can result from chronic use.	• Intense relaxation • Increased thirst • Euphoria, psychosis • Increased cravings for food • Dry mouth • Enhanced visual/color perception • Memory impairment • Giddiness, spontaneous laughter	Withdrawal symptoms may include: • Muscle tension • Memory loss • Respiratory distress and cardiac problems • Rage, euphoria, belligerence, and assaultive behavior • Dissociative states and visual hallucinations	• Observe any smoking-related issues and ability to make decisions. • Observe for any burns or head injuries. • Monitor for cough and respiratory function.
Stimulants (Snorted, injected, smoked or taken orally) Used primarily by teens due to availability.	Some short-term effects can include increased body temperature, heart rate, and blood pressure; sweating; loss of appetite; sleeplessness; dry mouth; and tremors.	Can precipitate immediate cardiac dysrhythmia. May result in death.	• Encourage rest periods. • Monitor hydration. • Offer food in small amounts. • Limit noise to reduce overstimulation. • Administer medication(s) to relieve symptoms associated with cessation of drug.
Club Drugs, Ecstasy, MDMA (Most notably taken orally, but some reports show certain drugs in this class can be and have been injected) There is no accepted medical use in the United States for this classification of drugs.	These drugs produce both stimulant and mind-altering effects. They can increase body temperature, heart rate, blood pressure, and heart wall stress. Ecstasy may also be toxic to nerve cells.	• Euphoric state can last up to 12 hours. • Mood swings and volatility in behavior. • Can produce a trance-like state; may present with psychotic-like symptoms.	• Encourage frequent rest periods. • Monitor vital signs. • Observe for mood changes and appetite changes. • Monitor temperature and fluid balance. • Offer small amounts of food. • Decrease environmental stimuli.
Steroids (Oral or injected) Substances that can be prescribed for certain medical conditions, but are also abused to increase muscle mass and improve athletic performance or physical appearance.	Serious consequences of abuse can include: • Severe acne • Heart disease • Liver problems • Stroke • Infectious diseases • Depression • Suicidality	Abrupt discontinuance may precipitate: • Convulsions • Tremors • Abdominal and muscle cramps • Vomiting • Sweating Abrupt cessation from long-term use can be dangerous or fatal.	• Observe behavior closely. • Medicate as needed to ameliorate symptoms of distress. • Provide emotional support during early period of drug cessation. • Encourage rest periods. • Monitor vital signs and temperature closely.
Inhalants (Inhaled, huffed) Gasoline or spray cans are used.	Profound changes in sensorium. Can cause respiratory depression.	• Spray cans used to "huff" with possibility of fatal reaction. • Cardiac and respiratory depression	• Observe vital signs closely. • Medicate as needed for presenting symptoms. • Observe cardiac and respiratory status. • Observe for cough and O_2 saturation. • Monitor for neurological changes. • Monitor fluid balance and temperature.

(Continued)

Overview of Commonly Abused Substances *(continued)*

table 20-3

Substance	Clinical Manifestations of Disease	Potential Adverse Effects of Withdrawal	Nursing Considerations
Hallucinogenics, LSD (Oral or sublingual)	• Altered states of perception and feelings • Synesthesia • May last for prolonged period of time (4–8 hours or longer).	• Increased body temperature • Increased heart rate and BP • Loss of appetite • Numbness and weakness • Tremors	• Monitor vital signs closely. • Observe fluctuations in BP and pulse. • Keep room quiet to decrease stimuli. • Observe for paranoia.
Sedatives/Hypnotics (Oral) Can be dangerous if mixed with alcohol.	Drowsiness, euphoria, slurred speech, nausea, vomiting, diarrhea (NVD), dizziness, memory deficits	May precipitate respiratory depression and ataxia. Abrupt discontinuance may precipitate convulsions, tremors, abdominal and muscle cramps, vomiting, and sweating. Abrupt cessation from long-term use can be dangerous or fatal.	• Observe closely for agitation. • Monitor for falls. • Monitor vital signs. • Provide supportive treatment if NVD is present. • Monitor fluid balance.
Nicotine (Chewed or smoked)	• Used in cigars, snuff, spit tobacco, chewing tobacco. • Burns and nicotine stains on fingers • Respiratory depression and altered pulmonary function tests (PFTs)	Adverse effects include: • Poor blood gas exchange; inability to inhale and exhale at full capacity • Pneumonias and cyanosis • Oral or lung cancers • Cancer of larynx and esophagus • Emphysema and chronic bronchitis	• Monitor vital signs closely. • Observe for cough and difficulty breathing. • Provide for safety. • Monitor fluid balance. • Medicate if required to ameliorate any anxiety. • O$_2$ as necessary. Observe closely if emphysemic.
Caffeine	With ingestion of more than 200 mg daily of caffeine, a person may experience tremulousness and agitation; rapid breathing, irritability, delirium, and/or panic; restlessness and paranoia.	• Cardiac fibrillation • Dehydration • Severe agitation and tremulousness • Gastrointestinal distress • Increased intraocular pressure in unregulated glaucoma • Increased plasma glucose and lipid levels	• Monitor vital signs and have emergency equipment available. • Provide education as to use and effects of caffeine, which may seem harmless. • Observe closely for signs of tremulousness or severe cardiac reaction. • EKG to assess cardiac status.

Based on National Institute of Drug Abuse. (2010b). *Drugs, Brains and Behavior: The Science of Addiction.* Available at http://www.drugabuse.gov/publications/science-addiction; Brick, J. & Erickson, C. (2006). *Drugs, the Brain and Behavior: The Pharmacology of Drug Use Disorders.* New York, NY: Routledge; Anderson, E., & McFarlane, J. (2004). *Community as Partner: Theory and Practice in Nursing.* New York, NY: Lippincott Williams & Wilkins; Carpenito, L. J. (2012). *Nursing Diagnosis: Application to Clinical Practice.* New York, NY: Lippincott Williams & Wilkins.

Medical Illness

As an individual progresses through addiction, changes in the body begin to occur. The individual begins to experience one or more medical concerns, and continued use of a substance may be identified as co-existing with mental health issues. The impact of substance use can include, but is not limited to, cardiovascular disease, increased risk for cerebrovascular accidents (CVAs), increased associated risk of cancers, all forms of hepatitis, HIV/AIDS, sexually transmitted diseases (STDs), pulmonary disease, eating disorders, and mental illness. Individuals experiencing addiction increasingly neglect their health, exacerbating the lack of timely diagnosis and treatment of resulting medical conditions.

Health concerns identified in individuals with substance dependency, including patients in recovery, are many and vary depending on the substance and route of administration. In particular, substance abuse can weaken the immune system. Weakened immunity combined with needle sharing and unsafe sexual behaviors increases risk of HIV and hepatitis C infection (NIDA, 2012a). Hepatitis C has emerged as the most prevalent health issue, affecting 50% to 90% of individuals battling with a co-morbid substance abuse issue (Evans et al., 2004). Hepatitis C has the potential to develop into cirrhosis of the liver and hepatocellular carcinoma (McGinnis et al., 2006).

The disease of alcoholism is associated with potentially severe health risks. The most widely identified are hepatocellular carcinoma, hepatitis C, and liver cirrhosis (McGinnis et al., 2006). Mertens et al. (2005) report that alcoholics are at higher risk for chronic illnesses such as bronchitis, pneumonia, and diabetes. It has been postulated that individuals who abuse alcohol have a higher incidence of chronic illnesses because they do not routinely use preventive medical care and typically have poor nutritional status (Zarkin, Bray, Babor, & Higgins-Bindle, 2004).

Cardiovascular Disease

Long-term substance abuse has been associated with increased risk of cardiovascular disease. Smoking has been shown to be a significant cause of atherosclerosis through inflammatory and oxidative processes (Perlstein & Lee, 2006). Smoking, abnormally high homocysteine levels, and elevated C-reactive protein constitute the major known risk factors for atherosclerosis (Porth, 2012). Chronic cocaine use can precipitate coronary artery atherosclerosis in young adults, which can result in myocardial infarction. Cocaine is implicated in approximately 25% of heart attacks occurring in individuals under age 45 (Patrizi et al., 2006). Depending on the extent and location of vascular obstruction, atherosclerosis can cause a variety of complications, including heart failure, stroke, and myocardial infarction (Porth, 2012). Environmental factors may contribute to an increased risk for atherosclerosis among homeless, substance-dependent individuals. Individuals with alcohol dependence have a high occurrence of hyperlipidemia and hyperhomocysteinemia related to nutritional deficiencies (for example, folate and vitamins B_6 and B_{12}) (Jarvis et al., 2007; Porth, 2012).

Other than atherosclerosis, infective endocarditis is an additional cause of cardiovascular disease seen among individuals who are substance dependent (though not necessarily homeless). A relatively uncommon disease in the general population, infective endocarditis involves an infection of the interior surface of the heart, usually stemming from bacteria in the bloodstream. Such infections invariably lead to destruction of cardiac tissue, causing irreparable damage to the valves of the heart and symptoms consistent with both systemic infection and cardiac dysfunction (Porth, 2012). Because they regularly expose their bloodstreams to bacteria, injection drug users are particularly susceptible to endocarditis infection. The incidence of infective endocarditis in this population is more than 300 times that of the general population (Mylonakis & Calderwood, 2001), and those who abuse cocaine are at increased risk for coronary atherosclerosis (Patrizi et al., 2006). Together, these factors render homeless, substance-dependent individuals especially susceptible to cardiovascular disease.

Psychological Domain

Individuals do not use substances in a vacuum. Often, regular use develops in response to stressors and events such as trauma, changing financial conditions, or deteriorating relationships or circumstances (Mignon, Marcoux-Faiia, Myers, & Rubington, 2009). Recent statistics demonstrate that more than 8.4 million people have coexisting issues that encompass use of substances and mental health problems (SAMHSA, 2013). It is important for the nurse to appraise the level of insight a patient has about the effects of substances on his or her life. This can directly affect acceptance of the diagnosis and response to treatment. A key behavior the nurse often witnesses is profound **denial**, in which the patient denies use of any substance or problems/consequences associated with it. A strong, intact denial system may prevent or interfere with the individual's realistic examination of consequences resulting from drug use. In addition, feelings of hopelessness, anxiety, and possible suicidal ideations may surface as the nurse begins the assessment (Figure 20-2). Depressive symptoms are often seen and may be associated with shame. Often ostracized and labeled, individuals with an addictive disorder may be coping with an inability to feel positive in any

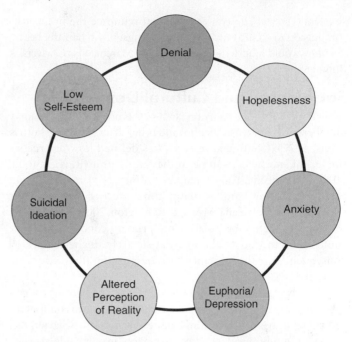

20-2   Psychological effects of substance use and abuse.

domain of health. Trying to wrestle with the chronicity of the disease and the negative view of others results in feelings of poor self-worth and low self-esteem. This can lead to further stigmatization by family members and the community (Oliver et al., 2012). Many individuals convince themselves that they are unable to function without the substance, and therefore exhibit extreme reactions of anxiety or fear when confronted about making changes in their lives (NIDA, 2011). Their ability to make informed, rational decisions is altered by neurochemical changes related to drug use. Individuals experience difficulty in the ability to focus, memory impairment, and difficulty with decisions and acceptance of changes. Their ability to think and focus toward a goal-oriented plan of a chemical-free lifestyle is impaired. Increased frustration and relapse into using the drug again initiates self-defeating behaviors and loss of purpose. Depressive symptomatology may be increased as neurotransmitters in the brain become unbalanced, and individuals may continue or increase their use of substances to ameliorate sad feelings or a sense of hopelessness. Studies have shown that with establishing healthy relationships, notably in self-help groups and through psychotherapy with a professional skilled in the treatment of addiction, individuals can begin the initial step in the recovery process. This step includes acceptance of who they are; recovery from the initial physical deterioration caused by the substance; sustaining abstinence; and learning to live with the chronic disease they now have.

Just as tolerance to the substance increases and the addictive cycle intensifies, the shame and stigma the individual faces may preclude seeking help for a life out of control. A concern shared by many health care professionals is that patients with a history of mental or emotional problems may view substance use as an easy solution to complex issues. Coexisting mental illness can confound the clinical presentation, as can concurrent use of multiple substances and potential medical sequelae of drug use.

One specific criterion seen in the progression of addiction is loss of control. The individual loses the ability to control use of the substance. This emerges as the substance alters both physical homeostasis and cognitive processes (Goode, 2007). The dependency on the substance creates lifestyle changes that reinforce the individual's compulsion to secure the drug, often by engaging in harmful behaviors they would otherwise avoid (Mignon, Marcoux-Faiia, Myers, & Rubington, 2009).

Sociological and Cultural Domains

Addiction is a process. Early research in this area shows that family members are affected by alcohol and other drug use (Klagsburn & Davis, 1977). Continued research has defined how destructive the use of substances can be to the family unit (Ruiz & Strain, 2011). The mechanism of adaptation manifests in a variety of ways, with some families being more successful than others (Mignon, Marcoux-Faiia, Myers, & Rubington, 2009). The inability to cope and increasing isolation are primary concerns. Uninterrupted substance abuse almost always leads to financial and legal consequences, as the substance becomes the prevailing priority in the individual's life.

Family relationships can both complicate and become complicated by drug use. Family members often feel unable to confront the individual who is dependent, and may even engage in behaviors that support the substance use. These behaviors may include allowing use of substances in the home, calling in sick for a family member who is using substances, keeping secrets about drug use in the family, and/or tolerating behavior that is dangerous or intimidating when drug use is involved. When friends or family members engage in these behaviors, they are **enabling** the individual to continue abusing drugs. When family members fail to address the behavior of the individual who is using substances, they are engaging in **codependency** (Mignon, Marcoux-Faiia, Myers, & Rubington, 2009). In other words, the family is dependent on maladaptive behaviors, just as the person using substances is dependent on the drug use. A hallmark behavior of codependency occurs when family members shield those using substances from the consequences of their actions. Other codependent behaviors include controlling and caretaking (Figure 20-3). Often, family members will lie to protect the individual with an addiction from the outside world. For example, a child whose parent is too intoxicated to answer the phone may tell a caller that "Mom is sick. She's sleeping right now." Although most professionals working in the field of substance abuse recognize codependency, there is a paucity of scientific research related to codependency.

Children who are raised in a family with alcohol or other drug use exhibit specific behaviors associated with the role they assume in their family as a result of destructive patterns. Pioneer work in this area defined what is commonly referred to as adult children of alcoholics or adult children of addicts (ACOA). The premise of this movement is that children bring the early pathology of the family into their adulthood and carry dysfunction into their own lives. The belief is that these adults do not have a sense of "normalcy" in a family and may exhibit their own patterns of destructive tendencies and dysfunction. Although this holds true for many families, continued research is necessary to support the construct that a high percentage of those individuals who grow up in a dysfunctional home suffer into adulthood. Nurses and clinicians working with families will do well to remember that the relationship between children and parents includes a shared history that is much more than that of the family's history of substance abuse (Mignon, Marcoux-Faiia, Myers, & Rubington, 2009).

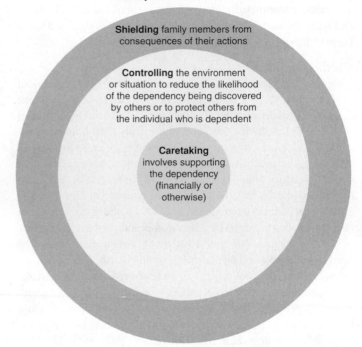

Codependent Behaviors

Shielding family members from consequences of their actions

Controlling the environment or situation to reduce the likelihood of the dependency being discovered by others or to protect others from the individual who is dependent

Caretaking involves supporting the dependency (financially or otherwise)

20-3 Codependent behaviors associated with substance use disorders.

There also is a cultural interplay when examining substance use and abuse. Researchers studying ethnicity related to use of substances continue to review patterns of similarities and differences. Different cultures address the use of substances in various ways based on religious use, expression, social impact, and belief systems. Some Native Americans, for instance, use hallucinogens in tribal and religious ceremonies, with very little abuse documented. However, further research of this group defines inhalant abuse and alcohol as primary concerns in this culture. One of the early landmark studies that reviewed data in Irish and Jewish cultures showed marked differences in the drinking habits of people and laid the groundwork for study in this area (Bales, 1946). The agricultural Irish used alcohol as a social outlet, whereas Jewish men drank at home in a religious context and demonstrated animosity toward drunkenness. Subsequent research documented the use of wine among Italian families. Many replicated studies support this early work and continue to examine why and how culture plays such a significant role in aspects of our society as it relates to substance use. Ethnologists are now examining the impact that culture brings to substance use and how the use of the substance affects the cultural community. Social scientists and anthropologists stress that in a blended society with a mix of cultures, it is misleading at best to apply extreme and definitive constructs when examining culture and how it relates to substance use and abuse for that group (SAMHSA, 2008).

Spiritual Domain

In the treatment of any addictive disorder, discussion in treatment often takes place regarding spiritual growth in recovery. Encouraging development of strategies that support healthy behaviors lends itself to strengthening the spiritual core for an individual. The outcome of this is connectedness and improved emotional well-being. It is important for nurses to be cognizant of the individual patient's attitudes toward spirituality and to support a plan for growth with which the patient feels comfortable. Some patients may seek a return to previous spiritual practices, whereas others may seek new outlets or may find other aspects of recovery as more essential.

Many patients find connectedness through participating in self-help groups. **Self-help groups** are both composed of and led by individuals who share the same or similar illness or addiction. The most popular self-help groups are Alcoholics Anonymous (AA) and Narcotics Anonymous (NA). AA/NA describe themselves as fellowships, although both encourage members to derive strength from a *Higher Power*, which some view in a religious context. Although some individuals in recovery choose to call their higher power in their deity's name, many others view the power of the group as their spiritual core. Thus, the spiritual connection in the group is their moral barometer. It speaks to a sense of self-worth, and meaning and purpose in their lives (Rosenblatt, 2007).

In the context of recovery, a Higher Power is viewed as the power outside the person that is greater than the individual. Thus, it could be a Higher Power, the power of the group, the love of family, the support of colleagues, or the fellowship of AA that assists individuals to understand the core values in their life and what is meaningful. Research has demonstrated that interventions promoting initial increases in spirituality appear to result in sustained AA affiliation, which results in sustained recovery over time (Tonigan, 2007). It is important to recognize the valuable role AA has, with more than 2 million members worldwide; studies have indicated that spirituality in AA membership seems to play a role in promoting remission of alcoholic symptoms (Galanter, 2008).

It is important to reflect that not all individuals who seek recovery will respond to a program that offers a spiritual connection in its format. Many do well in cognitive-based programs that examine thought and behavior without a moral construct to study (Perfas, 2004).

Pause and Reflect

1. *How is the brain involved in the development of substance use disorders?*
2. *What is the relationship between long-term substance abuse and cardiovascular diseases?*
3. *How can substance abuse affect family processes and relationships?*

Substance-Related and Addictive Disorders

The DSM-5 (APA, 2013) divides substance use disorders into two groups: substance-related disorders and substance-induced disorders. Substance-related disorders encompass 10 separate classes that address use and abuse of the following substances:

- Alcohol
- Cannabis
- Hallucinogens (with separate categories for phencyclidine and similarly acting hallucinogens)
- Inhalants
- Opioids
- Sedatives, hypnotics, and anxiolytics
- Stimulants (amphetamine-type substances, cocaine, and other stimulants)
- Caffeine
- Tobacco
- Other (or unknown) substances

In addition, the DSM-5 recognizes the new diagnosis of *gambling disorder*, which reflects evidence that behaviors associated with gambling activate the brain's reward center in ways similar to those of addictive drugs (APA, 2013). Diagnostic criteria for a substance use disorder are based on a pathological pattern of behaviors that are grouped under four general clusters: impaired control, social impairment, risky use, and pharmacological criteria (APA, 2013). Clinicians also apply the specifiers *mild, moderate,* and *severe* based on the number of symptoms present upon diagnosis.

Substance-induced disorders are characterized by the following conditions: intoxication, withdrawal, and other substance/medication-induced mental disorders. The essential feature of this classification is that the patient has developed a reversible substance-specific syndrome related to recent ingestion of a substance. Categories of substance/medication-induced mental disorders include psychotic disorders, bipolar and related disorders, depressive disorders, anxiety disorders, obsessive–compulsive and related disorders, sleep disorders, sexual dysfunctions, delirium, and neurocognitive disorders (APA, 2013).

The use of substances to change a feeling or affective state has a long history. **Substance abuse** can simply be defined as the harmful use of any substance for the purposes of improving or altering mood. **Drug abuse** may be defined as the use of any drug (illicit, prescription, or over-the-counter) for purposes other than those for which they are intended or in amounts or by methods other than as directed (NIDA, 2012a).

Drug use comprises both legal and illegal substances. Alcohol and tobacco are legal with age restrictions but are commonly used and abused. Prescription medications and steroids, although often prescribed for legitimate pain or medical conditions, can become problematic when unmonitored or overused. Other substances that are illegal for human consumption, such as inhalants, solvents, and designer drugs, have been shown to be lethal when used. Caffeine, although legal, is now being studied for the overuse and cardiac effects when consumed in large quantities (Yew, 2013). Nurses play an important role in identifying individuals experiencing substance abuse and in assisting them in recovery. As such, nurses must be aware of commonly abused substances, symptoms of use and withdrawal, and important considerations for nursing care (see Table 20-3).

Alcohol

Excessive use of alcohol can damage the brain and most body organs. Areas of the brain that are especially vulnerable to alcohol-related damage are the cerebral cortex (largely responsible for higher brain functions, including problem solving and decision making), the hippocampus (important to memory and learning), and the cerebellum (important for movement coordination) (NIDA, 2011) (Figure 20-4). Ethyl alcohol, or ethanol, is an intoxicating ingredient found in beer, wine, and liquor. Alcohol is a central nervous system depressant that

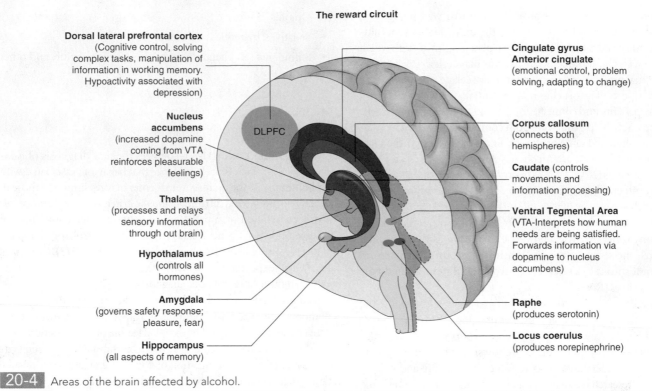

20-4   Areas of the brain affected by alcohol.

is rapidly absorbed from the stomach and small intestine into the bloodstream. A standard drink—12 ounces of beer, 8 ounces of malt liquor, 5 ounces of wine, or 1.5 ounces (a "shot") of 80-proof distilled spirits or liquor (such as gin, rum, vodka, or whiskey)—equals 0.6 ounces of pure ethanol (NIDA, 2012b) (Figure 20-5). Ninety to ninety-five percent of the alcohol ingested is metabolized by the ADH–ALDH enzymatic system and eliminated as water and CO_2. A small portion can be measured in urine, and the remainder is excreted unchanged in the urine, sweat, and breath (Ruiz & Strain, 2011). Intoxication also impairs brain function and motor skills. Most states recognize a blood alcohol content (BAC) level of 0.08% as a threshold for determining intoxication, especially related to driving privileges, although physiological and psychological responses that can impair coordination and judgment typically occur before an

individual reaches that threshold (Figure 20-6). Continued and chronic use may increase risk of certain cancers, stroke, and liver disease. Alcoholism or alcohol dependence is a diagnosable disease characterized by a strong craving for alcohol, and/or continued use despite harm or personal injury. Alcohol abuse, which can lead to alcoholism, is a pattern of drinking that results in harm to one's health, interpersonal relationships, or ability to work (NIDA, 2012b; SAMHSA, 2013). Specific patterns of alcohol use include heavy drinking and binge drinking (Box 20-2).

Caffeine

Caffeine is available in both liquid and pill form. Coffee, tea, and energy drinks are the primary methods by which people use caffeine. Excessive consumption of caffeine may result in cardiac effects,

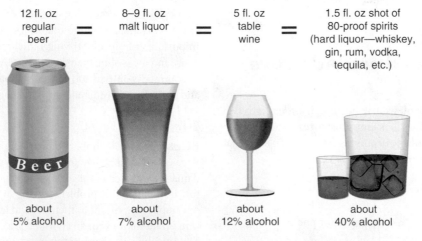

20-5   One standard drink = ½ ounce of ethyl alcohol.

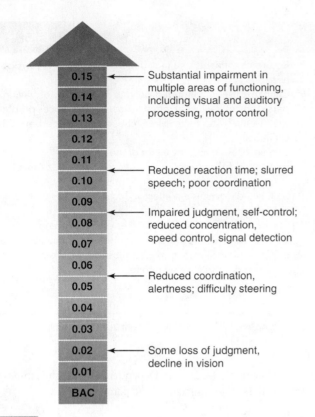

Substantial impairment in multiple areas of functioning, including visual and auditory processing, motor control

Reduced reaction time; slurred speech; poor coordination

Impaired judgment, self-control; reduced concentration, speed control, signal detection

Reduced coordination, alertness; difficulty steering

Some loss of judgment, decline in vision

20-6 Some of the typical effects of drinking alcohol by blood alcohol content (BAC), the percentage of alcohol by volume in the blood. Note that some decline in vision and loss of judgment appears as early as 0.02% BAC.

including palpitations, sweating, headache, and severe tremulousness. It may take a prolonged period of time for an individual's body to process the caffeine sufficiently to see a reduction in symptoms. Although typically tea has the least amount of caffeine of the three types of drinks mentioned previously, caffeine amounts can vary widely. This is especially true for energy drinks, which may contain more caffeine than advertised. A study conducted by *Consumer Reports* found that the amount of caffeine in energy drinks ranged from 6 mg to 242 mg per serving, as compared to an 8-ounce cup of coffee, which typically contains 100 mg per serving (Consumer Reports, 2012). Energy drinks can be particularly dangerous when mixed with alcohol (CDC, 2014).

Marijuana (Cannabis)

Typically ingested through smoking, marijuana comes from the plant *Cannabis sativa*, and usually appears as shredded parts of the plant.

Marijuana is the single most commonly abused illicit substance (SAMHSA, 2013). This is in part because the resulting euphoria may last as long as 3 hours or more, depending on the potency and amount used (NHTSA, 2013). Individuals abusing marijuana typically have bloodshot eyes and an elevated heart rate. Marijuana also impairs short-term memory and learning, the ability to focus attention, and coordination (NIDA, 2012c). Hallucinations and paranoia may be present in individuals who use large quantities. Marijuana users may experience lung irritation and are at increased risk for respiratory illness. See DSM-5 Diagnostic Criteria for Cannabis Use Disorder.

Hallucinogens

Hallucinogens are drugs that alter perception. Lysergic acid diethylamide (LSD) is one of the most potent hallucinogens. Its effects are unpredictable; those who abuse it may see vivid colors and images, hear sounds, and feel sensations that seem real but do not exist (synesthesia). LSD is also associated with traumatic experiences and emotions that can last for many hours. Biophysical symptoms include rapid mood swings, increase in heart rate and blood pressure, dilated pupils, loss of appetite, sweating, and tremors. **Flashbacks**—hallucinations or altered perceptions occurring well after an individual has used—are common in LSD users, even after long periods of abstinence.

Inhalants

Inhalants are volatile substances found in many household products, such as oven cleaners, gasoline, spray paints, and other aerosols. Most inhalants act as central nervous system depressants, causing euphoria, drowsiness, lightheadedness, impaired coordination, and loss of inhibition. Additional effects vary depending on the chemicals contained in the inhalant used. Heart failure can occur with either first or later use. Chronic use of inhalants may include liver damage, hearing loss, and diminished cognitive functioning (Stoppler, 2013; NIDA, 2012d).

Opioids/Opiates

Opioids include prescription medications used to treat severe pain, as well as the street drug commonly known as heroin. Opioids/opiates produce euphoria and feelings of relaxation. They also slow respiration and can increase risk of serious infectious diseases, especially when taken intravenously. Examples of opioids include morphine, methadone, oxycodone (Oxycontin), hydrocodone with acetaminophen (Vicodin), and oxycodone with aspirin (Percodan), all of which have legitimate medical uses; however, their nonmedical use or abuse can result in the same harmful consequences as abusing heroin (NIDA, 2011). Heroin is a semisynthetic drug made by treating morphine with acetic anhydride to yield diacetylmorphine. When it enters the brain,

Risks of Binge Drinking   box 20-2

Heavy drinking generally is defined as a pattern of drinking that consists of more than two drinks per day for men and more than one drink per day for women. **Binge drinking** is defined as the consumption of five or more drinks for men or four or more drinks for women within a 2-hour period (CDC, 2012a).

Binge drinking is a serious issue, especially for women. The CDC reports that binge drinking increases the risk for a number of illnesses and complications, including breast cancer, sexually transmitted infections, and unintended pregnancy. More than 90% of the alcohol drunk by youth is consumed while binge drinking. Binge drinking is greatly associated with risky behaviors, such as drinking and driving (CDC, 2012b).

Diagnostic Criteria for Cannabis Use Disorder | DSM-5

A. A problematic pattern of cannabis use leading to clinically significant impairment or distress, as manifested by at least two of the following, occurring within a 12-month period:
1. Cannabis is often taken in larger amounts or over a longer period than was intended.
2. There is a persistent desire or unsuccessful efforts to cut down or control cannabis use.
3. A great deal of time is spent in activities necessary to obtain cannabis, use cannabis, or recover from its effects.
4. Craving, or a strong desire or urge to use cannabis.
5. Recurrent cannabis use resulting in a failure to fulfill major role obligations at work, school, or home.
6. Continued cannabis use despite having persistent or recurrent social or interpersonal problems caused or exacerbated by the effects of cannabis.
7. Important social, occupational, or recreational activities are given up or reduced because of cannabis use.

8. Recurrent cannabis use in situations in which it is physically hazardous.
9. Cannabis use is continued despite knowledge of having a persistent or recurrent physical or psychological problem that is likely to have been caused or exacerbated by cannabis.
10. Tolerance, as defined by either of the following:
    a. A need for markedly increased amounts of cannabis to achieve intoxication or desired effect.
    b. Markedly diminished effect with continued use of the same amount of cannabis.
11. Withdrawal, as manifested by either of the following:
    a. The characteristic withdrawal syndrome for cannabis.
    b. Cannabis (or a closely related substance) is taken to relieve or avoid withdrawal symptoms.

Source: Reprinted with permission from the *Diagnostic and Statistical Manual of Mental Disorders*, Fifth Edition, (Copyright 2013). American Psychiatric Association.

---

heroin converts to morphine and acts on the opioid receptors. Routes of administration of heroin include injection and inhalation.

Symptoms of intoxication include drowsiness and slurred speech. Overdose may result in respiratory depression or even death. Prolonged use of opioids in individuals who do not have any legitimate medical use for them may result in an opioid use disorder. Indications that an individual has developed an opioid use disorder include spending an inordinate amount of time trying to obtain the substance or recover from its effects; failure to fulfill major role functions due to the effect of the substance; continued use despite detrimental effects on interpersonal relationships or physical health; and symptoms of tolerance and/or withdrawal (APA, 2013).

Stimulants

Stimulants produce feelings of euphoria and alertness. They include both amphetamine-like substances and cocaine. Amphetamines include an array of both illegal and prescription drugs. Methylphenidate (Ritalin) is an example of a stimulant frequently prescribed for attention-deficit/hyperactivity disorder. Stimulants are highly addictive; abuse of them carries risk of long-term adverse effects, particularly on brain function and the cardiovascular system. Common symptoms of stimulant use include increased heart rate, elevated blood pressure, confusion, restlessness and agitation, and muscular weakness. With heavy use, respiratory depression, arrhythmias, or seizures may occur (APA, 2013).

Amphetamines

The most popular stimulant is methamphetamine ("meth"), a form of amphetamine. Methamphetamine is highly addictive, and is manufactured as a white crystalline powder that can be smoked or injected. Its production involves dangerous, potentially explosive chemical processes. Amphetamines are associated with increased heart rate, blood pressure, and metabolism. Even casual use is associated with reduced appetite and weight loss. Amphetamines can cause high body temperature and can lead to serious heart problems and seizures. Methamphetamine's effects are particularly long lasting and harmful to the brain as a result of its ability to alter the activity of the

dopamine system (NIDA, 2010a). Dependence on amphetamines is associated with hostility, aggression, and paranoia.

Cocaine

Cocaine is one of the most powerful central nervous stimulants of natural origin. It is a white crystalline powder derived from coca leaf paste. It is often mixed with other white powders, such as lactose and mannitol, when sold on the street. Even though cocaine is a stimulant, it was classified as a narcotic in 1922 in the United States to apply the same controls to it as with opiates. Cocaine can be injected, inhaled, or snorted. *Crack* is a form of cocaine that is made from ammonia, baking soda, and water. The name "crack" describes the sound that occurs when this type of cocaine is smoked. It is considered highly addictive (NIDA, 2009b).

As a powerful CNS stimulant, cocaine can cause a wide variety of responses in addition to euphoria, including hypervigilance, restlessness and irritability, increased heart rate, nausea or vomiting, respiratory depression, impaired judgment, and confusion.

Two symptoms of cocaine use that can be especially alarming to family and friends are seizures and psychosis, the latter often presenting as paranoia. Impaired functioning, in personal relationships and at work, can occur with either acute or chronic use of cocaine. Cocaine withdrawal syndrome can occur within a few hours of cessation and is characterized by an intense craving for the drug as well as dysphoria and physiological changes, such as fatigue and increased appetite.

Tobacco

Tobacco use disorder is recognized as a substance use disorder because tobacco products contain *nicotine*, an addictive stimulant. Tobacco products include cigarettes, cigars, and chewing tobacco. Tobacco smoke increases a user's risk of cancer, emphysema, bronchial disorders, and cardiovascular disease. Use of tobacco rises to the level of a disorder when the individual has a persistent desire or craving for the substance and spends increasing time on activities related to obtaining or using tobacco to the extent of reducing or eliminating other activities or failing to meet obligations in major roles (e.g., work, home) (APA, 2013). The mortality rate associated with tobacco addiction is extremely high. Tobacco use has been attributed to approximately 100 million deaths during the 20th century and, if current smoking trends continue, the cumulative death toll for this century has been projected to reach 1 billion (NIDA, 2011).

> **PRACTICE ALERT** A particularly dangerous and not uncommon practice is the combining of two or more drugs. The practice ranges from the co-administration of legal drugs such as alcohol and nicotine, to the dangerous random mixing of prescription drugs, to the deadly combination of heroin or cocaine with fentanyl (an opioid pain medication). Whatever the context, it is critical to realize that because of drug–drug interactions, such practices often pose significantly higher risks than use of the already harmful individual drugs.

Factors Affecting Use and Addiction

A number of factors affect use and addiction. Routes of administration, for example, may affect how quickly a drug reaches the bloodstream, cost, and potential adverse effects. Coexisting mental or physical illness may also affect substance abuse and dependence.

Routes of Administration

Psychoactive substances are consumed by mouth (in capsules, tablets, or liquid form), injection, smoking, or inhalation. Individuals often begin using a substance in one form and increase their use by a different method as tolerance develops. Tolerance is a key indicator that the body is adapting to the use of the substance. The individual's method of use is directly related to the drug itself and how fast it can be delivered with the desired effect. Smoking and injection deliver drugs quickly and thus are considered more addictive than other routes (Figure 20-7). This may explain the popularity of smoking tobacco and using heroin among individuals who use substances (Samaha & Robinson, 2005).

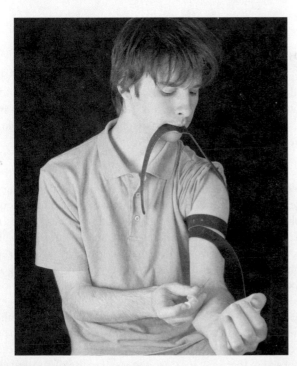

20-7 Injection and smoking allow for faster delivery of a drug and are more addictive than other routes of administration.

Source: Malyshev Maksim/Shutterstock

Co-Morbid Mental Illness

The National Institute on Drug Abuse estimates that six out of ten people with addictive disorders also have mental health problems. More often, people with coexisting mental health and addictive disorders may have multiple drug, alcohol, mental health, and medical health issues, referred to as co-occurring disorders (CODs) (Dennison, 2011). The problem is not insignificant: Those with mental illness (any mental illness and serious mental illness) experience substance abuse or dependence at three to four times the rate of the general population (SAMHSA, 2013).

Patients with both substance abuse disorders and mental illness often exhibit more severe symptoms and are in need of specialized treatment programs. Treatment of only one of the disorders often results in inadequate treatment and relapse, whereas programs that treat both disorders simultaneously have the best treatment results. For patients suffering from depression, posttraumatic stress disorder (PTSD), bipolar disorder, or other psychiatric conditions, substances may serve as a way to self-medicate and ease the pain and discomfort from their symptoms. Abstinence does not resolve the underlying mental health issues; in fact, many patients may feel and experience a great deal of pain once substance use is discontinued. This vulnerability to the re-experience of past trauma and the emergence of strong emotions and psychiatric symptoms can lead to relapse of the addictive behavior and continued use of substances (Hoff & Morgan, 2011).

The co-morbid problem of addictive disorders and mental illness has major implications for social and economic issues as well as the prognosis for treatment of those with both disorders. Issues such as poverty, homelessness, risk for violence, risk for accidental and homicidal deaths, and risky sexual behavior are often increased in the population with both disorders (Dennison, 2011).

Use of tobacco is also highly correlated with substance abuse, relapse, and early dropout from treatment. Despite research regarding lethality issues and smoking, for decades psychiatric inpatient and outpatient settings continued to allow—and even encourage—the use of tobacco as a way to gain compliance with other treatments. Over the past 10 to 15 years, as knowledge of early death rates of those with severe mental illness (SMI) 20 to 25 years earlier than that of the general population has increased, the need for a focus on smoking cessation in the population of people with mental illness has developed. Smoking cessation programs, as well as medication assistance in smoking cessation, should be offered to all people with mental illness in inpatient and outpatient treatment. The use of multiple strategies rather than a single intervention may be necessary with this population.

Pain

Chronic pain is one of the most common reasons that people seek health care (Kleiber, Jain, & Trivedi, 2005). A significant number of people who have chronic pain also have co-morbid psychiatric disorders. Unrecognized pain in psychiatric illness, and unrecognized psychiatric illness in chronic pain, can diminish the treatment response of individuals and worsen clinical outcomes. Undertreatment of either pain or psychiatric illness can have a serious impact on quality of life and the ability to function in work and social settings.

Portenoy (2011) and many others have examined the complex relationship between pain management and drug addiction. The increased use of opioids in the United States has led to concerns regarding development of an addiction among those with chronic pain conditions and concerns about treating those with an identified addictive disorder, as well as problems with drug diversion. Individuals with addictive disorders who have multiple medical problems often have pain as a result of those medical problems.

The focus for health care professionals begins with a thorough assessment of any painful problem, no matter what the patient's diagnosis may be. McCaffery's definition of pain as "whatever the experiencing person says it is, existing whenever s/he says it does" (McCaffery, 1968, p. 95) is the nursing approach to begin the assessment. Understanding the terms commonly used with pain management and addictive disease is also essential for differentiating the problems that patients present.

Important considerations for treating individuals with co-morbid disorders that cause chronic pain include the following:

- *Tolerance:* A tolerance or addiction to opiates needs to be considered before treatment begins, as this may affect the amount of opiate needed to achieve pain relief.

- *Pseudoaddiction:* Pseudoaddiction is defined as a syndrome caused by the undertreatment of pain. It is characterized by patient behaviors such as anger and escalating demands for more or different medications. It may appear that the patient is "drug-seeking," when in reality the patient is being undertreated for pain. When pain is treated adequately, the symptoms of pseudoaddiction resolve (Weissman & Haddox, 1989).

In the past two decades, the problem of pain and addictive disorders in the United States has been examined from different perspectives. Patients who have chronic pain may be at risk for developing an addictive disorder, and patients with addictive disorders may have chronic painful conditions for which they need pain relief. Much of the research in this area has focused on the patient with chronic pain and the risk for developing an addictive disorder. Many studies have attempted to define or interpret problematic behaviors in the chronic pain population as they relate to use of opiates primarily. Research is lacking, however, in the area of pain management for patients with addictive behaviors. Examination of the behaviors in the chronic pain population that indicate a problem with opiate use has termed these behaviors aberrant behaviors. These same behaviors may indicate when a person with a known addictive disorder is having difficulty managing the use of opiates for pain relief. Aberrant behaviors that are more predictive of addiction include forgery, selling of prescriptions, stealing or using someone else's drugs, obtaining prescriptions from more than one source, concurrent use of alcohol or other drugs, multiple dose increases, and decreased participation in or ability to work or function socially.

Behaviors that are less indicative of addiction include complaining or the need for more of a drug, requests for specific drugs, or dose escalation on one or two occasions (Fleming, Davis, & Passik, 2008).

The American Society of Pain Management Nurses (ASPMN), in its *Position Statement: Pain Management in Patients with Addictive Disease*, has stated, "Too often a patient's request for more or different medications is erroneously assumed to be addiction, and the possibility of under-treated pain is not explored" (2003, p. 2). To ensure that patients with addictive disease receive adequate pain treatment, it is recommended that a team of providers work together to treat the pain, while increasing services and supports for the addictive disorders. Use of treatment agreements, urine toxicology screening, and regular assessment of the pain scores with assessment of the patient's ability to function and activity level, as well as assessment of adverse effects of the pain medications, are important issues to be included in the treatment plan of a patient with pain and an addictive disorder (Cheatle & O'Brien, 2011).

Co-Morbid Medical Conditions

Other commonly seen medical conditions in patients with substance abuse problems include HIV/AIDS and hepatitis C, in large part because IV drug use is one of the main modes of transmission of both HIV and hepatitis C. In fact, the highest rates of HIV are found in individuals with substance abuse problems and serious mental illness (Goforth et al., 2011). Alcohol, IV drug use, and amphetamine use have been linked to an increased risk for HIV and hepatitis C.

Treatment programs for people with substance abuse problems should include medical care and education about risk for related medical conditions. Harm reduction programs will assist individuals with addictive diseases in caring for their health when they are not ready to stop using drugs. Treatment programs also need to include care for individuals with HIV and hepatitis C that recognizes that these patients will not be able to navigate care on their own while dealing with their addictive disease. A thorough understanding of some of the neuropsychological complications of HIV is necessary for those providing care to this population, as some of the neuropsychological problems may mimic substance intoxication, withdrawal, or psychiatric problems.

Pause and Reflect

1. *To what extent do you think substance use is acceptable? Why?*

2. *Do you know anyone who engages in binge drinking? Are you willing to talk to him or her about it after reading this chapter? What would you say?*

3. *What precautions are necessary when treating someone with an addictive disorder for pain?*

Vulnerable Populations

Certain populations may be more vulnerable to or at greater risk for the development of addictive disease and may experience greater negative consequences of drug use. The following section examines selected groups of individuals who may be at special risk of developing addictive disorders.

Adolescents

Adolescence is generally thought of as a time of experimentation. The effect of peer pressure on adolescents to try something new often involves the use of drugs and/or alcohol. Although many adolescents experiment, some individuals are at risk for developing lifelong problems with drugs and alcohol. Research has identified factors relevant to this age group. For example, adolescents who begin drinking alcohol before the age of 17 are at greater risk for developing an alcohol problem than those who started drinking at ages 18 through 25. Whether the substance is prescription medications such as Ritalin or alcohol used by adults in the home, children and adolescents in high-risk categories may initiate their use of substances at much earlier ages. Factors that may increase the risk for use of substances in children and adolescents include trauma, violence in the home or community, poverty, living with a family member who has a mental health disorder, and chronic illness (SAMHSA, 2011a).

Substances used by adolescents tend to vary with age. In 2012, almost 10% of youths ages 12 to 17 reported using illicit drugs The rate of alcohol use in adolescents appears to increase steadily with age with rates of use reported as follows: 11.1% among youth ages 14 and 15, 24.8% among adolescents ages 16 and 17, and 45.8% among young people ages 18 to 20 (SAMHSA, 2013).

The National Survey on Drug Use and Health conducted in 2012 sheds further light on drinking among adolescents. Binge drinking (see Box 20-2) among adolescents is reported at 7.2% but increases to 45.1% in the 18-to-25 age group. Heavy drinking rates are also higher in older youth (SAMHSA, 2013). Driving under the influence was reported by 11.2% of those surveyed, with the 18-to-25-year-old group reporting the highest rates of driving under the influence of alcohol or other drugs.

Prescription drug use among adolescents is on the rise. Prescription drug abuse involves use of a medication that was prescribed for someone else or use of one's own prescription in a manner or dose different from what was prescribed. Most of the adolescents surveyed indicated that they obtained these drugs from family or friends and viewed the drugs as safe because they were prescribed by a professional. Prescription drugs commonly used by adolescents include opioids; central nervous system depressants, such as alprazolam (Xanax); stimulants, such as atomoxetine (Adderal) and methylphenidate (Concerta); and dextromethorphan, a cough suppressant found in many over-the-counter cough and cold medications (NIDA, 2011).

Prevention programs focus on educating adolescents about the risks of use of illicit and prescribed medications and attempt to identify and prevent risky behavior before the use begins. Work with adolescents who have already begun substance use focuses on prevention of further use and addiction (NIDA, 2003). Community involvement is essential in developing effective prevention programs for this population.

Women

More than 12 million women annually report problems with substance abuse (SAMHSA, 2010). The disease in women often co-occurs with domestic violence; risky sexual behavior and abuse; unwanted pregnancy; mental illness, including depression and PTSD; fetal alcohol syndrome; and other medical illness (SAMHSA, 2010).

Women are at higher risk than men for developing physical problems related to alcohol. Women often begin heavy drinking later in life than men (in their 20s to 30s) and experience consequences of their drinking in a shorter period of time than men. This phenomenon has been referred to as **telescoping**, a quick progression from the start of substance use to dependence and problematic use requiring treatment (Brady & Randall, 1999). Additionally, gender differences related to the body's response to certain drugs and to relapse have been demonstrated. Hormonal fluctuation across time related to changes in the menstrual cycle is an area that may affect the difference in response experienced by women. Women may be more affected by alcohol owing to their lower rate of body water by percentage, as well as decreased amounts of alcohol dehydrogenase in the gastric mucosa, thereby slowing first-pass metabolism, and metabolism of alcohol in general (Greenfield, Back, Lawson, & Brady, 2011).

Nicotine, in particular, has severe consequences for women. Women who smoke are twice as likely to have a heart attack as men who smoke, and they also experience faster lung deterioration and greater risk for COPD and lung cancer (Figure 20-8). Smoking can also

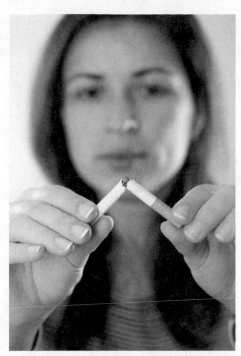

20-8 Substance use has wide-ranging implications for health and wellness. For example, women who smoke experience greater risk for heart attack and faster lung deterioration than men.

Source: Bojan Pavlukovic/Fotolia

increase the risk of spontaneous abortion, increase difficulty becoming pregnant, and increase the likelihood of early menopause. Risk to children born of mothers who smoke includes early sudden death, low birth weight, and other complications (Greenfield et al., 2011).

Women are less likely to seek treatment, drop out of treatment more often, and attend fewer treatment sessions than men (Greenfield et al., 2011). Issues that affect these responses to treatment are often focused around the role issues for women. Women often place themselves last in order of priorities following care of children, partners, and others. Issues such as domestic violence, financial constraints, and lack of transportation also affect women's ability to fully participate in treatment.

Much research is needed in terms of gender-specific diagnosis and treatment for women with addictive disorders. Treatment programs that link and connect women to care for the co-morbid mental illness and physical illnesses, and that address social and economic challenges, are essential to encouraging women to adhere to treatment. Trauma-informed care is often essential in the treatment of women with addictive diseases owing to the co-morbid problems related to violence in women's lives.

Perinatal Substance Use

Despite widespread knowledge that alcohol and other drugs may affect the developing fetus, some women continue to use or abuse substances during pregnancy. Use of alcohol during pregnancy can cause complications such as early labor, spontaneous abortion, and fetal alcohol spectrum disorder (FASD). Children born with FASD may have multiple problems in the physical, cognitive, and psychiatric arenas. Physical problems can include facial and ear malformation, heart defects, decreased muscle tone, and poor coordination. Cognitive and behavioral problems can include delayed development in thinking, speech, movement or social skills, impulse control problems and ADHD, and psychiatric issues such as mood, conduct and behavior disorders can occur (Greenfield et al., 2011).

Use of other substances during pregnancy can also result in complications for the fetus and in the birth process. Nicotine use during pregnancy, for example, has been associated with hypertension, vitamin deficiencies in the mother, congenital malformations, low birth weight, and cognitive deficits.

Older Adults

Clear documentation of the problem of substance abuse in older adults is not readily available. SAMHSA studies related to substance abuse group all adults over the age of 26 together, so actual information about adults over the age of 65 is difficult to determine. Recent literature, however, suggests that alcohol abuse and prescription drug abuse are increasing in the over-65 age group, at least in part due to the aging of the baby boomer generation, many of whom have long used substances recreationally (Morgan, White, & Wallace, 2011). Societal attitudes, as well as professional biases and stereotyping, may lead to underidentification and inadequate assessment of the problem of alcohol and substance abuse in older adults.

Screening tools used with other populations may not be accurate in assessing substance abuse among older adults. A thorough history and health assessment are always essential in screening for use of alcohol or other drugs in this population. The most commonly used screening tool, the CAGE questionnaire (discussed later in this chapter), has been used with older adults; however, a score of 1 or more (as opposed to a score of 2 or more with the general population) is considered a positive screen for those over the age of 60 (Dekker, 2002). The Michigan Alcoholism Screening Test-Geriatric (MAST-G), an adaptation of the original MAST, consists of 24 (long form) or 10 (shortened version) questions for older adults (Blow et al., 1992). Shulman (2003) developed a tool that attempted to address some of the shortcomings of screening tools for older adults. Also, the Impressions of Medication, Alcohol, and Drug Use in Seniors (IMADUS), screens for problems with alcohol, prescription drugs, and over-the-counter drugs, and also attempts to reduce the shame experienced by older adults who may misuse or abuse substances. Three or more positive answers indicate the need for further assessment.

Research has indicated that older adults have better treatment outcomes if treated in programs geared for older adults that include one-on-one counseling, nonconfrontational approaches, and attention to both medical and psychiatric co-morbid conditions (Atkinson, 1995; Blow, 2000; Morgan, White, & Wallace, 2011). Cognitive–behavioral interventions have been shown to be helpful in this population as well (Loukissa, 2007). Older adults may be more adherent to treatment recommendations than younger adults (Oslin, Pettinati, & Volpicelli, 2002).

Veterans

Veterans, particularly those who served in combat, are prone to PTSD. Experts are predicting a precipitous increase in the problems with substance use and abuse in military personnel who experienced active duty in Iraq and/or Afghanistan. Additionally, combat exposure increases the risk for mental and cognitive disorders, PTSD, and substance abuse and dependence. High rates of sleep problems, traumatic brain injuries, and relationship violence have also been identified in active and recently retired military personnel (NIDA, 2009a).

The military establishment, in conjunction with NIDA (2009a), has recently developed an increased focus on prevention and early identification of problems to assist in dealing with these problems. Diminishing the stigma associated with mental health and substance abuse issues among military personnel is essential in increasing the number of military personnel who seek treatment for these problems. Screening of all personnel prior to release will help identify at-risk veterans as they reenter civilian life. Trauma-informed care has an important role in the development of treatment programs for veterans with PTSD.

Gay, Lesbian, Bisexual, and Transgender Individuals

Research has indicated that many factors cause an increased risk for development of substance abuse among gay, lesbian, bisexual, and transgender (GLBT or LGBT) adolescents and adults (Jordan, 2000). The estimated incidence of substance abuse in this population ranges from 28% to 35%, as compared to 10% to 12% for the general population (Cabaj, 2011). Risk factors that may affect this increased rate of substance abuse include issues such as race, age of introduction to substances, depression, and peer risk behaviors. Additionally, the risk for suicide and suicide attempts is often increased in GLBT individuals who misuse/abuse substances, and GLBT youth are at very high risk (Cabaj, 2011).

The additional stress during adolescence of coping with sexual orientation or gender identity issues may lead to feelings of marginalization, depression, and isolation. GLBT youth may socialize in clubs and bars, and this access may lead to early drinking and substance use. Adequate assessment of GLBT patients should include questions about coming-out experiences, social support and activities, school difficulties, teasing, bullying, or violence history, as well as relationships with their family of origin.

Treatment facilities that are specifically oriented to GLBT individuals may be important in the identification and treatment of substance abuse problems in this population. If such facilities are not available, referral to an accepting, culturally sensitive provider or a specialized AA/NA group may be helpful. Countertransference issues in a provider can cloud treatment and add to stigma and traumatization of GLBT patients; thus, education and support for providers may be a very important aspect of caring for this population. Trauma-informed care may be an essential component of the treatment programs needed for this population because of the increased level of violence in the lives of individuals who identify as GLBT.

Homeless Individuals

Individuals who become homeless are at increased risk for co-morbid addiction and mental illness; this risk is even higher in those who are chronically homeless. Individuals who are homeless have more difficulty accessing treatment and other supports (such as housing, access to financial support, and meals). Issues of stigma and discrimination are especially potent in this population and lead to fragmented and inadequate medical and psychiatric care. Additionally, homeless individuals are susceptible to a variety of health problems. Lee et al. (2005) found that cardiovascular risk factors associated with homelessness are more difficult to address and attributed cardiovascular risk among the homeless to greater use of cocaine and cigarettes than in the general population. Homelessness is associated with a much greater risk of trauma, with 88% of homeless mothers studied reporting a history of violent trauma (Bassuk, Buckner, Perloff, & Bassuk, 1998).

Harm reduction and relapse prevention are strategies that are useful in engaging homeless individuals in treatment. Treatment models that provide comprehensive medical, psychiatric, and addictive disease care as well as housing and other supports have been demonstrated to improve outcomes in this population; however, funding remains a major hurdle in the provision of this care (Feldman, 2011).

Incarcerated Individuals

Individuals in prison have a higher incidence of substance use and abuse than those in the general population. Opiate, cocaine, and polysubstance abuse are common among prisoners, increasing their risk for health problems such as HIV and hepatitis C (Kinlock, Gordon, & Schwartz, 2011). Continued drug use is possible in prison settings, but more often individuals will go through drug or alcohol withdrawal upon entering the prison, with or without treatment of the withdrawal symptoms. Treatment programs are not always available in prisons, increasing the risk of relapse and re-incarceration for inmates when they leave the prison setting. This risk of relapse, the risks of developing HIV and hepatitis C, and crimes related to substance abuse make prisons an ideal place for prevention programs and active treatment of addictive diseases. Harm reduction education, HIV and hepatitis C testing, as well as linkages with programs prior to release from prison, are all public health issues that are crucial for the success of recovery for prisoners.

Pause and Reflect

1. *What challenges do you think you would face in caring for a woman who is pregnant and abusing alcohol? Abusing cocaine?*

2. *How would you go about providing this woman with safe, evidence-based care?*

3. *What are some of the challenges for the nurse working with patients who are homeless? How could you work to address these challenges?*

Collaborative Care

Collaborative care for patients seeking treatment for substance abuse depends on a number of factors, including the substance used, amounts and length of time used, presence of co-morbid conditions, and individual (such as health insurance) and community resources (variety and nature of programs) available. Many individuals initiate sobriety and recovery alone or in conjunction with participation in self-help groups. Because patients who use and abuse substances can interact with the health care system at various points on a continuum, nurses in all settings should know what resources are available in their community and should be familiar with the referral or entry paths for those resources.

Treatment for addictive disorders is considered to be most effective when delivered in a comprehensive manner that encompasses all facets of care that support recovery (SAMHSA, 2012). A well-integrated program will coordinate medical, social, psychological, vocational, and possible pharmacological strategies that are useful in laying the groundwork for early abstinence from a substance and thus promoting sustained recovery. This type of care emphasizes education as well as recreation so that the person develops cognitive and social skills for a drug-free lifestyle. In addition, stress reduction, relaxation, and creative therapy have been found to be useful components in providing an overall approach to recovery that promotes adherence and structure with an individualized plan (Mignon, Marcoux-Faiia, Myers, & Rubington, 2009). Treatment of patients with co-morbid or co-occurring disorders (COD) can be particularly challenging. Many of these patients will need pharmacotherapy combined with other forms of therapy. Treatment for COD is discussed in Box 20-3. The goal of all treatments for individuals who suffer from addictive disorders is to assist them in improving their quality of life, hopefully with the participation of family members and significant others.

Screening, Brief Intervention, and Referral to Treatment (SBIRT)

Screening, brief intervention, and referral to treatment (SBIRT) is an approach to substance abuse intervention and treatment designed to be sustainable in all venues of health care. It is the avenue that providers,

---

Treatment Considerations for Patients with Co-Occurring Disorders	box 20-3

Comprehensive treatment of COD involves using best practices in the field. Development of programs that involves integrated treatment of COD must focus on treatment that is flexible, provides long-term support for patients, and involves use of medication as well as a variety of therapeutic approaches (Dennison, 2011). Earlier models of treatment designated different and separate approaches for psychiatric disorders and addictive disorders. Over the past decade or two, this thinking has changed in many settings, and with increased evidence from data now suggesting that treatment needs to include both problems (psychiatric and addictive disorders) at the same time. Although much progress has been made, many programs and providers still adhere to the "old" way of thinking and may give patients incorrect information. Educational models have also been developed to include both disorders and their treatment for new clinicians entering either of these fields. Changing the approach for "more seasoned" providers may be more difficult and take more evidence and time.

Currently, the use of medication as a part of the treatment for patients with COD is more widely accepted, but certain issues are important to consider when choosing a medication for this patient population. Dennison (2011) lists principles for the use of such medications, primarily that the medication:

- Does not induce euphoria, even in higher doses than those prescribed.
- Does not cause dependence.
- Is effective even among those who may be actively using substances.
- Is safe in the actively using individual.

Treatment models that indicate superiority for successful treatment of COD have not consistently been identified in research, although this is an area in which much research activity has been focused in recent years.

educators, and clinicians can use to help individuals identify and address problems in life that arise from substance use/misuse or abuse. In addition to the usual route of health care providers, university campuses are using this approach to stem the tide of adverse effects from substance use in the lives of students. Gryczynski et al. (2011) reviewed the following programs and define SBIRT in the following manner:

- *Screening:* A health care professional assesses a patient for risky substance use behaviors using standardized screening tools.
- *Brief intervention:* A health care professional engages a patient showing risky substance use behaviors in a short conversation, providing feedback and advice.
- *Referral to treatment:* A health care professional provides a referral to therapy or additional treatment to patients who screen in need of additional services.

Beyond connecting individuals with substance dependence to treatment options, using SBIRT as an early intervention can reduce risky alcohol and drug use before they lead to more severe consequences or dependence. The effectiveness of brief interventions with patients can promote significant, lasting reductions in risky use of alcohol and other drugs. This outcome was demonstrated in a review of New Mexico's SBIRT program, which found that participants in the SBIRT program reported a significant decrease in drug and alcohol use within 6 months of receiving services (Gryczynski et al., 2011).

Madras et al. (2009) found significant reduction in illicit drug use (approximately 68% after 6 months) among patients receiving SBIRT services, and a lower rate of heavy alcohol use (nearly 39%) at the 6-month mark as well. In addition, patients participating in SBIRT services reported other positive outcomes, including fewer interactions with law enforcement and increasingly stable housing and employment situations, as well as improved emotional health. SBIRT has shown that early engagement in a conversation that addresses substance use in a nonjudgmental way can empower the individual to make decisions in his or her own life. By promoting reduction of use of a substance or a negative behavior, an individual can improve his or her long-term health and quality of life. Research is also proving SBIRT to be a cost-effective program (SAMHSA, 2011a).

Stages of Change Model

To effectively define a person's needs, clinicians often use a recently accepted format to assess where the person is on the continuum in the *stages of change*. This information helps clinicians assess where patients are in recognizing the impact of drug use on their lives and their willingness to change the related behaviors in that lifestyle (see Chapter 4 for a discussion of Prochaska's change theory). Application of this model to the therapeutic process affords a humane and empowering approach for an individual who may feel intense ambivalence about relinquishing a coping strategy (such as use of a substance) that provided relief (however temporary). An example for a nurse to support a person's early changes would be to ask, "Do you attend AA or NA or any other support group?" A follow-up question would be, "How does this help you . . . and what works best for you?" This supportive questioning allows the person struggling with addiction to make personal choices rather than be forced to comply with an externally imposed rule. It also lays the groundwork for increased self-esteem and wellness, states that support abstinence rather than abuse.

Motivational interviewing (Chapter 8) is used frequently with all approaches to treatment. Its strength lies in examining core ambivalence that patients may present regarding changing behavior and cessation of drug use. It addresses denial in a humane manner by use of five core principles that build on a patient's strength and willingness to change as well as examine the individual's self-determination.

Abstinence-Based Recovery

Abstinence is loosely defined as a physiological state in which an individual remains free from using a substance or engaging in a behavior that is clearly harmful (Mignon, Marcoux-Faiia, Myers, & Rubington, 2009). Engaging in recovery requires patients to be abstinent so cognitive processes can be engaged in the work of lifestyle change. In programs that promote abstinence (typically, self-help groups such as AA), life issues are confronted in a very direct manner so individuals are unencumbered by external reasoning or excuses. Clinicians as well as sponsors in the fellowship of self-help groups often use this approach, which is felt to ensure the best outcomes when done in a nonjudgmental manner with care and compassion.

Remaining substance-free (abstinent) is considered a key state to promote wellness. The brain recovers, behaviors stabilize, health patterns improve, sleeping disruptions lessen, and the individual is able to turn toward health.

SMART (Self-Management and Recovery Training) Recovery is an abstinence-based model that employs the cognitive approach utilizing rational emotive behavior therapy (REBT). This model has no spiritual base of discussion, but rather asks individuals to examine their own actions and accept responsibility. This is done using a variety of tools in a group format with a facilitator skilled in the use of SMART techniques and REBT.

All these approaches use the direct approach, which may seem confrontational but is most commonly used to present the destructive patterns in the person's life in the hopes that the person will self-decide to make changes and improve the quality of his or her own life. Direct approach programs, such as SMART and AA, may be held in a variety of settings.

Harm Reduction

The term *harm reduction* was coined by public health officials in the late 1970s and early 1980s as they began to study the spread of HIV in Europe and the United States. When they came to the conclusion that HIV could be spread by use of contaminated needles, a concentrated approach to care that began with sterile needle exchange programs and substitution treatment (referral to methadone maintenance programs) began. A criticism of this approach is that it encourages drug use. In reality, the goal is to assist individuals to examine their drug-related behaviors as a poor choice of health patterns. Use of motivational interviewing questions can assist the individual to consider abstinence as a primary option for the initial stage of recovery. Acceptance of the person and close examination of the behaviors is the hallmark of the harm reduction model.

Intervention

In an intervention, a trained professional, often in conjunction with family and friends, works to facilitate an individual's entry into treatment. The term *intervention* is often used when the process is conducted in an orchestrated manner in a group session that can be supportive as well as confrontational. At the point of intervention, the individual is engaging in self-destructive behavior and, often, behaviors that are actively harming others. The goal of the intervention is to help the person enter treatment.

Key issues to address when using the intervention approach are preparation of those involved, available supports, seating during the session, and being prepared for unknown sequelae of the event (such as anger eruptions, loss of custody, suicidality) (Mignon, Marcoux-Faiia, Myers, & Rubington, 2009). The focus in this type of clinical work is to use the family or friends as a caring cohort. Whether using a direct or indirect intervention format, it is vital to the therapeutic process of intervention to prepare those who are assisting with the intervention.

In a *direct intervention,* family and/or friends are prepared to address the person with letters, statements, and conditions. Examples of conditions may include withdrawal of emotional or financial support, housing, and custody. The facilitator conducts the process with the goal that the intervention will encourage the individual who is the focus of the strategy to accept help and/or treatment.

Often called the *systemic family model, indirect intervention* uses an invitational approach. It encourages those peripheral to the individual using substances to seek help for themselves as well.

There are many concerns surrounding the use of intervention techniques. For example, it is critical that a clinically trained therapist conduct the proceedings. Interventions conducted without skilled facilitators can result in negative outcomes and increased relapse rates.

Although there is some controversy regarding the long-term effectiveness of intervention and the person feeling "ambushed" by family, friends, and/or clinicians, the results can be extraordinary in facilitating a person to enter a form of treatment. When motivational interviewing techniques are employed during the intervention and less draconian methods are used, the outcome has the potential to be healing and less traumatic. Thus, use of interventions to facilitate wellness and recovery requires an evidence-based knowledge program and a skilled facilitator.

Pharmacotherapy

For some patients, medication-assisted therapy may be appropriate, although proponents are quick to point out that pharmacological interventions are only a support to recovery, not the total format for recovery. The newer body of research (NIDA, 2011) supports pharmacological intervention to promote abstinence, address changes, and support recovery (see Medications Used to Treat Addictive and Co-Occurring Disorders). Use of pharmacotherapy depends greatly on the needs of the individual patient. For example, benzodiazepines are sometimes used to assist patients during detoxification (withdrawal) from alcohol. SSRIs may be used in conjunction with therapy to treat coexisting anxiety or depression.

An important focus of medication-assisted therapy is treatment of cravings. Although cravings may occur at any time, they are more likely to occur when the individual is in an environment associated with use of the substance or when he or she is with others who use the substance (APA, 2013). Craving is a powerful force, in part because of the involvement of classical conditioning associated with craving. Pharmacotherapy for substance abuse often includes the use of anti-craving medications, whose goal is to alter the reward circuitry in the brain and lessen the desired effect of drinking alcohol or using opioids. Initially, anti-craving medications were developed to support abstinence from alcohol, and studies support its use: Patients who

return to drinking no longer achieve the desired effect, thus negating the intoxicating effect of alcohol. This strategy has been applied to address dependence on opiates and other substances.

Methadone

Methadone is a central nervous system depressant that was developed initially to assist patients in recovering from dependency on opiates. It is an opioid agonist and Schedule II controlled substance that has a gradual onset and a long half-life. The extended half-life is what may increase its potential for toxicity. Additionally, there are safety issues related to QT interval prolongation, respiratory depression, and possible sedation. Induction of methadone requires careful assessment and monitoring as the dosage is increased. Methadone has potential for major drug–drug interactions through metabolism via the CYP 450 enzyme. The key message for a nurse administering methadone is that there are tremendous variations in metabolism, absorption, and elimination among people, as well as in the same person over time.

Methadone maintenance programs address the psychological underpinning of the drug use and promote positive lifestyle changes in addition to the prescription use of methadone. Clinics offer daily dosing at a prescribed amount. Careful increasing of the dose and utilization of the treatment offered are heavily regulated by government standards. Consideration of an individual's ability to attend the methadone clinic on a daily basis, wait in line, and submit to urine drug screens is weighed by the treatment staff. In addition, when an individual is taking hepatitis C or HIV medication or has a preexisting psychiatric disorder, careful assessment is made to adjust methadone dosing. How long a patient remains on methadone maintenance is a decision made by the treatment team in consultation with the patient. Methadone may also be used for pain management, but the dosage varies from that used for methadone maintenance.

Buprenorphine

More recently, buprenorphine (Buprenex) or buprenorphine plus nalone (Suboxone) is being widely used to address opiate/opioid dependence. Buprenorphine is a partial opioid agonist/antagonist (Wilson, Shannon, & Shields, 2014). It is administered sublingually and has a slightly bitter taste. It occupies receptor sites and blocks the effects of opiate/opioid use, including preventing the associated euphoric state. At this writing, the medication can be prescribed legally only by a physician with a specialized education in administration of buprenorphine. It has been shown to be extremely efficacious in supporting recovery from individuals who seek help from either a clinic or from their primary care provider. This is known as *office-based opioid therapy* (OBOT). The newest form of buprenorphine is being administered in a film taken sublingually.

Antabuse

Disulfiram (Antabuse) offers an individual an ability to sustain abstinence from alcohol because of strong physical reactions to alcohol that are associated with this medication. Using alcohol while taking Antabuse will precipitate a severe response, including nausea, cardiac palpitations, headache, and possible vasovagal response. This is known as *aversion therapy,* because the patient knows he or she will become ill if he or she chooses to drink. The aversion encourages abstinence toward recovery.

Injectable Naltrexone

Injectable naltrexone (Vivitrol) is the newest method of pharmaceutical support that is widely gaining favor among treatment providers. Initially developed to support abstinence from alcohol, research supports its use

Addictive and Co-Occurring Disorders

medications commonly used to treat

Medications	Usual Adult Daily Dosage (mg)	Nursing Considerations
Benzodiazepines		**Used for detoxification/withdrawal from alcohol**
chlordiazepoxide (Librium)	50–100 mg PRN up to a maximum of 300 mg per day	• Avoid drinking lemon juice with Librium because it decreases the drug's effectiveness.
diazepam (Valium)	IV: 10 mg initially, then 5–10 mg in 3–4 hr	• Avoid heavy machinery and driving. • Doses may need to be titrated based on symptoms.
lorazepam (Ativan)	2–6 mg/day in divided doses up to a maximum of 10 mg	• Caution about dependency, confusion, memory loss, drowsiness. • Assess for co-morbid medical conditions. Some medications prescribed for medical conditions may potentiate the effects of benzodiazepines.
oxazepam (Serax)	Geriatric: 0.5–1 mg/day up to a maximum of 2 mg per day 15–30 mg 3–4 times per day	• Avoid alcohol and other CNS depressants that potentiate the effects of benzodiazepines because respiratory depression/apnea can result.
(Benzodiazepines are used in withdrawal/detoxification programs for short-term use only to prevent seizures during withdrawal.)		• Avoid abrupt discontinuation if a patient has been on these medications for a while; when terminating, taper doses to avoid precipitating withdrawal symptoms, especially seizures. • Observe closely for paradoxical reactions. • Short half-life of specific benzodiazepines (lorazepam) may require increased doses to control withdrawal symptoms. • Oxazepam (Serax) is used for individuals with liver function impairment or with older adults in withdrawal. • Medications to enhance sleep are generally used only during treatment for detoxification. Long-term use is discouraged owing to dependence potential. • Determine normal liver functioning prior to administering medication. • Assess for withdrawal symptoms. • Inform patient that treatment of withdrawal may take 4–7 days with sustained impaired functioning for a few weeks to months.
Antidepressant Medications	**Dosages**	**Nursing Considerations**
SSRIs		**For all SSRIs**
fluoxetine (Prozac)	20–80 mg per day Geriatric: Start with 10 mg/day	May be used in conjunction with therapy when anxiety and/or depression coexist with alcohol/drug dependence.
sertraline (Zoloft)	50–200 mg per day Geriatric: Start with 25 mg/day	May benefit individuals with late-onset alcohol dependence. Provide patient education regarding: • GI distress • Sexual dysfunction • Nausea or diarrhea • Tremors • Insomnia • Daytime drowsiness and driving ability
Partial Agonist–Antagonist Agents		
buprenorphine (Subutex contains buprenorphine only; Suboxone contains naloxone in addition to buprenorphine)	Therapy initiation: 8–16 mg SL once daily Maintenance dose: 4–24 mg/day Transdermal patch is worn for 7 days; rotate sites	• Medication is taken sublingually (SL) and is used in office-based settings. Has been used for pain in the past but efficacy limited for pain due to ceiling effect. • Suboxone contains naloxone (a narcotic/opiate antagonist) to prevent abuse. Can produce withdrawal in opioid-dependent patients. • Pregnant women may be prescribed Subutex without naloxone, but typically are referred to methadone clinics for treatment. • Caution regarding side effects such as grogginess, lethargy, or fatigue in relation to driving or operating machinery. • Inform patient of the dangers of relapsing back into using opioids/opiates.
Injectable Opioid Antagonist		
naltrexone (Vivitrol)	380 mg q 4 weeks Deep IM	• Long-acting antagonist that provides treatment of alcohol or opioid dependence. • Patient must be opioid-free for 7–10 days at time of administration to avoid precipitating withdrawal; may confirm with urine screen for opioids.

Antidepressant Medications	Dosages	Nursing Considerations
		• Inform patient of mild pain at the site of injection. • Monitor liver function. • Inform patient of the risks of attempting to overcome opioid blockade by relapsing with opioids/opiates. • Encourage patients to use this medication in conjunction with therapy.
Alcohol-Sensitizing Medication-Aversive Agents disulfiram (Antabuse)	**Dosage** 500 mg per day for 1–2 weeks, then 125–500 mg daily; maximum dose: 500 mg/day	• Binds to ALDH, the enzyme that metabolizes alcohol. It increases acetaldehyde concentration and causes an aversive reaction if alcohol is consumed. • Patient must have abstained from alcohol for 12–24 hours before therapy is initiated. • Caution patient that the disulfiram–ethanol reaction (DER) is flushing of the skin, nausea, vomiting, and severe headache. • Severe adverse effects with alcohol ingestion: hypotension to shock level arrhythmias; acute congestive failure. • Severe adverse reactions: marked respiratory depression, unconsciousness, convulsions, sudden death. • Side effects include drowsiness, lethargy, and fatigue. More serious side effects are peripheral neuropathy, hepatotoxicity, and mood disorders. • Potential exists for addiction and withdrawal.
Anti-Craving Medications For alcohol: acamprosate (Campral)—*glutament receptor modulator* For alcohol/opioids: oral naltrexone (ReVia)—*opioid antagonist*	666 mg TID Renal dose: 333 mg TID 50–150 mg daily; maximum 800 mg/day	• Do not use if patient is on opioid pain medications. • Monitor liver function. • May experience nausea, diarrhea, headache, and fatigue. • Inform patient of potential for upper respiratory infections and pneumonia. • Monitor renal functioning when using Campral. Decrease dosage by 50% if renal impairment is evident.
Opiate Agonists methadone	Usual dose may be anywhere from 20–120 mg per day. Renal dose: 50–75% of dose May be titrated up or lowered based on clinical assessment. Doses may be divided if individual is a rapid metabolizer of the medication.	• Goal of maintenance treatment is to address the craving associated with withdrawal from opioids/opiates. • Inform patient about the danger of driving and operating machinery until dose is titrated and well tolerated. • Caution patient about relapsing and the synergistic effect of using any other sedating medications (benzodiazepines, pain medications, etc.) • Rapid metabolizers may need a split dose to sustain a constant blood level of the medication. • Methadone is considered the "gold-standard" at this time if a woman is opioid dependent, seeking help, and pregnant.

Based on Hulse, G. K., Morris, N., Arnold-Reed, D., and Tait, R. J. (2009). Improving clinical outcomes in treating heroin dependence: Randomized, controlled trial of oral or implant naltrexone. *Archives of General Psychiatry, 66*(10) 1108–1115; Krupitsky, E., Nunes, E., Ling, W., Illeperuma, A., Gastfriend, D., & Silverman, B. (2011). Injectable extended-release naltrexone for opioid dependence: A double-blind, placebo-controlled, multicentre randomised trial. *Lancet, 377*(9776), 1506–1513; Mattick, R. P., Kimber, J., Breen, C., & Davoli, M. (2008). Buprenorphine maintenance versus placebo or methadone maintenance for opioid dependence. *Cochrane Database of Systematic Reviews, 16*(2), CD 002207; Wilson, B. A., Shannon, M. T., & Shields, K. M. (2014). *Pearson Nurse's Drug Guide 2014.* Upper Saddle River, NJ: Pearson Education.

in promoting abstinence from opiate/opioid dependence. Injectable naltrexone is administered in a single monthly dose. The most common concern is how to address pain management if required, because naltrexone is an opiate/opioid antagonist. Any form of override to this medication should be done in a controlled environment by trained professionals. The other criticism of this treatment is the cost of the medication, but insurance providers are beginning to provide coverage for naltrexone as a mechanism to support recovery.

Thiamine and Folic Acid

Thiamine (Vitamin B$_1$) and folic acid supplementation are important in the treatment of alcoholism. Thiamine helps prevent Wernicke syndrome, a constellation of symptoms including severe confusion, abnormal gait, and paralysis of some eye muscles; folic acid helps prevent anemia that may occur when the number of oxygen-carrying red blood cells are lowered from heavy drinking (Chick, 2009; Freeman, 2013).

Wernicke encephalopathy and Korsakoff syndrome are two conditions of brain damage caused by a deficiency of Vitamin B$_1$. Korsakoff syndrome, or Korsakoff psychosis, tends to develop as Wernicke symptoms go away. Wernicke encephalopathy causes brain damage in the thalamus and hypothalamus, and lower parts of the brain. It can progress to irreversible dementia or Korsakoff psychosis, affecting areas of the brain involved with memory (Wernicke-Korsakoff Syndrome, 2012).

Care Settings

Individuals who have become dependent on a substance often have tried many times to stop using on their own. The craving for the drug can be so profound, and the physiological and psychological dependence so intense, that they cannot complete cessation of the drug, and a vicious cycle ensues. Entry to treatment is based on the length and severity of dependence on the drug. Thus, various levels of care may be prescribed. Inpatient care may be necessary to address the most critical cases of addiction, especially for patients with co-morbid conditions. Less intensive options include structured outpatient addiction progams (SOAP), intensive outpatient programs (IOP), other outpatient programs, and referrals to halfway houses and sober living communities. It is recognized that patients who need treatment programs that allow them to return to their own home may be faced with items, places, and rituals that may trigger a response and a craving for their substance, as well as return to family or friends who either condone or encourage their addiction. Thus, programs are selected carefully to promote the most positive outcome.

The American Society of Addiction Medicine (ASAM) has identified five levels of care in the treatment of addiction disorders (ASAM, 2001). These guidelines have been adopted nationwide to help care providers distinguish appropriate levels of care for patients struggling with addiction. The five levels of care are:

- Level 0.5 Early Intervention
- Level I Outpatient Services
- Level II Intensive Outpatient/Partial Hospitalization
- Level III Residential/Inpatient Treatment
- Level IV Medically Managed Intensive Inpatient Services

While inpatient care requires admission to a hospital or treatment facility, other levels of care may be offered in a variety of settings, as described in the following sections.

Inpatient Settings

Inpatient settings are often located in or near a hospital. Length of stay depends on the severity of an individual's addiction. Specific therapy is prescribed based on the patient's history, drug use, acuity, and the presence of other physical or mental health issues. Prior to entry to inpatient treatment, the individual should be completely detoxified from substances of use and dependence. Inpatient hospitalization programs typically require participation in individual therapy, group therapy, and support sessions, as well as AA/NA and/or SMART Recovery meetings. Pharmacotherapy may or may not be prescribed, based on individual patient needs.

Detoxification

When individuals are referred for help, they are usually screened to see whether they require detoxification from the abused drug. This is often done in a Level IV hospital-based detoxification unit with medical management for the potentially unstable state. It also can take place under Level III medically monitored care for individuals with less complex health concerns. Once a patient completes the detoxification process, referral is often made to a lower level of care. Detoxification programs should include the following guiding principles:

- Evaluation
- Stabilization
- Promoting patient readiness for and entry into treatment

Where the patient is to undergo detoxification depends on the individual patient's level of need. The success of a detoxification program is determined by the individual's ability to enter, participate in, and remain compliant with the treatment/rehabilitation program protocols after detoxification (SAMHSA, 2006).

Rehabilitation

In rehabilitation units, length of stay depends on the patient's motivation, ability to have time off if employed, insurance coverage, and program availability. As a patient progresses through treatment, the treatment team periodically reviews established goals and objectives for treatment with the patient. Patient participation in this process encourages self-responsibility. The goals of rehabilitation programs are to improve patients' life patterns and decrease the potential for relapse.

Outpatient Programs

Structured outpatient addiction programs (SOAP) are often referred to by different names, depending on the geographic locale. The length of time spent in the program is determined by the individual's motivation and insurance coverage. Outpatient care options range from group therapy sessions to support programs to residential programs designed to promote recovery, such as halfway homes and sober houses (Table 20-4). Two widely used models of support groups include Alcoholics Anonymous and the SMART Recovery model.

Outpatient Treatment Options   table 20-4

Program/Option	Description
Group living arrangements • Halfway houses • Three-quarter houses • Sober houses	Residential options that provide a structured environment beyond the inpatient setting and require strict adherence to rules regarding abstinence, urine drug screenings, and program requirements. Halfway houses generally provide the most structure and have the greatest requirements. Funding varies, as does length of stay.
Homeless shelters	Some shelters offer substance abuse programming and require abstinence; these are known as "dry shelters." Shelters that accept individuals who are under the influence of substances and are not violent are referred to as "wet shelters." Safety is always the priority in the shelter setting because individuals who are intoxicated or under the influence of a substance may display risky or dangerous behaviors.
Support groups	Groups formed by individuals seeking to recover from addiction. Alcoholics Anonymous and Narcotics Anonymous follow the 12-step model and are widely available throughout the world. Many other groups that support people in recovery exist, formally and informally, with or without use of the 12-step model. Often these groups support a specific population with commonalities, such as health care professionals, attorneys, or working women. Usually, there is a skilled facilitator and groups meet on a weekly basis.

Alcoholics Anonymous and the 12-Step Model

Alcoholics Anonymous (AA) is a support group in which participants share their stories of addiction and recovery and offer strength and hope to each other. AA does not promote or endorse any methodology or treatment. All meetings are free and are rooted in the concept of volunteerism. The basic philosophy of the organization is defined in the Twelve Steps and Twelve Traditions, which were designed to help participants overcome the need to drink and return to full participation in life (Alcoholics Anonymous, 1976). This organization has laid the groundwork for Narcotics Anonymous (NA) and more than 200 other groups that ascribe to a 12-step model. Meetings are available online and in church halls, empty meeting rooms, hospitals, prisons, and treatment centers. AA and its counterparts are clearly self-help groups, with participants helping one another recover.

No other movement has spawned such success in helping the person with alcoholism or addiction toward recovery. The positions of AA and NA do not endorse or refute use of medications to treat alcoholism and/or addiction, but recognize that some individuals require medications to treat medical conditions. Many members participate throughout their lives and attribute the changes in their life to their spiritual concept of a Higher Power, which is an essential part of the 12-step model. Other critical aspects of the 12 steps include maintaining sobriety and making amends to those whom the individual recovering from addiction has wronged "except when to do so would injure them or others" (A. A. World Services, Inc., 2002).

SMART Recovery

A group known as SMART Recovery has grown from a small beginning to strong acceptance. SMART stands for Self-Management and Recovery Training (SMART Recovery, 2013). It is a group that is abstinence based, with a cognitive approach. It does not promote a spiritual core or use the concept of a Higher Power. Proponents of SMART Recovery often prefer this approach if they do not integrate into the AA philosophy. In SMART Recovery, a skilled group facilitator works with a small number of participants in group sessions. The facilitator uses principles of REBT. This approach decreases the emotional display when a member discusses behaviors and actions associated with his or her lifestyle. SMART Recovery promotes acceptance and offers an alternate for people seeking recovery who are not spiritual in nature.

Pause and Reflect

1. *What are the essentials that clinicians must bear in mind when developing treatment plans for patients with substance abuse disorders?*
2. *What are the benefits of halfway houses and other shared living arrangements?*
3. *Do you know anyone who attends a support group? What are the benefits? Drawbacks?*

Nursing Management

Patients who suffer from substance use disorders are unable to control their use or abstain from use. They experience significant cravings, a decreased ability to control other behaviors, cognitive impairment, and a decreased ability to recognize how their behavior affects relationships and situations. Like other chronic diseases, addiction often involves cycles of relapse and remission. Without treatment or engagement in recovery activities, addiction is progressive and can result in disability or premature death. Regardless of medical setting, the nurse usually is the first person the patient will meet to begin the assessment process.

Typically, admission criteria are identified in six dimensions: acute intoxication/withdrawal potential; biomedical, emotional, behavioral, or cognitive conditions and complications; readiness to change; relapse, continued use, or continued problem potential; and recovery environment. The severity of the patient's substance use disorder affects decisions related to treatment and admission. The presence of the following number of symptoms determines severity:

- Mild: 2 or 3 symptoms
- Moderate: 4 or 5 symptoms
- Severe: 6 or more symptoms (APA, 2013)

Gerald Kraymore Recovery Phase

APPLICATION

1. What are the priorities for Mr. Kraymore's care at this time?
2. According to the levels of care as outlined by the American Society of Addiction Medicine, what level of care is Mr. Kraymore receiving now? To what extent is it appropriate?
3. When Mr. Kraymore is ready for discharge, will it be appropriate to discharge him home to his mother's house? To his girlfriend's? Why or why not?

It has been three days since Mr. Kraymore's admission. His bacterial infection is resolving with the antibiotics, as are his related symptoms. Mr. Kraymore's primary provider has diagnosed him with anxiety and depression. Mr. Kraymore denies any history of mental health treatment, despite a history of three short-term drug-related arrests and subsequent incarcerations. A thorough nursing assessment has revealed that his girlfriend also is actively using drugs and "is trying to get help." Mr. Kraymore's mother is alive and he reports that she is his primary support. He has been unable to stay employed for any length of time because of his substance abuse.

Although Mr. Kraymore has had no previous involvement in AA or NA, he says he is willing to consider attending meetings while hospitalized. Mr. Kraymore expresses frustration over his addiction, his unsatisfactory work history, and how much he relies on his mother.

It is important to establish the patient's level of severity early in the assessment process. The process of a structured interview with a patient who is experiencing profound shame and stigma can precipitate extreme stress reactions, including the possibility that the patient will abandon the process. A primary step at this juncture is the therapeutic relationship. Patients respond to authentic offers of help to change their lives but often resist ordered or mandated treatment. Nurses who take the time to begin the therapeutic relationship before starting the assessment are likely to elicit a more positive response in patients. An acronym to use to help understand this process is RECOVER:

Respect for the individual

Empathy

Compassion

Observe for biological symptoms of withdrawal

Value the individual's strengths in his or her decisions

Expect success

Remember to acknowledge positive gains

Assessment

Assessment begins with thorough history taking that includes the patient's use of drugs from the first point of use to the present. Various assessment tools that include items directed at assessing the patient's activities of daily living and impact of the substance on daily functioning are available (Box 20-4). Whatever tool is used, it is important that the nurse ask questions that are most likely to elicit a response related to the patient's use of substances. Questions such as "How have you been sleeping?" and questions related to

eating patterns and nutrition will provide information related to the effects of substance abuse on the patient's sleeping patterns and appetite. In addition, a review of all symptoms using a systems approach and continuing the process of establishing a therapeutic relationship may provide a comprehensive picture of the person's current state of health.

During assessment and at all times when working with a patient, it is important to remain nonjudgmental. Patients suffering from substance abuse and addiction may relay information of a disturbing nature due to their prioritizing of their addiction above other facets of their lives. Nurses working with patients suffering from addiction are likely to hear a range of stories, from forgetting to pick up children from school to engaging in dangerous sexual behaviors. At all times, nurses must convey support and concern for the patient.

Observation and Physical Assessment

Nurses assessing patients who admit to or are suspected of substance use or abuse observe carefully for behaviors associated with pending withdrawal states and central nervous system vulnerability. Observe for any major presenting symptom, such as tremors, pain, headache, cough, or vomiting. Observe for changes in mental status, including fear and anxiety, and complaints of pain in any form. In addition, inquire about or monitor vital signs on admission and at periodic intervals; allergies; concurrent health issues; signs of depression and suicidality; history of head trauma; fluid balance; and neurological signs.

Nurses should also include a comprehensive systems review to assess for changes in homeostasis. Reviewing the patient's pattern of daily living will help assess how the patient functions on a daily basis (for example, eating, work, relationships, coping).

Screening for Substance Use   box 20-4

Use of a screening tool in primary care settings to reduce substance use and misuse by individuals at risk has been recommended by the U.S. Preventive Services Task Force (USPSTF). This recommendation will serve to help illuminate areas of need for those who use substances despite potential or adverse consequences. There are several screening tools to assist identification of individuals with a risk for alcoholism/addiction, notably the Addiction Severity Scale, the Michigan Alcohol Screening Test (MAST), the Substance Abuse Subtle Screening Inventory (SASSI), and the CAGE questionnaire. First developed in 1984, the CAGE is an extremely reliable and well-validated screening instrument that is easy to use and effective in gleaning information that would reflect the need for further assessment. It is still widely used today and is recommended as a primary screening tool to begin to assess for substance abuse concerns in an individual (Ewing, 1984). The CAGE format consists of four questions:

C: Have you ever felt you should *cut* down on your drinking? (or drug use)

A: Have people ever *annoyed* you by criticizing your drinking? (or drug use)

G: Have you ever felt bad or *guilty* about your drinking? (or drug use)

E: Have you ever had a drink (*eye opener*) first thing in the morning to steady your nerves or get rid of a hangover?

A positive answer to at least one question suggests a concern for substance misuse. Positive answers to two or more questions suggest problematic areas in a person's life and require further assessment.

Among the clinical professions that treat addictive disorders, there is often disagreement in the wording used by providers. Crafting of counseling screening techniques and wording of instruments is often debated. One researcher commented that use of the word "misuse" implies intent, is pejorative, and is an inappropriate term for dependence. Others, however, feel that consistency of language helps to "avoid any misinterpretation" (USPSTF, 2004).

The overall goal of the screening tools and intervention techniques is to reduce the harm associated with continued use of substances and/or destructive behaviors in a person's life. In screening for risk, which facilitates further clarification with health assessment and drug use history, the belief is predicated from the evidence that identification will help facilitate recovery, improve health, and lessen risk-related behavior.

Patient Interview

By using a series of structured questions, the nurse can elicit important information regarding the patient's drug of choice, the last time the patient used, the amount used, and the route of administration. As part of the assessment, the nurse should also inquire about previous attempts to abstain from use and elicit what helps the patient refrain from use and whether the patient is able to identify any situations or feelings that trigger use. Many hospitals and clinics use commercial screening and assessment tools to help determine a patient's risk for abuse or the extent of a patient's history with substances (see Box 20-4). Questions intended to elicit information about the extent of a patient's use may include the following:

- Have you ever been hospitalized for drug or alcohol use?
- How often do you abuse [substance]?
- Have you ever not been able to remember what you did?
- Have you ever been arrested related to use? (e.g., driving under the influence)

The Centers for Medicare and Medicaid Services recommends that primary care practitioners use the behavioral counseling interventions known as the 5 As approach, which has been adopted by the USPSTF (USPSTF, n.d.):

1. *Assess:* Ask about/assess behavioral health risk(s) and factors affecting the choice of behavior change goals/methods.
2. *Advise:* Give clear, specific, and personalized behavior change advice, including information about personal health harms and benefits.
3. *Agree:* Collaboratively select appropriate treatment goals and methods based on the patient's interest in and willingness to change the behavior.
4. *Assist:* Using behavior change techniques (self-help and/or counseling), aid the patient in achieving agreed-upon goals by acquiring the skills, confidence, and social/environmental supports for behavior change, supplemented with adjunctive medical treatments when appropriate.
5. *Arrange:* Schedule follow-up contacts (in person or by telephone) to provide ongoing assistance and support and to adjust the treatment plan as needed, including referral to more intensive or specialized treatment.

Difference in Assessment—Initial/Relapse, Recovery, Rehabilitation

When reviewing their progression in the disease of addiction, patients may experience a sense of loss or hopelessness for the future. In addition, they may experience situational depression and anxiety. As health issues increase, denial can begin to erode and patients may require close observation for mood changes and potential for suicidality. Continued assessment of triggers, responses, and coping mechanisms is necessary to determine a patient's readiness and strength to move forward through recovery. Patients who progress through detoxification and begin to think clearly may be more receptive to patient teaching and interventions designed to promote coping. Stress management techniques and, for some patients, pharmacotherapy may be helpful in supporting successful early recovery that will lead to sobriety and a more sustained form of recovery (NIDA, 2009b). Helping patients acknowledge and celebrate even small milestones can help build motivation and hope through recovery.

Diagnosis and Planning

Nursing diagnoses appropriate for patients with addictive disorders vary according to symptoms and circumstances. For example, a patient with alcoholism who is high functioning will present very differently from a patient who is experiencing hallucinations related to crack cocaine use. Despite this, there are two nursing diagnoses that nurses will find consistently appropriate for patients with addictive disorders:

- Health Maintenance, Ineffective
- Coping, Ineffective
  (NANDA-I, © 2014)

Individual patient circumstances that inform the process of identifying and prioritizing nursing diagnoses vary greatly. The patient's immediate safety (and the safety of those in immediate proximity) is the most important consideration. Additionally, the patient's ability to participate in and motivations for treatment are important factors. A patient experiencing active hallucinations or who is in a panic state and has an elevated heart rate will participate at a different level and have very different motivations from a patient who has just discovered she is pregnant and is asking for help to stop smoking.

Plans and Goals

Defining objectives for care with related interventions requires careful thought. Although this process improves with skill level and competency, the patient first requires acceptance for the decision to seek treatment, which demonstrates responsibility for personal behavior. As in any nursing situation, it is important to design measurable goals with patient input.

Patient Education

In planning education for patients with substance use disorders, it is important to keep in mind that patients who are still intoxicated have limited memory capacity and limited ability to focus. Education for these patients is a process, not a single session. Initially, nurses focus on helping patients understand how their presenting symptoms relate to their substance abuse. As the patient begins to progress from withdrawal to recovery, nurses can begin to plan patient education related to other areas, including exercise and wellness.

Revising the Care Plan during Recovery and Rehabilitation

Patients who are experiencing severe addiction with serious co-morbid health issues will require a continual review of their progress or inability to grasp the concept of recovery. The nurse is positioned to assess achievement of short-term goals in treatment and examine a patient's level of understanding of life processes. This often requires intense education, support, and referral to various programs that will address sustaining early successes and recovery.

When required, close monitoring of withdrawal protocols and the patient's health status can assist patients to begin the process of wellness and a life without substances. Appropriate goals include that the patient will accomplish the following:

- Complete a withdrawal protocol to ameliorate symptoms of acute abstinence syndrome (withdrawal).
- Improve health patterns of nutrition, sleep, and bodily functions.
- Stabilize social networks of sponsors in recovery, supportive friends, and recovery coaches and therapists if required.
- Increase capacity for goal setting and positive life-altering decisions as longer-term abstinence is achieved.

Implementation

Nurses provide an array of interventions for patients with substance use disorders, ranging from modeling and teaching communication skills to arranging referrals for housing and financial assistance. As with any patient, nurses begin their work with patients through therapeutic communication and keeping in mind how to help alleviate the patient's suffering.

Promote Safety during the Detoxification Period

According to SAMHSA, the purpose of supervised detoxification is to manage acute intoxication and withdrawal to prevent life-threatening complications (Center for Substance Abuse Treatment [CSAT], 2006). Detoxification is a form of palliative care because it lowers the intensity of the disorder for those wanting to become abstinent or who are forced to observe mandatory abstinence as a result of hospitalization or legal involvement. Supervised detoxification may be the patient's first introduction to the treatment system and the first step to recovery. Treatment and rehabilitation involve various therapeutic services and disciplines intended to promote recovery for substance abuse patients (CSAT, 2006).

Careful assessment and monitoring is required of patients going through withdrawal. The Clinical Institute Withdrawal Assessment Scale for Alcohol (CIWA-Ar) is a helpful tool for determining severity of alcohol withdrawal syndrome (AWS). This 10-item scale measures severity of nausea, sweating, agitation, headache, anxiety, tremor, orientation, and tactile, visual, and auditory disturbances. Scores provide guidance for treatment and may vary from institution to institution (Freeman, 2013).

Withdrawal symptoms typically cause significant distress and impairment of functioning in a number of domains (APA, 2013). Specific signs and symptoms may vary according to the substance. In the case of alcohol withdrawal, for example, an individual might experience some combination of diaphoresis (pulse rate above 100 bpm), hand tremors, nausea or vomiting, psychomotor agitation, anxiety, seizure activity, and delirium tremens within a few hours to several days after cessation of alcohol (APA, 2013). **Delirium tremens** (DT) consists of temporary visual, auditory, or tactile hallucinations and is characteristic of abrupt withdrawal from alcohol. It typically develops 48 to 72 hours after withdrawal begins (Alcohol Withdrawal, 2013). DT differs from *alcoholic hallucinosis,* which can develop within 12 to 24 hours of abstinence and typically resolves within 48 hours (Hoffman & Weinhouse, 2013).

DT, or alcohol withdrawal delirium, involves hypertension, tachycardia (rapid heart rate), tachypnea (rapid breathing), and tremens (shaking). Untreated DT can lead to cardiac and respiratory arrest. Early assessment of such potentially fatal symptoms is critical,

and the situation needs to be considered a medical emergency and requires close monitoring. Alcohol withdrawal occurs in 5% to 20% of the general population found in primary care and hospital settings (Chick, 2009; Alcohol Withdrawal, 2013).

Regardless of the substance, detoxification involves (1) evaluation, (2) stabilization, and (3) promoting patient readiness to begin and enter treatment. All these steps must occur, and they must occur in sequence.

Individuals with severe dependence may experience risk to homeostasis as their bodies adjust to reduction of the substance. Nursing interventions focus on alleviating whichever symptoms are exhibited and are dependent on the used substance (see Table 20-3). However, general interventions always include the following:

- Careful monitoring of vital signs and body systems
- Assessment and monitoring of existing medical conditions and medications
- Observation of neurological changes, especially the possibility of seizures
- Maintenance of fluid and electrolyte balance

Provide Therapeutic Communication

Therapeutic communication is important in all areas of nursing, but there is probably no specialty in which it is more important than in addictions nursing. Patients with substance use disorders often have had very negative experiences with judgmental providers in the health care system, due in part to societal stigma associated with addiction. Many health care providers have not had adequate education and supervision to assist patients in dealing with addictive disorders, as well as other chronic disorders in which relapse is common. As a result, many providers become frustrated and develop negative attitudes toward patients. Howard and Chung (2000a, 2000b) studied nurses' attitudes toward patients with addictive disorders over three decades and found that attitudes did improve over the course of the three decades, but that a significant number of nurses continued to maintain negative attitudes toward this population. Additionally, their research found that nurses were more negative and punitive and had more authoritarian orientations toward substance users than were other professional groups. Additional research has indicated that nurses spend less time and provide a decreased quality of care to patients whom they view negatively. Labels and stigmatization can result in premature discharge and neglect, and cause patients to feel frustrated, depressed, angry, and upset (Corley & Goren, 1998). For these reasons and many others, patients with addictive disorders are in need of best-practice therapeutic communication.

Skillful interviewing and the ability to build therapeutic relationships are essential skills in working with this population (Chapter 8). Beginning with the first contact with a patient, the nurse should set ground rules with the patient, including honest communication. The nurse can simply state that honesty about substance use will allow both patient and nurse the opportunity to understand what is not working in the treatment program and develop further strategies. This is particularly important because of the propensity of patients to deny or minimize their problems with substances.

When working with patients who are in denial, the principles of motivational interviewing can be helpful. As nurses build the

Nursing Interventions to Promote Effective Health Maintenance table 20-5

Actions/Interventions	Rationales
Assist the patient with identifying factors contributing to health maintenance change through value clarification strategies and one-to-one interviewing.	Healthy living habits reduce risk behaviors. Assistance is needed to identify factors that can help change long-term behaviors.
Assist the patient with developing a list of assets and deficits as he or she perceives them. From this list, assist the patient in deciding what lifestyle adjustments will be necessary to make changes.	Helps patient to establish control over self and situation. Increased control keeps patients from becoming overwhelmed.
Help the patient identify possible solutions to cope with each adjustment.	The more involved the patient is with the solutions, the more likely he or she is to stick to the adjustments.
Develop a plan that shows both short-term and long-term goals with the patient. For each goal, specify the time in which the goal is to be reached.	Establishing goals is an effective way of setting priorities and measuring accomplishments. It also keeps patients hopeful regarding the future versus focusing on past failures.
Assist the patient with developing a list of the benefits and disadvantages to behavior changes. Discuss each item with the patient as well as the strength and motivation the patient has toward achieving each goal.	Placing a priority according to the patient's motivation increases success rates.
Teach the patient appropriate information to improve health maintenance.	Adult learners will be able to synthesize information that is pertinent to their situation.
Provide the patient with appropriate positive feedback on goal achievement.	Appropriate positive feedback helps to establish rapport and helps patients to feel good about positive outcomes.

therapeutic relationship, they will begin to see opportunities to help patients address the discrepancies between their beliefs about their current situation and its realities. Two important aspects of motivational interviewing include asking open-ended questions to determine what is important to the individual and providing validation or affirmation of the individual's effort and feelings. Questions that may assist the nurse to help individuals clarify discrepancies include the following:

- What is important to you in your life?
- How would you like things to be different?
- What will change if you give up using _____?
- What do you want to do now?
- How can I help?

Promote Effective Health Maintenance

Substance abuse can have devastating consequences on patient health, in some cases from the very first use. As patients progress through treatment, nurses help them understand the consequences of substance use on their physical and mental health. Specific interventions include assisting patients to identify factors that adversely affect their health, such as neglecting to take prescribed medications for medical conditions and engaging in risky behaviors when under the influence of their addiction. By helping patients to identify issues, strategies, and possible solutions, nurses empower patients to take responsibility for their own health and behaviors (Table 20-5). This, in turn, can promote the hope that patients need to believe they can live a life free of abusing substances.

Promote Healthy Coping

Inadequate or nonexistent coping strategies contribute to patient addiction. Nurses can promote healthy coping among patients with

addictive disorders in a variety of ways (Table 20-6). Key interventions in this area include:

- Help patients to identify and interpret stressful situations
- Help patients identify their current means of dealing with stress and determine what methods have been successful or detrimental
- Model and offer healthy strategies for coping with stressors

Patients with addictive disorders are often starting from "zero" when it comes to coping strategies. Possibly more than any other population of patients, they need professional intervention to be able to replace maladaptive coping behaviors with successful ones.

Additional Strategies

Nurses typically recognize whether patients are in a state of acceptance or denial. Nurses play a key role in educating the individual that treatment only *begins* with detoxification and that life changing strategies require a commitment that can be fulfilled on a daily basis. In recovery terminology, this is referred to as "keeping it in the day." It lessens the fear of living "forever" without a substance. This daily coping strategy ameliorates anxiety and positions individuals to be able to live their lives "One day at a time" (AA, 2014).

In addition, the collateral effects of drug use on family members require concerted effort by all health care members. Interventions to support the family include referrals to and initiation of services. The nurse also can provide information on types of therapies that are most often prescribed for treatment of an addictive disorder. These various therapies may encompass pharmacological interventions, group sessions, complementary therapies, 12-step programs, outpatient programs, psychotherapy, and possible referral to an inpatient facility for extended care.

Nursing Interventions to Promote Healthy Coping Styles
table 20-6

Actions/Interventions	Rationales
Assist patients with identifying and interpreting stressful situations and people and determining new, more adaptive means of coping with them.	Identifying stressors and recognizing previously unsuccessful patterns of responding to them promotes creative problem solving.
Help patients to evaluate their methods for dealing with stressful situations and determining which methods have been successful or partially successful.	Empowers the patient to identify, develop, and reinforce effective coping methods and eliminate ineffective methods.
Monitor for and reinforce positive behaviors that suggest patterns of effective coping.	Psychologically strengthens and enhances coping skills. Increases confidence with regard to using new coping methods.
Maintain consistency with approach and teaching when interacting with the patient.	Provides structure, reduces stress, and promotes a trusting relationship.
Encourage patients to participate in care by assisting with activities of daily living as needed and able.	Promotes self-care, enhances coping, builds self-esteem, and increases motivation and compliance.
Encourage participation of significant others and family members in the development process by answering questions and allowing expression of feelings.	Builds a trusting support system and reduces stress.
Promote alternative techniques for self-expression and relaxation, such as journal writing, art projects, exercise, meditation, deep breathing, and/or volunteering.	Reduces stress and develops alternative coping methods.
Assist patients with identifying and using available support systems.	Broadens support network to reach short-term and long-term goals.
Initiate referrals to further psychological, psychiatric, and/or medical professionals as needed.	Provides support and a refined continuum of care.

Evaluation

Patients begin improving their lives by ceasing substance use and dependence and recognizing that addiction has played a major role in destructive patterns in their life. As patients progress through treatment, they will need to continue to examine their overall health across the domains and see how substances may continue to affect their health. Nursing evaluation includes reviewing the patient's health status, ability to sustain abstinence after withdrawal, daily compliance with medication protocols, use of support mechanisms, and adherence to other treatment recommendations, such as therapy (NIDA, 2009b).

PRACTICE ALERT It is important that nurses working with patients who abuse substances continue to engage in supervision with peers and supportive supervisors. Reactions to patients with addictive disorders can be intense and may precipitate emotional feelings in the health care provider. Recognition of personal awareness is a key strategy for nurses to provide ethical and humane treatment for those who suffer from an addictive disorder.

Pause and Reflect

1. *Why is it imperative to provide careful assessment and monitoring to patients experiencing substance withdrawal syndrome?*
2. *What nursing interventions can be used to promote effective health maintenance in patients with substance use disorders?*

From Suffering to Hope

Substance-related and addictive disorders may affect any individual, regardless of cultural or socioeconomic status. The ways in which individuals experience substance use disorders vary according to the individual as well as the substance. For example, in relation to alcohol, Benton has coined the term "high-functioning alcoholics" to describe individuals (including herself) who suffer silently because they and those around them deny any problem with alcohol (Benton, 2013). These are individuals who maintain success in their personal and professional lives while they and their families and friends remain in denial about their problem with alcohol.

Because many individuals turn to substances to alleviate physical or psychological suffering, assessment and treatment of underlying disorders are critical. As patients begin to develop hope that things can get better, they may begin to realize the effects of the substance on their physical and mental health. An individual's beliefs about hope may play a positive and significant role in substance abuse recovery (Matthis, Ferrari, Groh, & Jason, 2009). Nurses often are the care providers for individuals at different points of substance use and addiction, such as craving or withdrawal.

Nurses promote hope by ensuring safety, working with patients to reduce denial and become motivated to recover, providing education, and promoting appropriate coping mechanisms. Newer treatments, such as computer-based training for cognitive–behavioral therapy (CBT4CBT) modules supplemented with traditional counseling, offer hope by demonstrating improved outcomes for those with substance use disorders (Joel, 2009). Nursing care in combination with a comprehensive, collaborative treatment plan is more likely to be successful than any single intervention will be.

Gerald Kraymore—A Patient with Substance Use Disorder	NURSING CARE PLAN

Nursing Diagnosis: Anxiety Related to Withdrawal

Short-Term Goals *Patient will:* (include date for short-term goal to be met)	Intervention *Nurse will:*	Rationale
Short-term goal: Identify anxiety-producing states when person is in early stages of abstinence or withdrawal. (Within first 8 hours of acute hospitalization)	• Reduce anxiety by encouraging verbalization about a life without substances. Explore the effects of a new diagnosis and the patient's understanding of the diagnosis. • Review the patient's daily routine and the interplay of substance use in that routine. • Assess for withdrawal state and related symptomatology. • Assess for fluid balance and homeostasis. • Monitor closely for craving for substance of choice. • Medicate with appropriate withdrawal protocol as necessary, using the CIWA score. Provide additional nonpharmacological intervention to improve anxiety (e.g., warm baths, cool compresses, meditation, mindfulness strategies). • Allow grieving for the drug lifestyle. • Discuss the elements of stress and maladaptive coping.	• Allowing the person to maintain control by expressing fears can lessen anxiety in early stages of recovery. • With continued abstinence and use of appropriate medications if warranted for withdrawal state, the person will experience a calming effect as he proceeds through early recovery. • Development of healthy patterns of coping will replace the destructive drug using coping strategies. • Cessation of the drug requires patients to acknowledge that their relationship to the substance is ending; they will experience a sense of loss related to emotions, rituals, and lifestyle associated with the substance. • Examining stressors and how use of substances that provided relief can be replaced with healthy coping strategies.
Long-Term Goal Patient will address the fear and anxiety experienced when faced with cessation of use of their substance of choice (upon discharge and on a daily basis).	• Encourage the patient to use stress reduction techniques. • Encourage participation in support groups.	• Stress reduction techniques can help alleviate fear and anxiety, which may curb the patient's desire to return to substance use. • Support provided in therapy or self-help groups can assist patients to address fear and anxiety and maintain sobriety.

Clinical Reasoning

1. What other nursing diagnoses might the nurse working with Mr. Kraymore consider?
2. In addition to promoting a change in lifestyle for Mr. Kraymore, why might it be helpful to encourage him to consider medication-assisted treatment?
3. As the nurse, what will you need to include in Mr. Kraymore's discharge plan?

Gerald Kraymore Rehabilitation Phase

Mr. Kraymore has decided to accept extended post-hospitalization treatment at a residential treatment facility. He has been on the antidepressant medication citalopopram (Celexa) 40 mg PO daily to treat his depressive symptoms for about 4 weeks. His eating, sleeping, tearfulness, and moodiness have improved, although he still is struggling with feelings of guilt and shame. Mr. Kraymore has been attending AA meetings and meets regularly with his counselor. His endocarditis has improved. It has been noted by the staff that Mr. Kraymore is doing his best to comply with the program. He voices concern that he will relapse and be "a failure once again."

APPLICATION

1. What are the most immediate priorities for Mr. Kraymore at this stage of his care?
2. What major safety concerns should the nurse be mindful of at this stage of Mr. Kraymore's treatment and observable symptoms?

critical thinking

Chapter Highlights

1. Substance use disorders are a primary, chronic brain disease in which individuals engage in repetitive use of a substance despite negative consequences.

2. Substance-related and addictive disorders affect individuals across domains and may have long-lasting, adverse consequences.

3. Substance use disorders carry particular risk to cognitive and cardiovascular function. Some substances, such as opioids and marijuana, also carry risk to respiratory function.

4. As tolerance to a substance increases, the individual will need greater amounts of the substance to achieve the same effect, further increasing the risk for adverse effects.

5. Treatment may involve a variety of modalities, including pharmacotherapy, behavioral therapy, and self-help groups. Observation and assessment includes observing for withdrawal states, CNS vulnerability, and changes in mental status.

6. A targeted patient interview is necessary to elicit a full patient history of substance use.

7. Nursing interventions include those that promote communication, effective health maintenance, healthy coping, and hope.

NCLEX®-RN Questions

1. The nurse is working with the parents of a 16-year-old patient who has just begun treatment for alcohol use disorder. The parents state they still do not understand what could have caused their child to have this problem. Which response by the nurse is most appropriate?
   a. "Children usually carry on dysfunction that they have witnessed in their family lives."
   b. "Substance abuse is a complex problem believed to be influenced by a variety of factors."
   c. "In most cases parents have engaged in behaviors that shield their child from responsibility."
   d. "Many people who abuse substances have never really recognized the importance of a belief in a higher power."

2. The nurse is caring for a patient receiving treatment for a substance use disorder. Which statement by the patient best predicts a positive treatment response?
   a. "Everyone in my family wants me to get help."
   b. "My behavior may be because I have never felt loved."
   c. "I realize now I have a problem that is very destructive."
   d. "I am confident that I am ready to move on with my life."

3. The nurse is assessing the patient who has a history of substance use. Which finding indicates the presence of dependency?
   a. The patient is overcome by cravings and urges leading to use of the substance.
   b. The patient has a physiological withdrawal response when substance use ceases.
   c. The patient experiences physical and psychological changes after using the substance.
   d. The patient's addictive behavior continues despite a variety of negative consequences.

4. The nurse is planning care for a patient using methadone (Dolophine) therapy for the management of addiction. Which outcome is most appropriate for the nurse to identify?
   a. The patient will adhere to the treatment regimen for self-administration at home.
   b. The patient will develop an aversion to the use of substances of abuse.
   c. The patient will experience decreased severity of withdrawal symptoms.
   d. The patient will be free of symptoms of co-morbid depression and anxiety.

5. The nurse is evaluating readiness for discharge with a patient who is in a locked inpatient unit for the management of substance use/abuse and detoxification. The patient is no longer substance dependent and does not pose a danger to self or others. However, the patient has few resources, requires external structure, and would benefit from ongoing group intervention during recovery. Which treatment option is most appropriate?
   a. A sober house
   b. A "dry" shelter
   c. Continued inpatient treatment
   d. Participation in a 12-step program

6. The nurse is planning care for a patient in the recovery stage of alcohol abuse and dependency. The patient states that he does not want a treatment program that focuses on a strong spiritual component or offers groups in which members talk about their experiences and feelings. Which recovery option would the nurse explore with the patient?
   a. A 12-step group
   b. SMART Recovery
   c. A self-help group
   d. Alcoholics Anonymous

Answers can be found on the Pearson student resources site: nursing.pearsonhighered.com

References

A. A. World Services, Inc. (2002). The twelve steps of Alcoholics Anonymous. Available at http://www.aa.org/en_pdfs/smf-121_en.pdf

Adamson, D., and Ahmed, G. (2011). Addiction and Co-Occurring Disorders from a SMART Recovery Perspective: A Manual for Group Therapists. SMART Publications. Available at http://www.smartrecovery.org/professionals/

Addiction Intervention. (2014). Understanding the reasons people abuse drugs or alcohol. Available at http://www.addiction-intervention.com/addiction/addiction-research/understanding-the-reasons-people-abuse-drugs-or-alcohol/

Alcoholics Anonymous. (1976). *Alcoholics Anonymous*. New York, NY: Alcoholics Anonymous World Services, Inc.

Alcoholics Anonymous. (2014). Letter to anyone new to A.A. Available at http://www.alcoholics-anonymous.org/subpage.cfm?page=45

Alcohol Withdrawal. (2013). Available at http://www.webmd.com/mental-health/alcohol-abuse/alcohol-withdrawal-symptoms-treatments

American Academy of Pain Medicine (AAPM), American Pain Society (APS), & American Society of Addiction Medicine (ASAM). (2001). *Definitions Related to the Use of Opioids for the Treatment of Pain*. Glenview, IL: American Pain Society.

American Nurses Association (ANA). (1984). *Addictions and Psychological Dysfunctions in Nursing: The Profession's Response to the Problem*. Kansas City, MO: American Nurses Association.

American Nurses Association (ANA). (1997). ANA response to PEW Commission Report. Available at http://nursingworld.org/readroom/pew.htm#recommendations

American Psychiatric Association (APA). (2000). *Diagnostic and Statistical Manual of Mental Disorders* (4th ed., Text Revision). Washington, DC: American Psychiatric Association.

American Psychiatric Association (APA). (2012). Substance use and addictive disorders. Available at http://www.dsm5.org/proposedrevision/Pages/SubstanceUseandAddictiveDisorders.aspx

American Psychiatric Association (APA). (2013). *Diagnostic and Statistical Manual of Mental Disorders* (5th ed.). Washington, DC: American Psychiatric Publishers.

American Society of Addiction Medicine (ASAM). (2001). Patient placement criteria for the treatment of substance disorders (2nd ed., revised). Available at http://www.ncdhhs.gov/dma/lme/UMASAM.pdf

American Society of Addiction Medicine (ASAM). (2011). Definition of addiction. Available at http://www.asam.org/for-the-public/definition-of-addiction

American Society of Pain Management Nurses. (2003). *ASPMN Position Statement: Pain Management in Patients with Addictive Disease*. Pensacola, FL: American Society of Pain Management Nurses.

Anderson, D., Mizzari, K., & Kain, V. (2006). The effects of a multimodal intervention trial to promote lifestyle factors associated with the prevention of cardiovascular disease in menopausal and postmenopausal Australian women. *Health Care for Women International, 27*(3), 238–253.

Anderson, E., & McFarlane, J. (2008). *Community as Partner: Theory and Practice in Nursing*. Philadelphia, PA: Lippincott Williams & Wilkins.

Atkinson, R. M. (1995). Treatment programs for aging alcoholics. In T. P. Beresford & E. S. L. Gomberg, (Eds.). *Alcohol and Aging*. New York, NY: Oxford University Press, pp. 186–210.

Bales. R. F. (1946). Cultural differences in rates of alcoholism. *Quarterly Journal of Studies on Alcohol 6*, 489–499.

Bassuk, E. L., Buckner, J. C., Perloff, J. N., & Bassuk, S. S. (1998). Prevalence of mental health and substance use disorders among homeless and low-income housed mothers. *American Journal of Psychiatry, 155*, 1561–1564.

Bellack, A. S. & DiClemente, C. C. (1999). Treating substance abuse among patients with schizophrenia. *Psychiatric Services, 50*(1), 75–80.

Benton, S. A. (2013). The high functioning alcoholic. *Psychology Today*. Available at http://www.psychologytoday.com/blog/the-high-functioning-alcoholic/201308/alcoholism-does-not-discriminate-0

Blow, E. C., Schulenberg, K. J., Demo-Dananberg, L. M., Young, J. L., & Beresford, T. I. (1992). The Michigan Alcoholism Screening Test-Geriatric Version (MAST-G): A new elderly specific screening instrument. *Alcoholism: Clinical and Experimental Research, 16*, 372.

Blow, F. (2000) Treatment of older women with alcohol problems: Meeting the challenge for a special population. *Alcoholism: Clinical and Experimental Research, 24*(8), 1257–1266.

Boston University. (2007). Alcohol consumption linked to HIV disease progression, study shows. *Science Daily*. Available at http://www.sciencedaily.com/releases/2007/08/070820105240.htm

Brady, C., Becker, K., Bingham, L. E., Goldman, J., Wilson, B. B., & George, E. (2001). The case for mandatory certification. *Journal of Nursing Administration, 31*(10), 466–467.

Brady, K. T. (1998). Comorbidity of substance use and axis I psychiatric disorders. *Medscape Psychiatry & Mental Health ejournal, 3*(4). Available at http://www.medscape.com/viewarticle/430610

Brady, K. T., & Randall, C. L. (1999). Gender differences in substance abuse disorders. *Psychiatric Clinics of North America, 22*(2), 241–252.

Brick, J., & Erickson, C. (2006). *Drugs, the Brain and Behavior: The Pharmacology of Drug Use Disorders*. New York, NY: Routledge.

Brown, R. L., & Rounds, L. A. (1995). Conjoint screening questionnaires for alcohol and drug abuse. *Wisconsin Medical Journal, 94*(3), 135–140.

Cabaj, R. P. (2011). Gays, lesbians and bisexuals. In P. Ruiz & E. Strain, (Eds). *Lowinson and Ruiz's Substance Abuse: A Comprehensive Textbook* (5th ed.). Philadelphia, PA: Wolters/Kluwer/Lippincott Williams & Wilkins, pp. 871–880.

Carpenito, L. J. (2012). *Nursing Diagnosis: Application to Clinical Practice*. New York, NY: Lippincott Williams & Wilkins.

Carroll, C. R. (1989). *Drugs in Modern Society* (2nd ed.). Dubuque, IA: Wm. C. Brown Publishers.

Cary, A. H. (2001). Certified registered nurses: Results of the study on the certified work force. *American Journal of Nursing, 101*(1), 44–52.

Center for Substance Abuse Treatment (CSAT). (2004). Clinical guidelines for the use of buprenorphine in the treatment of opioid addiction. TIP Series 40. DHHS Publication No. (SMA) 04-3939. Rockville, MD: Substance Abuse and Mental Health Service Administration.

Center for Substance Abuse Treatment (CSAT). (2006). Detoxification and Substance Abuse Treatment. Treatment Improvement Protocol (TIP) Series, No. 45. Rockville, MD: Substance Abuse and Mental Health Services Administration. Available at http://www.ncbi.nlm.nih.gov/books/NBK64119/

Centers for Disease Control and Prevention. (2002). Drug-associated HIV transmission continues in the United States. Available at http://www.cdc.gov/hiv/resources/factsheets/idu.htm

Centers for Disease Control and Prevention. (2010). Basic information about HIV and AIDS. Available at http://www.cdc.gov/hiv/topics/basic/index.htm

Centers for Disease Control and Prevention. (2011). CDC health disparities and inequalities report—United States, 2011. *Morbidity and Mortality Weekly Report, 60*, 87–89. Available at http://www.cdc.gov/mmwr/pdf/other/su6001.pdf

Centers for Disease Control and Prevention. (2012a). Alcohol and public health: Frequently asked questions. Available at http://www.cdc.gov/alcohol/faqs.htm#heavyDrinking

Centers for Disease Control and Prevention. (2012b). Vital signs: Binge drinking. Available at http://www.cdc.gov/vitalsigns/bingedrinking/

Centers for Disease Control and Prevention. (2014). Alcohol and Public Health: Fact Sheets – Caffeine and Alcohol. Available at http://www.cdc.gov/alcohol/fact-sheets/cab.htm

Cheatle, M. D. & O'Brien, C. P. (2011). Opioid therapy in patients with chronic noncancer pain: Diagnostic and clinical challenges. In M. R. Clark & G. J. Treisman, (Eds.). *Chronic Pain and Addiction*. Basel, Switzerland: Karger, pp. 61–90.

Chick, S. L. (2009). Pharmacological management of the alcohol withdrawal syndrome. Available at http://www.michiganpharmacists.org/news/article.php?x=400.

Consumer Reports. (2012). The buzz on energy-drink caffeine. Available at http://www.consumerreports.org/cro/magazine/2012/12/the-buzz-on-energy-drink-caffeine/index.htm

Corley, M. C. & Goren, S. (1998). The dark side of nursing: Impact of stigmatizing responses on patients. *Scholarly Inquiry for Nursing Practice, 12*(2), 99–122.

Cryer, C., Jenkins, L., Cook, A., Ditchburn, J., Harris, C., Davis, A., & Peters, T. (1999). The use of acute and preventative medical services by a general population: Relationship to alcohol consumption. *Addiction 94*(10), 1523–1532.

Dekker, A. H. (2002). *Alcoholism in the Elderly*. Program and abstracts presented at the 33rd Annual Meeting and Medical-Scientific Conference. Atlanta, GA: American Society of Addiction Medicine, April 26, 2002.

Dennison, S. J. (2011). Substance use disorders in individuals with co-occurring psychiatric disorders. In P. Ruiz & E. Strain, (Eds.). *Lowinson and Ruiz's Substance Abuse: A Comprehensive Textbook* (5th Ed.). Philadelphia, PA: Wolters/Kluwer/Lippincott William & Wilkins, pp. 721–729.

DeVries, H., & Mudde, A. N. (1998). Predicting stage transitions for smoking cessation applying the attitude-social influence-efficacy model. *Psychology & Health, 13*(2), 369–385.

DiClemente, C. C. (1986). Self-efficacy and the addictive behaviors. *Journal of Social and Clinical Psychology, 4*(3), 302–315.

Ehrenstein, D. (1995). LA Times Book Review: All About Faye. *Los Angeles Times.* Available at http://articles.latimes.com/1995-01-22/books/bk227431nicole-brown/2

Erickson, C. (2007). *The Science of Addiction: Neurobiology to Treatment.* New York, NY: W.W. Norton & Company.

Evans, M., Stotts, A., Graham, S., Schmitz, J., & Grabowski, J. (2004). Hepatitis C knowledge assessment and counseling within the context of substance abuse treatment. *Addictive Disorders and their Treatment, 3*(1), 18–26.

Ewing, J. A. (1984). Detecting alcoholism: The CAGE questionnaire. *Journal of the American Medical Association, 252*(14), 1905–1907.

Feldman, J. M. (2011). The homeless. In P. Ruiz & E. Strain, (Eds.). *Lowinson and Ruiz's Substance Abuse: A Comprehensive Textbook* (5th Ed.). Philadelphia, PA: Lippincott Williams & Wilkins, pp. 901–907.

Fetal alcohol syndrome. (2012). Available at http://www.ncbi.nlm.nih.gov/pubmedhealth/PMH0001909/

Fingerhood, M. (2002). Substance abuse in older people. *Journal of the American Geriatrics Society, 48*(8), 985–995.

Finnell, D. (2002). White Paper. Certification in Addictions Nursing: Promoting and protecting the health of the public. International Nurses Society on Addictions. Available at http://www.intnsa.org/docs/certifications_addictions.pdf

Fishbain, D., Cutler, R., & Solomon, H. (1998). Comorbid psychiatric disorders in chronic pain patients with psychoactive substance abuse disorders. *Pain Clinics, 11*, 79–87.

Fleming, M., Davis, J., & Passik, S. (2008). Reported lifetime aberrant drug-taking behaviors are predictive of current substance abuse and mental health problems in primary care patients. *Pain Medicine, 9*(8), 1098–1106.

Freeman, D. (2013). Alcohol Abuse Health Center: 12 health risks of chronic heavy drinking. Available at http://www.webmd.com/mental-health/alcohol-abuse/features/12-health-risks-of-chronic-heavy-drinking

Galanter, M. (2008). Spirituality, evidence-based medicine, and Alcoholics Anonymous. *American Journal of Psychiatry, 165*(12), 1514–1517. Available at http://ajp.psychiatryonline.org/article.aspx?articleID=100364

Gastfried, D. R. (2004). Addiction treatment matching: Research Foundations of the American Society of Addiction Medicine (ASAM) Criteria. Binghamton, NY: The Haworth Medical Press.

Gastfried, D. R., & Mee-Lee, D. (2010). Patient Placement Criteria. In M. Galanter & H. D. Kleber (Eds.). *Psychotherapy for the Treatment of Substance Abuse* (4th ed.). Washington, DC: American Psychiatric Publishing, Inc., pp. 99–123.

Goforth, H. W., Caram, L. B., Maldonado, J., Ruiz, P., & Fernandez, F. (2011). Psychiatric complications of HIV-1 infection and drug abuse. In P. Ruiz & E. Strain, (Eds.). *Lowinson and Ruiz's Substance Abuse: A Comprehensive Textbook* (5th ed.). Philadelphia, PA: Lippincott Williams & Wilkins, pp. 682–694.

Goode, E. (2007). *Drugs in American Society* (7th ed.). New York, NY: McGraw-Hill Publishing Co.

Greenfield, S. F., Back, S. E., Lawson, K., & Brady, K. T. (2011). Women and addiction. In P. Ruiz & E. Strain, (Eds.). *Lowinson and Ruiz's Substance Abuse: A Comprehensive Textbook* (5th ed.). Philadelphia, PA: Lippincott Williams & Wilkins, pp. 847–870.

Grycynski, J., Mitchell, S. G., Peterson, T. R., Gonzales, A., Moseley, A., & Schwartz, R. P. (2011). The relationship between services delivered and substance use outcomes in New Mexico's screening, brief intervention, referral, and treatment (SBIRT) initiative. *Drug and Alcohol Dependence, 118*(2–3), 152–157.

Heath, D. B. (1992). Prohibition or liberalization of alcohol and drugs? In M. Galanter, (Ed.). *Recent Developments in Alcoholism: Alcohol and Cocaine.* New York, NY: Plenum, pp. 129–133.

Henningfield, J. E., Santora, P. B., & Bickel, W. K., (Eds.) (2007). *Addiction Treatment: Science and Policy for the Twenty-first Century.* Baltimore, MD: Johns Hopkins University Press.

Hoff, L. A., & Morgan, B. (2011). *Psychiatric and Mental Health Essentials in Primary Care.* New York, NY: Routledge.

Hoffman, R. S., & Weinhouse, G. L. (2013). Management of moderate and severe alcohol withdrawal syndromes. Available at http://www.uptodate.com/contents/management-of-moderate-and-severe-alcohol-withdrawal-syndromes

Howard, M. O., & Chung, S. S. (2000a). Nurses' attitudes towards substance misusers. I: Surveys. *Substance Use and Misuse, 35*(3), 347–365.

Howard, M. O., & Chung, S. S. (2000b). Nurses' attitudes towards substance misusers. II: Experiments and studies comparing nurses to other groups. *Substance Use and Misuse, 35*(4), 503–532.

Huether, S. E., & McCance, K. L. (2008). *Understanding Pathophysiology* (4th ed.). St. Louis, MO: Mosby.

Hulse, G. K., Morris, N., Arnold-Reed, D., & Tait, R. J. (2009). Improving clinical outcomes in treating heroin dependence: Randomized, controlled trial of oral or implant naltrexone. *Archives of General Psychiatry 2009, 66*(10), 1108–1115.

Iso, H., Baba, S., Mannami, T., Sasaki, S., Okada, K., Konishi, M. & Tsugane, S. (2004). Alcohol consumption and risk of stroke among middle-aged men: The JPHC Study Cohort I. *Stroke, 35*(5), 1124–1129.

Jaimes, C. M., DeMaster, E. G., Tian, R. X., & Raij, L. (2004). Stable compounds of cigarette smoke induce endothelial superoxide anion production via NADPH oxidase activation. *Arteriosclerosis Thrombus Vascular Biology, 24*(6), 1031–1036.

Jarvis, C. M., Hayman, L. L., Braun, L. T., Schwertz, D. W., Ferrans, C. E., & Piano, M. R. (2007). Cardiovascular risk factors and metabolic syndrome in alcohol and nicotine dependent men and women. *Journal of Cardiovascular Nursing, 22*(6), 429–435.

Jellinek, E. M. (2010). *The Disease Concept of Alcoholism.* New Haven, CT: New College and University Press.

Joel, L. A. (2009). *Advanced Practice Nursing: Essentials for Role Development* (2nd ed.). Philadelphia, PA: F. A. Davis.

Jordan, K. M. (2000). Substance abuse among gay, lesbian, bisexual, transgender and questioning adolescents. *School Psychology Review, 29*(2), 201–206.

Kinlock, T. W., Gordon, M. S., & Schwartz, R. P. (2011). Incarcerated populations. In P. Ruiz & E. Strain, (Eds.). *Lowinson and Ruiz's Substance Abuse: A Comprehensive Textbook* (5th ed.). Philadelphia, PA: Lippincott Williams & Wilkins, pp. 881–891.

Kinney, K. (1991). *Clinical Manual of Substance Abuse.* St. Louis, MO: Mosby.

Klagsburn, M., & Davis, D. (1977). Substance abuse and family interaction. *Family Process, 16*(2), 149.

Kleiber, B., Jain, S., & Trivedi, M. H. (2005). Depression and pain: Implications for symptomatic presentation and pharmacological treatments. *Psychiatry 2*(5), 12–24.

Krupitsky, E., Nunes, E., Ling, W., Illeperuma, A., Gastfriend, D., & Silverman, B. (2011). Injectable extended-release naltrexone for opioid dependence: A double-blind, placebo-controlled, multicentre randomised trial. *Lancet, 377*(9776), 1506–1513.

Lee, T. C., Hanlon, J. G., Ben-David, J., Booth, G. L., Cantor, W. J., Connolly, P. W., & Hwang, S. W. (2005). Risk factors for cardiovascular disease in homeless adults, *Circulation, 111*(20), 2629–2635.

Levin, B. R., Bull, J. J., & Stewart, F. M. (2000). *Epidemiology, Evolution and Future of the HIV/AIDS Pandemic.* Available at http://www.cdc.gov/ncidod/eid/vol7no3supp/levin.htm

Loneck, B., Garrett, J. A., & Banks, S. M. (1996). The Johnson intervention and relapse during outpatient treatment. *American Journal of Drug and Alcohol Abuse, 22*(3), 363–375.

Loukissa, D. (2007). Underdiagnosis of alcohol misuse in the older adult population. *British Journal of Nursing, 16*(20), 1254–1258.

Lowinson, J. H., Ruiz, P., Millman, R. B., & Langrod, J. G. (2005). *Substance Abuse* (4th ed.). Philadelphia, PA: Lippincott Williams & Wilkins.

Madras, B. K., Compton, W. M., Avula, D., Stegbauer, T., Stein, J. B., & Clark, H. W. (2009). Screening, brief interventions, referral to treatment (SBIRT) for illicit drug and alcohol use at multiple healthcare sites: Comparison at intake and 6 months later. *Drug and Alcohol Dependence, 99*(1–3), 280–295.

Matthis, G. M., Ferrari, J. R., Groh, D. R., & Jason, L. A. (2009). Hope and substance abuse recovery: The impact of agency and pathways within an abstinent communal-living setting. *Journal of Groups and Addiction Recovery, 4*(1/2), 42–50.

Mattick, R. P., Kimber, J., Breen, C., & Davoli, M. (2008). Buprenorphine maintenance versus placebo or methadone maintenance for opioid dependence. *Cochrane Database of Systematic Reviews, 16*(2), CD 002207.

Maurer, F. A., & Smith, C. M. (2009). *Community/Public Health Nursing Practice: Health for Families and Populations* (4th ed). St. Louis, MO: Saunders Elsevier.

McCaffery, M. (1968). *Nursing Practice Theories Related to Cognition, Bodily Pain, and Man Environment Interactions.* Los Angeles, CA: University of California at Los Angeles Students' Store.

McGinnis, K., Fultz, S., Skanderson, M., Conigliaro, J., Bryant, K., & Justice, A. (2006). Hepatocellular carcinoma and non-Hodgkins lymphoma: The roles of HIV, hepatitis C, and alcohol abuse. *Journal of Clinical Oncology, 24*(31), 5005–5009.

McIlvain, H., Bobo, J., Leed-Kelly, A., & Sitorius, M. (1998). Practical steps to smoking cessation for recovering alcoholics. *American Academy of Family Physicians.* Available at http://www.aafp.org/afp/980415ap/mcilvain.html

McMurran, M. (1994). *The Psychology of Addiction.* New York, NY: Taylor & Francis.

Meade, C. S., McDonald, L. J., Graff, S. F., Fitzmaurice, G. M., Griffin, M. L., & Weiss, R. D. (2009). A prospective study examining the effects of gender and sexual/physical abuse on mood outcomes in patients with co-occurring bipolar and substance use disorders. *Bipolar Disorders, 11*(4), 425–433.

Mee-Lee, D. (2006). Development and implementation of patient placement criteria, in "New Developments in Addiction Treatment." Academic Highlights, *Journal of Clinical Psychiatry, 67*(11), 1805–1807.

Mee-Lee, D., & Gastfried, D. R. (2008). Patient placement criteria. In M. Galanter & H. D. Kleber, (Eds.). *Textbook of Substance Abuse Treatment* (4th ed.). Washington, DC: American Psychiatric Publishers, pp. 79–91.

Mee-Lee D., & Shulman, G. D. (2009). The ASAM placement criteria and matching patients to treatment. In R. K. Ries, S. Miller, D. A. Fiellin, & R. Saitz, (Eds.). *Principles of Addiction Medicine* (4th ed.). Philadelphia, PA: Lippincott Williams & Wilkins, pp. 387–399.

Meichenbaum, D. (1994). *A Clinical Handbook/Practical Therapist Manual for Assessing Adults with Post-Traumatic Stress Disorder.* Ontario, Canada: Institute Press.

Mertens, J., Weisner, C., Ray, T., Fireman, B., & Walsh, K. (2005). Hazardous drinkers and drug users in primary care: Prevalence, medical conditions, and costs. *Alcoholism: Clinical and Experimental Research, 29*(5), 989–998.

Mignon, S., Marcoux-Faiia, M., Myers, P., & Rubington, E. (2009). *Substance Use and Abuse: Exploring Alcohol and Drug Issues.* Boulder, CO: Lynne Rienner Publishers.

Miller, W. R., & Rollnick, S. (2002). *Motivational Interviewing: Preparing People to Change.* New York, NY: Guilford Press.

Morgan, B., White, D., & Wallace, A. (2011). Substance abuse in older adults. In K. D. Melillo & S. C. Houde, (Eds.). *Geropsychiatric and Mental Health Nursing* (2nd ed.). Sudbury, MA: Jones & Bartlett Learning, pp. 227–252.

Mylonakis, E., & Calderwood, S. (2001). Infective endocarditis in adults. *New England Journal of Medicine, 345*(18), 1318–1330.

Najavits, L. (2002). *Seeking Safety: A Treatment Manual for PTSD and Substance Abuse.* New York: Guilford Press.

National Alliance on Mental Illness (NAMI). (2013). Dual diagnosis: Substance abuse and mental illness. Available at http://www.nami.org/Content/NavigationMenu/Inform_Yourself/About_Mental_Illness/By_Illness/Dual_Diagnosis_Substance_Abuse_and_Mental_Illness.htm

National Drug Prevention Alliance. (2007). Alcohol and Drug Dependence Is Not a Mental Illness. Position Paper. Available at http://www.cms.gov/medicare-coverage-database/details/nca-decision-memo.aspx

National Highway Traffic and Safety Administration (NHTSA). (2013). Drugs and human performance fact sheets: Cannabis/marijuana (Δ^9-Tetrahydrocannabinol, THC). Available at http://www.nhtsa.gov/people/injury/research/job185drugs/cannabis.htm.

National Institute on Drug Abuse (NIDA). (2003). Preventing drug use among children and adolescents: A research based guide for parents, educators and community leaders. NIH Publication No. 04-4212(A). Available at http://www.drugabuse.gov/publications/preventing-drug-use-among-children-adolescents

National Institute on Drug Abuse (NIDA). (2008). Drugs, brains, and behavior: The science of addiction. U.S. Department of Health and Human Services. NIH Pub. No. 08-5605. Available at http://www.drugabuse.gov/publications/science-addiction

National Institute on Drug Abuse (NIDA). (2009a). NIDA notes. Available at http://www.drugabuse.gov/NIDA_notes/NNvol22N5/DirRepVol22N5.html

National Institute on Drug Abuse (NIDA). (2009b). Principles of drug addiction treatment: A research-based guide. U.S. Department of Health & Human Services. NIH publication No. 09-4180. Available at http://www.drugabuse.gov/publications/principles-drug-addiction-treatment

National Institute on Drug Abuse (NIDA). (2010a) Drugfacts: Methamphetamine. Available at http://www.drugabuse.gov/publications/drugfacts/methamphetamine

National Institute of Drug Abuse (NIDA). (2010b). *Drugs, Brains and Behavior: The Science of Addiction.* Available at http://www.drugabuse.gov/publications/science-addiction

National Institute on Drug Abuse (NIDA). (2011). Comorbidity: Addiction and other mental disorders. NIDA Info Facts. Available at http://www.drugabuse.gov/tib/comorbid.html

National Institute on Drug Abuse (NIDA). (2012a). Medical consequences of drug abuse. Retrieved from http://www.drugabuse.gov/related-topics/medical-consequences-drug-abuse

National Institute on Drug Abuse (NIDA). (2012b). The science of drug abuse and addiction. Available at http://www.drugabuse.gov/publications/media-guide/science-drug-abuse-addiction

National Institute on Drug Abuse (NIDA). (2012c). Drug facts: Marijuana. Available at http://www.drugabuse.gov/publications/drugfacts/marijuana

National Institute on Drug Abuse (NIDA). (2012d). Drug facts: Inhalants. Available at http://www.drugabuse.gov/publications/drugfacts/inhalants

Newfield, S., Hina, M., Tilley, D., Sridaramont, K., & Maramba, P. (2007). *Cox's Clinical Applications of Nursing Diagnosis.* Philadelphia, PA: F.A. Davis.

North, C. S., Eyrich, K. M., Pollio, D. E., & Spitznagel, E. L. (2004). Are rates of psychiatric disorders in the homeless population changing? *American Journal of Public Health, 94*(1), 103–108.

Ochberg, F. M. (1995). Post-traumatic therapy. In G. S. Everly & J. M. Lating (Eds.). *Psychotraumatology: Key Papers and Core Concepts in Post-Traumatic Stress.* New York: Plenum, pp. 245–265.

Oliver, J., Coggins, C., Compton, P., Hagan, S., Matteliano, D., Stanton, M., St. Marie, B., Strobbe, S., & Turner, H. N. (2012). American Society for Pain Management nursing position statement: Pain management in patients with substance use disorders. *Pain Management Nursing, 13*(3), 169–183.

Oslin, D. W., Pettinati, H., & Volpicelli, J. R. (2002). Alcoholism treatment adherence: Older age predicts better adherence and drinking outcomes. *American Journal of Geriatric Psychiatry, 10*(6), 740–747.

Patrizi, R., Pasceri, V., Sciahabasi, A., Summaria, A., Rosano, G., & Lioy, E. (2006). Evidence of cocaine-related coronary atherosclerosis in young patients with myocardial infarction. *Journal of the American College of Cardiology, 47*(10), 2120–2122.

Perfas, F. (2004). *Therapeutic Community: Social Systems Perspective.* Lincoln, NE: iUniverse Inc.

Perlstein, T. S., & Lee, R. T. (2006). Smoking, metalloproteinases, and vascular disease. *Arteriosclerosis, Thrombosis, and Vascular Biology, 26,* 250–256.

Portenoy, R. K. (2011). Acute and chronic pain. In P. Ruiz & E. Strain, (Eds.). *Lowinson and Ruiz's Substance Abuse: A Comprehensive Textbook* (5th ed.). Philadelphia, PA: Lippincott Williams & Wilkins, pp. 695–720.

Porth, C. (2012). *Pathophysiology: Concepts of Altered Health States* (8th ed.). Philadelphia, PA: Lippincott Williams & Wilkins.

Reid, S., & Juma, O. (2009). Minimum infective dose of HIV for parenteral dosimetry. *International Journal of STD & AIDS, 20*(12), 828–833. Available at http://cabdirect.org/abstracts/20103014898.html

Ries, R. K., Miller, S. C., Fiellin, D. A., & Saitz, R., (Eds.). (2009). Appendix 1: ASAM addiction terminology. In *Principles of Addiction Medicine* (4th ed.). Chevy Chase, MD: American Society of Addiction Medicine, pp. 552–558.

The Role of Spirituality in Addiction Treatment and Recovery: A Qualitative Research Study. (2006). Burtonville, MD: 9th Sign Communications.

Rosenblatt, R. (2007). Investigating the role of spirituality in recovery from addiction. Available at http://www.rwjf.org/en/research-publications/find-rwjf-research/2007/12/spirituality-has-a-role-in-substance-abuse-treatment-programs--m.html

Ruiz, P., and Strain, E. (2011). *Lowinson and Ruiz's Substance Abuse: A Comprehensive Textbook.* New York, NY: Lippincott Williams & Wilkins.

Samaha A-N., & Robinson, T. E. (2005). Why does the rapid delivery of drugs to the brain promote addiction? *Trends in Pharmacological Sciences, 26*(2), 82–87.

Schultz, L. M., & Videbeck, S. L. (2008). *Manual of Psychiatric Nursing Care Plans.* Boston, MA. Lippincott Williams & Wilkins.

Screening Brief Intervention Referral to Treatment: Assessment Orders. (2012). Kettering, OH: Kettering Health Network.

Shulman, G. (2003). Senior moments: Assessing older adults. *Addiction Today, 15*(82), 7–19.

SMART Recovery. (2013). SMART Recovery—Self management for addiction recovery. Available at http://www.smartrecovery.org/

Smeltzer, S., Bare, B., Hinkle, J., & Cheever, K. (2008). *Brunner and Suddarth's Textbook of Medical-Surgical Nursing* (11th ed.). Philadelphia, PA: Lippincott Williams & Wilkins.

Solomon, S., Gerrity, E. T., & Muff, A. M. (1992). Efficacy of treatments for post traumatic stress disorder: An empirical review. *Journal of the American Medical Association, 268*(5), 633–638.

Sorajjakool, S., Thompson, K., Aveling, L. & Earl, A. (2006). Chronic pain, meaning, and spirituality: A qualitative study of the healing process in relation to the role of meaning and spirituality. *The Journal of Pastoral Care and Counseling, 60*(4), 369–378.

Stoppler, M. C. (2013). Is your child or teen "huffing"? Medicine.net. Retrieved from http://www.medicinenet.com/script/main/art.asp?articlekey=47975

Substance Abuse and Mental Health Services Administration (SAMHSA). (2006). Detoxification and substance abuse treatment. Available at http://www.ncbi.nlm.nih.gov/books/NBK64115/

Substance Abuse and Mental Health Services Administration (SAMHSA). (2010). *Adults with Mental Illness: Findings from the 2008 National Survey on Drug Use and Health.* HHS Publication No. SMA 10-4614, Analytic Series A-31. Rockville, MD: Center for Behavioral Health Statistics and Quality and Center for Mental Health Services.

Substance Abuse and Mental Health Services Administration (SAMHSA). (2011a). *Identifying Mental Health and Substance Use Problems of Children and Adolescents: A Guide for Child-Serving Organizations.* HHS Publication No. SMA 12-4670. Rockville, MD: Center for Behavioral Health Statistics and Quality and Center for Mental Health Services..

Substance Abuse and Mental Health Services Administration (SAMHSA). (2011b). *Results from the 2010 National Survey on Drug Use and Health: Summary of National Findings,* NSDUH Series H-41, HHS Publication No. (SMA) 11-4658. Rockville, MD: Substance Abuse and Mental Health Services Administration.

Substance Abuse and Mental Health Services Administration (SAMHSA), (2013). *Results from the 2012 National Survey on Drug Use and Health: Summary of National Findings,* NSDUH Series H-46, HHS Publication No. (SMA) 13-4795. Rockville, MD: Substance Abuse and Mental Health Services Administration.

Substance Abuse and Mental Health Services Administration, Center for Behavioral Health Statistics and Quality. (2011). *The NSDUH Report: Illicit Drug Use among Older Adults.* Rockville, MD: Substance Abuse and Mental Health Services Administration.

Substance Abuse and Mental Health Services Administration, Office of Applied Studies. (2009). *The NSDUH report: trends in non-medical use of prescription pain relievers: 2002–2007.* Rockville, MD: Substance Abuse and Mental Health Services Administration Office of Applied Studies.

Tonigan, J. S. (2007). Spirituality and Alcoholics Anonymous. *Southern Medical Journal, 100*(4), 437–440. Available at http://www.ncbi.nlm.nih.gov/pubmed/17458419.

U.S. Census Bureau. (2009). *State & Country Quick Facts.* Available at http://quickfacts.census.gov/gfd/states/25/2507000.html

U.S. Department of Justice. (2013). *Situation report, synthetic cathinones (bath salts): An emerging domestic threat.* Available at http://www.justice.gov/archive/ndic/pubs44/44571/44571p.pdf

U.S. Preventive Services Task Force (USPSTF). (2004). *Screening and behavioral counseling interventions in primary care to reduce alcohol misuse.* Available at http://www.uspreventiveservicestaskforce.org/uspstf12/alcmisuse/alcmisusefinalrs.htm

U.S. Preventive Services Task Force (USPSTF). (n.d.). *Evidence-based methods for evaluating behavioral counseling interventions.* Available at http://www.uspreventiveservicestaskforce.org/3rduspstf/behavior/behsum2.htm

van Wormer, K. & Davis, D. R. (2008). *Addiction Treatment: A Strengths Perspective* (2nd ed.). Belmont, CA: Thomson.

Verdiun, M. L., Tolliver, B. K., & Brady, K. T. (2005). Substance abuse and bipolar disorder. *Medscape Psychiatry & Mental Health ejournal.* Available at http://www.medscape.com/viewarticle/515954.

Watson, J. (1996). Art, caring, spiritual and humanity. In E. Farmer, (Ed.). *Exploring the Spiritual Dimension of Care.* Wiltshire, UK: Mark Allen, pp. 29–40.

Weissman, D. E., & Haddox, J. D. (1989). Opioid pseudoaddiction-an iatrogenic syndrome. *Pain, 36*(3), 363–366.

Wernicke-Korsakoff Syndrome. (2012). Available at http://www.nlm.nih.gov/medlineplus/ency/article/000771.htm

Wilson, B. A., Shannon, M. T., & Shields, K. M. (2014). *Pearson Nurse's Drug Guide 2014.* Upper Saddle River, NJ: Pearson Education.

Yew, D. (2013). Caffeine toxicity. Available at http://emedicine.medscape.com/article/821863-overview

Zarkin, G., Bray, J., Babor, T., & Higgins-Bindle, J. (2004). Alcohol drinking patterns and health care utilization in a managed care setting. *Health Services Research, 39*(3), 553–570.

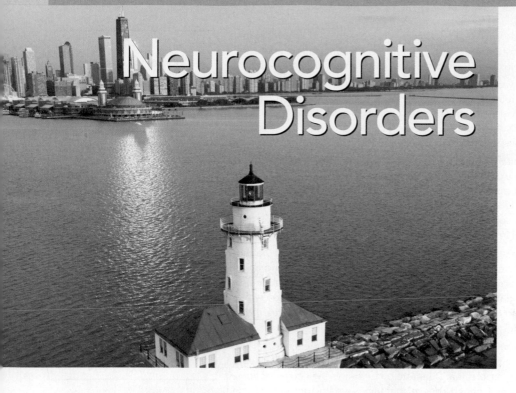

Neurocognitive Disorders

21

Maureen Gaynor

Learning Outcomes

1. Examine the etiology of neurocognitive disorders.

2. Analyze the impact of biological, psychological, sociological, cultural, and spiritual domains on neurocognitive disorders.

3. Differentiate the clinical characteristics, onset, and course of delirium and dementia.

4. Compare the different types of dementia.

5. Contrast the different stages of Alzheimer disease.

6. Evaluate various treatment modalities used in the treatment of patients with delirium and dementia.

7. Plan evidence-based nursing care for patients diagnosed with neurocognitive disorders.

Key Terms

Donnette Initial Onset

Donnette Kolb is a 72-year-old, well-dressed Jewish woman who comes to an outpatient private mental health practice accompanied by her husband of 52 years. When Ann, a psychiatric nurse practitioner, invites Donnette into the office, her husband joins her. Donnette uses a cane as she walks into the office.

During the interview, Ann learns that Donnette was a professor at a small college, where she taught microbiology and chemistry for 27 years. Donnette retired 5 years ago and has found the transition difficult. "My husband is always busy—he loves to woodwork and spends hours in the basement doing that. I don't know what to do with myself." Donnette informs Ann that she voluntarily surrendered her driver's license about a year ago, stating, "I didn't want to be responsible for hurting someone in an accident."

Donnette has been referred by her geropsychiatrist for therapy to help her cope with her diagnosis of Alzheimer disease. Donnette reports symptoms of forgetfulness, short-term memory loss, lack of motivation, sadness, poor appetite, apathy, boredom, and loss of interest in doing anything. She has become increasingly worried about what the future is going to bring and that she is going to end up like her mother, who died at 92. "My mother suffered for the last 15 years of her life with dementia. She didn't recognize me or my sister and died in a nursing home all alone."

Donnette also discloses that she doesn't understand what she is not doing right at home and that her husband, Jim, is becoming increasingly frustrated with her memory issues. She reports feeling down and sad a lot, and says, "Why am I here? What's the point?" She denies having suicidal ideation or a plan. Her husband shares that their 42-year-old married daughter has recently been diagnosed with a brain tumor and is currently undergoing chemotherapy and radiation. Donnette tearfully states, "Why her? She's so young—it should be me instead."

Jim reports that he is concerned for Donnette's safety in the house. "I went for a walk the other day. I was only gone about an hour, but when I got back, a pot was burning on the stove. Donnette had put some water on to boil and forgotten about it." He also reports that Donnette often forgets their conversations, and will ask Jim the same questions over and over. Donnette denies that things are that bad. During the interview Ann observes that Donnette is resistant to any suggestions that further limit her independence.

Jim has taken over the upkeep of the house: all the food shopping, cooking, and financial matters. Prior to Donnette's diagnosis with Alzheimer disease, Donnette and Jim had led a very active social life. Now it seems as if the only places they ever go are the doctor's office and the grocery store. Jim states that he doesn't know what to do and that he frequently feels overwhelmed, angry, and impatient with Donnette.

During the interview, Ann listens to both Donnette's and Jim's concerns. At the end of the joint session, Ann asks Donnette how she feels about coming to see her on a regular basis for individual therapy, and having Jim join her at times. Donnette agrees, stating, "Well, my doctor wanted me to come, and I feel comfortable with you." Ann asks Donnette to sign a release of information that will allow her to speak with Donnette's geropsychiatrist about any concerns. Ann sets up another appointment, for the following week, to start working with her.

APPLICATION

1. Address the five domains for Donnette:
   a. Biological
   b. Psychological
   c. Sociological
   d. Cultural
   e. Spiritual

2. In what ways do you think Donnette may be suffering? Why?

3. In what ways do you think Jim is suffering? Why?

4. How would you prioritize Donnette's needs during this encounter, and why?

5. In what ways does Ann convey hope to Donnette? What might be done differently to offer hope?

Introduction

Cognition involves processes to gain knowledge and comprehension, such as thinking, knowing, remembering, judging, and problem solving (Cherry, 2013). It involves one's perception of reality and understanding of its representations. Additionally, other cognitive functions include acquisition and use of language and orientation to time and space. Cognition is the basis of judgment, reasoning, attention, comprehension, concept formation, planning, and the use of symbols, such as letters and numbers, used in writing and mathematics.

Memory, a component of cognition, refers to the ability to recall or reproduce what has been learned or experienced. It is more than simple storage and retrieval; it is a complex cognitive mental function that includes most areas of the brain, especially the hippocampus, which is believed to be essential for the transfer of some memories from short-term to long-term storage (Swenson, 2006). Memory is the brain function that makes possible retaining, storing, and retrieving information (Cherry, 2013).

Deficits in cognition can result from a variety of causes: changes in neurological adaptation within the brain due to disease or illness;

modifications as the result of substance use, prescribed or illicit; and trauma. Deficits of memory, such as **amnesia**, the loss of recent and remote memory, are an essential feature of many cognitive disorders, particularly dementia. Both memory deficits and impairments in cognitive functioning, whether mild or severe, transient or chronic, can cause great distress to patients and their family members. This chapter covers specific disorders recognized in the DSM-5 characterized by deficits in cognition or memory and representing a clear-cut deterioration from a previous level of functioning.

The DSM-5 identifies several types of neurocognitive disorders (NCDs). The NCDs include delirium as well as other NCDs considered either mild or major, with etiological subtypes listed. A decline from a previous level of functioning may indicate the presence of an NCD (American Psychiatric Association [APA], 2013).

Delirium typically is an abrupt, short-term change in mental state marked by confused thinking, disorientation, perceptual disturbances, agitation, and mood swings. Delirium results from an underlying medical condition, substance intoxication or withdrawal, exposure to a toxin, or other etiology. Delirium often resolves with treatment of the condition.

Dementia, a progressive disorder characterized by gradual loss of cognitive functioning (including memory, language, and executive function), is classified in the DSM-5 as a neurocognitive disorder, with specifiers as to etiology. Some clinicians consider the term "dementia" as stigmatizing and favor the term "neurocognitive disorder" (Stetka & Cornell, 2013). The most common form of dementia is **Alzheimer disease,** which affects more than 5 million adults in the United States (Alzheimer Association, 2014). The term *neurocognitive disorder* may be used when discussing various types of dementia, but also may be used when discussing neurocognitive issues that affect a younger population, such as HIV-related dementia (APA, 2013). The DSM-5 differentiates the severity of NCDs and whether behavioral disturbances are a feature of the patient's presentation. *Major neurocognitive disorders* are characterized by a significant decline in cognitive ability to the extent that the individual requires assistance with daily activities. Individuals with *mild neurocognitive disorder* may need more time or may need to make accommodations to engage in daily activities, but are able to continue to do them independently (APA, 2013).

Amnestic disorders were included in earlier editions of the DSM. The category was excluded from the DSM-5. These disorders were characterized by an inability to learn new information (short-term memory deficit) despite normal attention, and an inability to recall previously learned information (long-term memory deficit). Profound amnesia may result in disorientation to place and time, but rarely to self (APA, 2000). An individual with amnesia may engage in **confabulation**, the creation of imaginary events to fill in memory gaps. The onset of symptoms may be acute or insidious, depending on the pathological process. Now, however, an amnestic disorder is categorized as a neurocognitive disorder due to another medical condition, with an onset and course progressing along the lines of the causative illness (APA, 2013).

Nurses often are the first and most frequent contacts that patients with NCDs and their families have within the health care system. This is true across multiple settings, from the emergency department to home health care, and from primary care clinics to assisted living and memory care facilities. Because of the widespread impact of NCDs on family members, nurses in every setting need to understand these disorders and be able to promote hope and healing to those affected by them.

Theoretical Foundations

Cognition affects every aspect of an individual's life and has real implications for health and wellness. A patient's ability to access health care, take medications, report symptoms and adverse effects, and participate in health promotion activities depends on and has an impact on cognitive ability. Even the slightest change in physiological homeostasis can affect cognition. In turn, the slightest cognitive change can affect physiological homeostasis, increasing the patient's risk for illness or injury. Nurses working with patients with cognitive deficits must understand the relationship between cognition and the wellness domains (Table 21-1).

Biological Domain

Delirium, dementia, and other cognitive disorders may share some clinical manifestations in common, but the onset and course of these disorders vary widely. Identifying etiology quickly can assist in determining appropriate treatment and improving patient outcomes.

Impaired Cognitive Responses by Domain	table 21-1

Domain	Responses
Biological	• Sleep disturbances, e.g., insomnia or hypersomnia • Psychomotor agitation • Restlessness • Aphasia • Apraxia • Agnosia • Incontinence • Sundowning • Hypervigilance
Psychological	• Confusion • Extreme distractibility • Rambling speech • Disorientation to time, place, person • Fear • Anxiety • Crying • Depression • Irritability • Anger • Apathy • Mood swings • Disturbance in executive function • Recent/remote memory loss • Delusions and hallucinations • Withdrawal • Psychosis • Impaired judgment/difficulty making decisions • Suspiciousness • Disinihibition • Hypersexuality
Sociological	• Lack of connections; feelings of isolation • Lack of sense of relatedness; feelings of loneliness • Challenged in relation to community resources
Cultural	• Loss of connectedness, sense of belonging to others from the same race, religion, or culture • Loss of connectedness to those who share values, language, or experience • Lack of access to services due to language or other cultural barriers
Spiritual	• Feeling a lack of connectedness to God or Higher Power and/or with others who share beliefs • Struggles with faith, meaning, and purpose • Expressing feelings of guilt related to symptoms

Delirium

The DSM-5 (APA, 2013) differentiates between the disorders of delirium by etiology. Changes in the mental status of a person with delirium generally occur because of one or more organic factors. The hallmark characteristics of delirium are a change in attention, such as inability to direct or focus attention, and cognition disturbances, such as memory deficits or disorientation. Delirium also develops over a short period of time and fluctuates in severity. Delirium may be acute (lasting hours or days) or persistent (lasting weeks or months) (APA, 2013). The following are some types of delirium:

Substance-intoxication delirium: These symptoms may arise within minutes or hours of taking high doses of certain drugs, such as alcohol, marijuana, phencyclidine (PCP), cocaine, inhalants, or hallucinogens, or exposure to toxins such as pesticides and carbon monoxide. The substance may be unknown. If a patient is experiencing symptoms from stopping use of substances such as recreational drugs, the clinician will instead diagnose *substance-withdrawal delirium*.

Medication-induced delirium: This disorder develops after reduction or termination of sustained or unusually high doses of certain medications, such as opioids, sedatives, hypnotics, anxiolytics, or amphetamines. Other medications that could precipitate a substance-induced delirium include analgesics, anticonvulsants, antihistamines, antihypertensives, lithium, and psychotropic medications with anticholinergic side effects. Polypharmacy, especially in older adults, can predispose an individual to developing delirium. The duration of the delirium is directly related to the half-life of the substance involved, lasting from a few hours to up to 2 weeks, and to the renal and hepatic function of the patient, among other factors.

Delirium due to another medical condition: Evidence must exist from the individual's history or lab findings to indicate that the symptoms of delirium are the direct result of physiological consequences of a general medical condition. Examples include infections, metabolic disorders, fluid or electrolyte imbalance, renal or hepatic disease, postoperative states, and head trauma.

Clinicians may also diagnose *delirium due to multiple etiologies* when multiple medical and/or substance etiologies are present.

Delirium occurs frequently among hospitalized older adults and may affect up to 24% of that population (APA, 2013). The presence of delirium in community settings is relatively low, but incidence increases with age. Other triggers of delirium include psychosocial stressors, such as relocation or sudden changes within a person's environment; sensory deprivation or sensory overload; injury due to a fall or accident; and sleep deprivation.

The most important fact about delirium is that it signals the presence of an underlying condition that potentially can be reversed. Without prompt diagnosis and treatment, however, the condition may become life threatening.

Neurocognitive Disorders

The etiology and pathology for dementia determine the type of dementia, although clinical manifestations and nature of onset play a role in diagnosis. For example, severe head trauma, HIV, Huntington disease, and Parkinson disease are types of injury or illness that may, for some patients, result in dementia (APA, 2013) (Table 21-2). The presence of a cognitive disorder can affect patient function within the biological domain. For example, patients experiencing the progressive effects of dementia are at greater risk for injury due to falls, medication errors (including forgetting to take prescribed medication), malnutrition, and elder abuse (Reinhard, Given, Petlick, & Bemis,

2008). For patients at a high level of acuity, patient education will be insufficient to protect them if they are living at home.

Alzheimer Disease

Alzheimer disease (AD) is the most common form of dementia, accounting for more than 50% of dementia cases (APA, 2013; Alzheimer's Association, 2014). At the turn of the 20th century, Alois Alzheimer, a German neuropsychiatrist, observed changes in the brain of a woman with clinical signs of what was regarded then as "senile" dementia (Page, 2011). A combination of genetics and biology is thought to play a role in the development of AD: There is clearly a familial pattern with some forms of the disease. Some studies indicate that early-onset cases are more likely to be familial than late-onset cases, and that from one-third to one-half of all cases may be of the genetic form. The International Genomics Alzheimer Project consortium has discovered 11 confirmed genes that are implicated in the development of AD (Lambert et al., 2013).

The exact cause of AD is still uncertain, but scientists have discovered several theories related to the cause of the disease. The pathological theory states that the decline in brain function is related to the buildup of plaques and tangles in the brain (Figure 21-1). Plaques are made up of fragments of a protein called *beta amyloid*. Plaques are formed when these fragments clump together; they accumulate in the spaces between neurons and interfere with neuron communication, metabolism, replenishment, and repair. Another protein, *tau*, is chemically altered in patients with AD; strands of the protein become tangled together, interfering with neuronal transport (National Institute on Aging, 2009). It is thought that the plaques and tangles contribute to the death and destruction of neurons, leading to memory failure, personality changes, and inability to carry out activities of daily living (ADLs). The genetic theory asserts that at least four isolated genes are responsible for the transmission of AD. The neurochemical theory postulates that the reduction of **acetylcholine**, an enzyme essential to memory, concentration, and attention, can contribute to the symptoms exhibited by patients with AD. An increase in the neurotransmitter glutamate can also cause the symptoms associated with AD.

Vascular Dementia

In **vascular dementia**, patients suffer the equivalent of small strokes that destroy many areas of the brain. Onset is abrupt, resulting in rapid changes to functioning (Yuhas, McGowan, Fontaine, Czech, & Gambrell-Jones, 2006). Computed tomography or magnetic resonance imaging usually shows multiple vascular lesions of the cerebral cortex and subcortical structures, resulting from the decreased blood supply to the brain. In addition to declining cognitive functioning characteristic of dementia, patients with vascular dementia commonly exhibit weakness of the limbs, small-stepped gait, and difficulty with speech.

Dementia Due to Prion Disease

Rarely, dementia may result from transmissible spongiform encephalopathies that are caused by the infectious form of a normally harmless type of protein, called a *prion* (National Institute of Neurological Disorders and Stroke [NINDS], 2014). The most common of these is Creutzfeldt–Jakob disease, which typically develops in adults 40 to 60 years of age. It involves altered vision, loss of coordination or abnormal movements, and dementia that usually progresses rapidly, with most individuals dying within a year.

Selected Neurocognitive Disorders Resulting in Dementia

table 21-2

Disorder	Etiology	Clinical Manifestations	Onset/Course
Dementia due to HIV	Infection with HIV-1 produces a dementing illness called HIV-1–associated cognitive/motor complex.	Symptoms vary widely from person to person. Severe cognitive changes, particularly confusion, changes in behavior, and sometimes psychosis, are not uncommon in the later stages.	At first, symptoms are subtle and may be overlooked. The severity of symptoms is associated with the extent of the brain pathology.
Dementia due to traumatic brain injury (TBI)	Any type of head trauma may result in symptoms of dementia. The most common forms of TBI are from falls, motor vehicle accidents, and head injuries.	Amnesia is the most common neurobehavioral symptom following head trauma.	A degree of permanent disturbance may persist.
Dementia due to Parkinson disease	Parkinson disease is a neurological condition resulting from the death of neurons, including those that produce dopamine, the chemical responsible for movement and coordination. It is characterized by tremor, rigidity, bradykinesia, and postural instability.	Dementia has been reported in approximately 20% to 60% of people with Parkinson disease and is characterized by cognitive and motor slowing, impaired memory, and impaired executive functioning.	Onset and course are slow and progressive.
Dementia due to Huntington disease	Huntington disease is an inherited, dominant gene, neurodegenerative disease. The first symptoms typically are choreic movements that involve facial contortions, twisting, turning, and tongue movements.	Cognitive symptoms include memory deficits, both recent and remote, as well as significant problems with frontal executive function, personality changes, and other signs of dementia.	The disease begins in the late 30s or early 40s and may last 10 to 20 years or more before death.
Lewy body dementia	This disorder is distinctive by the presence of Lewy bodies—eosinophilic inclusion bodies—seen in the cortex and brainstem.	Clinically, Lewy body disease is similar to AD; however, there is an earlier appearance of visual hallucinations and Parkinsonian features.	Irreversible and progressive; tends to progress more rapidly than AD.

Based on Andreasen, N. C., & Black, D. W. (2006). *Introductory Textbook of Psychiatry* (4th ed.).Washington, DC: American Psychiatric Publishing; Sharon, I. (2010). Huntington disease dementia. Available at http://emedicine.medscape.com/289706; Bourgeois, J. A., Seaman, J. S., & Servis, M. E. (2008). Delirium, dementia, and amnestic disorders. In R. E. Hales, S. C. Yudofsky, & G. O. Gabbard, (Eds.). *Textbook of Clinical Psychiatry* (5th ed). Washington, DC: American Psychiatric Publishing; American Psychiatric Association. (2013). *Diagnostic and Statistical Manual of Mental Disorders* (5th ed.). Washington, DC: American Psychiatric Publishers.

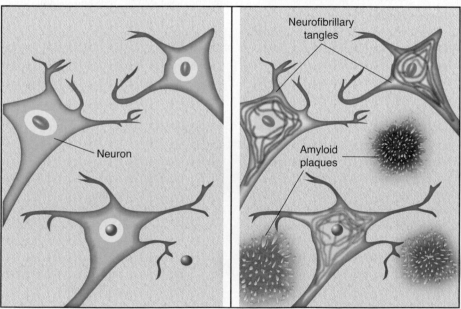

Normal Brain

Brain with Alzheimer Disease

Neurofibrillary tangles

Neuron

Amyloid plaques

21-1   A buildup of beta amyloid plaques and tangled strands of tau protein interferes with neuronal health, communication, and transport functions, resulting in the symptoms of Alzheimer disease. As plaques and tangles continue to form, symptoms become more severe.

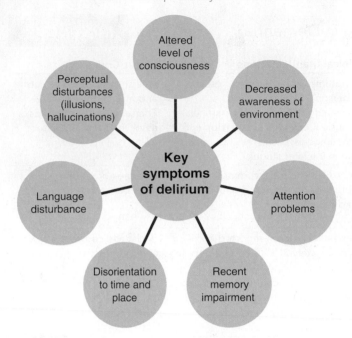

21-2   Delirium is characterized by rapid changes in cognitive function.

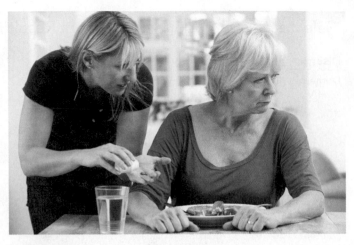

21-3   Symptoms of neurocognitive disorders can include memory loss, withdrawal, extreme distractibility, mood swings, and feelings of isolation. Helping patients manage these symptoms can be challenging for caregivers and nurses.

Source: Monkey Business/Fotolia

Psychological Domain

Psychological assessment of the individual with NCDs focuses on cognitive changes revealed through the mental status examination, as well as the resulting behavioral manifestations. The nurse must be cognizant of the critical differences in the onset and course between delirium and dementia. In the patient with delirium, a mental status evaluation reveals several rapid changes (Figure 21-2): alterations in the level of consciousness with reduced awareness of the environment; difficulty focusing and sustaining or shifting attention; recent memory impairment; disorientation to time and place; and language and perceptual disturbances.

Perception is the ability to process information from the internal and external environment. These perceptual disturbances may take the form of illusion or hallucinations. *Illusions* are false perceptions of sensory stimuli in the environment. *Hallucinations* are defined as sensory perceptions for which there is no external stimulus. Patients who experience perceptual disturbances respond with fear and anxiety.

In the patient with dementia, a mental status examination may not initially reveal a cognitive deficit, but will show a slow but progressive change if administered at given intervals over time. In the early stages of dementia, the patient may not report having any difficulty. Early reports of clinical manifestations may come from family members who witness changes or become frustrated with the patient, similar to the frustration Jim expressed in the case example. Cognitive changes associated with dementia are progressive and are marked by deterioration in intellectual functioning, memory, and the ability to learn new skills and to solve problems (Figure 21-3).

Symptoms in the psychological domain can be some of the most discouraging for family members. Confusion, agitation, apathy, sleep disturbances, and mood swings characteristic of dementia can frustrate, and even frighten, family members. In the early stages of dementia, memory loss can be annoying. As the dementia progresses, however, real safety concerns arise: The patient may begin

wandering and may become suspicious of family members and caregivers. The patient's communication skills begin to deteriorate, making caring for the patient a daily challenge. With advanced dementia, the patient may come to no longer recognize even close family members.

Individuals with an NCD may experience depression related to frustration with changes in functioning or to the pathology of the disorder. For example, Parkinson disease affects areas of the brain responsible for mood regulation. Up to 60% of patients with Parkinson disease may experience depressive symptoms (Parkinson's Disease Foundation, n.d.). Because AD shares several characteristic symptoms with depression (for example, social withdrawal, anhedonia, excess or insufficient sleep, and difficulty concentrating), it can be difficult to diagnose depression in individuals with AD, especially as the disease progresses and patients are less able to verbalize their feelings. Nevertheless, patients with AD can, and do, experience depression. As dementia progresses, patients may experience additional psychological symptoms, including paranoia. As they struggle to maintain as much independence as possible, anger and frustration with the disease, themselves, and caregivers is common.

Sociological Domain

For the patient experiencing an NCD, a hallmark symptom is loss of connections. This can have a negative impact on the patient and the functioning of the family unit. The relationships within the family unit can play an integral part in the patient's ability to participate and complete treatment. Nurses working with patients with cognitive disorders must be able to assess the level of family functioning, even when the disorder is suspected to be transient. In addition to the loss of ability to maintain connections, gradual impairment of executive function can affect family relationships as patients become increasingly unable to manage finances, recognize safety risks, and care for themselves. As this occurs, patients become increasingly discouraged by their lack of independence, which can give rise to conflicts between patients and family members.

Because cognitive disorders occur most frequently in older adults, it is especially important to determine the impact on financial resources and access to health care. Because dementia often goes unrecognized and is not treated adequately, this may lead to a poorer outcome for the patient, resulting in a further impact on health and financial expenditures (Ali et al., 2011). One study found that 49% of family and other caregivers of patients with AD had caregiving-related, out-of-pocket expenditures that averaged $219 a month (National Institute on Aging, 2009). Nurses planning care with older adults must also be able to assist patients with limited resources, and their caregivers, in maximizing those resources and finding new resources and support systems.

The progressive nature of dementia makes it important for critical conversations to occur early in the course of the disease. This includes discussing the need for patients to establish general health care powers of attorney and to ensure that their bills (including insurance premiums and copayments) continue to be paid once they are no longer able to perform that critical task. A health care power of attorney will be necessary once the patient is no longer able to make decisions on his or her own behalf (Chapter 10).

Cultural Domain

Culture affects how both families and providers interpret the signs and symptoms associated with cognitive responses. It is essential for nurses to acknowledge and respect patients' beliefs in the context of their illness, and for nurses to be aware of the impact of their own belief systems on the provision of patient care.

In poorer countries, dementia goes unrecognized or is poorly understood, which complicates efforts to improve earlier diagnosis. For example, in India, terms such as "tired brain" or "weak brain" are used for Alzheimer symptoms amid the widespread belief that dementia is a normal part of aging, which it is not. This mistake is not confined to the developing world. In Britain, just over half of families caring for someone with dementia held the same belief (Alzheimer's Disease International, 2011).

Regardless of the patient's cultural background, it is critical to identify the patient's stressors and ability to cope. Cultural variation may affect what is perceived as stressful, and perceptions of patient coping and comfort measures also may vary.

Spiritual Domain

Suffering is one of the core issues and mysteries in life. It occurs in and affects all domains (biological, psychological, sociological, cultural, and spiritual). Despite their cognitive deficits, older adults with cognitive impairment undergo similar types of grieving as those who are cognitively intact, although the process may be more complex (Potter, 2011). For the nurse providing care to a patient with a cognitive disorder, having knowledge of the patient's culture, religious traditions, and family background helps the nurse understand the nature and meaning of suffering for a particular individual. Nurses providing care to the cognitively impaired patient need to be fully present with those who are suffering. This presence supports the individual's spiritual journey toward discovering the meaning within the experience.

The diagnosis of dementia, consistent with other chronic and terminal illnesses, can lead a patient to take stock of life and explore its deeper meaning and purpose. A growing body of research supports the notion that both spirituality and religion play important roles in health and healing (Carr, 2008). The spiritual needs of patients with cognitive disorders include contextual factors that must be taken into consideration. These include the experience of being disconnected from others, which occurs when the patient cannot remember places, names, or faces and experiences declining memories (Jolley & Moreland, 2011).

Spiritual care definitions recognize that spirituality refers to the processes of seeking and/or finding meaning and purpose in life. Bell and Troxel (2001) suggested that staff concerned with the spiritual needs of people with dementia should address six main areas:

- Valuing and respecting the person
- Celebrating the person's religious heritage, where appropriate
- Embracing simplicity
- Seeking involvement of the person, when possible
- Using the creative arts to support spiritual needs and outpourings
- Providing spiritual care throughout the person's life, including end of life (based on Bell and Troxel, 2001)

Spiritual issues are core life issues that often draw people to look into the deepest places in their beings. These issues are often expressed as questions or mysteries that cannot be explained. Considerations of mystery, love, suffering, hope, forgiveness, grace, peacemaking, and prayer are all inherent in the spiritual domain.

Nurses are expected to assume a significant role in assessing spiritual needs of patients and providing spiritual care to both patients and their significant others (Carr, 2003). Doing so can positively affect the individual's sense of personhood and therefore nurture the spirit of the cognitively impaired and vulnerable (Carr, Hicks-Moore, & Montgomery, 2011). This may be particularly important for patients suffering from dementia, because there is no cure. By providing spiritual support and finding ways to help patients participate in familiar, comforting spiritual rituals, such as certain types of prayer or meditation, nurses can help patients and families maintain a sense of spiritual community, connectedness, and hope.

Pause and Reflect

1. *Referring to Table 21-1, under the psychological, sociological, and spiritual domains, what specific impaired cognitive responses can you identify that would most affect a patient's ability to function? Why might these be significant?*

2. *Imagine you have symptoms of short-term memory loss, forgetfulness, and loss of independence. How would you feel?*

3. *Why is the potential impact of delirium or dementia on family members so great?*

Delirium

As stated earlier, delirium is characterized by acute onset. Diagnosis is primarily clinical and is based on careful observation of key features. In addition to acute onset and language and perceptual disturbances, features associated with delirium include the following:

- Association with a serious underlying condition
- Reduced ability to focus, sustain, or shift attention
- Sleep–wake cycle disturbances
- Recent memory impairment
- Psychomotor retardation and agitation
- Disorganized thinking (Blazer & van Nieuwenhuizen, 2012)

Delirium may result from one of many possible etiologies or a combination of etiologies, including trauma or injury; illness; exposure to an excess amount of a substance, medication, or toxin; or sudden withdrawal of a substance or medication. Delirium can occur under a number of conditions, but is of particular concern in the hospital setting: During hospitalization for acute medical illnesses, the incidence of delirium ranges from 11% to 42% (Vidan et al., 2009). Delirium is associated with poor short-term and long-term prognosis, higher mortality and morbidity rates, functional decline, and more frequent institutionalization of patients in nursing homes or rehabilitation facilities, with the consequent increases in health care costs. Delirium can occur in seriously ill patients of all ages (Turkel, Jacobsen, Munzig, & Tavaré, 2012). It is frequently associated with older adults, but it is important to distinguish that it may occur in seriously ill children or adolescents as well (Table 21-3).

Risk Factors

There are several risk factors for delirium, including preexisting cognitive impairment, older age, cerebral damage, illness, certain medications, and functional impairment (Dharia, Verilla, & Breden, 2011). Older adults are at increased risk for delirium because of age-related changes in pharmacokinetics and pharmacodynamics and because of high levels of medication use. Studies have shown that risk of cognitive impairment increases with the number of prescription medications a person is taking. Specifically, anticholinergic medications may be a common risk factor in delirium-susceptible patients. In a study of hospitalized older adults, 25% of the delirium cases were caused by drug toxicity (Dharia, Verilla, & Breden, 2011).

Infections are also a common precipitant of delirium in the older patient. In a retrospective study, 69% of 87 acutely ill geriatric patients presenting with delirium were diagnosed with an infection (Laurila et al., 2008).

Dementia is the leading risk factor for delirium, with fully two-thirds of cases of delirium occurring in patients with dementia. The underlying vulnerability of the brain in patients with dementia may predispose them to the development of delirium as the result of acute medical illnesses, medications, or environmental changes (Fong et al., 2009). Recent studies suggest that delirium persists much longer than previously believed.

Preventing delirium is the most effective strategy for reducing its frequency and complications, and a multicomponent approach has been shown to be the most effective (Inouye, 2006). Delirium represents one of the most common preventable adverse events among older adults during hospitalization (Box 21-1).

Factors That May Result in Delirium Across the Lifespan		table 21-3

Age Group	Factors
Children	Infections and sepsis
	Febrile states
	Neoplasm/cancer
	Chemotherapy
	Mental retardation
	Closed head injury
	Seizures
	Hypoxia
	Trauma
	HIV/AIDS
	Emergence from anesthesia
	Use of anticholinergic agents
	Environmental toxins, such as paint
Adolescents	Infections and sepsis
	Drug/substance abuse
	Trauma, such as head injury
	Seizures from withdrawal
	Overdose
	Neoplasm
	Autoimmune disorders
	Environmental toxins, such as paint
Older Adults	Infections (respiratory/urinary)
	Drug toxicity
	Age > 65
	Fluid and electrolyte imbalance
	Hypoxemia due to medical conditions
	Drug withdrawal (sedative/alcohol)
	Urinary retention
	Intracranial events (stroke/bleeding)
	Acute myocardial/pulmonary events
	Use of anticholinergic medications
	Environmental toxins, such as paint

Clinical Manifestations

The hallmark characteristic of delirium is a fluctuation in the individual's state of consciousness that may range from that of hypervigilance to a drowsy, stuporous, or semi-comatose state. In addition to symptoms outlined earlier, other symptoms of delirium include extreme distractibility; disorganized thinking; speech that is rambling, irrelevant, pressured, and incoherent; and reasoning and goal-directed behavior that is rambling or inconsistent.

Delirium and Hospitalization	box 21-1

Many aspects of hospital care contribute to the development of delirium, including adverse effects of medications, sleep deprivation, complications of invasive procedures, immobilization, and dehydration (Inouye, 2006; Nelson, 2010). This needs particular consideration, as delirium is associated with prolonged hospitalization and poorer patient outcomes. Delirium is currently included as a marker of quality of care and patient safety by the National Quality Measures Clearing House of the Agency for Healthcare Research and Quality (Fong, Tulebaev, & Inouye, 2009). Higher delirium rates would be expected to correlate with lower quality of care. Every hospitalized patient should undergo brief but formal cognitive testing with the use of instruments such as the Mini Mental State Examination and the Confusion Assessment Method, as subtle delirium is often missed (Inouye, 2006).

Comparison of Delirium, Dementia, and Depression

table 21-4

	Delirium	Dementia	Depression
Onset	Acute, sudden, rapid	Slow, progressive	Variable
Duration	Hours to days	Months to years	Episodic
Cognitive impairment	Memory, consciousness	Abstract thinking, memory	Memory, concentration
Mood	Rapid mood swings	Depression, apathy	Sadness, anxiety
Delusions/hallucinations	Both; often visual	May present in later stages	Delusions only
Outcome	Recovery possible	Poor	Recovery possible

Nurses and caregivers also may observe manifestations such as vivid dreams or nightmares, or psychomotor activity that may fluctuate between agitation (for instance, restlessness, hyperactivity, striking out at nonexistent objects) to a vegetative state resembling a catatonic stupor. Emotional instability may be manifested by fear, anxiety, depression, irritability, anger, euphoria, or apathy. These varying emotions may be evidenced by crying, muttering, calls for help, cursing, moaning, acts of self-harm, fearful attempts to flee, or attacks on others.

A number of autonomic manifestations occur with the development of delirium. These include tachycardia, sweating, flushed face, dilated pupils, and elevated blood pressure. The symptoms of delirium usually begin quite abruptly but may be preceded by several hours or days of prodromal symptoms, including restlessness, difficulty thinking clearly, insomnia or hypersomnia, and nightmares. The slower onset is more common of an underlying systemic illness or metabolic imbalance. The duration of delirium is quite brief; on recovery from the underlying cause, symptoms usually diminish over a 3-to-7-day period, but may take as long as 2 weeks to resolve. The age of the patient and the duration of the delirium influence the rate of symptom resolution. Delirium may transition into a more permanent cognitive disorder and is associated with a high mortality rate (Bourgeois, Seaman, & Servis, 2008).

Distinguishing Delirium

Symptoms of delirium can be mistaken for those of dementia or depression. A delayed or missed diagnosis can have serious implications, especially if delirium is not diagnosed in a timely manner (Table 21-4). In delirium, the change that will be observed is a marked disturbance in consciousness. The changes in cognition are usually recent and include immediate memory impairment, fluctuations in attention span, disorientation to time and/or place, or language disturbances, such as rambling speech. In dementia, there are multiple cognitive deficits, including impairment in abstract thinking or a disturbance in executive functioning (the ability to think abstractly and to plan, initiate, sequence, monitor, and stop complex behavior), recent and remote memory loss, and either aphasia, apraxia, or agnosia. In depression, the sensorium is clear, but individuals may experience distractibility, difficulty concentrating, and selective memory impairment.

The individual with delirium may experience emotional disturbances: fear, anxiety, irritability, anger, euphoria, and/or apathy. In dementia, the mood is depressed, apathetic, and uninterested. Symptoms of depression include a depressed appearance, tearfulness, feelings of anxiety, irritability, fear, brooding, excessive concern with physical health, panic attacks, and phobias.

In delirium, both delusions and hallucinations are present. There is reduced clarity of awareness of the environment. Simple or complex perceptual disturbances may include misinterpretations, illusions, or hallucinations. Hallucinations may be visual, auditory, or tactile. Patients may become terrified if they perceive giant spiders crawling over their bedclothes or feel bugs crawling on their bodies. When perceptual disturbances occur, the emotional responses are fear and anxiety. In dementia, delusions and hallucinations are present. In individuals with depression, delusions related to self-worth are frequently evident.

In patients with delirium, recovery is possible if the underlying disease is corrected or self-limiting. If the disorder persists, delirium can shift to another, more stable, organic brain syndrome, such as dementia (Dwolotsky, 2009). Untreated or unresolved delirium may result in death. In dementia, the disease generally is irreversible. Slowing of deterioration depends on underlying pathology, timely diagnosis, and treatment. The more widespread the structural damage to the brain, the less likely the clinical improvement. Depression can be treated successfully. Recovery in depression is expected. Severe depression, however, may end in suicide. See Box 21-2 for information on depression in older adults.

Assessment Guidelines

Diagnostic assessment is integral to treating the underlying causative factor. A physical and neurological assessment should be completed to explore evidence of disease or other organs that could be affecting the individual's mental function. The neurological exam may include a mental status exam and assessments of muscle strength, reflexes, sensory perception, language skills, and coordination. Laboratory exams may include blood and urine samples to test for various infections, renal or hepatic dysfunction, metabolic and endocrine disorders, nutritional deficiencies, and the presence of toxic substances. Other diagnostic exams may include X-rays and computed tomography (CT) scans.

Intervention and Treatment

Treatment objectives for patients with delirium include identification of the immediate cause, correction of the underlying cause, symptom management, supportive care, and safety measures. Safety measures are particularly important, as the patient with delirium is unable to anticipate or respond to safety risks. Interventions include the following:

- Monitoring vital and neurological signs, including pain
- Reinforcing orientation to time, place, and person at each contact
- Maintaining face-to-face contact using short, simple sentences

Late-Life Depression	box 21-2

Depression occurring in adults older than 60 years of age is often referred to as *late-life depression*. "Depression in this age group has been diagnosed in 2% to 4% of community dwelling elderly, 6% to 9% of those seen in primary care clinics, 10% to 12% of hospitalized elderly, and 12% to 14% of elders residing in nursing facilities," state Dharia, Verilla, and Breden (2011, p. 575). Hospitalized or institutionalized medically ill patients older than 70 years of age are more likely to experience major depression, with incidences of 25% of those recently hospitalized to 45% of older individuals who are hospitalized (Dharia, Verilla, & Breden, 2011).

Depression in older adults continues to be underdiagnosed and undertreated. Older adults with depression frequently present complaining of cognitive impairment or with cognitive deficits. Depression in this population may present as a **pseudodementia**, in which cognitive changes arise secondary to depression. In the case of pseudodementia, depressive symptomatology, including loss of interest, decreased concentration, and memory difficulty, may lead to misdiagnosis. It is not uncommon for depression to coexist with a number of conditions, but it is particularly prevalent in patients with Parkinson disease, AD, and history of stroke (Dharia, Verilla, & Breden, 2011).

In addition to the complications of concurrent medical illness, depression in older adults may be difficult to diagnose when patients are unwilling to report symptoms of depression or do not recognize them as important. In addition, symptoms such as psychomotor slowing, fatigue, and increased pain may be attributed to medical illness instead of depression.

A tolerant, calm, matter-of-fact approach by the nurse has proven to be helpful. Lowering the level of noise in the environment can also help prevent startling and further confusion for the patient.

Breaking down instructions and activities into short time frames prevents confusion and fatigue. Limit the number of choices given to the patient when dressing or eating. Enlist the aid of significant others to stay with the patient experiencing delirium to avoid chemical or physical restraints, which should be used only as options of last resort.

Clarify reality when hallucinations are present. With perceptual disturbances, do not argue with the patient. Ask the patient directly, "Do you see something that is upsetting to you?" Validate the patient's feelings: "I don't see anything, but I am sorry you are upset." Distract the patient. Do not attempt to reason with the patient. Do not ignore the symptoms or force the patient into a situation that is frightening.

Promote adequate sensory input through having the patient use glasses or hearing aids, if necessary. Keep the room well lit and free of clutter to promote safety. Provide continuity of care as much as possible. After the patient's recovery, education is key. It is important to assess the patient's understanding of the nature of the problem to prevent a recurrence.

A multicomponent intervention integrated into daily clinical practice can prevent delirium in at-risk older patients hospitalized for acute disease. A controlled study (Vidan et al., 2009) evaluated the Hospital Elder Life Program (HELP), which was developed to prevent delirium in older medical patients. Interventions based on simple actions in different risk areas that are repeated daily for all patients at risk on a geriatric unit were compared with usual care in two internal medicine services. These actions included avoiding medication during sleep time, avoiding physical restraints, and encouraging the use of glasses and hearing aids and daily mobilization (Vidan et al., 2009). In summary, the incidence of delirium during hospitalization in older adults can be reduced with an intervention protocol aimed at reducing the number of precipitating factors. Nurses and staff should remain with the patient at all times to monitor behavior and provide reorientation.

Pause And Reflect

1. *What clinical manifestations of delirium do you think would be most challenging for nurses? Why? How would you handle these?*

2. *Why is it important to monitor the vital and neurological signs of the patient with delirium?*

3. *What nursing diagnoses might be appropriate for a patient with delirium?*

Alzheimer Disease

More than 35 million people around the world are living with AD or other types of dementia. There are currently more than 5 million Americans with AD, and the prevalence increases with age (Dharmarajan & Gunturu, 2009). The disease affects one in eight people ages 65 and older and nearly one in two people over the age of 85. The new count is about 10% higher than what scientists predicted just a few years ago. Earlier research underestimated the growing impact of the disease in developing countries.

Predictions are that by 2050, there will be between 11 million and 16 million persons with AD—unless medical breakthroughs identify ways to prevent or effectively treat the disease (National Institute on Aging, 2009; Tiedeman et al., 2011).

AD poses significant threats to health; in fact, it is a major cause of increased mortality and morbidity in older adults (Penrod et al., 2007). After initial diagnosis, patients with AD have a significantly decreased survival rate, with men having a median survival of 4.2 years, compared with women's median survival of 5.7 years (National Institute on Aging, 2005).

AD is characterized by an acquired intellectual impairment in multiple areas of mental activity: attention, memory, cognition, language, visual spatial skills, abstraction, judgment, personality, and emotions. AD features a loss of intellectual abilities that interferes with the patient's usual social or occupational activities. These intellectual abilities involve impairment in memory, judgment, and abstraction. Patients also lose executive functioning, which involves organizing and planning.

The diagnosis of AD is based on a combination of cognitive deficits and the degree to which those deficits impair function. In the early stages of AD, dementia symptoms are confused with normal signs of aging and patients often go undiagnosed until severe symptoms are present, which ultimately leads to a poor prognosis (Leifer, 2009). A number of warning signs are not part of the normal aging process and can help alert families, caregivers, and practitioners to when a loved one may have the disease. These warning signs include the following:

- Difficulty accomplishing daily, familiar tasks
- Difficulty with mental tasks, such as calculating a tip and totaling a bill or using a checkbook
- Memory loss that disrupts daily life
- Asking the same question or telling the same story over and over
- Confusion with time or place
- Trouble understanding visual images and spatial relationships
- Growing difficulty finding the right words or following directions
- Losing or misplacing items
- Decreased or poor decision making
- Withdrawal from work or social activities
- Mood or personality changes (Alzheimer's Association, 2010; NIH Medline Plus, 2010; Alzheimer's Foundation of America, n.d.)

AD may be diagnosed in a number of settings. In 2011, the National Institute of Aging and the Alzheimer's Association published new guidelines for the diagnosis of AD. This is the first update since the original guidelines were created nearly three decades earlier. The new guidelines include several significant changes. First, they describe three disease stages: asymptomatic (preclinical), thinking difficulties (mild cognitive impairment), and dementia (AD). Second, the guidelines propose—for research purposes only—using biomarker tests in conjunction with clinical assessments to determine whether someone might be at an early stage of AD, although these tests are not routinely used (National Institute on Aging, 2011). Investigators, clinicians, and policy makers are hoping that the new guidelines will help accelerate research on ways to prevent or at least slow the progression of AD (Figure 21-4).

Stage 1: Asymptomatic

The earliest stage of the AD process is preclinical, when symptoms such as memory loss are absent or so subtle as to go undetected. At this stage, however, pathological changes are probably already under way in the brain. This section of the guidelines describes how

researchers might use five biomarkers to estimate the chances of whether someone might be at the preclinical stage. Some of the biomarkers measure beta amyloid accumulation in the brain, which is an early sign of AD pathology that suggests that the disease process has begun. The new recommendations suggest that researchers use biomarkers not only to help determine whether someone might be in the preclinical stage of AD, but also to learn what factors might predict a transition to mild cognitive impairment.

Stage 2: Mild Cognitive Impairment

"Mild cognitive impairment is an intermediate state between the normal forgetfulness that occurs with age and the more pronounced memory and thinking deficits that occur in Alzheimer's," according to the *Harvard Mental Health Letter* (Harvard Medical School, 2011, p. 2). Within 5 years, about half of those with mild cognitive impairment develop dementia—most often, AD. A pattern of findings that may suggest mild cognitive impairment includes deterioration in thinking ability noticed by either the patient, a loved one, or a clinician; impairment of one or more abilities, including memory, attention, language, and ability to plan; ability to function independently, although perhaps less efficiently or more slowly than before; and an absence of dementia.

Stage 3: Dementia

The new criteria emphasize that memory impairment, although the most common initial symptom, may not be the only one. After stroke, delirium, and other possible causes of dementia are ruled out, a diagnosis of AD is probable when cognitive or behavioral impairment develops gradually, increases over time, and involves at least two of the following cognitive domains (Harvard Medical School, 2011).

- *Memory:* This is the most common problem area and typically involves episodic memory (difficulty learning or remembering new information). In day-to-day life, this might cause an individual to misplace personal belongings, repeat the same question or conversation, forget things, or get lost while walking or driving in familiar areas.
- *Executive function:* This type of thinking includes planning, reasoning, judgment, and problem solving. Impairment of executive function might manifest as difficulty with finances, failure to appreciate safety risks, or inability to organize meals.
- *Visuospatial ability:* This refers to the ability to interpret visual information and see how objects fit into surroundings. Impairments in visuospatial ability may manifest in many different

Mild Dementia
- Intermittent memory loss, confusion
- Difficulties with problem solving

Moderate Dementia
- Increasing cognitive impairment
- Sleep disturbances
- Apathy
- Mood swings

Severe Dementia
- Inability to maintain ADLs
- Wandering
- Paranoia
- Pronounced communication difficulties

21-4 Symptoms of dementia associated with Alzheimer disease are progressive.

ways, such as trouble recognizing familiar people, or the inability to find objects such as eating utensils (even when in plain view).

- *Language:* Impairments in language may manifest as hesitation in speaking, problems coming up with the right word, or spelling errors.
- *Behavior and personality:* Uncharacteristic changes in behavior and personality include agitation, apathy, mood swings, obsessive or compulsive behavior, or socially unacceptable behavior.

Hallmark Symptoms

Symptoms characteristic of AD include amnesia, aphasia, apraxia, and agnosia (Table 21-5). Patients may also experience wandering behaviors, incontinence of bladder and bowel, and self-deficits in all major areas. Patients may exhibit socially inappropriate behavior, and will often neglect hygiene, nutrition, and safety issues. There are also disturbances in the area of executive functioning, including problems with organizing, planning, sequencing, and abstracting (APA, 2013). Mood and emotional reactions will often be out of sync with environmental stimuli.

The most difficult symptoms for patients to handle are the neuropsychiatric symptoms that present in the later stages. These include apathy, agitation, aggression, depression, and anxiety. The presence and severity of neuropsychiatric symptoms are significantly correlated with the degree of cognitive impairment in patients with AD (Dechamps et al., 2008). Data from a large sample of 59 dementia special care units indicated that more than 81% of patients had clinically relevant neuropsychiatric symptoms (Zuidema et al., 2007)

Neuropsychiatric symptoms can be triggered by the patient's surrounding environment. Factors include excess noise, lack of structure, loneliness, and boredom. Sundowning may also be triggered by environmental stimuli. **Sundowning**, which represents a destabilization of cognitive abilities (for example, confusion, lability of mood), usually occurs during the late afternoon, early evening, or night (Gauthier et al., 2010).

Appropriate environmental stimuli, such as making conversation and smiling, can increase positive behaviors. Lack of stimuli, however, can increase negative behaviors, such as wandering, fidgeting, and showing aggression toward others. The symptoms of dementia may affect the patient's ability to articulate needs, which, in turn, may cause the patient to react with adverse behaviors. Dementia can decrease a patient's tolerance for stress. Patients may become more confused and present with delusions, psychosis, agitation, and aggression. Patient safety becomes a major concern for caregivers and health care workers as the patient's condition continues to deteriorate over time.

Patients with AD often experience mood lability, anxiety, and depression. Apathy is a distressing neuropsychiatric symptom for patients, caregivers, and family members. The symptom often hinders a patient's ability to express emotions and feelings, establish meaningful relationships, and effectively cope with the diagnosis of AD and decreased quality of life (Gauthier et al., 2010). Anxiety can be a debilitating symptom for patients with AD. The patient may present with a flat affect or appear to be in distress, depending on how the anxiety manifests. Anxiety may also stem from depression, a common symptom of AD.

Pause and Reflect

1. *How does delirium differ from Alzheimer disease?*
2. *What aspects of the symptoms of Alzheimer disease do you think are the most challenging?*
3. *Do you know anyone who has Alzheimer disease? How are that person and family members coping with the disorder?*

Common Symptoms of Alzheimer Disease   table 21-5

Symptom	Definition	Effects/Signs
Amnesia	Loss of recent and remote memory	• Inability to form new memories; may believe dead relatives are alive • Misplacing, losing items; may accuse others of taking them • Becoming lost during routine tasks—stopping in the middle or forgetting how to do it—or forgetting to begin a task • Repeating questions numerous times
Aphasia	Inability to speak or understand language	• Inability to remember names of things, people • Failing to understand directions • Becoming frustrated easily • Becoming upset when multiple people talk simultaneously • Saying "yes" when meaning "no"
Apraxia	The loss of purposeful movement in the absence of motor/sensory impairment	• Inability to perform motor functions, such as dressing, using utensils to eat • Difficulty sitting down, getting up • Falling more easily/frequently • Difficulty opening containers of food, beverages
Agnosia	Loss of sensory ability to recognize objects; may include *auditory agnosia*, the inability to recognize sounds	• Fails to recognize familiar environments. May wander, trying to find something familiar. • Rummages in drawers looking for something that is "lost." • May not recognize food as edible, may not eat anything. • May not recognize own reflection in a mirror. • May think people on TV are really there.

Collaborative Care

Collaborative care is a way in which health care professionals work together with patients and their families to provide the best quality care in complex situations, such as dementia and delirium. The patient and the family have a central role in establishing goals and the plan of care. The members of the collaborative interdisciplinary team must be able to share their decision making and communicate effectively. For patients with dementia or delirium, collaborative care may involve the nurse, physician, physical therapist, occupational therapist, the family, volunteers, personal care assistants, social workers, clinical care managers, and spiritual care providers.

Community-based care for the patient with dementia may involve appointments in an outpatient office setting, a day program (depending on the level of functioning), and/or a support group for both the patient and the caregivers. Psychotherapy assists the patient with dementia to develop more effective coping in regard to the loss of cognitive function. As the dementia progresses, many patients may need to be placed in a nursing facility for care.

Many older adults with AD and other forms of dementia receive most of their care from a primary care provider. This may not be the best setting for the patient with AD. In the case study in this chapter, Donnette received care from specialists—a geropsychiatrist and an advanced practice nurse.

As discussed throughout this chapter, many patients with dementia will experience behavioral and psychological symptoms. Nurses need to be aware that collaborative care includes communication among health care providers in the health care system and community. It also involves treatment for depression, anxiety, psychoses, and behavioral disturbances; active monitoring; and support of the patient's and the caregivers' emotional and psychological well-being.

Psychopharmacology

Cholinesterase inhibitors and *N*-methyl-d-aspartate (NMDA) receptor antagonists are currently the only approved therapies for treatment of mild to severe AD (see Medications Commonly Used to Treat Patients with Dementia). There are no medications to cure or provide meaningful relief from the symptoms of AD. Typically, medications are prescribed to alleviate symptoms, and efficacy may wane as the dementia progresses. For some patients, anxiolytics and other medications may be prescribed to address specific symptoms. This may depend on the presence of other medical conditions, such as asthma or COPD, hypertension, or diabetes. Nurses can provide support by encouraging patients to always use the same pharmacy, providing medication education to patients and caregivers, and taking other precautions to reduce a patient's risk for adverse effects related to polypharmacy.

> **PRACTICE ALERT** As dementia progresses and memory impairments increase, patients will be less able to be responsible for taking their own medications, even with alarms or other reminders. Nurses must help patients identify family and caregivers who can ensure consistent medication administration. Failure to take medications on time generally results in an increase in symptom severity and frequency.

Cholinesterase Inhibitors

Some of the clinical manifestations of AD are thought to be the result of a deficiency of the neurotransmitter acetylcholine. In the brain, acetylcholine is inactivated by the enzyme acetylcholinesterase.

Cholinesterase inhibitors (ChEIs) act by slowing the degradation of acetylcholine, thereby increasing concentration of the neurotransmitter in the cerebral cortex. This has shown to produce a therapeutic response that results in the patient's improved ability to perform self-care, and slow cognitive deterioration of AD for patients with mild to moderate Alzheimer dementia. In 2010, donepezil (Aricept) was approved by the FDA for moderate-to-severe AD based on clinical trials (Davis, Hendrix, & Superville, 2011). Of this class of medications, donepezil is considered first-line therapy because of its once-daily dosing, narrow adverse effect profile, and efficacy.

Side effects of ChEIs include nausea and diarrhea, which occurs in approximately 10% of patients. In addition, ChEIs are known to increase the risk of gastrointestinal bleeding. Nursing interventions and patient education include monitoring for gastrointestinal side effects and fluid volume deficits, and promoting adequate fluid intake. Gastrointestinal disturbances can usually be minimized by starting with low doses and increasing them gradually. Nonsteroidal anti-inflammatory drugs (NSAIDs) should be avoided. Both categories of medication may cause stomach ulcers and the combination may increase risk. Headache, dizziness, fatigue, and insomnia also have been reported. Another adverse effect of this classification of medications is bradycardia. Nursing interventions include teaching the family to monitor the patient's pulse rate when he or she is home; the patient also should be screened for underlying heart disease.

Before initiating medication treatment, the patient needs education in several areas:

- Dosage should start low and gradually be increased until side effects are no longer tolerable or the medication is no longer beneficial. Monitor for adverse effects and educate the patient and family about these effects.

- Taper medications when discontinuing to prevent abrupt progression of symptoms.

- Most of the medications are available in tablets and oral solutions. Donepezil is available in an orally disintegrating tablet. Monitor the patient for the ability to swallow tablets.

- Administer with or without food.

- Donepezil has a long half-life, and is administered once daily at bedtime. The other ChEIs are usually administered twice daily.

NMDA Receptor Antagonists

The second classification of medications used to treat the cognitive symptoms of AD is the *NMDA receptor antagonists*. These can be used as stand-alone symptomatic therapy or combined with a cholinesterase inhibitor to treat moderate to severe AD (Adams, Holland, & Urban, 2014). Memantine (Namenda) affects the NMDA receptor, another chemical and structural system involved in memory. In normal neurotransmission, glutamate plays a critical role in learning and memory by triggering NMDA receptors to regulate the amount of calcium that flows into a nerve cell (Alzheimer's Association, 2006). Memantine may protect cells against excess glutamate by partially blocking NMDA c-receptors. Memantine has shown in clinical trials to be effective in improving cognitive function and the ability to perform ADLs in patients with moderate to severe AD. It has been shown to slow the decline in functionality (Reisburg et al., 2003). Memantine can be used alone or taken in combination with one of the ChEIs for a possible synergistic effect.

Side/adverse effects include headache, dizziness, constipation, and confusion. Contraindications and precautions include avoiding use during pregnancy because memantine's effects during lactation have not been determined. It may also cause drowsiness or dizziness; patients should use caution while driving or performing other activities requiring mental alertness.

Nursing considerations for NMDA receptor antagonists include the following:

- Instruct caregivers in the recommended administration (twice per day with food for doses above 5 mg) and dose escalation (minimum interval of 1 week between dose increases).

- Advise the patient or caregiver that this drug does not alter the Alzheimer process and that the efficacy of the medication may decrease over time.

- Instruct the patient or caregiver to continue using other medications for dementia as prescribed by the health care provider.

- Advise the patient or caregiver that doses greater than 5 mg are taken twice a day, without regard to meals, but the patient should take them with food if GI upset occurs. Teach preparation of oral solution (attach the cap and plastic tube to new bottles or oral solution, withdraw prescribed dose using the dosing syringe, and administer the dose).

- Advise the patient or caregiver not to discontinue the drug or change the dose unless advised by the health care provider.

- Caution the patient or caregiver not to increase the dose of memantine if Alzheimer symptoms do not appear to be improving or appear to be getting worse, but rather to notify the health care provider.

- Caution the patient that memantine may cause drowsiness or dizziness and to use caution while driving or performing other activities requiring mental alertness or coordination until tolerance is determined.

- Instruct the patient or caregiver not to use any prescription or over-the- counter (OTC) medications, dietary supplements, or herbal preparations unless advised by the health care provider.

- Advise the patient and caregiver that follow-up visits may be required to monitor therapy and to keep appointments.

The hope for the future is that new treatments will not just improve symptoms, but also slow the progression of the disease or even lead to a cure.

Anxiolytics

The progressive loss of mental functioning is a significant source of anxiety in the early stages of dementia. Antianxiety medications may be helpful, but should be used for only a short time. Many providers prefer buspirone (Buspar) to benzodiazepines because it does not produce many unwanted side effects, such as psychomotor impairment, drowsiness, or cognitive impairment. Although benzodiazepines may be used, special consideration should be given when administering benzodiazepines to older adults. The drugs with shorter half-lives (such as lorazepam [Ativan] and oxazepam [Serax]) are preferred to longer-acting medications (such as diazepam [Valium]), which promote a higher risk for oversedation and falls in this vulnerable population. This is due to a slower rate of clearance as a result of a slower metabolism.

This can cause additional difficulties in patients who are already experiencing cognitive impairment.

Antidepressants

Antidepressant medication is sometimes used in treatment of depression in patients with AD. The selective serotonin-reuptake inhibitors (SSRIs) are considered by many to be the first-line treatment for depression in older adults because of their favorable side effect profile (Davis, Hendrix, & Superville, 2011). If patients experience anxiety, then paroxetine (Paxil), which has a greater sedative effect, can be used. In addition to its antidepressant effect, citalopram (Celexa) has been shown to improve certain emotional symptoms of AD, including panic, bluntness, irritability, and restlessness. Tricyclic antidepressants (TCAs) are often avoided because of cardiac and anticholinergic side effects. However, the TCA trazodone (Desyrel) may be a good choice for depression and insomnia, if used at bedtime.

Antipsychotics

Antipsychotic medications are used to control agitation, aggression, hallucinations, thought disturbances, and wandering in patients with dementia. The newer atypical antipsychotics carry less risk of anticholinergic and extrapyramidal side effects. Haloperidol (Haldol) is still commonly used because of its proven efficacy in the behaviors associated with dementia. Extrapyramidal side effects (EPS) are common in this drug class and can be particularly distressing to patients and families (Chapter 23). EPS can develop within days of initiating treatment, as well as any time throughout the course of therapy. The usual adult dosage of any antipsychotic must be decreased in older adults.

In 2005, the FDA required drug manufacturers to issue a "black box" warning about the risk of increased mortality in older adults being treated with second-generation antipsychotics for behavioral symptoms of dementia (Davis, Hendrix, & Superville, 2011). Three years later, this warning was extended to include the use of typical or first-generation antipsychotics.

Sedative–Hypnotic Medications

Sleep problems are common in patients with dementia and often intensify as the disease progresses. Wakefulness and nighttime wandering create much distress and anguish in family members who are charged with protection of their loved one. Sleep disturbances are among the problems that most frequently initiate placement of the patient in a long-term care facility.

Benzodiazepines may be useful for some patients, but are indicated for relatively brief periods only. Examples include flurazepam (Dalmane), temazepam (Restoril), and oxazepam (Serax). Daytime sedation and cognitive impairment, in addition to paradoxical agitation in older patients, are of particular concern with these medications (Beers & Jones, 2004). The nonbenzodiazepine sedative–hypnotics zolpidem (Ambien) and zaleplon (Sonata) and the antidepressant trazodone (Desyrel) are also prescribed.

Because of the potential for adverse drug reactions in older adults, many of whom are already taking multiple medications, nonpharmacological strategies should be attempted first. Sleep hygiene measures that may be helpful include rising at the same time each morning; minimizing sleep during the day; regular exercise; proper nutrition; avoiding alcohol, caffeine, and nicotine; and going to bed at the same time each night. These behavioral approaches to sleep problems may eliminate the need for sleep aids, particularly in the early stages of dementia.

Patients with Dementia — medications commonly used to treat

Acetylcholinesterase Inhibitors	Usual Adult Dosage (mg)	Nursing Considerations
donepezil (Aricept)	5, 10 mg	For all cholinesterase inhibitors:
donepezil (Aricept ODT)	23 mg daily	• Provide patient education regarding dizziness, headache, GI upset, fatigue.
rivastigmine (Exelon)	3–6 mg twice daily	• Promote adequate fluid intake.
(also available as a patch)		• Monitor patient's pulse rate.
galantamine (Razadyne)	4–12 mg twice daily	• Use with caution in patients with respiratory conditions (e.g., asthma, COPD).
galantamine (Razadyne ER)	8, 16, 24 mg	• Avoid use of tricyclics and anticholinergics due to antagonistic effects.
tacrine (Cognex)	10 mg four times daily Max 160 mg/day	

NMDA Receptor Agonists	Usual Adult Dosage	Nursing Considerations
memantine (Namenda)	5–10 mg twice daily	Provide patient education regarding:
memantine (Namenda XR)	7–14 mg daily	• Headache • Dizziness • Constipation • Confusion

Anxiolytic Medications	Usual Adult Dosage	Nursing Considerations
lorazepam (Ativan)	1–2 mg	Caution about dependency, drowsiness, hypotension, tolerance, dizziness, GI upset
oxazepam (Serax)	10–30 mg	

Antipsychotics	Usual Adult Dosage	Nursing Considerations
olanzapine (Zyprexa)	5 mg (increase dose cautiously)	Provide patient education regarding hypotension, dizziness, sedation, weight gain, constipation
risperidone (Risperdal)	1–4 mg (increase dose cautiously)	Provide patient education regarding agitation, insomnia, headache, EPS
quetiapine (Seroquel)	Initial dose 25 mg (titrate slowly)	Provide patient education regarding hypotension, tachycardia, dizziness, drowsiness, headache
haloperidol (Haldol)	1–4 mg (increase dose cautiously)	Provide patient education regarding blurred vision, orthostatic hypotension, extrapyramidal symptoms, sedation

Antidepressant Medications: SSRIs	Usual Adult Dosages	Nursing Considerations
sertraline (Zoloft)	25–100 mg	For all SSRIs:
citalopram (Celexa)	10–40 mg	Provide patient education regarding: dizziness, insomnia, somnolence, GI upset, nausea or diarrhea
fluoxetine (Prozac)	10–60 mg	
paroxetine (Paxil)	20–60 mg	

Sedative–Hypnotics	Usual Adult Dosage	Nursing Considerations
Benzodiazepines		For all sedative–hypnotics, provide patient education regarding:
temezepam (Restoril)	15 mg	• Avoid alcohol, other CNS depressants
Nonbenzodiazepines		• Warning against using heavy machinery and driving
zolpidem (Ambien)	5 mg	• Recognize potential for dependence and withdrawal
zalephon (Sonata)	5 mg	• Watch for dizziness, hypotension, drowsiness

Based on Wilson, B. A., Shannon, M. T., & Shields, K. M. (2014). *Pearson Nurse's Drug Guide.* Upper Saddle River, NJ: Pearson; Vallerand, A. H., Sanoski, C. A., & Deglin, J. H. (2011). *Davis's Drug Guide for Nurses* (13th ed.). Philadelphia, PA: F.A. Davis; Adams, M. P., Holland, L. N., & Urban, C. Q. (2014). *Pharmacology for Nurses: A Pathophysiologic Approach* (4th ed.). Upper Saddle River, NJ: Pearson.

Exercise

A study by Rolland et al. (2007) provided evidence that a moderate exercise program conducted twice a week significantly slowed, by one-third, the progressive deterioration in ability to perform ADLs in people with AD living in nursing homes. Exercise has been found to have the largest effect on executive function (planning, coordination, working memory, abstract thinking, initiating appropriate activities and inhibiting inappropriate ones). Patients with early AD who exercised showed less brain atrophy than those who did not (Burns et al., 2008). Regular exercise has been found to promote brain function. Researchers continue to study exercise as a neuroprotective mechanism, and evidence is emerging that it may play a role in preventing or reducing the symptoms of NCDs (Radak et al., 2010).

Reality Orientation

Both 24-hour and structured reality orientation can prevent confusion and keep patients oriented to time, place, person, and situation. A **reality orientation** discussion is a conversational aid designed to help orient the patient; it is not meant to be a "do you know?" test. The environment, when it is kept simple and focused, reinforces contact with reality—the here and now. Helpful physical props include pictures, photographs, clocks, calendars, and orientation boards (for instance, seasons of the year, weather).

Reality orientation groups can provide an opportunity to reinforce time, place, and person orientation with patients who have short attention spans and need extra verbal and visual stimulation. Reality orientation, along with a discussion of current events, stimulates patients to maintain contact with the real world and their place in it. The scope of the group depends on the patients' abilities and the other therapeutic modalities at hand.

Validation Therapy

Validation therapy is an alternative approach that was developed several decades ago by Naomi Feil in response to working with patient who do not respond to reality orientation. This approach involves searching for the emotion and meaning in the patient's disoriented or confused words and behavior (such as wandering) and validating them verbally with the patient (Feil, 2007). What is sometimes identified by caregivers as meaningless or incoherent conversation may often have significant meaning for the patient and can be related to current or past events. An example of this may be seen in a resident in a dementia care center who is found walking down the hallway, crying and asking staff if they have seen his mother. The nurse, using validation, would say, "Tell me about your mother—what did she look like?" The outcome of validation therapy is that the individual is able to express his or her feelings, and these feelings are acknowledged by an empathetic, trusted caregiver (Feil, 2007). Validation is being used successfully with both mildly and moderately impaired older adults, providing an effective avenue for reaching those experiencing cognitive dysfunction.

Reminiscence Therapy

Throughout the literature, reminiscence therapy has been regarded as a therapeutic intervention. Reminiscence is a process of reflection that involves remembering or thinking about a past event through which the individual has lived. Patients with AD retain long-term memory, especially in the earlier stages of the disease. Helping patients access older memories may provide comfort to those who are frustrated by deficits in short-term memory. **Reminiscence therapy** has been implemented as a means of promoting self-esteem and identity in older adults and to stimulate communication with patients who have AD. It is also an effective intervention for decreasing isolation and withdrawal.

Complementary and Alternative Therapies

Several complementary and alternative therapies provide relief from many of the neuropsychiatric symptoms experienced by those who suffer with cognitive disorders. In addition to the therapies discussed in Chapter 22, art therapy, music therapy, and healing touch and Reiki may be beneficial to patients with NCDs when provided by licensed providers experienced with working with this population.

Art Therapy

Art is defined as "any medium used for creative expression" (Basting, 2006, p. 16). The use of the arts to promote well-being in people with AD has increased across disciplines such as nursing. Patient well-being and staff members' satisfaction have been shown to increase with individualized interventions that include art and recreational therapy with a trained therapist (Walsh et al., 2011).

Music Therapy

As a complementary and alternative therapy, music provides an integrated body–mind experience that encourages patients to become active participants in their own health care (Morris, 2009). Music therapy is an exceptional and effective alternative therapy for health and managing the symptoms of AD (Tow, 2006). The use of music therapy for AD has evolved into evidence-based practice for nurses to use when caring for patients.

Incorporating music into patient care can help decrease anxiety, aggression, depression, and agitation. Nurses can help patients improve independent daily living and promote healthy sleeping habits and effective coping through the use of music as an intervention. Music is an effective intervention because of its ability to "act as a distracter, focusing the patient's attention away from negative stimuli to something pleasant and encouraging" (Nilsson, 2008, p. 782).

Music intervention can decrease the need for chemical or physical restraints. Research has shown that music has the ability to improve cognitive functioning; therefore, patients can maintain their autonomy and stay independent for a longer period (Goodall & Etters, 2005). The integration of music into the plan of care for patients with AD is a simple nursing intervention that can produce positive results and improve patient outcomes with minimal risks or side effects involved.

Healing Touch and Reiki

Complementary and alternative modalities that involve touching include healing touch (HT) and Reiki, which both are categorized as energy touch therapies. A pilot study investigated the effects of HT on patients with dementia who were experiencing agitated behaviors. Those who received HT were significantly less agitated, and the researchers recommended further investigation with large groups (Wang, 2006). In a 1-year study of nursing home residents who were offered Reiki, it was found that all participants experienced positive effects from the ongoing treatments (Jackson & Keegan, 2009). Residents with AD and other forms of dementia improved in symptoms related to stress and depression.

Pause and Reflect

1. *What are important nursing considerations associated with cholinesterase inhibitors?*
2. *How can music therapy be an effective intervention for patients with AD?*
3. *What do you think about using some of these complementary and alternative measures for yourself?*

Nursing Management

Nursing care of patients with delirium and neurocognitive alterations focuses on patient safety, as symptoms of these disorders can increase risk for injury, medication errors and adverse effects,

Donnette Recovery Phase

APPLICATION

1. Address the five domains for Donnette.

2. What are the criteria for Stage 3—dementia due to AD?

3. Why do think Donnette has been prescribed citalopram?

4. What other approaches/ strategies might be beneficial for Donnette? For Jim?

Donnette returns the following week for her therapy appointment with Ann, the PMH-APRN. Ann has spoken to Donnette's geropsychiatrist about the plan of care and to obtain more information about Donnette's treatment. Donnette is currently being prescribed rivastigmine (Exelon) patch 4.6 mg/24 hour, memantine (Namenda) 5 mg twice a day, and citalopram (Celexa) 20 mg once daily.

Donnette shares with Ann that she has been exercising by walking when the weather is nice. When conditions do not permit, she goes to the recreation center at the adult community she lives in and uses the treadmill. Donnette also has been participating in yoga twice a week.

Donnette shares that her husband, Jim, continues to become angry at her for minor things. "I don't know what I'm doing wrong," she says. Donnette feels that she is a burden to her husband and to her children. She states, "A lot of my friends have no idea what this is all about—no idea what I'm going through, I don't even want to tell them, it's embarrassing." Donnette is not able to cook dinner anymore, an activity that she used to perform regularly. Donnette has tried to prepare dinner, but she becomes confused about what ingredients to use and often forgets the steps to take in preparation.

Ann, using the new clinical guidelines for AD, recognizes that Donnette would fulfill the criteria for Stage 3—dementia (Alzheimer disease). Ann formulates a plan to begin working with Donnette to enhance her coping skills, to improve her sense of self, and to decrease her level of helplessness/hopelessness. Ann recommends that Donnette join a support group at the local medical center for those diagnosed with AD.

Donnette returns to the mental health office two weeks later for her follow-up appointment. She is accompanied by her husband, Jim. Donnette reports that she and Jim attended the monthly support group for patients with AD the previous week: "I didn't realize that there were people worse off than me." Donnette and Ann decide to meet on a bimonthly basis to continue their work.

and illness as a result of self-neglect (for instance, poor nutrition and inadequate fluid intake). Careful assessment is necessary to determine the patient's physical and psychological status, to confirm the underlying source of the symptoms, and to reduce manifestations that impair functioning.

Assessment

Assessment of patients with neurocognitive disorders includes a mental status exam and a functional assessment, as well as a history, physical, and diagnostic studies. Laboratory and diagnostic tests typically include chest and skull X-rays, electroencephalography (EEG), electrocardiography (ECG), liver and thyroid function studies, neuroimaging (CT, PET), and urinalysis and serum electrolytes.

Standardized screening tools may include the Functional Dementia Scale (Figure 21-5). Use of this tool will give the nurse information regarding the patient's ability to perform self-care, the extent of the patient's memory loss, mood changes, and the degree of danger to self and/or others.

The nurse should use standardized screening instruments on admission and at periodical intervals. These screening instruments should be used if there is any change in baseline to trigger further assessment. Common methods of cognitive screening include the Mini-Mental Status Exam (MMSE). The main focus of the exam is cognitive functioning. A total of 11 questions cover the scope of a patient's thinking and reactions. The maximum score is 30 points. Usually a score of 18 or higher is seen in the early stages of AD; a score between 12 and 18 is seen in moderate AD; and a score lower than 12 is characteristic of the severe stage of the illness. Clinical studies have shown that early detection and treatment of AD may help to improve outcomes such as cognition and behavior. Early detection may help to reduce costs associated with the treatment of AD.

Diagnosis and Planning

Safety needs play a substantial role in providing nursing care to a confused patient, but fear and anxiety are the most common of all nursing diagnoses in delirium and dementia. This may be related to illusions, delusions, or hallucinations, as evidenced by verbal and nonverbal expressions of anxiety and fearfulness. These neuropsychiatric symptoms can also be triggered by the patient's surrounding environment—factors that could include excess noise, lack of structure, loneliness, and boredom. Although a number of nursing diagnoses address various aspects of cognitive responses, some specific nursing diagnoses are more commonly seen in patients with cognitive disorders. Nursing diagnoses for patients with cognitive disorders are identified and prioritized based on patient and caregiver needs. These include:

- Injury, Risk for
- Fear
- Anxiety
- Confusion, Acute or Chronic
- Self-Care Deficit (specify: bathing, dressing, feeding, toileting)
- Nutrition, Imbalanced: Less than Body Requirements
- Memory, Impaired
- Communication: Verbal, Impaired
- Hopelessness
- Social Interaction, Impaired
- Caregiver Role Strain

(NANDA-I © 2014)

In developing the plan of care, the nurse will consider with the patient how the five domains are involved. In patients with dementia, this can be quite challenging. Nurses must consider whether the patient is capable of collaborating with the nurse on a care plan, as well as the

Functional Dementia Scale

Circle one rating for each item:

   1. None or little of the time

   2. Some of the time

   3. Good part of the time

   4. Most or all of the time

Client _____

Observer _____

Position or relation to patient _____

Facility_____

Date _____

1 2 3 4	1. Has difficulty in completing simple tasks on own (e.g. dressing, bathing, doing math)
1 2 3 4	2. Spends time either sitting or in apparently purposeless activity
1 2 3 4	3. Wanders at night or needs to be restrained to prevent wandering
1 2 3 4	4. Hears things that are not there
1 2 3 4	5. Requires supervision or assistance in eating
1 2 3 4	6. Loses things
1 2 3 4	7. Appearance is disorderly if left to own devices
1 2 3 4	8. Moans
1 2 3 4	9. Cannot control bowel function
1 2 3 4	10. Threatens to harm others
1 2 3 4	11. Cannot control bladder function
1 2 3 4	12. Needs to be watched so doesn't injure self (e.g., by careless smoking, leaving the stove on, falling)
1 2 3 4	13. Destructive of materials around him/her (e.g., breaks furniture, throws food trays, tears up magazines.)
1 2 3 4	14. Shouts or yells
1 2 3 4	15. Accuses others of doing him bodily harm or stealing his/her possessions – when you are sure the accusations are not true
1 2 3 4	16. Is unaware of limitations imposed by illness
1 2 3 4	17. Becomes confused and does not know where he/she is
1 2 3 4	18. Has trouble remembering
1 2 3 4	19. Has sudden changes of mood (e.g., gets upset, angered, or cries easily)
1 2 3 4	20. If left alone, wanders aimlessly during the day or needs to be restrained to prevent wandering

21-5 Functional Dementia Scale.

Source: Moore, J. T., Bobula, J. A., Short, T. B., & Mischel, M. (1983). A functional dementia scale. *Journal of Family Practice 16*, 499–503.

degree of participation of caregivers and significant others in the treatment plan. It also is important to consider what the most distressing symptoms are for both the patient and immediate family members.

- **Biological:** Does the patient have any other medical conditions that may affect the patient's ability to manage the disease state? Does the patient have any co-morbid medical condition that may be affected by the patient's dementia?

- **Psychological:** What are some distressing triggers that typically exacerbate the patient's symptoms? What strategies could be used to reduce the impact of such triggers?

- **Sociological:** What are the significant relationships in this patient's life? Are they positive or negative influences?

- **Cultural:** Are there family traditions or rituals that help or detract from the patient's level of health?

- *Spiritual:* Are there any spiritual concerns that could be affecting the patient's cognitive state negatively? Are there spiritual support systems in place in the patient's life that can be accessed to assist the patient?

As dementia progresses, the focus of nursing care shifts toward the physical body and related medical problems, such as feeding, hydration, injury, incontinence, weight loss, dysphagia, falls, fractures, pneumonia, sepsis, and skin breakdown (Penrod et al., 2007).

Implementation

Nursing interventions vary according to the nature of the illness and the symptoms that are most problematic. Patients with both delirium and dementia require interventions related to safety, self-care, orientation in space and time, and communication. Nurses also assist patients by addressing feelings of hopelessness and depressive symptoms (see the Nursing Care Plan). Patients with dementia and their families will benefit from education and additional support as needed.

Providing care for patients with dementia can challenge even the most experienced nurse. It can be particularly challenging for nursing students and new nurses whose experience with patients with dementia is limited. Careful attention to the development of communication skills, including the use of reminiscence therapy, may help nursing students and new nurses as they develop therapeutic relationships with their patients with dementia (see Evidence-Based Practice: Nursing Students Providing Care to Patients with Dementia).

Promote Safety

With the onset of confusion, whether attributable to delirium or dementia, patient risks related to safety increase. In a hospital or care facility, the following interventions will be helpful:

- Assign the patient to a room close to the nurses' station for close observation.
- Provide a room with a low level of visual and auditory stimuli.
- Provide for a well-lit environment, minimizing contrasts and shadows.
- Encourage use of identification bracelets, monitors, and bed alarms.
- Administer medications PRN for agitation or anxiety.
- Ensure safety in the physical environment generally, such as using a lowered bed.

Promote Orientation to Time and Space

Patient orientation in time and space is important regardless of the severity of illness, but may present differently at different times. Patients with mild confusion or memory impairment may simply miss occasional appointments. Patients with more severe impairment will begin to confuse day with night, have difficulty sitting down or standing without using furniture or assistive devices, and may experience a change in gait. Nursing interventions

---

Nursing Students Providing Care to Patients with Dementia   evidence-based practice

Clinical Problem

The aging U.S. population will generate a demand for nurses to be prepared to care for older adults. The prevalence of dementia is rapidly increasing in this population. What strategies can nursing faculty use to support and enhance nursing students' learning experiences?

Evidence

A phenomenological study explored the meaning of spiritual care from the perspectives of patients living with moderate to severe dementia, their families and their care providers. Providers and acts of caring were found to be meaningful if they contributed to a sense of personhood and fostered a connection to self and others (Carr, Hicks-Moore, & Montgomery, 2011).

Robinson and Cubit (2007) reported their findings from two qualitative projects that were aimed at improving nursing students' experiences of providing care to people with dementia within elder care settings. Two projects were conducted involving 87 second-year bachelor of nursing students who participated in 3-week clinical placements in eight residential elder care facilities. Through the use of weekly focus group discussions with mentors, nursing students were able to share their experiences of providing care to dementia patients.

The researchers identified several issues that have relevance to nurse educators that can affect teaching and learning:

- Students' unfamiliarity with dementia
- Nurse mentors' familiarity with dementia
- Communication problems

The researchers found that student nurses need far more extensive education about the condition of dementia and, more importantly, effective nursing intervention strategies. Researchers also identified that student nurses need to have a better understanding of the complex behavioral manifestations of dementia and its etiology.

In another qualitative study, Shellman (2006) examined a sample of 41 baccalaureate nursing students' participation in a reminiscence education program during their community health practicum working with older adults. Student nurses received reminiscence education, and students had 13 weeks to reminiscence with older adults during home visits. The researcher found that three themes emerged in relation to the students' experiences of reminiscing with older adults: making a connection; seeing the world through the patient's eyes; and the benefits of reminiscence.

Implications for Nursing Practice

Nurse educators may find that reminiscence, as a nursing intervention, may be helpful in the development of communication skills between student or new nurses and older adult patients. Students in this study described increased confidence in caring for older adults, as well as a therapeutic effect of reminiscence (Shellman, 2006). This has implications for nurse educators as they prepare student nurses to care for this challenging and complex population.

Critical Thinking Questions

1. Identify strategies that enhanced nursing students' learning in the studies cited.
2. What are your thoughts and feelings related to working with older adults?

that will help patients orient themselves in time and space include the following:

- Provide compensatory memory aids, such as clocks, calendars, photographs, memorabilia, seasonal decorations, and familiar objects.
- Reorient as necessary.
- Provide eyeglasses and assistive hearing devices, as needed.
- Keep a consistent daily routine.
- Maintain consistent caregivers.
- Ensure adequate food and fluid intake.
- Allow for safe pacing and wandering.
- Cover or remove mirrors to decrease fear and agitation.

Promote Self-Care

As a patient's cognitive function decreases, the ability to perform basic ADLs is affected. This can be particularly challenging, as the patient's awareness for the need for these activities also decreases. Appropriate nursing interventions include performing tasks based on the patient's condition, labeling the patient's clothes, monitoring food and fluid intake, initiating bowel and bladder training, weighing the patient weekly, and giving the patient step-by-step instructions.

Promote Communication

Dementia impairs an individual's ability to communicate effectively. It reduces the ability to decode and understand information (receptive language) and the ability to encode and therefore express information (expressive language). These language deficits are compounded by other dementia-related impairments, including memory loss, decreased attention span, and impairments in judgment, insight, abstraction, and visuospatial abilities.

Due to the patient's language deficits and other cognitive impairments, the responsibility to facilitate communication lies with the nurse. For persons with dementia, behavior is frequently a form of communication. Nurses should try to interpret the meaning of behaviors rather than dismissing them as symptoms of dementia.

Specific interventions that will promote communication include the following:

- Communicate in a calm, reassuring tone.
- Do not argue or question hallucinations or delusions.
- Reinforce reality.
- Reinforce orientation to time, place, and person.
- Introduce yourself to the patient with each new contact.
- Establish eye contact and use short, simple sentences when speaking to the patient.
- Acknowledge the patient's feelings; use distraction.
- Have clocks, calendars, and personal items in clear view.
- Have the patient wear glasses and/or hearing aids as necessary.
- Encourage reminiscence about happy times; talk about familiar things.
- Break instructions and activities into short time frames.
- Limit the number of choices when dressing or eating.

- Minimize the need for decision making and abstract thinking to avoid frustration.
- Avoid confrontation.
- Encourage family visitation, as appropriate.

Provide Support for Families

The stress of providing care, termed *caregiver burden*, must be considered in the management of an individual with dementia. More than 40% of family and other unpaid caregivers of people with Alzheimer and other dementias rate the emotional stress as high or very high (National Institute on Aging, 2009). The majority of caregivers outside nursing facilities are family members who often are untrained, are unpaid, have little prior knowledge of the disease, and therefore are vulnerable to being overwhelmed by caring for an individual with AD (Burns, 2000). Caregivers of people with dementia experience high rates of clinically significant anxiety (10–35%) and depression (10–34%) (Cooper, Balarmurali, & Livingston, 2007).

Interventions related to family teaching and support include the following:

- Assess the family's knowledge of the disease and resources and further re-assess patient and family needs and resources as the patient's health declines.
- Teach the family specific interventions regarding safety and communication.
- Teach the family strategies for handling problematic behaviors.
- Help the family to make the home safe.
- Encourage the family to follow family traditions.
- Provide support for caregivers.
- Teach caregivers stress management techniques.
- Recommend and encourage caregivers to use respite care.
- Establish routines.
- Attempt to have consistency in caregivers.

Because approximately two-thirds of patients with dementia live at home, it is critical to provide patient and family education related to safety. This includes education related to medication safety. Patient and family education should include the following:

- Remove scatter rugs.
- Install door locks that cannot be opened easily.
- Lock water heater thermostats and turn water temperature down to a safe level.
- Provide good lighting, especially on stairs.
- Install a handrail on stairs, and place colored tape on the edges of steps.
- Remove clutter, keeping clear, wide pathways for walking through a room.
- Secure electrical cords to baseboards.
- Store cleaning supplies in locked cupboards.
- Install handrails in bathrooms.

Baby monitors or intercom systems can promote communication and may relieve the anxiety of caregivers who are reluctant to be too far away from the patient while doing daily tasks. Bells can be installed on doors to alert caregivers when the patient is awake and

Donnette—A Patient with Alzheimer Disease | NURSING CARE PLAN

Nursing Diagnosis Hopelessness, related to perceived helplessness and powerlessness, as manifested by her verbalization, "What's the point?"; lack of motivation; loss of interest; feeling like a burden to her husband; decreased problem solving; and loss of independence.

Short-Term Goals *Patient will:*	Intervention *Nurse will:*	Rationale
Identify two alternatives for one life problem during the first interview.	Assist Donnette in recognizing two strategies to solve problems.	Determine what coping strategies may or may not be effective.
Identify three things that she is capable of doing right during the first interview.	Work with Donnette to identify strengths.	When people are feeling overwhelmed, they no longer view their lives or behavior objectively.
Name one community service resource that she has accessed at least twice by the third interview.	Provide referral to support group for patients diagnosed with Alzheimer disease.	Meaningful activity and establishing networks of social support assist patients in feeling more connected.
State that she believes that her life has value and she has an important role to play, by the second interview.	Identify things that give meaning and joy to life. Discuss how these things can be incorporated into her present lifestyle.	Creative activities give people intrinsic pleasure and joy and a great deal of satisfaction.
Make two decisions related to her care.	Assist Donnette in identifying what is important to her about her care.	Identify areas to target in providing care can help patients feel more empowered.
Long-Term Goal Donnette will come to accept her diagnosis and will report feeling more hopeful about her day-to-day life.	Support Donnette and husband Jim as they learn about AD and adapt their lifestyles as needed.	Patients and family members need assistance to help the patient remain as functional and hopeful as possible.

Clinical Reasoning

1. What other nursing diagnoses might the nurse working with Donnette consider?
2. Do you think that the selection of hopelessness as the priority diagnosis is appropriate? Why or why not?
3. In addition to promoting social interaction, what else might it be helpful to get Donnette to increase her socialization?

---

ambulating. Nurses should know what resources are available in the areas in which they live and practice and be able to provide referrals. Local departments of aging and chapters of the Alzheimer's Association and the National Family Caregivers Association are available in many areas.

Evaluation

Evaluation of the patient with cognitive disorders is based on a series of short-term outcomes rather than on long-term outcomes (see Perceptions, Thoughts, and Feelings). For patients with dementia, outcomes must be measured in terms of slowing down the process rather than stopping or curing the problem. Frequent evaluation and reformulation of outcome criteria also help to diminish patient and family frustration, as well as minimize the patient's anxiety. The overall goals in treatment are to promote the patient's optimal level of functioning and to prevent any further regression, when possible.

From Suffering to Hope

Patients who are suffering from disturbing cognitive responses often lose hope. They frequently feel alone, isolated, and in despair. Family members also experience hopelessness, finding themselves in situations for which they feel completely unprepared. Hope is a significant factor in overcoming illness and living through difficult situations. It helps people deal with fear and uncertainty. Hope can be an affirming quality for both patients with dementia and their families.

As discussed throughout this chapter, nursing interventions that promote safety, orientation, self-care, and communication can ease the suffering and burden that patients with dementia and their families experience. Supportive care for patients and families, including promoting a healthy diet, sufficient rest, and exercise, can help reduce levels of frustration and lift mood. Helping family members negotiate and share caregiving duties may help reduce interfamily conflicts that can arise when caring for a loved one with significant dementia. Connecting families to respite care, adult care programs, home health services, and counseling can assist in reducing caregiver burden and promote safety for patients and their family members.

Empowering patient independence for as long as possible and supporting patients and their families are essential to nursing care of patients with NCDs and their family members. Affirming what individuals with dementia can do, rather than focusing on what they cannot do, is a positive and hopeful strategy. Honoring the person for who he or she is can be powerful for families, as well as commending family members who attend to and spend time with the patient. Careful assessment to help determine the underlying cause of the disorder, as well as listening and observing for interventions and activities that improve health and awareness, can be beneficial. For example, if a family member says things such as "Dad seems to have a better day if we sit outside in the morning," or "Dad does not like it when the TV is on too loud," the nurse can encourage the family member to share that information with other caregivers and can relay that information to other staff in care settings such as hospitals and assisted living centers. Taking time with patients and their families to make and act on careful assessments is a significant nursing activity that can provide clear benefits to patients and instill trust and hope in their family members.

Pause and Reflect

1. *How can the nurse help alleviate patient suffering and promote healing for patients with cognitive disorders?*
2. *How does loss of memory affect a patient's functioning?*
3. *How does cognitive decline affect the family's functioning?*

PERCEPTIONS, THOUGHTS, & FEELINGS: Validating the Needs of a Patient Diagnosed with Dementia

Patient's behaviors	Nurse's perceptions, thoughts, and feelings	Exploration with patient
Donnette is seen in an outpatient mental health office. She arrives and sits on the couch, sighing loudly. Her face is drawn and her eyes are teary.	*Perceptions:* Donnette looks sad. *Thoughts:* I wonder what that sigh is about.	*Nurse:* Hello, Donnette. Your eyes are teary. What's going on?

VALIDATION Ann senses that Donnette is sad and wants Donnette to verbalize her feelings to Ann.

Patient's behaviors	Nurse's perceptions, thoughts, and feelings	Exploration with patient
Donnette: I don't know. What's the point?	*Perceptions:* Donnette seems sad, and sounds hopeless. *Thoughts:* I need to find out what's going on with her.	*Nurse:* Donnette, what do you mean by "What's the point?"

VALIDATION Clarifying exactly what Donnette means by "What's the point?"

Patient's behaviors	Nurse's perceptions, thoughts, and feelings	Exploration with patient
Donnette: Well, look at me. I used to teach, I loved teaching, now what do I do—nothing.	*Thoughts:* Hmm, I need to explore this more. I get the sense that Donnette feels useless.	*Nurse:* Well, you've told me that you do yoga, take walks, and do aerobics.

VALIDATION Continuing to enlist Donnette in the process of getting the help she needs.

Patient's behaviors	Nurse's perceptions, thoughts, and feelings	Exploration with patient
Donnette: Yes, but that only takes up a few mornings. Jim is always busy. I want to be busy like that—like when I was teaching.	*Thoughts:* Donnette is bringing up her teaching again. She really misses that role, and feeling productive and busy. *Feelings:* I feel sorry that Donnette is going through such a difficult transition. I want to help her.	*Nurse:* Donnette, it sounds like you enjoyed teaching and now that you are retired, you miss that role and feeling productive. Does that sound like an accurate assessment of what's going on with you?

VALIDATION Inviting Donnette to acknowledge or disagree with the assessment

Patient's behaviors	Nurse's perceptions, thoughts, and feelings	Exploration with patient
Donnette: I did enjoy teaching and I always loved having the students in my class. But I can't teach now, my mind is gone. Donnette puts her hands up in the air. *Donnette:* Where did my mind go?	*Thoughts:* Donnette is struggling with this role transition and loss of her abilities with memory. *Feelings:* This must be so frustrating for her, and sad.	*Nurse:* Donnette, this sounds like it is difficult for you. I suppose that's what you meant earlier when you said, "What's the point?" because you felt productive and fulfilled in your job and now you don't. It sounds disheartening for you.

VALIDATION Seeking to clarify what Donnette is feeling

Patient's behaviors	Nurse's perceptions, thoughts, and feelings	Exploration with patient
Donnette: I feel sad about it. I know that I need to do something, but I don't know what it is, because Jim has to drive me everywhere.	*Thoughts:* Donnette doesn't know where to start, she's lost her independence, and she feels that she has to depend on Jim for everything. I would like to develop some strategies to help Donnette feels more fulfilled.	*Nurse:* Well, Donnette, I've met Jim and he seems willing to take you places.

VALIDATION Continuing to enlist Donnette in the process of getting the help she needs

Patient's behaviors	Nurse's perceptions, thoughts, and feelings	Exploration with patient
Donnette: Yes, but he is so busy at work. I feel guilty to interrupt his time.	*Thoughts:* I'm thinking that Donnette often feels guilty and doesn't want to burden her husband. I need to address how this behavior is affecting her functioning.	*Nurse:* Donnette, do you think your feeling guilty is stopping you or preventing you from asking for help and joining activities?

VALIDATION Validating with Donnette her feelings to assess whether they are interfering with her behavior

Patient's behaviors	Nurse's perceptions, thoughts, and feelings	Exploration with patient
Donnette: Well, yes, I feel bad that I have to ask Jim to take me places. I used to be so independent. *Donnette:* I'm so frustrated! Donnette shakes both her fists.	*Thoughts:* I've never seen Donnette so upset. She does seem frustrated and angry about her life. I need to continue to see her to address her emotional and cognitive issues.	*Nurse:* Donnette, I hear that you are frustrated. Let's talk about strategies that could help you with your feelings of frustration.

VALIDATION Affirming to Donnette her feelings of frustration and enlisting her participation in getting her to ask for help

Patient's behaviors	Nurse's perceptions, thoughts, and feelings	Exploration with patient
Donnette: Okay, I'd like that.	*Thoughts:* At least she is willing to try. She also sounds receptive to discussing some strategies, so she can feel more empowered in her life.	*Nurse:* You mentioned that you feel bad or guilty about interrupting Jim's time, but you're also feeling frustrated about not being busy enough. I think it would be helpful if we can identify one activity that you would like to do.

VALIDATION Empowering Donnette by giving her choices

Based on Orlando, I. J. (1972). *The Discipline and Teaching of Nursing Process (An Evaluative Study)*. New York, NY: G. P. Putnam's Sons.

critical thinking

Donnette Rehabilitation Phase

Over the next few months, Donnette continues to meet with Ann. Donnette continues to attend the monthly support groups, accompanied by her husband. Donnette tells Ann that she feels happy that her husband attends the support groups with her. Donnette also adds that Jim is attending a monthly caregivers' support group. She tells Ann that she found a neighbor who wanted to try knitting classes with her, and this has helped ease the burden on Jim taking her to all her activities.

Donnette updates and shares with Ann that a former colleague had called her recently and they talked about her time at the college where she used to work. Donnette seems surprised that someone would remember her. Donnette spends the session disclosing and reminiscing about her former role as a professor. Ann observes that Donnette seems relaxed and at ease when speaking about how much she enjoyed teaching all her students.

Donnette also shares that she has been attending Sabbath services at a nearby community center. Donnette reports that she knows that at some point her symptoms will get worse, but she is trying to do the best she can until that happens. Ann notes that Donnette seems to be more at peace with her diagnosis and is coping more effectively with her day-to-day life. Donnette and Ann agree to continue to meet on a bimonthly basis.

APPLICATION

1. What are Donnette's needs during this encounter?

2. What steps has Donnette taken to cope more effectively?

3. Knowing that Donnette's improvement is merely temporary until her dementia progresses further, how do you anticipate that her care needs will change?

Chapter Highlights

1. Neurocognitive disorders constitute a large and growing public health concern.

2. Neurocognitive disorders include delirium and dementia.

3. Delirium is a disturbance of consciousness.

4. The symptoms of delirium usually begin quite abruptly and are often reversible and brief.

5. Delirium may be caused by a general medical condition, substance intoxication or withdrawal, or ingestion of a medication or toxin.

6. Dementia is a syndrome of acquired, persistent intellectual impairment with compromised function in multiple spheres of mental activity, such as memory, language, visuospatial skills, emotion, personality, and cognition.

7. Symptoms of dementia are insidious and develop slowly over time.

8. Objectives of care for the patient experiencing an acute syndrome are aimed at eliminating the etiology, promoting patient safety, and a return to the highest possible level of functioning.

9. Objectives of care for the patient experiencing a chronic, progressive disorder are aimed at preserving the dignity of the individual, promoting deceleration of the symptoms, and maximizing functional capabilities.

10. Nursing interventions are directed toward encouraging independence, ensuring safety, and helping the patient's family or primary caregivers learn about a chronic, progressive cognitive disorder.

NCLEX®-RN Questions

1. The nurse is admitting an 82-year-old adult presenting to the acute care setting with sudden onset of confusion. Which is the priority nursing action?
   a. Determining whether there is a family history of Alzheimer disease
   b. Evaluating the safety of the home/living environment
   c. Initiating assessments to rule out an underlying physiological cause
   d. Assessing for any missed signs of progressive functional decline

2. The nurse is providing education to the adult children of a patient diagnosed with late-onset Alzheimer disease. One of the children asks, "Does this mean that we will get this disease too?" Which response is accurate?
   a. "Research shows that only early-onset Alzheimer disease runs in families."
   b. "Not unless you have been exposed to the same environmental toxins."
   c. "A familial pattern may increase the likelihood of developing the disease."
   d. "If we live long enough, eventually we will all develop some form of the disorder."

3. The emergency department nurse is assessing an older adult patient who presents disoriented, with rambling speech and disorganized thinking. Which additional findings would support the nurse's suspicion that the patient is suffering from delirium? Select all that apply.
   a. Hallucinations
   b. Insidious onset
   c. Hypervigilance
   d. Depressed affect
   e. Altered consciousness

4. The nurse is caring for a patient with dementia. The patient is undergoing a comprehensive medical evaluation to determine the primary disorder. Which clinical manifestations suggest a condition other than Alzheimer disease? Select all that apply.
   a. Difficulty with speech
   b. Abnormal movements
   c. Rapid onset and progression
   d. Socially inappropriate behavior
   e. Disturbance in executive function

5. The nurse is caring for a patient in stage 2 of Alzheimer disease. Which interventions are appropriate at this time? Select all that apply.
   a. Installing door locks
   b. Providing memory aids
   c. Encouraging regular exercise
   d. Covering or removing mirrors
   e. Establishing advance directives

6. The nurse is caring for the patient in the early stages of Alzheimer disease. Which evaluation finding indicates that treatment with citalopram (Celexa) has been effective?
   a. Improved mood
   b. Continued independence in performing ADLs
   c. No symptoms of psychosis
   d. Restored memory

7. The nurse is planning care for the patient with Alzheimer disease. Which rationale best supports spending time with the patient, reviewing photo albums and talking about important life events?
   a. Life review activities can promote the patient's comfort and sense of connectedness.
   b. "Remembering" exercises have been shown to improve both short- and long-term memory.
   c. Reminiscence therapy can assist the nurse to overcome burnout and see the patient as an individual.
   d. Discussing life events provides a nonintrusive way for the nurse to gather critical assessment data.

Answers may be found on the Pearson student resource site: nursing.pearsonhighered.com

Pearson Nursing Student Resources Find additional review materials at **nursing.pearsonhighered.com**

References

Adams, M. P., Holland, L. N., & Urban, C. Q. (2014). *Pharmacology for Nurses: A Pathophysiology Approach.* Upper Saddle River, NJ: Prentice Hall.

Ali, S., Patel, M., Jabeen, S., Bailey, R. K., Patel, T., Shahid, M., . . . Arain, A. (2011). Insight into delirium. *Innovations in Clinical Neuroscience, 8*(10), 25.

Alzheimer's Association. (2006). Fact sheet: About memantine. Available at http://www.alznyc.org/aboutalz/pdf/fsmemantine.pdf

Alzheimer's Association. (2010). Alzheimer's disease: Facts and figures. *Alzheimer's Dementia,* 158–194.

Alzheimer's Association. (2014). What is Alzheimer's? Available at http://www.alz.org/alzheimers_disease_what_is_alzheimers.asp

Alzheimer's Disease International. (2011). World Alzheimer Report 2011: The benefits of early diagnosis and intervention. Available at http://www.alz.co.uk-research-WorldAlzheimerReport2011

Alzheimer's Foundation of America. (n.d.) About Alzheimer's: Warning signs. Available at http://www.alzfdn.org/AboutAlzheimers/warningsigns.html

American Psychiatric Association. (2000). *Diagnostic and Statistical Manual of Mental Disorders* (4th ed., Text Revision). Arlington, VA: American Psychiatric Association.

American Psychiatric Association. (2013). *Diagnostic and Statistical Manual of Mental Disorders* (5th ed.). Washington, DC: American Psychiatric Publishers.

Andreasen, N. C., & Black, D. W. (2006). *Introductory Textbook of Psychiatry.* (4th ed.). Washington, DC: American Psychiatric Publishing.

Arcangelo, V. P., & Peterson, A. M. (2005). *Pharmacotherapeutics for Advanced Practice: A Practical Approach.* Philadelphia, PA: Lippincott Williams & Wilkins.

Ballard, C., O'Brien, J., & Reichelt, K. (2002). Aromatherapy as a safe and effective treatment for the management of agitation in severe dementia: The results of a double-blind, placebo-controlled trial with Melissa. *Journal of Clinical Psychiatry, 63*(7), 553–558.

Basting, A. D. (2006). Arts in dementia care: "This is not the end . . . it's the end of this chapter." *Generations, Spring,* 16–20.

Beers, M. H., & Jones, T. V. (Eds.). (2004). Drugs and aging. *The Merck Manual of Health and Aging.* Whitehouse Station, NJ: Merck Research Laboratories.

Bell, V., & Troxel, D. (2001). Spirituality and the person with dementia: A view from the field. *Alzheimer's Care Quarterly, 2*(2), 31–45.

Blazer, D. G., & van Nieuwenhuizen, A. O. (2012). Evidence for the diagnostic criteria of delirium: An update. *Current Opinion in Psychiatry, 25*(3), 239–243.

Bourgeois, J. A., Seaman, J. S., & Servis, M.E. (2008). Delirium, dementia, and amnestic disorders. In R. E. Hales, S. C. Yudofsky, & G. O. Gabbard, (Eds.). *Textbook of Clinical Psychiatry* (5th ed.). Washington, DC: American Psychiatric Publishing, pp. 221–250

Burns, A. (2000). The burden of Alzheimer's disease. *Journal of Neuropsychopharmacology, 3*(17), 31–38.

Burns, J. M., Cronk, B. B., Anderson, H. S., Donnelly, J. E., Thomas, G. P., Harsha, A., Brooks, W. M., & Swerdlow, R. H. (2008). Cardiorespiratory fitness and brain atrophy in early Alzheimer disease. *Neurology, 71*(3), 210–216.

Butler, R. N. (1963). The life review: An interpretation of reminiscence in the aged. *Psychiatry, 26,* 65–76.

Carr, T. J. (2003). The spirit of nursing: Ghost of our past or force for the future? In M. R. McIntyre & E. H. Thomlinson, (Eds.). *Realities of Canadian Nursing: Professional, Practice, and Power Issues.* Philadelphia, PA: Lippincott Williams & Wilkins, pp. 470–492.

Carr, T. (2008). Mapping the processes and qualities of spiritual nursing care. *Qualitative Health Research 18*(5), 686–700.

Carr, T. J., Hicks-Moore, S., & Montgomery, P. (2011). What's so big about the "little things": A phenomenological inquiry into the meaning of spiritual care in dementia. *Dementia, 10*(3), 399–414.

Catic, A. G. (2011). Identification and management of in-hospital drug-induced delirium in older patients. *Drugs and Aging, 28*(2), 737–748.

Cherry, K. (2013). Memory—Psychology definition of the week. Available at http://psychology.about.com/b/2013/12/20/memory-psychology-definition-of-the-week.htm

Cherry, K. (2014). What is cognition? Available at http://psychology.about.com/od/cindex/g/def_cognition.htm

Cooper, C., Balamurali, T., & Livingston, G. (2007). A systematic review of the prevalence and associates of anxiety in caregivers of people with dementia. *International Journal of Geriatric Psychiatry, 22,* 181–188.

Cooper, C., Katona, C., Orrell, M., & Livingston, G. (2008). Coping strategies, anxiety and depression in caregivers of people with Alzheimer's disease. *International Journal of Geriatric Psychiatry 23*(9), 929–936.

Davis, N. J., Hendrix, C. C., & Superville, J. G. (2011). Supportive approaches for Alzheimer disease. *The Nurse Practitioner, 36*(8), 22–28.

Dechamps, A., Jutand, M. A., Onifade, C., Richard-Harston, S., & Bourdel-Marchasson, I. (2008). Co-occurrence of neuropsychiatric syndromes in demented and psychotic institutionalized elderly. *International Journal of Geriatric Psychiatry, 23*(9) 1182–1190.

Dharia, S., Verilla, K., & Breden, E. L. (2011). The 3 D's of geriatric psychiatry: Depression, delirium, and dementia. *The Consultant Pharmacist, 26*(8), 566–578.

Dharmarajan, T. S., & Gunturu, S. G. (2009). Alzheimer's disease: A healthcare burden of epidemic proportion. *American Health and Drug Benefits, 2*(1), 39–47.

Dwolotsky, T. (2009). When does delirium become dementia? *Aging Health, 5*(1), 1–2. Available at http://www.futuremedicine.com/doi/pdfplus/10.2217/1745509X.5.1.1

Feil, N. (2007). It is never good to lie to a person who has dementia. The Validation Training Institute, Inc. Available at http://www.vfvalidation.org/web.php?request=article5

Folstein, M., Folstein, S., & McHugh, P. (1975). Mini-mental state: A practical method for grading the cognitive state of patients for the clinician. *Journal of Psychiatric Residents, 12,* 189.

Fong, T. G., Jones, R. N., Shi, P., Marcantonio, E. R., Yap, L., Rudolph, J. L., Yang, F. M., Kiely, D. K., & Inouye, S. K. (2009). Delirium accelerates cognitive decline in Alzheimer's disease. *Neurology, 72*(18), 1570–1575.

Fong, T. G., Tulebaev, S. R., & Inouye, S. K. (2009). Delirium in elderly adults: Diagnosis, prevention, and treatment. *National Review of Neurology, 5*(4), 210–220.

Galek, K., Flannelly, K. J., Vane, A., Galek, R. M. (2005). Assessing a patient's spiritual needs: A comprehensive instrument. *Holistic Nursing Practice, 19*(2), 62–69.

Gauthier, S., Garcia, A., Sano, M., Robert, P., Senanarong, V., Woodbury, M., & Brodaty, H. (2010). Priorities for research consortia on Alzheimer's disease. *Alzheimer Dementia, 6*(4), 359–362.

Goodall, D., & Etters, L. (2005). The therapeutic use of music on agitated behaviors in those with dementia. *Holistic Nursing Practice, 19*(6), 258–262.

Grossman, H., Bergmann, C., & Parker, S. (2006). Dementia: A brief overview. *Mount Sinai Journal of Medicine, 73*(7), 985–992.

Hall, G. R., Gallagher, M., & Dougherty, J. (2009). Integrating roles for successful dementia management. *The Nurse Practitioner, 34*(11), 35–41.

Harvard Medical School. (2011). New diagnostic criteria for Alzheimer's disease. *Harvard Mental Health Letter, 28*(2), 1–3.

Henry, J. (1994). Lavender for night sedation with people with dementia. *International Journal of Aromatherapy, 6,*(2), 28–30.

Inouye, S. K. (2006). Current concepts: Delirium in older persons. *New England Journal of Medicine, 354,*(11), 1157–1165.

Jackson, C., & Keegan, L. (2009). Touch. In B. Dossey & L. Keegan, (Eds.). *Holistic Nursing: A Handbook for Practice.* Sudbury, MA: Jones & Bartlett, pp. 347–366.

Jolley, D. & Moreland, N. (2011). Dementia care: Spiritual and faith perspectives. *Nursing and Residential Care, 13*(8), 388–399.

Lambert, J. C., Ibrahim-Verbaas, C. A., Harold, D., Naj, A. C., Sims, R., Bellenguez, C., . . . Evans, D. (2013). Meta-analysis of 74,046 individuals identifies 11 new susceptibility loci for Alzheimer's disease. *Nature Genetics, 45*(12), 1452–1458.

Laurila, J. V., Laakkonen, M. L., Laurila, J. V., Timo, S. E., & Reijo, T. S. (2008). Predisposing and precipitating factors for delirium in a frail geriatric population. *Journal of Psychosomatic Research, 65*(3), 249–254.

Leifer, B. P. (2009). Alzheimer's disease: Seeing the signs early. *Journal of the American Academy of Nurse Practitioners, 21*(11), 588–595.

Linton, A. (2005). The benefits of cholinesterase inhibitors: Managing the behavioral and neuropsychiatric symptoms of Alzheimer's disease. *Journal of Gerontological Nursing, 31*(12), 4–10.

Lyketsos, C. G., DelCampo, L., Steinberg, M., Miles, Q., Steele, C. D., Munro, C., Baker, A. S., Sheppard, J. E., Frangakis, C., Brandt, J., & Rabins, P. V. (2003). Treating depression in Alzheimer's disease. *Archives of General Psychiatry, 60*(7), 737–746.

Morris, D. (2009). Music therapy. In B. Dossey & L. Keegan, (Eds.). *Holistic Nursing: A Handbook for Practice.* Sudbury, MA: Jones & Bartlett, pp. 327–346.

National Institute of Neurological Disorders and Stroke. (2014). Transmissible spongiform encephalopathies information page. Available at http://www.ninds.nih.gov/disorders/tse/tse.htm

National Institute on Aging. (2005). Progress report on Alzheimer's Disease: 2004–2005. Available at http://www.nia.nih.gov/sites/default/files/progress_report_on_alzheimers_disease_20042005small.pdf

National Institute on Aging. (2009). Alzheimer's disease facts and figures. Available at http://www.alz.org/national/documents/report_alzfactsfigures2009.pdf

National Institute on Aging. (2011). Alzheimer's Research Information News Release. *Alzheimer's & Dementia: The Journal of the Alzheimer's Association.* Available at http://www.nia.nih.gov/Alzheimers/ResearchInformation/NewsReleases/PR20110419gui

National Institutes of Health: Medline Plus. (2010). 7 Warning Signs of Alzheimer's. Available at http://www.nlm.nih.gov/medlineplus/magazine/issues/fall10/articles/fall10pg20-21.html

Nelson, J. M. (2010). Recognizing, preventing, and managing delirium in hospital patients. *American Nurse Today, 5*(11), 43–45.

Nilsson, U. (2008). The anxiety and pain reducing effects of music interventions: A systematic review. *AORN Journal, 87*(4), 780–807.

Orlando, I. J. (1972). *The Discipline and Teaching of Nursing Process (An Evaluative Study).* New York, NY: G. P. Putnam's Sons.

Page, S. (2011). Understanding dementia, the medications and new guidelines. *Nursing & Residential Care, 13*(3), 117–120.

Parkinson's Disease Foundation. (n.d.) Depression. Available at http://www.pdf.org/en/depression_pd

Penrod, J., Yu, R., Kolanowski, A., Fick, D. M., Loeb, S. J., & Hupcey, J. E. (2007). Reframing persons-centered nursing: Care for persons with dementia. *Research and Theory for Nursing Practice: An International Journal, 21*(1), 57–72.

Potter. M. L. (2011). Suffering special populations. In K. Perrin, C. Sheehan, M. Potter, & M. K. Kazanowski, (Eds.). *Palliative Care Nursing: Caring for Suffering Patients.* Sudbury, MA: Jones & Bartlett, pp. 25–52.

Radak, Z., Hart, N., Sarga, L., Koltai, E., Atalay, M., Ohno, H., & Boldog, I. (2010). Exercise plays a preventive role against Alzheimer's disease. *Journal of Alzheimer's Disease 20*(3), 777–783.

Reinhard, S. C., Given, B., Petlick, N. H., & Bemis, A. (2008). Supporting family caregivers in providing care. In R. G. Hughes, (Ed.). *Patient Safety and Quality: An Evidence-based Handbook for Nurses.* Rockville, MD: Agency for Healthcare Research and Quality, pp. 341–402.

Reisburg, B., Doody, R., Stoffler, A., Schmitt, F., Ferris, S., & Mobius, H. J. (2003). Memantine in moderate-to-severe Alzheimer's disease. *New England Journal of Medicine, 348*, 1333–1341.

Robinson, A., & Cubit, K. (2007). Caring for older people with dementia in residential care: Nursing students' experiences. *Journal of Advanced Nursing, 59*(3), 255–263.

Rolland, Y., Pillard, F., Klapouszcak, A., Reynish, E., Thomas, D., Andrieu, S., Riviere, D., & Vellas, B. (2007). Exercise program for nursing home residents with Alzheimer's Disease: A 1-year randomized, controlled trial. *Journal of the American Geriatrics Society, 55*(22), 158–165.

Sadock, B. J., & Sadock, V. A. (2003). *Synopsis of Psychiatry: Behavioral Sciences/Clinical Psychiatry* (9th ed.). Philadelphia, PA: Lippincott Williams & Wilkins.

Sadock, B. J. & Sadock, V. A. (2007). *Synopsis of Psychiatry: Behavioral Sciences/Clinical Psychiatry* (10th ed.). Philadelphia, PA: Lippincott Williams & Wilkins.

Sharon, I. (2010) Huntington disease dementia. Available at http://emedicine.medscape.com/289706

Shellman, J. (2006). "Making a connection": BSN students' perceptions of their reminiscence experiences with older adults. *Journal of Nursing Education, 45*(12), 497–503.

Snyder, L. (2001). The lived experience of Alzheimer's: Understanding the feelings and subjective accounts of persons with the disease. *Alzheimer's Care Quarterly, 2*(2), 8–22.

Stetka, B., & Cornell, C. (2013). A guide to DSM-5: Neurocognitive disorder. Available at http://www.medscape.com/viewarticle/803884_13

Swenson, R. (2006). Review of clinical and functional neuroscience. Dartmouth Medical School. Available at http://www.dartmouth.edu/~rswenson/NeuroS

Tiedeman, M., Kim, C., Flurie, R., Korch-Black, K., & Brandt, N. J. (2011). Alzheimer's disease: Current treatment options and future developments. *Formulary, 46*, 268–284.

Tow, D. (2008). Music is magic for residents with Alzheimer's. *Nursing Homes, 55* (11), 40–41.

Turkel, S. B., Jacobson, J., Munzig, E., & Tavaré, C. J. (2012). Atypical antipsychotic medications to control symptoms of delirium in children and adolescents. *Journal of Child and Adolescent Psychopharmacology, 22*(2), 126–130.

Vallerand, A. H., Sanoski, C. A., & Deglin, J. H. (2011). *Davis's Drug Guide for Nurses* (13th ed.). Philadelphia, PA: F.A. Davis.

Vidan, M., Sanchez, E., Alonso, M., Montero, B., Ortiz, J., & Serra, J. A. (2009). An intervention integrated into daily clinical practice reduces the incidence of delirium during hospitalization in elderly patients. *Journal of the American Geriatrics Society, 57*, 2029–2036.

Walsh, S. M., Lamet, A. R., Lundgren, C. L., Rillstone, P., Little, D. J., Steffey, C. M., Rafalko, S. Y., & Sonshine, R. (2011). Art in Alzheimer's care: Promoting well-being in people with late-stage Alzheimer's disease. *Rehabilitation Nursing, 36*(2), 66–72.

Wang, K. (2006). Pilot study to test the effectiveness of healing touch on agitation in people with dementia. *Geriatric Nursing, 27*(1), 34–40.

Wilson, B. A., Shannon, M. T., & Shields, K. M. (2014). *Pearson Nurse's Drug Guide.* Upper Saddle River, NJ: Prentice Hall.

Yuhas, N., McGowan, B., Fontaine, T., Czech, J., Gambrell-Jones, J. (2006). Interventions for disruptive symptoms of dementia. *Journal of Psychosocial Nursing, 44*(11), 31–42.

Zuidema, S. U., de Jonghe, J. F., Verhey, F. R., & Koopmans, R. T. (2007). Neuropsychiatric symptoms in nursing home patients: Factor structure invariance of the Dutch nursing home version of the neuropsychiaric inventory in different stages of dementia. *Dementia and Geriatric Cognitive Disorders, 24*(3), 169–176.

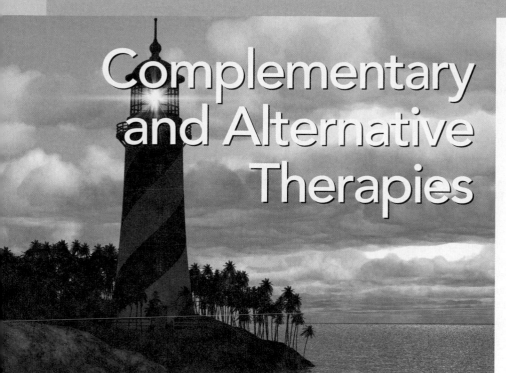

Complementary and Alternative Therapies

22

Joyce K. Anastasi
Bernadette Capili
Michelle Chang

Learning Outcomes

1. Define the term *complementary and alternative medicine* (CAM).

2. Discuss general principles of CAM.

3. Differentiate the main categories of CAM and list examples.

4. Evaluate potential adverse effects of CAM therapies.

5. Examine the evidence base for use of CAM therapies in treatment of selected psychiatric–mental health disorders.

6. Summarize the nurse's role in working with patients who use CAM therapies.

Key Terms

acupuncture, 500
allopathic medicine, 498
alternative medicine, 498
biofeedback, 502
complementary and alternative medicine, 498
complementary health approaches, 498
complementary medicine, 498
integrative medicine, 498
meditation, 500
mind and body practices, 498
tai chi, 500
yoga, 500

Alicia Initial Onset

Alicia Ramirez is a 45-year-old Hispanic woman who cannot sleep and recently has been getting headaches. She takes acetaminophen (Tylenol) to relieve her headaches. Stephen, a registered nurse, examines her at the outpatient clinic. During the health history, Alicia tells Stephen that she is a single mother of two and works full time. She immigrated to the United States from Mexico at age 15 and is bilingual in Spanish and English. Her mother passed away last year from kidney disease related to diabetes, and now her 76-year-old father lives with her. She also has a younger brother who lives nearby.

Alicia tells Stephen that work and family are sometimes very stressful and she comes home feeling exhausted. She falls asleep, but always wakes up several times in the middle of the night, worrying about things such as "Did I send in the permission slip for the field trip? I think I forgot to buy the folders for school! Did I mail that package for my boss at work? Is my brother going to remember to take Papi to the doctor?" Alicia also tells Stephen, "My head just can't stop. I feel so tired lately, but I just can't sleep."

On further assessment, Stephen learns that Alicia has to get up by 6 a.m. to get her school-age children ready for school before she goes to work. She drinks two cups of coffee per day, as well as soda. She does not smoke and is a social drinker only. Stephen inquires as to whether she takes any vitamins or "*hierbas*." Alicia says she sometimes drinks "*té de hierbas*," or herbal tea, at night. Her mother used to make a tea "*pasionaria*," or passionflower, for what she calls "*nervios*." Alicia buys the herb at her local market and drinks a cup at night. She tells Stephen that drinking the tea helps to calm her.

Stephen observes that Alicia's symptoms include difficulty sleeping, fatigue, persistent worrying, difficulty concentrating, and tension headache. Stephen recommends that Alicia keep a daily sleep diary for the next 2 weeks, recording her sleep patterns and how she feels upon waking. He suggests that she try to go to bed at the same time each day, not to eat a large meal before bedtime, to stop caffeine at least 6 hours before bedtime, and to make her bedroom environment accomodating for sleep (dark, quiet, comfortable temperature). He also suggests that if she cannot sleep after 15 minutes, that she get out of bed and do something relaxing. Stephen also advises her to stop drinking the passionflower tea until her next visit, to see if there is a change in any of her symptoms. He schedules a follow-up visit in 2 weeks and refers her to the clinic's PMH-APRN to help her deal with issues of stress and anxiety.

APPLICATION

1. Which of the five domains of wellness is a nursing priority for Alicia?

2. How significant are Alicia's symptoms of not being able to sleep, frequent headaches, and constant worrying?

3. Given Alicia's history, what questions related to culture should the nurse ask?

Introduction

The increasing use of complementary and alternative medicine (CAM) by the American public reflects consumer demand and shifting interest in approaches to health care. In 2007, the most recent year for which data are available, 38% of adult Americans used a CAM therapy in the past 12 months, with the most commonly used therapy being nonvitamin, nonmineral, natural products (Figure 22-1) (Barnes, Bloom, & Nahin, 2008). The National Center for Complementary and Alternative Medicine (NCCAM), established in 1998, is the federal government's lead agency for scientific research on CAM. NCCAM defines **complementary and alternative medicine**, or **complementary health approaches**, as a group of diverse medical and health care systems, practices, and products that are not generally considered part of **allopathic**, or conventional, medicine (NCCAM, 2013). How people use CAM therapies varies widely:

- **Complementary medicine** refers to the use of CAM in conjunction with conventional medicine.

- **Alternative medicine** refers to the use of CAM in place of conventional medicine.

- **Integrative medicine** refers to a practice that combines both conventional and CAM treatments for which there is high-quality scientific evidence of safety and effectiveness.

NCCAM has identified two broad categories of CAM. Natural (or biologically based) products include vitamins, herbs, and supplements (such as omega-3 fatty acids) (Figure 22-2). **Mind and body practices** are techniques and practices that require a certified practitioner or teacher (NCCAM, 2013). These include everything from yoga to chiropractic medicine. See Box 22-1 for examples of therapies from each of these four categories.

Patients choose CAM therapies for a variety of reasons, including the following:

- Dissatisfaction with conventional treatments due to unpleasant side effects and/or ineffectiveness

- Lack of health care coverage and the ability to afford conventional treatments

- Feeling that CAM is more congruent with personal values and beliefs about health

- CAM therapies are part of their cultural background

- Feeling that CAM is a "natural" and safer alternative

- Desire to reduce the need for medications

- Recommendation of family or friends

- Interest after reading something about CAM on the internet or in a magazine or newspaper

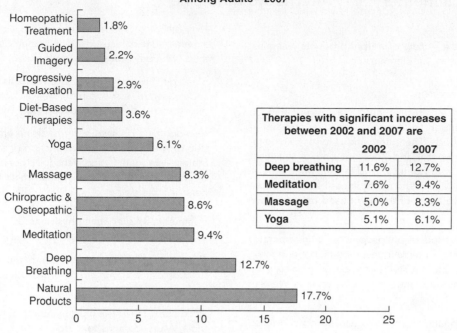

10 Most Common CAM Therapies Among Adults—2007

Therapy	Percentage
Homeopathic Treatment	1.8%
Guided Imagery	2.2%
Progressive Relaxation	2.9%
Diet-Based Therapies	3.6%
Yoga	6.1%
Massage	8.3%
Chiropractic & Osteopathic	8.6%
Meditation	9.4%
Deep Breathing	12.7%
Natural Products	17.7%

Therapies with significant increases between 2002 and 2007 are	2002	2007
Deep breathing	11.6%	12.7%
Meditation	7.6%	9.4%
Massage	5.0%	8.3%
Yoga	5.1%	6.1%

22-1 CAM therapies most commonly used by adults.

Data from Barnes, P.M., Bloom, B., Nahin, R. (2008). CDC National Health Statistics Report #12. Complementary and Alternative Medicine Use Among Adults and Children United States, 2007.

The number of reasons for which patients choose to try CAM underscores the importance of nurses asking about CAM use during the assessment process. Understanding if and why patients use CAM (and what therapies they use, and why) will help nurses assess patients for possible contraindications with pharmacologic therapies, potential issues with treatment compliance, and overall patient desire for health and wellness. Nursing assessment should include consideration of each of the domains: biological, psychological, sociological, cultural, and spiritual (Table 22-1). For many patients, cultural and spiritual background and beliefs may inform CAM usage, which will be discussed later in this chapter.

As CAM use in the general population continues to be prevalent, rates of use in people with mental disorders is common, particularly among those with depression and anxiety (Eisenberg et al., 1998; Kessler et al., 2001; Unutzer et al, 2000). According to the 2002 and

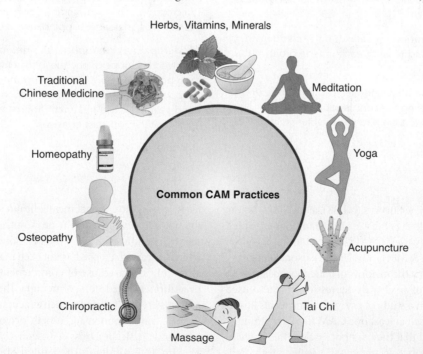

22-2 Select types of complementary and alternative medicine.

Types of Complementary and Alternative Medicine   box 22-1

Natural Products

This category includes a variety of herbal products, vitamins, minerals, and other dietary supplements.

Mind and Body Practices

Meditation: This practice cultivates internal awareness through contemplation or attention to thoughts, feelings, and sensations of the mind and body. There are various forms of meditation, such as transcendental and Zen, but one of the most commonly studied is *mindfulness meditation*. Mindfulness-based stress reduction (MBSR) and mindfulness-based cognitive therapy (MBCT) are two types of therapy based on meditative practices.

Yoga: Based on ancient Indian philosophy, yoga incorporates physical postures, breathing techniques, meditation, and relaxation. There are eight different styles of yoga, with hatha yoga being the most commonly practiced type of yoga in Western countries.

Acupuncture: A traditional Eastern practice involving stimulation of specific points on the body, acupuncture uses a variety of techniques to restore balance and maintain health. Acupuncture has been practiced for thousands of years in Asian countries such as China, Japan, and Korea.

Tai chi and qigong: Qigong refers to Eastern practices that incorporate postures, and meditation to cultivate the flow of vital energy or "qi." **Tai chi**, considered a form of qigong, focuses on slow, gentle, linked movement and awareness of the breath, often referred to as "moving meditation" (Figure 22-3).

Guided imagery: A technique that uses suggestions and directs thoughts to help the mind relax. Studies show that guided imagery may reduce some measures of psychological distress and improve relaxation.

Progressive muscle relaxation: A relaxation technique that involves slowly releasing and tensing each muscle group in the body.

Biofeedback: A technique that uses instruments measuring body functions and providing sensory feedback (for example, blood pressure, heart rate) to train patients to voluntarily control certain bodily processes.

Hypnotherapy: Through exercises and guidance, hypnosis induces a mental state of focused attention that allows individuals to affect their own body processes and physiological responses.

Massage: This body therapy involves manipulation of muscle layers and connective tissue to promote well-being and relaxation. Various styles include Swedish, deep tissue, and shiatsu.

Osteopathy: This system of medicine emphasizes the relationship between structure and function of the body. In the United States, osteopathic physicians (doctors of osteopathy, with DO degrees) are licensed physicians similar to allopathic practitioners with the doctor of medicine (MD) degree. Therefore, they use the same or similar diagnostic procedures and medical treatments as allopathic physicians but also are trained in and use manipulative techniques.

Chiropractic: A hands-on therapy that focuses on the health and function of the spine and other body structures and their effect on health.

Ayurveda: One of the oldest systems of medicine, originating in India, Ayurveda aims to integrate the body, mind, and spirit to prevent and treat illness and may employ herbs, massage, meditation, diet, and lifestyle modifications.

Reiki: This practice originated in Japan and uses light touch to access universal (or source) energy to support the body's innate healing abilities.

Homeopathy: A medical system developed in Germany about 200 years ago, following the principle of similars, or "like cures like." It seeks to stimulate the body's ability to heal itself by giving very small doses of highly diluted substances that, in larger doses, would produce symptoms or illness.

Traditional Chinese medicine (TCM): A medical system originating in China whose philosophy views the human body as a microcosm of the surrounding universe. TCM employs acupuncture, herbs, massage, cupping, and dietary and other therapies.

Naturopathy or *naturopathic medicine:* This system, which evolved in Europe during the 19th century, is guided by the healing power of nature and treating the whole person. It aims to support the body's inherent ability to maintain and restore health, and prefers to use treatment approaches considered to be the most natural and least invasive.

2007 National Health Interview Surveys (NHIS), anxiety/depression, stress, and insomnia or trouble sleeping were the conditions for which adult patients most frequently used CAM (Barnes, Bloom, & Nahin, 2008; Bertisch, Wee, Phillips, & McCarthy, 2009; Pearson, Johnson, & Nahin, 2006). Data suggest that the majority of patients who have seen a psychiatrist for treatment of anxiety or depression have also used CAM (Kessler et al., 2001). In a study of psychiatric inpatients hospitalized for acute care, 63% used at least one CAM therapy within the past year and most indicated that they did not disclose this use with their psychiatrist (Elkins, Rajab, & Marcus, 2005). Patients with mental disorders who have reported using alternative medicine were as likely to use conventional mental health services as respondents who did not use alternative medicine (Unutzer et al., 2000). Self-reported mental conditions (those which respondents report having but for which a formal diagnosis has not been made or confirmed) are associated with increased use of complementary treatments, and use of practitioner-based complementary therapies (therapies that are administered by a provider, such as acupuncture or chiropractic medicine) is fairly common and usually occurs without the knowledge or input of a physician (Druss & Rosenheck, 2000).

In 2007, adults in the United States spent $33.9 billion on CAM. Nearly two-thirds of the total out-of-pocket costs were for self-care purchases of CAM products, classes, and materials (Nahin, Barnes, Stussman, & Bloom, 2009). The increased concurrent use of CAM therapies with conventional treatments is of concern because the safety and efficacy of some therapies have not yet been firmly established. Because patients often fail to disclose herbal and dietary supplement use to their physicians (Kennedy, Wang, & Wu, 2008), nurses need to ensure open communication and possess the knowledge required to discuss the risks and benefits of CAM use with patients.

Pause and Reflect

1. *What are some reasons patients may choose to use CAM?*
2. *Referring to Box 22-1, what CAM therapies are you familiar with, or which ones have you tried? If you tried them, in what ways were they helpful?*

CAM and Mental Health

Some major CAM treatments for anxiety, depression, mania, schizophrenia, substance use disorders, and sleep disorders are reviewed briefly in this section. Using an evidence-based approach, key data from randomized controlled trials (RCTs), meta-analyses, and systematic reviews of RCTs have been synthesized. Information in regard to effectiveness is based on current evidence. Research on CAM therapies is relatively recent; thus, knowledge and understanding of these therapies is increasing and changing. As stated earlier, many of the therapies discussed require additional research to confirm safety and efficacy. Some may be more helpful as adjuvant, or complementary, therapies than as alternatives to conventional treatment. Mind–body practices

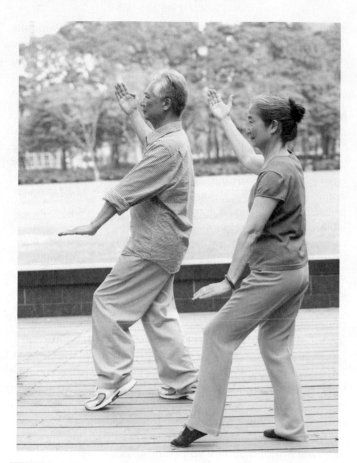

22-3 Tai chi focuses on slow, gentle, linked movement and awareness of the breath.

Source: Monkey Business/Fotolia

Nursing Considerations Related to CAM Therapies by Wellness Domain — table 22-1

Domain	Nursing Considerations
Biological	Does the patient have any medical conditions that may contradict use of certain herbs or supplements? If so, has the patient discussed use of CAM therapies with the primary health care provider?
	If the patient is currently using one or more natural products, what is the potential for toxicity or adverse effects?
Psychological	What is the meaning of CAM therapies as compared to traditional prescription medication for the patient?
	Does the patient's level of cognitive functioning at this time suggest that the patient can successfully participate and/or manage CAM therapies?
	If the patient is considering using one or more CAM therapies as an alternative to conventional therapy, what are the possible consequences for the patient, and is the patient able to understand these?
Sociological	Are the therapies the patient is considering or using available in the local area from properly licensed or certified providers?
	What is the family's level of support for the patient's use of CAM therapies?
Cultural	Is mental illness recognized in the patient's culture?
	Are there any CAM therapies that are a regular part of the patient's cultural practices for health maintenance? What impact do they have on the patient's mental health status currently?
	Does the patient's culture rely on CAM therapies as a primary treatment because there is an innate distrust of conventional medicine?
	Does the culture include traditional healers that rely on CAM treatments first?
Spiritual	Is mental illness viewed as a spiritual condition?
	Are there any CAM therapies that are a regular part of the patient's spiritual practices?
	Does the spiritual leader in the community recognize abnormal behavior as something that can be treated, or is the patient ostracized and sent away?

and exercise may be particularly helpful in patients who seek to lower stress and anxiety levels and improve their overall quality of health. In each case, nurses should be open-minded about patient use of CAM, seek to learn how and why patients choose to use CAM therapies to address their mental health needs, and be informed as to best-practice approaches.

Sleep–Wake Disorders

Given the prevalence of insomnia and other sleep–wake disorders, it is not surprising that patients are choosing to try CAM therapies to improve their sleep (Chapter 12). Commonly seen CAM treatments for sleep–wake disorders include two natural products—melatonin and valerian root—and mind–body therapies (Table 22-2).

Melatonin

Melatonin, a hormone found naturally in the body, is produced by the pineal gland, which regulates circadian rhythm and sleep–wake cycles. As darkness falls, endogenous melatonin levels rise, sending signals to the body to sleep. Light reduces melatonin production and signals the body to awaken. When taken at night, melatonin may decrease the time it takes to fall asleep (sleep latency) in circadian rhythm sleep disorders, but with variable effects on sleep duration (Brzezinski et al., 2005; Morgenthaler et al., 2006). Melatonin administration in sleep onset insomnia in children with autism spectrum disorders has been associated with improved sleep parameters (Andersen, Kaczmarska, McGrew, & Malow, 2008; Malow et al., 2012; Rossignol & Frye, 2011). However, the role of melatonin in primary or secondary insomnia is less well established.

Practice alerts/precautions: Synthetic melatonin is available in different formulations such as controlled time-released tablets, capsules, and lozenges. Doses of melatonin have ranged from 0.3 to 5 mg/day. The most common side effect is daytime drowsiness. Melatonin use appears to be safe for short-term periods of days or weeks, up to 2 months (Natural Standard Database, 2011). Melatonin should be used with caution by women who are pregnant or nursing because risks to the fetus/infant have not been evaluated. Melatonin can increase blood pressure in patients treated with antihypertensive medications. Concomitant administration of melatonin and nifedipine has resulted in elevations in blood pressure and heart rate (Lusordi, Piazza, & Fogari, 2000). Fluvoxamine (Luvox) may increase circulating plasma levels of melatonin, resulting in sedation (Härtter, Grözinger, Weigmann, Röschke, & Hiemke, 2000). Patients taking anticoagulant medications should use melatonin with caution, as it may increase the risk of bleeding.

Valerian (*Valeriana officinalis*)

This herb, native to Europe and Asia, is a common ingredient in products promoted as sedatives and sleep aids. However, clinical studies for the efficacy of valerian are inconsistent, owing to small sample sizes, varying amounts and sources of valerian, and different measurement outcomes (Bent et al., 2006; Fernández-San-Martín et al., 2010; Taibi, Landis, Petry, & Vitiello, 2007). Without further research, the current evidence is inconclusive.

Practice alerts/precautions: Headaches, dizziness, and gastrointestinal (GI) disturbances are the most common adverse effects reported. Valerian may cause a modest increase in levels of alprazolam but is unlikely to produce significant effects on CYP3A4 or CYP2D6 metabolic pathways (Donovan et al., 2004) (Chapter 23).

Animal studies have shown valerian to enhance the sedation time induced by barbiturates (Taibi et al., 2007). It may have synergistic effects with benzodiazepines and other sedating agents. Valerian should be used with caution by pregnant and nursing women because risks to the fetus/infant have not been evaluated.

Mind and Body Practices

Although some patients may choose to try acupuncture, a traditional Eastern practice involving stimulation of specific points on the body, the current evidence for acupuncture is not sufficiently extensive or rigorous to support its use for the treatment of insomnia (Cheuk, Yeung, Chung, & Wong, 2007; Huang, Kutner, & Bliwise, 2009). Larger, high-quality RCTs are needed to further investigate the usefulness of acupuncture.

In a limited number of preliminary trials, mind–body interventions such as meditation and tai chi have shown promise in improving sleep quality or duration. *Meditation* refers to a group of techniques that use strategies such as focused attention and posture to help relax the body and the mind. Mindfulness-based meditation and stress-reduction techniques may be associated with improved sleep or reduction in sleep-interfering cognitive processes such as worry (Gross et al., 2011; Shapiro et al., 2003; Winbush, Gross, & Kreitzer, 2007). A novel treatment combining mindfulness meditation with cognitive–behavioral therapy for insomnia found sleep-related benefits that continued one year after treatment (Ong, Shapiro, & Manber, 2009). Tai chi may be an effective nonpharmacological approach to improving sleep quality in older adults with moderate sleep complaints (Li et al., 2004; Irwin, Olmstead, & Motivala, 2008). Further studies are needed in exploring the full potential of these techniques as nonpharmacologic treatment options.

Other CAM therapies that may be effective for sleep disorders are cognitive–behavioral therapies such as progressive muscle relaxation and biofeedback (Morgenthaler et al., 2006). **Biofeedback** is a technique that uses instruments that measure body function and provide sensory feedback (for example, blood pressure, heart rate) to train patients to control certain bodily functions voluntarily. These therapies provide patients with nonpharmacological options that offer advantages over the long term, particularly for the common co-morbidity of insomnia and other chronic medical and/or psychiatric illnesses (Box 22-2).

Disorders of Anxiety, Stress, and Trauma

Patients with disorders of anxiety, stress, and trauma (Chapter 13) or who are experiencing symptoms of anxiety related to a general medical condition may benefit from using a variety of CAM therapies (Ekor, Adeyemi, & Otuechere, 2013). Assessment of the patient's current level of anxiety, history of use and success with CAM therapies, and current treatment regimen will guide the nurse in helping the patient determine whether a CAM therapy may be beneficial and will decrease the likelihood of any contraindications between CAM therapies and the patient's individual treatment regimen. In particular, patients with anxiety may benefit from regular exercise or incorporation of mind and body practices, such as meditation or yoga (Table 22-3).

Kava (*Piper methysticum*)

Kava is a plant indigenous to the Pacific Islands, where it is used as a social beverage. Its anxiolytic activity is primarily attributed to the

Selected Natural Products

table 22-2

	Product	Use/Possible Benefit	Potential Adverse Effects	Nursing Implications
Sleep Disorders	Melatonin	• Effective in circadian rhythm sleep disorders • Effective in reducing sleep latency • Variable effects on sleep duration • Possibly useful for insomnia in children with autism spectrum disorders	• Daytime drowsiness	• Use with caution in patients taking nifedipine, fluvoxamine, anticoagulants. • Safety in pregnant/nursing women has not been established.
	Valerian	• Current evidence inconclusive, but common ingredient in products promoted as sedatives and sleep aids	• Headaches • Dizziness • GI disturbances	• Use with caution in patients taking barbiturates, benzodiazepines, alcohol and other sedatives. • Safety in pregnant/nursing women has not been established.
Anxiety Disorders	Kava	• May provide anxiolytic activity for short-term treatment for symptoms of mild anxiety.	• Hepatotoxicity	• Use with caution in patients taking barbiturates, benzodiazepines, or other sedatives; patients with liver conditions; patients who drink alcohol; pregnant and nursing women.
	Chamomile	• May provide modest benefits to patients with mild to moderate generalized anxiety disorder. • May be helpful as a sleep aid in patients with insomnia due to underlying anxiety disorder.		• Contraindicated in patients with allergies to ragweed, chrysanthemum. • Use with caution in patients using anticoagulants, sedatives.
Mood Disorders	St. John's wort	• May be beneficial as short-term treatment for mild to moderate depression. • May be similarly effective to standard antidepressants for depression mild to moderate in severity.	• May cause increased photosensitivity. • Side effects similar to SSRIs. • May result in serotonin syndrome if used concomitantly with SSRIs.	• Interacts with a large number of medications. • Use with caution in patients taking immunosuppressants, HIV medications, antidepressants, anticoagulants, statins, calcium channel blockers, oral contraceptives, benzodiazepines, digoxin, and certain cancer drugs. • May also interact with fexofenadine, chlorzoxazone, lopinavir, methadone, and theophylline.
	Omega-3 fatty acids	• May have antidepressant or mood stabilizing effects when used as an adjunctive therapy. • Low doses safe and generally well tolerated.	• Doses > 3 g per day may decrease platelet aggregation.	• Caution against children, pregnant and nursing women eating fish high in mercury. • FDA recommends no more than 12 oz per week of fish with lower mercury levels (e.g., canned light tuna).
	SAMe	• May be beneficial for patients with MDD	• Common side effects: mild GI symptoms, sweating, dizziness, anxiety. • May result in serotonin syndrome if used concomitantly with SSRIs.	• Long-term safety data are limited.
	DHEA	• Possible potential for midlife-onset MDD and treatment of depressive symptoms in patients with HIV-related illness.	• May cause androgenic events, especially when taken at high doses. • Hormone-related side effects may include increased blood sugar levels, insulin resistance, altered adrenal function. • Reports of mania with high doses in some patients with suspected mood disorders.	• More research is needed to prove efficacy and long-term use. • Some concern that it may increase risk for hormone-sensitive cancers and conditions. • Not recommended for use by children, pregnant and nursing women.

(Continued)

Selected Natural Products (*continued*)

table 22-2

	Product	Use/Possible Benefit	Potential Adverse Effects	Nursing Implications
Cognitive Disorders	Folate	• May be beneficial as adjunctive therapy, as folic acid deficiency has been associated with depression and linked to poorer and slower responses to antidepressant treatment,	• Safe and well tolerated in recommended doses of 200 to 500 mcg daily.	• Very high doses may have CNS effects and exacerbate seizures in people with seizure disorders.
	Ginkgo	• Current evidence is conflicting and inconsistent for dementia and cognitive function.	• GI complaints. • Prolonged bleeding. • Can increase anticoagulant/antiplatelet effects.	• Use with caution in patients using antiepileptics, thiazide diuretics, ibuprofen, risperidone, efavirenz, trazodone, midazolam, warfarin.
	DHEA	• Some reports have suggested that DHEA may have neuroprotective effects, but clinical research to date does not support improvement of cognitive function with DHEA supplementation.	• May cause androgenic events, especially when taken at high doses • Hormone-related side effects may include increased blood sugar levels, insulin resistance, altered adrenal function.	• More research is needed to prove efficacy and long-term use. • Some concern that it may increase risk for hormone-sensitive cancers and conditions. • Not recommended for use by children, pregnant and nursing women
Substance Use Disorders	Little information available on the use of natural products with substance use disorders			• Assess patients for use of "natural products," including marijuana and peyote.

Relaxation Techniques

box 22-2

Relaxation techniques may be used as part of an overall treatment plan for disorders including insomnia, anxiety, and depression. In addition to the techniques listed here, certain mind–body practices such as meditation and yoga may also be considered.

Biofeedback

Biofeedback uses sensors applied to different parts of the body and monitors physiological responses. The feedback is used to teach and train patients to control their thoughts, emotions, and behaviors. By becoming aware of the physiological responses that occur when patients are anxious or under stress, patients can learn to relax and modify their behavior. The number of sessions can vary based on the condition and the learning pace of the patient. Ultimately, patients learn techniques to use on their own without the instruments. Some common types of biofeedback include thermal or temperature feedback, in which sensors on the fingers or feet measure skin temperature; electromyography, which measures muscle tension; and neurofeedback (electroencephalography), which measures brain wave activity.

A biofeedback therapist may be licensed as a provider in another field, such as nursing, psychology, physical therapy, or social work, and then also be board certified by the Biofeedback Certification International Alliance (BCIA). Regulations vary by state.

Deep Breathing or Breathing Exercises

Individuals who feel anxious or stressed often experience rapid, shallow breathing, shortness of breath, muscle tension, and an increased heart rate. Simple, slow breathing enhances parasympathetic activity and, by slowing down the breathing rate, it may help to relax and ease anxiety. By focusing on the inhalation and exhalation, awareness of the breath develops.

Some exercises to try: First, find a quiet and comfortable position sitting or lying down. Place your hands on your abdomen and begin to inhale deeply and feel your chest and belly rise. Try breathing deeply from the abdomen rather than taking shallow breaths. Then, as you exhale, feel your abdomen fall. Repeat a few times. Another exercise is to close your mouth and inhale through the nose for a mental count of 3, hold the breath for a count of 3, and then exhale through the nose for a count of 6. Repeat a few times.

Progressive Muscle Relaxation

The essence of this technique involves tensing and releasing muscle groups. While a patient is sitting or lying down in a comfortable position with eyes closed, the whole body is covered in a sequential pattern, either starting with the upper body first and then the lower body, or vice versa. For example, the patient is instructed to tense the right foot, hold it for a few seconds, and then relax it. Then, the left foot is tensed and released, and the patient continues with the right calf, left calf, thighs, hips, buttocks, stomach, back, chest, shoulders, arms, neck, and head. This technique may be accompanied by deep breathing exercises or guided imagery.

Selected Mind and Body Practices

table 22-3

Type of CAM	Description	Potential Benefits	Nursing Implications
Acupuncture	Traditional Eastern practice involving stimulation of specific acupuncture points of the body.	May reduce anxiety. May reduce anxiety and depression due to cancer and related treatments.	Generally considered safe. Practice laws vary from state to state; encourage patients to seek licensed practitioners with certification from NCCAM.
Biofeedback	Technique that uses instruments that measure body function and provide sensory feedback, allowing patients to learn to control certain bodily functions voluntarily.	Sleep disorders, anxiety, stress.	Generally considered safe.
Exercise	Type of exercise may vary depending on individual preferences, but typically regular, aerobic exercise is thought to confer benefit in multiple areas.	May help reduce anxiety, elevate mood. May improve physical and mental well being of patients with schizophrenia. May enhance cognitive functioning in older adults.	Exercise should be tailored to individual's need, abilities, and physical status.
Meditation	Mind–body practice that uses techniques to focus attention and cultivate internal awareness.	May decrease sleep-interfering processes (e.g., worry). May reduce anxiety, stress. May lower relapse/recurrence rates for patients with MDD.	Generally considered safe.
Music therapy	Therapeutic method which uses musical interaction involving active and receptive techniques as a means of communication and expression.	May assist in relieving anxiety. May improve global state, mental state, and function in patients with schizophrenia.	Generally considered safe.
Tai chi	Eastern practice focusing on slow, linked movements and an awareness of breath.	May benefit older adults with depression and moderate sleep complaints. May provide benefit to patients with mild to moderate depression.	Practice should be tailored to age, physical limitations, and health status.
Yoga	Mind–body practice that incorporates physical postures, breathing, meditation, and relaxation.	May reduce anxiety.	Yoga practices vary from gentle to more vigorous. Practice should be tailored to age, physical limitations, and health status.

kavalactones, which may produce skeletal muscle relaxation, sedative, and local anesthetic effects. Compared with placebo, kava may be effective in the symptomatic treatment for mild to moderate anxiety (Pittler & Ernst, 2003; Witte, Loew, & Gaus, 2005). Most clinical trials have used kava extract standardized to 70% kavalactone content.

Practice alerts/precautions: Safety concerns have been raised about potential hepatotoxicity from kava-containing dietary supplements, which may be due to poor quality/contamination, prolonged use (more than 24 weeks), high doses (more than 300 mg/day), or co-medication. More studies are needed to be certain of kava's possible potential adverse effects. Kava is banned in the United Kingdom, Germany, France, Switzerland, and Canada. Kava has never been banned in the United States, where it continues to be sold as a dietary supplement, although at much lower levels since the U.S. Food and Drug Administration advised consumers on the potential liver hepatotoxicity issue in 2002. Kava may have enhanced sedation effects if taken concurrently with barbiturates, benzodiazepines, or sedatives. Caution is needed if the patient has an underlying liver condition or drinks alcohol, as well as use in pregnant and nursing women because risks to the fetus/infant have not been evaluated.

Chamomile

Chamomile (*Matricaria recutita*) is a common herbal tea extracted from a daisy-like plant known as *Asteraceae*; it is consumed in many cultures for various health benefits. Preliminary animal studies suggest it may have effects on the central nervous system (McKay & Blumberg, 2006). An RCT suggests chamomile may have modest anxiolytic activity in patients with mild to moderate generalized anxiety disorder (GAD) (Amsterdam et al., 2009). It may also be helpful as a sleep aid for patients whose insomnia is due to an underlying anxiety disorder (Zick, Wright, Sen, & Arnedt, 2011).

Practice alerts/precautions: Chamomile is available as a tea, liquid extract, and capsules. It may cause allergic reactions in individuals sensitive to the Asteraceae/Compositae family, which includes ragweed and chrysanthemum. It may possibly increase anticoagulant effects of drugs such as warfarin and increase the effects of sedatives (Segal & Pilote, 2006).

Mind and Body Practices

In a systematic review and meta-analysis it was reported that meditative therapies may be an effective option for patients with anxiety symptoms

(Chen et al., 2012). Although the exact biological or psychological mechanism is not completely understood, it has been suggested that meditation cultivates the ability to moderate attention, modifies maladaptive cognitive styles such as negative attribution, and encourages a nonjudgmental stance (Lang et al., 2012). Mindfulness meditation therapies may effectively reduce anxiety and mood symptoms in generalized anxiety disorder (Evans et al., 2008; Hofmann, Sawyer, Witt, & Oh, 2010; Kabat-Zinn et al., 1992). Another form of meditation, transcendental meditation, was found to be comparable with other kinds of relaxation therapies in reducing anxiety (Krisanaprakornkit, Krisanaprakornkit, Piyavhatkul, & Laopaiboon, 2006). A report prepared for the Department of Veterans Affairs found that meditation techniques were associated with moderate improvements in posttraumatic stress disorder (PTSD) severity and health-related quality of life compared to usual care (Strauss et al., 2011).

Yoga

Yoga is a mind–body practice that incorporates physical postures, breathing techniques, meditation, and relaxation. Limited research evidence exists for the efficacy of yoga in anxiety, but it may improve mood and decrease anxiety by increasing γ-aminobutyric acid (GABA) levels, which are found to be reduced in mood and anxiety disorders (Kirkwood et al., 2005; Streeter et al., 2010). The controlled breathing and meditative components of yoga may also lead to a reduction in sympathetic and an increase in parasympathetic activity, and is possibly linked to decreasing levels of cortisol (Brown & Gerbarg, 2009; Meyer et al., 2012). As yoga includes attention control, meditative practices, and breath awareness, it is also being studied as a potential intervention for patients with PTSD.

Practice alerts/precautions: Yoga practices can range from gentle (restorative) to more vigorous types. Nurses should instruct patients to seek out appropriately trained instructors and to inform yoga instructors of any physical injuries, limitations, or illnesses that may require they avoid or modify certain types of yoga or specific moves or poses.

Acupuncture

Acupuncture may be effective for the treatment of anxiety. In one study, auricular acupuncture and intranasal midazolam (Versed) were similarly effective for the treatment of dental anxiety (Karst et al., 2007). Cancer patients receiving acupuncture reported improvement immediately after treatment and significant improvement over time for anxiety and depression (Dean-Clower et al., 2010). Research is very limited in evaluating acupuncture for posttraumatic stress disorder (PTSD), but it may be helpful in improving symptoms of anxiety, sleep disruption, and depression. A single RCT of 12 weeks of acupuncture found that participants experienced a change in PTSD symptoms and health-related quality of life similar to group CBT and greater than waitlist control, and that clinical improvement persisted for at least 3 months after completion of treatment (Hollifield, Sinclair-Lian, Warner, & Hammerschlag, 2007).

Practice alerts/precautions: Acupuncture generally is considered safe. Most states require a license to practice acupuncture and successful completion of the National Certification Commission for Acupuncture and Oriental Medicine (NCCAOM) exam; however, practice laws vary from state to state.

Other CAM

Music therapy is a therapeutic method that uses musical interaction involving active and receptive techniques as a means of communication and expression. Music therapy is used for reducing anxiety in a variety of clinical settings. Listening to music may provide benefit in reduction of heart rate and blood pressure in patients with coronary heart disease and reduction of anxiety in myocardial infarction patients upon hospitalization (Bradt & Dileo, 2009). Music interventions and verbal relaxation have also been shown to have a beneficial effect on anxiety, mood, and quality of life in patients with cancer (Bradt et al., 2011; Lin et al., 2011). Even though the music employed is usually calming, it is unclear which specific style or type of music, duration, and frequency are most effective. Music therapy may offer benefits as an inexpensive, nonpharmacological, and noninvasive adjunct therapy.

Research suggests that various types and levels of exercise may have anxiolytic effects, depending on the physical fitness level and interests of the individual patient. It may reduce anxiety symptoms among sedentary patients who have a chronic illness. Exercise training programs lasting no more than 12 weeks, using session durations of at least 30 minutes, and an anxiety report time frame greater than the past week resulted in the largest anxiety improvements (Herring, O'Connor, & Dishman, 2010). Exercise, a nonpharmacological approach with minimal adverse effects, also promotes healthy lifestyle behavior (Box 22-3).

Exercise   box 22-3

Regular exercise helps to promote and improve health. In addition to the multiple physical fitness benefits, exercise can be beneficial to mental and emotional well-being (Bertish, Wells, Smith, & McCarthy, 2012). Exercise affects the production of endorphins and neurotransmitters, such as serotonin and norepinephrine, which may improve mood. There is an association between exercise and a reduction in depressive symptoms. In addition, there is growing literature demonstrating that exercise, particularly aerobic exercise, impacts the structure and function of the brain and improves cognition (Ahlskog, Geda, Graff-Radford, & Petersen, 2011; Erickson et al., 2011). Exercise enhances neurogenesis in the hippocampus and increases gray matter in the cortex and levels of brain-derived neurotrophic factor (Ahlskog, Geda, Graff-Radford & Petersen, 2011).

Exercise includes working out at the gym, bicycling, running, and tennis, but walking the dog, dancing, gardening, mopping the floor, and other household activities also constitute exercise. Nurses can provide suggestions for patients to find ways to keep active and moving. Some suggestions may include taking the stairs instead of the elevator, getting off one subway/bus stop early and walking to work, or parking the car farther away and walking the extra distance.

The Centers for Disease Control and Prevention (CDC) recommends that adults should do 2 hours and 30 minutes a week of moderate-intensity, or 1 hour and 15 minutes (75 minutes) a week of vigorous-intensity, aerobic physical activity, or an equivalent combination of moderate- and vigorous-intensity aerobic physical activity. Aerobic activity may be performed in episodes of at least 10 minutes, preferably spread throughout the week (CDC, 2011). Nurses can help guide exercise programs according to the patient's age, individual needs, physical limitations, and health status.

Alicia Recovery Phase

APPLICATION

1. Given Alicia's lifestyle, what are some CAM options to recommend that are not costly or time consuming?

2. Why is it important to involve Alicia in her care plan?

3. In what ways does Linda offer hope to Alicia?

Alicia returns to the clinic 2 weeks later for a follow-up appointment with Linda, the PMH-APRN. Linda reviews her sleep diary. Alicia reports that she tried some of the suggestions, such as cutting down on soda in the late afternoon and going to sleep at the same time each night. These have helped, but she still feels stressed and tired. During the interview, Alicia reveals that she was feeling "*nervios*" and started drinking the passionflower tea again the previous week and that it helps her feel "*calme.*" Linda searched two CAM resources, MedlinePlus and the Natural Standard, for information about passionflower's safety, effectiveness, and possible interactions with medications. Linda determines that the tea is not likely harmful and may confer benefit to the patient, counseling Alicia that she may continue to drink the tea, although she advises Alicia to stop drinking the tea if it causes too much sleepiness and/or drowsiness. Linda offers to set up a counseling schedule, but Alicia says she doesn't have the time, between her work, children, and caring for her father. Linda then suggests some self-help strategies that Alicia can practice regularly. Linda demonstrates a simple breathing exercise that can be done in 5 minutes. Linda emphasizes that meditation, which is also a part of Alicia's church service, can be done wherever she is—while walking, commuting on the subway or bus, or when waiting in the doctor's office. Linda offers Alicia options for meditating, such as repeating a calming word or thought, or listening to the sounds of her breath. She also shows Alicia a progressive muscle relaxation technique to do while lying in bed. Linda also makes some lifestyle suggestions, such as cutting down on coffee and having tea instead, and trying not to drink coffee or caffeinated beverages after lunchtime. Other suggestions Linda makes include exercise, such as brisk walking up to 20 to 30 minutes each day, and incorporating activities Alicia enjoys for herself. Alicia says she likes to listen to music to relax. When she was younger, she loved to go dancing. But now she says, "No time for me." Linda recommends that Alicia integrate these strategies into her life and return in 6 months.

Depressive and Bipolar Disorders

Many people with mood disorders use a variety of CAM therapies, mind–body therapies, or natural products to reduce suffering and promote health. Patients with mood disorders may try several natural products, including St. John's wort, omega-3 fatty acids, *S*-adenosyl methionine (SAMe), dehydroepiandrosterone (DHEA), and folate (Qureshi & Al-Bedah, 2013).

St. John's Wort

Native to Europe, Asia, and northern Africa, St. John's wort (*Hypericum perforatum*) is an herb also commonly found in the United States and Canada. Active constituents that have been isolated include hypericin and hyperforin, with hyperforin as the major constituent (Bouron & Lorrain, 2014), responsible for its antidepressant activity by selectively inhibiting serotonin, dopamine, and norepinephrine reuptake in the central nervous system. Scientific studies suggest that St. John's wort may be useful for short-term treatment of mild to moderate depression (Kasper et al., 2010), but studies have been inconsistent. A Cochrane review (Linde, Berner, & Kriston, 2008) suggested that St. John's wort is superior to placebo in nonpsychotic major depression, similarly effective as and with fewer side effects than standard antidepressants. However, a meta-analysis did not find a difference in response rates between St. John's wort and selective serotonin-reuptake inhibitors (SSRIs) (Rahimi, Nikfar, & Abdollahi, 2009).

Practice alerts/precautions: St. John's wort is available as capsules, tablets, tinctures, and teas; most products are standardized to contain 0.3% hypericin. Similar to the side effects of SSRIs, St. John's wort may cause GI discomfort, dry mouth, dizziness, rashes, fatigue, and headache (Natural Standard, 2011). It may also cause increased photosensitivity. If taken concurrently with SSRIs, St. John's wort may interact and result in serotonin syndrome. Its ability to induce the cytochrome P450 3A4 system has the potential to reduce the plasma concentrations of a large number of drugs,

including certain immunosuppressants, such as cyclosporine and tacrolimus; HIV medications; antidepressants; anticoagulants, such as warfarin and phenprocoumon; statins, such as simvastatin and atorvastatin; calcium channel blockers; oral contraceptives; benzodiazepenes; digoxin; and certain cancer drugs. It may also have P450 interactions with fexofenadine, chlorzoxazon, lopinavir, methadone, and theophylline (Borrelli & Izzo, 2009). Use with caution in women who are pregnant or nursing because risks to the fetus/infant have not been evaluated.

Omega-3 Fatty Acids

The main omega-3 fatty acids in the brain, docosahexaenoic acid (DHA) and eicosapentaenoic acid (EPA), are associated with cell membrane fluidity and phospholipid composition affecting serotonin and dopamine transmission. Low levels of omega-3 fatty acids have been hypothesized in the pathogenesis of depression (Lin, Huang, & Su, 2010; McNamara et al., 2007). Because omega-3 fatty acids are not synthesized efficiently in the body, they must be obtained from dietary sources (Mahaffey et al., 2011). Research has suggested that supplementation with DHA and EPA may have antidepressant or mood-stabilizing effects. Adjunctive EPA or the combination of EPA and DHA (the combination found in most commercially available brands) appears most useful for mild to moderate major depressive disorder (MDD), with less evidence for DHA as a monotherapy (Freeman & Rapaport, 2011; Mischoulon, 2007). Until further research is completed, current studies suggest a potential role as an adjunctive treatment for major depressive disorder (MDD) and possibly bipolar depression (Parker et al., 2006). Patients with a mood disorder might benefit from the addition of omega-3 fatty acids to their diet. Dietary sources of omega-3 fatty acids include cold-water fish, such as salmon, mackerel, halibut, sardines, tuna, and herring; flaxseeds, pumpkin seeds, and walnuts; and canola oil, soybean oil, and cod liver oil.

Practice alerts/precautions: Doses of 1 to 9 grams per day have been studied in mood disorders, with most evidence supporting use of lower doses (Freeman et al., 2010). Omega-3 fatty acids are considered safe and are generally well tolerated when taken in low doses (3 grams or less per day) (Natural Standard, 2011). The side effects of fish oil supplements may include fishy taste, nausea, belching, and loose stools. Doses greater than 3 grams per day may decrease platelet aggregation. Children and pregnant and nursing women should avoid eating fish with the highest levels of mercury concentration (e.g., shark, mackerel, swordfish, and tilefish). In addition, the FDA recommends eating no more than 12 ounces a week of fish with lower mercury levels, such as canned light tuna, salmon, pollock, and catfish.

| **PRACTICE ALERT**   Patients with a chronic medical condition, such as asthma, diabetes, or hypertension, should be encouraged to consult their primary care provider or pharmacist before trying CAM or products labeled as "natural."

S-Adenosyl Methionine

S-adenosyl methionine (SAMe) is a naturally occurring compound synthesized from methionine and adenosine triphosphate (ATP) found throughout the body and involved in many biochemical reactions, including the synthesis of neurotransmitters in the brain. The specific antidepressant mechanism remains unclear. Low levels of SAMe have been reported in the cerebrospinal fluid (CSF) of severely depressed patients (Bottiglieri et al., 1990). The antidepressant efficacy of SAMe has been studied in numerous randomized controlled trials involving adults with depression in Europe and the United States (Hardy et al., 2002; Papakostas, 2009). However, despite evidence indicating a potential antidepressant role for SAMe, literature is limited for its efficacy as a monotherapy. SAMe may be beneficial as an adjunctive treatment strategy for patients with MDD and/or those who do not respond to antidepressants (Papakostas et al., 2010).

Practice alerts/precautions: A number of clinical studies have found SAMe to be efficacious in oral doses that range from 800 mg/day to 1,600 mg/day, for up to 6 weeks (Natural Standard, 2011). It is available in enteric-coated supplement form and appears to be safe and generally well tolerated, but long-term safety data are limited. It may result in an increased risk of serotonin syndrome if taken concomitantly with SSRIs. Common side effects include mild gastrointestinal symptoms, sweating, dizziness, and anxiety.

Dehydroepiandrosterone (DHEA)

DHEA is a hormone secreted by the body's adrenal glands. It is a precursor to the male and female sex hormones, androgen and estrogen. Levels of DHEA peak at around age 20 and decline with age. Limited small studies suggest the potential of DHEA for treatment of midlife-onset major depressive disorder (MDD) and depressive symptoms in patients with HIV-related illness (Rabkin et al., 2006, Schmidt et al., 2005). However, the role of DHEA in regulation of mood is unclear and inconsistent. Future research is required to confirm its efficacy and tolerability for long-term use.

Practice alerts/precautions: DHEA is available in liquid, capsules, tablets and injections, with commonly used doses ranging from 30 to 90 mg daily for up to 6 weeks (Natural Standard, 2011). At high doses of 200 mg/day, it may cause androgenic effects. Androgenic effects, including irreversible hair loss, hirsutism, and deepening of voice, have occasionally been reported in women. There is concern that DHEA could increase the risk of hormone-sensitive cancers and

conditions. Hormonal-related side effects may include increased blood sugar levels, insulin resistance, altered cholesterol and thyroid hormone levels, and altered adrenal function. In addition, reports of mania with high doses of DHEA have been reported in some patients with suspected mood disorders (Natural Standard, 2011). It is not recommended to use DHEA during pregnancy or breastfeeding, or in children.

Folate

Folate is a water-soluble B vitamin that occurs naturally in food, with folic acid as the synthetic form. Foods that provide folate include leafy green vegetables, fruits (melons, citrus), cereals/grains, legumes, and organ meats. Folic acid deficiency has been associated among people with depression and has been linked to poorer and slower response to antidepressant treatment (Papakostas et al., 2004). Limited clinical research suggests that folic acid is not effective as a replacement for conventional antidepressant therapy, but it may have a potential role as a supplement to other treatments for depression (Fava & Mischoulon, 2010; Morris, Trivedi, & Rush, 2008; Taylor, Carney, Geddes, & Goodwin, 2003).

Practice alerts/precautions: Doses of 200 to 500 micrograms daily have been used for augmenting treatment response to antidepressants (Natural Standard, 2011). Folate appears to be safe and well tolerated in recommended doses. Supplemental folic acid in very high doses may have central nervous system (CNS) effects and might exacerbate seizures in patients with seizure disorders.

Mind and Body Practices

Mindfulness meditation-based therapies may be beneficial in reducing negative psychological states such as stress, anxiety, and depression (Hofmann, Sawyer, Witt, & Oh, 2010). Mindfulness-based cognitive therapy (MBCT), which combines cognitive–behavioral therapy with mindfulness meditation, may provide benefit in lower relapse or recurrence rates in patients with recurrent MDD (Chiesa & Serretti, 2011; Piet & Hougaard, 2011).

Acupuncture shows some promise for depression, but results are mixed and limited (Smith, Hay, & Macpherson, 2010; Wang et al., 2008). For MDD, it showed greater effects than control on depressive symptoms but did not improve response or remission rates; however, for patients with poststroke depression, acupuncture was more effective than short-term use of antidepressants (Williams et al., 2011). An RCT for depression during pregnancy demonstrated symptom reduction with acupuncture with a response rate comparable to those observed in standard depression treatments of similar length, suggesting that acupuncture could be a possible treatment option for depression during pregnancy (Manber et al., 2010). Future research is warranted to assess whether acupuncture yields benefit, perhaps not as a monotherapy but as an adjunctive therapy (Yeung et al., 2011).

Mind–body exercise, such as tai chi with its gentle slow movements, may provide benefit in geriatric depression (Lavretsky et al., 2011). Yoga shows promise and has been investigated in small studies for depression. These limited trials suggest that yoga may offer potential as an adjunct treatment, but findings from larger scale studies are needed (Meyer et al., 2012; Uebelacker et al., 2010). A systematic review assessed six RCTs that evaluated meditative exercises such as yoga, tai chi, and qigong for treating depression. All six studies showed a positive response to treatment, with five studies reporting a statistically significant reduction in depression scores (Tsang, Chan, & Cheung, 2008).

Bright light therapy (BLT) is exposure to bright artificial light using a device that mimics natural light. The mechanism of action of BLT is to stop the secretion of melatonin by the pineal gland during the day. Melatonin is continually secreted in low levels if a person is not exposed to bright sunlight in the morning, and this contributes to fatigue and ongoing sleep disruption.

BLT, which has been used for seasonal affective disorder, appears also to be effective for nonseasonal depression with effect sizes comparable to those found in antidepressant drug trials (Golden et al., 2005). BLT has shown potential in treatment of antepartum depression (Wirz-Justice et al., 2011) and in elderly patients with nonseasonal MDD (Lieverse et al., 2011).

Practice alerts/precautions: Doses required for efficacy include daily exposure to at least 10,000 lux (equivalent to bright sunlight) for 20 to 30 minutes in the morning during the fall and winter for seasonal affective disorder (SAD) and throughout the year for nonseasonal depression. Light therapy is generally safe, but some patients may experience headaches, eye strain, or nausea, which often subside after a few days of treatment. Case studies have been reported of light-induced agitation and hypomania in patients with bipolar disorder. The proper duration, timing, and intensity of light exposure should be monitored and adjusted for safety and effectiveness. It is important that the patient does not sit closer than 12 inches to the light source.

Regular exercise, ranging from daily walking to aerobics and resistance training, may improve the symptoms of depression. Studies have shown an association between exercise and a reduction in depressive symptoms (Freeman et al., 2010; Rimer et al., 2012). Regular exercise may reduce the prevalence of depressive symptoms in the general population with specific benefit in older adults and individuals with concomitant medical problems. Exercise alone may reduce patient-perceived symptoms of depression as effectively as cognitive–behavioral therapy or drugs (Gill, Womack, & Safranek, 2010). One study reported that 90 minutes of exercise per week for 16 weeks was comparable to antidepressant medication (Blumenthal et al., 2007) and maintenance of 60 minutes per week of exercise reduced the risk of relapse over a 1-year follow-up period in adults with MDD (Hoffman et al., 2011).

The American Psychiatric Association's clinical practice guidelines for treatment of MDD suggest at least a modest improvement in mood symptoms for patients who engage in aerobic exercise or resistance training (Gelenberg et al., 2010). Although the optimal amount of exercise for benefit is uncertain, it probably needs to be continued in the longer term for benefits to be maintained.

Studies have suggested that music therapy is associated with improvements in mood, but these studies limited by size and methodological quality (Maratos, Gold, Wang, & Crawford, 2008).

Schizophrenia and Other Psychotic Disorders

Because of the severity of these disorders, use of CAM as an alternative to conventional treatment is not recommended. With the exception of exercise, which is highly recommended for patients with schizophrenia owing to the increased risks for obesity and diabetes in these patients, further research is needed to determine the extent to which CAM therapies may be helpful as complementary or adjuvant treatments for this population of patients.

Omega-3 Fatty Acids

Preliminary research suggested that supplementation of diet with polyunsaturated fatty acids may have a positive effect on the symptoms of schizophrenia (Joy, Mumby-Croft, & Joy, 2006) but results are conflicting (Fusar-Poli & Berger, 2012). The data for omega-3 fatty acids in the treatment of bipolar disorder have also been limited and mixed (Amminger et al., 2010; Montgomery & Richardson, 2008). A Cochrane review concluded that there was little evidence that these supplements help manic symptoms, but suggested they might help depressive symptoms in bipolar patients (Montgomery & Richardson, 2008).

Mind and Body Practices

Meditation may hold potential in treating the negative symptoms of schizophrenia (Johnson et al., 2011) or reducing anxiety symptoms in bipolar patients, particularly MBCT (Chiesa & Serretti, 2011). However, research is preliminary and further studies are needed to confirm findings in larger studies compared with control groups.

A Cochrane review concluded that music therapy as an addition to standard care may help individuals with schizophrenia to improve their global state, mental state, and social functioning over the short to medium term (Mössler, Chen, Heldal, & Gold, 2011). However, further research is needed to address the duration, frequency, and long-term effects.

Regular exercise and physical activity can help individuals with schizophrenia improve both physical and mental health and well-being (Gorczynski & Faulkner, 2010). As discussed in Chapter 17, the lack of motivation typical of patients with schizophrenia can impair patients' abilities to maintain an exercise regimen, despite the many benefits of exercise to these patients.

Neurocognitive Disorders

With more than 5 million patients with Alzheimer disease worldwide, and more than 14 million caregivers, there is ever-increasing pressure to find new methods of reducing risk, treating symptoms, and ultimately curing Alzheimer disease, the most common form of dementia (Alzheimer's Association, 2011). Increasingly, certain natural products and exercise are thought to play a protective role in cognitive function, although more research is needed to determine the extent of the benefit to the patient.

Ginkgo (*Ginkgo biloba*)

Ginkgo is native to Asia and one of the oldest species of trees in the world, with distinctive fan-shaped leaves. Standardized extracts are usually taken from the ginkgo leaf, which contains flavonoids and terpenoids. Despite the popularity of ginkgo's use for dementia and cognitive impairment, the evidence is inconsistent (Birks & Grimley Evans, 2009). Most clinical studies have been conducted with a standardized extract of ginkgo, EGb761. Early studies indicated that ginkgo may improve cognitive performance in patients with dementia (LeBars et al., 1997), but more recent studies have shown conflicting evidence. The NCCAM-funded Ginkgo Evaluation of Memory (GEM) study concluded that use of ginkgo did not result in less cognitive decline in older adults with normal cognition or with mild cognitive impairment (Snitz et al., 2009) and was not effective in reducing either the overall incidence rate of dementia or Alzheimer disease incidence in older adults with normal cognition or those with mild cognitive impairment (DeKosky et al., 2008).

Practice alerts/precautions: Ginkgo's adverse effects include GI complaints and prolonged bleeding. It can increase anticoagulant/antiplatelet effects. Pharmacokinetic trials have shown it reduces plasma concentrations of alprazolam (Xanax, Niravam), omeprazole (Prilosec), ritonavir (Norvir), and tolbutamide (Tol-Tab). Case reports indicate that it may interact/react with antiepileptics, thiazide diuretics, ibuprofen, risperidone (Risperdal), efavirenz (Sustiva), trazodone (Desyrel, Oleptro), midazolam (Versed), and warfarin (Coumadin, Jantoven) (Natural Medicines Comprehensive Database, 2012).

DHEA

Reports have suggested that the decline of DHEA with aging is associated with cognitive impairment and that DHEA may have neuroprotective effects. However, clinical evidence does not support improvement in cognition with DHEA supplementation (Bradley, McElhiney, & Rabkin, 2012; Kritz-Silverstein, von Mühlen, Laughlin, & Bettencourt, 2008; Wolkowitz et al., 2003). Previous trials in healthy, middle-aged to elderly women have not demonstrated beneficial effects with supplementation. A Cochrane review of three studies did not find a beneficial effect of DHEA supplementation in middle-aged or older adults without dementia, although the authors noted a need for long-term studies with an adequate number of subjects (Grimley Evans, Malouf, Huppert, & van Niekerk, 2006).

Mind and Body Practices

There is growing evidence for exercise as a potential intervention to decrease the risk of developing aging-related cognitive impairment. Animal studies suggest that exercise may induce neuroplasticity with improved learning outcomes (Ahlskog, Geda, Graff-Radford, & Petersen, 2011). Exercise, particularly aerobic exercise, may enhance cognitive functioning in older adults. Significant increases in brain volume were found in older adults who participated in aerobic fitness training but not for those who participated in stretching and toning (nonaerobic) (Colcombe et al., 2006). Aerobic exercise increases hippocampal volume and improves spatial memory (Erickson et al., 2011; Jedrziewski, Ewbank, Wang, & Trojanowski, 2010). Gentle exercise such as yoga or tai chi may attenuate cognitive impairment and reduce dementia risk (Lam et al., 2011).

As science confirms that neural networks are modifiable, there is growing interest in meditation for possibly improving cognitive function such as memory (Newberg et al., 2010). Studies have shown meditation experience to be associated with increased cortical thickness (Lazar et al., 2005). Results suggest that participation in mindfulness-based stress reduction (MBSR) is associated with changes in gray matter concentration in brain regions involved in learning and memory processes, emotion regulation, self-referential processing, and perspective taking (Hölzel et al., 2011).

Substance-Related and Addictive Disorders

Little information is available regarding the use of natural products for substance-related disorders, and there is insufficient evidence to support the primary use of CAM therapies. St. John's wort was investigated for efficacy in smoking cessation, but it did not significantly increase tobacco abstinence rates or decrease nicotine withdrawal compared with placebo (Sood et al., 2010). Nurses may note that chronic alcohol users and patients experiencing alcohol withdrawal may be at risk of deficiency of B vitamins such as thiamine.

The nurse must assess for the use of "natural products" by the patient being treated for a substance use disorder because many substances, such as marijuana and peyote, are considered "natural." The treatment of substance-related disorders with CAM holds some promise for the future, as acupuncture, herbal therapies, and mind–body interventions have shown some positive results in human trials (Behere, Muralidharani, & Benegal, 2009).

Mind and Body Practices

CAM interventions commonly used as supportive therapies for substance withdrawal and stress management include mind–body practices such as meditation, relaxation, acupuncture, and yoga.

Early support for acupuncture use began in the 1970s. Auricular acupuncture is the most common form used for substance addiction. Acupuncture has been integrated into more than 400 substance use disorder treatment programs in the United States and Europe in the form of auricular acupuncture, which has been suggested to reduce cravings and anxiety levels. However, several RCTs investigating auricular acupuncture for cocaine dependence as a sole or stand-alone treatment have not yielded consistent positive results (Margolin et al., 2002; Gates, Smith, & Foxcroft, 2006). Despite limited research evidence, its use continues owing to perceived clinical benefits reported from patients and treatment staff in residential and outpatient programs. A Cochrane review also reported a lack of consistent evidence for acupuncture as an effective intervention for smoking cessation; the authors concluded that because of the lack of evidence and methodological problems, further studies are warranted (White et al., 2011).

Meditation and/or mindfulness based practices are increasingly used in substance use clinics and show promise in reducing psychiatric symptoms and effecting behavioral change, but evidence is preliminary (Brewer et al., 2009; Dakwar & Levin, 2009; Zgierska et al., 2009). Mindfulness training, which focuses on acknowledging momentary and nonjudgmental awareness, has been used for relapse prevention. In an 8-week outpatient mindfulness-based relapse prevention program, participants demonstrated greater decreases in craving, and increases in acceptance and acting with awareness, as compared with treatment as usual (Bowen et al., 2009). A small pilot study that evaluated mindfulness training as a stand-alone treatment for smoking cessation also shows promise (Brewer et al., 2011).

Pause and Reflect

1. *Has a patient under your care ever discussed a CAM therapy that you felt was harmful? If so, what made you feel this way?*
2. *Are you aware of any personal or cultural biases you may have toward certain CAM therapies? Please explain.*
3. *How can CAM therapies potentially support or potentially compromise a patient's biological health?*
4. *What benefits do mind–body therapies offer to a patient's psychological health?*

Implications for Nursing

As stated earlier, it is essential for nurses to be aware of current evidence-based CAM to be able to answer patients' questions and concerns honestly, knowledgeably, and safely. Nurses play a pivotal role in the assessment of CAM use, and therefore need to be nonjudgmental, unbiased in attitude, and informed about each patient's choices to use CAM (Box 22-4). Through open communication and

Is Passionflower Useful in Treating Anxiety?   evidence-based practice

Clinical Question
Passionflower is a traditional folk remedy known for its sedative properties. Is it useful for anxiety?

Evidence
Akhondzadeh et al., (2001) compared passionflower (*Passiflora incarnata*) with oxazepam (Serax) in a randomized controlled trial (RCT) for the treatment of generalized anxiety disorder (GAD). Each group had 18 subjects with a diagnosis of GAD and had a score of 14 or more on the Hamilton Anxiety Rating Scale. One group received 45 drops of passiflora extract per day plus placebo tablets and another group received oxazepam at 30 mg/day plus placebo drops over 4 weeks. Both groups ended with a significant reduction in scores, suggesting that passionflower is as effective as benzodiazepine. However, subjects in the oxazepam group showed a more rapid onset of action. Subjects from the passionflower group also reported lower job impairment performance (44%) than those in the oxazepam group (61%), but this finding did not reach statistical significance and there was no significant difference between the two treatments in terms of the overall frequency of side effects. Adverse effects reported included dizziness, drowsiness, and confusion. A systematic review of passiflora for anxiety disorder (Miyasaka, Atallah, & Soares, 2007) found only two studies, involving 198 participants, that were eligible for inclusion. The reviewers concluded that the RCTs were too few in number to permit any conclusions on its effectiveness or safety in the treatment of anxiety disorders. Movafegh et al., (2008) conducted an RCT comparing the effect of passiflora with placebo for preoperative anxiety in ambulatory surgery patients. Sixty patients were randomly assigned to two groups. One group ($n = 30$) received passiflora 500 mg tablets orally 90 minutes before surgery. The other group ($n = 30$) received placebo. A numeric rating scale (NRS) was used to evaluate anxiety and measured before, and 10, 30, 60, and 90 minutes after, administration. NRS anxiety scores were significantly lower in the passiflora group.

These findings seem to suggest efficacy and safety, but are limited by the number of studies and the small sample sizes.

These findings need to be confirmed in larger placebo controlled studies.

Implications for Nursing Practice
Herbs, particularly in the form of folk or home remedies, are used in many cultural traditions. Folk remedies have often been associated with lack of access to health care, cultural and language barriers, and socioeconomic status. For many patients, folk remedies passed down through generations become part of their culture and are often used along with allopathic medicine. A number of modern drugs are derived from ethnomedical or folk uses of plants, such as atropine (*Atropa belladonna*), digoxin (*Digitalis lanata*), and salicin (*Salix alba*, more commonly known as willow bark).

Despite a long history of use, limited research evidence exists that passionflower may be helpful in decreasing anxiety. The active constituents and its effects on the central nervous system are unclear. However, it has been used for many years and has not been associated with chronic toxicity. There is one case report of a 34-year-old female who developed nausea, vomiting, drowsiness, QTc prolongation, and episodes of nonsustained ventricular tachycardia using a passionflower product and recovered after discontinuation of the supplement (Fisher, Purcell, & Le Couteur, 2000).

As this chapter's case study of Alicia illustrates, in some situations combining folk remedies with allopathic medical care may be acceptable, as long as the practice is not harmful to the patient and the patient is benefiting from the therapy. For nurses, the challenge lies in recognizing and incorporating knowledge of cultural influences, such as folk medicine with effective and safe counseling.

Critical Thinking Questions
1. Is there any folk remedy use in your family or culture? What thoughts or feeling do those memories have for you?
2. Is there any evidence to support its use? Please explain.
3. Name other modern medications that are derived from traditional medicine use.

Recommendations for Nursing Practice   box 22-4

Key Nursing Assessment Questions
- Please list any types of complementary or alternative practices you are currently using and why you are using it/them.
- Which herbal or dietary supplements are you taking?
- Who recommended you to try these?
- When and why did you start taking these?
- How often and how much are you taking?
- What effects do you notice?
- Have you ever had a bad reaction to an herbal or vitamin supplement?

Key Nursing Interventions Related to CAM
- Use open-ended questions to inquire about current and past CAM use, and be sure to include home remedies.
- Document all CAM usage in the patient's record.
  ### *Advise patients:*
- To consult with their health care provider if they take herbal supplements and to discontinue them at least 2 weeks prior to any surgery.

- To consult with their health care provider about use of herbal and dietary supplements if they are pregnant or nursing.
- Not to take herbs and psychiatric medications together or at the same time without the advice of their prescriber of psychiatric medications.
- To take the smallest amount possible when starting herbal therapy to determine whether allergies or other adverse effects occur.
- To read and follow carefully the label instructions on herbal and dietary supplements and vitamins.
- To look for the symbols GMP (Good Manufacturing Practices), NSF (National Safety Foundation), or USP (United States Pharmacopoeia) on product labels.
- Not to exceed recommended dosages or take the herbal or dietary supplement for longer than recommended.
- To talk with their health care provider if they have any questions, particularly about the best dosage to take.

Alicia Rehabilitation Phase

Alicia returns 6 months later and reports to Linda that she is sleeping better and feels more "*calme*." She hasn't had any headaches recently. Sometimes she wakes up once in the night, but generally she wakes in the morning feeling more rested. Alicia still drinks her passionflower tea and reports no adverse effects. At night before she goes to bed, Alicia closes her door and does the breathing exercise Linda showed her. When the weather is nice, she gets off one bus stop early and walks. Alicia and her brother agreed to alternate every other weekend accompanying their father so she has some time for herself. Last weekend, she enjoyed a free music festival in the park with her cousins. Alicia and Linda acknowledge that Alicia has taken steps to manage her stress and she is feeling less anxious and tired all the time. She will return in a year's time for her annual physical exam; Linda advises Alicia to contact her if she has any other concerns before then.

> ### APPLICATION
> 1. What steps has Alicia taken to manage the stress and worry in her life? How have they been helpful across the domains of wellness?
> 2. What further CAM therapies or lifestyle suggestions would you recommend for Alicia?

by developing a rapport, nurses will help patients feel comfortable sharing information. When inquiring about current medications and taking the health history, it is vital for nurses to ask about herbal and dietary supplement use. Almost two-thirds of adults using commonly consumed herbs did not do so in accordance with evidence-based indications (Bardia et al., 2007). Therefore, nurses must be able to advise their patients about potentially dangerous drug–herb combinations. They must be aware of potential interactions with a supplement(s) or other CAM when patients are taking psychiatric medications. If there is uncertainty, it is important to do further research and/or contact a pharmacist.

With the increasingly diverse immigrant population in the United States and the need for culturally competent care, nurses need to respect and understand the influence of ethnic and cultural traditions on the health care beliefs and practices of patients. It is important to obtain knowledge about geographic, cultural, social, and health practices for various patient populations. For example, in Hispanic cultures, a *curandero/a* or folk healer is often sought for illnesses. *Susto* (fright sickness), with symptoms similar to the Western definition of anxiety, is considered a separation of the soul and body; traditional treatment may involve integrating spiritual and symbolic interventions. In some Asian cultures, an individual with emotional/mental distress may refer to problems with the "liver," differing from the Western biomedical definition of the liver, as traditional Asian medicine often associates regulation of emotions with the energy of this organ. Numerous cultures, from Asian and Middle Eastern to African, associate mental illness with possession of "the evil eye" and embrace the use of protective amulets. Many cultural communities and rural populations embrace herbal and spiritual interventions, which may provide comfort, hope, and positive expectations for patients and health care practitioners need to respect these practices.

In summary, CAM therapies are increasingly being used by patients to address suffering related to symptoms of mental health illnesses. CAM therapies may be particularly interesting to patients who do not initially respond to treatment or who have achieved only limited success with treatment. Nurses play an important role in assessing CAM therapies, discussing use, and providing guidance to patients, helping patients manage their expectations, while at the same time conveying a sense of hope that patients' symptoms and functioning will improve. A better understanding of evidence-based CAM therapies is important for the planning of patient-centered collaborative nursing care. For nurses, being able to discuss, engage in patient teaching, and make appropriate referrals for CAM therapies ensures patient safety and enhances quality of care.

Chapter Highlights

1. Complementary and alternative medicine is a group of diverse medical and health care systems, practices, and products that are not generally considered part of allopathic, or conventional, medicine.

2. There are two categories of CAM: natural (or biologically based) products and mind and body practices.

3. Use of CAM therapies is increasing generally, and particularly among patients with sleep disturbances and anxiety.

4. The National Center for Complementary and Alternative Medicine is the federal government's lead agency in terms of research and information about CAM therapies.

5. Careful assessment of patient use of CAM therapies is essential, especially to identify potential interactions with pharmacologic therapies.

6. St. John's wort, a natural product sometimes used by patients to relieve symptoms of depression, can cause serotonin syndrome when taken in conjunction with SSRIs.

7. Omega-3 fatty acids may provide benefit to patients with mild to moderate mood disorders. It may also play a protective role in cognitive function.

8. Most natural products have not been studied to determine safety and efficacy for use in pregnant and nursing women.

9. Exercise may benefit patients in a variety of areas; research is beginning to indicate that regular exercise confers cognitive benefits as well as serving to lower stress and anxiety levels.

NCLEX®-RN Questions

1. The nurse is caring for a patient who has been using cognitive–behavioral therapy in conjunction with selective serotonin-reuptake inhibiters (SSRIs) to manage anxiety. The nurse recognizes that the patient's treatment is most consistent with which type of medicine?
   a. Allopathic
   b. Alternative
   c. Complementary
   d. Integrative

2. The nurse is applying principles of complementary and alternative medicine (CAM) to ensure that a patient in the outpatient mental health setting is receiving safe, effective care. Which question by the nurse best addresses the need to assess the sociological domain of wellness activities?
   a. How do you feel about the use of conventional medical services?
   b. Is traditional medicine consistent with your spiritual or religious beliefs?
   c. Does your primary care physician know that you use nonconventional therapies?
   d. What systems and providers do you use to access your alternative treatments?

3. The nurse is admitting a patient with depression to the mental health unit. The patient states that she has been using light therapy instead of antidepressant medication. Which category of clinical guidelines would the nurse refer to understand implications of this practice?
   a. Mind–body therapies
   b. Biologically based products
   c. Manipulative body-based medicine
   d. Other nonpharmacological treatments

4. The nurse is caring for a patient with a history of chronic alcohol abuse. The patient states that a friend recommended the use of kava to manage the symptoms of anxiety. Which response by the nurse is best?
   a. "You need to stop drinking if you want to take kava."
   b. "Patients with a history of dependence should not take kava."
   c. "Kava can increase the likelihood of liver toxicity or failure."
   d. "Kava has not been shown to be effective in treating anxiety."

5. The nurse is caring for a patient who has been taking St. John's wort for the treatment of depression and theophylline (Elixophylline) for chronic obstructive pulmonary disease (COPD). Which evaluation finding indicates that the patient is experiencing adverse effects resulting from the interactions of these two agents?
   a. Worsening sedation
   b. Respiratory distress
   c. Excitability and agitation
   d. Tachycardia and hypotension

6. The nurse is admitting a child with a mental health disorder to a psychiatric treatment facility. The parents state that they primarily use complementary and alternative medicine (CAM) to manage the symptoms of the child's disorder. Which nursing action is most essential?
   a. Determine the exact nature of all treatments being used.
   b. Assess the parents attitudes toward traditional medical treatment.
   c. Inform the parents of allopathic treatments that may be more effective.
   d. Ensure that all treatments can be continued while the patient is hospitalized.

Answers to questions may be found on the Pearson student resource site: nursing.pearsonhighered.com

Pearson Nursing Student Resources Find additional review materials at **nursing.pearsonhighered.com**

References

Ahlskog, J. E., Geda, Y. E., Graff-Radford, N. R., & Petersen, R.C. (2011). Physical exercise as a preventive or disease-modifying treatment of dementia and brain aging. *Mayo Clinic Proceedings, 86*(9), 876–884.

Akhondzadeh, S., Naghavi, H. R., Vazirian, M., Shayeganpour, A., Rashidi, H., & Khani, M. (2001). Passionflower in the treatment of generalized anxiety: A pilot double-blind randomized controlled trial with oxazepam. *Journal of Clinical Pharmacy and Therapeutics, 26*(5), 363–367.

Alzheimer's Association. (2011). 2011 Alzheimer's disease facts and figures. Available at http://www.alz.org/downloads/Facts_Figures_2011.pdf

Amminger, G. P., Schäfer, M. R., Papageorgiou, K., Klier, C. M., Cotton, S. M., Harrigan, S. M., . . . Berger, G. E. (2010). Long-chain omega-3 fatty acids for indicated prevention of psychotic disorders: a randomized, placebo-controlled trial. *Archives of General Psychiatry, 67*(2), 146–154.

Amsterdam, J. D., Li, Y., Soeller, I., Rockwell, K., Mao, J. J., & Shults, J. (2009). A randomized, double-blind, placebo-controlled trial of oral *Matricaria recutita* (chamomile) extract therapy for generalized anxiety disorder. *Journal of Clinical Psychopharmacology, 29*(4), 378–382.

Andersen, I. M., Kaczmarska, J., McGrew, S. G., & Malow, B. A. (2008). Melatonin for insomnia in children with autism spectrum disorders. *Journal of Child Neurology, 23*(5), 482–485.

Bardia, A., Nisly, N. L., Zimmerman, B., Gryzlak, B. M., & Wallace, R. B. (2007). Use of herbs among adults based on evidence-based indications: Findings from the national health interview survey. *Mayo Clinic Proceedings, 82*(5), 561–566.

Barnes, P. M., Bloom, B., & Nahin, R. L. (2008). Complementary and alternative medicine use among adults and children: United States, 2007. National Health Statistics Reports, no. 12. Hyattsville, MD: National Center for Health Statistics. Available at http://www.cdc.gov/nchs/data/nhsr/nhsr012.pdf

Behere, R. V., Muralidharani, K., & Benegal, V. (2009). Complementary and alternative medicine in the treatment of substance use disorders—a review of the evidence. *Drug and Alcohol Review, 28*, 292–300.

Bent, S., Padula, A., Moore, D., Patterson, M., & Mehling, W. (2006). Valerian for sleep: A systematic review and meta-analysis. *American Journal of Medicine, 119*(12), 1005–1012.

Bertisch, S. M., Wee, C. C., Phillips, R. S., & McCarthy, E. P. (2009). Alternative mind-body therapies used by adults with medical conditions. *Journal of Psychosomatic Research*, 66(6), 511–519.

Bertisch, S. M., Wells, R. E., Smith, M. T., & McCarthy, E. P. (2012). Use of relaxation techniques and complementary and alternative medicine by American adults with insomnia symptoms: Results from a national survey. *Journal of Clinical Sleep Medicine*, 8(6), 681–691.

Birks, J., & Grimley Evans, J. (2009). Ginkgo biloba for cognitive impairment and dementia. *Cochrane Database of Systematic Reviews*, Issue 1. Art. No. CD003120.

Blumenthal, J. A., Babyak, M. A., Doraiswamy, P. M., Watkins, L., Hoffman, B. M., … Sherwood, A. (2007). Exercise and pharmacotherapy in the treatment of major depressive disorder. *Psychosomatic Medicine*, 69(7), 587–596.

Borrelli, F., & Izzo, A. A. (2009). Herb-drug interactions with St. John's wort (*Hypericum perforatum*): An update on clinical observations. *AAPS Journal*, 11(4), 710–727.

Bottiglieri, T., Godfrey, P., Flynn, T., Carney, M. W., Toone, B. K., & Reynolds, E. H. (1990). Cerebrospinal fluid S-adenosylmethionine in depression and dementia: Effects of treatment with parenteral and oral S-adenosylmethionine. *Journal of Neurology, Neurosurgery, and Psychiatry*, 53(12), 1096–1098.

Bouron, A., & Lorrain, E. (2014). Cellular and molecular effects of the antidepressant hyperforin on brain cells: Review of the literature. *L'encéphale*, 40(2), 108–113.

Bowen, S., Chawla, N., Collins, S. E., Witkiewitz, K., Hsu, S., Grow, J., … Marlatt, A. (2009). Mindfulness-based relapse prevention for substance use disorders: A pilot efficacy trial. *Substance Abuse*, 30(4), 295–305.

Bradley, M., McElhiney, M., & Rabkin, J. (2012). DHEA and cognition in HIV-positive patients with non-major depression. *Psychosomatics*, 53(3), 244–249.

Bradt, J., & Dileo, C. (2009). Music for stress and anxiety reduction in coronary heart disease patients. *Cochrane Database of Systematic Reviews*, Issue 2. Art. No. CD006577.

Bradt, J., Dileo, C., Grocke, D., & Magill, L. (2011). Music interventions for improving psychological and physical outcomes in cancer patients. *Cochrane Database of Systematic Reviews*, Issue 8. Art. No. CD006911.

Brewer, J. A., Mallik, S., Babuscio, T. A., Nich, C., Johnson, H. E., Deleone, C. M., …. Rounsaville, B. J. (2011). Mindfulness training for smoking cessation: Results from a randomized controlled trial. *Drug and Alcohol Dependence*, 119(1–2),72–80.

Brewer, J. A., Sinha, R., Chen, J. A., Michalsen, R. N., Babuscio, T. A., Nich, C., … Rounsaville, B.J. (2009). Mindfulness training and stress reactivity in substance abuse: results from a randomized, controlled stage I pilot study. *Substance Abuse*, 30(4), 306–317.

Brown, R. P., & Gerbarg, P. L. (2009), Yoga breathing, meditation, and longevity. *Annals of the New York Academy of Sciences*, 1172, 54–62.

Brzezinski, A., Vangel, M. G., Wurtman, R. J., Norrie, G., Zhdanova, I., Ben-Shushan, A., & Ford, I. (2005). Effects of exogenous melatonin on sleep: A meta-analysis. *Sleep Medicine Reviews*, 9(1), 41–50.

Centers for Disease Control and Prevention. (2011). How much physical activity do adults need? Available at http://www.cdc.gov/physicalactivity/everyone/guidelines/adults.html

Chen, K. W., Berger, C. C., Manheimer, E., Forde, D., Magidson, J., Dachman, L., & Lejuez, C. W. (2012). Meditative therapies for reducing anxiety: A systematic review and meta-analysis of randomized controlled trials. *Depression and Anxiety*, 29(7), 545–562.

Cheuk, D. K., Yeung, W. F., Chung, K. F., & Wong, V. (2007). Acupuncture for insomnia. *Cochrane Database of Systematic Reviews*, Issue 3. Art. No. CD005472.

Chiesa, A., & Serretti, A. (2011). Mindfulness based cognitive therapy for psychiatric disorders: A systematic review and meta-analysis. *Psychiatry Research*, 187(3), 441–453.

Colcombe, S. J., Erickson, K. I., Scalf, P. E., Kim, J. S., Prakash, R., McAuley, E., … Kramer, A. F. (2006). Aerobic exercise training increases brain volume in aging humans. *Journals of Gerontology Series A: Biological Sciences and Medical Science*, 61(11), 1166–1170.

Dakwar, E., & Levin, F. R. (2009). The emerging role of meditation in addressing psychiatric illness, with a focus on substance use disorders. *Harvard Review of Psychiatry*, 17(4), 254–267.

Dean-Clower, E., Doherty-Gilman, A. M., Keshaviah, A., Baker, F., Kaw, C., Lu, W., … Rosenthal, D. S. (2010). Acupuncture as palliative therapy for physical symptoms and quality of life for advanced cancer patients. *Integrative Cancer Therapies*, 9(2),158–167.

DeKosky, S. T., Williamson, J. D., Fitzpatrick, A. L., Kronmal, R. A., Ives, D. G., Saxton, J. A., … Ginkgo Evaluation of Memory (GEM) Study Investigators. (2008). Ginkgo biloba for prevention of dementia: A randomized controlled trial. *Journal of the American Medical Association*, 300(19), 2253–2262.

Donovan, J. L., DeVane, C. L., Chavin, K. D., Wang, J. S., Gibson, B. B., Gefroh, H. A., & Markowitz, J. S. (2004). Multiple night-time doses of valerian (*Valeriana officinalis*) had minimal effects on CYP3A4 activity and no effect on CYP2D6 activity in healthy volunteers. *Drug Metabolism and Disposition*, 32(12),1333–1336.

Druss, B. G., & Rosenheck, R. A. (2000). Use of practitioner-based complementary therapies by persons reporting mental conditions in the United States. *Archives of General Psychiatry*, 57(7), 708–714.

Eisenberg, D. M., Davis, R. B., Ettner, S. L., Appel, S., Wilkey, S., Van Rompay, M., & Kessler, R. C. (1998). Trends in alternative medicine use in the United States, 1990–1997: Results of a follow-up national survey. *JAMA*, 280(18), 1569–1575.

Ekor, M., Adeyemi, O. S., & Otuechere, C. A. (2013). Management of anxiety and sleep disorders: Role of complementary and alternative medicine and challenges of integration with conventional orthodox care. *Chinese Journal of Integrative Medicine*, 19(1), 5–14.

Elkins, G., Rajab, M. H., & Marcus, J. (2005). Complementary and alternative medicine use by psychiatric inpatients. *Psychological Reports*, 96(1), 163–166.

Erickson, K. I., Voss, M. W., Prakash, R. S., Basak, C., Szabo, A., Chaddock, L., … Kramer, A F. (2011). Exercise training increases size of hippocampus and improves memory. *Proceedings of the National Academy of Sciences U S A*, 108, 3017–3022.

Evans, S., Ferrando, S., Findler, M., Stowell, C., Smart, C., & Haglin, D. (2008). Mindfulness-based cognitive therapy for generalized anxiety disorder. *Journal of Anxiety Disorders*, 22(4), 716–721.

Fava, M., & Mischoulon, D. (2010). Evidence for folate in combination with antidepressants at initiation of therapy. *Journal of Clinical Psychiatry*, 71(11), e31.

Fernández-San-Martín, M. I., Masa-Font, R., Palacios-Soler, L., Sancho-Gómez, P., Calbó-Caldentey, C., & Flores-Mateo, G. (2010). Effectiveness of valerian on insomnia: A meta-analysis of randomized placebo-controlled trials. *Sleep Medicine*, 11(6), 505–511.

Fisher, A. A., Purcell, P., & Le Couteur, D. G. (2000). Toxicity of *Passiflora incarnata* L. *Journal of Toxicology and Clinical Toxicology*, 38(1), 63–66.

Freeman, M. P., Fava, M., Lake, J., Trivedi, M. H., Wisner, K.L., & Mischoulon, D. (2010). Complementary and alternative medicine in major depressive disorder: The American Psychiatric Association Task Force report. *Journal of Clinical Psychiatry*, 71(6), 669–681.

Freeman, M. P., Mischoulon, D., Tedeschini, E., Goodness, T., Cohen, L.S., Fava, M., & Papakostas, G. I. (2010). Complementary and alternative medicine for major depressive disorder: A meta-analysis of patient characteristics, placebo-response rates, and treatment outcomes relative to standard antidepressants. *Journal of Clinical Psychiatry*, 71(6), 682–688.

Freeman, M. P., & Rapaport, M. H. (2011). Omega-3 fatty acids and depression: From cellular mechanisms to clinical care. *Journal of Clinical Psychiatry*, 72(2), 258–259.

Fusar-Poli, P., & Berger, G. (2012). Eicosapentaenoic acid interventions in schizophrenia: Meta-analysis of randomized, placebo-controlled studies. *Journal of Clinical Psychopharmacology*, 32(2),179–185.

Gates, S., Smith, L. A., & Foxcroft, D. R. (2006). Auricular acupuncture for cocaine dependence. *Cochrane Database of Systematic Reviews*, Issue 1. Art. No. CD005192.

Gelenberg, A. J., Freeman, M. P., Markowitz, J. C., Rosenbaum, J. F., Thase, M. E., Trivedi, M. J. H., & Van Rhoads, R. S. (2010). *Practice Guideline for the Treatment of Patients with Major Depressive Disorder* (3rd ed.). Arlington, VA: American Psychiatric Association Press. Available at http://psychiatryonline.org/pdfaccess.ashx?ResourceID=243261&PDFSource=6

Gill, A., Womack, R., & Safranek, S. (2010). Clinical inquiries: Does exercise alleviate symptoms of depression? *Journal of Family Practice*, 59(9), 530–531.

Gold, C., Heldal, T. O., Dahle, T., & Wigram, T. (2005). Music therapy for schizophrenia or schizophrenia-like illnesses. *Cochrane Database of Systematic Reviews*, Issue 2. Art. No. CD004025.

Golden, R. N., Gaynes, B. N., Ekstrom, R. D., Hamer, R. M., Jacobsen, F. M., ... Nemeroff, C. B. (2005). The efficacy of light therapy in the treatment of mood disorders: A review and meta-analysis of the evidence. *American Journal of Psychiatry, 162*(4), 656–662.

Gorczynski, P., & Faulkner, G. (2010). Exercise therapy for schizophrenia. *Cochrane Database of Systematic Reviews,* Issue 5. Art. No. CD004412.

Grimley Evans, J., Malouf, R., Huppert, F., & van Niekerk, J. K. (2006). Dehydro-epiandrosterone (DHEA) supplementation for cognitive function in healthy elderly people. *Cochrane Database of Systematic Reviews,* Issue 4. Art. No. CD006221.

Gross, C. R., Kreitzer, M. J., Reilly-Spong, M., Wall, M., Winbush, N. Y., Patterson, R., Mahowald, M., & Cramer-Bornemann, M. (2011). Mindfulness-based stress reduction versus pharmacotherapy for chronic primary insomnia: A randomized controlled clinical trial. *Explore (NY), 7*(2), 76–87.

Hardy, M., Coulter, I., Morton, S. C., Favreau, J., Swamy, V., Chiappelli, F., . . . Shekelle, P. (2002). S-Adenosyl-l-methionine for treatment of depression, osteoarthritis, and liver disease (publication number 02-E04). Rockville, MD: Agency for Healthcare Research and Quality, U.S. Department of Health and Human Services.

Härtter, S., Grözinger, M., Weigmann, H., Röschke, J., & Hiemke, C. (2000). Increased bioavailability of melatonin after fluvoxamine coadministration. *Clinical Pharmacology and Therapeutics, 67,* 1–6.

Herring, M. P., O'Connor, P. J., & Dishman, R. K. (2010). The effect of exercise training on anxiety symptoms among patients: A systematic review. *Archives of Internal Medicine, 170*(4), 321–331.

Hoffman, B. M., Babyak, M. A., Craighead, W. E., Sherwood, A., Doraiswamy, P. M., Coons, M. J., & Blumenthal, J. A. (2011). Exercise and pharmacotherapy in patients with major depression: One-year follow-up of the SMILE study. *Psychosomatic Medicine, 73*(2),127–133.

Hofmann, S. G., Sawyer, A. T., Witt, A. A., & Oh, D. (2010). The effect of mindfulness-based therapy on anxiety and depression: A meta-analytic review. *Journal of Consulting and Clinical Psychology, 78,* 169–183.

Hollifield, M., Sinclair-Lian, N., Warner, T. D., & Hammerschlag, R. (2007). Acupuncture for posttraumatic stress disorder: A randomized controlled pilot trial. *Journal of Nervous and Mental Disorders, 195*(6), 504–513.

Hölzel, B. K., Carmody, J., Vangel, M., Congleton, C., Yerramsetti, S. M., Gard, T., & Lazar, S. W. (2011). Mindfulness practice leads to increases in regional brain gray matter density. *Psychiatry Research, 191*(1), 36–43.

Huang, W., Kutner, N., & Bliwise, D. L. (2009). A systematic review of the effects of acupuncture in treating insomnia. *Sleep Medicine Review, 3*(1), 73–104.

Ihl, R., Bachinskaya, N., Korczyn, A. D., Vakhapova, V., Tribanek, M., Hoerr, R., & Napryeyenko, O. (2011). Efficacy and safety of a once-daily formulation of *Ginkgo biloba* extract EGb 761 in dementia with neuropsychiatric features: A randomized controlled trial. *International Journal of Geriatric Psychiatry, 26*(11), 1186–1194.

Irwin, M. R., Olmstead, R., & Motivala, S. J. (2008). Improving sleep quality in older adults with moderate sleep complaints: A randomized controlled trial of Tai Chi Chih. *Sleep, 31*(7), 1001–1008.

Jedrziewski, M. K., Ewbank, D. C., Wang, H., & Trojanowski, J. Q. (2010). Exercise and cognition: Results from the National Long Term Care Survey. *Alzheimer's Dementia, 6,* 448–455.

Johnson, D. P., Penn, D. L., Fredrickson, B. L., Kring, A. M., Meyer, P. S., Catalino, L. I., & Brantley, M. (2011). A pilot study of loving-kindness meditation for the negative symptoms of schizophrenia. *Schizophrenia Research, 129*(2–3), 137–140.

Joy, C. B., Mumby-Croft, R., & Joy, L. A. (2006). Polyunsaturated fatty acid supplementation for schizophrenia. *Cochrane Database of Systematic Reviews,* Issue 3. Art no. CD001257.

Kabat-Zinn, J., Massion, A. O., Kristeller, J., Peterson, L. G., Fletcher, K. E., Pbert, L., Lenderking, W. R., & Santorelli, S. F. (1992). Effectiveness of a meditation-based stress reduction program in the treatment of anxiety disorders. *American Journal of Psychiatry, 149*(7), 936–943.

Karst, M., Winterhalter, M., Münte, S., Francki, B., Hondronikos, A., Eckardt, A., ... Fink, M. (2007). Auricular acupuncture for dental anxiety: A randomized controlled trial. *Anesthesia and Analgesia, 104*(2), 295–300.

Kasper, S., Caraci, F., Forti, B., Drago, F., & Aguglia, E. (2010). Efficacy and tolerability of *Hypericum* extract for the treatment of mild to moderate depression. *European Neuropsychopharmacology, 20*(11), 747–765.

Kennedy, J., Wang, C. C., & Wu, C. H. (2008). Patient disclosure about herb and supplement use among adults in the US. *Evidence Based Complementary and Alternative Medicine, 5,* 451–456.

Kessler, R. C., Soukup, J., Davis, R. B., Foster, D. F., Wilkey, S. A., Van Rompay, M. I., & Eisenberg, D. M. (2001). The use of complementary and alternative therapies to treat anxiety and depression in the United States. *American Journal of Psychiatry, 158*(2), 289–294.

Kirkwood, G., Rampes, H., Tuffrey, V., Richardson, J., & Pilkington, K. (2005). Yoga for anxiety: A systematic review of the research evidence. *British Journal of Sports Medicine, 39*(12), 884–891.

Krisanaprakornkit, T., Krisanaprakornkit, W., Piyavhatkul, N., & Laopaiboon, M. (2006). Meditation therapy for anxiety disorders. *Cochrane Database of Systematic Reviews,* Issue 1. Art. No. CD004998.

Kritz-Silverstein, D., von Mühlen, D., Laughlin, G. A., & Bettencourt, R. (2008). Effects of dehydroepiandrosterone supplementation on cognitive function and quality of life: The DHEA and Well-Ness (DAWN) Trial. *Journal of the American Geriatric Society, 56*(7), 1292–1298.

Lam, L. C., Chau, R. C., Wong, B. M., Fung, A. W., Lui, V. W., Tam, C. C., ... Chan, W. M. (2011). Interim follow-up of a randomized controlled trial comparing Chinese style mind body (tai chi) and stretching exercises on cognitive function in subjects at risk of progressive cognitive decline. *International Journal of Geriatric Psychiatry, 26*(7), 733–740.

Lang, A. J., Strauss, J. L., Bomyea, J., Bormann, J. E., Hickman, S. D., Good, R. C., & Essex, M. (2012). The theoretical and empirical basis for meditation as an intervention for PTSD. *Behavior Modification,* published online June 5.

Lavretsky, H., Alstein, L. L., Olmstead, R. E., Ercoli, L. M., Riparetti-Brown, M., Cyr, N. S., & Irwin, M. R. (2011). Complementary use of Tai Chi Chih augments escitalopram treatment of geriatric depression: A randomized controlled trial. *American Journal of Geriatric Psychiatry, 19*(10), 839–850.

Lazar, S. W., Kerr, C. E., Wasserman, R. H., Gray, J. R., Greve, D. N., Treadway, M. T., ... Fischl, B. (2005). Meditation experience is associated with increased cortical thickness. *Neuroreport, 28*(16–17), 1893–1897.

Le Bars, P. L., Katz, M. M., Berman, N., Itil, T. M., Freedman, A. M., & Schatzberg, A. F. (1997). A placebo controlled double-blind randomized trial of an extract of ginkgo biloba for dementia. *JAMA, 278,* 1327–1332.

Li, F., Fisher, K. J., Harmer, P., Irbe, D., Tearse, R. G., Weimer, C. (2004). Tai chi and self-rated quality of sleep and daytime sleepiness in older adults: A randomized controlled trial. *Journal of the American Geriatric Society, 52*(6), 892–900.

Lieverse, R., Van Someren, E. J., Nielen, M. M., Uitdehaag, B. M., Smit, J. H., & Hoogendijk, W. J. (2011). Bright light treatment in elderly patients with nonseasonal major depressive disorder: A randomized placebo-controlled trial. *Archives of General Psychiatry, 68*(1), 61–70.

Lin, M. F., Hsieh, Y. J., Hsu, Y. Y., Fetzer, S., & Hsu, M. C. (2011). A randomised controlled trial of the effect of music therapy and verbal relaxation on chemotherapy-induced anxiety. *Journal of Clinical Nursing, 20*(7–8), 988–999.

Lin, P. Y., Huang, S. Y., & Su, K. P. (2010). A meta-analytic review of polyunsaturated fatty acid compositions in patients with depression. *Biological Psychiatry, 68*(2),140–147.

Linde, K., Berner, M. M., & Kriston, L. (2008). St John's wort for major depression. *Cochrane Database of Systematic Reviews,* Issue 4. Art. No. CD000448.

Lusordi, P., Piazza, E., Fogari, R. (2000). Cardiovascular effects of melatonin in hypertensive patients well controlled by nifedipine: A 24 hour study. *British Journal of Clinical Pharmacology, 49,* 423.

Mahaffey, K. R., Sunderland, E. M., Chan, H. M., Choi, A. L., Grandjean, P., Mariën, K., ... Yasutake, A. (2011). Balancing the benefits of n-3 polyunsaturated fatty acids and the risks of methylmercury exposure from fish consumption. *Nutrition Review, 69*(9), 493–508.

Malow, B., Adkins, K. W., McGrew, S. G., Wang, L., Goldman, S. E., Fawkes, D., & Burnette, C. (2012). Melatonin for sleep in children with autism: A controlled trial examining dose, tolerability, and outcomes. *Journal of Autism and Developmental Disorders, 42*(8), 1729–1737.

Manber, R., Schnyer, R. N., Lyell, D., Chambers, A. S., Caughey, A. B., Druzin, M., ... Allen, J. J. (2010). Acupuncture for depression during pregnancy: A randomized controlled trial. *Obstetrics and Gynecology, 115*(3), 511–520.

Maratos, A. S., Gold, C., Wang, X., & Crawford, M. J. (2008). Music therapy for depression. *Cochrane Database of Systematic Reviews,* Issue 1. Art. No. CD004517.

Margolin, A., Kleber, H. D., Avants, S. K., Konefal, J., Gawin, F., . . . Vaughan, R. (2002). Acupuncture for the treatment of cocaine addiction: A randomized controlled trial. *JAMA, 287*(1), 55–63.

McKay, D. L., & Blumberg, J. B. (2006). A review of the bioactivity and potential health benefits of chamomile tea (*Matricaria recutita* L.). *Phytotherapy Research, 20*(7), 519–530.

McNamara, R. K. Hahn, C. G., Jandacek, R., Rider, T., Tso, P., Stanford, K.E., & Richtand, N. M. (2007). Selective deficits in the omega-3 fatty acid docosahexaenoic acid in the postmortem orbitofrontal cortex of patients with major depressive disorder. *Biological Psychiatry, 62,*17–24.

Meyer, H. B., Katsman, A., Sones, A. C., Auerbach, D. E., Ames, D., & Rubin, R. T. (2012). Yoga as an ancillary treatment for neurological and psychiatric disorders: A review. *Journal of Neuropsychiatry and Clinical Neuroscience, 24*(2), 152–164.

Mischoulon, D. (2007). Update and critique of natural remedies as antidepressant treatments. *Psychiatric Clinics of North America, 30*(1), 51–68.

Miyasaka, L. S., Atallah, Á. N., & Soares, B. (2007). Passiflora for anxiety disorder. *Cochrane Database of Systematic Reviews,* Issue 1. Art. No. CD004518.

Montgomery, P., & Richardson, A. J. (2008). Omega-3 fatty acids for bipolar disorder. *Cochrane Database of Systematic Reviews,* Issue 2. Art. No. CD005169.

Morgenthaler, T., Kramer, M., Alessi, C., Friedman, L., Boehlecke, B., Brown, T., … Swick, T. (2006). Practice parameters for the psychological and behavioral treatment of insomnia: An update. An American Academy of Sleep Medicine report. *Sleep, 29*(11), 1415–1419.

Morris, D. W., Trivedi, M. H., & Rush, A. J.(2008). Folate and unipolar depression. *Journal of Alternative and Complementary Medicine, 14*(3), 277–285.

Mössler, K., Chen, X., Heldal, T. O., & Gold, C. (2011). Music therapy for people with schizophrenia and schizophrenia-like disorders. *Cochrane Database of Systematic Reviews,* Issue 12. Art. No. CD004025.

Movafegh, A., Alizadeh, R., Hajimohamadi, F., Esfehani, F., & Nejatfar, M. (2008). Preoperative oral *Passiflora incarnata* reduces anxiety in ambulatory surgery patients: A double-blind, placebo-controlled study. *Anesthesia and Analgesia, 106*(6), 1728–1732.

Nahin, R.L, Barnes, P. M., Stussman, B. J., & Bloom, B. (2009). Costs of complementary and alternative medicine (CAM) and frequency of visits to CAM practitioners: United States, 2007. National Health Statistics Reports, No. 18. Hyattsville, MD: National Center for Health Statistics.

National Center for Complementary and Alternative Medicine (NCCAM). (2013). *Complementary, Alternative, or Integrative Health: What's in a Name?* Available at http://nccam.nih.gov/health/whatiscam

Natural Medicines Comprehensive Database. (2012). *Ginkgo,* Stockton, CA: Therapeutic Research Faculty; ©1995–2012. Available at http://www.naturaldatabase.com

Natural Standard Database. (2011). Available at http://www.naturalstandard.com

Newberg, A. B., Wintering, N., Khalsa, D. S., Roggenkamp, H., & Waldman, M. R. (2010). Meditation effects on cognitive function and cerebral blood flow in subjects with memory loss: A preliminary study. *Journal of Alzheimer's Disease, 20*(2), 517–526.

Ong, J. C., Shapiro, S. L., & Manber, R. (2009). Mindfulness meditation and cognitive behavioral therapy for insomnia: A naturalistic 12-month follow-up. *Explore, 5,* 30–36.

Papakostas, G. I. (2009). The role of S-adenosyl methionine in the treatment of depression. *Journal of Clinical Psychiatry, 70*(suppl 5), 18–22.

Papakostas, G. I., Mischoulon, D., Shyu, I., Alpert, J. E., & Fava, M. (2010). S-adenosyl methionine (SAMe) augmentation of serotonin reuptake inhibitors for antidepressant nonresponders with major depressive disorder: A double-blind, randomized clinical trial. *American Journal of Psychiatry, 167*(8), 942–948.

Papakostas, G. I., Petersen, T., Mischoulon, D., Ryan, J. L., Nierenberg, A. A., Bottiglieri, T., … Fava, M. (2004). Serum folate, vitamin B12, and homocysteine in major depressive disorder, Part 1: Predictors of clinical response in fluoxetine-resistant depression. *Journal of Clinical Psychiatry, 65*(8), 1090–1095.

Parker, G., Gibson, N.A., Brotchie, H., Heruc, G., Rees, A. M., & Hadzi-Pavlovic, D. (2006). Omega-3 fatty acids and mood disorders, *American Journal of Psychiatry, 163*(6), 969–978.

Pearson, N. J., Johnson, L. L., & Nahin, R. L. (2006). Insomnia, trouble sleeping, and complementary and alternative medicine: Analysis of the 2002 national health interview survey data. *Archives of Internal Medicine, 166*(16), 1775–1782.

Piet, J., & Hougaard, E. (2011). The effect of mindfulness-based cognitive therapy for prevention of relapse in recurrent major depressive disorder: A systematic review and meta-analysis. *Clinical Psychology Review, 31*(6), 1032–1040.

Pittler, M. H., & Ernst, E. (2003). Kava extract for treating anxiety. *Cochrane Database of Systematic Reviews,* Issue 1. Art. No. CD003383.

Qureshi, N. A., & Al-Bedah, A. M. (2013). Mood disorders and complementary and alternative medicine: A literature review. *Neuropsychiatric Disease and Treatment, 9,* 639–658.

Rabkin, J. G., McElhiney, M. C., Rabkin, R., McGrath, P. J., & Ferrando, S. J. (2006). Placebo-controlled trial of dehydroepiandrosterone (DHEA) for treatment of nonmajor depression in patients with HIV/AIDS. *American Journal of Psychiatry, 2006, 163*(1), 59–66.

Rahimi, R., Nikfar, S., & Abdollahi, M. (2009). Efficacy and tolerability of *Hypericum perforatum* in major depressive disorder in comparison with selective serotonin reuptake inhibitors: A meta-analysis. *Progress in Neuropsychopharmacology and Biological Psychiatry, 33*(1), 118–127.

Rimer, J., Dwan, K., Lawlor, D. A., Greig, C. A., McMurdo, M., Morley, W., & Mead, G. E. (2012). Exercise for depression. *Cochrane Database of Systematic Reviews,* Issue 7. Art. No. CD004366.

Rossignol, D. A., & Frye, R. E. (2011). Melatonin in autism spectrum disorders: A systematic review and meta-analysis. *Developmental Medicine and Child Neurology, 53*(9), 783–792.

Schmidt, P. J., Daly, R. C., Bloch, M., Smith, M. J., Danaceau, M. A., St. Clair, L.S., … Rubinow, D. R. (2005). Dehydroepiandrosterone monotherapy in midlife-onset major and minor depression. *Archives of General Psychiatry, 62*(2), 154–162.

Segal, R., & Pilote, L. (2006). Warfarin interaction with *Matricaria chamomilla. CMAJ, 174*(9), 1281–1282.

Shapiro, S. L., Bootzin, R. R., Figueredo, A. J., Lopez, A. M., & Schwartz, G. E. (2003). The efficacy of mindfulness-based stress reduction in the treatment of sleep disturbance in women with breast cancer: An exploratory study. *Journal of Psychosomatic Research, 54*(1), 85–91.

Smith, C. A., Hay, P. P., & Macpherson, H. (2010). Acupuncture for depression. *Cochrane Database of Systematic Reviews,* Issue 1. Art. No. CD004046.

Snitz, B. E., O'Meara, E. S., Carlson, M. C., Arnold, A. M., Ives, D. G., Rapp, S. R., … Ginkgo Evaluation of Memory (GEM) Study Investigators. (2009). Ginkgo biloba for preventing cognitive decline in older adults: A randomized trial. *JAMA, 302*(24), 2663–2670.

Sood, A., Ebbert, J. O., Prasad, K., Croghan, I. T., Bauer, B., & Schroeder, D. R. (2010). A randomized clinical trial of St. John's wort for smoking cessation. *Journal of Alternative and Complementary Medicine, 16*(7), 761–767.

Strauss, J. L., Coeytaux, R., McDuffie, J., Nagi, A., & Williams, J. W., Jr., (2011). Efficacy of complementary and alternative therapies for posttraumatic stress disorder. VA-ESP Project #09-010. Washington, DC: Department of Veterans Affairs.

Streeter, C. C., Whitfield, T. H., Owen, L., Rein, T., Karri, S. K., Yakhkind, A., … Jensen, J. E. (2010). Effects of yoga versus walking on mood, anxiety, and brain GABA levels: A randomized controlled MRS study. *Journal of Alternative and Complement Medicine, 16*(11), 1145–1152.

Taibi, D. M., Landis, C. A., Petry, H., & Vitiello, M. V. (2007). A systematic review of valerian as a sleep aid: Safe but not effective. *Sleep Medicine Reviews, 11,* 209–230.

Taylor, M. J., Carney, S., Geddes, J., & Goodwin, G. (2003). Folate for depressive disorders. *Cochrane Database of Systematic Reviews,* Issue 2. Art. No. CD003390.

Tsang, H. W., Chan, E. P., & Cheung, W. M. (2008). Effects of mindful and nonmindful exercises on people with depression: A systematic review. *British Journal of Clinical Psychology, 47,* 303–322.

Tuunainen, A., Kripke, D. F., & Endo, T. (2004). Light therapy for non-seasonal depression. *Cochrane Database of Systematic Reviews,* Issue 2. Art. No. CD004050.

Uebelacker, L. A., Epstein-Lubow, G., Gaudiano, B. A., Tremont, G., Battle, C. L., & Miller, I. W. (2010). Hatha yoga for depression: Critical review of the evidence for efficacy, plausible mechanisms of action, and directions for future research. *Journal of Psychiatric Practice, 16*(1), 22–33.

U.S. Department of Health and Human Services. Physical Activity Guidelines Advisory Committee. (2008). *Physical Activity Guidelines Advisory Committee Report, 2008.* Washington, DC: U.S. Department of Health and Human Services. Available at http://www.health.gov/paguidelines/guidelines

Unutzer, J., Klap, R., Sturm, R., Young, A. S., Marmon, T., Shatkin, J., & Wells, K. B. (2000). Mental disorders and the use of alternative medicine: Results from a national survey. *American Journal of Psychiatry, 157*(11), 1851–1857.

Wang, H., Qi, H., Wang, B. S., Cui, Y. Y., Zhu, L., Rong, Z. X., & Chen, H. Z. (2008). Is acupuncture beneficial in depression? A meta-analysis of 8 randomized controlled trials. *Journal of Affective Disorders, 111*(2–3), 125–134.

White, A. R., Rampes, H., Liu, J. P., Stead, L. F., & Campbell, J. (2011). Acupuncture and related interventions for smoking cessation. *Cochrane Database of Systematic Reviews*, Issue 1. Art no. CD000009.

Williams, J. W., Jr., Gierisch, J. M., McDuffie, J., Strauss, J. L., & Nagi, A. (2011). An overview of complementary and alternative medicine therapies for anxiety and depressive disorders: Supplement to efficacy of complementary and alternative medicine therapies for posttraumatic stress disorder. VA-ESP Project #09-010. Washington, DC: Department of Veterans Affairs.

Winbush, N. Y., Gross, C. R., & Kreitzer, M. J. (2007). The effects of mindfulness-based stress reduction on sleep disturbance: A systematic review. *Explore* (NY), *3*(6), 585–591.

Wirz-Justice, A., Bader, A., Frisch, U., Stieglitz, R. D., Alder, J., Bitzer, J.,… Riecher-Rössler, A. (2011). A randomized, double-blind, placebo-controlled study of light therapy for antepartum depression. *Journal of Clinical Psychiatry, 72*(7), 986–993.

Witte, S., Loew, D., & Gaus, W. (2005). Meta-analysis of the efficacy of the acetonic kava-kava extract WS1490 in patients with non-psychotic anxiety disorders. *Phytotherapy Research, 19*, 183–188.

Wolkowitz, O. M., Kramer, J. H., Reus, V. I., Costa, M. M., Yaffe, K., Walton, P.,… DHEA-Alzheimer's Disease Collaborative Research. (2003). DHEA treatment of Alzheimer's disease: A randomized, double-blind, placebo-controlled study. *Neurology, 60*, 1071–1076.

Yeung, A. S., Ameral, V. E., Chuzi, S. E., Fava, M., & Mischoulon, D. (2011). A pilot study of acupuncture augmentation therapy in antidepressant partial and non-responders with major depressive disorder. *Journal of Affective Disorders, 130*(1–2), 285–289.

Zgierska, A., Rabago, D., Chawla, N., Kushner, K., Koehler, R., & Marlatt, A. (2009). Mindfulness meditation for substance use disorders: A systematic review. *Substance Abuse, 30*(4), 266–294.

Zick, S. M., Wright, B. D., Sen, A., & Arnedt, J. T. (2011). Preliminary examination of the efficacy and safety of a standardized chamomile extract for chronic primary insomnia: A randomized placebo-controlled pilot study. *BMC Complementary and Alternative Medicine, 22*(11), 78.

23

Psychopharmacology

Vanessa Genung

Key Terms

Learning Outcomes

1. Distinguish the ABCs of psychiatry.

2. Discuss the nurse's role and responsibility in managing a psychotropic medication order.

3. Summarize the pharmacokinetic drug process of absorption, distribution, metabolism, and elimination.

4. Describe the protective role of the blood–brain barrier.

5. Discuss the pharmacodynamic process between a ligand and receptor.

6. Differentiate the actions of drug agonists, antagonists, and partial agonist/antagonists.

7. Examine the pharmacodynamic process of drug reactions, such as target effects and side effects.

8. Explain the pharmacodynamic process involved in drug and food interactions in the liver, including inhibitor and inducer actions.

9. Contrast the pharmaco-therapeutic function of antidepressants, anxiolytics, antiepileptics, antipsychotics, anticholinesterase medications, and sleep–wake promoters.

Introduction

Pharmacology involves understanding the principles of **pharmacokinetics** (how the body processes medications), **pharmacodynamics** (how medications affect the body), and **pharmacotherapeutics** (the clinical application of medications to brain circuit and neurotransmitter–receptor dysfunction). **Psychopharmacology** is the study of the use of medications in the treatment of psychiatric–mental health disorders and conditions. Psychopharmacology applies pharmacological principles to the understanding of how medications affect the brain, primarily, and the body in ways that influence an individual's perception, experiences, and behavior. The use of medications in the treatment and management of mental illness is relatively new (Chapter 2). It is critical that nurses working with patients with psychiatric disorders have a solid understanding of the drugs used to treat psychiatric disorders and their effects on the ABCs of psychiatry: Affect, Attitude, Behavior, and Cognition (Table 23-1). This chapter identifies the necessary elements of a psychotropic medication order and provides a detailed review of basic medication pathways (how a medication travels through the body) and the pharmacokinetic and pharmacodynamics processes. The pharmacotherapeutics of psychotropic medication classes (antidepressants, anxiolytics, antiepileptics, antipsychotics, anticholinergics, and sleep–wake medications) also will be discussed, as well as the essentials of providing nursing care for patients taking psychotropic medications.

ABCs of Psychiatry: Affect, Attitude, Behavior, and Cognition   table 23-1

Observation	Descriptors/Elements
Assessment Domain: A = Affect/Mood	
Affect • Objective: observed by others • Emotion felt/expressed now • Fluctuating feelings in response to current event	**Terms to Describe Affect** • Mad, sad, glad, scared (fear), surprised, hurt **Types of Affect** • Appropriate/inappropriate • Constricted, flat, blunted, labile, full range
Mood • Subjective: felt by individual • How individual feels overall through the day • Consistent internal state of experience	**Mood Continuum** • High: Euphoric, elated, anxious, angry • Middle: Calm/stable, sad/hurt, irritable/edgy • Low: Depressed, melancholic, indifferent, ambivalent **Mood Intensity** • Mild, moderate, severe **Types of Mood** • Stable/unstable • Dysphoric/euphoric • Dysthymic/euthymic • Angry, irritable, anxious, elevated, expansive **Mood Consistent With Affect, Thought, and Circumstances** • Congruent /incongruent
Assessment Domain: A = Attitude	
Interaction • Approach/avoidance	**Terms to Describe Interaction** • Cooperative /oppositional • Friendly/hostile, belligerent • Involved/apathetic • Open/motivated vs. evasive/secretive
Orientation • Awareness (as opposed to consciousness)	**Types of Orientation** • Oriented/disoriented • Person, place, time, situation
Attention • Alertness • Level of consciousness • Eye contact	**Terms to Describe Attention** • Clear, confused, preoccupied, distractible, drowsy
Grooming, Hygiene	**Terms Used to Describe Grooming and Hygiene** • Clean, tidy, dirty, unclean
Assessment Domain: B = Behavior	
Presentation Appearance • Demeanor toward self and other • How individual relates socially	**Terms to Describe Demeanor and Social Engagement** • Approaching/avoidant • Social/antisocial • Tolerant/intolerant • Sense of humor, smiling, animated • Joking, sarcastic

(Conitnued)

ABCs of Psychiatry: Affect, Attitude, Behavior, and Cognition (*continued*)   table 23-1

Observation	Descriptors/Elements
	• Tactful, gracious, sensitive, supportive, engaging • Agitated/aggressive • Argumentative/oppositional • Intrusive/persistent • Spontaneous/apprehensive, guarded • Dependent, compliant • Flexible, forceful, impulsive, seductive, sexual, threatening • Deferring, detached, distrustful • Superficial, indifferent
Psychomotor Activity • Psychomotor function, dysfunction	**Types of Psychomotor Activity** • Normal, agitation, retardation • Calm, energetic, hyperactive, akathisic • Tics, tremors, rigidity, involuntary movements
Coping Attributes • Capacity to cope with illness, change	**Types of Coping Attributes** • Strengths, limitations, weaknesses
	Assessment Domain: C = Cognition
Thought Processes • Observed in flow of speech and in speech quality, quantity, fluidity, tone	**Terms to Describe Speech** • Volume, rate, flow, articulation • Pressured speech • Thought blocking • Echolalia, clanging, parroting • Perseveration, neologisms, word salad
Thought Content • What individual thinks about • Observed in substance of thought	**Terms to Describe Thought Content** • Poverty of content • Suicidal or homicidal: ideation, intention, plan • Self-harm: ideation, intention, plan, occurrences • Derealization: feeling disconnected from flow of time • Depersonalization: feeling disconnected from self • Obsessions, compulsions, ruminations, phobias • Illusion: sensory stimulation misperceived • Hallucination: sensory stimulation not present • Delusion: fixed false belief **Types of Delusions** • Persecutory, erotomanic, grandiose, somatic, jealous, religious, mixed **Types of Hallucinations** • Auditory, visual, tactile, gustatory, olfactory
Memory • Ability to recall information	**Types of Memory** • Short-term (recent), long-term (remote)
Fund of Knowledge • Development of normal intelligence	**Terms to Describe Fund of Knowledge** • Intelligence quotient (IQ) • Borderline intelligence • Trauma loss
Insight • Ability to understand problems, process, and consequences	**Terms to Describe Insight** • Limited, good, fair, poor, impaired
Capacity • Medical term describing the ability to make decisions for self	**Key Elements** • Individual is capable of understanding information, reasoning, and making decisions. • Capacity may fluctuate. For example, an individual who is heavily sedated does not have the capacity to give informed consent.
Competency • Adjudication of competence by a court	**Key Elements** • A court has determined the individual does not have the capacity to make health care decisions. • Competency does not fluctuate; only a court hearing can restore competency.
Judgment • Ability to make good choices	**Types of Judgment** • Limited, good, fair, poor, impaired

Psychotropic Medication Orders

The nurse's authority and responsibility to administer medications has grown in response to changes in federal, state, and institutional policies. This evolution in health care has also expanded prescriptive authority. State laws and hospital codes dictate that medications must be ordered by a licensed prescribing health care provider acting within the scope of professional training. Advanced practitioners who prescribe psychotropic medications (drugs used specifically for psychiatric symptoms) are generally referred to as psychopharmacologists. These include psychiatrists and other physicians (MDs, DOs), advanced practice registered nurses (APRNs), physician assistants (PAs), and (in some states) doctorally prepared licensed psychologists.

The registered nurse may receive different types of orders to administer psychotropic medication. There are four typical medication order classifications: (1) standing orders, (2) emergency or STAT orders, (3) single orders, and (4) PRN orders. Certain elements are required to be provided for all prescription orders to be filled (Table 23-2). Additional details may accompany the order for specific clarification—for example, the timing of a dose in relationship to food intake.

The nurse has a legal responsibility to exercise good professional judgment in carrying out the tasks of verifying that there is a match between the right patient and medication, dose, route, and time, and making note of the patient's reactions when administering ordered medications. (These are often referred to as the "five rights" of medication administration: right patient, right medication, right dose and route, right time, and right documentation.) Every effort should be made to review for accuracy details of medication orders, medication protocols, labs, drug therapeutic levels, and patient response to medication for both desired and untoward effects.

Pharmacokinetics

The process of chemically transforming a medication to a form that the body can use is referred to as *pharmacokinetics*. Four chemical processes occur to bring a drug to the point of utilization by the body: absorption, distribution, metabolism, and excretion, often referred to as ADME (Figure 23-1).

Absorption

The first stage, *absorption*, involves the way a medication enters the body through the administration site and its passage into the fluids and tissues via circulation. The medication is absorbed through diffusion, filtration, and osmosis. For a medication to be absorbed by tissues, it must first be dissolved in body fluid. This is referred to as *solubility*. Psychotropic medication administration routes include *enteral* (through GI tract—oral, nasogastric, and rectal), *parenteral* (through skin or bloodstream—subcutaneous, intramuscular, and intravenous), and *percutaneous* (through skin topically, under tongue, in cheek, or through the lungs—transdermal, sublingual, buccal, and inhaled). The speed of absorption depends on the route of administration, the solubility of the drug, and the degree of circulation to tissues. Liquid medications are more soluble than tablets, whereas sublingual medications are more soluble than capsules. Where there is greater blood flow, there is faster absorption. For example, most medications are water soluble; drinking a little water with the medication will facilitate the dissolving of the medication and thus increase the speed of its absorption in the gut. Other medications, such as ziprasidone (Geodon) are absorbed better when taken with food, which helps break down the medication in different chemical reactions through the digestive process.

Overview of Psychotropic Medication Orders — table 23-2

Prescribers

Physicians: DO, MD
Advanced Practice Registered Nurses: (APRN)-PMHNP-BC, PMHCNS-BC, FNP, PNP, WHNP
Physician Assistants: PA
Licensed Psychologists: (PhD) in some states

Required Elements in Orders

Patient's full name, age, address
Date
Name of drug, route of administration, dose, frequency, duration, reason for medication Signature of prescriber

Types of Medication Orders	Example
STANDING ORDER Administer until discontinued or administer for a certain number of doses.	fluoxetine 20 mg PO once a day for depression
STAT ORDER One-time order to be given immediately.	haloperidol 5 mg IM now for agitation lorazepam 1 mg IM now for agitation diphenhydramine 25 mg IM now for agitation
SINGLE ORDER One-time order to be given at a specific time.	diazepam 5 mg PO q 30 min before CT scan procedure
PRN ORDER Administer on an as-needed basis. Involves nurse judgment regarding patient's need and safety.	temazepam 30 mg PO PRN qhs for insomnia

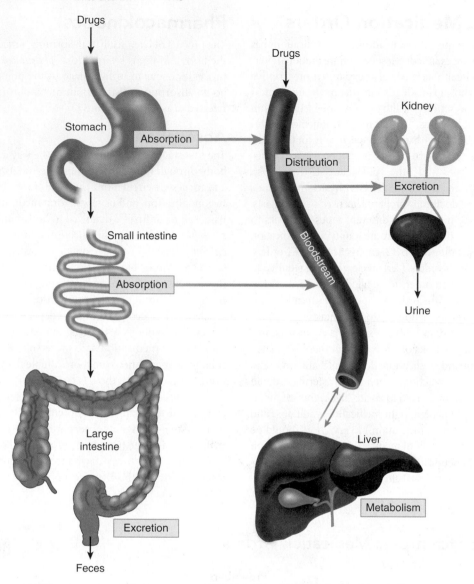

23-1 The four processes of pharmacokinetics: absorption, distribution, metabolism, and excretion.

Distribution

Once a medication is absorbed, it begins its *distribution* journey through circulation in the bloodstream and lymphatic systems to body tissues, where it is expressed in target and side effects in sites of action. Medications are designed to have targeted effects in the body and brain; however, other receptors throughout the body may communicate with a medication. For example, a selective serotonin-reuptake inhibitor (SSRI) targets the serotonin receptors in the brain. There are also serotonin receptors in the gut, which cause some individuals to experience gastrointestinal disturbances when taking serotonin medications. In many cases, a small modification may resolve a side effect. In the example of SSRIs, taking the medication with a small amount of food usually resolves gastrointestinal side effects.

Protein binding within blood plasma is a key factor in the distribution and efficiency of medication in the body. Common blood proteins available for drug binding include albumin, lipoprotein, glycoprotein, and α, β, and γ globulins. A specific drug's affinity for a plasma protein determines what proportion of the drug becomes plasma protein bound. A drug exists in the blood in bound and unbound forms. The unbound drug can more efficiently diffuse out of the cell, or travel through cell membranes, to exert its pharmacologic effects, be metabolized by the liver, and then excreted. The plasma protein bound portion holds the drug and allows for a controlled dissociation from the plasma protein for slower release to the unbound and useful form. Two events increase the amount of unbound drug. A higher drug concentration leads to saturation of available plasma proteins with the drug, which, in turn, leads to more unbound medication for pharmacological effect. For example, aspirin can increase the free concentration of valproate many times over, while the total valproate levels often do not change appreciably (Sandson, Marcucci, Bourke, & Smith-Lamachia, 2006). Liver disease, renal disease, malnutrition, or catabolism decrease the amount of plasma proteins in the blood. This results in less drug plasma protein binding and increases the amounts of unbound drug available.

Other factors can influence the distribution of medication in the body. Properties of a drug influence drug dispersion into the brain and body. The size of the drug molecule can determine its capacity to

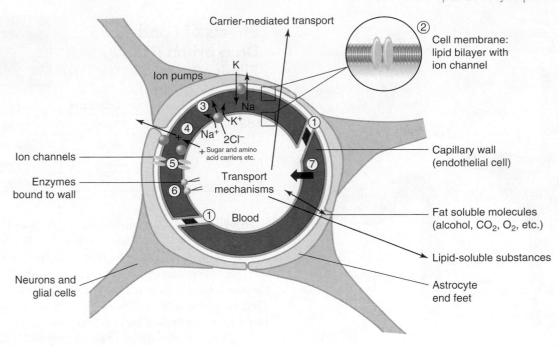

Carrier-mediated transport

Ion pumps

K

Na

K⁺

Na⁺

2Cl⁻

Sugar and amino acid carriers etc.

Ion channels

Enzymes bound to wall

Transport mechanisms

Blood

Neurons and glial cells

② Cell membrane: lipid bilayer with ion channel

Capillary wall (endothelial cell)

Fat soluble molecules (alcohol, CO_2, O_2, etc.)

Lipid-soluble substances

Astrocyte end feet

23-2 The blood–brain barrier.

pass through very small capillary membranes in the brain. This can have the protective effect of keeping a particular environment stable and safe, as in the cases of the placenta and the brain. These are referred to as placental and brain barriers. The **blood–brain barrier** (BBB) is a semipermeable membrane that protects the brain and the spinal cord by preventing substances in the blood from diffusing out of cerebral capillaries (Figure 23-2).

Special conditions are required for entrance to and exchange in the brain. Large molecules cannot pass through the densely packed endothelial cells in the brain's capillary linings. Molecules with strong electrical charges are decelerated from entering. A lipid–protein membrane separates intracellular and extracellular cerebral fluids. The brain is *lipophilic,* preferring fat-soluble molecules for slower diffusion and using protein to regulate solute movement across the membranes. Some exchanges occur through ion channels and others through more active transport systems.

Psychotropic medications gain entrance and leave the protected brain environment by being lipophilic, through transport systems, through ion channels, or through second messenger systems. High blood pressure can open the BBB. In addition, particularly high concentrations of a substance (hyperosmolarity) in general circulation, radiation, infection, and brain injury also can open the BBB. It is important to note that the BBB is not fully developed at birth; thus, the infant is particularly vulnerable to brain insult. Similarly, the process of aging weakens the BBB and, most certainly, the progression of dementia causes a weakening of the BBB, increasing the risk of insult or injury to the brain.

Metabolism

After a medication has been absorbed, distributed, and reached the target receptors, it begins the process of *metabolization*. This is the enzymatic process, primarily accomplished by the liver, of transforming and deconstructing (breaking down) a medication until it becomes chemically inactive and is eliminated. Children with young,

healthy livers metabolize drugs quickly, meaning that they flush out medications faster. Older adults metabolize medications more slowly, resulting in medications staying in their systems longer. Some drugs, such as inhaled or some parenteral medications, are able to pass directly from the bloodstream to the site of action. However, most drugs require repeated chemical reactions to be metabolized, called **biotransformation**. A medication continues to exert biochemical influence until it is eliminated from the body.

Enzymes play an important role in the metabolism of medications. Medications taken orally travel through the digestive tract to the liver and are broken down by metabolic enzymes in what is referred to as the *first pass effect*, which often inactivates the medicine on the first pass (Figure 23-3). Metabolic liver enzymes contained in the **cytochrome P450 system** (CYP450) greatly influence how the body will respond to the medication, medication sensitivity, drug–drug or drug–food interactions, and how much of the medication the body will receive. Genetic differences influence this enzymatic process and can create idiosyncratic or individualized responses to medications (Kaplowitz, 2005). **Metabolites** are the products of this enzymatic breakdown and are typically far less chemically potent than the original drug. Still, a metabolite can be an active drug and produce a response effect of its own. This is taken into account when prescribing a drug. For example, propranolol 1 mg IV is considered a bioequivalent to propranolol 40 mg PO. When given orally, the medication will be broken down in a first pass effect in the liver. When given intravenously, it will go directly to the bloodstream and then to the target site. For this reason, most clinicians prefer to prescribe propranolol via IV for its immediate effect rather than having to wait for the gastrointestinal metabolism process.

Elimination

Once the medication has undergone the process of being deactivated by the liver enzymes, the chemical by-products are now ready for *elimination* via *excretion*. Quite simply, insolubles are excreted through

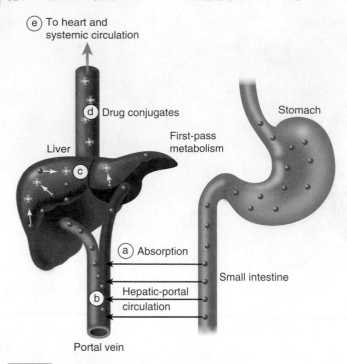

23-3   First-pass effect.

Effects of Food and Drug pH on Drug Elimination			table 23-4
Drug pH	**GI pH**	**Urine pH**	**Drug Elimination**
Acid	Acid	Base	Increased
Acid	Base	Acid	Decreased
Base	Acid	Base	Decreased
Base	Base	Acid	Increased

taken will about equal the amount leaving the body (Kramer, 2003). This is referred to as **steady state**, which is typically achieved in about five half-lives of medication. There is a standard calculation process for determining the diminishing effect of a medication. **Half-life** is the time it takes a drug to journey from metabolism to excretion, eliminating 50% of the drug from the body. Many tests and trials go into determining the half-life of medications.

Figure 23-4 offers a view of how a drug builds in serum blood concentration over a series of dosing until it achieves a steady state. Methadone dosing is used to demonstrate the concept. Average once a day dosing of methadone is in the range of 60 to 100 mg/day based on body weight. The serum blood level concentration of methadone (serum methadone level, SML) is 100 to 1000 ng/mL, with the average trough level eliciting the clinical effect of no withdrawal and sufficient blockade of the opioid receptor being 400 to 500 ng/mL. At SML 200 to 400 ng/mL, the individual may not get sufficient opioid blockade and may experience opioid withdrawal. At SML 500 to 800 ng/mL, the individual is unlikely to experience opioid withdrawal but may be clinically overmedicated. After four or five daily doses, a steady state of the medication is achieved and the individual maintains a steady amount of the medication in the blood stream (Fareed et al., 2010).

How a drug is dosed, its frequency of administration, its expected duration in the body, and the anticipated duration of targeted effects are all decided based on this information. Taking too much of a drug with a longer half-life means that its effects will last longer. Drug metabolism and elimination may also be affected by liver or kidney dysfunction. In some cases, such as with children, an individual can be a swift metabolizer and the medication can pass through the drug pathways and be eliminated from the body quickly. Reducing the amount of medication in the body in this manner diminishes the effects of the medication and makes dosing a challenge. These are the reasons that liver function tests, renal function tests, and drug therapeutic blood levels are monitored closely.

the GI tract as waste; water-soluble chemicals are excreted through the kidneys in urine; and some chemicals are exhaled through the lungs during the normal process of breathing, whereas others eliminated through skin evaporation, tears, saliva, or mother's milk. For some drugs, the excretion process is swift, while other drugs take longer. With the majority of drugs being eliminated via the GI tract and kidneys, the acid–base balance of the body becomes critically important because a diet that is highly acidic can increase the rate of elimination of acidic drugs, and vice versa (see Tables 23-3 and 23-4).

The rate of elimination of a medication has great importance: As long as a medication is in the body, it can have an effect. When a medication is taken on a regular basis, it eventually will achieve a steady state in the body. This means that the amount of the drug

Pause and Reflect

1. *What factors affect the distribution of medication in the body?*
2. *What implications does the first-pass effect have for the assessment and monitoring of patients taking psychotropic drugs?*

Pharmacodynamics

As stated earlier, *pharmacodynamics* refers to the actions drugs have on the body. These include both the direct action of a drug and the subsequent reaction of the body once the pharmacokinetic process begins.

Foods That Contribute to Acid or Alkaline Urine		table 23-3
FOODS	**ACID**	**ALKALINE**
Meats	Fish, shellfish, fowl, eggs, cheese, peanut butter	
Vegetables	Corn, lentils	All vegetables
Fat	Bacon Nuts: Brazil, hazelnuts, peanuts, walnuts	Almonds, chestnuts, coconut
Fruit	Cranberries, plums, prunes	Citrus fruits
Breads	All breads, crackers, pasta	
Desserts	Cakes, cookies	
Dairy products		Milk, cream, buttermilk

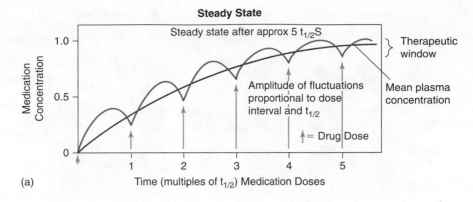

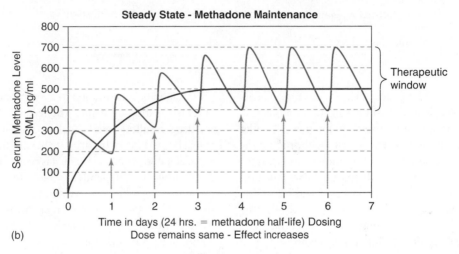

23-4 Drug elimination: half-life to steady state.

Drug Actions

For a drug to have an action, it must have a target. Research in neurochemistry has revealed the targets of psychoactive medications to be the neuronal pathways in the central nervous system of the brain and spinal cord. However, a drug does not target the entire central nervous system. A psychoactive drug targets specific neuronal cells and neuronal synapses (junctions between neurons) in the central nervous system, creating chemical reactions that change the physiologic activity at the specific site. The activity occurs at the presynaptic neuron, the synaptic cleft, or on the postsynaptic neuron. The site on the postsynaptic neuron where the neurotransmitter or the medication chemically bonds and neurochemical reaction occurs is called a **receptor**. The drug molecule that binds to the receptor is a **ligand**. The receptor is a protein embedded in the cell's plasma membrane. Like a key (drug ligand molecule) fitting into a lock (receptor protein in the neuron cell), the drug molecule ligand tells the protein receptor in the neuron cell to do something (open the gate). The drug's ability to bind to a particular receptor site is referred to as its *selectivity*. It selects that particular receptor to bind to and not the others around it. A drug's **affinity** refers to how strong an interest or attraction it might have for a particular receptor. The drug's ability to produce a response once it has been bound or attached itself to the receptor is called its *intrinsic activity*.

Presynaptic Transporters

Some drugs (such as reuptake inhibitors) target the BBB transporters in the presynaptic portion on the neuronal cell. It is the responsibility

of the BBB transporters to shuttle away neurotransmitters and their metabolites from entering the brain (Marc et al., 2011). Once the neurotransmitter has been released from the presynaptic nerve cell into the synaptic cleft, the neurotransmitter floats in the synaptic cleft, awaiting the opportunity to sit on a postsynaptic receptor. If it is not taken into the postsynaptic receptor and used to affect the postsynaptic nerve, it will eventually be taken back up into the presynaptic nerve cell by transporters and be destroyed by enzymes and recycled. Each neurotransmitter has such a presynaptic transporter site. Some examples include serotonin transporter (SERT), norepinephrine transporter (NET), dopamine active transporter (DAT), GABA transporter (GAT), and glutamate excitatory amino acid transporter (EAAT) (Stahl, 2013; Zhou, 2006). Medications designed to block these presynaptic transporters are called *transport reuptake inhibitors*, or just **reuptake inhibitors**. Their responsibility is to stop the reuptake of the neurotransmitter, thereby increasing the amount of the neurotransmitter available in the extracellular synaptic cleft, making more neurotransmitter available for the receptors on the postsynaptic neuron. Some examples include selective serotonin-reuptake inhibitors (SSRIs), serotonin-reuptake inhibitors (SRIs), norepinephrine-reuptake inhibitors (NRIs), and norepinephrine–dopamine-reuptake inhibitors (NDRIs).

Receptor Agonists and Antagonists

Drugs are designed to have chemical properties that mimic the body's own drug-to-receptor process. There are three known outcomes

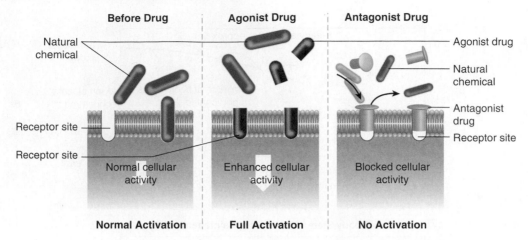

23-5   Receptor agonist and antagonist activity.

when a drug ligand attaches itself to activate a cell receptor protein. When a drug ligand molecule is most similar in chemical shape to that which is naturally produced by the body for that particular receptor, the drug–receptor attachment activity will produce the same response in the cell. This drug acts as an **agonist**, producing the same response the body would. As the body has natural ways of turning things on and off, there is also a neurobiological off switch. Another drug ligand molecule shape, similar to one the body itself produces as an off switch, can sit on a neural receptor cell protein and block the response of the receptor cell. This drug acts as an **antagonist** (inhibitor, blocker), in that it causes there to be no chemical action. Antagonists compete with agonists for a receptor protein cell site position. If the antagonist can secure the position, it can prevent the agonists from getting the site, thereby blocking the agonist from activating the protein receptor on the cell site (Figure 23-5). To clarify, it is not the drug that creates the neurological response—that is the receptor's responsibility. The receptor opens the door to a particular response. Some receptors are in place to activate a cell, others to deactivate it. The agonist or antagonist drugs only tell the cell to do its job or stop doing its job. A third possible activity occurs when a drug ligand molecule has a weaker chemical action on the receptor and elicits only a modest response from the cell. This drug is referred to as a *partial agonist* or *partial antagonist*. It is important to remember that the term "neurotransmitter ligand molecule" can be substituted for "drug ligand molecule" and used to describe the body's own natural activity on its receptor sites.

Therapeutic Efficacy

The ability of a drug to produce the desired response is referred to as its **efficacy**. Is the drug effective for the purpose it is intended? Will it occupy enough receptor sites to get the job done? The amount (dose) of the drug necessary to produce the desired response is its **potency**. One drug delivered at a lower dose achieving the same effect as another delivered at a higher dose can be considered to have the same efficacy. However, the drug given at the lower dose would be more potent. When the concentration of the amount of drug in the body becomes harmful to the individual, it is considered **toxic**. For that reason, some medications have a defined **therapeutic range** (the range at which therapeutic efficacy can be achieved without risking harm to the patient) that is closely monitored. The repeated

presentation of a medication to a receptor can lead to a diminished effect of the drug over time. The receptor becomes desensitized to the drug, resulting in a loss of responsiveness to the medication. When larger doses of the drug are needed to achieve the same results as smaller doses previously did, it is referred to as building **tolerance** to the drug. Drug **dependence** and **addiction** are terms used synonymously to refer to a developed compulsive need to use a substance to function normally. In such cases, in the absence of the particular drug, the person experiences physical or psychological withdrawal symptoms (Genung, 2012; NIH, 2010). Different medication categories lend themselves to these drug action attributes, discussed further in this and other chapters.

Drug Reactions

Target effects occur when a medication reaches the target site and produces the desired effect or the expected or intended response. For example, when a patient in pain receives a nonsteroidal anti-inflammatory drug (NSAID) and experiences pain relief. In addition to target effects, each drug carries the potential for causing **side effects**, which occur when a medication produces additional actions by interacting with neurotransmitters other than those at the target site. In most cases, side effects are limited to common, expected symptoms that are mild and that resolve within a few doses or with some modification, as in the earlier example of eating food when taking an SSRI. However, because all individuals are different, there is always the possibility that a patient may exhibit a less likely and more serious response to a medication. For this reason, nurses monitor patients closely to determine both expected and untoward responses (Table 23-5). There are several medication-caused uncomfortable, harmful, unexpected, or emergent reactions for which to observe (Edmunds, 2010; Woo & Wynne, 2011). These are called **adverse effects** because of their greater level of severity. For example, EKG findings are monitored in patients who are given ziprasidone (Geodon) to monitor for cardiac arrhythmia or torsade de pointes–ventricular tachycardia, which can occur as a result of the medication's adrenergic properties. A **teratogenic effect** is an extreme adverse effect that disturbs the development of an embryo or fetus, as can occur with the use of antiepileptics, such as phenytoin (Dilantin) or valproic acid (Depakote), or when taking benzodiazepines during pregnancy.

Target Effects, Side Effects, and Adverse Effects of Medications
table 23-5

Target, Side, and Adverse Effects	
Target effect (desired action)	The intended or expected response of a medication (e.g., fluoxetine [Prozac] resolving depression)
Side effect (additional action)	The effects of the medication as it interacts with other neurotransmitters (e.g., desyrel [Trazodone] causing sedation)
Adverse effect (harmful action)	The development of severe symptoms or complications following use of the drug (e.g., an antiepileptic used during pregnancy resulting in a birth defect or the development of cardiac problems when the use of ziprasidone [Geodon] results in the prolongation of the QT$_c$ interval)
Unexpected Responses	
Idiosyncratic response (unpredicted reaction)	A unique and strange response to medication resulting in pain, bleeding, over response, or organ failure (e.g., valproate [Depakote] causing hepatotoxicity)
Paradoxical response (opposite reaction)	The development of a contradictory reaction to the medication (e.g., use of a benzo-diazepine causing hyperactivity, agitation, aggression, or rage)
Emergency Reactions	
Allergic reaction (hypersensitivity response)	Typically, an unexpected antibody–antigen response (e.g., lamotrigine [Lamictal] causing a Stevens-Johnson rash)
Anaphylactic reaction (medical emergency)	Life-threatening severe, whole-body allergic response to medication (e.g., morphine or codeine causing pain and respiratory distress)

Other unanticipated outcomes can be observed. An *idiosyncratic response* is an unexpected reaction or a unique or strange response to medication, resulting in pain, bleeding, over response to the medication, or even organ failure, such as hepatotoxity from the use of valproic acid (Depakote). A *paradoxical response* is a response that is contrary to the expected target effect of a particular medicine. An example of this occurs when use of benzodiazepines causes hyperactivity, agitation, aggression, or rage instead of calming.

Perhaps the most severe responses to medications are hypersensitive, or allergic, responses. An allergic hypersensitive reaction occurs when there is an antibody–antigen response that causes an extreme reaction in the body. For example, lamotrigiene (Lamictal) has been observed to cause Stevens-Johnson rash, which can be fatal. The most extreme allergic response is an *anaphylactic reaction*. This is a life-threatening, whole-body allergic response to a medication and is considered a medical emergency. It is a critical part of assessment to ask patients about their history of food and drug responses and to consistently assess and report any side effects, unusual responses, or allergic reactions to foods and medications.

Side effects of medications are frequently given as a reason for nonadherence. Because of this, it is essential that nurses provide patient education related to the need to take psychotropic medications as ordered. Patients taking psychotropic medications who suddenly stop taking them may experience discontinuation symptoms, uncomfortable physical or emotional symptoms that occur once the medication is no longer in their system. These patients may also face a re-emergence of the symptoms for which they were being treated (Ramaswamy, Malik, & Dewan, 2013).

It is also critical to carefully chart responses of patients taking medications that carry black box warnings, which are assigned by the FDA for medications with reported serious adverse reactions. This information can be found easily in medication inserts, at pharmacies, or on the FDA website. If a medication is ordered for a purpose that is not approved by the FDA, it is referred to as an *off-label* use. Many medications are employed quite safely for off-label purposes, but should also be monitored carefully. Examples of medications that are provided for off-label use include doxepin (Sinequan) topical for pruritus/itching or hydroxyzine (Atarax or Vistaril) for insomnia or anxiety.

PRACTICE ALERT Careful assessment regarding patient use of over-the-counter medications, other prescription medications, and herbs and supplements (Chapter 22) is necessary prior to patients beginning a course of psychotropic medication, as use of certain medications, herbs, or supplements may reduce efficacy or increase the potential for adverse effects.

Drug and Food Interactions

Medications are processed or metabolized typically through the intestine or liver, and broken down to other compounds. The process of metabolism is often that of converting a lipophilic compound (food or drug) into a more excretable hydrophilic product. How fast this occurs determines how long the medication is in the body and how intense the response to the medication will be. An enzyme system is in place in the liver to facilitate these chemical biotransformations. The reactions in these enzymatic pathways contribute to drug resistance, drug tolerance, and drug toxicity.

A *substrate* is a molecule on which the enzyme acts in a particular pathway in the liver. The pertinent substrates are CYP450 1A2, 2B6, 2C19, 2D6, and 3A4. Every food and drug has a particular substrate destination, where the enzymes will work to transform them. Moreover, there is some competition for these CYP450 substrate sites in the liver, as more than one food or drug can be present and awaiting the opportunity to be broken down by the enzyme in the same substrate pathway. When one substance competes with another for these CYP450 sites, it can create drug interactions. Two such interactions are of particular importance: induction and inhibition. In some cases, a food or drug is a potent inhibitor of another in a particular pathway. For example, ciprofloxacin (Cipro) is a potent inhibitor of the CYP 1A2 enzyme, whereas olanzapine is a substrate of the CYP 1A2 enzyme. This inhibitive competition of one substance (ciprofloxacin) interferes with the ability of the enzyme to breakdown the other substance (olanzapine). The outcome is an increase in the blood level of the latter substance (olanzapine), increasing its bioavailability (how much of a drug is available in the body) when it needed to be broken down and excreted. This creates an opportunity for toxicity. Grapefruit is an inhibitor of CYP450-3A4, which affects the metabolism of a great number of drugs. It also causes other medications to be chemically inactivated. Therefore, many psychiatric medications (including alprazolam (Xanax), buspirone (Buspar), triazolam (Halcion), carbamazepine (Tegretol), diazepam (Valium), sertraline (Zoloft), and methadone) should not be taken with grapefruit juice because they will potentially build up to toxic levels.

In some cases, a food or drug is a potent inducer of another in a particular pathway. For example, carbamazepine is an inducer of the CYP 3A. This induction accelerates the production of enzymes available to break down the substrates requiring the CYP 3A enzyme, such as alprazolam. The outcome is a decrease in the latter substance (alprazolam) as it is broken down faster, decreasing its bioavailability. The patient who is receiving alprazolam and is also taking carbamazepine will experience a minimal effect of the alprazolam. Another example occurs when carbamazepine (Tegretol) is given to a patient who is taking haloperidol (Haldol), which is converted more quickly and there is less in the blood available for the targeted purpose (Sandson, 2013). A particular case of food–drug interaction occurs when processed or aged cheeses, wines, or processed foods are combined with monoamine oxidase inhibitors (MAOIs) used in the treatment of depression, such as phenelzine (Nardil) or tranylcypromine (Parnate), resulting in severe reactions including death from a hypertensive crisis (Edmunds, 2010). A list of substrates, inhibitors, and inducers of CYP450 can be found at the FDA website.

Pause and Reflect

1. What is the difference between a receptor agonist and a receptor antagonist?
2. What information about food and drug interactions would you want to provide to someone taking psychotropic drugs?

Pharmacotherapy

Pharmacotherapy refers to the clinical application of medications to disorders. Recognition and treatment of mental health issues has progressed from treating a specific disease to addressing neurotransmitter–receptor issues, brain circuits, genetics, and signal transduction cascades. The outcome is that as more intricate details of the neurological workings of the brain are discovered, individual medication categories may be used to treat more than one dysfunction process. The FDA has evaluated research and given approval for medications to treat mental health issues, but as medications become available, it takes time to build a body of research, so medications are often prescribed off-label, based on clinical knowledge and support in the absence of FDA approval. In the sections that follow, clinical application principles for use of medications across disease states are discussed. A medication category may be prescribed for the treatment, management, or resolution of several symptoms or disease states.

Antidepressants

Antidepressants are medications used to treat a variety of disorders, including depression, anxiety, symptoms of depression associated with eating disorders, bipolar disorder, and psychosis. They may also be used to treat pain, headaches, neuropathy, sleep apnea, and dermatologic disorders. Depression is associated with affective, behavioral, cognitive, and somatic symptoms. The prominent symptoms of depression include sleep disturbance, lack of interest, feelings of guilt or worthlessness, decreased energy, poor concentration, reduced appetite, a slowing of movement as in fatigue, or acceleration as in restlessness, anhedonia, irritability, anxiety, and, in some cases, suicidal ideation (APA, 2013; Carlat, 2011). These symptoms are related to the dysregulation of the serotonin, norepinephrine, and dopamine neurotransmitters.

Medications prescribed to treat depressive symptoms target the serotonergic, noradrenergic, and dopaminergic brain circuit pathways. Several categories of antidepressants are available to address the dysregulation of these neurotransmitter brain circuits: tricyclic antidepressants (TCAs), SSRIs, SNRIs, NRI/NDRIs, alpha-2 antagonists and serotonin/norepinephrine disinhibitors (SNDIs), serotonin antagonist/reuptake inhibitiors (SARIs), and MAOIs (Stahl, 2011). Although their precise mechanism is unknown, what is recognized is that SSRIs, SNRIs, NRI/NDRIs, and TCAs all work by preventing the presynaptic reuptake of serotonin, norepinephrine, and/or dopamine by blocking the presynaptic transporter (dopamine transporter [DAT], norepinephrine transporter [NET], or serotonin transporter [SERT]). MAO is an enzyme that participates in the presynaptic breakdown of serotonin, norepinephrine, and dopamine *after* it has been released to the synaptic cleft and returned to the presynaptic neuron by the reuptake valve. MAOIs work by interfering with the enzyme that would breakdown these three neurotransmitters, thereby keeping more of these three neurotransmitters available for release for postsynaptic receptor activation. SARIs both inhibit the presynaptic SERT and activate the postsynaptic serotonin receptor (Stahl, 2011; Stern et al., 2008; Schatzberg & Nemeroff, 2009; Sadock & Sadock, 2007).

In some cases, SSRIs can increase anxiety or produce agitation, restlessness, sexual dysfunction, insomnia, nausea, and, occasionally, weight gain. Some modifications to address or reduce side effects of SSRIs include the following:

- Adding a noradrenergic medication such as bupropion (Wellbutrin) can reduce sexual dysfunction.

- Adding a benzodiazepine or an adrenergic beta antagonist (such as propranolol) can reduce anxiety, agitation, or restlessness.

- Trazodone may be useful in treating resulting insomnia. If the patient becomes somnolent, a reduction in the medication should be considered.

An excess of serotonin can result in **serotonin syndrome**, observed as agitation, sweating, fever, tachycardia, hypotension, rigidity, and/or hyperreflexia (Boyer, Traub, & Grayzel, 2012). Serotonin syndrome can be fatal. Although it may occur with use of a single medication that increases serotonin levels, serotonin syndrome typically occurs when two or more medications are used concurrently. In addition to some psychotropic medications, certain medications used to treat migraines (for example, triptans such as sumatriptan [Imitrex], and valproic acid [Depakote]) and pain (such as cyclobenzaprine [Flexeril] and fentanyl [Duragesic]) may increase serotonin levels. Concurrent use of St. John's wort and/or medications that contain dextromethorphan (a common cough suppressant) with other medications that increase serotonin levels may result in serotonin syndrome.

Side effects typically associated with TCAs include those stated previously, as well as symptoms that occur as a result of cholinergic receptor blockade. *Anticholinergic effects* include a series of "dry-up" type symptoms such as constipation, urinary hesitancy or retention, dry mouth, and blurred vision. Additionally, patients on TCAs should be monitored for orthostatic hypotension, sedation, weight gain, and tachycardia. This side effect profile is often reported as the reason for medication discontinuance.

Patients taking MAOIs should be cautioned against taking other antidepressants, stimulants, opiates, or sympathomimetic medications. They should also be cautioned against consuming foods containing tyramine (processed milk, cheeses, aged meats, beans, beers and wines, soy, sauerkraut, and yogurt), which could pose a potential life-threatening hypertensive crisis. MAO breaks down tyramine in certain foods. When MAO is unavailable, elevated serum tyramine levels can lead to serious problems with hypertension, hyperpyrexia, tachycardia, diaphoresis, trembling, and cardiac dysrhythmias.

Anxiolytics

Antianxiety medications are used to treat a variety of disorders and symptoms, including anxiety, somatoform disorders, depression, insomnia, agitation, and extrapyramidal symptoms. Medications used to treat anxiety disorders include antidepressant SSRIs, SNRIs, and TCAs; benzodiazepines; and alpha-adrenergic agonists.

Anxiety is a normal human emotion that exists on a continuum from mild to severe, and whose responsibility is to alert the individual to the need for safety or the need to make some life adjustment. In some cases, however, anxiety may not simply be experienced as a general sense of uneasiness, but rather be experienced disproportionately to life events. Enduring symptoms can be sufficient to interfere with functioning. Anxiety is a neurochemical signaling in the brain that can become excessive and cause significant distress, or impairment in normal functioning influencing perceptions, memory, judgment, and motor responses (Guess, 2008). Several medical conditions (such as cardiovascular, respiratory, endocrine, neurologic and metabolic conditions, as well as substance abuse/dependency) mimic anxiety disorders and should be ruled out as potential causes of the anxious condition (Guess, 2008). Obtaining CBCs, chem studies, thyroid function tests, B_{12} levels, drug toxicity screening, CO_2, bicarbonate, and pH levels, as well as MRI, PET brain scans, and cerebrospinal fluid tests, can assist in ruling out metabolic causes of anxiety.

Anxiety can be experienced both in the mind, as anxiety disorders, and in the body, as somatoform disorders; thus, there are many symptoms and subtypes, as detailed in Chapters 13 and 14. The neurobiological cause of anxiety is largely considered to be a dysregulation of the gamma-aminobutyric acid (GABA) neurotransmitter–receptor complex found throughout the brain, the serotonergic and noradrenergic brain circuits, and the neuropeptide cholecystokinin. Structures of the brain recognized to be involved in anxiety symptoms include the limbic, thalamic, and hypothalamic structures of the central nervous system, as well as,

more specifically, the hippocampus in PTSD; the prefrontal cortex, caudate nuclei, and amygdala in OCD; and the temporal lobe in panic disorders (Sadock & Sadock, 2007; Schatzberg & Nemeroff, 2009; Stahl, 2013; Stern et al., 2008).

Dysregulation of the serotonergic brain circuit as a potential contributor to anxiety is treated with SSRIs. SSRIs (fluoxetine, fluvoxamine, paroxetine, certraline, citalopram, and escitalopram), which are considered first-line treatment for anxiety disorders, carry no risk of dependency and may take 2 to 4 weeks to reach symptom control; best results occur in combination with psychotherapy. These medications prevent the neurotransmitter serotonin (5HT) from being taken back up into the presynaptic neuron to be destroyed. This allows more serotonin to remain in the synaptic cleft between the pre- and postsynaptic neurons to be available for use on the serotonin postsynaptic neuron receptor. It is believed that allowing the serotonin brain circuit to function normally with sufficient serotonin can reduce anxiety disorder symptoms.

The locus ceruleus, located in the brainstem, is a noradrenergic site that has demonstrated the potential to initiate panic when stimulated, and calm when blocked. The associated neurotransmitter is norepinephrine. Tricyclic antidepressants have shown efficacy in quieting this circuit (Sadock & Sadock, 2007). Their side effects typically affect medication compliance. Other noradrenergic medications, such as the alpha-agonists clonidine and guanfacine, work on alpha-adrenergic sites to reduce norepinephrine activation. These are often used in children. Antidepressant SNRIs (venlafaxine, duloxetine) affect both the serotonergic and noradrenergic brain circuit pathways and thus can reduce anxiety symptoms through two pathways. SNRIs may take several weeks for symptom resolution, but typically have tolerable side effect profiles and do not cause dependence.

The GABA complex is the brain's inhibiting or quieting system in which the benzodiazepine receptor is found. Medications such as benzodiazepines potentiate GABA, thereby opening chloride channels and inhibiting brain excitement or activity. Because of their short half-life, benzodiazepines such as alprazolam and lorazepam require more frequent dosing, carry a risk for withdrawal symptoms or rebound anxiety, and are accompanied by a greater risk for addiction. Benzodiazepines with longer half-life (for example, clonazepam and diazepam), require less frequent dosing, and patients experience less withdrawal or rebound anxiety but still can develop dependence (Baldwin et al., 2013; Stahl, 2011). Because of their cerebral inhibition properties, anxiolytic medications, primarily benzodiazepines, are also used to reduce agitation and treat or terminate seizures, and also combine with typical antipsychotic D_2 antagonist medications to reduce extrapyramidal symptoms.

Medications used to reduce anxiety disorders should be considered short-term interventions while other remedies can be found. They typically do not prevent the cause of anxiety, but offer a temporary solution. Nonpharmacologic management includes behavioral therapies such as systematic desensitization, exposure therapy, relaxation therapy, biofeedback, cognitive–behavioral therapy, interpersonal therapies, and self-help groups.

Mood Stabilizers

Mood disturbances—extremes of emotional highs and lows, sometimes exhibiting in sudden swings or rapid cycles—are seen in treatment-resistant depression, bipolar disorder, and schizoaffective disorder. Mood stabilizers include antiepileptics and lithium.

Antiepileptics

Antiepileptics, also known as anticonvulsants or mood stabilizers, work to balance neurotransmission, thereby maintaining a consistent mood. Antiepileptics raise the seizure threshold to reduce the opportunity or occurrence of seizure activity in the brain, which is associated with an excitotoxic effect that can damage the brain. Similarly, cerebral excitement can lead to a **kindling** process in which cerebral voltage channels become overexcited and overfire, resulting in excesses of neurotransmission. Kindling can lead to the exaggerations of affect, behavior, and cognitive alterations recognized in bipolar disorder and psychosis. Multiple theories exist regarding the cause of mood cycling shifts. Most theorists agree that there is general neurotransmitter dysregulation resulting in an increase of noradrenergic activity, dysregulation of GABA, abnormalities in voltage-gated ion channels, irregularities in intracellular and extracellular levels of neurotransmitters, dysfunction in the neuronal membrane sensitivity thresholds, and neuronal firing without stimuli (Guess, 2008).

The antiepileptics prescribed for mood and seizure stabilization include valproic acid, carbamazepine, oxcarbazepine, lamotragine, gabapentin, topiramate, levatiracetam, and zonisamide. Benzodiazepines have also been used for mild antiepileptic action and include diazepam and clonazepam. In general, antiepileptic medications exert their effects by primarily blocking the sodium channel or some calcium channels, or enhancing GABA. They target $GABA_A$ receptors, GAT-1 GABA transporters, and GABA transaminase (Stahl, 2011; Stern et al., 2008).

Valproic acid should be monitored for trough serum blood levels between 50 and 125 mcg/mL because of the potential for toxicity. Liver and pancreatic functions should be monitored. Commonly reported side effects include weight gain, alopecia, and hand tremors. Carbamazepine should be monitored for trough serum blood levels between 6 and 12 mcg/mL. Routine CBCs should be examined for agranulocytosis and aplastic anemia, low white blood count (WBC), and low platelets, and liver function tests should be done. Side effects common to both valproic acid and carbamazepine include nausea, drowsiness, dry mouth, and blurred vision. Lamotrogine does not require a serum blood level, but should be monitored for leukopenia and the life-threatening Stevens-Johnson rash. Patients taking topiramate should be monitored for kidney stones and glaucoma, patients taking oxcarbazepine for hyponatremia, patients taking levatiracetem for anemia and leukopenia, and patients taking zonisamide for kidney stones, elevated creatinine and BUN, anemia, agnranulocytosis, and Stevens-Johnson rash. Antiepileptic and benzodiazepine medications are considered teratogenic and should be avoided, especially during the first trimester of pregnancy. Patients should be warned that these medications may interfere with the effectiveness of oral birth control.

Lithium

Lithium is an established gold standard for the treatment of mania in bipolar disorder. It is a salt ion that works intracellularly on G proteins and enzymes, stabilizing serotonin, dopamine, and acetylcholine and decreasing norepinephrine. Routine serum lithium levels are required owing to the high incidence of toxicity. The trough serum blood level of the medication should range between 0.5 and 1.0 mEq/L. Thyroid (hypothyroidism) and kidney (creatinine, BUN) functions should be routinely monitored, as lithium can be toxic to these organ systems. Lithium can also interfere with sodium and water regulation in the body, as the kidney cannot distinguish between dietary sodium and lithium. Patients should be counseled to drink sufficient water and avoid overheating. Sweating, dehydration, and vomiting can lead to elevated levels of lithium, which can lead to lithium toxicity as the body retains the lithium to maintain normal fluid and electrolyte balance. Signs of lithium toxicity include thirst, diarrhea, vomiting, drowsiness, muscle weakness, slurred speech, confusion, and alterations in coordination. These symptoms can occur with a lithium level of 1.5 mEq/L and above. Lithium toxicity can lead to coma, renal failure, and death. Always assess for symptoms; do not rely solely on lab values.

Antipsychotics

Antipsychotics are used to treat the instability of affect and cognition in disorders such as depression, bipolar disorder, schizophrenia, other types of psychosis, delirium, dementia, agitation, and aggression. Psychosis may be manifested by illusions, hallucinations, delusions, disorganized thinking, disorganized speech, paranoid or grandiose self-referential thinking, and disorientation from reality. The current scientific thought is that during psychosis there is a dysfunction primarily in the dopamine brain circuit pathway, as well as dysregulation in other brain circuits, including glutamate. There are currently no medications to regulate glutamate in the brain, but a few are being investigated in the pharmaceutical pipeline. Excessive dopamine neurotransmitter in the dopamine mesolimbic pathway is believed to cause positive psychotic symptoms, whereas a depletion of dopamine in the mesocortical pathway, and a general decrease in serotonin in serotonin pathways, can cause negative depressive symptoms. An excess of glutamate plays a role in the excitation experienced, and decreased GABA prevents the brain from being able to calm or still itself.

First-Generation Antipsychotics

First-generation antipsychotics are known by many names: D_2 antagonists, D_2 blockers, D_2 inhibitors, conventional antipsychotics, neuroleptics, and typical antipsychotics. These include, but are not limited to, haloperidol, chlorpromazine, fluphenazine, perphenazine, loxapine, and thiothixene (Stahl, 2011; Wilson, Shannon, & Shields, 2013). The action of a D_2 antagonist is to decrease dopamine along all dopamine pathways. The anticipated result is that once the excessive dopamine is reduced in the mesolimbic pathway, symptoms of psychosis will decrease, and thoughts will be more clearly based in reality.

Antipsychotic medication doses sometimes must be raised to adequately reduce dopamine level in the mesolimbic dopamine pathway to assist the patient with clarity of thought. Along the way, as the D_2 antagonist is blocking dopamine in the mesolimbic pathway to resolve psychosis, it is also blocking dopamine along the other pathways. As dopamine is blocked on the mesocortical pathway, the reduction in dopamine in this pathway can cause increased depressive symptoms. There is a reciprocal relationship between dopamine and acetylcholine in the nigrostriatal dopamine pathway in the basal ganglia. As dopamine is blocked on the nigrostriatal pathway, there can be an acetylcholine surge, resulting in **extrapyramidal symptoms** (EPS) (akathisia, akinesia, dystonia, tardive dyskinesia [TD], or pseudoparkinsonism). There is also a reciprocal relationship between dopamine and prolactin in the tuberoinfundibular dopamine pathway in the hypothalamus. Dopamine released at this location regulates secretion of prolactin from the anterior pituitary gland in the brain. As dopamine is blocked in the tuberoinfundibular dopamine pathway in the hypothalamus, the anterior pituitary is signaled to release prolactin, which results in hyperprolactinemia. This leads to galactorrhea (lactation in both men and women), gynocomastia (breast enlargement), amenorrhea, and sexual side effects. It is also important to watch for anticholinergic side effects of antipsychotic medications, such as constipation, urine retention, dry mouth, dizziness, and blurred vision.

Extrapyramidal side effects include the following:

- *Akathisia* is the inability to sit still, and includes rocking, pacing, and/or restlessness. Individuals with akathisia will report this as emanating from the body. Akathisia is a drastically uncomfortable feeling and often very difficult to endure.

- *Akinesia* is the absence of movement, difficulty initiating movement, or the lack of motivation to move; it is not the same as disinterest in moving or laziness.

- *Dystonia* is a spasticity of a muscle group, a muscle spasm of typically a back or neck muscle, and is quite painful.

- *Pseudoparkinsonian* symptoms look just like those of Parkinson disease, as both occur for the same neurological reason, but each has a different root cause. In Parkinson disease, the cause is organic disruption in the basal ganglia. In **pseudoparkinsonism** EPS, the disruption is caused by the antipsychotic medication blockade of dopamine in the basal ganglia, resulting in acetylcholine increases. The symptoms will look the same as those of Parkinson disease and include motor slowing or tremors, pill rolling, muscle rigidity, masklike facial expressions, shuffling gait, and slowing of speech. Patients typically do not recognize these symptoms coming on and are not particularly bothered by the symptoms.

- *Tardive dyskinesia (TD)* is an involuntary and potentially irreversible abnormal muscle movement of the mouth, tongue, face, and jaw areas, which may progress to the limbs. TD can be extremely disfiguring and create problems with social interactions.

When patients are taking psychotropic medications, it is important to evaluate them regularly using a scale to detect unusual movements. The Abnormal Involuntary Movement Scale (AIMS) was designed in the 1970s to measure involuntary movements and is still in use today (Chapter 17). All EPS can be treated with anticholinergics (benztropine and trihexyphenidyl). Diphenhydramine may be used for all of these symptoms except akathisia, as it may increase this. Beta-blockers such as propranolol or the alpha-2 agonist clonidine may be useful in treating akathisia. The dopamine agonist amantadine may be useful in treating akinesia and pseudoparkinsonism. The anxiolytic benzodiazepines clonazepam and lorazepam may be useful for their skeletal muscle relaxant properties in reducing akathisia and dystonia. TD can occur at any point in antipsychotic medication treatment, and there is no pharmacologic treatment except to switch to another antipsychotic (Guess, 2008; Sadock & Sadock, 2007; Schatzberg & Nemeroff, 2009; Stahl, 2011; Stern et al., 2008).

Another side effect of antipsychotic medications is **neuroleptic malignant syndrome** (NMS), a rare but potentially life-threatening neurological response to medications that can occur at any point in treatment. Lithium, anticholinergics, and serotonergic agents can lead to NMS as well (Wijdicks, Aminoff, & Wilterdink, 2013).

Symptoms include an alteration in sensory process, cognitive changes that may look like delirium, hyperthermia, hyperreflexia, muscle rigidity, autonomic instability, hypotension, tachycardia, tachypnea, diaphoresis, and sialorrhea (hypersalivation). NMS and serotonin syndrome are difficult to distinguish. Patients with serotonin syndrome are typically found on an antidepressant and demonstrate shivering, myoclonus, and ataxia, and perhaps some nausea, vomiting, and diarrhea (Boyer, Traub, & Grayzel, 2012; Wijdicks, Aminoff, & Wilterdink, 2013). In NMS, look for the four Ts: temperature (elevated), tone (muscle rigidity/exaggerated reflexes), tension (hypotension), and tachy (tachycardia, tachypnea) (Ramaswamy, Malik, & Dewan, 2013). Rapid recognition and treatment is essential. Labs are drawn to look for elevated creatine phosphokinase (CPK), elevated white blood count (leukocytosis), elevated liver functions (lactate dehydrogenase, alkaline phosphatase, liver transaminase), electrolyte abnormalities (hypocalcemia, hypomagnesemia, hypo/hypernatremia, hyperkalemia), and metabolic acidosis and anemia (low iron). NMS is typically treated with dantrolene (direct-acting skeletal muscle relaxant), bromocriptine (dopamine agonist), amantadine (NMDA receptor antagonist with dopamine agonist and anticholinergic effects), and, anecdotally, with apomorphine, carbamazepine, and the benzodiazepines lorazepam or clonazepam (Wijdicks, Aminoff, & Wilterdink, 2013).

Second-Generation Antipsychotics

Progression in psychopharmacology has led to the evolution of second-generation antipsychotics (SGAs), also known as *atypical antipsychotics* or *serotonin–dopamine antagonists*. First introduced in the 1990s, these have fewer neuromuscular side effects than conventional D_2 blockers and treat both negative and positive psychotic symptoms. They include clozapine, quetiapine, olanzapine, risperidone, ziprasidone, aripiprazole, iloperidone, asenapine, and lurasidone. SGAs work on the dopamine pathways, just as D_2 inhibitors do. SGAs block dopamine in the mesolimbic pathway, where there are fewer serotonin receptors, thereby reducing psychosis and returning mental clarity. As serotonin inhibits dopamine in some areas of the brain, blocking the ability of serotonin to inhibit dopamine in the mesocortical dopamine pathway in the prefrontal cortex will allow more dopamine to be present in these areas, thereby reducing depressive symptoms and improving mood. It is also believed that SGAs work similarly in the nigrostriatal dopamine pathway by limiting the reduction in dopamine, preventing the cholinergic surge responsible for EPSs. It is also believed that SGAs work similarly in the tuberinfundibular dopamine pathway by limiting the reduction in dopamine, preventing the release of prolactin responsible for endocrine sexual side effects (Kuroki, Nagao, & Nakahara, 2008). Unfortunately, when higher doses of an SGA are required for effective treatment of psychosis, the advantage to using the SGA may be lost, as the side effect profile may become much like that of first-generation antipsychotics.

Anticholinesterases

For degenerative cognitive processes, in particular the major neurocognitive disorders (such as the various dementias, including Alzheimer disease, vascular dementia, and Lewy body dementia), multiple neurotransmitter dysfunctions occur. The results include impaired executive functioning, global intellect, problem solving, and organizational skills, as well as alteration in memory. Diagnosis involves determining the presence of both cognitive and memory impairment in the presence of aphasia, apraxia, agnosia, or the more global disturbance of executive functioning and investigating possible biological etiologies (for example, head trauma, HIV, or Parkinson disease). In addition to these cognitive symptoms, the individual may experience personality changes and require symptomatic treatment for depression, anxiety, insomnia, psychosis, and agitation.

No therapies are currently available to reverse or retard the progression of any dementia. Each of the dementias involves a unique neurological insult and has a different time progression profile, but they all share similar end results. As acetylcholine, norepinephrine, dopamine, and serotonin neurotransmitter levels diminish, brain functioning capacity also diminishes. A deficiency in cholinergic activity (muscarinic and nicotinic receptors; acetylcholine neurotransmitters) has been shown to impair memory (Stahl, 2013). If this trend can be recognized early, neurotransmitter support can be provided with medications that replenish diminishing neurotransmitters. The most common drugs are the cholinesterase inhibitors tacrine (Cognex), donepezil (Aricept), revastigmine (Exelon), and galantamine (Reminyl). These drugs have been used to cause several effects: presynaptically increase acetylcholine; postsynaptically activate the cholinergic receptor; and reduce the presynaptic reuptake and breakdown of acetylcholine. The result is to provide more acetylcholine in the synapse to be available for the postsynaptic acetylcholine receptor (Stahl, 2011, 2013; Wilson, Shannon, & Shields, 2013). Another line of thinking considers that cognitive deficiency may be the result, in part, of plaque and neurofibrillary tangles igniting glutamatergic excitation, which results in a neurotoxic inflammatory response. N-methyl d-aspartate glutamate receptor antagonist (NMDA) (memantine [Namenda]) accomplishes this by reducing activation of glutamate neurotransmission (Sadock & Sadock, 2007; Schatzberg & Nemeroff, 2009; Stahl, 2011; Stern et al., 2008). The introduction of these medications can slow, but not stop, the progression of the disease.

Antidepressants may be used to treat emerging depression or anxiety in patients with dementia. To treat emerging psychotic symptoms such as hallucinations, delusions, and paranoia, antipsychotics may be prescribed. Mood stabilizers may be prescribed to reduce affective instability and abate aggressive episodes. Although benzodiazepines can be useful in calming, sedating, and reducing anxiety, they may also induce delirium or worsen already diminishing cognitive capacities.

Sleep–Wake and Attention Promoters

Managing the balance between drowsy and alert or sleep and wake states is a delicate effort involving brain circuits, lobes of the brain, and the endocrine system. A sleep–wake disturbance is often reported as a problematic symptom in several mental health disease processes (Chapter 12).

Sleep is an active process of neuronal circuit exchanges initiated and terminated in different areas of the brain. Higgins and George (2013) state that the brain's ascending arousal circuits that govern sleep and wakefulness was first identified in 1949. The reticular activating system houses a group of neurons in the midline of the brainstem that arouse and sedate. The research that followed further identified five important cell body nuclei and neurotransmitters involved: cholinergic neurons, noradrenergic neurons, serotoninergic

neurons, dopaminergic neurons, and histaminergic neurons (Schatzberg & Nemeroff, 2009; Stahl, 2013; Stern et al., 2008). All five types of neurons are active during periods of wakefulness and arousal. The cholinergic neurotransmitters are quiet during the first four stages of sleep and activate during stage-five REM sleep. The other four monoamine neurotransmitter systems remain quiet during all five stages of sleep. Also playing a prominent role is GABA, the chief inhibitory neurotransmitter in the brain, which is responsible for opening and closing potassium-chloride ion channels in the brain. When the tuberomammilary nuceleus (TMN) of the hypothalamus is activated, histamine is released in the cortex to awaken, and in the ventrolateral preoptic (VLPO) nucleus of the hypothalamus to inhibit sleep. When the VLPO of the hypothalamus is activated, GABA is released in the TMN and VLPO and sleep is induced (Stahl, 2013).

Before medications are considered for sleep restoration, behavioral interventions for maintaining good sleep hygiene habits should be established (Chapter 12). Good sleep hygiene behaviors inform neurotargets in the brain to follow their natural circadian rhythm. Other behavioral methods include cognitive–behavioral therapy, relaxation training, and sleep restriction therapy (Chanin, 2012). Although these routines influence neurotransmitter activity, behavioral interventions should always be implemented before medications are considered for sleep cycle restoration.

When medication is necessary to induce or maintain sleep, the cause of sleep disturbance is examined. Medications are used to create drowsiness so one can fall asleep, ameliorate a cause of sleep interference, target a particular aspect of sleep, or induce sleep. Nonselective benzodiazepines, such as triazolam (Halcion) and temazepam (Restoril), bind to four of the six $GABA_{A1,2,3,5}$ subunits, causing sedation, a reduction in anxiety, muscle relaxation, and addictive side effects (Stahl, 2011; Wilson, Shannon, & Shields, 2013). Because of the multiciplicity of these effects, tolerance, dependence, and withdrawal effects can occur. The more popular and expensive nonbenzodiazepine–benzodiazepine A agonist medications, such as eszopiclone (Lunesta) and zolpidem (Ambien), work by selectively binding to the $GABA_{A1}$ receptors to induce sleep (Stahl, 2011; Wilson, Shannon, & Shields, 2013). They are reported to be good at inducing sleep, but less effective in sleep maintenance unless given in a sustained-release form. These do not appear to be habit or tolerance forming, but psychological reliance can occur. Side effects include hallucinations and amnesia, so precautions should be taken that the patient be directed to take the medication immediately upon going to bed and not a time before. Flumazenil, a benzodiazepine receptor antagonist, can reverse the side effects of selective and nonselective benzodiazepines (Stahl, 2011; Wilson, Shannon, & Shields, 2013).

Ramelteon (Rozerem), a newer medication on the market and the first melatonin receptor agonist, promotes sleep by selectively binding to the melatonin receptor sites in the superchiasmatic nucleus (SCN). TCAs, SNRIs, and SSRIs accomplish the task of sleep promotion through their effect on the adrenergic, serotonergic, dopaminergic, and histaminic neurotransmitter circuits. Because of their adrenergic properties, the TCAs must be closely monitored. Trazodone has strong antihistaminic effects that induce sedation. Serotonin–dopamine antagonists (SGAs), such as quetiapine (Seroquel), can also have a strong histaminic sleep-inducing effect (Stahl, 2011; Wilson, Shannon, & Shields, 2013). SSRIs stabilize the melatonin and serotonin balance, thereby balancing the sleep–wake circadian rhythm. Over-the-counter (OTC) antihistamines can be used to promote sleep by inducing drowsiness or by increasing melatonin (a hormone typically produced by the pineal gland in the brain in response to darkness). These medications have not shown dependence or abuse potential. Antihistamines can sometimes cause behavioral disinhibition in some individuals and may cause excitation or insomnia. It should be remembered that melatonin is a hormone and interacts with other endocrine functions.

When the VPLO circuit is overactive, the individual experiences reduced alertness, poor concentration, excessive drowsiness, narcolepsy or attention deficit hyperactivity disorder, When this happens agents to promote alertness and attention may be useful. It is thought that modafinil stimulates histamine, dopamine, serotonin, and norepinephrine in the brain, having prominent effects in the TMN. Stimulants (such as caffeine, modafinil [Provigil], and methylphenidate [Ritalin, Adderall]) affect the same neurotransmitter systems, each a little differently. Specifically, for the treatment of attention deficit hyperactivity disorder, dextroamphetamine, methylphenidate, amphetamine, or atomoxetine is prescribed. Methylphenidate and amphetamine accomplish their mission by initiating the presynaptic release and reuptake of norepinephrine, dopamine, and serotonin purported to result in a stabilization of brain circuits. Atomoxetine is a nonstimulant SNRI. For those who do not fully respond, an antidepressant may also be prescribed.

Nursing Management

Nursing management of patients taking psychotropic drugs varies according to the medication prescribed and the patient's personal history. Psychotropic medications are powerful molecules that change brain function and affect every body system. Some principles hold true across patient populations and regardless of medications prescribed. The nurse must assess the patient's past and current medication history, including history of adherence to previous treatment regimens, drug reactions and interactions, presence of co-morbid illnesses, and presence of any known contraindications or allergies. The nurse must also assess for use of other prescribed, OTC, and complementary medications and supplements to identify possible risks for adverse effects. Assessing for substance use and abuse is essential to prepare for potential withdrawal symptoms.

Diagnosis and planning incorporate the patient's priority needs as assessed by the nurse and reported by the patient or caregiver. The nurse must be alert for potential erroneous diagnoses that may affect the success of a given medication regimen. Often, patients receive five to seven diagnoses before the correct one is identified. In the meantime, patients suffer with needless side effects that could have been prevented. The nurse needs to be diligent in uncovering collateral information that will assist in proper diagnosis.

Interventions incorporated in the care plan for patients participating in psychopharmacotherapy include patient education related to the reasons for taking the medication, mechanism of action, potential side effects and adverse effects, drug–drug and drug–food interactions, and issues related to adherence (including modifications to reduce side effects and discontinuation syndrome). Side effects that need to be reported immediately include all types of allergic responses, changes in gastrointestinal functioning, changes in mental status, and changes in behavior and ability to participate in therapeutic interactions.

Most important, the nurse is the last person to provide a check and balance between diagnosis, prescription, and the pharmacy filling the prescription. The nurse should never hesitate to question any aspect about any psychiatric medication prescribed for a patient in any setting prior to administering the medication. The nurse is the link between the patient and the prescriber and, as such, has a tremendous responsibility for the welfare of patients who are prescribed psychotropic medications.

Pause and Reflect

1. *As a nurse, what is your responsibility when you have a question about a medication that is prescribed for a patient?*
2. *What information should patient education related to psychotropic medications include?*

Chapter Highlights

1. The ABCs of psychiatry (affect, attitude, behavior, and cognition) play an important role in the assessment and treatment of patients with psychiatric disorders.

2. The nurse has a legal responsibility to exercise good professional judgment in carrying out psychotropic medication orders.

3. Absorption refers to the way a medication enters and passes through the body. Distribution describes a medication's journey through the circulatory system to body tissues, where target and side effects are expressed. Metabolism is the enzymatic process of breaking down a medication until it becomes inactive and is eliminated. Elimination refers to the excretion of a drug's chemical by-products as waste.

4. The blood–brain barrier protects the brain and spinal cord by preventing substances in the blood from diffusion out of cerebral capillaries.

5. Drug molecule ligands bind to protein receptors in neuron cells to initiate the drug's chemical reactions.

6. An agonist is a drug that is intended to produce the same natural response as that of the body. A drug antagonist inhibits or blocks a natural response or chemical action. A drug ligand molecule that has a weaker chemical action and elicits only a modest or partial response is referred to as a partial agonist or partial antagonist.

7. Drug reactions include target effects, which occur when a medication reaches the target site and produces a desired or intended response; side effects, which are additional actions that occur when a medication interacts with neurotransmitters at sites other than the target site; and adverse effects, which are harmful, unexpected, or emergent reactions to a drug.

8. Medications taken orally travel through the digestive tract to the liver and are broken down in the first pass effect, which may inactivate the medication.

NCLEX®-RN Questions

1. The nurse is documenting an evaluation of a patient who has been taking psychotropic medications using an assessment template that includes the ABCs of psychiatry. Under which domain would the nurse enter observations related to the finding of akathisia?
   a. A: Attitude
   b. A: Affect/mood
   c. B: Behavior
   d. C: Cognition

2. The registered nurse is working in an acute care inpatient psychiatric setting. With regard to psychotropic medications, which aspects of role function would the nurse be prepared to carry out? Select all that apply.
   a. Monitoring diagnostic findings, such as therapeutic drug levels
   b. Reviewing medication orders to ensure the accuracy of details
   c. Exercising appropriate judgment in the administration of medication
   d. Selecting appropriate therapies based on an assessment of diagnostic findings
   e. Evaluating and documenting patient response for desired and untoward effects

3. The nurse is administering a selective serotonin-reuptake inhibitor (SSRI) to the patient experiencing anxiety. The patient complains of gastric distress following the administration of the medication. The nurse recommends that the patient take a small amount of food with the medication. Which best represents the rationale for this action?
   a. Food contains lipids that enhance the breakdown of fat-soluble medications.
   b. Food reduces the impact of the SSRI-targeting serotonin receptors in the gut.
   c. Food contains proteins required to facilitate efficient gut-to-plasma absorption.
   d. Food contains enzymes that are necessary for the proper elimination of the drug.

4. The nurse is caring for a patient who has been self-medicating with an herbal agent. The patient states that the product claims to have natural agents that regulate neurotransmitter function in the brain. The nurse researches the agent and learns that clinical studies demonstrate that the oral formulation does not cross the blood–brain barrier. Based on this finding, which information would be best for the nurse to provide to the patient?
   a. The agent cannot be properly metabolized and may build up in the body.
   b. The agent cannot be transported to the target site and will be ineffective.
   c. The agent cannot be effectively eliminated and may cause injury to the brain.
   d. The agent may need to be taken in larger doses to cross the semipermeable membrane.

5. The nurse educator is explaining the role of the ligand molecule in activating a cell receptor protein. Which statement is accurate?
   a. Drug receptor proteins are activated by the ligand.
   b. The ligand is responsible for doing the job of the cell.
   c. The ligand usually acts as a neurobiological off switch.
   d. All ligands are intended to elicit a similar cellular response.

6. The nurse is caring for a patient who is receiving an opioid agonist. Which principle(s) would the nurse consider when caring for the patient? Select all that apply.
   a. As long as receptor sites are free, the drug will maintain efficacy over time.
   b. The action of the drug may be reversed by the administration of an antagonist agent.
   c. The number of available receptor sites may determine the efficacy of the agonist agent.
   d. The ligand molecule will act on the receptor to block the natural neurochemical response.
   e. The repeated presentation of the drug to the receptor may lead to a diminished effect of the drug over time.

7. The nurse is administering psychotropic medications to a patient hospitalized in an inpatient unit. Which evaluation finding is most likely to indicate that the target effect of the medication has been achieved?
   a. The patient taking antianxiety medication experiences a paradoxical response.
   b. The patient taking antianxiety medication uses the medication only when needed.
   c. The patient taking an atypical antidepressant for insomnia experiences sedation at night.
   d. The patient taking antipsychotic medication for schizophrenia reports that symptoms of dry mouth have resolved.

8. The nurse is caring for the patient who is taking a medication that is a substrate of the CYP 1A enzyme. The nurse understands that the patient taking this medication with grapefruit juice is at increased risk for which outcome?
   a. Diminished efficacy of the medication
   b. Chemical inactivation of the medication
   c. Increased bioavailability of the medication
   d. An acceleration in the breakdown of substrates

9. The nurse is caring for a patient experiencing the early neurocognitive changes associated with dementia. The nurse anticipates that which class of medication would be used to support the function of neurotransmitters involved in memory?
   a. Cholinesterase inhibitors
   b. Tricyclic antidepressants
   c. Second-generation antipsychotics
   d. Benzodiazepine receptor agonists

Answers can be found on the Pearson student resource site: nursing.pearsonhighered.com

Pearson Nursing Student Resources Find additional review materials at **nursing.pearsonhighered.com**

References

American Academy of Child & Adolescent Psychiatry (AACAP). (2012). Facts for Families. Children's Sleep Problems. Publication #34. Available at http://www.aacap.org/galleries/FactsForFamilies/34_childrens_sleep_problems.pdf

American Psychiatric Association (APA). (2013). *Diagnostic and Statistical Manual of Mental Disorders* (5th ed.). Washington, DC: American Psychiatric Publishers.

American Psychiatric Association (APA). (2013). DSM-5: The Future of Psychiatric Diagnosis. Available at http://www.dsm5.org/

Baldwin, D. S., Aitchison, K., Bateson, A., Curran, H. V., Davies, S., Leonard, B., … Wilson, S. (2013). Benzodiazepines: Risks and benefits. A reconsideration. *Journal of Psychopharmacology, 27*(11), 967–971.

Bliwise, D. L. (1993). Sleep in normal aging and dementia. *Sleep, 16,* 40–81.

Boyer, E. W., Traub, S. J., & Grayzel, J. (2012). Serotonin syndrome. *UpToDate*, April 12. Available at http://www.uptodate.com/serotinin-syndrome

Carlat, D. J. (2011). *The Psychiatric Interview* (3rd ed.). Philadelphia, PA: Lippincott Williams & Wilkins.

Chanin, L. R. (2012). Drug treatments for sleep problems. Available at http://www.webmd.com/sleep-disorders/drug-treatments

Davies, S. J. C., & Nutt, D. (2007). Pharmacokinetics for psychiatrists. *Psychiatry*, 6(7): 268– 272.

Dawson, P. (2005). Sleep and adolescents. *Counseling, 101*, 11–15. Available at http://www.nasponline.org/resources/principals/Sleep%20Dosprders%20WEB.pdf

Dijk, D.-J. (2013). Sleep in children, sleep spindles, and the metrics of memory. *Journal of Sleep Research, 22*, 119–120.

Edmunds, M. W. (2010). *Introduction to Clinical Pharmacology* (6th ed.). St. Louis, MO: Mosby.

Fareed, A., Casarella, J., Amar, R., Vayalapalli, S., & Drexler, K. (2010). Methadone maintenance dosing guideline for opioid dependence. A literature review. *Journal of Addictive Diseases, 29*(1), 1–14.

Genung, V. (2012). Understanding the neurobiology, assessment, and treatment of substances of abuse and dependence: A guide for the critical care nurse. *Critical Care Nursing Clinics of North America, 24*(1), 117–130.

Guess, K. (2008). *Psychiatric-Mental Health Nurse Practitioner: Review and Resource Manual* (2nd ed.). Silver Spring, MD: American Nurses Credentialing Center. Available at www.nursecredentialing.org

Herlihy, B. (2010). *The Human Body in Health and Illness* (4th ed.). St. Louis, MO: W.B. Saunders Co.

Higgins, E. S., & George, M. S. (2013). *The Neuroscience of Clinical Psychiatry*. Philadelphia, PA: Wolters Kluwer-Lippincott Williams & Wilkins.

Kaplowitz, N. (2005). Idiosyncratic drug hepatotoxicity. *Nature Reviews-Drug Discovery, 4*, 489–499. Available at www.nature.com/reviews/drugdisc/

Kramer, T. A. (2003). Side effects and therapeutic effects. *Medscape General Medicine, 5*(1). Available at www.medscape.com/viewarticle/448250

Kuroki, T., Nagao, N., & Nakahara, T. (2008). Neuropharmacology of second-generation antipsychotic drugs: A validity of the serotonin-dopamine hypothesis. *Progress in Brain Research, 172*, 199–212. doi: 10.1016/S0079-6123(08)00910-2

Marc, D. T., Ailts, J. W., Ailts-Campeau, D. C., Bull, M. J., & Olson, K. L. (2011). Neurotransmitters excreted in the urine as biomarkers of nervous system activity: Validity and clinical applicability. *Neuroscience and Biobehavioral Reviews, 35*, 635–644.

National Institute of Health. (2010). Drug dependence. Available at http://www.ncbi.nlm.nih.gov/pubmedhealth/PMH0002490/

National Sleep Foundation. (2013a). Aging and sleep. Available at http://www.sleepfoundation.org/article/sleep-topics/aging-and-sleep

National Sleep Foundation. (2013b). Children and sleep. Available at http://www.sleepfoundation.org/article/sleep-topics/children-and-sleep

National Sleep Foundation. (2013c). Teens and sleep. Available at http://www.sleepfoundation.org/article/sleep-topics/teens-and-sleep

Neubauer, D. N. (1999). Sleep problems in the elderly. *American Family Physician, 59*(9), 2551–2558.

Neubauer, D. N., Smith, P. L., & Earley, C. J. (1999). Sleep disorders. In L. R. Barker, J. R. Burton, & P. D. Zieve, (Eds.). *Principles of Ambulatory Medicine*. Baltimore, MD: Williams & Wilkins, pp.1314–1328.

Ramaswamy, S., Malik, S., & Dewan, V. (2013). Tips to manage and prevent discontinuation syndromes. Neuroleptic Malignant Syndrome Information Service. Available at http://www.nmsis.org/content.asp?type=publications&src=pages/preventdiscontinuationsyndromes.asp&title=Tips+to+manage+and+prevent+discontinuation+syndromes

Sadock, B. J., & Sadock, V. A. (2007). *Kaplan & Sadock's Synopsis of Psychiatry* (10th ed.). New York, NY: Wolters Kluwer Lippincott Williams & Wilkins.

Sandson, N. B. (2013). Neurological and psychiatric drug interactions: The cytochrome P450 system and beyond. Available at http://www.aacc.org/SiteCollectionDocuments/ResourceCenters/ResourceLibrary/PharmacogenomicsResources/sandson__presentation.pdf

Sandson, N., Marcucci, C., Bourke, D. L., & Smith-Lamacchia, R. (2006). An interaction between aspirin and valproate: The relevance of plasma protein displacement drug–drug interactions. *American Journal of Psychiatry, 163*,1891–1896.

Schatzberg, A. F., & Nemeroff, C. B. (2009). *Textbook of Psychopharmacology* (4th ed.). Arlington, VA: American Psychiatric Publishing.

Scott, N., Blair, P. S., Emond, A. M., Fleming, P. J., Humphrey, J. S., Henderson, J., & Gringras, P. (2013). Sleep patterns in children with ADHD: A population-based cohort study from birth to 11 years. *Journal of Sleep Research, 22*, 121–128.

Selim, K., & Kaplowitz, N. (1999). Hepatotoxicity of psychotropic drugs. *Hepatology Concise Review, 29*(5), 1347–1351. Available at http://www.hepatitis-central.com/hcv/drugs/hepatotoxicity/cause.html

Stahl, S. (2011). *The Prescriber's Guide* (4th ed.). New York, NY: Cambridge University Press.

Stahl, S. (2013). *Stahl's Essential Psychopharmacology. Neuroscientific Basis and Practical Applications* (4th ed.). New York, NY: Cambridge University Press.

Stern, T. A., Rosenbaum, L. F., Fava, M., Biederman, J., & Rauch, S. L. (2008). *Comprehensive Clinical Psychiatry*. Philadelphia, PA: Mosby Elsevier.

U.S. Department of Health and Human Services, National Institutes of Health, National Institute of General Medical Sciences. (2011). *Medicines by Design*. NIH Publication No. 06474. Available at http://publications.nigms.nih.gov/medbydesign/chapter1.html

Wijdicks, E., Aminoff, M. J., & Wilterdink, J. L. (2013). Neuroleptic malignant syndrome. *UpToDate*, May 3. Available at http://www.uptodate.com/contents/neuroleptic-malignant-syndrome

Wilson, B. A., Shannon, M. T., & Shields, K. M. (2013). *Pearson Nurse's Drug Guide*. Upper Saddle River, NJ: Pearson Education.

Woo, T. M., & Wynne, A. L. (2011). *Pharmacotherapeutics for Nurse Practitioner Prescribers* (3rd ed.). Philadelphia, PA: F.A. Davis.

Zhou, J. (2006). Norepinephrine transporter inhibitors and their therapeutic potential. *Drugs Future, 29*(12): 1235–1244. Available at http://www.ncbi.nlm.nih.gov/pmc/articles/PMC1518795/

24 Group and Family Therapy

Vanya Hamrin

Key Terms

Learning Outcomes

1. Evaluate the curative factors that make group psychotherapy effective.

2. Compare different types of therapeutic groups.

3. Distinguish the stages of group development.

4. Examine the roles and responsibilities of group therapy leaders.

5. Differentiate among various roles assumed by members of therapeutic groups.

6. Describe some of the major theoretical frameworks from which to approach family therapy.

7. Plan a family assessment to identify family strengths and needs.

8. Contrast evidence-based family approaches to specific psychiatric disorders.

Introduction

Emotional healing happens in the context of meaningful interpersonal relationships. People need meaningful, reciprocal, positive interpersonal bonds for survival and emotional health. As a result, people participate in a variety of groups in formal and informal contexts: family and kinship relationships; groups of friends; social and spiritual groups, such as bands, choirs, supper groups, and reading groups; and work groups and committees. Each individual—nurse, patient, family member, or other health care professional—brings his or her own history of family and group relationships to the context of the health care environment.

Psychiatric disorders and their symptoms can be very stressful both for the individual experiencing symptoms and for family members and friends. Patients with mental illness often feel increasingly isolated, one of the many factors that increase their feelings of suffering and hopelessness. By engaging in psychotherapy with others, individuals with mental illness can begin to restore their abilities to engage in meaningful relationships, decreasing their sense of isolation and increasing feelings of hope and confidence. **Psychotherapy** refers to the treatment of mental illness using different types of therapies, as outlined in Chapter 4. **Group therapy** is a form of psychotherapy in which a group of individuals meet together under the guidance of a professionally trained therapist. The purpose of group therapy is to help group members learn about themselves and others in the group, improve their quality of life, learn to cope with illness, and develop improved interpersonal relationships (American Group Psychotherapy Association, 2011). **Family therapy** is a specific form of group therapy in which the group is the family unit.

Participation in group or family therapy may be voluntary or required. Required participation in psychotherapy typically occurs under a court order. Examples include required individual and family psychotherapy for parents who are struggling with their abilities to care for their children, or required group therapy for an individual with a substance use disorder who has resorted to engaging in criminal activity to pay for his or her addiction.

This chapter provides an overview of the theories behind and evidence supporting group and family psychotherapy, frequent issues that arise during therapy sessions, and the role of the nurse in group and family therapy.

Group Therapy

Group psychotherapy is an effective therapeutic intervention for a number of psychiatric disorders. Currently, group therapy is used in many contemporary inpatient hospital and outpatient settings because of both its demonstrated efficacy in the treatment of various mental health issues and its cost effectiveness (Burlingame, McKensie, & Strauss, 2004). Depending on the setting and the nurse's credentials and experiences, the nurse's role may be that of a leader or co-leader of group psychotherapy.

Emotional healing occurs in the context of interpersonal relationships developed in group psychotherapy. The goals of interpersonal group psychotherapy include the following:

- Creating a social microcosm to explore the way one relates to others in his or her world
- Developing distortion-free, gratifying interpersonal relationships
- Decreasing isolation

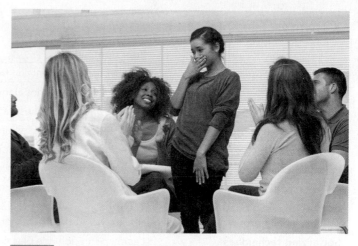

24-1 Group therapy is unique from other types of social groups in that direct, honest, open feedback is encouraged and explored in a safe, supportive environment.

Source: Wavebreakmedia/Shutterstock

- Obtaining feedback about oneself from multiple perspectives
- Learning new skills
- Decreasing psychiatric symptoms

Group therapy provides participants with both the opportunity to learn about the way they relate to others and the opportunity to make changes in the way they relate to others so they may have more meaningful interpersonal encounters (Yalom & Leszcz, 2005). Group therapy is unique from other types of social groups in that direct, honest open feedback is encouraged and explored in a safe, supportive environment (Figure 24-1). This helps participants make changes in the way they relate to others in their lives based on the feedback they receive from group members. The social microcosm of the group reflects that individuals will behave toward members of the group in the same way they relate to others in their world.

Curative Factors of Group Therapy

Irvin Yalom describes the important therapeutic factors that enhance healing in interpersonal relationships that can occur through group psychotherapy (Yalom & Leszcz, 2005). These include instilling hope in the patients that therapy will be helpful and imparting a sense of **universality** to all patients so they understand that they are not alone or unique in their suffering (Table 24-1).

Cohesiveness, the extent to which group members share a common sense of belonging or purpose, has been shown to be an important therapeutic factor in various types of groups (see Evidence-Based Practice: Cohesion). In addition to cohesiveness and other curative factors, the strengths of the group leader and the motivation of individual group members affect the group's trajectory. Group therapy has proven to be successful in a variety of settings, as evidenced by a meta-analysis of the differential effect of group psychotherapy in 111 experimental studies. Studies that compare active group treatment to wait-list controls have demonstrated that the average recipient of group treatment is better off than 72% of the untreated controls. Homogeneous groups attained more improvement than heterogeneous groups, outpatient groups outperformed inpatient groups, and mixed-gender groups had higher gains than all-male groups. In looking at diagnostic categories, the researchers

Curative Factors of Group Therapy

table 24-1

Factor	Function
Instillation of hope	A belief that treatment can be effective
Universality	The idea that one is not alone or unique in suffering
Cohesiveness	A sense of connectedness among group members and the group leader
Imparting meaningful information	Members benefit from helping others by sharing meaningful information
Altruism	The effect of feeling good about having something to offer or helping other members of the group
Imitative behavior	Members learning how to cope by observing others modeling new behaviors or skills
Interpersonal learning	The process of learning about oneself based on the feedback of other group members
Corrective recapitulation of the primary family group	The process in which individuals may act out their relationship with members of the group in a similar way to their behavior in their own family system
Socializing techniques	Learning through role play or learning from the way another group member handles a situation
Catharsis	Being able to share feelings and experiences and not hold them in
Existential factors	Being able to take full responsibility for one's own actions regardless of the level of support one has or receives

Adapted from Yalom, I. D., & Leszcz, M. (2005). *The Theory and Practice of Group Psychotherapy* (5th ed.). New York, NY: Basic Books.

found that patients with depression or eating disorders improved significantly more from group therapy than patients with other medical or stress-related conditions (Burlingame, Fuhriman, & Mosier, 2003).

Types of Therapeutic Groups

As stated earlier, psychotherapy groups (sometimes referred to as psychodynamic groups) provide members with a forum to work through common issues such as substance abuse, anger management, parenting skills, and grief, and provide the opportunity to practice new skills together. Group members learn how to share information and respond to each other appropriately, provide positive feedback, identify behavioral triggers, and gain insight into behaviors that impair their relationships with others. The length of time an individual participates in group psychotherapy varies. Sessions typically are targeted to last a specific time (for example, the typical length of an

Cohesion

evidence-based practice

Clinical Question
To what extent is cohesion important to the quality of therapeutic groups?

Evidence
Burlingame, Theobald-McClendon, and Alonso (2011) evaluated the therapeutic concept of group cohesion in both quality and structure. Researchers evaluated the cohesion between the members and the leader and between members and other members, as well as the members' relationship toward the group as whole. The researchers found that the theoretical orientation of the leader affected the level of group cohesion. The leader who had an interpersonal orientation, such as emphasizing member-to-member interaction, discussing group rules and the responsibilities of members, creating here-and-now discussions, balancing positive and corrective feedback, creating nonjudgmental language and attitudes with members, creating an atmosphere of both support and challenge, and responding to the meaning of group members' comments demonstrated the highest cohesion outcomes compared with a psychodynamic or cognitive–behavioral leader orientation. Cohesion was also stronger in groups with five to nine members and in groups lasting more than 12 sessions. It was noted that younger group members had larger outcome changes when cohesion was present in the group. A sense of group cohesion positively decreased symptom distress and improved interpersonal functioning (Burlingame, Theobald-McClendon, & Alonso, 2011).

Hamrin, Weycer, Pachler, and Fournier (2006) evaluated the learning opportunities of leaders, group themes, and curative and therapeutic factors in nine-week, peer-led support groups for first-year graduate nursing students at a major school of nursing. Student group leaders had to pass the group psychotherapy course to become leaders. Student leaders who participated in the peer support groups ranked the most observed curative and therapeutic factors as universality (mean = 1.67), followed by cohesiveness (mean = 2.78) and catharsis (mean = 5.44). Student participants felt that the benefits of the group were building confidence in their nursing identity, adjusting to their roles as nurses, and learning skills to navigate relationships with hospital and educational systems as well as with relationships with preceptors and faculty. Students also felt that a benefit of the group was having a place to process their experiences involving patient care decisions and relationships with patients.

Implications for Nursing
By fostering opportunities to build group cohesiveness, group leaders can have a positive impact on patients' overall functioning, target specific skills to build within the group, and lower patient levels of distress.

Critical Thinking Questions
1. What kinds of support groups for students exist within your school or program? Do you participate? Why or why not?
2. What do you see as barriers to group cohesiveness? How would you try to address these barriers if you were the member of a support group? If you were the leader?

admission stay in an inpatient unit, 6 to 8 weeks in an outpatient setting, or a year or more for some self-help groups). Duration of group psychotherapy may depend on the setting, the goals of treatment, or other factors such as length of participation in the program or the extent to which a patient's health insurance will cover participation. Psychodynamic groups require a group leader with an advanced degree and specific training in group psychotherapy, such as an Advanced Practice Nurse with specialized training.

Many types of group settings may offer a therapeutic benefit without providing psychotherapy. Modern group treatments may include task groups, psychoeducational groups, and support and self-help groups (Table 24-2). Activity therapy groups are offered in a variety of inpatient and outpatient settings. The nature of the leadership of these groups varies, as do duration and setting.

Task groups are usually inclusive of task forces, committees, planning groups, social action groups, study circles, and learning groups. Task groups are found in the community, business, and educational settings. Task groups demonstrate a clear purpose, a balance of process and content, an appreciation of differences, and a climate of cooperation, collaboration, and mutual respect. Task groups address conflict, give feedback in clear and immediate terms, and reflect on here and now issues. Members in the group are viewed as resources, and members are given time to reflect on their work (Hulse-Killacky, Killacky, & Donigian, 2001). Task groups typically are formed for a clear purpose (for instance, to improve safety or to resolve some form of conflict), and may terminate once that purpose has been accomplished.

Psychoeducational groups give members the opportunity to gain increased knowledge on a certain topic. Often, psychoeductional groups will use cognitive, affective, and behavioral techniques. Information

or skills related to a specific topic are taught in a group setting with other individuals sharing the same problem, such as a coping skills group for children who are grieving the death of a parent. Other topics appropriate for psychoeducation include stress or anger management skills, assertiveness training, management of symptoms of anxiety or depression, and medication administration and adherence. Psychoeducational groups can also occur in nontraditional psychotherapy settings, such as schools, churches, or community centers. Leaders must receive specific training in the area in which they are delivering the educational content (Corey, Corey, & Corey, 2010). Psychoeducational programs may be offered in a single session or over multiple sessions depending on the setting, the purpose of the program, and the target participants. When leading psychoeducational groups, nurses still must attend to the elements of group dynamics, such as setting norms of attendance, identifying roles members play, and encouraging members to discuss with one another how they are applying newly learned skills. Nurses will demonstrate unconditional positive regard for patients while setting the stage of anticipated change.

Support groups, or self-help groups, are run by the members themselves, who encourage one another to maintain compliance with treatment and continue to develop interpersonal skills. Support groups may follow formal or informal rules for membership and gathering. Groups such as Alcoholics Anonymous, Narcotics Anonymous, and Overeaters Anonymous meet in a variety of settings, including churches and community centers. Individuals usually may participate in self-help or support groups as long as they feel they continue to gain benefit from them.

Activity therapy groups offer creative, low-stress environments in which individuals can explore their emotions under the guidance

Types of Therapeutic Groups

table 24-2

Type of Group	Description	Nurse's Role
Psychotherapy/ psychodynamic group	Therapy group led by a trained/licensed clinician or therapist designed to help participants identify triggers, work through issues, and develop new skills.	• Refer or encourage participation as part of the overall treatment plan. • RNs may participate as co-leaders or facilitators in addition to the group leader. • APRNs with specialized training may serve as group leaders.
Psychoeducational group	Group setting that provides instruction related to a specific topic, such as medication administration or anger or stress management.	• Refer patients as appropriate. • RNs may design and lead psychoeducational groups.
Task group	Groups convened with the purpose of accomplishing a given task, such as determining how to increase safety on a unit, raising funds for a particular event, or studying the benefits of a community wellness effort.	• RNs may participate in and/or lead task groups at the organizational level.
Support or self-help group	Groups led by members motivated to seek help from their peers to improve progress or receive support related to a health or mental health issue. Examples include AA/NA groups, cancer survivor groups, and support groups for parents of children with serious illnesses.	• RNs provide referrals as appropriate. • Groups are typically led by members, although RNs may provide leadership or assistance to these groups depending on setting and structure of the group.
Activity group	Offer creative, low-stress opportunities for individuals to explore their emotions or gain some type of health benefit in a small group setting. Typically led by an experienced therapist. Examples include art and music therapy groups and water therapy or other exercise-related groups.	• RNs provide referrals as appropriate. • RNs may facilitate a group alongside the experienced/licensed therapist as appropriate to patient group and setting.

of an experienced therapist. Art therapy has been shown to be effective when used in the group setting for a variety of types of patients. Poetry therapy, music therapy, and dance therapy groups are offered in numerous settings. Length and number of sessions vary.

The Group Leader

The group leader is responsible for laying the foundation for maximizing interpersonal exchanges in the group. The leader must be able to do the following:

- Establish solid relationships with and among the members of the group
- Be committed to reflection and growth in his or her own life
- Encourage group members to engage in personal growth (Corey, Corey, & Corey, 2010)

Characteristics of effective group leaders include the ability to be present with members' struggles, pain, and successes. An effective leader will also have a genuine interest in the welfare of the group members and demonstrate commitment to helping members achieve their goals. The leader must believe in the group process, be able to tolerate and work through conflict, not become defensive when confronted, and be able to foster a sense of group cohesiveness (Corey, Corey, & Corey, 2010).

Leaders of therapeutic groups begin by establishing the type and purpose of the group, the duration of the group from formation to termination, and the selection of participants. Particularly for group psychotherapy, leaders must establish norms from the group's inception, emphasizing the importance of good attendance, honest and open communication, gradual self-disclosure, and respect for one another's ideas. The leader can create a safe and trusting environment by modeling empathy toward all the members, ensuring confidentiality, and creating dialogue that allows for direct member-to-member feedback. The leader may want to meet with each member individually before the group begins to explain the purpose of the group and to help each individual identify personal goals he or she wants to accomplish from attending the group. Initially, the leader is active in orienting the group to its purpose and modeling high-quality interactions. As time progresses, the leader encourages the group to take ownership of its functioning with greater member discussion. The leader will ask questions to encourage the group to reflect on the quality of its functioning (Yalom & Leszcz, 2005). The leader may do this by asking the group open-ended questions, such as:

- "What was the most engaging part of the group for you today?"
- "With which members did you feel most comfortable speaking?"
- "What was the least engaging part of the meeting?"
- "What was your role in the meeting today?"

The leader will also discourage out-of-session subgrouping if the subgrouping has a negative effect, such as excluding particular members or keeping secrets from the rest of the group.

In most therapeutic groups, the leader also takes on the role of group historian, tracking the themes and bringing those themes back to the group from one session to the next. The leader is aware that he or she is creating the culture of the group by establishing norms that will help the group function in a productive manner, such as coming on time, learning to self-disclose, learning to identify and express emotions, and learning to give and receive support and constructive

feedback. If the group has an interpersonal growth focus, the leader observes interactions among members and encourages open discussion of the interactions by following a process of helping members see what their behavior is like, how their behavior affects the other group members, how their behavior affects others' opinions of them, and eventually how the individual's behavior influences the opinions he has of himself (Yalom & Leszcz, 2005).

Experienced leaders also mentor other professionals in developing their leadership skills. Students and new professionals bring energy, creativity, a fresh perspective, and a wish to be helpful to their patients. They learn about group psychotherapy by first being a co-leader of a group with someone who has specific training and experience and has a reputation as a good group therapist. Students and new nursing graduates should engage in weekly supervision with a respected group leader to gain good group leadership skills by processing the events in the group with the supervisor.

Stages of Group Development

Most longer-term groups go through stages of development, beginning with the *orientation stage,* during which members size up one another, evaluate their ability to fit in the group, and evaluate potential connections with other members (Table 24-3). At this stage, group members may try to determine the relevance of the group's activity to their personal therapy goals. The group members look to the group leader for structure, approval, and acceptance, thus demonstrating more dependent behavior in this initial orientation stage. Behaviors observed in the orientation stage may include giving and seeking advice, searching for similarities, defining roles within the group, and sharing superficial personal information.

Following the orientation stage, group members may enter a *conflict stage.* At this stage, members' behavior revolves around creation of a social hierarchy, including challenging the authority of the group leader. Dominance, control, and power are themes of the conflict stage. Negative or critical comments can be observed. Rivalry among members over the attention of the leader or therapist may occur. In psychotherapy groups, the therapist's role in helping patients deal with conflict is to assist them in providing feedback accurately and sensitively and to help the listener become an ally in the process. The therapist will help the members learn to keep conflict within constructive bounds. The therapist can use techniques such as role switching to help members gain empathy for others' perspectives. The group therapist never retaliates with anger or defensiveness if anger is expressed toward him or her; instead, the therapist models exploration of the members' feelings, listening to members' feedback and obtaining other group members' perspectives on issues raised by individual members.

The therapist may ask a patient whether he or she has ever had the same reaction to others as he or she is having toward the therapist currently; this method can help the therapist to explore issues of **transference** the patient may be having. Such feelings can be either positive or negative, and should be explored with patients to enhance therapy. **Countertransference** also can occur when the therapist projects or transfers his or her own emotions to a patient. For example, a therapist who has repressed feelings of anger toward her own mother may find herself feeling angry at a patient who reminds her of her mother. Countertransference can interfere with the therapist–patient relationship and is something that therapists must work through if it has a negative impact on the work of the group.

Stages of Group Development

table 24-3

Stage of Group Development	Member Behaviors	Leader Strategies/Responsibilities
Orientation stage	• Determine relevance of group to individual treatment plan. • Seek approval, acceptance. • Search for similarities. • Share only superficial information.	• Establish norms of structure, communication, behaviors. • Ensure a safe, honest environment.
Conflict stage	• Challenge authority of leader. • Make negative, critical comments toward leader or others. • Engage in rivalries for attention.	Therapist helps patients/members deal with conflict by: • Providing feedback. • Engaging listeners as allies. • Teaching conflict resolution. • Using techniques that promote empathy—e.g., "role switching." • Avoiding retaliation and/or countertransference.
Cohesiveness stage	• Self-disclosure increases. • Greater sense of trust, cooperation among members. • Increased problem solving, ownership of process.	• Continue providing leadership. • Address regression to early stages if it occurs. • Orient new members.
Termination stage	• Some regression may occur as members anticipate separation. • Acknowledge progress, recognize loss.	• Facilitate group termination. • Provide further referral or follow-up as appropriate.

Once conflict is worked through, a *cohesive stage* typically follows. In this stage, intimacy between members is observed and more self-disclosure occurs. There is a greater sense of group pride, cooperation, mutual trust, common goals, problem solving in conflicts, and ownership over the process of the group by the members. Occasionally, such as when a new member joins the group, a group may regress to earlier stages.

The *termination stage* typically follows the cohesiveness stage. Termination occurs because members can transfer the meaningful connections made in the group to outside relationships. The group in the termination stage may regress to earlier stages to deal with the ambivalence they might feel about separating from important connections they have made in the group. Acknowledging progress made is an important step in the termination process, as is recognizing the loss of group and individual experiences. Reflecting on past group events and meaningful interactions can be helpful during the termination process (Corey, Corey, & Corey, 2010; Yalom & Leszcz, 2005). A useful termination teaches patients that they were meaningful to other members, the importance of processing and feeling the emotions associated with the end of a relationship, and how to take what they have learned about relating to others in the group and apply it to their relationships outside the group. Discussing termination before the event is imperative to help members cope and process the loss of the group and how this loss may remind them of past losses. The nurse may serve as a role model to group members as to how to have closure, by saying what each member contributed to the group and what the member meant to the group leader. The nurse may also encourage the members to think about who they will connect with outside the group to support their continued journey of healing.

Group Member Roles

Group members may take on both functional roles and problem behavior roles. Functional classifications of member roles include task roles, group building, and maintenance roles. Group task roles (Table 24-4) can include the initiator–contributor, who proposes new ideas to a group problem or goal. The information seeker looks for clarification of suggestions; the opinion seeker seeks clarification of values pertinent to the group's task.

Group Member Task Roles

table 24-4

Group Member Task Role	Description
Initiator–contributor	Proposes new ideas to a group problem or goal
Information seeker	Looks for clarification of suggestions
Opinion seeker	Seeks clarification of values pertinent to the group's task
Information giver	Offers facts relevant to the group's problem
Opinion giver	Offers beliefs and alternate suggestions
Elaborator	Offers rationale for suggestions
Coordinator	Clarifies relationships between various ideas
Orienter	Defines the position of the group with respect to its goals
Evaluator/critic	Reviews the accomplishments of the group
Energizer	Prompts the group toward action
Procedural/technical contributor	Expedites group movement by performing tasks such as distributing material or arranging seating
Recorder	Writes down suggestions and serves as the group memory

Group building and maintenance roles evolve as the group moves past the conflict stage. Building and maintenance roles include the following:

- The *encourager* encourages the contributions of others.
- The *harmonizer* may mediate tensions or group conflicts.
- The *compromiser* may discipline himself or herself to maintain group harmony.
- The *gatekeeper* will facilitate participation of others and keep the flow of communication open.
- The *standard setter* reminds the group of its norms and standards.
- The group *observer* keeps records of group process and provides interpretations.
- The group *follower* tries to go along with the movement of the group. (Benne & Sheats, 1948)

Not every patient assumes a helpful role in the group process. Some problematic roles patients in the group may assume include those of the monopolizer, the silent patient, and the help-rejecting complainer. The *monopolizer* usually talks incessantly to cope with anxiety. Other members may become angry at the monopolizer, and this may have a negative impact on group cohesiveness. The goal of intervention is not to shut down the patient, but to evaluate the group in terms of why the group allows one person to carry the burden of the meeting. The nurse or group leader may help the monopolizer become aware of sacrificing the opportunity for meaningful interpersonal relationships for the need for attention and control. The nurse may also show the monopolizer how to engage with others in a way that shows empathy. The nurse might help the monopolizer communicate more succinctly by saying something such as, "In one sentence, tell us what you want us to hear" (Corey, Corey, & Corey, 2010; Yalom & Leszcz, 2005).

Another challenging role presented in the group is that of the *silent patient*. There are multiple reasons that a patient may remain silent, including feeling that he or she has nothing meaningful to contribute, uncertainty about the group process, fear of not knowing what to say, fears of members or the authority figure, or fears of rejection, trust, and confidentiality (Corey, Corey, & Corey, 2010). The group leader should take time to discuss with this patient the fact that the more the patient invests and participates in the group, the more he or she will get out of it. The leader observes the patient's nonverbal behavior as well, and explores the reasons for the silent behavior. Questions to help bring in the silent patient could include, "What is the ideal question we could ask that might help you participate in the group today?" (Yalom & Leszcz, 2005).

The *help-rejecting complainer* will request help from the group members and then reject the solutions they offer. This individual may take pride in the inability to solve his or her problems and may find comfort in keeping the group in conflict as a result of his or her own personal, conflicted feelings about dependency. Unfortunately, this behavior can drain the group's energy and create an atmosphere of frustration and despair. Retaliation and resentment toward this group member should be avoided, as it just fuels core feelings of abandonment. The group leader will acknowledge the help-rejecting complainer's sense of hopeless about his or her problems and encourage ways for the member to attach to the group to enable the patient to value the members' feedback about his or her behavior, which in turn could bring a change in the way he or she relates to others (Yalom & Leszcz, 2005).

Pause and Reflect

1. *What aspects of group therapy do you find interesting? Intimidating? What aspects do you think are most helpful to patients?*
2. *Think about groups in which you have participated—therapy groups, student organizations, study groups, community organizations, or committees. Which of the following group roles did you see: Harmonizer? Help-rejecting complainer? Monopolizer? How did other group members interact with those individuals? What did you do to make an effort to work with them?*
3. *Referring to Chapter 5, what cultural considerations might affect individual participation in group therapy?*

Group Interventions for Specific Psychiatric Disorders

Whereas the principles of interpersonal group psychotherapy have just been described, numerous forms of group treatment have demonstrated success for various patient populations. These include dialectical behavior therapy, group therapy designed for individuals with trauma history, and group therapy in the treatment of depression.

Dialectical Behavior Therapy

Developed by Marsha Linehan, dialectical behavioral therapy (DBT) has a psychoeducational group component designed to supplement the individual DBT (Linehan, 1993). Through DBT groups, patients are taught skills to decrease chaos, improve impulsiveness and distress tolerance, improve cognitive and emotional dysregulation, and improve their sense of self. These groups have norms that promote attendance and confidentiality; prohibit members from coming to group under the influence of substances; discourage members from developing private relationships with members outside the group; and ask members to call the leader if one is late or ill and cannot attend. Other skills taught within the framework of the group include mood monitoring with diary cards, mindfulness skills, and interpersonal skills. Group sessions also focus on building interpersonal effectiveness, emotion regulation, and distress tolerance (Linehan, 1993). DBT has been successful for patients with borderline personality disorder in decreasing anxiety and depression, creating hope for the future, decreasing self-harm, and improving social functioning (Perseius et al., 2003). DBT also has demonstrated reductions in self-mutilation, depression, and anxiety. DBT can also improve interpersonal functioning and social adjustment (Bohus et al., 2004).

Group Therapy and Trauma

Individuals with a history of trauma, including childhood sexual abuse, can benefit from interpersonal, cognitive–behavioral, and psychoeducational group therapy to decrease isolation, shame, and posttraumatic stress symptoms, and to improve skill-building competencies (Campanini et al., 2010; Dorrepaal et al., 2010; Ginzburg et al., 2009). Additional examples of the positive impact of group therapy on individuals who have experienced trauma include the following:

- Exposure-based cognitive–behavioral group therapy has been shown to improve anxiety, somatic, depressive, and PTSD symptoms in military veterans with PTSD (Rademaker, 2009).

Sally Tollerson

APPLICATION

1. In what stage of development is the group?

2. What behaviors might she observe in the first meeting?

3. What additional orientation tasks will the therapist want to address in this first meeting?

Sally Tollerson is a 45-year-old woman with a history of depression. She has been in treatment for 6 months, receiving medication management and individual cognitive–behavioral therapy. Sally's therapist encourages her to attend a group therapy session with six other individuals from the outpatient clinic who also have mood disorders, with the goal of increasing her social support and decreasing her isolation. She just attended her first group therapy meeting, in which the leader explained the purpose of the group, length of the group, and confidentiality of the group. The members were introduced to one another and asked to describe their goals for attending the group. Sally was evaluating whether the group was safe, to whom she might feel connected in the group, and whether the other members had similar symptoms of depression to her own.

- Group-based interpersonal psychotherapy has been demonstrated to improve interpersonal functioning, PTSD, and depression, and to reduce anger and stress levels in veterans with PTSD (Ray & Webster, 2010).

Group Therapy and Depression

A meta-analysis of 48 studies was conducted to evaluate the effectiveness of group therapy for both male and female adult patients with the diagnosis of depression, with an average of 12 sessions (McDermut, Miller, & Brown, 2001). Types of group therapy included cognitive, psychodynamic, interpersonal, and social support groups. Patients who received these treatments were compared with patients without treatment, wait-list controls, or patients who underwent individual therapy. Patients were evaluated using the Beck Depression Inventory. Forty-three of the 46 studies found that group therapy significantly reduced depression, compared with the control groups. Four studies found no difference between group therapy and individual therapy, cognitive–behavioral therapy, or psychodynamic therapy. Group therapy was also found to be more cost effective compared with other treatments (McDermut, Miller, & Brown, 2001).

Other types of educational groups include anger management groups, social skills groups, medication teaching groups, and parenting groups.

Pause and Reflect

1. *How can dialectical behavior therapy be used in the treatment of individuals with mental illness?*

2. *How or why might group psychotherapy be helpful in the treatment of patients with posttraumatic stress disorder?*

Family Therapy

Family therapy is an effective form of group therapy that helps family members to have more satisfying interpersonal relationships with one another. Typically, family therapy serves the family of origin (parents and their biological offspring), but it may include extended family members or stepparents and stepchildren, depending on how the individual family defines itself. The goals of family therapy include helping members to:

- Adjust to new family life stages
- Cope with a family member's physical or mental health problem
- Explore family-of-origin issues and how they affect current family relationships
- Improve communication and family problem-solving skills

One of the most challenging aspects for the nurse working with families is to maintain a collaborative and trusting relationship with all the members of the family. It is helpful to maintain eye contact with all family members, get each individual's perspective on the problem, and maintain a nonjudgmental attitude toward the family. The nurse must be careful not to ally with one family member against another. In the initial assessment, the nurse discusses the confidentiality of the treatment, assesses whether the family is in crisis, and determines whether there is any physical, sexual, or emotional abuse. The nurse should demonstrate an attitude of empathy and warmth, and highlight the family's strengths. One of the most import aspects of the initial interview is to convey a sense of confidence and hope for change that the treatment can provide. The nurse might make a statement such as, "With some hard work,

John Sims

APPLICATION

1. What stage of development might the group be in?

2. What types of interventions should the therapist make to explore John's reaction to him and the pattern of John's late behavior?

John Sims is a 29-year-old man attending his sixth interpersonal group therapy session. He becomes very angry and reactive to the therapist when the therapist points out that he has been 15 minutes late to the past three sessions. John accuses the therapist of acting just like his boss at work.

critical thinking

I believe we can make some good progress on the problem that you identified."

Family Assessment

Conducting a thorough family assessment can be helpful in a variety of settings in which nurses work with families, such as pediatric clinics and cancer units in hospitals, as well as in mental health treatment settings. A thorough family assessment is critical to choosing the type of family therapy and designing an individualized family treatment plan. Often, families want immediate advice on how to fix their problems. It is important not to offer advice until after completing the assessment and obtaining all the facts about the problem and the family history (Box 24-1).

Family Assessment   box 24-1

(A) **Who Is in the Family:** obtain data on three generations (names/ages/genders)
  1. List pregnancies, adoptions, abortions, deaths (date and cause).
  2. Determine how each person is related to the others.
  3. Obtain marital status, partner status (list marriages, separations, divorces, unmarried relationships).
  4. Obtain information about the personalities of family members.
  5. Determine the level of intellect, education, presence of learning problems or other mental disabilities.
  6. Assess physical health of all members (acute/chronic health conditions, hospitalizations, illnesses).
  7. Assess psychiatric health of all members, including substance abuse (alcohol, drugs, tobacco use).
  8. Identify cultural and ethnic background (language spoken, rituals around death, other commemorative ceremonies).
  9. Determine the number of persons living in the home.
  10. Inquire about extended family (names, ages, dates of births of siblings and parents, parents' marriages and divorces).
  11. Determine the whereabouts of family members who have left home.

(B) **Material Dimensions and Life Events**
  1. Income and family resources (source, amount, management, socioeconomic status)
  2. Occupation of immediate family members and extended family
  3. Type and size of living quarters (e.g., house or apartment, are family members sharing bedrooms)
  4. Type of neighborhood
  5. Military service or retirement
  6. Moves, job changes, job satisfaction
  7. Life events—both happy and traumatic (a timeline is a good way to obtain this information)
  8. How the family spends leisure time (together, apart, some of both)

(C) **Family and Community Interface**
  1. Educational history (achievements, problems)
  2. Spiritual/cultural beliefs and activities
  3. Recreational and other activities
  4. Relationships with friends and neighbors
  5. Triangles within current family and family of origin
  6. Legal problems/history

(D) **Relationships Among Family Members** (central, family of origin, and extended)
  1. Type of relationship (close, cut off, conflicted, distant)
  2. Subgroups or special alliances
  3. Trust among family members

  4. Degree of expression of warmth/affection/love, hostility, violence
  5. Stage in the family life cycle
  6. Physical, verbal, or sexual abuse
  7. Marriage relationships, parent–child relationships
  8. Dominance or submissive patterns, pursuer/distancer patterns
  9. Attitudes about gender
  10. Family secrets

(E) **Psychological**
  1. Power: Who has it, is it shared, who makes decisions about what aspects of family life?
  2. Roles of members (caretaker, sick role, successful, cold, distant)
  3. Boundary issues, such as autonomy, differentiation, enmeshment
  4. Adaptability, flexibility, rigidity
  5. Conflict management skills
  6. Decision-making processes
  7. Family strengths (loyalty, hope, humor, intelligence)
  8. Behaviors that indicate resilience

(F) **Communication Style**
  1. Active or passive
  2. Ability to express self.
  3. Defense mechanisms
  4. Tone, cadence, rhythm
  5. Affect
  6. Ability to listen
  7. Ability to validate one another
  8. Ability to take ownership for own behavior
  9. Nonverbal communication

(G) **Social Functioning**
  1. Marital patterns
  2. Patterns from family of origin (sibling positions, history of sibling relationships, relationships with parents)
  3. Family norms
  4. Relationships with teachers, community members, church members, etc.

(H) **Reasons for Entering Treatment**
  1. Why are they coming now?
  2. Who is motivated for treatment?
  3. What is the presenting problem and when did it begin?
  4. Who noticed it?
  5. How does each family member view the problem?
  6. How has each family member responded?
  7. What were their relationships like prior to the problem?
  8. Has the problem changed?
  9. What will happen if the problem continues?
  10. Has the family ever experienced problems like this before?
  11. What solutions did they try? What was the result?

Selected Domain Considerations—Group and Family Therapy
table 24-5

Domain	Nursing Considerations
Biological	What is the biological status of the family or group members? Does a patient or family member have a medical illness that may affect participation (e.g., dialysis 2 days a week)?
Psychological	Does a patient's or family member's level of anxiety or cognitive functioning at this time impair participation (e.g., delusions, risk for violence)? What is the patient's or family's previous history of participation in therapy?
Sociological	Are there any impediments to therapy, such as cost, transportation, legal considerations (e.g., restraining order)?
Cultural/spiritual	Are there any cultural or spiritual practices that might impede or promote participation among family members? In a group setting? (e.g., dominant male head of household, prayer schedules, attributing mental health issues to external factors)

In the summary, the nurse will assess the presenting problem, biological status of family members, psychological status of members, cultural considerations, members' social functioning within the society, nuclear family patterns, including patterns of family functioning, patterns of relationships and communication, patterns related to position in the family, family of origin family patterns, stage in the family life cycle, current stressors, current family strengths and resources, role of spiritual life, and potential barriers to treatment (Table 24-5).

Family Genogram

The family **genogram** (Figure 24-2) is a visual display of the current and extended family and the types of relationships the members have with one another. It can also be used to obtain and track family medical and psychiatric history. The genogram can be used early in the assessment phase to gather facts about a family and decrease emotional reactivity. It can help individuals think about their relationships and their family of origin patterns, rather than reacting emotionally to charged topics. The genogram is useful for evaluating the stage in the family life cycle and its developmental challenges, such as transition to marriage or parenthood, stepfamilies, families at midlife, and families later in life. The genogram also is helpful in identifying relationship, health, and psychiatric patterns that have been carried from one generation to the next (McGoldrick, Gerson, & Petry, 2008).

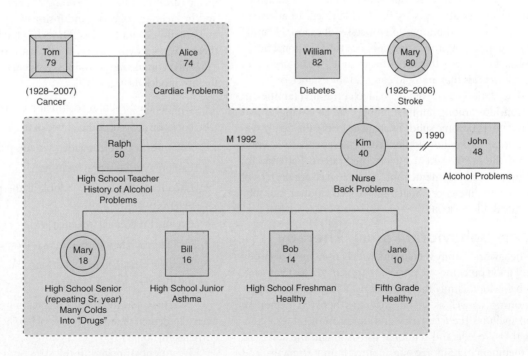

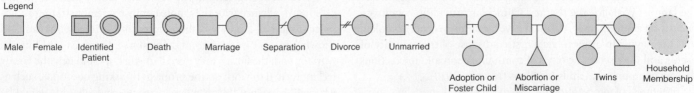

24-2 Example of a family genogram with accompanying legend (symbols used in genograms).

Understanding the family's culture is critical to the family therapy process. Cultural practices can influence family dynamics and decision-making processes and may also affect the level of trust that family members have in the process of family therapy. Spiritual beliefs and practices may also affect a family's willingness to participate in therapy. By assessing cultural and spiritual practices early, the nurse can identify any issues that need to be addressed prior to beginning therapy.

Pause and Reflect

1. *When planning or organizing a family assessment, what areas are most important for the nurse to assess?*
2. *How might constructing a family genogram help the nurse identify priorities for care?*

Theoretical Approaches to Family Therapy

Most family therapies incorporate systems theory principles. One of the major concepts of systems theory includes taking the focus away from the individual's problem in isolation and considering the problem in the context of one's relationships and one's culture (White & Klein, 2008). Family systems theory views the presenting problem from a holistic perspective, considering how family members' responses affect the presenting problem (**mutual causality**), how individual family members influence the family system, and how the family system influences the individual family members. Family systems theory evaluates attempts by family members to adjust to change and the flow of communication processes. It examines family **boundaries**, barriers that protect and enhance the functional integrity of families. Boundaries that are clear promote separateness and belonging; boundaries that are rigid can lead to distance or disengagement. Boundaries that are diffuse lead to **enmeshed families**, in which relationships among family members are so entangled that individual members become subordinate to or lost in the family system. Systems theory takes into account that a system affects its environment and the environment affects the system. Patterns are repetitive and predictable interactions. All systems have degrees of tolerance for norm differences. Systems have levels, power, and subsystems (White & Klein, 2008).

Cognitive–Behavioral Family Therapy

Cognitive–behavioral family therapy is a widely used form of family therapy with good outcomes in numerous areas of family treatment. Cognitive–behavioral family therapy is derived from classical operant conditioning, as well as social exchange theory (Chapter 4). Assessment includes the frequency and duration of the problem, conditions that precede and reinforce the problem, the ability of the family members to reinforce one another, family strengths, and the family's goals for the therapy. Clinicians providing cognitive–behavioral family therapy will often have the family reenact a problem they are having in order to get a firsthand sense of the sequence of events and to observe the types of communication and interactions that occur among the family members (Nichols, 2010).

Methods of intervention include role rehearsal, modeling, shaping new interactions, token economies to reward positive behaviors, assertiveness training, contingency contracting, thought stopping

and replacement, and homework assignments to practice new skills. For example, the therapist may instruct family members to share with one another when something upsets them (increasing assertiveness), or may instruct family members to affirm another family member when that person does something well (rewarding positive behaviors). To ensure success, it is helpful to have the family practice the skills in session to gain mastery prior to trying the new skills at home. This treatment has proven useful for parent management training, behavioral couples therapy, and treatment of sexual dysfunctions. This model focuses more on the current problem versus the evaluation of historical problematic patterns from the family of origin (Nichols, 2010).

Structural Family Therapy

Structural family therapy focuses on the current organization of the family as demonstrated through repeated patterns of interactions, usually rules that govern family interactions and decisions. This method of family therapy was designed by Salvador Minuchin. In structural family therapy, family members' interactions are evaluated as either promoting or inhibiting the tasks the family needs to accomplish through the various stages of the life cycle. The goal of structural family therapy is to change the family structure so the family can solve its own problems and support the goals of individual members, while preserving mutual support of family members. Interventions may include hierarchical change in the executive subsystem, such as putting parents in charge and teaching parents co-parenting skills (Minuchin, 1974). Other possible goals of structural family therapy include creating differentiation and boundaries in enmeshed families and/or creating cohesion and intimacy by softening rigid rules in emotionally distant families. Minuchin found that structural family therapy was very effective for youths with conduct disorders.

After completing a family assessment using the structural family therapy model, the nurse will:

- Explore the presenting complaint in depth.
- Focus on areas of competence of the identified patient.
- Reframe the problem with a systems perspective.
- Explore symptom presentation.
- Encourage the family to look at the problem from multiple perspectives.
- Explore the context in which symptoms appear.
- Evaluate each family member's response to the problem.
- Have the identified patient discuss the symptoms and the meaning they have for the family.

Structural family therapy also explores how the parents have been raised, their views and beliefs of family, and how those affect the current situation.

Treatment strategies in the structural family method include creating an alliance with the whole family by demonstrating acceptance toward all family members, accommodating their styles, and showing respect to the parents. The nurse, therapist, or clinician working with the family may need to instill hope and help the family feel motivated to work on the problem by asking questions, such as what will happen if this problem continues and what life would be like if this problem were not central to the family's functioning. The clinician may encourage the family to reenact a problem to assess the problematic sequence. The clinician will then create a structural map with the family that highlights and modifies interactions and creates boundaries and flexibility where needed. Unproductive assumptions or thoughts will be challenged and replaced with accurate and useful thoughts; problem-solving skills will be taught. Throughout the therapy, the clinician will highlight what the family is doing right, as well as empower the family to feel confident in implementing solutions (Minuchin, 1974).

Bowenian Family Therapy

Another influential family therapy model is Bowenian family therapy, based on the work of Murray Bowen (Bowen, 1978). Bowenian family therapy assumes that the family is an emotional relationship system with the goals of promoting engagement, fostering differentiation, and avoiding fusion. Therapy is aimed at promoting individuation, understanding current conflicting interactions, and understanding intergenerational patterns of behavior. An important goal in this model is balancing individuality with togetherness. Bowen believes that working on unresolved emotional reactivity to parents is the most important unfinished business in life. Bowenian family therapy fosters individuation by encouraging family members to use logic when dealing with other members rather than making decisions based on emotional reactions to one another.

Concepts of Family and Family Processes

Concepts from Bowenian therapy include differentiation of the self, emotional triangles, nuclear family emotional process, the family projection process, multigenerational transmission process, sibling position, emotional cutoff, and the societal emotional process (Nichols, 2010).

Differentiation of the Self

Differentiation is the capacity to think and reflect without responding automatically to emotional pressures, regardless of whether those pressures are internal or external. Well-differentiated individuals have the ability to be flexible in the face of anxiety, whereas those who are undifferentiated are more reactive emotionally and more impulsive. Differentiated individuals can think things through, decide what they believe, and act on those beliefs.

Emotional Triangles

Emotional triangles describe relationships that may involve a third party. This may be a person, an activity, a memory, alcohol or other substance, or a job that functions to defuse anxiety between two individuals. Drawing in a third person or element functions to decrease anxiety or conflict between two individuals (Box 24-2).

Family Projection Process

The term **family projection process** refers to a process in which parents develop unrealistic fears and behaviors that promote the idea that something is wrong with their child. These fears may relate to the parents' own problems. These fears may shape the child's schemas, so the child believes that the parents' fears and perceptions are true. For example, parents who develop a view of their daughter as being irresponsible or lazy may attribute any successes their daughter has to luck or external factors, rather than recognizing their daughter's attributes and legitimate efforts. As a result, their daughter may begin to believe in their perceptions, and consequently see herself as being without talent or worth.

Nuclear Family Emotional System

The nuclear family emotional system is a pattern of responses that a family uses when it encounters a significant stressor. The goals of the system include healthy adaptation to the stressor. The family may or may not use social networks or extended family during these times of stress. The goal is for the family to use extended resources to adapt and grow stronger as a group due to the stressor, rather than depending on a single family member to absorb all the stress and reduce or eliminate the stressor without the help of other members.

Sibling position may affect roles members may take within the family system. Birth order affects personality development. Firstborn children may identify with power and authority and demonstrate a sense of great responsibility and conscientiousness, as well as provide care to younger siblings. Younger children may identify with the

---

Emotional Triangles   box 24-2

Emotional triangles describe relationships that may involve a third party. Some examples of emotional triangles include the following scenarios:

- A parent complains to a child about the other parent.
- A spouse works increasingly longer hours to avoid being home with the other spouse.
- A parent turns to alcohol to reduce stress after arguing with his teenage son.

Triangles postpone conflict by creating alliances, but over the long term may increase anxiety levels, especially for the third member of the triangle, who is excluded from the alliance. As anxiety increases, family members seek emotional closeness or distance, resulting in pursuer and distancer roles within relationships. The greater the level of anxiety or enmeshment, the less tolerant individuals can become of one another's differences (Nichols, 2010).

Emotional triangles can facilitate **fusion**, the projecting of one's needs onto another, which can lead to enmeshed relationships. For example, a wife who feels unappreciated or unloved by her father seeks her husband's attention and approval to fill the void. Results of fusion can include emotional distancing or cutoff, emotional overinvolvement, physical or emotional problems in one partner, marital conflict, or projection of problems onto the children. Fusion can result in members taking on roles of either under- or overfunctioning. An example of overfunctioning is one family member taking on more responsibilities in the family that could be (and perhaps should be) distributed among other members—for example, the oldest child in a family who begins to take on more and more of the parenting responsibilities, such as getting the other children ready for school in the morning, helping with homework, preparing meals, and doing housework. Family fusion can lead to states of chronic emotional anxiety and exhaustion in the overfunctioning family members (Nichols, 2010).

oppressed, question the status quo, and demonstrate strong creativity. Younger children are often more open to new experiences. Middle children may learn to be good negotiators. Only children may be socially independent and more comfortable in relationships with adults than with peers (McGoldrick, Gerson, & Petry, 2008). Gender roles may also affect family functioning and should also be evaluated.

Emotional Cutoff

Emotional cutoff refers to the process by which people disconnect from one another to manage anxiety between and within the generations. The more fusion that exists within the relationship or the more unresolved differentiation from the family of origin, the greater the likelihood that emotional cutoff will occur. Individuals who are cut off may struggle with feelings of helplessness due to unresolved family conflicts and feelings of rejection. Teaching families conflict resolution skills and agreeing to respect one another even if they disagree on an issue can help prevent cutoff situations.

Societal Emotional Process

The societal emotional process refers to the relationship between society and the family. It takes into consideration how sexism, classism, and racism, as well as educational, peer, work, and legal systems, interface with the family. The more differentiated one is, the more he or she is able to resist destructive social influences and shape positive social society values.

Goals and Aspects of Bowenian Family Therapy

A goal of Bowenian family therapy is for individuals to learn more about themselves and their relationships so they can assume responsibility for their own problems. Another goal is to evaluate the process of emotional reactivity and the family structure, such as interlocking networks of triangles (Nichols, 2010).

Detriangulation occurs when parents are able to manage their own anxiety and not transfer it onto their children or other family members. Treatment goals include assisting the family members to operate in their family of origin with less anxiety. This can occur when individuals take steps to be true to themselves, despite either approval or rejection by family members. Obtaining a genogram will help to evaluate the triangles in the immediate family and the family of origin. The nurse will also encourage family members to develop a relationship with individuals in the extended family to diffuse the intensity of the relationships that are involved in triangles. Last, the family will create a therapeutic triangle with the therapist to diffuse anxiety.

Therapy techniques include asking questions that get family members to evaluate in what way they contribute to problems in the relationship. Initial questions that may elicit information that will help the nurse target further questions may include the following:

- How much time does each family member spend with other members? With the family as a whole?

- What do family members do when they spend time together?

- What family members assume which tasks that promote the success of the family (such as earning income, cleaning house, preparing meals)?

- How does each family member view the presenting problem of the patient (the reason that brought the family to therapy)?

The clinician's interaction style consists of asking questions to encourage self-discovery rather than giving advice. The clinician will assign tasks to get people out of triangles, such as practicing managing

conflict within the dyadic relationships (specific relationships between two family members) without bringing in other family members to take sides. Family members will benefit from learning positive coping skills that help reduce anxiety, such as deep breathing and positive self-talk, and by practicing not seeking approval from others for their own identity. Last, treatment will help individuals to set relationship boundaries so they refrain from absorbing or attempting to fix the anxiety of other family members. This occurs when family members stop feeling a sense of responsibility for the happiness of others.

The Bowenian therapist asks questions that stimulate the patient and family members to think cognitively rather than react emotionally. Educational interventions include teaching individuals to make statements and teaching listening strategies to partners. Displacement stories are used in this type of treatment. Examples of a displacement story would be: "I wonder what couples do when they cannot get through to each other." "What do you think might make that step of change difficult for people?" The clinician will ask process questions, such as, "When your boyfriend neglects you, how do you deal with it?" or "How do your problems affect others?"(Bowen, 1978). The clinician focuses on the process of the interaction, not always on the content. In the Bowenian framework, patients are encouraged to figure out how they typically respond to other family members' behaviors and to develop plans for healthy responses to anticipated family interactions (Nichols, 2010).

Integrated Problem-Solving Family Therapy

Integrated problem-solving therapy was developed by Feldman and Pinsof (1982) and Catherall (1988). It is an integration of systems theory, social learning theory, psychodynamic theory, behavioral family therapy, strategic family therapy, and structural family therapy. This model is student friendly, as it relies less on the personality of the therapist and has a very specific problem focus, clear direction for assessment, and focused interventions and steps of treatment. One of the premises of the model is that the family is healthy until proven otherwise. The clinician or therapist works with the patient system, the presenting problem, and the intervention, and evaluates any blocks that might impede successful resolution of the problem. In the assessment phase, the therapist establishes an alliance with all the family members, exploring emotions connected to the problem and identifying with the family the nature of the presenting problem, its onset, and its course. The therapist inquires why the family is seeking treatment at this time. The therapist will clarify each person's perspective and each person's role within the family, including what efforts each family member has made in an effort to try to solve the presenting problem. The therapist empathizes with the entire family while collecting the data and frames problems from a systems perspective. Making a genuine connection with the family is one of the most important tasks during the assessment phase (Feldman & Pinsof, 1982).

One of the core elements of the integrated problem-solving model is a focus on the presenting problem, with an understanding that other problems will not be addressed until the initial problem is resolved. A contract can be made to work on other problems after the initial problem is resolved. Integrated problem-solving therapy has an educational emphasis on teaching families problem-solving and communication skills to give them the skills to solve their own problems. The model focuses on recognizing family patterns and family pattern modification.

Seven Steps of Integrated Problem-Solving Family Therapy   table 24-6

Step	Action
1. Pattern identification	Evaluation of repeated transactions that establish patterns of how, when, and to whom individuals relate within the family system.
2. Emotion identification	Increasing awareness of family members of their own affective reactions to the problematic situation, including the first time they felt that way.
3. Adaptive solution identification	Identifying all potential solutions to the problem, choosing a solution to implement, trying the solution, and evaluating the effectiveness of the solution.
4. Interpersonal block identification	Evaluating the family system's power distribution, communication of affect, quality of structural boundaries, and assignment of roles.
5. Catastrophic expectation identification	Exploring real or irrational fears that block change.
6. Intrapersonal block identification and modification	Identifying and working on unresolved conflicts from earlier relationships and personality defects that interfere with present functioning.
7. Termination	Highlighting the family's strengths and ability of family members to change their own family system. Successful resolution of the problem and ending treatment. This can be a time to negotiate working on a new problem.

Based on Catherall, D. (1988). *Interviewing in Family Therapy: The Problem Centered Approach.* Unpublished manuscript; Feldman, L., & Pinsof, W. (1982). Problem maintenance in family systems: An integrative model. *Journal of Marital and Family Therapy, 8*(3), 295–308.

Careful evaluation of the solution attempts and outcomes are reviewed. There are seven steps to treatment, as noted in Table 24-6.

A unique feature of the integrated problem solving model is *block identification*, which occurs when the family cannot implement an adaptive solution. Feelings of anxiety are what often cause problem-solving blocks; these feelings may include catastrophic expectations or individual or collective fantasies of a feared thought, feeling, or behavior. The clinician looks at maladaptive patterns in problem solving and evaluates the roles, communication, emotions, and boundaries. Factors such as individual physical health, psychopathology, and power within the family system are also explored to determine the block. Blocks are evaluated in terms of whether they are from the past or present, interpersonal or intrapsychic, biological in nature, problems of power distribution or communication, or structurally related. Block interventions include surfacing suppressed emotions, resolving interpersonal conflicts, identifying and reducing catastrophic fears, weakening rigid boundaries and strengthening weak boundaries, separating historical issues from the current situation, confronting irrational fears, and building ego strength.

In the termination phase of therapy, the family can contract to work on a new problem once the original problem is resolved. It is important to recognize the family's success in family treatment and get closure on the original presenting problem. The clinician can schedule a follow-up meeting one month after treatment to evaluate the sustaining power of the solution.

The therapist using this model must know effective problem-solving strategies and be able to teach them to the families. These include helping family members identify specific problems without blaming and identify potential solutions (Figure 24-3).

The therapist must be able to identify the problem maintenance structure and use role play in the session to help the family employ new solutions. The therapist also encourages family members to solve problems by speaking directly to one another. Some useful teaching guidelines for families on communication skills are listed in Box 24-3.

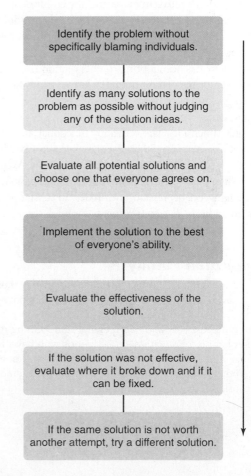

24-3   Family teaching: problem solving skills.

Based on Catherall, D. (1988). *Interviewing in Family Therapy: The Problem Centered Approach.* Unpublished manuscript; Feldman, L., & Pinsof, W. (1982). Problem maintenance in family systems: An integrative model. *Journal of Marital and Family Therapy, 8*(3), 295–308.

| Strategies for Teaching Communication Skills to Families | box 24-3 |

1. Teach members to make "I" statements to communicate how they feel about a problem, rather than blaming other family members for the problem.
2. Have family members practice reflective listening by verbally paraphrasing what they hear each other say.
3. Encourage family members to be direct and specific, which helps other members to know what they need.
4. Help family members learn to listen to one another with good eye contact, and allow each other to finish an idea without interrupting.

5. Suggest that family members limit or reduce distractions so they can better focus on the speaker's message.
6. Teach family members to use a neutral tone of voice and facial expressions. Highly expressed emotions and eye rolling can inhibit good listening and make others defensive.
7. Teach family members to ask questions to make sure they understand what the other family member is saying.
8. Encourage family members to stay on one topic.
9. Encourage family members to increase opportunities to communicate with one another.

Based on Bloomquist, M. (2005). *Skills Training for Children with Behavioral Disorders: A Parent and Therapist Guidebook.* New York, NY: Guilford Press; Park, E. (2012). Communication skills for you and your family. In P. T. Nelson (Ed.). *Families Matter: A Series for Parents of School-Age Youth.* Newark, DE: Cooperative Extension of the University of Delaware; Peterson, R. & Green, S. (2009). Families First: Keys to Successful Family Function—Communication. Available at http://pubs.ext.vt.edu/350/350-092/350-092_pdf.pdf

Child-Focused Family Therapy

Knowledge of family therapy interventions is imperative when working with children and adolescents because the family system is critical to the child's mental health. There is substantial evidence that family therapy is an effective intervention for children and youth experiencing behavior and eating problems and for adolescents abusing substances. Family therapy has also been shown to reduce the risk of emotional and physical abuse.

Family therapy has been a primary intervention for youth with substance abuse problems, demonstrating improved family functioning and improved parenting behaviors and decreases in target symptoms of alcohol and drug use (Liddle, 2004). Several types of therapy—specifically, multidimensional family therapy, functional family therapy, and group cognitive–behavioral therapy—have been shown to be effective interventions for adolescents with substance abuse (Waldron & Turner, 2008). Family-based interventions often are effective in reducing delinquency, aggression, depression, and anxiety in substance-abusing adolescents. In addition, family treatments for adolescent substance abusers often result in improved parenting skills and family problem-solving techniques (Hogue & Liddle, 2009). Waldron and Turner (2008) found that the family etiology and antecedents for substance abuse that have been effectively targeted with family therapy interventions included parent and sibling use, parental attitudes toward use, parent–child communication and conflict skills, and parent–child bonding and relationship involvement. Additional research supports the following:

- Family-based behavioral therapies have been found effective in the treatment of sleep and eating problems in young children (Carr, 2009a).

- Functional family therapy (FFT) and multisystemic therapy (MST) have been found to significantly reduce jail time or re-arrest for children and adolescents with conduct disorders (Austin, Macgowan, & Wagner, 2005; Woolfenden, Williams, & Peat, 2002).

- Parent management training has been found to decrease internalizing symptoms in youth with attention deficit/hyperactivity disorder (Corcoran & Dattalo, 2006).

The Kellerman Family

Mary and Bob Kellerman have come to their first family therapy evaluation because their 14-year-old son Kyle's behavior has changed in the past year, culminating in recent a hospitalization for substance dependence. Until their son needed hospitalization, Mary and Bob had no idea he had been drinking alcohol during the last year and had recently started using marijuana. Kyle was also caught shoplifting and has been hanging out with a set of friends who have vandalized public property. He is currently failing his freshman year in high school, because he has been skipping school and not completing his homework. The parents reported that they began having more arguments with Kyle over the past year, and this is causing tension in their marriage.

APPLICATION

1. What types of questions will you want to ask about the presenting problem to get a better sense of this family's problem?

2. What types of family therapy have been identified in the research as being helpful for youth with conduct problems and substance use?

3. What programs or therapists in your area specialize in working with adolescents with substance abuse and their families?

critical thinking

- A meta-analysis of parent training programs found that parent training is effective in reducing risk for emotional maltreatment and physical abuse, although not for sexual abuse (Lundahl, Nimer, & Parsons, 2006). Additional systemic reviews found that family-based therapy for the treatment of physical abuse and neglect took at least six months. Types of family treatments for physical abuse that were found useful included cognitive–behavioral therapy, parent–child interaction therapy, and MST (Carr, 2009b).

- Family-based interventions have also demonstrated success in the treatment of youth with anorexia nervosa, bulimia, and obesity (Carr, 2009a).

Adult-Focused Family Therapy

Research on the outcomes of family therapy in adult psychiatric disorders indicated that couples who received couples therapy fared better than 80% of couples in control groups (Shadish &

The Alvarez Family

APPLICATION

1. What stressors, risk factors, and strengths can you identify in the immediate and extended family system, including biological, social, cultural, spiritual, and psychological realms?

2. What does Bowenian family theory say would be contributing factors to a relationship cutoff? How will you inquire as to the reasons for Emily's cutoff with her sister?

3. What treatment interventions might be helpful for this family?

Emily and Rick Alvarez married five years ago after dating for two years. Emily's family is Jewish and has been in this country for several generations; Rick's family is Roman Catholic and immigrated to the United States from Mexico when his parents were both young. They speak English in their home. Rick and Emily both earned college degrees, and they work in the same company, where they met. Emily is in sales, and Rick is in management. They earn similar salaries. They have a few close friends from work and in the community where they live. They have two sons, Scott (3 years old) and Gabriel (5 months old).

They came to see you because Emily feels overwhelmed and depleted with the responsibilities of work and mothering. She reports getting only about 4 hours of sleep a night owing to the baby not sleeping through the night. Emily feels that she must keep working, as they depend on her salary. They report that their sexual life is less fulfilling and they have less time for each other. Emily wishes that Rick would help with more of the domestic chores around the house as well as attending to the boys' needs; however, Rick feels that it is his job to be a breadwinner and he feels that Emily should attend to the role of parent and homemaker, as his mother did. Emily does not attend synagogue; Rick attends Catholic mass every weekend with his parents and the two boys. Emily says she is not comfortable attending the Catholic church but allows the boys to go with Rick, as it gives her some time to herself. Both Emily's and Rick's parents are married, with no divorces.

In obtaining the family psychiatric history, you learn that Rick's father is a recovering alcoholic and Rick's two brothers are alcoholics. Rick reports that he drinks only occasionally. Emily's mother had depression and was successfully treated with sertraline (Zoloft) and cognitive–behavioral therapy in the past year. Emily is concerned that she may have some symptoms of depression. Emily cut off her relationship with her only sister approximately 5 years ago. Emily's parents live several states away and Rick's family lives in the same town. Emily has hypertension, and her father has Crohn's disease. Rick and his parents are in good health. Rick's mother is a homemaker and had three children; Rick's father owns his own landscaping business. Emily's mother is a retired accountant and her father was an engineer before his health declined due to Crohn's disease and he could no longer work. You begin a family genogram (Figure 24-4).

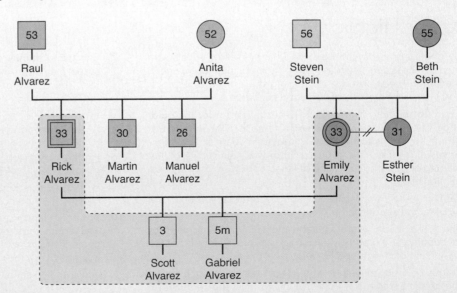

24-4 Family genogram of the Alvarez family. What needs to be added to complete the genogram?

Baldwin, 2003). Couples therapy using an emotionally focused framework involves improving insecure and anxious attachment bonds. The strength of the therapeutic alliance is critical in emotionally focused family therapy. Behavioral couples therapy works by creating fair and pleasing exchanges and responses between the couple (Carr, 2009b). Sex therapy has demonstrated improvement outcomes of patients with a variety of sexual dysfunctions (Duterte, Segraves, & Althof, 2007). Family-based therapy treatments have been successful in reducing domestic violence and improving agoraphobia and obsessive–compulsive disorder (Carr, 2009b). Partner-assisted cognitive behavioral exposure therapy was useful in patients with panic disorder. Various forms of couples therapy have been useful in decreasing depression in a partner or spouse. Behavioral couples therapy and community reinforcement with family training were found to be the most effective approaches to creating abstinence, having greater relationship satisfaction, and better child adjustment in adults with substance abuse problems (Carr, 2009b).

Pause & Reflect

1. *What are the benefits to having family members practice new skills in therapy before trying them at home?*

2. *Why do you think cognitive–behavioral therapy has been proven useful for parent management training?*

3. *Referring to Chapter 5, what cultural considerations are important when determining the appropriateness of different family interventions? How might completing the cultural formulation interview assist the nurse in helping identify appropriate family interventions?*

From Suffering to Hope

Group and family therapy provide safe, directed settings in which patients and family members can examine their suffering, explore feelings, learn to identify triggers, and practice appropriate and healthy behaviors. Appropriate therapy experiences depend on thorough assessment of the patient or family and require a leader experienced in setting boundaries and skilled at working with families and groups. The registered nurse provides support and encouragement to patients and families considering or participating in the group process. The RN also may lead task groups and psychoeducation groups, providing information about important topics such as medication administration and community resources. Advanced practice nurses with appropriate training and certification may lead psychotherapy groups. Regardless of the setting, nurses at all levels must be empowered to recognize the suffering of patients and families and be able to provide support and information to help patients and families recognize and cope with distress. As patients work through the group or family therapy process, they may find hope and healing as they begin to learn how to listen and respond appropriately to others, and as they receive positive feedback for their efforts. By participating in group or family therapy, patients can learn valuable skills that will have a positive impact on their experiences in all types of groups and relationships, promoting hope and increased confidence in their relationships with others.

Chapter Highlights

1. By engaging in psychotherapy with others, individuals with mental illness can begin to restore their abilities to engage in meaningful relationships, decreasing their sense of isolation and increasing feelings of hope and confidence.

2. In group therapy, individuals meet together under the guidance of a professionally trained therapist. The purpose of group therapy is to help group members learn about themselves and others in the group, improve their quality of life, learn to cope with illness, and develop improved interpersonal relationships

3. Family therapy is a specific form of group therapy in which the group is the specific family unit.

4. The group leader establishes the group's norms and rules for functioning and gradually encourages group members to take ownership of the group's function.

5. Stages of group development include the orientation stage, the conflict stage, the cohesive stage, and the termination stage.

6. Group members assume various roles within the group. Challenging roles that the leader must address include the monopolizer, the silent patient, and the help-rejecting complainer.

7. Successful family therapy depends on a thorough family assessment that includes data about the presenting problem, the biological and psychological status of individual family members, and established patterns of function and communication.

8. A family genogram is a visual display of the family and their relationships with one another.

9. Cognitive–behavioral family therapy provides opportunities for role rehearsal, assertiveness training, thought stopping and replacement, and practicing new skills before using them at home.

10. Bowenian family therapy promotes a balance of individuality and togetherness by promoting differentiation, resolving emotional triangles, and addressing family processes.

11. Family therapy promotes development of problem-solving and communication skills.

NCLEX®-RN Questions

1. The nurse is working with a patient experiencing an alteration in mental health. The nurse recognizes that group therapy has the potential to offer which curative factors? Select all that apply.
   a. Altruism
   b. Universality
   c. Individuality
   d. Heterogeneity
   e. Corrective recapitulation

2. The charge nurse is planning group activities for patients on an inpatient unit. Which type of group does the nurse identify as most appropriate for introducing nonpharmacologic approaches to treat depression?
   a. Task
   b. Activity
   c. Support
   d. Psychoeducation

3. The nurse is evaluating the progress of a weekly support group. The nurse recognizes that the group is in the cohesiveness stage when what occurs?
   a. Competition for the leader's attention increases.
   b. Participant self-disclosure begins to increase.
   c. Members actively evaluate their ability to fit in.
   d. Members look toward the leader for acceptance.

4. The nurse has been assigned the responsibility of leading a group. Which action would the nurse carry out first?
   a. Establishing norms
   b. Ensuring confidentiality
   c. Determining the purpose
   d. Encouraging self-disclosure

5. The nurse is evaluating group process and documenting emerging roles of individuals in a group. Which task role would be most appropriate for the nurse to use to describe the patient who consistently offers explanations for suggestions made by other group members?
   a. Energizer
   b. Elaborator
   c. Information giver
   d. Initiator-contributor

6. The nurse is explaining the types of activities a family is likely to engage in while participating in cognitive–behavioral family therapy. Which would be included in the discussion? Select all that apply.
   a. Exploring the conditions and antecedents that triggered the conflict and its outcomes
   b. Replacing negative patterns of behavior with problem solving strategies
   c. Encouraging positive reinforcement within the family
   d. Focusing on the history of the problem from family of origin
   e. Providing opportunities for catharsis and open-ended discussion

7. The nurse is completing a family assessment using the Bowenian family therapy model. Which finding indicates the presence of emotional triangles within the family system?
   a. Several family members become inflexible in the face of change.
   b. A spouse works longer hours to avoid being with another spouse.
   c. A first-born child identifies with power and authority in the family.
   d. Unrealistic parental fears promote the belief that something is wrong with a child.

8. The nurse is working in the mental health setting that employs various types of individual and group therapies depending on patient needs. The nurse understands that which type of treatment intervention is most likely to result in improvement outcomes for children or adolescents with conduct disorders?
   a. Parent management training
   b. Functional family therapy
   c. Emotionally focused frameworks
   d. Partner-assisted cognitive–behavioral therapy

Answers can be found on the Pearson student resource site: nursing.pearsonhighered.com

Pearson Nursing Student Resources Find additional review materials at **nursing.pearsonhighered.com**

References

American Group Psychotherapy Association. (2011). What is group psychotherapy? Available at http://www.agpa.org/home/practice-resources/what-is-group-psychotherapy-

Austin, A. M., Macgowan, M. J., & Wagner, E. F. (2005). Effective family-based interventions for adolescents with substance use problems: A systematic review. *Research on Social Work Practice, 15*(2), 67–83.

Benne, K. & Sheats, P. (1948). Functional roles of group members. *Journal of Social Issues, 4*(2), 41–49.

Berlin, L., & Ziv, Y. (2005). *Enhancing Early Attachment: Theory, Research, Intervention and Policy.* New York, NY: Guilford Press.

Bloomquist, M. (2005). *Skills Training for Children with Behavioral Disorders: A Parent and Therapist Guidebook.* New York, NY: Guilford Press.

Bohus, M., Haaf, B., Simms, T., Limberger, M., Schmahl, C., Unckel, C., Lieb, K., & Linehan, M. (2004). Effectiveness of inpatient dialectical behavioral therapy for borderline personality disorder: A controlled trial. *Behaviour Research and Therapy, 42*(5), 487–499.

Bowen, M. (1978). *Family Therapy in Clinical Practice.* New York, NY: Aronson Publishers.

Burlingame, G., Fuhriman, S., & Mosier, J. (2003). The differential effectiveness of group psychotherapy: A meta-analytic perspective. *Group Dynamics, Theory, Research and Practice, 7*(1), 3–12.

Burlingame, G. M., Mackenzie, K. R., & Strauss, B. (2004). Small group treatment: Evidence for effectiveness and mechanisms of change. In M. Lambert, (Ed.). *Bergin & Garfield's Handbook of Psychotherapy and Behavior Change* (5th ed.). New York, NY: Wiley, pp. 647–696.

Burlingame, G., Theobald-McClendon, D., & Alonso, J. (2011). Cohesion in group therapy. *Psychotherapy, 48*(1), 34–42.

Campanini, R., Schoedl, A., Pupo, M., Costa, A., Krupnick, J., & Mello, M. (2010). Efficacy of interpersonal therapy group format adapted to posttraumatic stress disorder: An open label add on trial. *Depression and Anxiety, 27*(1), 72–77.

Carr, A. (2009a). The effectiveness of family therapy and systemic interventions for child focused problems. *Journal of Family Therapy, 31*, 3–45.

Carr, A. (2009b). The effectiveness of family therapy and systemic interventions for adult focused problems. *Journal of Family Therapy, 31*, 46–74.

Catherall, D. (1988). *Interviewing in Family Therapy: The Problem Centered Approach.* Unpublished manuscript.

Corcoran, J., & Dattalo, P. (2006). Parent involvement in treatment of ADHD: A meta-analysis of the published studies. *Research on Social Work Practice, 16*(6), 561–570.

Corey, M., Corey, G., & Corey, C. (2010). *Groups: Process and Practice* (8th ed.). Belmont, CA: Brooks/Cole (Cengage Learning).

Dorrepaal, E., Thomas, K., Smit, J., van Balkom, A., van Dyck, R., Veltman, D., & Draijer, N. (2010). Stabilizing group treatment for complex posttraumatic stress disorder related to childhood abuse based on psychoeducation and cognitive behavioral therapy: A pilot study. *Child Abuse and Neglect, 34*(4), 284–288.

Duterte, E., Segraves, T., & Althof, S. (2007). Psychotherapy and pharmacology for sexual dysfunctions. In P. Nathan and J. Gorman, (Eds.). *A Guide to Treatments That Work* (3rd ed.). New York, NY: Oxford University Press, pp. 531–569.

Feldman, L., & Pinsof, W. (1982). Problem maintenance in family systems: An integrative model. *Journal of Marital and Family Therapy, 8*(3), 295–308.

Ginzburg, K., Butler, L., Giese-Davis, J., Cavanaugh, C., Neri. E., Koopman, C., Classen, C., & Spiegel, D. (2009). Shame, guilt and posttraumatic stress disorder in adult survivors of childhood sexual abuse at risk for human immunodeficiency virus: Outcomes of a randomized clinical trial of group psychotherapy treatment. *Journal of Nervous and Mental Disease, 197*(7), 536–542.

Hamrin, V., Weycer, A., Pachler, M., & Fournier, D. (2006). Evaluation of peer led support groups for graduate nursing students. *Journal of Nursing Education, 45*(1), 39–42.

Hogue, A., & Liddle, H. (2009). Family based treatments for adolescent substance abuse: Controlled trials and new horizons in service research. *Journal of Family Therapy, 31*(1), 126–154.

Hulse-Killacky, D., Killacky, J., & Donigian, J. (2001). *Making Task Groups Work in Your World.* Upper Saddle River, NJ: Prentice Hall/Pearson.

Jonsson, H., & Hugaard, E. (2009). Group cognitive behavioral therapy for obsessive-compulsive disorder: A systematic review and meta-analysis. *Acta Psychiatrica Scandinavica, 119*(2), 98–106.

Liddle, H. (2004). Family-based therapies for adolescent alcohol and drug use: Research contributions and future research needs. *Addiction, 99*(2), 76–92.

Linehan, M. (1993). *Skills Training Manual for Treating Borderline Personality Disorder.* New York, NY: Guilford Publications.

Lundahl, B., Nimer, J., & Parsons, B. (2006). Preventing child abuse: A meta-analysis of parent training programs. *Research on Social Work Practice, 16*(3), 251–262.

McDermut, W., Miller, I. W., & Brown, R. A. (2001).The efficacy of group psychotherapy for depression: A meta-analysis and review of the empirical research. *Clinical Psychology: Science and Practice, 8*(1), 98–116.

McGoldrick, M., Gerson, R., & Petry, S. (2008). *Genograms: Assessment and Intervention* (3rd ed.). New York, NY: W.W. Norton & Company.

McGoldrick, M., Giordano, J., & Garcia-Preto, N. (2005). *Ethnicity and Family Therapy* (3rd ed.). New York, NY: Guilford Press.

Minuchin, S. (1974). *Families and Family Therapy.* Cambridge, MA: Harvard University Press.

Nichols, M. (2010). *Family Therapy: Concepts and Methods* (9th ed.). Boston, MA: Allyn & Bacon.

Park, E. (2012). Communication skills for you and your family. In P. T. Nelson, (Ed.). *Families Matter: A Series for Parents of School-Age Youth.* Newark, DE: Cooperative Extension of the University of Delaware.

Perseius, K., Ojehagen, A., Ekadahl, S., Asberg, M., & Samuelsson, M. (2003). Treatment of suicidal and deliberate self-harming patients with borderline personality disorder using dialectical behavioral therapy: The patients' and the therapists' perceptions. *Archives of Psychiatric Nursing, 17*(5), 218–227.

Peterson, R. & Green, S. (2009). Families First: Keys to Successful Family Function—Communication. Available at http://pubs.ext.vt.edu/350/350-092/350-092_pdf.pdf

Pinsof, W. (1995). *Integrated Problem-Centered Therapy: A Synthesis of Family, Individual, and Biological Therapies.* New York, NY: Basic Books.

Rademaker, A. (2009). Multimodal exposure based group treatment for peacekeepers with PTSD: A preliminary evaluation. *Military Psychology, 21*(4), 482–496.

Ray, R., & Webster, R. (2010). Group interpersonal psychotherapy for veterans with posttraumatic stress disorder: A pilot study. *International Journal of Group Psychotherapy, 60*(1), 131–140. doi: 10.1521/ijgp.2010.60.1.131

Shadish, W., & Baldwin, S. (2003). Meta-analysis of MFT interventions. *Journal of Marital and Family Therapy, 29*(4), 547–570.

Waldron, H., & Turner, C. (2008). Evidence based psychosocial treatments for adolescent substance abuse. *Journal of Clinical Child and Adolescent Psychology, 37*(1), 238–261. doi: 10.1080/15374410701820133

White, J., & Klein, D. (2008). *Family Theories* (3rd ed.). Thousand Oaks, CA: Sage Publications, Inc.

Woolfenden, S., Williams, K., & Peat, J. (2002). Family and parenting interventions for conduct disorder and delinquency: A meta-analysis of randomized controlled trials. *Archives of Disorders in Children, 86*(4), 251–256.

Yalom, I. D., & Leszcz, M. (2005). *The Theory and Practice of Group Psychotherapy* (5th ed.). New York, NY: Basic Books.

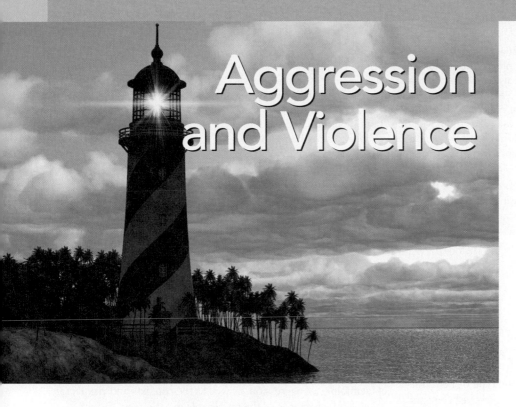

Aggression and Violence

25

Joanne DeSanto Ienacco

Learning Outcomes

1. Discuss the role that anxiety and anger play in the development of aggressive and violent behaviors.

2. Summarize the role of neurobiology in aggression and in perception of and response to aggression.

3. Identify societal and environmental contexts that contribute to aggression and violence.

4. Differentiate categories of workplace aggression and features of victims and perpetrators by type.

5. Identify factors that increase the risk of aggression in patients with mental illness and in health care settings.

6. Evaluate different interventions and therapies used in the care of patients with anxiety and aggression.

7. Describe standards of practice related to maintaining safety with aggressive behaviors and to safely using interventions that restrict patient freedoms, such as restraint and seclusion.

8. Examine factors important to the nurse's self-awareness and self-care when exposed to aggressive behavior.

9. Recognize signs and symptoms that indicate that an individual may be at risk for, or be a victim of, interpersonal violence or rape.

10. Summarize interventions appropriate to caring for patients who are victims of interpersonal violence or rape.

Key Terms

Joe Logan Relapse Phase

Joe Logan is involuntarily admitted to an inpatient psychiatric setting after being dropped off at the emergency department (ED). The police found him outside a convenience store pacing back and forth, swinging his arms as if boxing, and talking loudly to himself on the sidewalk in front of a store. Joe is homeless and has a history of substance abuse and schizoaffective disorder and is well known to the unit staff. The nurse finds Joe in the dayroom, playing with a Nerf football in front of the television. Several patients are in the dayroom trying to watch a sci-fi movie. Joe starts shouting, "I told you we were being invaded by them! The aliens will bring us back in their ships, we have to stop them!" He has not slept since his admission the night before, and he refuses to eat because of concerns that the aliens have drugged his food so they can abduct him. Joe has refused medications for the same reason.

A psychiatric technician approaches the nurse to explain that he plans to take the football and get Joe to settle down. The tech walks out to the dayroom and directly confronts Joe, stating, "Joe, give me the ball. You need to quiet down because you are scaring the other patients." Joe responds by getting very close to the tech's face, shaking his fist and yelling, "Oh, so you *are* part of it! You already have your implants and now you want to help them do this to the rest of us!"

APPLICATION

1. What do you think is the best action for the technician to take at this moment?

2. What are some alternate ways that the staff might have managed this problem?

3. What environmental factors may be promoting Joe's escalation?

Introduction

Nurses in every setting must be able to intervene to prevent aggressive and violent behavior and to provide care for patients manifesting these behaviors as well as for those who are victims of aggression and violence. **Aggression** may be defined as any type of behavior intended to intimidate, harm, or injure another. Aggressive behaviors may manifest in speech, as either subtle or direct verbal threats, or in action, as in holding another at knife- or gunpoint. **Violence** may be defined as the purposeful use of force, resulting in physical or psychological injuries or death. Violence includes force directed toward self or others.

It is difficult to capture aggression numerically. Aggression ranges from mild threats to more severe forms, including large-scale efforts at intimidation. Two very different examples of large-scale forms of aggression are (1) the "tagging" of buildings by neighborhood gangs in an attempt to influence neighborhood behaviors, and (2) voter intimidation. Many acts of aggression go unreported owing to fear of the aggressor. Violence, on the other hand, is more frequently reported, and can be more accurately estimated through aggregate reporting by law enforcement and emergency departments. Still, some acts of violence, including and especially interpersonal violence and rape, often go unreported (Rape, Abuse, and Incest National Network [RAINN], 2009a).

Violence is a significant problem in the United States (Box 25-1). Witnessing violent events is associated with 2.6 times greater risk of

depressive symptoms and 2.4 times greater risk of anxiety symptoms (Clark et al., 2007). The high rates of violence and the negative consequences of aggression exposure make aggression and violence a priority for intervention.

This chapter provides an overview of the pathophysiology and epidemiology of aggression, as well as the contexts and risk factors for violent behaviors and the nurse's role in acting to reduce the risk for aggressive and violent behaviors in psychiatric patients. In addition, the chapter provides an overview of two specific types of violent behaviors, interpersonal violence and rape.

In all settings, nurses must be prepared to identify early warning signs of aggression to intervene to prevent the escalation of anxiety, frustration, and anger to aggressive behavior. Psychiatric patients experience a variety of risk factors for aggression. Knowledge of these characteristics and risk factors helps nurses to better understand the potential for aggression and violent behavior and to intervene to prevent aggressive episodes.

Aggression and Violence

Aggressive behaviors can be thought of as existing on a continuum from least aggressive to most aggressive (Box 25-2). This continuum often can be observed in the clinical setting, where nurses may see a trajectory of behaviors that escalates over time to the point at which an aggressive act occurs. The episode may start with a patient muttering

Prevalence of Violence in the United States   box 25-1

- Death by violence (homicide or suicide) is among the top five causes of injury deaths in every age group.
- Assault is the most prevalent violent crime.
- Homicide is the least prevalent violent crime.
- It is estimated that slightly more than half of individuals who exhibit violent behavior have a psychiatric disorder.

- Of urban women receiving care at neighborhood health clinics, 66% report witnessing violence.
- Witnessing violent events puts individuals at greater risk for depressive and anxiety symptoms.

Based on Centers for Disease Control and Prevention (CDC). (2010a). 10 leading causes of injury deaths by age group highlighting violence-related injury deaths United States—2010. Available at http://www.cdc.gov/injury/wisqars/pdf/10LCID_Violence_Related_Injury_Deaths_2010-a.pdf; Federal Bureau of Investigation. (2012). Violent crime. Available at http://www.fbi.gov/about-us/cjis/ucr/crime-in-the-u.s/2011/crime-in-the-u.s.-2011/violent-crime/violent-crime; Clark, C., Ryan, L., Kawachi, I., Canner, M. J., Berkman, L., & Wright, R. (2007). Witnessing community violence in residential neighborhoods: A mental health hazard for urban women. *Journal of Urban Health, 85*(1), 22–38.

The Continuum of Aggression

box 25-2

Figure 25-1 identifies some of the common behaviors that occur in aggressive events and places them on a continuum from lowest to highest levels of aggressive behavior. Above the figure, a line extends, illustrating the continuum beginning at a lack of aggressive behavior all the way across the figure to the highest levels of aggressive behavior. The upper row denotes aggressive actions that are directed toward objects and the bottom row denotes actions that are aggressive toward other people or self-directed. Most of the behaviors identified in the upper row can be directed toward others or self. Nonverbal behaviors (such as loud noises) and verbal behaviors are considered less aggressive than physical behaviors, which can range from slamming things and spitting to physical contact and use of a weapon.

Continuum of Aggressive Behavior
4 No Harm Rules:
Pets
Property
People-Self
People-Others

Nonverbal-----------------------------Verbal--Physical

	Nonverbal	Verbal	(Physical)	Physical
Toward Objects	• Staring • Glaring • Making obscene gestures • Pacing	• Making loud noises • Shouting • Swearing • Insulting • Threatening	• Slamming doors • Slamming items	• Throwing • Kicking • Breaking
Toward self or others	• Staring • Glaring • Making obscene gestures • Pacing	• Making personal threats • Making personal insults • Spitting • Making loud noises • Shouting • Swearing • Insulting • Threatening	• Pushing • Slapping • Pinching • Striking/Hitting • Punching • Biting	• Attacking • Using a weapon • Cutting

25-1   Continuum of aggression. *Based on* an unpublished figure by Joanne DeSanto Iennaco.

expletives or raising his or her voice about a situation. This may be an expression of anxiety, fear, frustration, or anger. In most cases, aggressive behavior is a response to an unmet need, often combined with underlying anxiety and poor coping mechanisms. As the need continues to go unresolved and the patient's anxiety rises, frustration followed by anger can lead to an aggressive or violent outburst (Figure 25-2). If the patient's concern or need is not resolved, the patient may escalate to higher-level aggressive behaviors. Some forms of verbal aggression are considered more severe, such as threatening to harm others. Threats range from general statements, such as "You better watch out, because I might hurt someone," to very specific, such as "If I see Mary, I am going to bash her head through the wall." When threats become specific and personal, they are considered more severe.

Physical forms of aggression may include movements that are threatening, such as flexing the arms or pounding a fist in one's hand. These are less severe than actually throwing something or punching a wall. Aggression is most severe when it escalates to violence, such as hitting someone or throwing someone across a room. Individuals may also use weapons or objects to threaten or harm others, which is considered higher on the continuum of aggressive behaviors.

Generally, individuals progress from less severe behaviors to more severe behaviors. It is unlikely that an individual would move abruptly from a state of complete relaxation to physically assaulting others. Careful observation of patients and communication with them allows the nurse to observe changes in feelings that result in

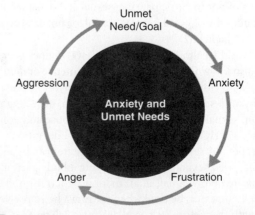

25-2   Anxiety rises as needs are not met. Without resolution, anxiety may lead to frustration, and then, in turn, to anger and aggression.

changing behaviors, such as fear or anxiety leading to agitation, or anger leading to verbal aggression. The key to managing aggressive behavior is to identify the cues or warning signals of feeling states and actions that suggest the potential for aggressive behavior. Intervention early in the continuum of aggressive behavior will help prevent further escalation of this behavior.

Types of Aggression

In general, two types of aggression are identified: predatory aggression and impulsive aggression (McEllistrem, 2004). The distinction is important to understanding the motivation, antecedents, and interventions that would be most effective. **Predatory aggression** refers to aggressive activity that is premeditated or planned. In predatory aggression, the aggressor usually is calm, unemotional, controlled, and has a goal (McDermott et al., 2008). Predatory aggression is also called *planned* or *instrumental aggression*.

Impulsive aggression refers to aggressive activity in which the individual is in a state of emotional arousal. This form of aggression is overt and reactive, and it may involve self-protection. Impulsive aggression is also called *reactive* or *affective aggression*. Some further identify a form of aggression that is psychotic in nature due to it being precipitated by psychotic symptoms. However, research reveals that this form of aggression has qualities similar to impulsive aggression, although it may originate from psychotic symptoms such as hallucinations, delusions, or paranoia (McDermott et al., 2008). Impulsive aggression is the most common type of aggression seen in psychiatric hospitals; it relates to anger management and psychiatric symptoms. This suggests that intervention for impulsive aggression should focus on effective treatment of symptoms, as well as treatment for anger regulation (McDermott et al., 2008).

Types of Violence

Violence ranges from simple assault to homicide. In between are a number of violent acts, including child abuse, elder abuse, interpersonal violence, and rape. Suicide is a form of self-directed violence. *Simple assault* is characterized as a physical attack by one individual against another, without the use of or display of a weapon and without any resulting serious or aggravated injury. *Child abuse* includes physical assault or violence, mental abuse (including intimidation and verbal threats), and child sexual abuse (which includes exposure to pornographic material or sexual acts as well as the coercion or forcing of a minor to participate in a sexual act) (Chapter 30). *Elder abuse* includes the physical, mental, sexual, or financial abuse of an older adult (Chapter 32).

The World Health Organization (WHO) defines *interpersonal violence* (also known as **intimate partner violence** or *domestic violence*) as "behaviour by an intimate partner or ex-partner that causes physical, sexual or psychological harm, including physical aggression, sexual coercion, psychological abuse and controlling behaviours" (WHO, 2012). Although the legal definitions of terms such as rape and sexual assault vary by state, **rape** generally is defined as forced sexual intercourse (using a body part or object). Rape may involve vaginal, anal, or oral penetration. The term *acquaintance rape* may be used when the rapist had a previous relationship with the victim, such as a classmate, lab partner, or friend (RAINN, 2009b).

As discussed throughout this text, the trauma associated with violent experiences can result in an individual developing one or more psychiatric illnesses. In particular, the trauma-related disorders

and dissociative disorders have their roots in traumatic violence such as child abuse and rape.

Neurobiology of Aggression

Several areas of the brain are involved in aggression and violence, including the frontal lobes and limbic structures. Limbic system involvement includes the amygdala, hippocampus, and hypothalamus, all of which play roles in the regulation of the fight-or-flight reaction and aggressive responses. When faced with a threat, the sensory system relays this message to the thalamus. The thalamus responds in one of two ways: relaying the information to the prefrontal cortex followed by the amygdala; or, if an immediate threat to safety is present, sending the message directly to the amygdala. The amygdala can be thought of as an alarm center, alerting the body to potentially life-threatening situations. With the amygdala, the hippocampus stores memories of threatening situations. When directly alerted through the thalamus, the amygdala response triggers the hypothalamic–pituitary–adrenal (HPA) axis, with the hypothalamus excreting corticotropin-releasing hormone [CRH]) that stimulates the pituitary to release adrenocorticotrophic hormone (ACTH), resulting in the release of cortisol and other hormones from the adrenal cortex. Simultaneous activation of the sympathetic nervous system results in activation of smooth muscles and resulting symptoms of the fight-or-flight response. This response prepares the body to react to threats (to fight or flee), increasing heart rate, blood pressure, and respirations, and reducing nonessential functions (such as digestion). When the body is working effectively, there is a feedback system that "shuts off" the HPA axis, so the body returns to normal function.

There are also differences in brain activity based on the kind of aggression, predatory or impulsive. The involvement of the frontal lobes involves the prefrontal cortex, which has an inhibitory effect on aggressive behavior. The prefrontal cortex can put the brakes on aggressive behavior, with this occurring in a top-down (frontal cortex → limbic) manner to reduce reactivity. Reduced activity in the medial and orbitofrontal cortex is associated with violence and aggression. Predatory aggression is associated with activity in the lateral hypothalamus, whereas impulsive aggression is associated with activity in the medial hypothalamus (Higgins & George, 2013).

The study of humans with diseases, head injuries, and mental illness have helped clinicians better understand brain functioning. For example, a case study identified a woman with hyperphagia, obesity, and overt aggression; on autopsy, it was found that she had a tumor in her ventromedial hypothalamus, which had been found in previous studies of cats to be related to impulsive aggression (McEllistrem, 2004; Reeves & Plum, 1969). One of the most famous examples is the case of Phineas Gage, who had an accident in which an iron rod was forced through his skull and caused damage to his left and right prefrontal cortex. Prior to his injury, Mr. Gage was responsible, efficient, and balanced. After his accident, he was described as fitful, impulsive, unfocused, and easily agitated. This provides validation of the role of the frontal cortex in inhibiting impulses (Higgins & George, 2013). Imaging results suggest that decreased frontal lobe function may result in poor executive functioning and lack of top-down inhibition of threatening stimuli (Bufkin & Luttrell, 2005).

Neurotransmitters also play a role in aggression, with serotonin and GABA function inhibiting both impulsive and predatory aggression, and norepinephrine and dopaminergic systems facilitating impulsive aggression (McEllistrem, 2004). Studies have shown lower levels of serotonin metabolites in those with a history of aggression (Antypa, Serretti, & Rujescu, 2013; Duke, Begue, Bell, & Eisenlohr-Moul, 2013). These connections are supported by results from studies of medication use to treat aggression, in which benzodiazepines and serotonergic agents have reduced aggressive behavior. Norepinephrine levels also play a role in aggression, with high levels exacerbating aggressive behavior. Drugs that reduce norepinephrine levels, such as the beta-adrenergic antagonists, have been used to inhibit aggression (Yanowitch & Coccaro, 2011). In addition, dopamine antagonism, using antipsychotic medications such as risperidone and haloperidol, has been used to reduce aggressive behavior for many years.

Evidence suggests that neurobiological, genetic, and environmental factors all play a role in aggression. For example, in studies of children with biologic family members having risk for aggression (antisocial behavior), the children were found to be influenced both by familial risk as well as by placement in disruptive adoptive homes, with greatest risk of aggression and conduct disorder in children with both risk factors (Gallardo-Pujol, Andres-Pueyo, & Maydeu-Olivares, 2013; McAdams, Gregory, & Eley, 2013; Pickles et al., 2013).

Pause and Reflect

1. *Have you ever witnessed someone escalating along the continuum of aggression? How did you respond?*
2. *How might an understanding of the neurobiology of aggression influence treatment of individuals who are prone to aggressive behavior?*

Epidemiology of Aggression

Unfortunately, the media portrayal of violence in those with mental illness tends to promote stigma and stereotypes of those with mental health problems, and promotes exaggerated perceptions of the problem. Of all media coverage, 39% focuses on the dangerousness of people with mental illness, rather than focusing on issues of mental health treatment, recovery, or public policy (Council of State Governments Justice Center, n.d.). It is important to recognize that some individuals with psychiatric disorders are at lower risk of violent behavior and others at higher risk than the general population (Choe, Teplin, & Abram, 2008; Sadeh, Binder, & McNiel, 2013). The prevalence of aggression will vary based on the sample and measures used. For example, if a community is interested in determining the prevalence of violent behavior by those with a mental illness, then a community-based sample must be used, and the study must not only identify the prevalence of violence, but it must also have a mechanism to determine whether individuals have mental disorders. In addition, it would be interesting to know how many of those individuals have also been identified and treated or whether they are suffering a disorder without treatment in the community. Very few community-based studies can provide this information.

Stigma (discrimination) also is an issue, as both the media and the public have fears about people with mental illness (Torrey, 2011). Even though individuals with disorders such as schizophrenia and mania have higher rates of violence than the general public, they contribute to only a fraction of total violence in society. Before considering the contribution of mental illness to violence, the contributions of violent criminal offenders must first be identified. In 2010, Yang, Wong, and Coid identified that the most violent crimes are committed by persistent male offenders. They state, "it is estimated that about 50% of all crimes are committed by 5–6%" of these offenders (Yang, Wong, & Coid, 2010, p. 740). Studies consistently report that less than 10% of violent crime is attributable to individuals with schizophrenia, which is one of the disorders most commonly thought to increase risk of violence (Walsh, Buchanan, & Fahy, 2002). Although studies show that those arrested are three times more likely to have a mental illness than the general population, the most common diagnoses of arrestees are substance use and personality disorders, as compared to diagnoses such as schizophrenia and bipolar disorder (Teplin et al., 2012). In reality, most episodes of violence committed by individuals with mental illness result from a failure to receive adequate treatment (Torrey, 2011).

Aggression and Mental Illness

The relationship between aggression and mental illness is complex. Certainly, many patients with mental illness do not exhibit aggressive behavior, or may exhibit only mild to moderate aggression during times of frustration or high acuity. The National Epidemiologic Survey on Alcohol and Related Conditions (NESARC) findings suggest that the role of mental illness in violent behavior is complex and part of a group of other factors that increase the risk of violence, including history of physical abuse, parental criminal acts, unemployment, and victimization (Elbogen & Johnson, 2009).

Differences in samples used to study the incidence and prevalence of violence in those with mental health problems are critical to understand. If only acute populations are studied, it is more likely that associations of mental illness with aggression prevalence will be overestimated, given that those hospitalized have more acute symptoms of psychosis and, typically, greater co-morbidity with substance use (Walsh, 2002). The only population-based epidemiologic study to describe violence in the United States was the 1990 Epidemiologic Catchment Area (ECA) Survey, which identified that 3.7% of all respondents reported at least one violent behavior in the year preceding the interview. The ECA study offers a community-based random sample of individuals who were asked about the presence of violent behavior, including hitting a spouse, partner, or child; having been in a fight as an adult; having used a weapon; or having fought while drinking (Swanson, Holzer, Ganju, & Jono, 1990). Prevalence of violent behavior in the overall ECA sample was 3.7%, and males had higher rates of violence than females: 5.29% versus 2.21%, a consistent finding. The highest prevalence of violent behavior was in younger men of lower socioeconomic status. Finally, this study found that rates of violent behavior were greater in men than women, and increased by number of psychiatric diagnoses (Swanson, Holzer, Ganju, & Jono, 1990). It should also be noted that violence by women toward men is increasing (Straus, 2005).

Prevalence of affective disorders and schizophrenia were three times higher in those who were violent compared with those who were not violent; however, violence was not significantly higher in those with schizophrenia compared to those with other disorders. When individual disorders were identified using diagnostic surveys, from 11% to 12% of those with psychiatric disorders (including schizophrenia, mania, and depression) identified experiencing one or more violent behaviors in the past year (Swanson, Holzer, Ganju, & Jono, 1990).

Based on rates of violence reported in the ECA study, the risk of violence in the entire population that can be attributed to schizophrenia is only 5.5% (Swanson, Holzer, Ganju, & Jono, 1990).

Internationally similar rates have been found; for example, 5.2% of the risk of violence in Sweden was attributed to those with serious mental illness (Fazel & Grann, 2006; Volavka & Citrome, 2008). This proportion of violence attributable to mental illness reflects those at greatest risk of violence when they are acutely experiencing symptoms and is reflected in the higher rates of aggression in those hospitalized for psychiatric symptoms.

In an early study of hospitalized patients, Tardiff and Sweillam (1982) found that only 7% of patients over a 3-month period were assaultive. Walsh, Buchanan, and Fahy (2002) identified two studies of patients with schizophrenia. Both studies demonstrated that 20% of patients had been violent prior to hospital admission. Other studies have found that 20% of assaults can be directly attributed to positive symptoms of schizophrenia (Nolan et al., 2003). Researchers have also found that a small number of patients with schizophrenia often account for a large number of assaults in a setting because they are persistently assaultive and have many repeated aggressive events while hospitalized (Volavka, 2013).

Mania and dementia are associated with an increased risk for violent behavior, although these patients typically do not choose a target, but rather strike at those who happen to be nearby (Rueve & Welton, 2008). Patients admitted to a public sector hospital should be evaluated for a history of aggression as a possible predictor of inpatient violence (Newton et al., 2012). Personality disorders are also a risk factor for violence—in particular, for repeated violence (Council of State Governments Justice Center, n.d.). A much higher risk group than those with schizophrenia are those with substance abuse, which greatly increases the risk of violence (Walsh, Buchanan, & Fahy, 2002). For example, alcohol reduces the inhibitions that may quell aggressive behavior by modifying neurotransmitter function, including decreasing serotonin function (Ciccarelli & White, 2013). In addition, the use of illicit substances increases the risk for being both a victim of interpersonal violence and a perpetrator of violence (WHO, 2009).

Risk Factors

One way to think about risk factors for aggression is to consider them based on whether the risk factor is static or dynamic. A *static* risk factor refers to one that does not change over time, such as gender. *Dynamic* factors are those that could potentially be changed (Box 25-3). Interventions may help decrease the risk of aggression when focused on changing these factors. Static risk factors for increased aggression include male gender, having a history of prior aggressive behavior,

Dynamic Risk Factors for Aggression and Violence	box 25-3

Younger age

Low socioeconomic status

Psychosis, psychiatric symptoms

Medication nonadherence

Involuntary hospitalization

Delayed gratification of needs in the inpatient setting

Substance use

low IQ, and history of head injury (Hamrin, Iennaco, & Olsen, 2009; Petit, 2005; Rueve, 2008). Volavka et al. (2013) identify that conduct problems in childhood double the rate of violent behavior in those with schizophrenia. Individuals who have been prior victims of violence also are at increased risk of aggressive behavior (Council of State Governments Justice Center, n.d.).

Dynamic factors that increase risk for aggression include younger age, low socioeconomic status, and substance use (Buckley et al., 2003; Hamrin, Iennaco, & Olsen, 2009). In addition, psychiatric symptoms such as psychosis or recurrence of psychiatric symptoms increase risk for aggressive behavior, as does nonadherence to medications in psychiatric patients (Council of State Governments Justice Center, n.d.). Patients who are hospitalized involuntarily are also at greater risk of being aggressive. Other dynamic risk factors relate to the environment, such as delaying gratification of needs, which can be common in inpatient settings where patients are not given complete freedom to eat, sleep, use particular belongings, or communicate with friends and family whenever they choose to (Dack et al., 2013; McDermott et al., 2008).

The Context of Violence

From a global perspective, violence is a significant problem. War, political unrest, terrorism, forced labor, and family violence commonly occur. Unfortunately, for most of human history, violence of this nature has resulted in recurrent loss of life. Although many nations may be free of internal disputes, there are often actions taken outside those countries' borders that involve warfare and loss of life. At times, these acts are done with the intent of preserving peace, or promoting freedom, yet violence, injury, and mortality can result. Worldwide, approximately 310,000 people died in 2000 from war-related reasons, which accounted for nearly 20% of all violence-related deaths, with a rate of 5.2 deaths per 100,000 population (WHO, 2002).

Violence in Communities

Local communities also experience violence, whether due to gang violence, road rage, domestic violence, substance abuse, or bullying at work or school. A number of factors increase the risk of violence to a community. For example, there is a disproportionate amount of violence in lower-income, impoverished neighborhoods. Many theories exist to attempt to explain the greater risk in one community versus another. One theory, the "broken windows" theory, suggests that when a neighborhood or area is run down and appears to be lacking engagement or investment by both community members and larger society, there will be a disproportionate amount of violence and crime, and further disorder will occur (O'Brien, 2013). The process results in people moving from the area. Disengagement occurs, as businesses and other resources also relocate in response to their consumers relocating. Without some reversal of the disengagement, the neighborhood declines. However, this theory has been disputed, suggesting that the association of "broken windows" with crime is not necessarily one of direct etiology, but that the etiology of community violence and crime is more complex and likely also relates to other factors, including community cohesion, collective action, inequality, and poverty (Gault & Silver, 2008; Sampson & Raudenbush, 2004). Other theories about community violence include the social contagion theory, which suggests that the presence and use of violence

Types of Workplace Violence

table 25-1

Type of Violence	Definition	Examples
Type I	• Criminal intent or activity results in violence. • The perpetrator has no relationship to the victim.	• A drive-through window clerk is injured by gunshots during a robbery. • A nurse is injured during a robbery at night on hospital property.
Type II	• Violence occurs while conducting business or being served by a worker. • The perpetrator has a legitimate relationship with the business.	• A police officer is injured while handcuffing an agitated person during an arrest. • A receptionist in the emergency department is threatened and assaulted by a father who is upset that other patients have been seen before his child.
Type III	• Violence by a worker or ex-worker directed toward another worker. • The perpetrator has or had a formal employment relationship with the victim.	• A computer programmer who was demoted by his boss brings a gun to work and shoots his boss and a co-worker. • A disgruntled physician threatens and verbally abuses a clinician who disagrees with him.
Type IV	• Violence occurs in the workplace to a worker or customer. • The perpetrator has a personal relationship to the victim, but no direct relationship to the business or workplace.	• A grocery store clerk is stalked and assaulted by a former boyfriend while at work. • A nursing assistant is murdered by her ex-husband in the hospital, related to a child custody dispute.

begets further violence (Bogat, Levendosky, & von Eye, 2005; Clark et al., 2007). Even though these are only theories, evidence shows that violence, whether interpersonal or at the community level, results in mental health problems in community members, including stress, anxiety, and depressive disorders.

Workplace Aggression and Violence

The workplace is not immune to violence; it is a microcosm of society, mirroring behaviors seen elsewhere. Aggression and violence in the workplace fall into four categories used by the National Institute for Occupational Safety and Health (NIOSH) to better understand the effects of violence on workers (Table 25-1). Type I violence involves criminal intent—for example, a robbery during which someone is injured or killed. Type II violence involves an individual who has a business or formal relationship to the workplace harming a worker—for example, a passenger on a delayed airplane assaults a flight attendant while trying to leave the plane. Type III violence is an event in which one worker assaults or murders another worker. These events may relate to changes in position, downsizing, or disciplinary action. Type IV violence is associated with a personal relationship between the victim and perpetrator—for example, a violent family member hunts down and assaults or murders a sibling in the workplace.

Recently attention has focused on bullying as a problem in the workplace. Whereas aggression relates to one event, **bullying** refers to repeated events or a pattern of behavior involving abuse or misuse of power. Although bullying typically is thought as occurring in school or among children, bullying can occur in a variety of contexts, including family, work, and social groups. **Workplace bullying** can be defined as deliberate, repeated mistreatment of a worker over time by another worker; it involves negative and aggressive behaviors such as harassment, social exclusion, or interference with job performance (Figure 25-3) (Namie, 2013; Samnani & Singh, 2012; Srabstein & Leventhal, 2010). Workplace bullying results in hostile work environments, and workers may feel isolated and unable to escape the situation (Lutgen-Sandvik, Tracy, &

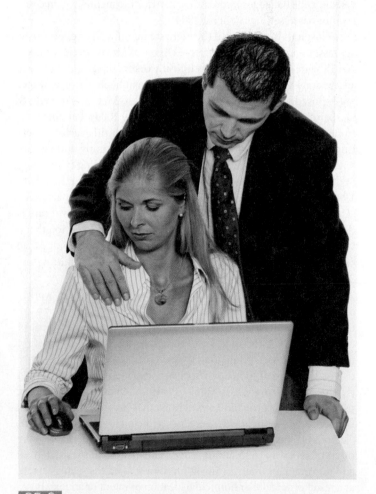

25-3 Workplace bullying involves negative and aggressive behaviors such as harassment, social exclusion, or interference with job performance. Sexual harassment is a form of workplace bullying.

Source: Gina Sanders/Fotolia

Alberts, 2007). Approximately 25% to 30% of U.S. workers report experiencing workplace bullying in the past year (Lutgen-Sandvik, Tracy, & Alberts, 2007; Namie, 2013). **Cyberbullying** (online bullying) in the workplace has also been studied, with reports of 10.7% of workers experiencing cyberbullying (Privitera & Campbell, 2009). Many workplaces have begun to address these issues, promoting improved communication skills, interpersonal relationships, and civility in the workplace. (See Chapter 30 for a discussion of bullying and children and adolescents.)

Violence in Health Care Settings

Violence in health care settings varies by type of setting and acuity of care delivered. Hospital settings are prone to conditions that increase risk for violence, such as when the public can freely move around or when workers are alone with patients and isolated from other workers (Occupational Safety and Health Administration [OSHA], 2004). Other risk factors for aggression and violence in health care settings include characteristics of the services delivered, such as the frequent presence of distraught patients and family members; individuals having to wait for services to be delivered; and low staffing levels that may exacerbate waiting times for those having to wait for care. Societal factors also affect the incidence of aggression in hospitals or health care settings, such as the use of services by the criminal justice system, and challenges in providing care for the mentally ill in community-based settings (OSHA, 2004).

Hospitals have some of the highest rates of worker exposure to aggression and violence (Iennaco, Dixon, Whittemore, & Bowers, 2013), with more than half of clinical workers reporting past-year aggression exposure, compared with approximately 6% of all workers exposed to physical aggression (Findorff, McGovern, Wall, & Gerberich, 2005; Winstanley & Whittington, 2004). Patients tend to be the most frequent perpetrators, although this varies by setting. For example, in obstetrics and pediatrics, family and visitors have higher rates of verbal aggression and threatening (Chapman, Styles, Perry, & Combs, 2009; Whittington, Shuttleworth, & Hill, 1996; Winstanley & Whittington, 2004). Emergency departments also experience family and visitor aggression, particularly if care is delayed, painful treatment is involved, or there a perception that a vulnerable patient needs protecting or is not receiving appropriate care (Gates, Ross, & McQueen, 2006; Winstanley & Whittington, 2004).

Psychiatric settings tend to have the highest rates of worker exposure to aggression. A variety of risk factors for aggression are common to both the populations served and the environment of care. Risk factors for aggression related to the patient population include psychosis and impaired thought processes, mania, substance use or withdrawal, personality disorder diagnosis, and dementia (Hamrin, Iennaco, & Olsen, 2009). Environmental risk factors in the psychiatric setting include restrictions that infringe on individual freedoms; for example, doors are locked, belongings (such as razors, electrical items, belts, and personal communication devices) are often taken away to maintain safety, and visitors are restricted. In addition, patients often are involuntarily admitted to psychiatric care as a result of suicidal or homicidal ideation or intent or an inability to care for themselves because of impaired judgment, thought processes (psychosis), and dangerous behavior (Kho, Sensky, Mortimer, & Corcos, 1998; Raja & Assoni, 2005). Unit-based routines and processes can help to prevent aggression. These include having a unit routine and structure, carefully managing transitions, and carefully assisting patients to maintain their own self-care and hygiene (Hamrin, Iennaco, & Olsen, 2009; Kling et al., 2009).

Although inpatient settings treat patients with the greatest overt symptoms and acuity, rates of aggression generally will be lower in community treatment settings owing to requirements for individuals to be well enough to be discharged or reside in the community. However, lower levels of staffing may be common and many clinicians work alone, which presents risk to workers if a patient is actively decompensating. In general, personnel in these settings must be alert to and actively monitor symptoms of decompensation or crises and stressors that occur in their patients' daily lives.

Assessment of Aggression and Violence

Many clinicians assess the risk of violence in daily practice using clinical judgment based on assessment information obtained from the patient, from the clinician's observations of the patient, and from knowledge of static and dynamic risk factors for violence. Risk assessment tools may also be used to inform the overall assessment of the patient's risk for violence.

Risk Assessment Tools

Some of the more commonly used violence risk assessment tools are the Brøset Violence Checklist (BVC), the Classification of Violence Risk (COVR), and the Historical Clinical Risk–20 (HCR-20). Unfortunately, there is a high rate of false positive results with these tools (Fazel, Singh, Doll, & Grann, 2012). Many individuals are identified and labeled as being at risk but never go on to become aggressive. One strategy may be to use prediction tools to identify those for whom the risk of aggression is low, identifying those not considered a safety risk. Evidence suggests that monitoring dynamic measures may be most effective in predicting aggression in those with serious mental illness such as schizophrenia (Grann, Belfrage, & Tengström, 2000; Vitacco et al., 2012). However, clinicians are cautioned to be careful regarding the contribution of psychiatric illness to aggression risk, as this may promote stigma rather than help in predicting risk (Corrigan & Watson, 2005; Norko & Baranoski, 2005; Rueve, 2008; Torrey, 2011). For example, predicting low-rate events is difficult and imprecise, and the expectation is that instruments will overidentify people at risk or identify many false positives (Yang, Wong, & Coid, 2010). Caution should be used in identifying individuals in this way, as negative repercussions may result, such as detaining or restricting the freedom of individuals based on assessments. Overall, risk assessment tools predict violence with moderate to very good accuracy, although differences exist based on scale and population studied. Some scales are designed for use in the inpatient psychiatric setting, whereas others are designed for use with forensic populations.

Some studies use identification of symptoms to identify high risk of aggression. The Positive and Negative Syndrome Scale (PANSS) has been used to assess poor impulse control and predict the development of aggressive behavior in patients with schizophrenia and schizoaffective disorders (Nolan et al., 2005).

Instruments also have been developed to assess violence risk in specific groups, such as forensic populations and children and

Interventions to Reduce Anxiety and Fear Associated with Aggression — table 25-2

Time Frame	Interventions
Daily	<ul><li>Show a calm, positive, friendly demeanor.</li><li>Employ casual behavioral observation, attention to behavioral changes.</li><li>Express compassion and concern for patients.</li><li>Assist patients without delay.</li><li>Provide needed food and drink.</li><li>Use redirection, distraction, and relaxation techniques.</li></ul>
Acute	<ul><li>Identify origin of anxiety, violence to inform treatment.</li><li>Assess and meet unmet needs.</li><li>Match specific interventions with patient anxiety level.</li><li>Use positive choices and least-restrictive interventions.</li></ul>
Long-term	<ul><li>Cognitive–behavioral interventions designed to reframe incorrect or negative thinking or perceptions of events.</li><li>Anger management interventions.</li><li>Social skills training focused on assertiveness and self-control.</li></ul>

adolescents. The Brief Rating of Aggression by Children and Adolescents (BRACHA), for example, is a tool developed to identify aggression risk during Emergency Department evaluation. Scores have been compared to the Overt Aggression Scale results during psychiatric unit admission, with the instrument being most predictive in older youth (13–19 yrs) (Barzman et al., 2011).

In most settings, nurses may not use specific scales to assess patients for violence. However, they should be alert to factors that may be revealed during history taking. In a review of 20 years of longitudinal data on aggressive events in psychiatric settings, Flannery et al. (2011) identified a triad of symptoms that are associated with aggression risk over time: history of violence toward others, personal victimization, and substance use disorder. These results suggest that a high level of awareness is needed when these factors are part of a patient's history.

Nursing Assessment

The first steps in responding to aggression are to understand the reasons that individuals become aggressive and to better understand the experience of aggression. From this knowledge, the nurse is more likely to be successful in intervening to resolve aggressive behavior. Intervention is based on time frame and can be used as follows:

Daily: on a day-to-day basis to set the culture of how staff and patients interact in the therapeutic milieu

Acute: for a patient who is experiencing acute anxiety and agitation

Long term: if anxiety, anger, and aggressive behavior have been identified as problems on which an individual patient needs to focus in therapy

In addition to understanding the cycle or trajectory of experiences from anxiety to aggression, nurses and clinicians can employ several universal interventions to help patients reduce the anxiety and fear associated with aggression (Table 25-2).

As stated earlier, aggressive behavior usually is a response to an unmet need, often combined with underlying anxiety and poor coping mechanisms. As the need continues to go unresolved and the individual's anxiety rises, frustration followed by anger can lead to an aggressive or violent outburst (see Figure 25-2). For example, a father may lash out at hospital staff when he is unable to get what he perceives as timely information about his child's condition. Aggressive behavior often is preceded by certain signs or symptoms, or warning signs (Box 25-4). When nurses and clinicians are able to identify warning signs and meet the underlying unmet need or anxiety when the individual is at a lower level of anxiety, they may reduce the risk for the anxiety or behavior escalating.

The first step in providing care is assessment of risk and identification of factors on which to focus for intervention (Table 25-3). Knowledge of the patient's history of aggression and violence, as well as an understanding of the subtypes of violence, can help to improve the likelihood that intervention will be successful. For example, when violence is caused by severity of positive symptoms of schizophrenia, such as command hallucinations and delusions or impulsive behavior, interventions should focus on managing psychotic symptoms.

Nurses must also be able to assess the patient's level of anxiety. Patients with severe anxiety or who are in a panic state will be unable

Warning Signs of Impending Aggressive Behavior — box 25-4

Nurses who are able to identify warning signs may be able to implement interventions when the patient is at a lower level of anxiety and reduce the patient's risk of escalating to aggression or violence. These psychological, emotional, and behavioral warning signs include:

- Pacing
- Agitation
- Guardedness
- Paranoia
- Emotional lability
- Irritability

Violence Assessment

table 25-3

Assessment Indicators	Nursing Implications
Patient history of aggression and violence	Helps identify underlying cause, such as symptoms of psychiatric illness, emotional triggers, poor coping mechanisms.
Patient risk factors: • Substance abuse • Impulsivity • Exposure to violence • History of violence in relationships	Helps identify threat level.
Appearance: • Facial expression • Muscles tense or relaxed • Hands relaxed, tense, held in a fist	Provides clues to the patient's anxiety level and mental status.
Behavior and cognition: • Quality of speech (loud, rapid, slurred) • Altered responses to stimuli (lack of reaction, hyperalertness) • Restlessness, agitation, pacing	Indicates the patient's ability to communicate needs and take in and process information.
Interactions with staff and others	Assists in determining patient attitudes, level of engagement.

to take in new information or engage in active problem solving. Specialized interventions are needed to assist these patients in lowering their anxiety levels. For patients with lower levels of anxiety or who are at risk for escalating behaviors, it is important to find out how the patient usually copes with anxiety and frustration. Being aware of what works for the patient historically can assist staff to help patients lower their anxiety levels when they are in crisis (Chapter 13).

As the nurse assesses the patient's anxiety, the nurse must also assess his or her own anxiety level to ensure that it does not interfere with the ability to intervene. Additionally, there must be some recognition that there is an aspect of anxiety that is contagious and can be transmitted from person to person. It is important for the nurse to monitor personal reactions to the patient and use coping mechanisms to be sure that anxiety does not overtake the nurse and escalate to a level at which nursing interventions are negatively influenced by anxiety, fear, frustration, or anger.

Interventions

Intervention begins with communication among nurses and clinicians caring for the patient, especially when team members identify symptoms of anxiety or changes in behavior or communication in the patient. Early awareness of a patient who is having difficulty or is in crisis allows team members to intervene to prevent escalating symptoms and negative outcomes (Wright, Duxbury, Baker, & Crumpton, 2014). Generally, interventions can be classified into four areas. Interventions that reduce anxiety are essential for all patients. Some patients will require the use of seclusion or restraints. Pharmacological interventions may be appropriate for some patients. Finally, environmental and organizational interventions assist nurses and clinicians in reducing patient anxiety and creating a healing environment in both inpatient and outpatient settings.

Reducing Anxiety

Team members who are aware of patients with greater risk for aggression can provide needed support to patients and other members of

the team who are affected. Interventions with a patient who is displaying anxiety, frustration, anger, and aggression are based on core principles of therapeutic communication used to establish therapeutic relationships with patients (see Chapter 8). Nurses should communicate interest in, respect for, and caring to the patient. Nurses must also convey a sense of confidence and competence in their ability to provide care. This can be difficult in situations in which a patient becomes angry and hostile. However, it is important for the patient to see staff as composed and able to provide support and care, despite difficult behaviors that arise. Staff members should focus on building rapport daily with all patients on their unit so patients feel safe and perceive that staff members are genuine in their caring and empathic to patient needs. In addition, having consistently positive interactions each day with patients provides a sense of reliability of staff members in caring about and for patients over time. These positive relationships that are built from the time of the patient's admission are key to being able to manage crisis situations well.

At mild to moderate levels of anxiety, interventions start from a level of verbal empathic communication. Patients at this level are usually able to discuss needs and to problem-solve to improve their ability to cope. It can help to reflect back feelings and ask patients to provide clarification on their experience. Identifying problem behaviors early on is important so intervention can occur when anxiety levels are lower and cognition is clearer.

As patient anxiety increases to moderate levels, verbal statements may need to be more specific and, if anxiety escalates further, statements may be concise and direct. To be effective and be heard at high levels of anxiety, the nurse may need to use the patient's name and shorter statements. Basic communication principles are important.

As patient anxiety reaches severe levels, nurses use several important interventions. The nurse should make contact with the patient, identify the behavior that is problematic, and engage in problem solving appropriate to the level of anxiety. At severe or panic levels of anxiety, the individual may not be able to identify his or her own options to better cope with the problem, but the nurse can offer acceptable options to the patient that will help the patient feel less anxious and more in control. It is important to do whatever is possible to remove the stimulus that is disturbing the patient. For example, if the patient is reacting to another patient or a particular staff member negatively, having the other person move to a different area will be helpful. Anxiety and agitation tend to escalate when there is an audience, particularly if the patient feels a need to "save face," so having other patients move to another area of the unit is a useful intervention. In addition, some attention should be paid to having a patient maintain self-esteem. Although the tension and anxiety associated with situations such as this are hard to manage, the situation should not be rushed to closure. Attention to environmental stimuli is helpful. Decreasing the level of noise and activity is important to helping calm an anxious or agitated patient. A final consideration is space. As anxiety levels increase, people need more space. During interventions, nurses provide space and do not crowd the patient.

Seclusion and Restraint

Seclusion and restraint are two potential interventions that may be used in the inpatient psychiatric setting to protect a patient who is a danger to self or to protect others from injury when imminent risk is present. *Current standards of practice suggest that these are measures of last resort that are used infrequently and only when all other interventions are not successful at maintaining the patient's or unit's safety.* In many ways, the need to resort to use of seclusion or restraint may be viewed as a failure of intervention. Nurses are wise to be mindful of the potential dangers of using restraint and seclusion, which can include psychological and physical injury and even death. Most settings have active programs to eliminate the use of seclusion and restraint. To be successful, programs involve all levels of the organization, from direct care providers to the highest leadership's view and commitment to changing organizational culture (American Psychiatric Nurses Association [APNA], 2007; Haimowitz, Urff, & Huckshorn, 2006). Important ethical and legal boundaries surround the use of these interventions, given the vulnerability of the patient and the risk for inappropriately confining individuals and restricting their autonomy.

Many criteria must be met for seclusion or restraint to be used. In particular, there must be evidence that the patient presents an imminent risk of danger to self or others and that other, less restrictive interventions have been tried successively and have been unsuccessful in addressing the patient safety issue. The direct assessment of a patient and order for the use of seclusion or restraint by a physician or licensed independent practitioner are required to use these interventions. Federal regulations exist on the use of these interventions by hospitals and are part of the conditions of participation in Medicare and Medicaid programs (Federal Register, 42 CFR Part 482: Centers for Medicare and Medicaid Services [CMS], 2006). Rules and requirements for use of these interventions also vary by state and local jurisdiction and by hospital or setting policies and procedures, all of which must be followed carefully. In addition, regulations require all staff with direct patient care activities to have education related to alternative interventions and safe use of restraint and seclusion.

Seclusion is the placing of a person in a locked room; this may be used if the patient requires a place where there is low stimulation and when it is not safe for the patient to be on the regular unit. Typically the seclusion room is a bare room, without furniture or any other items. Patients placed in seclusion usually are dressed in hospital clothing (pajamas or scrubs) and searched to ascertain that they do not have any other items on their person or in the room that may be unsafe. Patients held in seclusion are monitored constantly to ascertain their safety. It should be noted that the standards for use of seclusion specify that "seclusion may only be used for the management of violent or self-destructive behavior" (CMS, 2006).

Physical restraint is the immobilization of a patient either by staff (a physical hold) or by mechanical restraint using locked restraints. Historically, settings have used other devices, including restraint chairs, straitjackets, and "body bags," to physically immobilize patients. The only reason patients are restrained is to prevent them from harming themselves or someone else. When restraints are used, the patient is under constant observation to maintain the patient's physical safety (Box 25-5, Box 25-6). In recent years, the use of physical restraints has been reduced or eliminated in many settings. Further, the American Psychiatric Nurses Association (APNA) has taken the position that "psychiatric-mental health

---

Nursing Care of the Patient in Seclusion or Restraint   box 25-5

The nurse must be vigilant to ensure that a patient's basic safety and physiologic needs are met during the course of any confining intervention. A staff member is assigned to observe the patient so if an emergency arises the patient can be safely cared for, and to protect the patient from others, given the patient's vulnerable state. General nutrition and toileting of the patient must occur regularly during the course of use of seclusion or restraint. Patients should be asked whether they need to use the bathroom, and they should be offered fluids, snacks, and meals—generally, finger foods in small portions that can be consumed by the patient or fed to the patient if needed.

If physical or mechanical restraints are used, assessment of circulation, respiration, and skin integrity are required. Vital signs must be obtained and the patient assessed for risks such as asphyxiation. During mechanical restraint, patients are checked for skin integrity and circulation in each limb. In addition, turning

and passive range-of-motion exercises are provided until the patient is able to move about freely.

The length of confinement in seclusion or restraint should be as short as possible with the patient allowed free movement and full return of all rights and privileges as soon as the risk of danger has resolved. Federal regulations identify maximum time periods for which an individual can be restrained, by age (42 CFR §483.352). For those over the age of 18, the maximum length of an order for restraint is 4 hours; for youths 9 to 17 years old, the maximum is 2 hours; and for those under 9 years old, the maximum is 1 hour. Other requirements involve the need for a face-to-face evaluation of the individual within 1 hour by a physician or licensed independent practitioner, and staff must continually assess, monitor, and reevaluate the patient who is restrained or secluded (Haimowitz, Urff, & Huckshorn, 2006).

The Dangers of Seclusion and Restraint

box 25-6

It is well known that both seclusion and restraint can be dangerous to the patient and providers involved in the procedure. Psychological dangers include acute stress reactions and posttraumatic stress disorder. Physical dangers include injury to patient and staff and even death (most often by asphyxiation of the patient in restraint). In 1998, a team of reporters from the *Hartford Courant* compiled research on the risks associated with seclusion and restraint (Weiss et al., 1998). They compiled this information into the National Restraint Death Database, which documents 142 deaths over a series of 10 years (1988 to 1998).

This series of articles is now famous for reporting the dangers associated with the use of restraint, including asphyxiation, cardiac arrest, medication overdoses, and pulmonary emboli due to restriction of movement and lack of proper assessment of physical well-being. Since the publication of this investigation, federal rules and regulations have been implemented that require standards be met to protect patient rights in hospitals as well as residential settings.

Based on Weiss, E. M., et al. (1998). Deadly restraint: A Hartford Courant investigative report. *Hartford Courant*, October 11, p. 15; U.S. Department of Health and Human Services. (1999). Health Care Financing Administration, Interim Final Rule: Medicare and Medicaid Programs: Hospital Conditions of Participation: Patients' Rights. 42 CFR Part 482. Baltimore, MD: U.S. Department of Health and Human Services; U.S. Department of Health and Human Services. (2006). CMS Final Rule: Medicare and Medicaid Programs: Hospital Conditions of Participation: Patients' Rights. 42 CFR Part 482. Baltimore, MD: U.S. Department of Health and Human Services, December 8, 2006.

nurses provide leadership to create a culture that minimizes the use of seclusion or restraint while promoting a safe environment for persons served as well as staff" (APNA, 2007). All nurses have the responsibility to work toward a culture that promotes safety for both patients and staff while minimizing the use of seclusion and restraint.

Medications

One form of intervention is the pharmacologic management of aggression. For many years, pharmacologic agents have been used to manage symptoms associated with aggression, although there has been limited research (Rueve & Welton, 2008). Depending on the patient's symptoms, level of acuity, and urgency of treatment, careful consideration is made related to choice of medication and route of administration. If there is a risk of immediate harm to the patient or others, medication may be administered involuntarily or despite the patient's declining the medication. This can be considered a **chemical restraint**. Similar to other procedures that infringe on the rights of

patients, careful documentation and orders to provide the medication, even if the patient declines, are required. If involuntary medication is used outside a period of imminent risk to the patient, typically a guardian or health care proxy must provide consent, or a court order must be obtained to administer the medication despite the patient's declining.

In most situations in which a patient has symptoms of anxiety or agitation, medication will be ordered as needed (PRN), or regularly scheduled to begin to titrate the patient to a helpful dose of medication that will manage the presenting symptoms. As with other interventions, there are several time frames to consider in managing the anxious or aggressive patient with medications: the daily medication regimen; the acute medication needs; and the long-term medication regimen (Table 25-4).

Other agents playing a role in aggression management include mood stabilizers and beta-blockers to manage symptoms associated with aggression and violence. Lithium has been found to reduce volatility and irritability in both mental retardation and in bipolar

Use of Medications for the Treatment of Aggression

table 25-4

Time Frame	Purpose	Nursing Implications
Daily	Medication prescribed to manage primary symptoms, such as anxiety, depression, psychosis, or mood instability, that may contribute to risk of aggressive behavior.	SSRIs have been used to minimize impulsiveness, anxiety, and depression, but are not FDA approved specifically for aggression.
Acute	Immediate dose required to lower anxiety level. First-generation antipsychotics, often with a benzodiazepine, may be used to manage anxiety or aggression at this level. Second-generation antipsychotics that may be used include risperidone, olanzapine, and aripiprazole.	Haloperidol is relatively safe, even if little medical history is available, owing to its minimal cardiac effects and or effects on seizure threshold (Petit, 2005). However, some patients have had had acute dystonic reactions from the first introduction of haloperidol and need to be monitored carefully. The second-generation antipsychotics (e.g., aripiprazole, olanzapine, ziprasidone) are now available in injectable form and have much lower risk of extrapyramidal side effects,
Long-term	Medication recommended for patients who have a high risk of violence or repeated episodes over time.	Clozapine has been shown to have great effect when used over time. Perphenazine has shown to be effective on violent behavior in patients with schizophrenia (Buckley, Citrome, Nichita, & Vitacco, 2011; Swanson et al., 2008, Volavka & Citrome, 2008).

disorder (Rueve & Welton, 2008), and lithium improves impulse control and reduces aggression in those with personality disorders (Volavka & Citrome, 2008). Beta-blockers have been used in traumatic brain injury to reduce agitation (Stahl, 2011), and carbamazepine has had similar results in this population (Kavoussi, Armstead, & Coccaro, 1997). Valproate reduces aggression in a variety of disorders, as well (Lindenmayer & Kotsaftis, 2000), although not all results were positive, with evidence supporting only short-term effects in managing aggression (Volavka & Citrome, 2008). Although these agents have had some evidence to indicate their usefulness, additional evidence is needed (Volavka & Citrome, 2008).

Environmental and Organizational Interventions

Several conditions should be considered by team members in mental health settings, including the environment and unit norms and culture, as well as the culture of the organization. For example, a psychiatric setting should have a pleasant environment that is conducive to emotional healing. Serious consideration should be given to space, color, lighting, ambiance, and warmth of the physical environment used to provide psychiatric treatment. The environment should also be safe from potential dangers and free of objects that might be thrown or used as a weapon. In addition, use of space should be considered, including providing for a quiet, low-stimulation environment, and enough space to prevent crowding (Rueve & Welton, 2008; Buckley et al., 2003) One of the more important aspects of the environment in a psychiatric setting is the visibility, approachability, and demeanor of the staff members and other workers on the unit. The staff provides the core structure and care to meet the patient's mental health goals.

Aspects of the unit and team norms and culture include open communication, collaborative problem solving among members, and providing structure and activities. If the team members are not communicating well, this will translate into communication issues with patients. Staff members will not be adequately prepared or knowledgeable about the patients they are caring for if communication is not valued by team members. The unit and team are also responsible for maintaining the safety of the setting by alerting one another of changes in patient status and safety.

The unit context also varies by shift. The day shift tends to be more fast-paced, with many more clinicians visible and providing care. The evening shift typically operates at a slower pace, and the night shift is quiet, with generally lower lighting and a focus on helping patients to have a good night's sleep. Current inpatient unit acuity is generally high and admissions are accepted around the clock, despite lower staffing levels in the evening and night shifts. Methods to manage admissions without disrupting unit processes and culture are important to maintaining a therapeutic milieu.

The Nurse's Response to Violence

A difficulty of working in human services is that although nurses' intentions are to best serve their patients, they are not always appreciated by the patients and/or their family members. The nurse or clinician can be confronted with negative reactions to well-intentioned caregiving. This disturbs and produces anxiety for the nurse. The nurse must be aware of and actively address the emotional residue that can build up from interacting with individuals who are anxious, angry, or aggressive; otherwise, it can be detrimental to the nurse's health and well-being. A variety of strategies can help nurses to manage negative emotions. A key component is maintaining an active regimen of self-care that enables healthy functioning despite consequences inherent in the role. Self-awareness is the cornerstone to self-care. To gain awareness of the impact of work activities, the nurse can engage in a variety of activities that offer active reflection on experiences (Box 25-7). Whether by meditating, journaling, or reviewing experiences with colleagues prior to leaving work, it is important to take some time to review and reflect on interactions and experiences during the course of daily work. Including a scan of emotional well-being is also helpful in considering the feelings that may have been engendered during a shift and how those feelings have affected the nurse's state of mind. Regular practice of deep

---

Values Clarification	box 25-7

You enter a patient room with a glass of juice for Toni, as the report indicated that she was thirsty all night. You think this might be helpful, as you meet with the patient to find out how she is feeling this morning. When you approach and greet the patient, she screams at you, "Get out of my room, none of you know what you are doing! Get me a real nurse!"

1. How does it make you feel when you approach a patient to provide needed care and you are met with an angry or hostile response? How might you respond to the patient in this situation? After you leave an interaction like this, what feelings would you have?

2. Imagine returning later in the day or the next day to care for this same patient. How might you feel as you enter her room and greet her? What can you do to prepare yourself emotionally to interact with a patient who is hostile and potentially volatile?

You are called to another unit to help intervene with David, a young male patient who was paranoid and delusional and believed staff members were actually prison guards who were planning to incarcerate him without a trial. Earlier, David threw a chair across the room and overpowered one of the staff members from your unit. The team of staff that responded to the emergency ended up having to place him in a physical hold and mechanically restrain him so he was not a further danger. After securing the restraints, David continued to yell and scream because he believed his delusion was true and he was now being held in a prison.

1. What kind of thoughts run through your mind about this patient? How do you think you would feel if you were actually in this situation? Do you feel any differently about this situation because a staff member you work with was assaulted?

2. How do you make sense of this situation, where one perspective on the events could be that the staff did exactly what David feared?

3. How would you feel about providing care for this patient the following day on the unit? Should your coworker who was assaulted by the patient be required to care for this patient?

breathing and relaxation techniques or mindfulness meditation, spiritual activities, physical exercise, engaging with family and social supports, or hobbies and leisure activities are important for the nurse to maintain balance, given the stressful nature of being a caregiver (Chapter 7).

Protective factors that help the nurse to maintain resilience in stressful clinical settings include making good choices about work environments and taking steps to develop a strong working team. Work settings should address the need for staff to debrief after difficult interactions and interventions. Most settings debrief for purposes of improving processes of care delivery for individuals or groups of patients, but it is also important to attend to the strong feelings and attitudes that surface when staff members are subjected to disrespect or physical injury from a patient.

Models of intervention and debriefing have been developed to provide support to staff members after aggressive events. The Assaulted Staff Action Program (ASAP) is one model that shows positive response to intervention over time (Flannery, Farley, Rego, & Walker, 2007; Flannery, Farley, Tierney, & Walker, 2011). ASAP provides peer help to assist staff victims in coping with the aftermath of patient assault.

Pause and Reflect

1. *Why is reducing anxiety so important to reducing the risk for aggressive behavior?*
2. *What concerns do you have about working with patients who have a history of aggression? What strategies can you use to help address your concerns?*

Intimate Partner and Sexual Violence

Intimate partner and sexual violence occur across the spectrum of life. Although there are definitive risk factors that can increase the individual's risk of experiencing intimate partner or sexual violence, nurses in every setting should be able to recognize signs and symptoms and know how to support victims in getting help to recover from violence and in maintaining safety.

Intimate Partner Violence

Intimate partner violence (IPV), or domestic violence, involves aggressive behavior of many types between individuals in an intimate or dating relationship. IPV most often refers to violence toward women by men; however, some studies suggest that women may engage in an equal amount of violence toward men, although the results of male partner violence are stronger and more severe (Bensimon & Ronel, 2012). Despite increasing recognition of the need for services to address issues of IPV in same-sex relationships, research regarding IPV among same-gender partners remains limited (Baker et al., 2013). Most often, the behaviors in IPV relate to dynamics of power and control over a partner or significant other (Figure 25-4). Behaviors can include emotional or physical abuse or injury, sexual violence, coercion, or stalking (American College of Obstetricians and Gynecologists [ACOG], 2012). Psychological or emotional abuse may involve isolation or deprivation, intimidation, or coercion. IPV occurs regardless of gender, sexual orientation, or age. IPV has a great

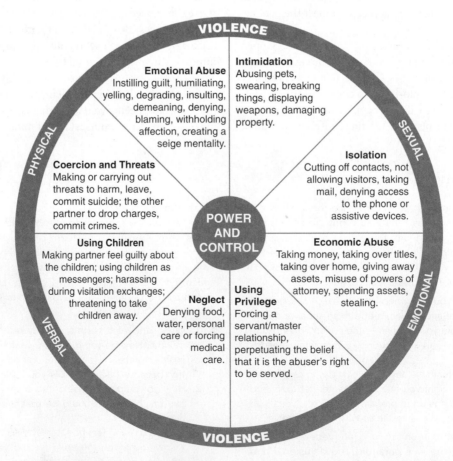

25-4   The power and control wheel illustrates the strategies that one partner may use to intimidate, control, and harm another.

impact on society from the costs of caring for the physical and mental health needs of victims of IPV and rape, with estimates of more than $8 billion per year for direct care and lost productivity (Family Violence Prevention Fund [FVPF], 2010; National Center for Injury Prevention and Control [NCIPC], 2003).

Walker (1984) describes a three-phase model depicting a cycle of violence. The first phase is one of tension building; this is the longest phase, during which tensions gradually increase and escalate between a couple (Bensimon & Ronel, 2012). In the second phase, the acute battering phase, violence erupts and the victim may be injured or even killed, as the batterer loses physical and emotional control. The final stage is the "honeymoon" phase, during which the batterer is contrite and fearful that the victim will leave and tries to make up for the violence, and the victim may feel some responsibility for the event—and the cycle begins again. Over time, cycles tend to be shorter, with more outbursts and with a shorter honeymoon phase (Bensimon & Ronel, 2012).

Sexual violence involves any unwanted sexual contact and can range from unwanted kissing or touching to rape (ACOG, 2012). It also includes any type of forced penetration with any body part or object. Sexual assault does not require completion of a sexual act to be considered assault. Forms of sexual violence include:

- Using force (including the threat of harm or death) to compel a person to engage in a sexual act
- Engaging in a sexual activity with a person who cannot consent or understand the act
- Abusive sexual contact (violence during or following consensual sex) (Centers for Disease Control and Prevention [CDC], 2010b)

Sexual violence also includes **stalking**, harassment, or other unwanted communication or contact (including following, phone calls, messages, and vandalizing property) that may instill fear or harm (CDC, 2010b; Mullen, Pathe, & Purcell, 2001; National Institute of Justice [NIJ], 2007). Unwanted communication or contact may occur in person or through social media and other means. Often, technology is used by abusers to control, coerce, or stalk victims (Connecticut Coalition Against Domestic Violence [CCADV], 2013).

Teen dating violence is one form of IPV and includes acts that occur when people are together or when apart via electronic media—for example, texting or posting sexual pictures online. Dating violence may begin with less obvious behaviors, such as teasing and name calling; however, these can lead to actual physical assaults as well as rape. The Youth Risk Behavior Surveillance System identifies that 9.4% of high school students reported being hit, slapped, or physically hurt by a boyfriend or girlfriend in the prior year (CDC, 2012).

Prevalence and Risk

Each year, an estimated 4.8 million incidents of physical or sexual assault to women are reported. Because many incidents are not reported, this is considered an underestimate of actual incidents (ACOG, 2012; Tjaden & Thoennes, 2000). Most research focuses on IPV perpetrated by males on their female partners, finding high rates of negative physical and mental health outcomes (Afifi et al., 2009; Coker et al., 2002; Seedat, Stein, & Forde, 2005; Zlotnick, Johnson, & Kohn, 2006). However, based on National Comorbidity Survey Replication results, 15.2% of women and 20.3% of men in heterosexual marital relationships experienced intimate partner violence (IPV) in their current relationship (Afifi et al., 2009). There are important differences in prevalence and risk for violence based on gender and age.

Youths are a high-risk group: surveys indicate that one out of 10 adolescents has experienced physical violence from a dating partner in the past year (ACOG, 2012; Silverman, Raj, & Clements, 2004). History of violence in adolescence is associated with later IPV as an adult. Suicide attempts and mental health problems are also associated with history of dating violence (ACOG, 2012). Pregnancy is also a risk factor for IPV. Annually 324,000 pregnant women are victims of IPV in the United States and their infants suffer from a variety of problems, including low birth weight and fetal injury (ACOG, 2012; Brown, 2009). History of child abuse or domestic violence may increase risk for IPV. Different theories exist as to why individuals with a history of child abuse are more at risk for IPV, including learned helplessness and perceiving violence as normal (Renner & Slack, 2006).

Access to a firearm significantly increases mortality rates in incidents of domestic violence. More than two-thirds of firearm homicides of women were perpetrated by an intimate partner (Violence Policy Center, 2012). Homicide is five times more likely in a violent relationship when an intimate partner has access to a firearm (Campbell et al., 2003). A victim may believe that having a firearm protects her; however, in most cases, purchase of a handgun increases a victim's risk for intimate partner homicide (Wintemute, Wright, & Drake, 2003). Firearms are the most frequently used weapon in IPV homicides (CCADV, 2013).

Prior history of being physically abusive and having been a victim of physical or psychological abuse are predictors of perpetration. Head injury may increase the risk of aggressive behavior due to impaired impulse control. Abusive men have higher rates of borderline personality disorder and antisocial personality disorder. Many studies find that alcohol abuse is a risk factor for perpetration of IPV, and the frequency and severity of violence were higher in men who were alcoholics compared with men who were not alcoholics (Ali & Naylor, 2013).

Signs and Symptoms

Warning signs of IPV include indicators of physical and psychological abuse. IPV is often about power and control in a relationship and involves many behaviors and patterns of control that often belittle and isolate victims. The following are considered warning signs of an abusive relationship:

- Isolation: not allowing a partner to see family or friends
- Extreme jealousy
- Threats to harm a partner, their children, relatives or friends, or themselves
- Aggressive behavior
- Control of access to finances, transportation, or children
- Criticism or humiliation of a partner
- Control or restriction of movement or activities
- Physical harm—hitting, punching, slapping, biting, kicking, pinching, pushing, or choking
- Overprotectiveness
- Sudden anger, volatility, or hostility
- Rigid sex roles; use of force during sex

The presence of any of these behaviors suggests that a risk for abuse may be present and that help and support may be needed.

Nursing Interventions

Nursing interventions focus on confidentiality, safety and protection, and empowerment, beginning with being able to recognize and screen for domestic violence. Victims of IPV often have difficulty extricating themselves from violent relationships. Reasons include love, loyalty, embarrassment, denial of abuse, to hold the family together for children, financial reasons, religious or cultural reasons, stigma, low self-esteem, and relationship conflicts. As with any kind of abuse, when the abuser plays an important role to the victim, the victim may experience fear, self-blame, shame, and anxiety related to identifying that violence and abuse are a part of the relationship. Often there is a dynamic in the relationship such that cycles of closeness and intimacy are followed by conflict and aggression and then followed by remorse and forgiveness. Screening is one way that nurses can help to provide information and resources to a person who may be suffering IPV. Hawley and Hawley Barker (2012) suggest that screening be implemented across health care settings using framing and direct questions, such as the following:

- I'm concerned that your symptoms might be caused by someone hurting you.
- Some of the patients we see here are being hurt by their partners. Is anyone hurting you?
- Did someone cause these injuries? Was it your partner/spouse/husband/wife?
- Do you ever feel afraid? Is it safe for you to go home?

There are many reasons that a victim stays with an abusive partner, and the dynamic that develops within the victim–abuser relationship is a hard one to change. Often, victims work for years to make changes so they can leave the relationship. It can be difficult as a nurse to stand by and support a person through cycles of violence. However, it is important to help victims of violence to develop plans for their safety (and for the safety of their family, if the victim has children or other dependents) and provide support until they are able to resolve this problem. Although child abuse and elder abuse are situations for which reporting is required of professionals who have knowledge of safety issues, IPV is not reportable in most jurisdictions.

Safety planning involves providing the victim with information about community resources available, including safe houses that provide shelter to victims of violence (Figure 25-5), crisis hotline services, and legal options available to victims for protection from violence (for example, obtaining restraining orders). The plan should contain a list of important phone numbers that may be needed in the event of a crisis or immediate safety threat, including the police or sheriff, friend or relative, counselor, shelter, probation officer, clergy, attorney, work, and school contact information. Victims should have a list of safe people they can contact, and they can identify a code with supportive friends, family, or co-workers so if the victim is in danger, the police can be notified and help sent. The plan should also include plans for what victims can do to safely respond or leave a situation with their abusers. Plans should also address what to do if the abuser arrives and a problem occurs when the victim is leaving work or arriving home and provide options for how to manage crisis situations. Victims also should keep important papers, such as Social Security cards, passports, birth certificates, marriage licenses, bank records, insurance cards, and other

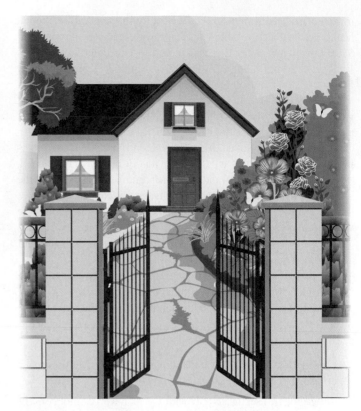

25-5 Domestic violence programs offer safe, transitional housing to victims of interpersonal violence that provides a gateway to help them rebuild their lives after they leave their abusive partners. Nurses should be knowledgeable about the shelters and services in their area, including which programs accept families, LGBT clients, and pets.

documentation. Victims should also find a safe place to keep a bag ready, which should include money, keys, and copies of important documents and phone numbers.

The time of greatest risk for victims of violence is when they attempt to end the violent relationship (CCADV, 2013). After leaving a violent relationship, a victim may need to plan for many changes that will help to maintain safety, including changing phone number(s), changing locks, and documenting all contact and incidents that involve the abuser.

Sexual Violence and Rape

As stated earlier, rape involves sexual violence or assault in which one individual forces another to engage in a sexual act without permission or consent. Rape occurs in intimate partner relationships (and is one form of IPV) and also between acquaintances or strangers. Rape is considered a crime by the legal system, although it is not always reported and often charges are not pressed against the perpetrator. When a sexual act is performed with an individual who is unable to give consent—for example, a child or an unconscious or intoxicated person—that also is considered sexual assault or rape. Consent is an important issue in defining sexual violence. For a person to consent to sexual contact, that person must be either legally or functionally competent to give informed consent. Generally individuals who are underage, ill, disabled, asleep, or under the influence of a substance such as alcohol or drugs are considered unable to give consent (Basile & Saltzman, 2009). The negative sequelae from rape include physical injury, sexually transmitted diseases, and pregnancy, as well as anxiety, depression, acute stress disorder, and posttraumatic stress disorder.

Prevalence

Although anyone can be a victim of rape, regardless of age, gender, or sexual preference, girls or women ages 16 to 24 are most often victims (Mollen, Goyal, & Frioux, 2012). It is difficult to know the actual prevalence of rape, as it is under-reported—in the United States, 54% of rapes are not reported (RAINN, 2009a). Even though 46% of rapes are reported, only 12% of rapists are arrested (RAINN, 2009a). Military sexual trauma is another source of rape that is often unreported (Burgess, Slattery, & Herlihy, 2013).

Signs and Symptoms

Typically, individuals will report to a health care setting if they sustain serious injuries in a sexual assault. However, many rape victims do not seek help because of fear of retaliation, shame, or self-blame. Despite not seeking help, many victims suffer physically and emotionally with injuries and psychological distress. Victims of rape should be encouraged to seek support or counseling to help them deal with the negative sequelae of sexual assault.

Rape results in severe trauma for many victims; many experience difficulty in daily functioning, including interference with thinking, working, socializing, eating, and sleeping. Some victims may present to a health care setting reporting sleep disturbances, depression, or anxiety symptoms and not disclose that they have been raped or assaulted until later in the therapeutic process (Carretta & Burgess, 2013). Victims may have traumatic memories associated with the event, and feel numb, detached, strange, or unreal, common symptoms of depersonalization or dissociation after traumatic events. They may re-experience the event from repeatedly thinking about it or through nightmares or flashbacks. For many victims, these acute stress disorder symptoms continue over time, and they are eventually diagnosed with PTSD. Pregnancy and sexually transmitted infections are potential physical sequelae.

One of the most difficult aspects of sexual violence is victim blaming. Victims may be subject to blame for their sexual assault or rape, particularly in instances in which the perpetrator is known to family and friends. Aspects of victim blaming include accusing the victim of "asking for" the sexual assault as a result of engaging in suggestive behaviors or wearing provocative clothing.

Nursing Interventions

Individuals may present to acute or emergency care after a sexual assault for treatment of injuries sustained during the assault. Most regions have sexual assault counseling teams who are able to attend to the psychological needs of victims. Given that rape is a crime, health care professionals caring for victims may be involved in the collection of forensic evidence from a victim. Sexual Assault Nurse Examiner (SANE) certification programs offer education and training specific to this circumstance. Although victims are encouraged to report rapes to the police, victims are not forced or required to do so. Victims should have access to testing and prophylaxis for sexually transmitted infections, HIV, and pregnancy. If the victim is a child or adolescent, the nurse may be mandated to report to child protective services if the injuries are due to maltreatment by a caregiver or someone who resides with the child.

As with victims of interpersonal violence, nursing care of sexual assault victims focuses on safety, confidentiality, and empowerment. Nurses empower victims by encouraging them to make their own decisions regarding medical and psychological care following the event. Ensuring that victims have safe transportation to a safe location is critical. Referrals to rape crisis centers, counselors, and other resources are essential.

Pause and Reflect

1. *What concerns do you have about working with a patient who has been sexually assaulted?*
2. *What resources are available in your area for individuals who are experiencing domestic violence or have been raped?*

Chapter Highlights

1. In most cases, aggressive behavior is a response to an unmet need. If the need continues to go unresolved, the individual's anxiety and anger may rise and result in an aggressive or violent outburst.

2. The frontal lobes and limbic structures are two areas of the brain involved in aggression and violence. Neurotransmitters are thought to play an important role in aggression.

3. Risk factors for aggression are either static (i.e., they do not change over time) or dynamic. Dynamic risk factors include younger age, low socioeconomic status, psychosis, medication nonadherence, delayed gratification of needs in the hospital setting, and substance use.

4. Violence takes place within contexts. Examples include global, community, workplace, and health care settings.

5. Violence in health care settings varies by the type of setting and acuity of care delivered. Hospital settings are prone to conditions that increase risk for violence. Psychiatric settings, in particular, have high rates of worker exposure to aggression.

6. The Brøset Violence Checklist, Classfication of Violence Risk, and Historical Clinical Risk–20 are three tools that are commonly used to assess patients' risk for violence.

7. Successful nursing assessment and intervention require determining the reasons that individuals become aggressive. Intervention is based on whether a response is required on a daily basis in the treatment setting, for acute anxiety and agitation, or to address behaviors over a long period of time.

8. Nursing assessment requires knowledge of the warning signs of impending aggressive behavior, as well as assessment of specific indicators, such as patient history of aggression and violence, risk factors, appearance, behaviors, cognition, and interactions with others.

9. Interventions may include actions to reduce anxiety, seclusion or restraint, the use of medications, and/or environmental or organizational modifications.

10. Nurses working with aggressive or violent patients must manage negative emotions appropriately through appropriate self-care strategies.

11. Intimate partner violence or domestic violence involves aggressive behavior of many types between individuals in an intimate or dating relationship.

12. Intimate partner violence typically exhibits in three stages: tension, acute battering, and a honeymoon phase.

13. Access to a firearm significantly increases the risk for death in an abusive situation.

14. Warning signs of intimate partner violence include both physiologic and psychological indicators, such as isolation, threats, restriction of movement or activities, and physical harm.

15. Rape involves sexual violence or assault in which a sexual act is forced on one person by another person without permission or consent.

16. One of the most difficult aspects of sexual violence is victim-blaming. Victims may be subject to blame for their sexual assault or rape, particularly when the perpetrator is known to family and friends.

17. Nursing interventions for victims of interpersonal or sexual violence focus on safety, confidentiality, and empowerment.

NCLEX®-RN Questions

1. The nurse is working on an inpatient psychiatric unit and notices a patient pacing with fists clenched. The nurse approaches the patient with the understanding that this behavior is usually a manifestation of which of the following?
   a. A lack of regard for others
   b. An unmet need with anxiety
   c. Poor environmental controls and limits
   d. Predatory instincts with cognitive deficits

2. The nurse is caring for a patient with a history of injury to the frontal lobe of the brain. The nurse recognizes that the impact of this injury on the ability to manage aggressive impulses results from an alteration in which key neurological function?
   a. Stimulation of the limbic axis
   b. Hypothalamic hormone release
   c. The responsiveness of the amygdala
   d. Executive function and inhibition of impulse

3. The community health nurse is working on an initiative to reduce the incidence of violence in an inner city, impoverished neighborhood. Which evaluation finding best indicates that a risk factor for community violence has been addressed?
   a. More affluent citizens begin to populate the area.
   b. Funding is obtained for neighborhood beautification.
   c. Disenfranchised youth are bused to better school systems.
   d. Members take advantage of opportunities for cohesion and engagement.

4. The nurse working on an inpatient mental health unit is attending to a colleague who was assaulted while caring for an agitated patient. The nurse recognizes that the colleague was a victim of which type of workplace violence?
   a. Type I
   b. Type II
   c. Type III
   d. Type IV

5. The nurse is completing an assessment of a patient being admitted to the inpatient mental health unit. Which initial assessment is most useful for identifying the risk that the patient will become violent or assaultive?
   a. Level of anxiety
   b. Reality orientation
   c. Past episodes of violence
   d. History of incarceration

6. The nurse is evaluating outcomes for a patient presenting in the emergency department for treatment after being sexually assaulted. The nurse understands that it is most essential that the care provided results in which outcome?
   a. The patient agrees to undergo counseling.
   b. The patient initiates a criminal complaint.
   c. The patient's physical safety is maintained.
   d. The patient identifies the perpetrator of the assault.

7. The nurse is implementing evidence-based practice to reduce the incidence of injuries related to restraint and seclusion on the inpatient mental health unit. Which approach to patient care is most likely to be effective?
   a. Providing for the direct supervision of any patient in restraints
   b. Ensuring that all personnel are properly trained in restraint techniques
   c. Emphasizing activities that build rapport and ensure that patient needs are met
   d. Warning patients frequently that if behaviors escalate, restraints will be used

8. The nurse is working with a population of anxious and potentially aggressive patients. Which intrapersonal factor is most essential to the nurse's capacity to promote a safe and effective care environment?
   a. Absence of fear or anxiety
   b. Composure and self-control
   c. Assertive communication style
   d. Ability to sacrifice safety for others

9. The nurse is caring for a patient who has been a victim of physical abuse at the hands of a domestic partner. The nurse recognizes that which action by the patient places the patient at the greatest risk for imminent violence?
   a. Begins planning for a safe exit
   b. Reports the abuse to authorities
   c. Tells the partner that the relationship is over
   d. Seeks treatment for physical injuries

10. The nurse is working with a pregnant adolescent patient and her partner in the prenatal clinic. Which behaviors would alert the nurse to the possibility that the patient is a victim of interpersonal violence? Select all that apply.
   a. The partner insists that they should get married after the baby is born.
   b. The patient states that her partner has made her cut off contact with all her friends.
   c. The patient states that her partner did not want to terminate the pregnancy.
   d. The partner is extremely jealous of the attention that the unborn child is getting.
   e. The partner makes frequent derogatory comments about the patient's physical appearance.

Answers can be found on the Pearson student resource site: nursing.pearsonhighered.com

References

Afifi, T. O., MacMillan, H., Cox, B. J., Asmundson, G. J. G., Stein, M. B., & Sareen, J. (2009). Mental health correlates of intimate partner violence in marital relationships in a nationally representative sample of males and females. *Journal of Interpersonal Violence, 24*(8), 1398–1417.

Ali, P. A., & Naylor, P. B. (2013). Intimate partner violence: A narrative review of the biological and psychological explanations for its causation. *Aggression and Violent Behavior, 18,* 373–382.

Almvik, R., & Woods, P. (1998). The Brøset Violence Checklist (BVC) and the prediction of inpatient violence: Some preliminary results. *Psychiatric Care, 5*(6), 208–211.

Almvik, R., Woods, P., & Rasmussen, K. (2000). The Brøset Violence Checklist (BVC): Sensitivity, specificity and inter-rater reliability. *Journal of Interpersonal Violence, 12,* 1284–1296.

American College of Obstetricians and Gynecologists (ACOG). (2012). Intimate partner violence. Committee Opinion Number 518. *Obstetrics & Gynecology, 119, 2*(1), 412–417.

American Psychiatric Nurses Association. (2007). Seclusion and restraint position paper. Available at http://www.apna.org/i4a/pages/index.cfm?pageid=3728

Antypa, N., Serretti, A., & Rujescu, D. (2013). Serotonergic genes and suicide: A systematic review. *European Neuropsychopharmacology, 23*(10), 1125–1142.

Archer, J. (2000). Differences in aggression between heterosexual partners: A meta-analytic review. *Psychological Bulletin, 126,* 651–680.

Arnetz, J. E. (1998). The Violent Incident Form (VIF): A practical instrument for the registration of violent incidents in the health care workplace. *Work & Stress: An International Journal of Work, Health & Organisations, 12*(1), 17–28.

Asnis, G. M., Kaplan, M. L., Hundorfean, G., & Saeed, W. 1997. Violence and homicidal behaviors in psychiatric disorders. *Psychiatric Clinics of North America, 20,* 405–425.

Baker, N. L., Buick, J. D., Kim, S. R., Moniz, S., & Nava, K. L. (2013). Lessons from examining same-sex intimate partner violence. *Sex Roles, 69,* 182–192.

Banyard, V. L., & Cross, C. (2008). Consequences of teen dating violence: Understanding intervening variables in ecological context. *Violence Against Women 14*(9), 998–1013.

Barzman, D. H., Brackenbury, L., Sonnier, L., Schnell, B., Cassedy, A., Salisbury, S., Sorter, M., & Mossman, D. (2011). Brief Rating of Aggression by Children and Adolescents (BRACHA): Development of a tool for assessing risk of inpatients' aggressive behavior. *Journal of the American Academy of Psychiatry and the Law, 39,* 170–179.

Basile, K. C., & Saltzman, L. E. (2009). Sexual violence surveillance: uniform definitions and recommended data elements version 1.0. Atlanta, GA: Centers for Disease Control and Prevention, National Center for Injury Prevention and Control. Available at http://www.cdc.gov/ViolencePrevention/pub/SV_surveillance.html

Bensimon, M., & Ronel, N. (2012). The flywheel effect of intimate partner violence: A victim-perpetrator interactive spin. *Aggression and Violent Behavior, 17,* 423–429.

Blomhoff, S., Seim, S., & Friis, S. (1990). Can prediction of violence among psychiatric inpatients be improved? *Hospital Community Psychiatry, 41,* 771–775.

Bogat, G. A., Levendosky, A., & von Eye, A. (2005). The future of research on intimate partner violence: Person-oriented and variable-oriented perspectives. *American Journal of Community Psychology, 36*(1–2), 49–70.

Borum, R., Bartel, P., & Forth, A. (2002). *Manual for the Structured Assessment of Violence Risk in Youth (SAVRY).* Tampa, FL: University of South Florida.

Borum, R., Bartel, P., & Forth, A. (2003). *Manual for the Structured Assessment of Violence Risk in Youth (SAVRY):* Version 1.1. Tampa, FL: University of South Florida.

Bowers, L., Brennan, G., Flood, C., Lipang, M., & Oladapo, P. (2006). Preliminary outcomes of a trial to reduce conflict and containment on acute psychiatric wards: City nurses. *Journal of Psychiatric Mental Health Nursing, 13*(2):165–172.

Bowers, L., Whittington, R., Nolan, P., Parkin, D., Curtis, S., Bhui, K., … Flood, C. (2006). The City 128 study of observation and outcomes on acute psychiatric wards: Report to the NHS SDO Programme. London, UK: City University London.

Brown, H. L. (2009). Trauma in pregnancy. *Obstetrics and Gynecology, 114,* 147–60.

Buckley, P. F., Noffsinger, S. G., Smith, D. A., Hrouda, P. R., & Knoll, J. L. (2003). Treatment of the psychotic patient who is violent. *Psychiatric Clinics of North America, 26*(1), 231–272.

Buckley, P., Citrome, L., Nichita, C., & Vitacco, M. (2011). Psychopharmacology of aggression in schizophrenia. *Schizophrenia Bulletin, 37*(5), 930–936. doi: 10.1093/schbul/sbr104

Bufkin, J. L., & Luttrell, V. R. (2005). Neuroimaging studies of aggressive and violent behavior: Current findings and implications for criminology and criminal justice. *Trauma, Violence and Abuse, 6*(2), 176–191.

Bureau of Justice Statistics. (2010). Criminal Victimization, 2009. Washington, DC: U.S. Department of Justice, p. 7. Available at http://bjs.ojp.usdoj.gov/content/pub/pdf/cv09.pdf

Burgess, A. W., Slattery, D. M., & Herlihy, P. A. (2013). Military sexual trauma: A silent syndrome. *Journal of Psychosocial Nursing and Mental Health Services, 51*(2), 20–26.

Campbell, J. C., Webster, D., Koziol-McLain, J., Block, C., Campbell, D., Curry, M. A., … Laughon, K. (2003). Risk factors for femicide in abusive relationships: Results from a multistate case control study. *American Journal of Public Health, 93*(7), 1089–1097.

Carretta, C. M., & Burgess, A. W. (2013). Symptom responses to a continuum of sexual trauma. *Violence and Victims, 28*(2), 248–258.

Centers for Disease Control and Prevention (CDC). (2003). Violence prevention: Intimate partner violence: Consequences. Available at http://www.cdc.gov/violenceprevention/intimatepartnerviolence/consequences.html

Centers for Disease Control and Prevention (CDC). (2010a). 10 leading causes of injury deaths by age group highlighting violence-related injury deaths United States—2010. Available at http://www.cdc.gov/injury/wisqars/pdf/10LCID_Violence_Related_Injury_Deaths_2010-a.pdf

Centers for Disease Control and Prevention (CDC). (2010b). Violence prevention: Intimate partner violence: Definitions. Available at http://www.cdc.gov/violenceprevention/intimatepartnerviolence/definitions.html.

Centers for Disease Control and Prevention (CDC). (2012). Youth risk behavior surveillance—United States. *MMWR,* Surveillance Summaries 2012; 61 (no. SS-4). Available at www.cdc.gov/mmwr/pdf/ss/ss6104.pdf

Centers for Medicare and Medicaid Services (CMS). (2006). CMS Final Rule: Medicare and Medicaid Programs: Hospital Conditions of Participation: Patients' Rights. 42 CFR Part 482. Baltimore, MD: U.S. Department of Health and Human Services, December 8, 2006.

Chapman, R., Styles, I., Perry, L., & Combs, S. (2009). Examining the characteristics of workplace violence in one hospital. *Journal of Clinical Nursing.19*(3–4), 479–488. doi: 10.1111/j.1365-2702.2009.02952.x

Cho, H., Hong, J. S., & Logan, T. K. (2012). An ecological understanding of the risk factors associated with stalking behavior: Implications for social work practice. *Affilia, 27*(4), 381–390. doi: 10.1177/0886109912464474

Choe, J. Y., Teplin, K. A., & Abram, K. M. (2008). Perpetration of violence, violent victimization, and severe mental illness: Balancing public health concerns. *Psychiatric Services, 59,* 153–164. doi:10.1176/appi.ps.59.2.153

Ciccarelli, S. K., & White, J. N. (2013). *Psychology: An Exploration* (2nd ed.). Upper Saddle River, NJ: Pearson Education.

Citrome, L., Volavka, J., Czobor, P., Sheltman, B., Lindenmayer, J. P., McEvoy, J., … Lieberman, J. A. (2001). Effects of clozapine, olanzapine, risperidone, and haloperidol on hostility among patients with schizophrenia and schizoaffective disorder. *Psychiatric Services, 52*(11), 1510–1514.

Clark, C., Ryan, L., Kawachi, I., Canner, M. J., Berkman, L., & Wright, R. (2007). Witnessing community violence in residential neighborhoods: A mental health hazard for urban women. *Journal of Urban Health, 85*(1), 22–38.

Coker, A. L., Davis, K. E., Arias, I., Desai, S., Sanderson, M., Brandt, H. M., & Smith, P. H. (2002). Physical and mental health effects of intimate partner violence for men and women. *American Journal of Preventive Medicine, 23*(4), 260–268.

Connecticut Coalition Against Domestic Violence (CCADV). (2013). Upon further examination: 2013 findings and recommendations of the Connecticut Domestic Violence Fatality Review Committee. Wethersfield, CT: Connecticut Domestic Violence Fatality Review Committee.

Corrigan, P. W., & Watson, A. C. (2005). Findings from the National Comorbidity Survey on the frequency of violent behavior in individuals with psychiatric disorders. *Psychiatry Research, 136*(2–3), 153–162.

Council of State Governments Justice Center. (n.d.). The literature on mental illness and violence: A toolkit for state mental health commissioners. Available at http://www.dbhds.virginia.gov/documents/130114ViolenceToolkit.pdf

Dack, C., Ross, J., Papadopoulos, C., Stewart, D., & Bowers, L. (2013). A review and meta-analysis of the patient factors associated with psychiatric in-patient aggression. *Acta Psychiatrica Scandinavica, 127*(4), 255–268.

DeVries, K. M., Mak, J. Y., Bacchus, L. J., Child, J. C., Falkder, G., Petzold, M., Astbury, J., & Watts C. H. (2013). Intimate partner violence and incident depressive symptoms and suicide attempts: A systematic review of longitudinal studies. *PLOS Medicine, 10*(5), e1001439. doi: 10.1371/journal.pmed.1001439

Duke, A., Begue, L., Bell, R., & Eisenlohr-Moul, T. (2013). Revisiting the serotonin-aggression relation in humans: A meta-analysis. *Psychological Bulletin, 139*(5), 1148–1172.

Eichelman, B. (1986). The biology and somatic experimental treatment of aggressive disorders. In P. A. Berger & H. K. Brodie, (Eds.). *The American Handbook of Psychiatry,* Vol. 8. New York, NY: Basic Books, pp. 651–678.

Eichelman, B. S. (1990). Neurochemical and psychopharmacologic aspects of aggressive behavior. *Annual Review of Medicine, 41,* 149–158.

Einarsen, S., Hoel, H., & Notelaers, G. (2009). Measuring exposure to bullying and harassment at work: Validity, factor structure and psychometric properties of the Negative Acts Questionnaire–Revised. *Work & Stress: An International Journal of Work, Health & Organisations, 23*(1), 24–44.

Elbogen, E. B., & Johnson, S.C. (2009). The intricate link between violence and mental disorder: Results from the National Epidemiologic Survey on Alcohol and Related Conditions. *Archives of General Psychiatry, 66*(2), 152–161.

Family Violence Prevention Fund (FVPF). (2010). The health care costs of domestic and sexual violence. San Francisco, CA: FVPF. Available at http://www.futureswithoutviolence.org/userfiles/file/HealthCare/Health_Care_Costs_of_Domestic_and_Sexual_Violence.pdf

Fazel, S., & Grann, M. (2006). The population impact of severe mental illness on violent crime. *American Journal of Psychiatry, 163,* 1397–1403.

Fazel, S., Singh, J. P., Doll, H., & Grann, M. (2012). Use of risk assessment instruments to predict violence and antisocial behaviour in 73 samples involving 24,827 people. *Medscape.* Available at www.medscape.com/viewarticle/768365

Federal Bureau of Investigation. (2012). Violent crime. Available at http://www.fbi.gov/about-us/cjis/ucr/crime-in-the-u.s/2011/crime-in-the-u.s.-2011/violent-crime/violent-crime

Fergusson, D. M., Boden, J. M., & Horwood, J. (2006). Examining the intergenerational transmission of violence in a New Zealand birth cohort. *Child Abuse and Neglect, 30*(2), 89–108.

Findorff, M. J., McGovern, P. M., Wall, M. M., & Gerberich, S.G. (2005). Reporting violence to a health care employer: A cross-sectional study. *AAOHN Journal, 53*(9), 399–406.

Flannery, R. B., Farley, E., Rego, S., & Walker, A. P. (2007). Characteristics of staff victims of psychiatric patient assaults: 15 year analysis of the Assaulted Staff Action Program (ASAP). *Psychiatric Quarterly, 78*(1), 25–37.

Flannery, R. B., Farley, E., Tierney, T., & Walker, A. P. (2011). Characteristics of assaultive psychiatric patients: 20-year analysis of the Assaultive Staff Action Program (ASAP). *Psychiatric Quarterly, 82*(1), 1–10.

Gallardo-Pujol, D., Andrés-Pueyo, A., & Maydeu-Olivares, A. (2013). MAO—a genotype, social exclusion and aggression: An experimental test of a gene-environment interaction. *Genes, Brain and Behavior, 12*(1), 140–145.

Gates, D. M., Ross, C. S., & McQueen, L. (2006). Violence against emergency department workers. *Journal of Emergency Medicine, 31*(3), 331–337.

Gault, M., & Silver, E. (2008). Spuriousness or mediation? Broken windows according to Sampson and Raudenbush (1999). *Journal of Criminal Justice, 36,* 240–243.

Goldstein, J. S. (2011). Think again: War. *Foreign Policy.* Available at http://www.foreignpolicy.com/articles/2011/08/15/think_again_war?page=full

Grann, M., Belfrage, H., & Tengström, A. (2000). Actuarial risk assessment in Sweden: Predictive validity of the VRAG and the historical part of the HCR-20. *Criminal Justice and Behavior, 27,* 97–114.

Haimowitz, S., Urff, J., & Huckshorn, K.A. (2006). Restraint and seclusion—a risk management guide. National Association of State Mental Health Departments. Available at http://www.power2u.org/downloads/R-S%20Risk%20Manag%20Guide%20Oct%2006.pdf

Hamrin, V., Iennaco, J., & Olsen, D. (2009). A review of ecological factors affecting inpatient psychiatric unit violence: Implications for relational and unit cultural improvements. *Issues in Mental Health Nursing, 30*(4), 214–226.

Hare, R. D. (1991). The Hare Psychopathy Checklist—revised (PCL-R). North Tonawanda, NY: Multi-Health Systems. Available at http://www.mhs.com/product.aspx?gr=saf&prod=pcl-r2&id=overview

Hare, R. D. (2003). The Hare Psychopathy Checklist—revised (2nd ed.). North Tonawanda, NY: Multi-Health Systems. Available at http://www.mhs.com/product.aspx?gr=saf&prod=pcl-r2&id=overview

Hawley, D. A., & Hawley Barker, A. C. (2012). Survivors of intimate partner violence: Implications for nursing care. *Critical Care Nursing Clinics of North America, 24*(1), 27–39.

Health Care Financing Administration. (2001). Use of restraint and seclusion in residential treatment facilities providing inpatient psychiatric services to individuals under age 21. Federal Register 42 CFR Parts 441 and 483. Washington, DC: U.S. Department of Health and Human Services.

Hermans, J., Kruk, M. R., Lohman, A. H., Meelis, W., Mos, J., Mostert, P. G., & van der Poel, A. M. (1983). Discriminant analysis of the localization of aggression-inducing electrode placements in the hypothalamus of male rats. *Brain Research, 260*(1), 61–79.

Higgins, E. S., & George, M. S. (2013). *The Neuroscience of Clinical Psychiatry: The Pathology of Behavior and Mental Illness* (2nd ed.). Philadelphia, PA: Lippincott Williams & Wilkins.

Holcomb, W., & Ahr P. (1988). Arrest rates among young adult psychiatric patients treated in inpatient and outpatient settings. *Hospital Community Psychiatry, 39*(10), 52–57.

Iennaco, J. D., Dixon, J., Whittemore, R., & Bowers, L. (2013). Measurement and monitoring of health care worker aggression exposure. *OJIN: The Online Journal of Issues in Nursing, 18*(1), Manuscript 3.

Jaber, F. S., & Mahmoud, K. F. (2013). Risk tools for the prediction of violence. *Journal of Psychiatric and Mental Health Nursing,* epub ahead of print. doi: 10.1111/jpm.12102

Janofsky, J. S., Spears, S., & Neubauer, D. N. (1998). Psychiatrists' accuracy in predicting violent behavior on an inpatient unit. *Hospital Community Psychiatry, 39*(10),1090–1094.

Kavoussi, R., Armstead, P., & Coccaro, E. (1997). The neurobiology of impulsive aggression. *Psychiatric Clinics of North America, 20*(2), 395–403.

Kelling, G., & Coles, C. (1998) *Fixing Broken Windows: Restoring Order and Reducing Crime in Our Communities.* New York, NY: Simon & Schuster/Touchstone.

Kelling, G. L., & Wilson, J. Q. (1982). Broken windows: The police and neighborhood safety. *The Atlantic.* Available at http://www.theatlantic.com/magazine/archive/1982/03/broken-windows/304465/

Kho, K., Sensky, T., Mortimer, A., & Corcos, C. (1998). Prospective study into factors associated with aggressive incidents in psychiatric acute admission wards. *British Journal of Psychiatry, 172,* 38–43.

Kling, R. N., Yassi, A., Smailes, E., Lovato, C. Y., & Koehoorn, M. (2009). Characterizing violence in health care in British Columbia. *Journal of Advanced Nursing, 65*(8), 1655–1663.

Lanza, M. (2009). An innovative intervention to reduce aggressive behavior in psychiatric inpatients: Violence prevention community meeting. Work, Stress, and Health 2009: Global Concerns and Approaches, 8th International Conference on Occupational Stress and Health, San Juan, PR, November 6, 2009.

Leymann, H. (1990). Mobbing and psychological terror at workplaces. *Violence and Victims, 5,* 119–126.

Lindenmayer, J., & Kotsaftis, A. (2000). Use of sodium valproate in violent and aggressive behaviors: A critical review. *Journal of Clinical Psychiatry, 61*(2), 123–128.

Lutgen-Sandvik, P., Tracy, S. J., & Alberts, J. K. (2007). Burned by bullying in the American workplace: Prevalence, perception, degree, and impact. *Journal of Management Studies, 44*(6), 837–862.

McAdams, T. A., Gregory, A. M., & Eley, T. C. (2013). Genes of experience: Explaining the heritability of putative environmental variables through their association with behavioural and emotional traits. *Behavior Genetics, 43*(4), 314–328.

McDermott, B. E., Quanbeck, C. D., Busse, D., Yastro, K., & Scott, C. L. (2008). The accuracy of risk assessment instruments in the prediction of impulsive versus predatory aggression. *Behavioral Sciences and the Law, 26*(6), 759–777.

McEllistrem, J. E. (2004). Affective and predatory violence: A bimodal classification system of human aggression and violence. *Aggression and Violent Behavior, 10,* 1–30.

Merriam-Webster. Aggression. Available at http://www.merriam-webster.com/dictionary/aggression

Mollen, C. J., Goyal, M. K., & Frioux, S. M. (2012). Acute sexual assault. *Pediatric Emergency Care, 28*(6) 584–593.

Monahan, J., Steadman, H., Robbins, P., Appelbaum, P. S., Banks, S., Grisso, T., … Silver, E. (2005). An actuarial model of violence risk assessment for persons with mental disorders. *Psychaitric Services, 56,* 810–815.

Mossman, D. (1994). Assessing predictions of violence: Being accurate about accuracy. *Journal of Consulting Clinical Psychology, 62*(4), 783–792.

Mullen, P. E., Pathe, M., & Purcell, R. (2001). Stalking: New constructions of human behaviours. *Australian & New Zealand Journal of Psychiatry, 35*(1), 9–16.

Mulvey, E. (1994). Assessing the evidence of a link between mental illness and violence. *Hospital Community Psychiatry, 45*(7), 663–668.

Namie, G. (2013). The WBI definition of workplace bullying. Workplace Bullying Institute. Available at http://www.workplacebullying.org/individuals/problem/definition/

Namie, G., & Namie, R. (2009). U.S. workplace bullying: Some basic considerations and consultation interventions. *Consulting Psychology Journal: Practice and Research, 61*(3), 202–219.

National Center for Injury Prevention and Control (NCIPC). (2003). Costs of intimate partner violence against women in the United States. Atlanta, GA: Centers for Disease Control and Prevention. Available at http://www.cdc.gov/violenceprevention/pdf/IPVBook-a.pdf

National Institute of Justice. (2007). Stalking. Available at http://www.nij.gov/topics/crime/stalking/welcome.htm

National Network to End Domestic Violence (NNEDV). (2013). The Violence Against Women Reauthorization Act of 2013: Safely and effectively meeting the needs of more victims. http://nnedv.org/downloads/Policy/VAWAReauthorization_Summary_2013.pdf

Newton, V. M., Elbogen, E. B., Brown, C. L., Snyder J., & Barrick, A. L. (2012). Clinical decision-making about inpatient violence risk at admission to a public-sector acute psychiatric hospital. *Journal of the American Academy of Psychiatry and the Law, 40*(2), 206–214.

Nijman, H. L. I., Muris, P., Merckelbach, H. L. G. J., Palmstierna, T., Wistedt, B., Vos, A., … Allertz, W. (1999). The staff observation aggression scale-revised (SOAS-R). *Aggressive Behavior, 25*(3), 197–209.

Nijman, H. L., Palmstierna, T., Almvik, R., & Stolker, J. J. (2005). Fifteen years of research with the Staff Observation Aggression Scale: A review. *Acta Psychiatrica Scandinavica, 111*(1), 12–21.

Nolan, K. A., Czobor, P., Roy, B. B. Platt, M. M., Shope, C. B., Citrome, L. L., & Volavka, J. (2003). Characteristics of assaultive behavior among psychiatric inpatients. *Psychiatric Services 54*(7),1012–1016.

Nolan, K. A., Volavka, J., Czobor, P., Sheitman, B., Lindenmayer, J. P., Citrome, L. L., McEvoy, J., & Lieberman, J.A. (2005). Aggression and psychopathology in treatment-resistant inpatients with schizophrenia and schizoaffective disorder. *Journal of Psychiatric Research, 39*(1), 109–115.

Norko, M., & Baranoski, M. (2005). The state of contemporary risk assessment research. *Canadian Journal of Psychiatry, 50*(1), 18–26.

O'Brien, D. (2013). Broken windows and low adolescent prosociality: Not cause and consequence, but co-symptoms of low collective efficacy. *American Journal of Community Psychology, 51*(3–4), 359–369.

Occupational Safety and Health Administration. (2004). Guidelines for Preventing Workplace Violence for Health Care & Social Service Workers. U.S. Department of Labor. OSHA 3148-01R 2004.

Participation: Patients' Rights. (1999). 42 CFR Part 482. Baltimore, MD: US Department of Health and Human Services.

Perlin, M. L. (n.d.). The regulation of the use of seclusion and restraints in mental disability law. National Association for Rights Protection and Advocacy. Available at http://www.narpa.org/regulation.of.seclusion.htm

Petit, J. (2005). Management of the acutely violent patient. *Psychiatric Clinics of North America, 28,* 701–711.

Pickles, A., Hill, J., Breen, G., Quinn, J., Abbott, K., Jones, H., & Sharp, H. (2013). Evidence for interplay between genes and parenting on infant temperament in the first year of life: Monoamine oxidase a polymorphism moderates effects of maternal sensitivity on infant anger proneness. *Journal of Child Psychology and Psychiatry and Allied Disciplines, 54*(12), 1308–1317.

Pinker, S. (2011). Violence vanquished. *The Wall Street Journal,* September 24. Available at http://online.wsj.com/article/SB10001424053111904106704576583203589408180.html

Powell, G., Caan, W., & Crowe, M. (1994). What events precede violent incidents in psychiatric hospitals? *British Journal of Psychiatry, 165*(1), 107–112.

Privitera, C., & Campbell, M. A. (2009). Cyberbullying: The new face of workplace bullying? *CyberPsychology & Behavior, 12*(4), 395–400. doi: 10.1089/cpb.2009.0025

Raja, M., & Assoni, A. (2005). Hostility and violence of acute psychiatric inpatients. *Clinical Practice and Epidemiology in Mental Health, 1*(11), 1–11.

Rape, Abuse, and Incest National Network (RAINN). (2009a). Statistics. Available at http://www.rainn.org/statistics

Rape, Abuse, and Incest National Network (RAINN). (2009b). Was I raped? Available at http://www.rainn.org/get-information/types-of-sexual-assault/was-it-rape

Reeves, A. G., & Plum, F. (1969). Hyperphagia, rage, and dementia accompanying a ventromedial hypothalamic neoplasm. *Archives of Neurology, 20,* 616–624.

Renner, L. M., & Slack, K. S. (2006). Intimate partner violence and child maltreatment: Understanding intra- and intergenerational connections. *Child Abuse and Neglect, 30,* 599–617.

Ridenour, M. (2009). Real-time assessment of aggressive behavior in psychiatric inpatients. Paper presented at Work, Stress, and Health 2009: Global Concerns and Approaches, 8th International Conference on Occupational Stress and Health, San Juan, Puerto Rico, November 6, 2009.

Rueve, M. E., & Welton, R. S. (2008). Violence and mental illness. *Psychiatry, 5*(5), 34–48.

Sadeh, N., Binder, R. L., & McNiel, D. E. (2014). Recent victimization increases risk for violence in justice-involved persons with mental illness. *Law and Human Behavior, 38*(2), 119–125.

Samnani, A. K., & Singh, P. (2012). 20 years of workplace bullying research: A review of the antecedents and consequences of bullying in the workplace. *Aggression and Violent Behavior, 17,* 581–589.

Sampson, R. J., & Raudenbush, S. W. (2004). Seeing disorder: Neighborhood stigma and the social construction of "broken windows." *Social Psychology Quarterly, 67,* 319–342.

Seedat, S., Stein, M. B., & Forde, D. R. (2005). Association between physical partner violence, posttraumatic stress disorder, childhood trauma, and suicide attempts in a community sample of women. *Violence and Victims, 20*(1), 87–98.

Serper, M. R., Goldberg, B. R., Herman, K. G., Richarme, D., Chou, J., Dill, C. A., & Cancro, R. (2005). Predictors of aggression on the psychiatric inpatient service. *Comprehensive Psychiatry, 46*(2), 121–127.

Siever, L. J. (2008). Neurobiology of aggression and violence. *American Journal of Psychiatry, 165*(4), 429–442.

Silverman, J. G., Raj, A., & Clements, K. (2004). Dating violence and associated sexual risk and pregnancy among adolescent girls in the United States. *Pediatrics, 114*(2): e220–e225.

Smith, P. H., White, J. W., & Holland, L. J. (2003). A longitudinal perspective on dating violence among adolescent and college-age women. *American Journal of Public Health, 93*(7),1104–1109.

Snowden, R. J., Gray, N. S., Taylor, J., & Fitzgerald, S. (2009). Assessing risk of future violence among forensic psychiatric inpatients with the Classification of Violence Risk (COVR). *Psychiatric Services, 60*(11), 1522–1526.

Srabstein, J. C., & Leventhal, B. L. (2010). Prevention of bullying-related morbidity and mortality: A call for public health policies. *Bulletin of the World Health Organization, 88*(6), 403.

Stahl, S. (2011). *Prescriber's Guide.* New York, NY: Cambridge University Press.

Stanton, B., Baldwin, R. M., & Rachuba, L. A. (1997). Quarter century of violence in the United States: An epidemiologic assessment. *Psychiatric Clinics of North America, 20,* 269–282.

Steadman, H. J., Mulvey, E. P., Monahan, J., Robbins, P. C., Applebaum, P. S., Gusso, T., Roth, L. H., & Silver, E. (1998). Violence by people discharged from acute psychiatric inpatient facilities and by others in the same neighborhoods. *Archives of General Psychiatry, (55)*5, 393–401.

Straus, M. A. (2005). Women's violence toward men is a serious social problem. In D. R. Loseke, R. J. Gelles, & M. M. Cavanaugh, (Eds.). *Current Controversies on Family Violence* (2nd ed.). Thousand Oaks, CA: Sage, pp. 55–77.

Sugden, S. G., Kile, S. J., & Hendren, R. L. (2006). Neurodevelopmental pathways to aggression: A model to understand and target treatment in youth. *Journal of Neuropsychiatry and Clinical Neuroscience 18*(3), 302–317.

Swanson, J. W., Holzer, C. E., Ganju, V. K., & Jono, R. T. (1990). Violence and psychiatric disorder in the community: Evidence from the epidemiologic catchment area surveys. *Hospital and Community Psychiatry, 41*(7), 761–770.

Swanson, J. W., Swartz, M. S., Van Dorn, R. A., Volavka, J., Monahan, J., Stroup, S., … Lieberman, J. A. (2008). Medication effects on reducing violence in persons with schizophrenia. *British Journal of Psychiatry, 193*(1), 37–43.

Tardiff, K., & Sweillam, A. (1982). Assaultive behavior among chronic inpatients. *American Journal of Psychiatry, 139*(2), 212–215.

Teplin, L. A., Welty, L. J., Abram, K. M., Dulcan, M. K., & Washburn, J. J. (2012). Prevalence and persistence of psychiatric disorders in youth after detention: A prospective longitudinal study. *Archives of General Psychiatry, 69*(10), 1031–1043.

Tjaden, P., & Thoennes, N. (2000). Extent, nature, and consequences of intimate partner violence: Findings from the National Violence Against Women Survey. Washington, DC: Department of Justice. Available at https://www.ncjrs.gov/pdffiles1/nij/181867.pdf

Torrey, E. F. (2011). Stigma and violence: Isn't it time to connect the dots? *Schizophrenia Bulletin, 37*(5), 892–896.

U.S. Department of Health and Human Services. (1999). Health Care Financing Administration, Interim Final Rule: Medicare and Medicaid Programs: Hospital Conditions of Participation: Patients' Rights. 42 CFR Part 482. Baltimore, MD: U.S. Department of Health and Human Services.

U.S. Department of Health and Human Services. (2006). CMS Final Rule: Medicare and Medicaid Programs: Hospital Conditions of Participation: Patients' Rights. 42 CFR Part 482. Baltimore, MD: U.S. Department of Health and Human Services, December 8, 2006.

Vaaler, A. E., Iversen, V. C., Morken, G., Flovig, J. C., Palmstierna, T., & Linaker, O. M. (2011). Short-term prediction of threatening and violent behaviour in an acute psychiatric intensive care unit based on patient and environment characteristics. *BMC Psychiatry, 11.* Available at http://www.ncbi.nlm.nih.gov/pmc/articles/PMC3068951/

Violence Policy Center. (2012). When Men Murder Women: An Analysis of 2010 Homicide Data. September 2012, p. 7. Available at https://www.vpc.org/studies/wmmw2012.pdf

Vitacco, M. J., Gonsalves, V., Tomony, J., Smith, B. E. R., & Lishner, D. A. (2012). Can standardized measures of risk predict inpatient violence?: Combining static and dynamic variables to improve accuracy. *Criminal Justice and Behavior, 39*, 589–606.

Volavka, J. (2013). Violence in schizophrenia and bipolar disorder. *Psychiatria Danubina, 25*(1), 24–33.

Volavka, J., & Citrome, L. (2008). Heterogeneity of violence in schizophrenia and implications for long-term treatment. *International Journal of Clinical Practice, 62(8)*, 1237–1245.

Volavka, J., Czobor, P., Nolan, K., et al. (2013). Overt aggression and psychotic symptoms in patients with schizophrenia treated with clozapine, olanzapine, risperidone, or haloperidol. *Journal of Clinical Psychopharmacology, 24*, 225–228.

Walker, L. E. A. (1984). *Battered Woman Syndrome.* New York, NY: Springer.

Walsh, E., Buchanan, A., & Fahy, T. (2002). Violence and schizophrenia: Examining the evidence. *British Journal of Psychiatry, 180*, 490–495.

Webster, C. D., Douglas, K. S., Eaves, S. D., & Hart, S. D. (1997). Assessing risk of violence to others. In C. D. Webster & M. A. Jackson (Eds.). *Impulsivity: Theory, Assessment, and Treatment.* New York, NY: Guilford, pp. 251–277.

Weiss, E. M., et al. (1998). Deadly restraint: A Hartford Courant investigative report. *Hartford Courant*, October 11, p. 15.

Whittington, R., Shuttleworth, S., & Hill, L. (1996). Violence to staff in a general hospital setting. *Journal of Advanced Nursing, 24*, 326–333.

Winstanley, S., & Whittington, R. (2004). Aggression towards health care staff in a UK general hospital: Variation among professions and departments. *Journal of Clinical Nursing, 13*, 3–10.

Wintemute, G. J., Wright, M. A., & Drake, C. M. (2003). Increased risk of intimate partner homicide among California women who purchased handguns. *Annals of Emergency Medicine, 41*(2), 282.

World Health Organization (WHO). (2002). World report on violence and health. Geneva, Switzerland: World Health Organization. Available at http://whqlibdoc.who.int/publications/2002/9241545615_eng.pdf?ua=1

World Health Organization (WHO). (2009). Interpersonal violence and illicit drugs. Available at http://www.who.int/violenceprevention/interpersonal_violence_and_illicit_drug_use.pdf

World Health Organization (WHO). (2012). Violence against women. Available at http://www.who.int/mediacentre/factsheets/fs239/en/index.html

Wright, K. M., Duxbury, J. A., Baker, A., & Crumpton, A. (2014). A qualitative study into the attitudes of patients and staff towards violence and aggression in a high security hospital. *Journal of Psychiatric and Mental Health Nursing, 21*(2), 184–188. doi: 10.1111/jpm.12108

Yang, M., Wong, S. C. P., & Coid, J. (2010). The efficacy of violence prediction: A meta-analytic comparison of nine risk assessment tools. *Psychological Bulletin, 136*(5),740–767.

Yanowitch, R, & Coccaro, E. F. (2011). The neurochemistry of human aggression. *Advanced Genetics, 75*, 151–169.

Zlotnick, C., Johnson, D. M., & Kohn, R. (2006). Intimate partner violence and long-term psychosocial functioning in a national sample of American women. *Journal of Interpersonal Violence, 21*(2), 262–275.

Crisis Intervention

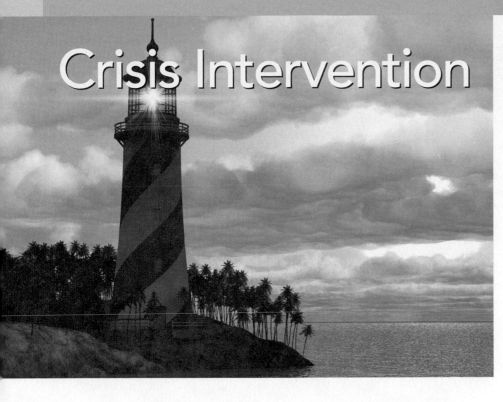

26

Brant Oliver

Learning Outcomes

1. Analyze the different categories of crisis.

2. Compare and contrast elements of crisis assessment.

3. Plan clinical approaches to crisis intervention.

4. Examine considerations for specific populations.

5. Summarize key elements of patient and family teaching during crisis intervention.

Key Terms

Rebecca Initial Onset

Rebecca Dormier is a 47-year-old woman who presents to her primary care clinic for her annual examination. During the intake portion of her visit, she meets with Bill, a registered nurse at the clinic. Bill immediately observes that Rebecca appears tense and withdrawn. She tells Bill that she was "forced out of her job" 6 months earlier because her employer learned that she had multiple sclerosis (MS). Rebecca explains that, after a relapse of her MS, her neurological status worsened and she was unable to resume her usual duties; she was unable to be transferred to a new position with the same employer. Since her termination, Rebecca has exhausted her short-term disability coverage, but she does not meet eligibility criteria for Social Security disability. Her attempts to find work with other employers have been unsuccessful. She has been unemployed for almost a month and is worried that she will soon be unable to provide for her two children. Rebecca laments that she does not have family in the area and her ex-husband is "not at all supportive." She feels trapped and has little hope that her situation will improve. She states, "I will probably have to sell my house."

Rebecca describes a number of new symptoms that she has developed over the past months, including worry, irritability, difficulty sleeping, and a sense of daytime heaviness, fatigue, and malaise. She has been exercising less and has gained 5 pounds, which she describes as being related to "more comfort eating." Rebecca also confides that she has not been taking her MS medication because "it is too expensive." She is worried that her MS may worsen as a result. Finally, she states a concern that her "depression might be coming back." She is worried about that because "it was bad when I had it in the past." Bill asks about her feelings about self-harm and learns that she is not experiencing suicidal ideation.

> ### APPLICATION
>
> 1. Address the five domains for Rebecca, identifying potential issues that may be present in each:
>   a. Biological
>   b. Psychological
>   c. Sociological
>   d. Cultural
>   e. Spiritual
> 2. In what ways might Rebecca be suffering? Why?
> 3. How would you prioritize Rebecca's needs during this encounter, and why?

Introduction

Crises can take many shapes and forms, ranging from individualized and population-based (for instance, injury or disease) to environmental (such as natural disasters). Some crises arise as a normal aspect of development, such as transitioning from college to employment or becoming a parent. Others arise out of circumstances that are not at all ordinary, normal, or expected, such as an automobile accident or a violent crime.

A **crisis** is often conceptualized as a state of disequilibrium, whereas *crisis intervention* refers to a means to help re-establish equilibrium. **Homeostasis**, or *equilibrium*, is demonstrated when the magnitude of stressors an individual experiences is matched by that of the coping response, and the individual's coping response is sufficient to resolve the stressors. When an individual's coping response becomes disproportionate to the stressors, **disequilibrium** results, and psychological and/or physiological symptoms can occur. Crises have three basic characteristics: (1) a perceived threat or danger; (2) an imbalance or disturbance in psychological functioning; and (3) no ready or feasible solution (Aguilera, 1998; Greenston & Leviton, 2002). Perceived threats, or stressors, may occur in any one or more of the domains: biological, psychological, sociological, cultural, or spiritual. In the critical thinking feature, Rebecca faces perceived sociological and psychological threats (workplace discrimination, unemployment) and a biological threat (MS exacerbations), and these affect her ability to support her children and purchase medications. Additionally, she lacks substantive supports and perceives that she must cope with the situation alone.

Individuals perceive threats differently, depending on a variety of factors. Financial resources, cultural beliefs, spiritual values, family support, and many other factors influence individual responses to stress. Rebecca, for example, might not achieve crisis state if she were in a supportive relationship and had additional financial resources. In another example, a man who has recently lost his job may perceive threats to his role identity as a successful husband and father (psychosocial) because he fears he may not be able to provide for his family (financial). He may also worry that his extended family, which possesses a strong work ethic, will shun him for failing at work and failing to provide for his family (cultural).

Because crises present suddenly and with acute intensity, causing significant disruption to daily living, they can quickly overwhelm people and generate a significant sense of hopelessness and suffering. An individual's perception of hopelessness and suffering can overshadow the fact that many crises resolve within a limited time. Nurses often are the first professionals to respond to crisis; they can offer hope to people who are suffering by providing timely and targeted educational and therapeutic interventions. Targeted interventions can help patients mitigate the immediate effects of crisis and assist them to achieve stability and prevent adverse sequelae.

Theoretical Foundations

Crisis has developed as a specific focus in mental health. Erich Lindemann (1944) first described acute grief reactions after treating the victims of a devastating fire at the Cocoanut Grove nightclub in Boston in 1944. His work described acute and anticipatory grief reactions and their presenting characteristics of perceived threat, functional disequilibrium, and lack of effective coping or resolution. He also observed that crisis intervention, which often was provided by nonclinical personnel such as clergy, helped to resolve acute crises and prevent them from developing into chronic conditions. In subsequent years, these "grief reactions" that Lindemann described became conceptualized as the crisis experience.

Following Lindemann's pioneering work, Tyhurst (1951, 1957, and in James, Gililand, & James, 2012) and Caplan (1961, 1964, and in James, Gililand, & James, 2012) built more detailed and articulated theoretical frameworks describing the crisis experience. Tyhurst's

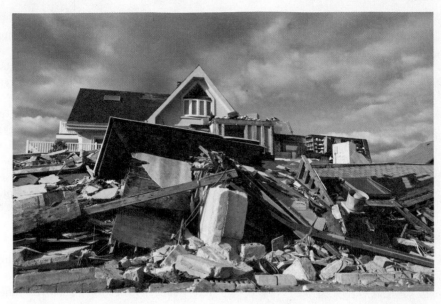

26-1   In the acute phase of a crisis experience, the focus is on immediate threats and needs. What needs and threats might the family who lived in this house face?

Source: Leonard Zhukovsky/Fotolia

Stages of Disaster model (Figure 26-1) established a stepwise progression through the crisis experience characterized by three stages:

1. *Impact:* The acute phase of the crisis experience, characterized by shock, panic, immobilization, and an immediate focus on immediate threats and needs.

2. *Recoil:* The phase following the resolution of the immediate threat and stressor, in which the injuries caused by the crisis event slowly become evident, and internal and external supports are rallied.

3. *Post-trauma:* The resolution phase of the crisis experience, in which the full extent of the damage caused by the crisis experience is realized, and emotional and behavioral signs and symptoms such as nightmares, grief, survivor guilt, and posttraumatic stress symptoms may occur. Without resolution at this stage, the individual may eventually become exhausted and unable to cope, resulting in development of despair.

Caplan's model also presents a stepwise progression that is somewhat similar to Tyhurst's, but differs in that that it focuses on problem solving and the concept of *internal tension* that is experienced by the crisis victim. In the initial experience of crisis, tension is generated and rises abruptly. This experience is quite similar to the *impact* phase of the Tyhurst model. In Caplan's second phase, the individual employs preexisting coping strategies in an attempt to problem-solve to reduce internal tension. If these coping strategies are adaptive and successful, internal tension reduces and eventually resolves. However, if coping is maladaptive or unsuccessful, internal tension rises further. In this case, the resulting rise in tension usually is adaptive and drives the individual to mobilize further internal and external resources to maximize the coping effort. This may include a strong motivation to learn and employ new approaches. Caplan sees this stage as a critical one for timely therapeutic intervention to help individuals mobilize effective problem-solving strategies, as doing so may reduce, and eventually resolve, internal tension. A failure to accomplish this can result in a phase similar to Tyhurst's *post-trauma*

phase, characterized by exhaustion, disorganization, and a continuing increase in tension.

As crisis became better understood and recognized as a specific mental health experience, specific approaches to crisis intervention were developed. Following the cognitive–behavioral revolution in psychotherapy in the 1970s and 1980s, and earlier observations that brief intervention was helpful for crisis, Donna Aguilera (1998) developed a short-term, problem-solving approach for crisis intervention for nurses and other mental health professionals. Derived from general cognitive–behavioral therapy methods, her approach facilitates development of an understanding of thoughts, beliefs, and perceptions of crisis events, emotions accompanying them, and facilitation of effective behavioral coping to restore the functional equilibrium that is disrupted during a crisis. The following is an overview of Aguilera's approach:

- *Assessment*
  - Assessment of the individual in the situation and of the presenting problem or crisis precipitant

- *Planning*
  - Planning the therapeutic intervention, with a focus on short-term management of the crisis and goal of restoring pre-crisis equilibrium

- *Intervention*
  - Helping the individual to develop an understanding of the crisis
  - Helping the individual to become aware of and articulate associated emotions
  - Helping the individual to explore and employ effective coping approaches
  - Helping the individual to re-engage and leverage the social world

- *Resolution and Anticipatory Planning*
  - Reinforcement for effective coping strategies and leveraging the resolution of the current crisis as a learning experience
  - Realistic planning for anticipated future stressors (Aguilera, 1998)

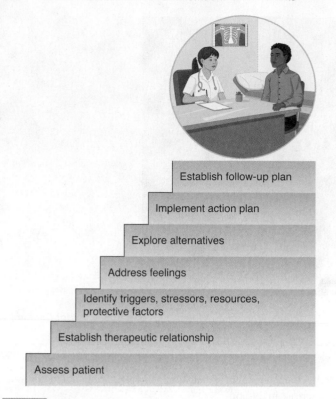

Establish follow-up plan

Implement action plan

Explore alternatives

Address feelings

Identify triggers, stressors, resources, protective factors

Establish therapeutic relationship

Assess patient

26-2 Roberts's Assessment, Crisis Intervention, and Trauma Treatment (ACT) model.

Other models have built upon Aguilera's general approach, such as the Assessment, Crisis Intervention, and Trauma Treatment (ACT) approach (Roberts, 2002). Roberts's stages often build on one another, but do not always follow in sequential order (Figure 26-2). The stages are:

- Assessing (including suicidality, medical conditions, protective factors)

- Establishing rapport

- Identifying problems (including crisis precipitants)

- Dealing with feelings (using active listening)

- Exploring alternatives (through identifying strengths and taking inventory of coping skills used in the past)

- Implementing an action plan (in the least restrictive manner possible)

- Establishing a follow-up plan (Roberts, 2002)

Roberts's model differs from Aguilera's in that it has a more pragmatic and less psychotherapeutic approach and does not emphasize insight-oriented aspects. Roberts's approach begins with a practical medical status and risk assessment (including presenting problems, co-morbidities, psychiatric history, and suicide risk) and an assessment of supportive and resiliency characteristics, which he terms "protective factors" (such as family supports or ready access to services). The approach follows with the establishment of general rapport and then moves immediately to the specification of the problem, its situational precipitants, and the development of an action plan using a problem-solving approach. The planning stage favors the use of strengths and adaptive coping skills already possessed by the person rather than developing new coping skills. These are leveraged to implement a "least restrictive," low-complexity intervention plan, which includes a short-term follow-up component.

It is significant to note that Roberts's approach favors a predominantly behavioral style, unlike Aguilera's, which features a more balanced cognitive–behavioral approach. Roberts's approach also does not emphasize anticipatory (preventive) planning for future problems, as Aguilera's does, but rather focuses entirely on the current presenting situation. However, the two approaches are very similar in that they both focus on the short-term management of the existing crisis experience and use a cognitive–behavioral style to facilitate the therapeutic intervention.

Categories of Crises

The experience of crisis differs among individuals and is affected by a variety of factors, including culture and socioeconomics. This makes it very difficult to develop a standard, unified understanding of crisis. However, some progress has been made in categorizing different types of crisis experiences, which has aided in the development of category-specific approaches to crisis intervention. Three major categories of crisis generally recognized are maturational, situational, and adventitious.

Maturational Crisis

The classification of maturational crises derives from a developmental psychology perspective, which assumes that there are key developmental tasks, challenges, or milestones that all individuals experience during a normal life cycle. A **maturational crisis** arises when an individual has difficulty achieving developmental tasks using available resources and coping strategies. Maturational crises may occur during milestones or developmental tasks, such as transitioning from home to college, entering into an intimate relationship, or experiencing menopause. This category of crisis experience has been described by Kulic (2005), who noted that "maturational–developmental" crises may also arise following the successful completion of a developmental task. In these situations, individuals may find themselves in novel situations in which previously effective coping techniques no longer apply or are no longer effective.

Try, Morken, and Hunskar (2001) established important epidemiologic trends related to maturational crises. They found that adolescents and young adults experience a disproportionate share of maturational crises, and that these often are due to educational (including college transitions), employment, relationship, and early parenting situations. They also noted that a majority of individuals experiencing maturational crises did not meet diagnostic criteria for psychiatric disorders.

Situational Crisis

Situational crises develop in response to sudden, unexpected traumatic life events. Situational crises are often beyond the established coping capabilities of the individuals experiencing them. Situational crises can arise from many kinds of precipitants, including medical (acute onset injury or new chronic illness diagnosis), psychosocial (divorce, legal problems, financial problems), and cultural (immigration). Situational crises may present concomitantly with or be exacerbated by maturational crises, especially in adolescents. For example, an adolescent who experienced a situational crisis (such as a car accident) resulting in significant injury may also suffer from maturational crises (body image, peer acceptance, and sexuality concerns) (Worthington, 1989). Interventions for situational crises focus on the development of new adaptive coping approaches targeted to the specific crisis.

Physical Illness

Individuals experiencing acute or chronic physical illness may experience situational crises. In a study by Iezzoni and Ngo (2007), more than 57% of individuals with MS were disabled. Given that MS has a typical age of onset in young adulthood (Noonan, Kathman, & White, 2002), it can cause both situational (onset of potentially disabling disease affecting functioning and employment) and maturational crises (impact on ability to establish a career and a family). Fortunately, psychosocial interventions for crises related to chronic or terminal illnesses, such as cognitive–behavioral therapy (CBT), behavioral stress reduction, and clinical case management, generally are effective (Malcomson, Dunwoody, & Lowe-Strong, 2007). However, no single type of intervention has yet proven superior to others (Meyer & Mark, 1995).

Mental Illness

Individuals with a predisposition to mental illness may experience onset of symptoms triggered by a situational crisis, and those with existing mental illness may experience symptom exacerbations while in crisis. For example, Post and Leverich (2006) described the role of psychosocial stress and crisis in the onset and progression of bipolar disorder. Additionally, a new diagnosis of mental illness, in and of itself, is usually a precipitant for a situational crisis.

Crisis intervention can help to minimize the psychiatric sequelae of crisis, and it can be tailored to specific psychiatric conditions. For example, a crisis intervention approach for individuals with borderline personality disorder has been found to be helpful in managing personality disorders (Laddis, 2010). Similarly, Hepp, Wittmann, Schnyder, and Michel (2004) reviewed a number of interventions for individuals who had recently made suicide attempts. Interestingly, they found that duration or type of treatment made no difference on outcomes, but that the establishment of "lifeline supports," people or services devoted to crisis support, appeared to be most helpful. This attachment to a therapeutic support also has been described by Fosha (2006) as a critical facilitator for stability, establishment of trust, reduction of fear associated with crisis, and promotion of healing.

Suicide, or recurrent risk of suicide, can generate crisis. For family and significant others, the loss of a relative, friend, or spouse by suicide can be a traumatic experience. Similarly, for those experiencing recurrent suicidal ideation, these experiences can present recurrent crises or result from ineffective coping with crisis. Especially in adolescents, the witnessing of a suicide or its aftermath can sometimes motivate suicidal behavior in others. Community-based trauma intervention programs, such as the Community Services Program (CSP), can be effective in helping adolescents cope and reduce the risk of suicide. The CSP provides organized community-based peer and paraprofessional outreach to at-risk adolescents, including education and 24-hour access to supports. This has decreased isolation, improved structure and connectedness, and reduced suicides for at-risk youth in Boston housing projects (Macy, 2003).

Impact on Significant Others

Crisis can have an impact on significant others. For example, a father witnessing a child experience a life-changing or life-limiting illness or injury may develop a situational crisis related to his perceptions of what the event might mean for the child and for him as a parent. He may experience a sense of loss for the child's future, perceive himself as unable to adequately parent the child in the setting of the new impairment, or feel guilt or responsibility for the event that has harmed the child. A similar type of situational crisis often results in women who experience miscarriages or in mothers who give birth to premature infants. They may perceive role failure as mothers owing to the adverse outcome of their pregnancies, even if they maintained healthy pregnancy behaviors. This perceived failure could challenge a mother's perceived ability to succeed as a parent in the future: "If I failed during the pregnancy, maybe it's just not in me to be a parent." Structured, short-term intervention initiated during the initial hospitalization of a premature infant has been found to be effective in reducing trauma symptoms for mothers of premature infants (Hepp, Wittmann, Schnyder, & Michel, 2004).

Adventitious Crisis

Adventitious crises arise from traumatic events that are well beyond the expected scope of normal human experience, such as violent crime, natural disasters, war, and terrorism. Adventitious crises are unlike maturational crises in that they do not relate to events expected to coincide with normal events that most people experience during a normal life cycle. Crises in this category are similar to situational crises in that they arise from traumatic events, but differ in that situational crises arise from events that are within the expected scope of normal human experience (such as illness or job loss), whereas adventitious crises do not. Another factor that is often (but not always) different between situational and adventitious crises is that adventitious crises often occur on a large scale, such as a terrorist attack on a large building or a tornado causing destruction of home and loss of life in an entire community, whereas situational crises tend to occur at an individual level. However, it is important to recognize that this trend does not always hold. For example, a person who has been traumatized by physical or sexual assault may experience an adventitious crisis at an individual level, whereas a group of workers laid off from a company during a workforce reduction campaign may experience a situational crisis at a group level.

Many interventions for adventitious crises have been developed for population-based applications. Hembree and Foa (2003) found a benefit to crisis intervention for individuals experiencing violent crime who developed posttraumatic stress disorder (PTSD). However, they also found that those developing PTSD were a minority of those who experience violent crime and that the intervention was not of benefit to those who did not develop PTSD. One-time *debriefing interventions*, which provide practical education regarding expectations, basic coping, and resource referral during or immediately following a trauma experience, have been found to be effective for survivors of natural disasters. Chemtob, Tomas, Law, and Cremniter (1997) found that one-time multihour sessions including either education regarding normal responses to trauma or situational, supportive counseling both reduced reported distress levels similarly.

Diaz (2008) described three critical aspects of an effective response to natural disasters: (1) dealing with "root shock" (loss of normal environment) of survivors; (2) mobilization of individuals and the community; and (3) community redevelopment after initial recovery. This model has been employed by the American Red Cross in its response to multiple national disasters. This three-component model may be necessary but insufficient, according to Ng et al. (2009). They argue that, especially in international crisis relief efforts, disasters tend to intensify preexisting social inequalities in communities and that the dominant social culture of relief teams may fail to take cultural factors of the disaster-stricken communities they serve into account when delivering interventions.

Pause and Reflect

1. *Think of a crisis that you or a family member has experienced. What type of crisis was it? How did you (or your family member) attempt to deal with it? In what ways was this successful?*

2. *Using the same crisis example, reflect on how this crisis affected the person's significant others. How were they affected? Were they supportive during the crisis?*

3. *Why do you think lifeline supports are helpful to individuals in crisis? What are some examples of services that can serve as lifeline supports?*

Assessment of Crisis

Nurses perform crisis assessments in diverse settings, including emergency departments, disaster sites, schools, medical and psychiatric hospital units, and outpatient clinics. Specific assessment techniques and methods are likely to differ depending on the setting and situations. However, the following basic elements of assessment apply in most crises:

- Ensuring safety
- Classifying the type of trauma
- Classifying the stage of adaptation displayed by the individual
- Articulating the individual's perceptions of the crisis
- Identifying coping skills and resources available to the individual
- Assessing the risks associated with the crisis
- Identifying treatment and referral needs
- Determining the likelihood of available treatments to support the individual effectively

The essential elements of crisis assessment are discussed in the following sections and are outlined in Box 26-1.

Safety First

The most critical portion of an initial crisis assessment is the determination of the safety of the individual. This involves assessing both the actual and potential safety of the patient. The assessment of actual safety includes a review of the current physical, emotional, and environmental safety of the patient and determining whether emergency services are required. This includes assessing for any physical or sexual injuries sustained, as well as emotional or behavioral sequelae. It also involves an assessment of the safety of the individual's home and work environments, including the safety of the physical structures and the people with whom the patient normally interacts. In some cases, patients experiencing crisis may be homeless or unable to return home. Availability, safety, and reliability of transportation also should be considered in this assessment, as should access to required life-sustaining medications for major health conditions.

Trauma Category

Assessment of the type of trauma and how the individual is adapting helps determine an appropriate approach to crisis care and the risk of psychiatric sequelae. In his commentary on crisis intervention following the 9/11 terrorist attacks, Roberts (2002) described two types of trauma that can contribute to adventitious crises, and their relative potentials for causing PTSD. **Type I trauma** experiences are one-time, limited experiences that generally are less likely to cause PTSD, whereas **type II trauma** experiences are recurrent or chronic (for instance, deployment to a war zone or recurrent victimization by an abusive partner), and are more likely to cause PTSD. However, Roberts argues that there are exceptions to this trend. Type I traumas that occur on a large scale and/or are associated with significant mortality and morbidity, such as the 9/11 World Trade Center terrorist attack, are more likely to cause PTSD than other type I traumas. Additionally, Elklit and Brink (2003) found that the magnitude of perceived loss of trust or feeling "let down" by a trusted other during a traumatic event is predictive of later development of PTSD. An example of this type of situation would be a woman who is raped by a person whom she knew well and greatly trusted prior to the rape.

Adaptation Stage

General Adaptation Syndrome (Seyle, 1956) describes the basic stages through which most individuals progress during attempts to

---

Essential Elements of Crisis Assessment   box 26-1

- **Safety:** Assess basic physical and environmental safety; conduct suicide assessment.
- **Category of crisis experience:** Assess trauma type (type I vs. type II) and associated risk for developing PTSD.
- **Stage:** Assess the stage of general adaptation (alarm, resistance, or exhaustion).
- **Lived experience:** Assess the patient's intellectual perception of the crisis and articulate associated emotions.
- **Coping skills:** Assess current and previous strategies and their effectiveness.
- **Resources:** Assess current social, financial, and environmental resources and supports that could be leveraged to help the patient.

- **Risks:** Assess for related risks in biological, psychosocial, cultural, and spiritual domains that might reasonably follow as sequelae to the crisis experience, such as physical/mental illness onset or exacerbation, increased risk of suicide, or decreased treatment adherence.
- **Treatment and adherence potential:** Assess the likelihood that the patient will participate in appropriate treatment and the availability of appropriate treatment.
- **Referral need and feasibility:** Assess whether referrals are required and whether appropriate referrals can be acquired in a timely manner.

cope with significant stressors. The progression of general adaptation is described in detail in Chapter 13 and includes three stages: alarm, resistance, and exhaustion. The alarm stage involves the fight-or-flight response that occurs during the initial experience of a stressor and is characteristic of early stage coping. The resistance stage is characterized by the mobilization of resources in an attempt to resolve the stressor and evidences later stage coping. The exhaustion stage represents a complete failure of coping to resolve the stressor and is often associated with a significant worsening in mental or physical health. Symptom exacerbations often are observed in chronic illness, and risk for acute episodic conditions (for example, a major depressive episode) and suicide is highest in the exhaustion stage. In the critical thinking feature, Rebecca has MS, a chronic neurological condition that is characterized by periodic exacerbations (relapses). During exacerbations, and especially while in the exhaustion phase (when her coping resources are low or depleted), Rebecca is more likely to experience a depressive episode secondary to the MS exacerbation (Mohr, 2006).

Assessment of an individual's stage of general adaptation can be very helpful in developing a crisis intervention approach that is specific to the individual's current lived experience. For example, for a patient demonstrating an alarm stage reaction to crisis, education regarding normal responses to trauma, available supports, and practical supports (such as shelter) may be sufficient, especially in the setting of a type I trauma experience. If a resistance stage reaction is observed, care should be taken to determine whether the patient is showing signs of success in resolving the stressor. If not, this may predict an eventual progression to the exhaustion stage if a different strategy to resolve the crisis is not employed. If a patient is exhibiting an exhaustion stage reaction, priority should be placed on ensuring basic stability of physical and mental health and providing for basic needs until the patient regains appropriate resources for individual coping.

Lived Experience

Most modern crisis intervention methods derive from CBT and depend on an accurate assessment of the lived experience of crisis (Aguilera, 1998; Roberts, 2002). A baseline understanding of the patient's perception of the crisis experience and an articulation of the patient's emotions about the crisis are necessary to develop an effective crisis intervention approach. In the treatment phase, nurses and therapists work to help patients modify or better cope with these perceptions and emotions. In developing such an assessment, the nurse first works to identify these elements, but then determines whether the perceptions and emotions being articulated are in proportion and appropriate in relationship to the crisis situation. For example, a patient who articulates fears for his safety after experiencing a terrorist attack would be assessed as displaying appropriate perceptions and emotions toward that crisis. In contrast, an individual who has recently lost his job but has not experienced a physical threat to his safety might not be exhibiting a proportionate perception of the crisis if he reports fearing direct physical harm.

Resources

Every crisis assessment should include a review of the physical, behavioral, emotional, and social resources available to the individual experiencing a crisis and if and how these resources are being used. Physical resources include finances, residence, transportation, health insurance coverage (which facilitates access to health care services), and employment (source of social support, sustainable finances, and insurance). Behavioral and emotional resources include an individual's resilience to stress as well as behavioral coping strategies, such as relaxation training, problem-solving skills, and general coping style. For example, one individual may exhibit a rational coping style, in which reason and logic are the primary mode of situational perception and reaction. Conversely, another individual may use an emotive coping style, in which feelings and intuition are the primary mode of situational perception and reaction. Social resources include people and programs that are available to provide support and reduce crisis-related isolative or avoidance behaviors.

After resources are identified, the next step is to determine whether and how resources are being used, and if they are effective. Patients with ample access to resources may not use them or may use them inconsistently. Some patients may not have access to resources, owing to lack of transportation or other factors. Others may focus on resources or strategies that have been helpful in the past but are ineffective for managing the current crisis. Understanding how the patient is using available resources is just as important as identifying which resources are available or necessary for the patient.

Risk and Adherence Potential

Because crisis can cause significant disruption in functioning, there is an increased risk of physical, psychological, and practical sequelae during a crisis period. As such, a crisis assessment should assess for risks in each of the five domains (biological, psychological, sociological, cultural, and spiritual) that are likely to follow the crisis experience. For example, a patient suffering from a chronic illness may experience acute stress related to decreased treatment adherence and increased relapse rate (Mohr, 2006; Fraser & Polito, 2007). A comprehensive crisis intervention plan for such a patient would include a component that safeguards against relapse and promotes adherence to treatment. The risk component of crisis assessment also should include a determination of possible applicable psychiatric and nursing diagnoses, as appropriate.

Crisis assessment should include review of an individual's prior adherence history (if known) and the likelihood that available treatment approaches will appropriately and actively engage the client in participation. For example, an individual who has developed strong rapport and has a strong prior adherence history is far more likely to engage in recommended treatments or follow referral recommendations than an individual who has not been successful at adhering to treatment. Similarly, if available resources lack cultural competence or lack a specific treatment capability that is essential to the individual's success, or if the patient cannot access the required services, the treatment and referral plan will need to be tailored with these considerations in mind.

The final element of an initial crisis assessment involves determining whether continued services or referrals are required and, if so, identifying services that are appropriate. The determination of service needs is assisted by earlier elements in the assessment process, including safety, trauma type, and adaptation stage. It also is influenced by the availability of resources and the individual's capacity to access care.

Rebecca Recovery Phase

Bill recognizes that Rebecca is in crisis owing to the presence of the following elements:

- Onset of situational life events that have caused significant disruptions to employment and financial stability

- Potential of the current situation to progress and adversely affect the patient and her family

- Chronological relationship to new psychological symptoms that the patient has been experiencing

- A sense of hopelessness and an apparent absence of an effective coping strategy

Bill consults with Janice, Rebecca's primary care APRN at the clinic, and recommends that she collaborate with Rebecca's neurology providers regarding her MS care. He also asks Janice to conduct a thorough mental health assessment during the office visit. While Rebecca is working with Janice, Bill arranges for a rapid mental health referral for crisis management supports and further mental assessment, and contacts a social worker to help with Rebecca's financial and employment predicaments. He describes to the social worker that collaboration with legal services and Rebecca's neurology providers may be necessary related to her inability to qualify for disability coverage or if it is discovered that she has suffered from workplace discrimination. Finally, after the office visit, Bill meets with Rebecca again to talk further about her situation, to review the plan of care, and to discuss additional supports that might be helpful to her. He assures her that he and the primary care team at the clinic will be there for her, that crisis situations like these commonly present, that she is not alone, that much can be done to help, and that she has options. They agree to check in by phone or use the secure online communication feature of the clinic's electronic medical record system once a week to make sure that Rebecca gets connected to the supports she needs and is making progress. They also agree on a crisis plan for use should her situation or symptoms worsen.

APPLICATION

1. What stage of adaptation is Rebecca in when she comes to the clinic?

2. What nursing diagnoses are appropriate for Rebecca at this time?

3. In what ways does Rebecca's medical diagnosis affect her ability to cope with stress? In what ways do you think stress has affected or might affect Rebecca's physical health?

Pause and Reflect

1. *Why is safety the most important part of a crisis assessment?*

2. *How can a nurse use an assessment of trauma experience type (type I vs. type II) and stage of general adaptation to guide crisis intervention planning?*

3. *Why do you think loss of trust or support from a significant other during trauma might increase an individual's risk for PTSD?*

Crisis Intervention

A variety of crisis intervention approaches are available, and many are designed to address specific crises or populations. However, the following general elements of crisis intervention are applicable to most crisis situations (Aguilera, 1998):

- Maintaining safety

- Managing mood symptoms associated with the crisis

- Developing coping skills

- Promoting connections with social and resource supports

- Taking a directive and instructional approach similar to interventions appropriate for patients with severe anxiety (see Chapter 13)

Similarly, Hobfoll et al. (2007) suggest that successful crisis interventions engender five essential outcomes: a sense of safety; a calming of anxiety; a strengthened sense of efficacy (coping); a strengthened sense of connectedness; and increased hope. The directive and instructional style, which differs from the patient-centric, collaborative nature of the general nursing approach, is of particular importance in crisis intervention because clients in acute crisis are often too overwhelmed to fully process the trauma experience, fully consider values and preferences, or make informed decisions.

Psychological Debriefing

Psychological debriefing (PD) methods, including critical incident stress debriefing (CISD), are brief, one-time interventions conducted within 72 hours of crisis onset. Debriefing interventions aim to (1) provide information regarding the crisis, (2) elicit feelings and perceptions related to the crisis, (3) provide education regarding normal responses to trauma, and (4) provide resources for treatment and support. Originally, PD methods were employed universally to all victims of severe trauma, especially in mass trauma situations. However, further research (Bisson, Brayne, Ochberg, & Everly, 2007; Devilly, Gist, & Cotton, 2006); has challenged the effectiveness of PD methods, noting a general lack of evidence support, and suggesting that PD approaches may not be an economically feasible or effective intervention.

Devilly, Gist, and Cotton (2006) suggest that CISD, which attempts to "normalize" responses to stress, may in fact "pathologize" them and worsen outcomes for those with the worst presenting symptoms. They also argue that many of the teaching interventions used in PD methods may not be necessary or improve outcomes. They recommend that individuals who are offered a PD intervention should be informed of the trade-offs involved in undergoing treatment and that clinicians use these interventions selectively instead of universally, weighing the risks and benefits of PD treatment. Bisson, Brayne, Ochberg, and Everly (2007) argue that CISD methods should not be used at all for trauma victims. However, the alternative method they recommend contains similar aspects to PD approaches, including education about normal reactions to trauma, and information about how to access support and treatment. Finally, Bryant (2005) argues that PD proceeds from an erroneous assumption that all individuals exposed to trauma will develop PTSD, when, in fact, only a small minority do.

Crisis Management

Clinical Question
What is the best approach for the clinical management of crisis?

Evidence
There are several options for individuals who are experiencing crisis and experiencing clinically significant symptoms or at risk of developing sequelae, including psychopharmacology and cognitive–behavioral therapy (CBT).

CBT approaches can be helpful in promoting hope. A key component of CBT focuses on an examination of the cognitive perceptions an individual has about the magnitude of the stressor, the capability to cope, and value of the experience. One CBT approach, *decatastrophizing*, involves an adjustment in the perceived magnitude of the trauma stressor to realistic proportions. For example, a patient who has experienced a car crash may perceive that he will never be able to drive again and that being in a car will result in future injury. By helping the patient adjust his perception to a more realistic understanding of the actual probabilities of auto-related injury, the nurse can help the patient reduce the magnitude of the perceived stressor and increase his confidence in his ability to cope with it. Another approach, *benefit finding*, involves the patient learning how to successfully cope with the stressor, and through experiencing a successful recovery from the traumatic experience, gaining greater self-esteem and feeling more prepared to deal with future problems. For example, an adolescent who learns to successfully cope with the end of a romantic relationship may feel more confident in pursuing future relationships because she perceives herself as more capable to cope with that experience and better able to select future relationships based on what she has learned.

Hobfoll et al. (2007) found that eclectic approaches can sometimes optimize crisis intervention outcomes. Pharmacological agents, such as antiadrenergic agents, antidepressants, and anxiolytics, may be useful in reducing anxiety. Promotion of self-efficacy may be achieved by short-term CBT, and collective group efficacy may be promoted through community-led rebuilding and redevelopment projects following disasters and terrorism. Community connectedness can be promoted by encouraging the use of existing supports and developing new supports and strategies.

Implications for Nursing Practice
Patients experiencing crisis may benefit from short-term use of cognitive–behavioral approaches that focus on modifying cognitive perceptions of the crisis and identifying and reinforcing successful coping behaviors.

Critical Thinking Questions
1. In addition to car accidents, what relatively common crisis events might be likely to cause patients to develop unrealistic perceptions of the event or possible recurrences of the event? How might you intervene to help patients decatastophize their unrealistic fears?
2. You are working with Pam, a middle-aged woman who has just lost her job and is facing an "identity crisis" as she discovers that she really doesn't like her chosen career. Would a "benefit-finding" approach be helpful to her? If so, how would you, as the nurse working with Pam, employ a basic benefit-finding intervention for her?
3. When and why might a combination of approaches be helpful to patients?

Psychological First Aid
Psychological first aid is a brief and practical intervention that is often used in the immediate aftermath of disasters and other large-scale trauma experiences (Brymer et al., 2006). Psychological first aid incorporates three aspects: provision of practical supports, ranging from food and shelter to information about tasks, such as how to plan a funeral; education regarding normal reactions to trauma/crisis; and coping skills training. Psychological first aid includes some aspects of PD, but differs in that it contains a coping skills training component. Evidence support for the effectiveness of psychological first aid is minimal, specifically regarding whether or not it can prevent psychiatric sequelae such as PTSD (Bisson, Brayne, Ochberg, & Everly, 2007). Unfortunately, a barrier to evidence development is that it is very difficult to conduct effective research in disaster situations.

Cognitive–Behavioral Therapy
Short-term CBT interventions are considered first-line treatment for individuals experiencing mood symptoms secondary to crisis experiences (Hembree & Foa, 2003). CBT interventions include exposure therapy, stress inoculation, and interventions that facilitate critical evaluation of cognitive perceptions of crisis and the development of adaptive coping skills. Eye movement desensitization and reprocessing (EMDR) is an exposure-deconditioning approach effective in treating PTSD. It is used only for individuals in crisis who are suffering clinically significant symptoms of PTSD or acute stress disorder

(Hembree & Foa, 2003). Aguilera's widely used short-term, problem-solving approach for crisis intervention also uses cognitive reappraisal techniques and coping skills training. CBT approaches are not recommend for universal use in preventing onset of PTSD (Roberts, Kitchiner, Kenardy, & Bisson, 2012), but rather for use in symptomatic individuals only (Bryant, 2005; Shu-Hsin, 2003).

Pharmacologic Interventions
Pharmacologic interventions are not commonly used for individuals experiencing crisis. However, short-term pharmacotherapy can be helpful for patients who are experiencing significant mood symptoms that are preventing CBT from succeeding. By reducing mood symptoms, pharmacologic interventions may enhance the effectiveness of psychotherapeutic interventions. Anxiolytic medications may help to decrease the physiologic discomforts of anxiety and tension that often accompany crisis. Benzodiazepines, such as lorazepam (Ativan), are used for management of acute anxiety. Selective serotonin-reuptake inhibitors (SSRIs), such as paroxetine (Paxil), and the nonbenzodiazepine anxiolytic buspirone (Buspar) are used for adjunctive management of persistent anxiety (Turnbull, 1998; Ravindran & Stein, 2010; Bandelow et al., 2012). There also has been investigation into the use of the beta-adrenergic blocker propanolol when given immediately after a traumatic experience to help block the formation of emotionally charged memories that might precipitate acute stress disorder or PTSD (Pitman & Delahanty, 2005). In

Basic Crisis Education and Health Counseling Recommendations box 26-2

- Facilitate a general basic understanding of the crisis experience, emphasizing that there are effective, short-term interventions and supports that can help.
- Help the individual to understand the basics about general adaptation syndrome, including self-monitoring for changes in the adaptation response stage.
- Facilitate an understanding of the common emotional responses that can accompany a crisis experience.
- Educate on basic coping skills (such as behavioral stress reduction techniques and exercise) and self-monitoring

training (for example, using a calendar or journal to track stress exposures and anxiety levels).
- Discuss the risks and benefits of different treatment options and facilitate appropriate referrals in a timely manner.
- Encourage social connectivity to help the individual understand that he or she is not alone.
- Educate on basic safety monitoring and status reporting, including surveillance for common illnesses and suicide prevention.

certain cases, antidepressant therapy with an SSRI or serotonin–norepinephrine-reuptake inhibitor (SNRI) may be indicated, especially if the individual suffers from a depressive or preexisting anxiety disorder or is experiencing chronic mood symptoms that impair functioning and progress in crisis therapy.

Patient Education and Health Counseling

Nurses often are the first point of contact for individuals in crisis, and frequently are required to provide general crisis education and health counseling. Specific education and health counseling approaches will vary based on the characteristics and situations being experienced by each individual. However, general educational recommendations, which are derived in part from aspects of the evidence-based crisis interventions previously discussed in this chapter, can be helpful in many crisis situations and can often be delivered during the initial clinical encounter (Box 26-2).

Pause and Reflect

1. *When is therapeutic intervention indicated for individuals experiencing a crisis?*
2. *Which crisis intervention is considered first-line for patients experiencing mood symptoms in the setting of a crisis experience?*
3. *When is pharmacotherapy appropriate to consider for patients in crisis?*

Crisis and Specific Populations

Thus far, general approaches to crisis assessment and intervention in adults have been emphasized. However, it is also important for nurses to understand that there are important differences in approaches that are relevant to specific populations. This section provides an overview of special considerations for children, adolescents, older adults, intercultural situations, men, and nurses and other health care providers. Please note that issues related to prevalence of certain conditions among specific populations are discussed in other chapters.

People respond to crisis via one or more of six major coping styles, as described by the *Basic Ph* coping model (National Association of School Psychologists, 2013). The first style, *belief*, is characterized by the use of core values and world views to place the crisis

in context—to frame the crisis experience in order to better understand and integrate it. The second style, *affect*, is characterized by the use of an outward expression of emotion to reduce internal stress. The third style, *social*, is characterized by the use of social support and relationships to process the crisis and to decrease isolation. The fourth style, *imagination*, is characterized by the use of creativity and sublimation to displace and/or process the crisis stressor, or to try to escape from it. The fifth style, *cognitive*, entails the use of reasoning and rationale dialogue to think through and problem solve the experience. The final style, *physiological*, entails the use of physical activity as a method of displacing, processing, or avoiding the stressor (Figure 26-3).

Children and Adolescents

Young children who have not yet developed substantial belief or cognitive structures may respond to crisis via the affective, social, physiological, or imagination pathways. In particular, they may look to adults for guidance and safety, and may display behavioral regressions (such as thumbsucking or bedwetting in school-age children), clinginess to adults, sleep disturbance, and withdrawal. In comparison, adolescents may leverage belief, cognitive, and physiological coping styles more than imagination, and are far less likely to seek adult support than younger children. Instead, adolescents may seek peer supports (Macy, 2003). Adolescents may demonstrate withdrawal similar to that of younger children, but they may also display aggressiveness, sleeping and eating disturbances, and physical symptoms.

Recommendations for crisis interventions in pediatric populations are somewhat different than those for adult populations, particularly in terms of the crisis intervention setting and the involvement of parents and families in the delivery of care. Cohen, Berliner, and Mannarino (2003) reviewed a number of pediatric crisis intervention approaches, including psychoeducation, psychological first aid, play therapy, psychoanalytic techniques, family therapy, traumatic bereavement therapy, EMDR, therapeutic preschool interventions, and pharmacologic treatment. They found a general superiority of CBT-related approaches over others, but were unable to specify what aspects of CBT are most helpful for children. Gaffney (2008) found a distinct advantage in school-based interventions (increased adherence and access) and parent-assisted interventions, especially in large-scale adventitious crisis situations.

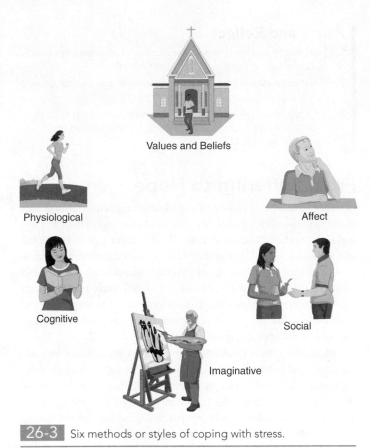

Values and Beliefs

Physiological

Affect

Cognitive

Social

Imaginative

26-3 Six methods or styles of coping with stress.

Adolescents differ from other populations in that they experience a number of critical developmental milestones and therefore are especially susceptible to maturational crises. These may present individually or in combination with situational or adventitious crises, resulting in a magnified effect on the adolescent. Additionally, adolescents may be more likely than those in other age groups to resist parental or health professional recommendations during crisis situations. Successful interventions for adolescents include similar strategies to those that are effective for adults, including coping skills training, but they differ in the delivery mechanism. Whereas adults and children under parental supervision may seek crisis care from providers in health care centers and schools, respectively, adolescents are more likely to seek advice from select peers or adult laypersons in the general community. For this reason, community-based interventions and trauma response networks that pair adolescents with peer or adult supports in the community have been effective for crisis intervention and suicide prevention (Macy, 2003).

Adults

Adults are less likely to use imagination styles of coping and often rely heavily on belief (influenced greatly by past experience) and cognitive styles, and in general may seek to resolve crises individually. Withdrawal and denial-based coping, in which attempts are made to minimize the crisis experience or simply avoid its effects, is common in adults, especially in men (Gilles & L'Heureux, 2005). This can limit their social coping potential. Men also tend to display less affective coping potential, which can worsen this deficit comparative to women.

Older Adults

Older adults (individuals age 60 and older) who are victims of crisis may also suffer diminished social coping potential due to lack of access to social supports and a tendency toward self-reliance and resilience learned through the experience of coping with numerous situational crises that accompany aging (Vernooij-Dassen et al., 2010). They also may have less access to or capability for exercise-based (physiological) coping. Belief-based coping may be strongest in this age group, especially in those with prior history of effective coping and/or religious or spiritual practices.

Older adults are more likely to experience situational crises than any other age group. Common situational crises affecting the elderly include personal illness or illness in a loved one; loss of friends, family, and spouses; financial scarcity; and retirement. However, the greater life experience possessed by individuals in this age category can often provide increased resilience. In addition, older adults often have a greater repertoire of coping strategies. One of the greatest threats to older adult functioning is dementia: It is both a situational crisis and a process that significantly affects cognitive functioning. Dementia substantially impairs perception and coping capacity, and it significantly reduces the ability of older adults to resolve situational crises (Vernooij-Dassen et al., 2010).

Situational crises also are common in caregivers of individuals with dementia. Spouses, close family members, and other caregivers may experience significant caregiver role strain over time while providing care. For example, consider adult children who care for parents with advancing dementia. As the cognitive impairment worsens, the parent requires more support from the adult children, which may require more visits to the parent's home, more direct time spent with the parent, or bringing the parent to live with one of his or her children. This increases the time commitment required of the caregiver and may interfere with or add to parenting or employment demands, consuming more energy and resources and generating a higher cumulative stress burden.

Intercultural Situations

There are special considerations for crisis care delivered in countries outside the U.S., including international relief efforts or other situations in which care providers and care recipients are from different cultures. In these intercultural situations, cultural competence and recognition and involvement of local communities in crisis intervention are of critical importance. Western organizations involved in international crises have drawn criticism for failing to thoroughly involve local community members in leading mental health interventions. This has led to revised training guidelines for international crisis relief teams, guidelines that emphasize cultural competence, and the facilitation of local community leadership (Kaul, 2002; Weine et al., 2002).

There is also substantial debate across cultures concerning the cultural applicability of Western psychiatric diagnoses such as PTSD, definitions of normal and abnormal expressions of emotional pain, and the definition of a crisis experience (von Peter, 2008). Individuals from different cultures perceive the lived experience of crisis very differently, and interventions must be modified accordingly to maximize applicability and effectiveness.

Men

Gilles and L'Heureux (2005) argue that men may compose a particularly vulnerable population in the setting of crisis. Men are far more likely to resist help because help-seeking behaviors may challenge social norms of masculinity and induce a sense of vulnerability. Some men may attempt to regain control in a crisis situation through the use of aggressive behavior. Men usually access intervention only when in acute crisis; for this reason, it is critical to initiate crisis intervention within 24 to 48 hours of initial contact. The most successful interventions for men include the utilization of peer-led men's support groups and the delivery of care by practitioners who resist developing negative biases toward the avoidant and aggressive coping styles exhibited by many men when experiencing a crisis (Gilles & L'Heureux, 2005).

> **PRACTICE ALERT**   Clinicians must remain aware at all times of how their unconscious biases may affect the care they provide to individuals experiencing crisis, and take great care not to allow these biases to sabotage their provision of crisis care.

Nurses and Health Care Providers

Working with individuals going through crisis can generate significant emotional strain for the professional nurse, as well as for other health care providers. Adequate supervision, maintenance of boundaries, appropriate use of therapeutic respites, and a regular practice of coping and self-care skills are necessary to avoid developing vicarious traumatization (also called **secondary trauma**), which is an experience of trauma developed via the repeated observance of others suffering from traumatic events. Another adverse result is **compassion fatigue,** a sense of exhaustion that can develop secondary to providing clinical crisis care repetitively over long periods of time (Kaul, 2002). **Compassion satisfaction**, which is a sense of fulfillment, value, and joy derived from helping others, can often buffer compassion fatigue (Kaul, 2002). One coping measure commonly used among nurses and health care providers is psychological debriefing (PD). Although PD is not well supported as a general crisis intervention for laypersons, there is some evidence supporting its use as a distress reduction and general crisis prevention method for crisis clinicians (Chemtob, Tomas, Law, & Cremniter, 1997).

Pause and Reflect

1. *How might you modify a general crisis intervention approach (for an adult) to best suit a pediatric client?*
2. *What strengths might you be able to leverage to help older adults better cope with situational crises?*
3. *Why do you think it is important for nurses working in crisis care to prevent vicarious (secondary) traumatization and compassion fatigue?*

From Suffering to Hope

Crises can cause acute and significant disruptions across the domains of a person's lived experience, and can lead to feelings of hopelessness and suffering. Crises can be situational, adventitious, or maturational and are characterized by a perceived threat or danger; an imbalance or disturbance in psychological functioning; and lack of a feasible solution. Health care professionals can significantly reduce crisis-related suffering, reduce the risk of crisis-related sequelae, and increase hope for people experiencing a crisis by providing timely assessment and appropriate intervention.

Basic elements of crisis assessment begin with assessing individual actual and potential safety and include activities such as identifying coping skills and resources, assessing risks, and determining the potential for adherence to treatment. Many crisis intervention approaches are available, including psychological first aid, debriefing, cognitive–behavioral interventions, and pharmacotherapy. There is conflicting evidence concerning the safety and effectiveness of many of these interventions, but CBT approaches are currently the most strongly supported by research evidence and most commonly used.

Crisis presentation and treatment considerations may differ in specific populations and may vary by gender, ethnicity, and age. Crisis may also be experienced by caregivers. Nurses and other health care professionals providing care for people in crisis can experience secondary trauma and compassion fatigue. They must maintain supervision supports, reflective practice, and appropriate clinical boundaries to optimize their wellness and avoid unconscious biases from affecting care delivery.

Nurses are often the initial point of contact for persons in crisis and can provide timely and effective intervention beginning in the initial clinical encounter. Appropriate assessment and timely intervention can have a significant impact on suffering and provide hope for people experiencing trauma and crisis.

Chapter Highlights

1. Crisis is commonly experienced and causes functional disequilibrium in individuals.
2. There are three general types of crises: maturational, situational, and adventitious.
3. Individuals demonstrate a general response to crisis that is described by the general adaptation syndrome.
4. Crises can increase the risk for physical and mental health problems.
5. Crisis assessment includes seven aspects: (1) safety status; (2) categorization; (3) adaptation staging; (4) perceptions and emotions related to the crisis; (5) assessment of potential risks; (6) resources and their current utilization; and (7) service needs and treatment adherence potential.
6. There are a number of methods currently utilized for crisis intervention. Short-term cognitive–behavioral therapy (CBT) approaches are most strongly supported by available research evidence.
7. Pharmacotherapy is not recommended as a first-line treatment for individuals in crisis, but may be helpful in managing severe mood symptoms.

8. There are specific considerations for crisis intervention applying to children, adolescents, older adults, intercultural situations, and men in crisis.

9. Nurses and clinicians engaged in crisis care must practice routine self-care, access regular supervision, maintain appropriate boundaries, and remain cognizant of their unconscious biases.

10. General education and health counseling recommendations derived from evidence-based crisis interventions can be delivered by a nurse during initial crisis encounters.

NCLEX®-RN Questions

1. A young adult patient is brought to a mental health center by his parents when he drops out of college at the end of the first semester. The patient reports living in a dorm that experienced a devastating fire that resulted in the death of several classmates and friends. The nurse recognizes that the patient is experiencing acute stress that is best categorized as which type of crisis?
   a. One in which an experience of others produces secondary trauma in the individual
   b. One arising from an event that is beyond the scope of normal human experience
   c. One that is a traumatic but inevitable, with death and loss of relationships
   d. One that occurred in relationship to a developmental period where previously used coping skills no longer apply

2. The nurse is performing an assessment of a patient who has just experienced an acute crisis. Which action is priority?
   a. Validating the patient's perception of what has just occurred
   b. Classifying the type of trauma that the patient has experienced
   c. Eliminating any immediate physiological and psychosocial threats
   d. Determining which type of treatment interventions will be necessary

3. The nurse is working with a patient who is coping with a situational crisis related to the unanticipated loss of a job. The patient states, "I am a failure and I will never be able to find another job." Which cognitive–behavioral approaches will best allow the nurse help the patient to optimize hope?
   a. Identifying any behaviors or attitudes that may have contributed to the job loss
   b. Suggesting that the patient try to be more positive by using this time to enjoy other aspects of life
   c. Encouraging the patient to identify other situations in which the patient has been able to successfully cope
   d. Assisting the patient to develop a more realistic appraisal of the situation by minimizing the importance having a job

4. The nurse is planning psychoeducational groups for patients. The nurse understands that the approach should be guided by which population-specific considerations? Select all that apply.
   a. Children and adolescents will generally look toward adults for guidance and safety.
   b. Adult men commonly withdraw from a crisis or simply avoid and or deny its effects.
   c. Older adults tend to focus on social supports when confronted with a crisis situation.
   d. In comparison to younger adults, older adults are at more risk for a variety of situational crises.
   e. Adults who care for aging parents are more susceptible to the effects of a high cumulative stress burden.

5. The nurse is providing teaching to the parents of a child who has just experienced a traumatic event. The parents note that the child denies that anything is wrong and spends lots of time engaged in imaginative play. Which response is most appropriate?
   a. "Your child is demonstrating a developmentally and psychologically typical response."
   b. "Denial is always a maladaptive response to stress that should be challenged right away."
   c. "There may be an issue with trust because children usually look to adults for guidance."
   d. "Children are much more resilient than adults and traumatic events do not have the same degree of impact on them."

Answers may be found on the Pearson student resource site: nursing.pearsonhighered.com

Pearson Nursing Student Resources Find additional review materials at **nursing.pearsonhighered.com**

References

Aguilera, D. C. (1998). *Crisis Intervention: Theory and Methodology* (8th ed.). St. Louis, MO: Mosby.

Bandelow, B., Sher, L., Bunevicus, R., Hollander, E., Kasper, S., Zohar, J., Möller, H-J., World Federation of Societies of Biological Psychiatry (WFSBP) Task Force on Mental Disorders in Primary Care, WFSBP Task Force on Anxiety Disorders, OCD and PTSD. (2012). Guidelines for the pharmacological treatment of anxiety disorders, obsessive compulsive disorder and post-traumatic stress disorder in primary care. *International Journal of Psychiatry in Clinical Practice, 16*(2), 77–84.

Bisson, J. I., Brayne, M., Ochberg, F. M., & Everly, G. S. (2007). Early psychosocial intervention following traumatic events. *American Journal of Psychiatry, 164*(7), 1016–1019.

Bryant, R. A. (2005). Conceptually driven psychosocial approaches of acute stress reactions. *CNS Spectrums, 10*(2), 116–122. Available at http://www.cnsspectrums.com/aspx/articledetail.aspx?articleid=311

Brymer, M., Jacobs, A., Layne, C., Pynoos, R., Ruzek, J., Steinberg, A., …Watson, P. (2006). *Psychological First Aid: Field Operations Guide* (2nd ed.). Available at http://www.ptsd.va.gov/professional/manuals/maual-pdf/pfa/PFA_2ndEditionwithappendices.pdf

Caplan, G. (1961). *An Approach to Community Mental Health.* New York, NY: Grune & Stratton.

Caplan, G. (1964). *Principles of Preventive Psychiatry.* New York, NY: Basic Books.

Chemtob, C. M., Tomas, S., Law, W., & Cremniter, D. (1997). Postdisaster psychosocial intervention: A field study of the impact of debriefing on psychological distress. *American Journal of Psychiatry, 154*(3), 415–417.

Cohen, J. A., Berliner, L., & Mannarino, A. P. (2003). Psychosocial and pharmacological interventions for child crime victims. *Journal of Traumatic Stress, 16*(2), 175–186.

Devilly, G. J., Gist, R., & Cotton, P. (2006). Ready! Fire! Aim! The status of psychological debriefing and therapeutic interventions: In the work place and after disasters. *Review of General Psychology, 10*(4), 318–345.

Diaz, J. O. P. (2008). Integrating psychosocial programs in multisector responses to international disasters. *American Psychologist, 63*(8), 820–827.

Dulmus, C. N., & Wodarski, J. S. (2002). Six critical questions for brief therapeutic interventions. *Brief Treatment and Crisis Intervention, 2*(4), 279–285.

Elklit, A., & Brink, O. (2003). Acute stress disorder in physical assault victims visiting a Danish emergency ward. *Violence and Victims, 18*(4), 461–472.

Fosha, D. (2006). Quantum transformation in trauma and treatment: Traversing the crisis of healing change. *Journal of Clinical Psychology: In Session, 62*(5), 569–583.

Fraser, C., & Polito, S. (2007). A comparative study of self-efficacy in men and women with multiple sclerosis. *Journal of Neuroscience Nursing, 39*(2), 102–106.

Gaffney, D. A. (2008). Families, schools, and disaster: The mental health consequences of catastrophic events. *Family Community Health, 31*(1), 44–52.

Gilles, T., & L'Heureux, P. (2005). Psychosocial intervention with men. *International Journal of Men's Health, 4*(1), 55–62.

Greenston, J., & Leviton, S. (2002). *Elements of Crisis Intervention: Crises and How to Respond to Them* (2nd ed.). Pacific Grove, CA: Brooks/Cole.

Hembree, E. A., & Foa, E. B. (2003). Interventions for trauma-related emotional disturbances in adult victims of crime. *Journal of Traumatic Stress, 16*(2), 187–199.

Hepp, U., Wittmann, L., Schnyder, U., & Michel, K. (2004). Psychological and psychosocial interventions after attempted suicide: An overview of treatment studies. *Crisis, 25*(3), 108–117.

Hobfoll, S. E., Watson, P., Bell, C. C., Bryant, R. A., Brymer, M. J., Friedman, M. J., … Ursano, R. J. (2007). Five essential elements of immediate and mid-term mass trauma intervention: Empirical evidence. *Psychiatry, 70*(4), 283–315.

Iezzoni, L. I., & Ngo, L. (2007). Health, disability, and life insurance experiences of working-age persons with multiple sclerosis. *Multiple Sclerosis, 13*, 534–546.

James, R. K., Gilliland, B. E., & James, L. (2012). *Crisis Intervention Strategies* (7th ed.). New York, NY: Cengage Learning.

Jotzo, M., & Poets, C. F. (2005). Helping parents cope with the trauma of premature birth: An evaluation of a trauma-preventative psychological intervention. *Pediatrics, 115*(915), 915–919.

Kaul, R. E. (2002). A social worker's account of 31 days responding to the Pentagon disaster: Crisis intervention training and self-care practices. *Brief Treatment and Crisis Intervention, 2*(1), 33–37.

Kulic, K. R. (2005). The crisis intervention semi-structured interview. *Brief Treatment and Crisis Intervention, 5*(2), 143–157.

Laddis, A. (2010). Outcome of crisis intervention for borderline personality disorder and post-traumatic stress disorder: A model for modification of the mechanism of disorder in complex post-traumatic syndromes. *Annals of General Psychiatry, 9*(1), 19.

Lindemann, E. (1944). Symptomology and management of acute grief. *American Journal of Psychiatry, 101*(2), 141–148.

Macy, R. (2003). Community-based trauma response for youth. *New Directions for Youth Development, 98*, 29–49.

Malcomson, K. S., Dunwoody, L., & Lowe-Strong, A. S. (2007). Psychosocial interventions in people with MS: A review. *Journal of Neurology, 254*, 1–13.

Meyer, T. J., & Mark, M. M. (1995). Effects of psychosocial interventions with adult cancer patients: A meta-analysis of randomized experiments. *Health Psychology, 14*(2), 101–108.

Mohr, D. C. (2006). The relationship between stress and MS relapses. *Brain Behavior and Immunology, 20*, 27–36.

National Association of School Psychologists. (2013). Online resource library: Crisis. Available at http://www.nasponline.org/resources/crisis_safety/ongoingthreat.aspx

Newfield, S. A., Hinz, M. D., Tilley, D. S., Sridaromont, K. L., & Maramba, P. J. (2007). *Cox's Clinical Applications of Nursing Diagnosis: Adult, Child, Women's, Psychiatric, Gerontic, and Home Health Considerations* (3rd ed.). Philadelphia: F.A. Davis.

Ng, C., Ma, H., Raphael, B., Yu, X., Fraser, J., & Tang, D. (2009). China-Australia training on psychosocial crisis intervention: Response to the earthquake disaster in Sichuan. *Australasian Psychiatry, 17*(1), 51–55.

Noonan, C. W., Kathman, S. W., & White, M. C. (2002). Prevalence estimates for MS in the United States and evidence of an increasing trend for women. *Neurology, 58*(1), 136–138.

Pitman, R. K., & Delahanty, D. L. (2005). Conceptually driven pharmacologic approaches to acute trauma. *CNS Spectrums, 10*(2), 99–106. Available at http://mbldownloads.com/0205CNS_Pitman.pdf

Post, R. M., & Leverich, G. S. (2006). The role of psychosocial stress in the onset and progression of bipolar disorder and its comorbidities: The need for earlier and alternative modes of therapeutic intervention. *Development and Psychopathology, 18*(4):1181–1211.

Ravindran, L. N., & Stein, M. B. (2010). The pharmacologic treatment of anxiety disorders: A review of progress. *Journal of Clinical Psychiatry, 71*(7), 839–854.

Roberts, A. R. (2002). Assessment, crisis intervention, and trauma treatment: The integrative ACT intervention model. *Brief Treatment and Crisis Intervention, 2*(1), 1–21.

Roberts, N. P., Kitchiner, N. J., Kenardy, J., & Bisson, J. I. (2012). Early psychological interventions to treat acute traumatic stress symptoms. *Cochrane Database of Systematic Reviews, 3*, Pub. no. CD007944.

Seyle, H. (1956). *The Stress of Life*. New York, NY: McGraw-Hill.

Shafiq, S., Matsenko, O., & Taneli, T. (2009). Play therapy with children in crisis. *Journal of the American Academy of Child Adolescent Psychiatry, 48*(10), 1043.

Shu-Hsin, L. (2003). Effects of using a nursing crisis intervention program on psychosocial responses and coping strategies of infertile women during in vitro fertilization. *Journal of Nursing Research, 11*(3), 197–208.

Try, E., Morken, T., & Hunskar, S. (2011). A personal crisis support team at an accident and emergency department. *Journal of the Norwegian Medical Association, 128*, 2056–2059.

Turnbull, G. J. (1998). A review of post-traumatic stress disorder. Part II: Treatment. *Injury, 29*(3), 169–175.

Tyhurst, J. S. (1951). Individual reactions to community disaster: The natural history of psychiatric phenomena. *American Journal of Psychiatry, 107*, 764–769.

Tyhurst, J. S. (1957). Psychological and social aspects of civilian disaster. *Canadian Medical Association Journal, 76*(5), 385–393.

Vernooij-Dassen, M., Vasse, E., Zuidema, S., Cohen-Mansfield, J., & Moyle, M. (2010). Psychosocial interventions for dementia patients in long-term care. *International Psychogeriatrics, 22*(7), 1121–1128. doi: 10.1017/S1041610210001365.

von Peter, S. (2008). The experience of "mental trauma" and its transcultural application. *Transcultural Psychiatry, 45*(4), 639–651.

Weine, S., Danieli, Y., Silove, D., Van Ommeren, M., Fairbank, J. A., & Saul, J. (2002). Guidelines of international training in mental health and psychosocial interventions for trauma exposed populations in clinical and community settings. *Psychiatry, 65*(2), 156–164.

Worthington, J. (1989). The impact of adolescent development on recovery from traumatic brain injury. *Rehabilitation Nursing, 14*(3), 118–122.

Preventing and Responding to Suicide

27

Pamela Marcus

Learning Outcomes

1. Identify populations with a high rate of suicide.

2. Examine the impact of biological, psychological, sociological, cultural, and spiritual domains on the individual who is at risk for suicide.

3. Summarize risk factors and protective measures for suicide.

4. Assess patient risk for a suicide attempt.

5. Plan evidenced-based nursing care for a patient who has attempted or is at risk for suicide.

6. Describe community services that a patient or family member can use to prevent a suicide attempt.

Key Terms

Brian Initial Onset

Brian Brown is a 43-year-old married man, the father of two children, who is an electrical engineer at a research company in Baltimore. As part of his job, he often travels to Boston to work with his research team. Brian's research group meets once a month for a week to review the status of the project. In the past couple of months, Brian and his wife, Jennifer, have been arguing regularly. Jennifer has been increasingly frustrated by Brian's frequent absences from home for work. When he is on the way to his hotel in Boston from the airport, Jennifer calls him and tells him that she has left the house, taking their children, and will be living with her parents until they can get a place to live separate from him. Brian becomes enraged, yelling at her over the phone. During the week's meetings, he has difficulty concentrating—he is unable to sleep at the hotel, his thoughts about his marriage and his family keeping him awake. Brian had no idea that there were marital problems, and Jennifer's decision to move out came as a complete surprise. On his third night in Boston, after a very intense meeting, Brian begins to think about dying and feeling relieved by the idea of not being here anymore. On the way to the hotel, he buys a fifth of gin, a bottle of cola, a bottle of acetaminophen (Tylenol), and a bottle of doxylamine (Unisom). Brian calls Jennifer and gets her voice mail. He leaves a message that he will no longer be here and that she and the children can go back to the house to live. He then writes a suicide note:

Dear Family,

By the time you get this letter, I will be gone. I loved all of you and did not realize that you were hurting like this. I hope you have a good life and enjoy life without me.

Love, Dad

Brian takes a handful of pills, drinks a gin and cola, and lies down on the couch. When Jennifer finally listens to her voicemail, she calls the hotel to ask security to check on Brian. Security finds him crying on the couch, with vomit all over him, and calls 911. The paramedics administer charcoal and transport Brian to the nearest hospital. After becoming medically stable, Brian is admitted to the behavioral health unit.

APPLICATION

1. Assess Brian in the five domains:
   a. Biological
   b. Psychological
   c. Sociological
   d. Cultural
   e. Spiritual
2. How would you prioritize Brian's needs during this encounter? What is your rationale?
3. How would you begin to help Brian find hope in his situation?

Introduction

Suicide is a very complex subject. It involves a level of personal suffering that is so great that the individual contemplates ending his or her life. Unable to reach out to others, the individual becomes isolated, often thinking that other people will judge his or her actions or thoughts. Profound feelings of hopelessness and worthlessness constrict the individual's thinking and prevent the ability to problem-solve. When this occurs, some individuals view suicide as a reasonable solution to bring relief to their suffering.

Suicide refers to death as a result of self-inflicted injury accompanied by an intent to die from the injury (Crosby, Ortega, & Melanson, 2011). It is estimated that 1 million individuals worldwide die from suicide annually (World Health Organization [WHO], 2013). In the United States, 38,364 individuals died of suicide in 2010—approximately 105 per day. This represents an annual rate of 12.43 suicides per 100,000 individuals (Centers for Disease Control and Prevention [CDC], 2012; American Association for Suicidology [AAS], 2013). Suicide is the 10th leading cause of death in the United States. Suicide occurs more in the intermountain states than other parts of the country: Wyoming, Alaska, Montana, and Nevada are the states with the highest rates of suicides (AAS, 2013). According to the CDC (2012) and AAS (2013):

- Men commit suicide 3.85 times more than women.
- Women have a higher rate of suicide attempts than men.
- Individuals ages 85 and older commit suicide at a rate 36% higher than adults younger than 85.
- Suicide is the third leading cause of death for individuals ages 15 to 24 years old.

Statistics are useful to understand trends in order to determine what population of individuals may be at risk for suicide. Caucasians have the highest rate of death by suicide in the United States. Out of the total 38,364 deaths by suicide in 2010, 34,690 were Caucasian: 27,422 men and 7,268 women. Native American and Alaskan Native American youth between 15 and 24 years of age have shown an increase in deaths by suicide. African American women have the lowest rate of suicide (AAS, 2013; CDC, 2012). In general, it has been found that death by suicide increases during periods of economic distress and decreases during times of war. Individuals who are divorced, separated, and widowed have a higher rate of suicide (CDC, 2012).

Individuals who have made unsuccessful suicide attempts provide an understanding of the suffering that led them to have thoughts of suicide (commonly called **suicidal ideation**) that led to their suicide attempt. A **suicide attempt** may be described as any self-directed injury with an intent to die that does not result in death. A study by the Substance Abuse and Mental Health Services Administration (SAMHSA) of nonfatal outcomes of suicide attempts found that health care providers reported 959,100 nonfatal attempts in 2010, approximately 25 attempts for each completed suicide (SAMHSA, 2012; AAS, 2013).

When an individual commits suicide, a psychological autopsy is often performed. A psychological autopsy is considered the best practice to determine the causal factors of the suicide. This is a comprehensive evaluation that is conducted by collecting information from the individual's family, friends, co-workers, and health care providers. The information is used not only to comprehend one individual's experience prior to death, but also to piece together common themes that are demonstrated by individuals who have committed suicide. This information can assist practitioners to develop the best method of preventing suicide (Aborido, Musson, & LeGueut, 2008; Batt, Belliver, Delatte, & Spreux-Varoquaux, 2006).

Shneidman's Ten Commonalities of Suicide   box 27-1

1. The common purpose of suicide is to seek a solution.
2. The common goal of suicide is cessation of consciousness.
3. The common stimulus in suicide is intolerable psychological pain.
4. The common stressor in suicide is frustrated psychological needs.
5. The common emotion in suicide is hopelessness–helplessness.

6. The common cognitive state in suicide is ambivalence.
7. The common perceptual state in suicide is constriction.
8. The common action in suicide is escape.
9. The common interpersonal act in suicide is communication of intention.
10. The common consistency in suicide is with lifelong coping patterns.

Sources: Shneidman, E. S. (1985). *Ten Commonalities of Suicide and Some Implications for Public Policy.* Washington, DC: ERIC Clearinghouse; Shneidman, E. (1992). A conspectus for conceptualizing the suicidal scenario. In R. Maris, A. Berman, J. Maltsberger, & R. Yufit, (Eds.). *Assessment and Prediction of Suicide.* New York, NY: Guilford Press, pp. 50–65.

Theoretical Foundations

Suicide has long been a part of human behavior. John Donne, a religious scholar in the early 1600s, wrote about it as he contemplated his own suicide due to relationship and professional failures in his life. He utilized a Christian framework to understand suicide and potential treatment (Minois, 1999). Centuries later, Emile Durkheim identified three types of suicides from a sociological perspective. *Egoistic suicide* occurs when an individual is isolated from others, emotionally and socially. *Altruistic suicide* takes place when there is a loyalty or identification with rules of a society, such as a suicide bomber who completes suicide for the cause of the greater political organization. *Anomic suicide* occurs when an individual feels estranged from the society in which he or she lives or when the individual's role in the society has radically changed. An example of an anomic suicide is an executive who has been caught embezzling money from his organization and completes suicide after the jury finds him guilty of the charges (Durkheim, 1897, 1951).

Edwin Shneidman (1918–2009) founded the American Association of Suicidology (AAS) in 1968. This organization studies suicide, including prevention, risks, and protective factors, and developed the psychological autopsy. Shneidman developed the Ten Commonalities for Suicide (Box 27-1).

Current research is geared toward understanding the causal factors for suicide, determining risk factors for suicide, and identifying protective measures that prevent suicidal action. The 2012 National Strategy for Suicide Prevention outlined a research-based, comprehensive report to assist legislators, communities, clinicians, individuals, and families in understanding and preventing suicide.

It is important to understand that individuals who are having suicidal ideation are suffering as a result of hopelessness, and that these individuals do not necessarily have mental illness. Suicidal ideation and completion are complex; the nurse must understand this to identify those that may be at risk. Risk factors for suicide attempt include difficulty in problem solving, social isolation, and feelings of hopelessness (Figure 27-1). Individuals with mental illness have an increased risk for a suicide attempt if they are experiencing depression. The risk of completed suicide by those who have major depression is approximately 20 times that of the general population (AAS, 2013). Use of alcohol also is a factor: The risk of suicide is 50% to 70% higher in individuals who are using alcohol than in the general population (CDC, 2012).

Protective measures are factors that can help the individual to feel hopeful and worthy enough to begin problem solving, even when he or she feels that there are no answers to the presenting problem. There are internal and external protective measures. Internal factors are related to the ability to problem-solve, think through conflict, and handle disputes without violence. Effective internal protective measures can help individuals identify personal, social, cultural, and spiritual beliefs that discourage suicide and violence. An individual with external protective measures relates to others and can request assistance when needed. This person has valued relationships that include responsibility for caring for another's basic needs. There are connections to family, friends, co-workers, and community support. There is restricted access to means for a suicide attempt. By assessing the individual for risk factors and protective measures, the nurse can help patients to begin to identify solutions to problems and dilemmas and resources to help them (WHO, 2013).

Within the domains of wellness, a number of behaviors and sociological and environmental factors can affect or indicate an individual's risk for suicide (Table 27-1).

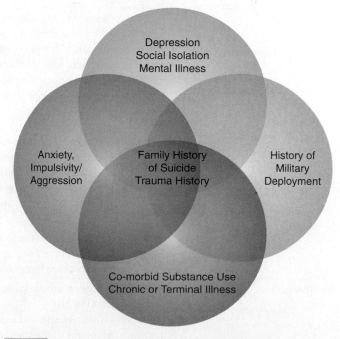

Depression
Social Isolation
Mental Illness

Anxiety,
Impulsivity/
Aggression

Family History
of Suicide
Trauma History

History of
Military
Deployment

Co-morbid Substance Use
Chronic or Terminal Illness

27-1   Risk factors for suicide.

Suicidal Behaviors and Risk Factors by Domain	table 27-1

Domain	Behaviors and Risk Factors
Biological	• Decreased appetite • Difficulty sleeping, changes in sleep pattern • Decreased concentration • Decreased energy • Decreased libido • Increase in physical manifestations of anxiety • Elevated pulse, blood pressure, respiration • Increase in somatic feelings, such as pain, headache, stomach pain, nausea • Agitation • Hypervigilance • Pacing • Chronic or terminal illness • Family history of suicide, especially if the individual who died is a first-degree relative • Family history of mental illness and substance use disorder
Psychological	• Being hypercritical • Confusion • Crying • Decreased interest • Decreased productivity • Depression • Difficulty concentrating • Expressing suicidal thoughts and feelings • Feelings of apprehension, helplessness, worthlessness • Focusing on past choices • Forgetfulness • Helplessness • History of psychiatric illness • Irritability • Lack of interest or apathy • Low self-esteem and self-worth • Persistent worrying • Preoccupation with negative thoughts • Withdrawal
Sociological	• Lacking a sense of relationships with others, feeling like a burden to others, feeling alone, isolating self from those who care about the patient, feeling estranged from family • Feeling not a part of a family or a friendship network or a peer at work or at school; no participation in community groups, such as church or hobby group • Identifying self as different from others, feeling a lack of understanding and trust with others • Lacking a sense of belonging to the whole of society, feelings of loneliness and worthlessness • Recent loss of a relationship • Intimate partner violence • Childhood sexual and/or physical abuse • Unemployment, including a change in socioeconomic status • Feeling hopeless in obtaining resources, including financial, housing, electric, water • Feeling unable to function at work or school; failing school or unable to carry out job due to lack of concentration and focus on thoughts of wanting to die
Cultural	• Lack of connectedness or sense of belonging to others from the same race, religion, or culture • Lack of connectedness to those with similar values, shared language, or similar experiences • Lack of access to services due to language or other cultural barriers • Feelings of shame, due to perceived affront to cultural values
Spiritual	• Feeling a lack of connectedness with God or Higher Power and/or with others of like-minded beliefs • Struggling with faith • Struggling with meaning and purpose of life • Expressing feelings of guilt and shame related to symptoms

Biological Domain

Current research on biological factors related to suicide focuses on understanding suicidal drive and some of the following questions:

- Which areas of the brain are affected by psychological pain?

- What behavioral patterns are predictable for a strong biological possibility of a suicide attempt? Does suicidal behavior have a genetic component? If so, how does that affect prevention of a suicide attempt?

- Is there a correlation between vitamin D status and an increase in suicidal drive?

Meerwijk, Ford, and Weiss (2013) performed an extensive literature review to determine whether there are specific areas in the brain that react to psychological pain as opposed to physiological pain. Several regions in the brain are hypothesized to be involved in psychological pain: the thalamus, anterior and posterior cingulated cortex, the prefrontal cortex, the cerebellum, and the parahippocampal gryus. Further research is needed to understand the implications for identifying areas in the brain that are affected by psychological pain and how this relates to a suicidal drive. Research involving postmortem studies and individuals who have attempted suicide and survived show decreased central serotonin activity in the ventromedial prefrontal cortex. This is exhibited in a higher level of aggression and impulsive behavior. Brent (2009) and McGirr et al. (2009) hypothesized that a decreased level of serotonin activity and a high level of impulsive aggression may account for an increased number of suicide attempts. Impulsive aggression is considered an endophenotype for suicidal behavior. An **endophenotype** is a genetic concept that takes into consideration the complexity, heterogeneity, and multigenetic disorders that make up psychiatric illnesses (Brent, 2009). McGirr et al. reported that relatives of their study group who had a family member who completed suicide demonstrated an increase in Cluster B personality disorder traits, such as impulsive aggression. Families that had major depression without Cluster B traits showed an overlapping but distinct phenotype of suicide (McGirr et al., 2009).

A recent study noted that there is an increase in suicides during spring, when there is a reduction in available vitamin D. Umhau et al. (2013) hypothesized that a low vitamin D level can be one reason for an increase in the suicide rate in the spring. They conducted a study utilizing serum samples collected by the Department of Defense Serum Repository of military personnel who had been deployed for active duty between 2002 and 2008. The vitamin D level was measured for each sample of the 495 military personnel who had completed suicide and in 495 control subjects. The authors determined that low vitamin D status was common in active duty service members. Although their research found that there is an increased risk for suicide with low levels of vitamin D, further research is indicated (Umhau et al., 2013).

Some individuals become suicidal when confronted with a chronic or terminal illness. Ongoing monitoring of these patients includes depression and suicide assessments, especially for individuals with diseases of the nervous system, cancer, HIV/AIDS, lung diseases such as COPD, chronic kidney failure, systematic lupus erythematosus, diabetes, chronic pain syndrome, and any functional impairment (American Psychiatric Association [APA], 2010; U.S. Department of Health and Human Services [DHHS], 2012).

Psychological Domain

Psychological factors associated with higher risk of suicide include depression, alcohol use, and impulsive behavior patterns. This has important implications for the nurse. All individuals who come into the health care setting should be screened for an affective disorder, substance use, and suicidal ideation (U.S. Preventive Services Task Force, 2013).

Anxiety has been implicated as a causal factor in most research that has focused on the study of suicide. The current APA Practice Guideline (2010) identifies anxiety that is fearful and filled with apprehension as the most severe psychic anxiety. This type of anxiety has a high probability of increasing the drive to commit suicide in individuals with anxiety disorders, obsessive–compulsive disorder, and posttraumatic stress disorder (PTSD). Individuals who have symptoms of depression, schizophrenia, and substance abuse along with severe psychic anxiety have an increased risk of a suicidal attempt (U.S. DHHS, 2012; APA, 2010).

As stated earlier, individuals who experience impulsive and aggressive behavior patterns are at a higher risk for a suicide attempt (APA, 2010). Individuals with personality disorders are at greater risk for suicide than the general population. Some of the diagnostic criteria for borderline personality disorder include an increase in suicidal drive due to the level of impulsive and aggressive behavior that is often manifested by individuals with this personality disorder. The National Strategy for Suicide Prevention states that between 3% and 10% of individuals with borderline personality disorder commit suicide (U.S. DHHS, 2012).

Teenagers have a higher level of suicidal drive than the general population owing to their level of impulsivity and lack of experience in handling complex stressors. The increase in stress often is due to changes in expectations of self and others and an increase in sexual hormones, which can cause stress in the individual as a result of new desires. The teen also may have increased responsibilities at home, in school, and in the community. Lentz, Coderre, and Wantanabe (2009) state that risk factors for adolescent depression include family history of depression, sustaining a loss, physical and sexual abuse, issues relating to sexuality, family conflicts, issues in school performance, and medical disorders. They also report that 60% of children with depression manifest suicidal ideation, with half of them attempting suicide (Lentz, Coderre, & Watanabe, 2009). A study of adolescents presenting to the emergency department for medical reasons found that these patients often tested positive for suicidal ideation (King, O'Mara, Hayward, & Cunningham, 2009).

Older, single Caucasian men have one of the highest rates of suicide (AAS, 2013). This may be due to perceiving themselves as a burden to others, viewing themselves as worthless, and experiencing emotional or social isolation. Older adult males with chronic physical or mental illness may have the perception that death is preferable to continuing to live (Kjølseth, Ekeberg, & Steihaung, 2010). This population typically has seen a primary practitioner within the last month or week of life, often without being screened for an affective disorder or suicidal ideation (Cornwell, 2009). In general, older, single men select more lethal methods, often using firearms (U.S. DHHS, 2012; Cornwell, 2009; AAS, 2013). It is important to screen older adults who come into the primary care setting for anxiety, mood disorders, and suicidal ideation (Figure 27-2).

It is a common assumption that suicide is a result of an untreated depression. Data from psychological autopsy studies state that 90%

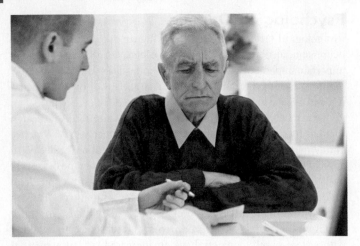

27-2 Older adults presenting for care for a medical illness benefit from screenings for depression and suicidal ideation.

Source: Igor Mojzes/Fotolia

of individuals who completed suicide had one or more psychiatric disorders (APA, 2010). The association between depression and suicide currently shows that 60% of individuals who committed suicide experienced depression (AAS, 2013). Several risk factors for suicide, such as isolation, a sense of worthlessness, and hopelessness occur as symptoms of depression. The risk for suicide increases when an individual with a major depressive disorder or bipolar disorder also exhibits severe psychic anxiety and substance abuse (APA, 2010). Substance abuse carries a high risk for suicide completion (U.S. DHHS, 2012). Because some patients use substances to alleviate anxiety, it is important for the nurse to assess patients experiencing affective disorders or suicidal ideation for substance use.

Individuals with schizophrenia are at risk for suicide, especially if they are young, early in the illness, have recently been discharged from the hospital, or have had multiple hospitalizations. The current APA Clinical Guidelines (2010) note that a psychotic state may account for an increase in suicidal drive in individuals with schizophrenia or schizoaffective disorder; however, command hallucinations account for a small number of suicides in this population. There is an increased probability of suicide in individuals who have a psychosis and symptoms of depression, especially if the individual is using alcohol. When caring for an individual with schizophrenia or schizoaffective disorder, it is important to assess for suicidal ideation as well as symptoms of depression, hopelessness, and substance use.

Sociological Domain

Understanding the sociological etiology of suicide goes back to Emile Durkheim's description of egoistic suicide, which occurs when an individual is isolated from others, emotionally and socially. Several types of isolation must be considered when assessing an individual who may be at risk for suicide. Vulnerable populations include individuals who are lesbian, gay, bisexual, or transgender (LGBT); active duty military personnel and veterans; individuals who are incarcerated; and individuals who experienced childhood trauma, such as sexual abuse.

D'Augelli et al. (2005) conducted a study to understand the types of circumstances that may increase suicidal drive in LGBT youth.

They found that youth who have been abused (verbally or physically) or rejected due to their sexual orientation have a higher probability of attempting and committing suicide. The 2012 National Strategy for Suicide Prevention (U.S. DHHS, 2012) notes that, worldwide, homosexual men have four times the number of suicide attempts than heterosexual men. Lesbian and bisexual women have twice as many suicide attempts as women who are heterosexual. There is a higher suicide attempt rate in LGBT individuals of African American, Latino, Native American, and Asian American heritage. The increase of suicidal attempts in the LGBT population may be due, in part, to "institutional discrimination," laws and policies that are discriminatory in nature. Media coverage of the suicide of individuals who died as a response to bullying, isolation, and a negative sexual and gender identity tend to highlight this behavior as a response to institutional discrimination (U.S. DHHS, 2012).

Active duty military personnel and veterans have demonstrated an increase in suicide rates since 2006. In particular, those who have served in Afghanistan and Iraq and veterans receiving care from the Veterans Health Administration carry a greater risk for suicide. Some common risk factors for suicide in military personnel include:

- Caucasian males under age 25 years
- Personnel ranked junior enlisted between E1 and E4
- Those with a high school or GED education
- Personnel experiencing relationship problems, financial difficulties, and legal and/or administrative problems
- Personnel engaging in substance abuse (Defense Centers of Excellence for Psychological Health and Traumatic Brain Injury [DCOE], 2013)

In this population, firearms are most frequently used to commit suicide, with drug overdose as the most common means of suicide attempt. Those committing suicide often did not communicate to others their intent and did not have a prior history of emotional problems. Veterans who committed suicide had higher rates of medical and mental illness as compared with the overall population of veterans (DCOE, 2013; U.S. DHHS, 2012). Because of the increasing rate of suicide among active duty military and recent veterans, the Veterans Health Administration and Department of Defense have developed suicide prevention programs that are specific to individuals currently serving in the military and those who are veterans. These programs highlight the sense of duty to one another that is an important component of military service. The DCOE has a website that encourages returning military members, veterans, and family members to understand some of the issues experienced by service members who are suffering with suicidal thoughts, how to seek help, and to promote a sense of resilience that can facilitate recovery (DCOE, 2013).

Individuals who are incarcerated also have a higher potential for suicide. Research demonstrates that suicide is one of the leading causes of death in correctional facilities. Inmates who present the most risk are Caucasian, young, and single, and have a problem with substance abuse. The highest risk for a suicide attempt is within the first 24 hours of incarceration, when there are legal concerns after incarceration (such as denial of parole), after receiving upsetting information about family and friends outside the institution, and after a sexual assault or trauma within the institution (APA, 2010).

There also is an increased potential for a suicide attempt after the individual has been discharged from a correctional facility (Zlodre & Fazel, 2012).

Individuals who were abused as children or who witnessed abuse of their parents or caregivers have a higher risk for suicide attempt and completion. Individuals who experienced sexual abuse are three times more likely to experience suicidal ideation than their peers (Calder, McVean, & Yang, 2010). Interpersonal violence also increases the risk for suicidal ideation. It is common for individuals who experience abuse to feel ashamed and isolate from others; confiding about abuse is rare. This shame and isolation may increase hopelessness and suffering, with suicidal ideation or a suicide attempt as a means of coping with the suffering. It is important for nurses to recognize the sociological issues and assess individuals who may be at risk for suicide as a result of their isolation from others.

Cultural Domain

Culture may specify behavior for the group of individuals who are members of that specific cultural group. Within the culture are the norms and history that can be seen in the behavior and value system of the people within that group (Chapter 5). Past traumas may influence the present behavior. When discussing suicide, it can be helpful to know which cultural groups carry a higher risk for suicide while understanding that cultural risk factors can vary from one individual to another. In particular, individuals from Native American tribes, China, or Japan may be at increased risk for suicide due to specific cultural factors.

An example of past trauma influencing present behavior can be seen in a study examining the high suicide rate in Native American youth. For these individuals, the history of the past trauma of the tribe endures, including reaction to the wars with the early settlers. Experiences over the years with forced boarding schools for men and boys have changed how men see their role in their family and their tribe. This can be seen in an increased use of alcohol, family abuse, gang membership, and an increase in homicide, accidents, and suicide (Yellow Horse Brave Heart, Elkins, Tafiya, & Bird, 2012). By understanding the cultural context, interventions that may be designed to decrease these behaviors combine the traditional role of males as Wicasa Was'aka ("strong man" in Lakota), along with how that role is exhibited in the community. The use of programs such as RezRIDERS, which combines extreme sports with the community's values, can strengthen the positive identity of the participants, decreasing their sense of isolation and increasing their sense of self-esteem. This program allows the participants to take risks that are monitored for safety and build relationships with one another that reflects the values of Wicasa Was'aka. Responsibility to the community, family, and membership in a health-promoting group assist in reducing isolation and suffering in the context of cultural tradition, which, in turn, reduces the suicidal drive in the individual.

The suicide rate in China is equal to one-quarter of all the suicidal deaths throughout the world. In China, more women than men commit suicide. Role expectations in China are high for women—they are expected to run the household and earn money outside the home, and there is the expectation that the home cannot function without them. Pesticide ingestion is a popular means of suicide, accounting for 62% of the completed suicides in China between the years 1996 and 2000. Pesticides are involved in approximately one-third of suicides worldwide (WHO, 2013). When providing care to a Chinese woman with depressive symptoms, history of suicidal ideation, or suicide attempt, it is important to understand how she sees her role within the family, as well as her concerns to assist the family financially by working outside the home.

Japan has experienced an increase in suicide rates within the past decade. There has been a shift from the traditional collective model of family and government to a democratic model, with changes in the traditional family roles. Following a series of economic changes in the late 1990s, many families who previously had a secure financial footing found themselves scrambling to meet their basic needs. In addition, bullying is on the rise among Japanese adolescents, who have begun resisting going to school or work. Psychotherapy, which has met with much success in developed Western countries, is new to Japan. For it to be an accepted modality, the therapy must be culturally congruent. Care for individuals from Japan is likely to require indirect, context-driven therapy that concentrates on nonverbal cues and holistic care to be successful (Grabosky, Ishii, & Mase, 2012).

Spiritual Domain

In many religious cultures, suicide is seen as going against life and against the Creator. Some religions have consequences for suicide, such as prohibitions against burial on sacred grounds for those who have completed suicide. For some individuals, concerns about these sanctions motivate them to obtain treatment to assist in reducing the suicidal drive.

As discussed in Chapter 6, spirituality has to do with appreciation of the world and understanding the individual's meaning in the world. Both religion and spirituality help to reduce suffering and increase hope, as well as provide protective measures. When an individual is suicidal, the sense of his or her role in the world becomes constricted and feelings of suffering increase. Assessing and exploring individuals' views on spirituality and religion can assist the patients to identify a meaning to their lives and increase the will to live and contribute.

Suicidal ideation occurs in a continuum, between no suicidal ideation and at the verge of death. By understanding risk and protective factors, as well as the severity of risk for suicide, nurses can better identify patients at risk and assist them in meeting their needs and finding hope for recovery.

Pause and Reflect

1. *Referring to the critical thinking feature at the beginning of the chapter, what psychological and sociological factors did Brian present on the day leading up to his suicide attempt?*

2. *How does past trauma affect an individual's risk for suicide?*

3. *Generally speaking, what populations are at greater risk for suicidal action? How can you use this knowledge to inform your nursing practice?*

Collaborative Care

Providing care for an individual who has suicidal thoughts and plans requires a multidisciplinary approach. Individuals who express suicidal thoughts may be in the community. Many communities have a suicide hotline that can be accessed by calling the National Suicide Prevention Lifeline, 1-800-273-TALK (8255). This lifeline is connected to crisis mobile teams or law enforcement personnel who are trained to go into the community and assess the individual for safety. When this occurs, the individual is often transported to the emergency department for evaluation. If the individual refuses and is imminently suicidal, law enforcement personnel or licensed members of a community's crisis mobile team may invoke an emergency involuntary hospitalization to prevent the suicide (Young, Fuller, & Riley, 2008). Evaluation in the emergency department (ED) will include a physical exam, patient health history to assess for history of mental illness and previous attempts, and a full psychological assessment. If the assessment reveals a risk for self-harm, the patient may either be admitted to an inpatient psychiatric unit or kept in the ED for further evaluation.

An ongoing collaboration between the Emergency Nurses Association and the American Psychiatric Nurses Association began in 2010 because of the increased numbers of patients being detained in EDs for suicidal ideation and plans, and because of the lack of referral sources available for patients determined not safe to be discharged. The concept of "boarding" in EDs is reaching crisis proportions across the country, as the nation's available inpatient psychiatric beds have been decreased by 90% since 1960. In a survey of more than 6,000 EDs, 70% reported boarding psychiatric patients for hours or days, and 10% reported boarding persons for several weeks (Glover, 2012).

Patients who have attempted suicide often benefit from psychotropic medications to reduce symptoms of emotional illness. For patients placed on antidepressants, it is important to monitor them for increased suicidal drive, particularly when the medication is first initiated. Sometimes patients experience an increase in energy and use this to facilitate a suicide attempt. It is important for the nurse to observe for changes in energy and suicidal drive, as well as provide support to continue treatment. Lithium carbonate has been shown to decrease suicidal thoughts and the motivation to attempt suicide in some patients with major depressive disorder and bipolar disorder. Clozapine has been shown to decrease suicidal ideation and drive in patients with schizophrenia or psychosis.

Electroconvulsive therapy (ECT) is useful for patients with psychotic depression who have not responded to a medication regimen. Other patients who may benefit from short-term use of ECT are pregnant women who are severely suicidal, individuals who refuse to eat, or those who are catatonic (APA, 2010).

The APA Clinical Practice Guideline (2010) indicates that individuals who have attempted suicide or are experiencing suicidal thoughts benefit from psychotherapy. The most common psychotherapy modalities that have been effective are cognitive–behavioral therapy, psychodynamic therapy, and interpersonal psychotherapy. As discussed in Chapter 18, dialectical behavioral therapy is often used with individuals with borderline personality disorder to decrease symptoms of difficulty with emotional regulation, impulse control, anger management, and interpersonal assertiveness.

Pause and Reflect

1. *What resources in your community are available to individuals who are depressed or having thoughts of suicide? Are there different resources for children? Teens? Older adults?*

2. *Why is it critical for emergency departments to be able to provide appropriate care or referral for patients with mental illness?*

Nursing Management

Nursing management of the patient who has expressed suicidal thoughts or intent focuses first on immediate safety. Because individuals experiencing suicidal ideation often experience a great deal of shame and low self-esteem, it is important to encourage them to express their concerns in an open, nonjudgmental manner.

Assessment

One of the principal roles of nursing practice is to gather information in a thorough assessment. This assessment can assist in preventing a suicide attempt because it gives patients the opportunity to talk about the problems they feel are overwhelming. Assessment begins with identifying the individual's risk for suicide and follows with assessment of the individual domains of wellness and an assessment of risk and protective factors. Much of nursing assessment for risk of suicide can be conducted through interviewing and observing the patient. Listening is a powerful problem-solving strategy. In addition, the Beck scales are available for nurses and other clinicians to use (Box 27-2).

critical thinking

Brian Recovery Phase

Shortly after Brian's admission to the behavioral health unit, he decides to telephone Jennifer and see whether she would be willing to talk to him. He feels strongly that he needs to figure out whether his marriage is really finished or whether Jennifer has room in her heart to work with him. Jennifer is glad to hear from him. She is feeling guilty about telling him that she and the kids were moving out without giving him any indication of her dissatisfaction with the marriage. Jennifer wants to come to Boston to see Brian, and asks him if he is ready for her visit. Brian wants to see her and discuss the issues that she identified in their relationship. He tells his primary nurse, Cynthia, that he is feeling stronger and more in control of his thoughts and feelings. Cynthia asks him if he can identify topics of conversation that he may have with Jennifer that could cause him to feel suicidal. He agrees to think about this. Cynthia recognizes this as an important step for Brian, as identifying triggers helps reduce the risk of a repeated suicidal gesture.

APPLICATION

1. What questions could Cynthia ask to determine Brian's readiness for the visit with Jennifer?

2. How can Cynthia support Brian to explore his marital issues?

3. What assessment questions would be helpful to determine Brian's level of risk for suicide at this point in his recovery?

The Beck Scales   box 27-2

Aaron T. Beck contributed to understanding and measuring the causal factors of suicide. He developed a theoretically based treatment modality: cognitive–behavioral therapy. Through research, it has been found that individuals who are suicidal are at most risk when feeling hopeless. Beck developed the Beck Hopelessness Scale (BHS), which measures three aspects of hopelessness:

1. Feelings the individual has about the future
2. Loss of motivation to do the usual and customary things in that person's life

3. Expectations the individual has for his or her life and those around them

This tool is predictive of suicidal intent.

Beck also developed two scales that are useful in determining what level of care the individual needs to prevent a possible suicide. The Beck Scale for Suicide Ideation (BSI), uses questions that elicit information about the individual's suicide plans and deterrents to committing suicide. The Scale for Suicide Ideation (SSI) measures the severity of the individual's suicidal ideation. These scales are used in research as well as in the clinical area.

Based on Beck, A. T., Steer, R. A., Kovacs, M., & Garrison, B. (1985). Hopelessness and eventual suicide: A 10-year prospective study of patients hospitalized with suicidal ideation. *American Journal of Psychiatry, 142*(5), 559 –563; Beck, A. T., & Weishaar, M. E. (1990). Suicide risk assessment and prediction. *Crisis, 11*(2), 22 –30; Department of Psychiatry, Penn Behavioral Health. (2013). Aaron T. Beck, MD. Beck Scales and Inventories. Available at http://www.med.upenn.edu/suicide/beck/scales.html?6

Assessment of Suicide Risk

The assessment must take place in a safe, quiet space where the individual can process the nurse's questions and the nurse can assess the resources that are available to the patient. Ask patients explicitly if they feel as though they want to commit suicide and want to die. Inquire about whether they have a means to harm themselves with a firearm, knife, or overdose, or by hanging themselves. Ask whether they have fantasies about hurting themselves, such as jumping to their death. Ask patients whether their thoughts are concentrated on how to commit suicide or whether there are other thoughts that reduce this risk. When the nurse asks these questions in an open manner, patients realize that the nurse can fully listen to their level of suffering.

It is important for nurses to recognize the warning signs of suicide and to provide immediate assistance when these manifest. Individuals who are suicidal are not seeking attention; rather, their state of mind is one of hopelessness, they see their problems as inescapable, and they feel out of control. Some warning signs of potential suicidal thoughts or behavior are the patient talking about death, dying, being a burden, feeling worthless, and looking for a means to commit suicide. Other warning signs include the patient talking about being trapped or being in unbearable pain, either physical or emotional. There is an increase in anxiety, mood swings, or demonstrating rage or vengeful behavior. The individual may be increasing use of alcohol or drugs and/or may be increasing risk-taking behavior. The American Association of Suicidology (2013) developed a mnemonic, IS PATH WARM, to remember the warning signs of suicide:

Ideation

Substance abuse

Purposelessness

Anxiety

Trapped

Hopelessness

Withdrawal

Anger

Recklessness

Mood change

It is important to ask questions about past history of suicide attempts and to determine how earlier attempts were resolved (Box 27-3). Patients who have one or more previous suicide attempts are at increased risk of another suicidal gesture that is more severe and may lead to death.

PRACTICE ALERT   There is a common myth that asking direct questions about suicide leads the patient to wanting to commit suicide. It has been demonstrated, however, that when an individual shows interest in helping someone who is suicidal, it reaffirms the patient's self-worth, reduces feelings of isolation, and increases the patient's desire to live (APA, 2010).

Assessment Across the Domains

After assessing the patient for suicidal thoughts, begin to ask questions in each of the five domains: biological, psychological, sociological, cultural, and spiritual. Remember to assess for risk and protective factors, such as the presence of co-morbid illness and trauma history.

Biological Domain

Assess for the presence of chronic illness. How has the illness affected the individual's life, family, friends, work, and school? How has it changed the individual's ability to meet his or her own needs? Ask questions related to the neurovegetative signs of depression: difficulty concentrating, decrease of energy, decrease in sexual libido/drive, and changes in sleeping patterns. Assess for increase in somatic complaints, such as headache and stomach pain, and whether those body sensations have increased with anxiety.

Psychological Domain

Assess for the psychological indicators of depression: feelings of sadness, hopelessness, inability to problem-solve, and feelings of worthlessness. How does the patient express emotional states? Is there a feeling of being overwhelmed or an inability to recognize the possibility of problem-solving the areas of grave concern? Is the patient constricted in the ability to visualize the future? Are there feelings of shame and low self-esteem? Is there a history of mental illness, such as an anxiety or mood disorder?

Questions to Elicit Suicidal Ideation and Level of Risk   box 27-3

Questions to establish empathy:

- How is your life now?
- What struggles in your life are upsetting you?
- How are you trying to solve some of these problems? (Use the words that the patient uses to describe problem areas.)

Questions directly asking about the suicidal ideation and intent:

- Have you ever felt like you want to hurt yourself?
- Do you have thoughts about how you would do that? (Use the language that the patient uses to describe desire to harm self.)
- Do you have any thoughts of hurting others?
- Do you have anything in your home or available to you that you could use to harm yourself? Do you have any firearms? If so, are they in a safe place? Is the ammunition locked away separately from the gun? Is the gun locked and is it stored in a locked place? (During the time that the patient is feeling suicidal, ask whether there is a possibility to give consent to present the gun to a trusted person to store while the feeling of wanting to die is frontmost in the person's thoughts.)
- Have you ever thought about how you would commit suicide and planned it out by rehearsing it either in your thoughts or by doing some of the act?
- What has prevented you from completing the act?
- Have you ever attempted suicide in the past?
- How did you do this?
- What things were happening in your life that were upsetting you at that time?
- Have you ever been hospitalized or participated in any other treatment? What helped you at the time? How can any of the past experiences help you stay safe now?
- Is there anything that you could do now to feel better?

Sociological Domain

Assess the patient's relationship with others in the home, at school and/or work, and in the community. Has there been a change in the usual pattern of relating? Is there an increase in isolation from others? Does the patient feel worthy of having relationships? Are there areas of disappointment, guilt, or vengeful anger that may be expressed by statements of wanting to commit suicide? Have there been any losses, such as ending a major relationship, increased conflict or abuse in a primary relationship, or anger at a significant person in the family or friendship network? Does the patient have a history of trauma, such as child abuse, neglect, or deployment to a war zone (Figure 27-3)?

Cultural Domain

Determine how the patient views his or her role in the family and within society. Often the role is determined by cultural influences. Are there culturally significant historical events that may have affected the individual, such as earlier cultural trauma, war, slavery, or intertribal conflict?

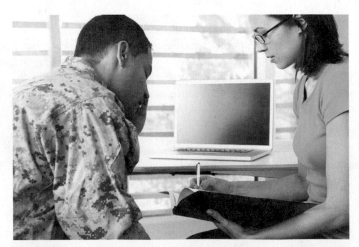

27-3   A history of military deployment in a war zone is a risk factor for suicide.

Source: Monkey Business/Fotolia

Spiritual Domain

Ask questions about the individual's belief system. Does the individual identify with a religious or spiritual group? Does the belief system of the group assist the individual in finding meaning and solace? Can the individual allow these spiritual values to provide hope to relieve the suffering being experienced now? How does the individual identify his or her self-worth and ability to contribute to family, work, and society?

Assessment of Suicide Severity

The next step in a comprehensive evaluation is to determine the Level of Suicidal Severity Index (Green, Katz, & Marcus, 1995). This index categorizes individual risk in one of five stages of severity:

- *Stage I:* The individual has no thoughts of suicide.
- *Stage II:* Mild thoughts of suicide. The individual begins to have fleeting thoughts of suicide, followed by thoughts that dismiss the idea of hurting himself or herself. The patient may disclose these thoughts to a nurse, but will specify that they are short-lived thoughts and that the individual would never act on them. At this stage, the individual can identify people to talk to and protective measures that emphasize the desire to live.
- *Stage III:* Moderate thoughts of suicide. This risk for suicide occurs when an individual begins to consider suicide as an option for problem solving. This may be a chronic thought that is comforting and a means of decreasing the individual's suffering. At stage III, generally the individual has no explicit plan in mind, nor are there readily available means.
- *Stage IV:* Advanced thoughts of suicide. The individual at this stage has a plan for suicide and a method to carry out the strategy. Sometimes, while in stage IV, the individual does make a nonlethal suicide attempt and is evaluated in the emergency department for further care.
- *Stage V:* Severe thoughts of suicide. An individual who is in stage V is **moribund** (on the verge of death). The individual has a plan and a means for committing suicide. He or she can no longer identify any protective measures or reason for

continuing to live. Often, the individual with stage V suicidal severity does not disclose the suicide plan or intent, to prevent being interrupted.

Staging the risk for suicide by using the Level of Suicidal Severity Index is helpful for both the clinician and patient to determine the best level of care to assist in maintaining safety. Individuals identified at stage I do not need any direct suicidal prevention intervention. However, at stage II, the individual's usual problem-solving abilities are overwhelmed. The individual may have fleeting thoughts of suicide, but no intention of acting on them. Nurses can assist individuals at this stage by helping them reduce feelings of anxiety, depression, or worry and helping them identify steps they can take to address issues that are overwhelming them.

Feelings of hopelessness permeate the individual who is at stage III. If there is a network of friends and relatives, this individual does not use their assistance. Although the individual has no specific plans for suicide, there is a desire to "go to sleep and never wake up." The person may use substances to facilitate coping. For some individuals, the thoughts of suicide and death are comforting. Individuals at stage III require professional evaluation to determine the extent of psychiatric symptoms and design an appropriate treatment plan. They may benefit from a combination of interventions, including pharmacotherapy and psychotherapy.

In stage IV, the individual has advanced thoughts of suicide. The individual has both a desire to die and a plan. There are thoughts about how to facilitate an attempt and, in some cases, the person makes an attempt. Individuals identified at stage IV need a thorough, multidisciplinary evaluation and may require hospitalization or inpatient care.

Stage V occurs when the individual has severe thoughts of suicide and makes a potentially lethal suicidal attempt or gathers lethal weapons, such as preparing a gun to fire or practicing knots with a rope for hanging. Brian, in the beginning of this chapter, was in stage V of the Level of Suicidal Severity Index. He planned and carried out a lethal attempt of an overdose with pills and alcohol. He wrote a suicide note to his family. He could not think of any other option to solve the marital discord other than death.

Nurses working in any setting should be familiar with the Level of Suicide Severity Index and know and be able to use their agency's policies and procedures for identifying, caring for, and referring individuals with suicidal ideation to appropriate care. Evaluation and care of patients with suicidal ideation may follow one of several protocols. The Suicide Prevention Resource Center suggests a five-step program: SAFE-T, Suicide Assessment Five-step Evaluation and Triage (Box 27-4). At all times, the nurse maintains a nonjudgmental attitude and begins by establishing the patient's trust in the nurse and the therapeutic alliance (see Perceptions, Thoughts, and Feelings near the end of this chapter).

Difference in Initial and Relapse Phases of Recovery

The patient in an initial or relapse phase is at high risk for attempting suicide. The patient is experiencing a stage IV or V Level of Suicidal Severity Index. The emphasis of patient care in this phase is to provide safety, promote problem solving, and instill hope. The patient may receive care on either a voluntary or an involuntary basis. It is not unusual for a patient who failed an attempt at suicide to feel angry about being alive. The initial assessment should include questions about the patient's desire to live and receive help. Answers to these questions will help the nurse formulate the care plan. Patients who are ambivalent about living or who are angry that their suicidal attempt failed need to be placed on strict observation. As the patient becomes more hopeful about living and begins to identify some protective measures, the intensity of the observation can be reduced.

The patient in recovery begins to learn more about personal precipitants that are triggers for suicidal ideation and a potential attempt. Strategies to avoid relapse may be employed, such as seeking psychotherapy or calling the National Suicide Prevention Lifeline (1-800-273-TALK [8255]), and reducing social isolation by interacting with family and friends. Understanding the dynamics of the suicidal drive empowers the patient to employ safety strategies more quickly and successfully.

Diagnosis and Planning

After the initial assessment, it is critical to develop a direction for providing comprehensive nursing care. Patients who have had a suicide

---

SAFE-T: Suicide Assessment Five-Step Evaluation and Triage   box 27-4

The SAFE-T assessment assists the nurse in determining the level of probability for a suicide attempt and provides a guide to implementing the most appropriate intervention for the individual. The first step in this program is to perform a thorough assessment, described earlier in this chapter. The second step in SAFE-T is to identify protective factors. The third step is direct inquiry about the person's intention to commit suicide. The fourth step is to determine the risk level and intervention. The fifth step is documentation of the assessment and the intervention.

This tool categorizes individual risk level in three stages: high, moderate, and low. An individual with a high risk factor has several serious risk factors, such as a history of severe psychiatric disorders or an acute precipitating event.

Using the Level of Suicidal Severity Index can help the nurse determine the risk for suicide and the appropriate level of care. Because Brian had a serious suicide attempt and continued

to state that he wanted to die, he was stage V, and considered high risk with the SAFE-T level of risk. Brian required hospitalization to prevent another suicide attempt. Individuals with a moderate level of risk may possess several risk factors identified by SAFE-T, such as a current or past psychiatric disorder, a family history of suicide, or a serious crisis.

When an individual with a moderate risk has a few protective factors, such as a spiritual belief system or the love of a child who needs parenting, the individual can generally be treated in a partial hospitalization or an outpatient setting, provided he or she has the ability to develop a crisis plan that includes seeking more intensive care if there in an increase in suicidal drive. An individual with a low risk of suicide as determined by SAFE-T is one who has a few risk factors, such as an interpersonal stressor, and both internal and external protective factors. Generally, these individuals can be treated in an outpatient setting (Suicide Prevention Resource Center, 2008).

attempt or are currently having suicidal ideation are at risk for safety and need interventions designed to prevent harm. Nursing diagnoses can provide guidance for the nurse to plan interventions to assist the patient in employing problem-solving skills.

Common Nursing Diagnoses

Nursing diagnoses for patients who have suicidal ideation or have recently attempted suicide are identified and prioritized based on the severity of the risk. Nursing diagnoses that may be appropriate for the individual who is experiencing suicidal thoughts include the following:

- Suicide, Risk for
- Violence: Self-Directed, Risk for
- Self-Mutilation, Risk for
- Impulse Control, Ineffective
- Hopelessness
- Self-Esteem, Situational Low
- Coping, Ineffective
- Denial, Ineffective
- Powerlessness

(NANDA-I, © 2014)

It is important to note that Risk for Suicide and Risk for Self-Directed Violence are not the same. Individuals who are at risk for suicide are experiencing a desire to die and have plans to take action on these thoughts. Patients who may cause harm to the physical, emotional, or sexual sense of self are at risk for self-directed violence. Self-mutilation refers to deliberate self-injury that is not life threatening but helps the individual to regulate mood when feeling overwhelmed with affect. As with any other nursing diagnoses, these are made based on information gained during assessment.

Prioritizing Nursing Diagnoses

Determining the primary nursing diagnosis is based on the patient's need for safety. Diagnoses related to risk for suicide or self-directed violence define the most important need for providing safe patient care. The nursing care varies between these two diagnoses, in that patients at risk for self-directed violence may not have death as the main goal. Both these nursing diagnoses involve providing a safe milieu for the patient to reduce the drive to harm himself. The diagnosis of Risk for Self-Mutilation is also important to consider. Sometimes a patient who is suicidal may also employ self-mutilation to reduce overwhelming emotions. Assessing patients who are suicidal for current risk for self harm and self-mutilation is important to determine the patient's needs and a plan for care. Algorithms to help the student differentiate the direction of care for the patient at risk for suicide and the patient who engages in self-directed violence are provided as Figures 27-4a and b.

The next area to consider is the ability for the patient to maintain impulse control. Individuals who manifest difficulty controlling their impulses will need to be placed in a milieu that is safe. These patients may require hospitalization until impulse control is regained in order to prevent a suicide attempt.

Once safety has been ensured and the individual is embraced in an environment with the potential to reduce harm and assist in gaining some level of impulse control, the patient's feelings of hopelessness can be addressed. Hope provides an individual with the ability to determine options for problem solving. When an individual is

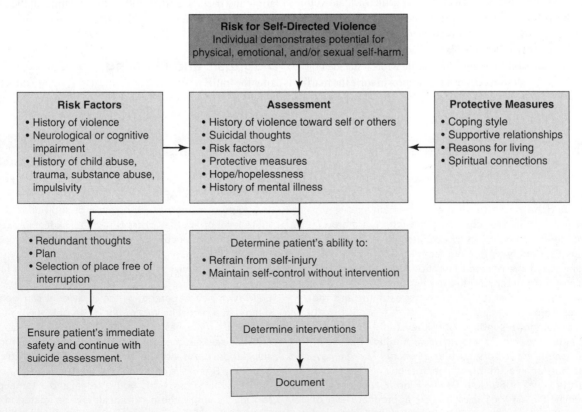

27-4a Algorithm for assessing a patient at risk for self-directed violence.

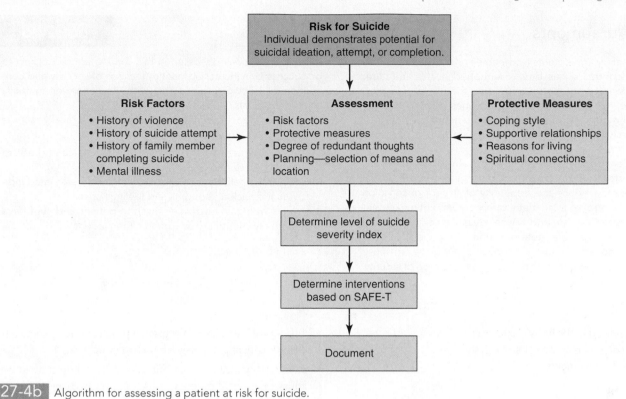

Risk for Suicide
Individual demonstrates potential for
suicidal ideation, attempt, or completion.

Risk Factors
- History of violence
- History of suicide attempt
- History of family member completing suicide
- Mental illness

Assessment
- Risk factors
- Protective measures
- Degree of redundant thoughts
- Planning—selection of means and location

Protective Measures
- Coping style
- Supportive relationships
- Reasons for living
- Spiritual connections

Determine level of suicide severity index

Determine interventions based on SAFE-T

Document

27-4b   Algorithm for assessing a patient at risk for suicide.

contemplating suicide, hopelessness is often part of the person's thought process and impairs problem-solving ability (Ackley & Ladwig, 2014).

Plans and Goals

The plans and goals for nursing care are based on the patient's need for safety. One goal is to begin to understand and work through the factors that precipitated the suicidal ideation or attempt. Collaborating with the patient by jointly discussing the nursing care plan strengthens the patient's ability to meet identified goals. Assist the patient in determining measurable and realistic goals that can be met in a reasonable time frame. For example, Brian is being admitted to the inpatient unit to prevent another suicide attempt, to maintain safety, and to promote problem solving. Considering the nursing diagnosis of Risk for Suicide, the following goals may be optimal for Brian's care:

- Brian will agree to voluntary admission to the behavioral health unit.
- Brian will seek assistance from staff members if he is experiencing an increase in suicidal thoughts.
- Brian will participate in group sessions provided in the milieu to promote problem solving and decrease isolation.

The expected outcome for individuals who have survived a suicide attempt or have had suicidal ideation is that there will be a reduction in drive to facilitate suicide. This outcome is complex, as the individual must decide to explore the causes of the desire to die. The patient also must have sufficient energy to believe that life is worth living and be able to recognize internal resources and support from others to decrease the feelings of hopelessness. Identification of the factors that precipitated the suicidal drive begins the

problem-solving process. As the patient identifies the possibilities toward working through the issues that caused the feelings of hopelessness, the suicidal drive will diminish. Expected outcomes for the patient who is at risk for suicide may include that the patient will be able to:

- Identify the factors that precipitated the suicidal ideation.
- Determine internal strengths and resources.
- Recognize a support system.
- Describe a reduction in suicidal drive.

Revising the Care Plan During Recovery and Rehabilitation

As the patient begins to embrace life and feel hope, it is important to adjust the nursing care plan. Less observation is needed as the thoughts of wanting to die recede. It is important for the patient to identify the precipitating events or thoughts that culminated into a desire to die. Understanding the dynamics of the hopelessness can lead to a deeper level of problem solving than the patient had prior to the suicidal gesture. The nurse–patient relationship can facilitate some of this exploration. By asking the patient open-ended questions, the nurse assists the patient to recognize and explore resources (for example, family, friends, and cultural or spiritual beliefs) that can be used in the future to prevent another suicide attempt and promote reassurance of the individual's worth.

Implementation

Each patient has his or her own needs for safety observation based on the severity of the suicidal thought process, risk factors, and personal isolation. Suicidal ideation often occurs when an individual does not use protective measures, including supportive relationships, when feeling overwhelmed with problems. Reducing isolation and providing

Safety Agreements

box 27-5

The use of safety agreements (sometimes referred to as *suicide prevention contracts*) has been mentioned in the literature. There has been some controversy about the use of this intervention. The APA Clinical Practice Guidelines (APA, 2010) indicates that the effectiveness of these agreements has not been proven in research and they are not legal documents. A safety agreement is not a protection in court if a patient were to complete suicide. The use of a safety agreement often decreases the nursing staff's anxiety about the patient's degree of suicidal drive, which may reduce the frequency of patient observation rounds. It is an error to think that a safety agreement means that the patient is feeling safe and will seek assistance if experiencing an increase of suicidal determination. The patient may still experience and act on suicidal thoughts. Reliance on these agreements also may give staff members a false sense of security.

Other interventions discussed in this chapter are more likely to be successful in increasing patient feelings of security and connection, as will working together with the patient on mutually established goals.

When safety agreements are used, they typically include the following elements:

- A commitment by the patient to remain safe and not to engage in self-harm
- A commitment by the patient to contact a designated individual if suicidal thoughts and feelings arise
- A list of healthy activities that the patient and staff have mutually identified to redirect the patient from suicidal thoughts

---

interventions related to the individual's severity index are essential to reducing the patient's risk for a suicidal gesture. Some agencies also implement safety agreements (Box 27-5).

Reduce Isolation

Developing a therapeutic alliance with the patient is a critical intervention, as it leads to problem solving and helps the patient to decrease isolation. In a psychiatric milieu, either inpatient or partial hospital program, group therapy sessions are held on a regular basis. These groups help to facilitate problem solving and reduce isolation by promoting a therapeutic community. Both one-to-one discussions with the nurse and attending group sessions assist individuals in reducing suicidal intent.

In other settings, the same principles discussed previously also apply. Nurses need to help patients identify social supports and referral resources. Patients who are estranged from family members may require a referral to a therapist to work through issues behind the estrangement or to role-play ways to reach out and repair the relationships. For older adults presenting to primary care for a medical illness, nurses should assess for depression at every health care interaction. Older adults who are isolated may benefit from referrals for transportation services or to adult day care centers or recreational facilities.

Interventions to Prevent Suicide

Nurses can take a number of actions to reduce suicidal ideation and assist individuals in preventing suicide. Generally, appropriate actions include the following:

- Ask directly whether the patient is thinking about suicide. Directly asking whether the patient is having any thoughts about suicide does not "put ideas in his or her head," but shows caring and understanding.
- Listen and encourage patients to express their feelings.
- Be nonjudgmental and available, remembering that the therapeutic alliance reduces the suicidal drive.
- Get involved; show interest and support for the patient.
- Offer hope by giving feedback about the patient's participation in care.

- Encourage the patient to engage in problem solving in the area that the patient previously felt was overwhelming.
- Remove any means to commit suicide, including guns, knives, ropes, or any medications of which an overdose can be taken. A safe milieu provides the individual with the opportunity to recover.
- For the patient who is imminently suicidal, call for help and stay with the patient until help arrives.

It also is critical to recognize that some actions may be harmful to patients experiencing suicidal ideation. In most cases, nurses engage in these actions inadvertently. The nurse's self-awareness is particularly important when working with patients who are suicidal (Box 27-6). It also is important to recognize what actions *not* to take, including the following:

- Do not judge or lecture the patient, or tell the patient what to do.
- Do not dare the patient to do the suicidal act.
- Do not act shocked or express surprise or discomfort when working with the patient; this may distress the patient and result in patient discomfort and unwillingness to participate. This may also reinforce feelings of worthlessness and isolation.
- Do not offer false reassurance, such as "It will get better," or "Hang on, you can do this." These types of statements are not helpful to patients who are feeling acutely suicidal.

In addition to varying interventions based on individual needs, interventions for patients with suicidal ideation or who have attempted suicide will vary based on their risk levels. Patients at stages IV and V will need a variety of interventions related to their immediate safety and mental health. They will not be able to take in new information at this time, so patient teaching must be postponed until the patients' level of anxiety and risk for self-harm are reduced. Patients at lower levels of risk benefit from patient education; support in developing new, healthy methods of coping; and encouragement to use community resources and follow recommended treatment protocols. Table 27-2 outlines nursing interventions for the different levels of suicide risk.

The Nurse's Self-Awareness

box 27-6

Self-awareness is important when working with individuals who exhibit suicidal thoughts and behaviors. Patients are very sensitive to the reactions of others. Clarification of the nurse's own feelings related to suicide is critical to being able to build a therapeutic alliance and provide best practice care.

- Assess your own feelings about suicide and suicidal ideation in patients.
- If you find that you tend to discount the suicidal threats of patients as acting out, attention-seeking, or manipulation,

or use terms such as "frequent flier" to describe these patients, you may miss a potentially lethal suicide threat.
- Assess your level of stress and evaluate your self-care practices. Nurses who maintain a positive life balance by integrating work, play, spiritual beliefs, and exercise in their lives are better equipped to deal with patients who are chronically depressed and hopeless about the quality of their lives.

Nursing Interventions According to Stage of Severity for Suicide Risk

table 27-2

Severity Index for Suicide Risk	Patient Perceptions	Nursing Interventions
Stage I	• No risk of suicide.	• Provide information on community resources. • Provide information in public areas or at health fairs. • Teach National Suicide Prevention Lifeline: 1-800-273-TALK (8255).
Stage II—mild thoughts of suicide	• Patient has fleeting thoughts of suicide that occur after several crises. • Patient has no plan or intent to carry out any suicidal action. • Patient feels the suicidal thoughts are "stupid," unlike usual coping patterns. • Patient has protective measures and uses them.	• Help the patient to define the problems that precipitated the thoughts and feelings of fleeting suicidal ideation. • Encourage the patient to plan options to solve one problem at a time. • Encourage using internal and external support systems. • Encourage coping skills, such as stress reduction. • Encourage the patient to seek short-term crisis counseling. • Teach the use of crisis intervention techniques. • Teach the patient to use support systems. • Teach the use of the National Suicide Prevention Lifeline.
Stage III—moderate thoughts of suicide	• Suicide is seen as an option to problem solving; sometimes the thoughts of suicide are comforting to the patient. • Patient may have physical illness, e.g., cancer, chronic pain, neurological illness. • Patient may have chronic mental illness, e.g., PTSD, major depressive disorder. • Patient has no clear plan for suicide, but thinks about death. • Patient has a support system, but does not disclose need for support. • Spiritual beliefs are a protective measure.	• Assist the patient to define problems that precipitated suicidal ideation. • Encourage the patient to plan options to solve one problem at a time. • Encourage the patient to attend psychotherapy. • Encourage coping skills, such as stress reduction. • Monitor use of medication; encourage use of medication to reduce target symptoms. • Teach about using protective measures to reduce isolation. • Teach use of National Suicide Prevention Lifeline.
Stage IV—advanced thoughts of suicide	• Patient's thoughts are focused on how to commit suicide. • Suicide is an option for problem solving due to feelings of hopelessness and powerlessness. • Patient may have auditory hallucinations that are commanding patient to facilitate a suicidal act. • Patient cannot identify internal or external protective measures. • Patient rationalizes that friends and family will be better off if the individual would be dead. • Patient has multiple high risk factors. • Patient will accept advice to go to ED for assessment and possibility of hospitalization. • Patient will allow a voluntary admission to a behavioral health unit.	• Assess level of risk for suicidal gesture. • Facilitate assessment in ED to determine level of care needs. • Encourage patient to call friend or family member to accompany to the hospital. • Once admitted, employ observation for safety. • Promote problem identification of the precipitating factors to facilitate problem solving and reduce hopelessness. • Encourage patient to attend all therapeutic groups on the unit. • Encourage patient to identify protective factors to use post-hospitalization. • Encourage patient to follow up with psychotherapy post-discharge.

(Continued)

Nursing Interventions According to Stage of Severity for Suicide Risk *(continued)*

table 27-2

Severity Index for Suicide Risk	Patient Perceptions	Nursing Interventions
	• Patient may use National Suicide Prevention Lifeline to obtain assistance.	• Patients at this stage are focused on death and cannot attend to new information.
Stage V—severe thoughts of suicide	• Moribund, patient cannot identify any reason to live. • Patient has selected and obtained lethal means of committing suicide. • Patient has multiple high risk factors. • Patient no longer communicates with family or friends and makes provisions for the care of children, pets, elderly relatives. • Patient writes a suicide note. • Patient may have auditory hallucinations commanding the patient to act on suicidal thoughts. • Patient questions self-worth, cannot identify internal or external protective measures. • Patient cannot identify spiritual or cultural factors to assist in affirming life.	• Be aware that the patient is likely to reject any attempt at intervention, including teaching. • Patient is in imminent danger of completing suicide. This individual needs immediate evaluation in the ED and likely needs admission to the behavioral health unit. • Place the patient on constant observation for safety. • Assess for risk for suicide every shift. • Encourage the patient to attend all therapeutic groups on the unit. • Meet with the patient on a one-to-one basis for 15 minutes every shift to assist with problem solving. • Promote problem identification of the precipitating factors to facilitate problem solving and reduce hopelessness. • Encourage the patient to take medications as prescribed, note the effect of the medication on the target symptoms. • Encourage use of stress reduction activities. • Encourage the patient to identify a family member or friend to provide support during and after hospitalization. • Encourage follow-up after hospitalization with partial hospitalization and outpatient psychotherapy.

Primary, Secondary, and Tertiary Interventions

Primary, secondary, or tertiary level of interventions are used to conceptualize ways of preventing and intervening to prevent a suicide attempt (Table 27-3). Primary intervention is used to reduce the risk of suicide or a suicide attempt. The goal is to prevent suicide by helping individuals to receive assistance before the hopelessness closes in and the person views the only option to problem solving as death. This is achieved by encouraging the individual to reach out for assistance by calling the National Suicide Prevention Lifeline (1-800-273-TALK [8255]) or by going to the nearest emergency department, crisis center, or urgent care clinic to obtain help. Children and teenagers may obtain assistance from their teachers, youth ministers, coaches, and other significant adults who can support and assist them in obtaining help. The goal of patient education during primary intervention is aimed at prevention of a suicide attempt.

Early intervention and treatment are the theme of secondary intervention. A secondary level of intervention involves awareness of an individual who may be at risk for suicide. This may involve teaching individuals in the community to become aware of the symptoms people display when they may be at risk. Teaching primary care practitioners in general medicine, law enforcement personnel and first responders, teachers, clergy, parents, and community leaders to recognize when an individual may need support and intervention may prevent a suicidal gesture from occurring. Community education is aimed at recognition and assistance. Patient education is focused on accepting the help and going for an evaluation of the level of risk for suicide and placement in the appropriate level of care.

Tertiary intervention involves interventions after the person has survived a suicide attempt and is on the road to recovery. The goal is to assist the individual in problem solving and connecting with a support system to prevent a recurrence of suicidal thoughts and enhance day-to-day functioning. Patient education is directed toward re-establishing a healthy sense of self, and understanding the dynamics that occurred that caused the suicidal thoughts and behavior.

Patient Education

Patients who have experienced suicidal thoughts and those who have attempted suicide often talk about feeling overwhelmed and having feelings of hopelessness. Individuals become stuck and constricted in their ability to solve problems. Their hopelessness complicates the ability to think through options toward dealing with the issues at hand. Patient education needs to include identification of the precipitating factors and assistance with problem-solving strategies. The Collaborative Assessment and Management of Suicidality (CAMS) approach to reducing suicidal drive provides an evidence-based clinical framework for problem solving. The CAMS is based on Shneidman's Ten Commonalities (see Box 27-1). This therapeutic intervention uses a Suicide Status Form (SSF) that assesses the patient's psychological pain, stress, agitation, hopelessness, self-hatred, and suicidal risk (Jobes & Drozd, 2004). During this assessment, the therapeutic alliance is developed, which decreases the patient's isolation and assists the patient and clinician in understanding the causal factors of the suicidal ideation and/or attempt. During each session, the patient identifies the level of suicidal drive and identifies a problem area that needs to be understood and addressed. The outline of CAMS emphasizes the importance of the patient's alliance with the clinician. Teaching the patient to request assistance and to collaborate with the nurse to problem-solve is a powerful means of combating hopelessness.

Often, individuals have become stuck in their ability to identify options that can be taken to reduce the precipitating factors.

Brian—A Patient at Risk for Suicide | NURSING CARE PLAN

Nursing diagnosis: Risk for suicide related to marital conflict and difficulties at work. Previous suicide attempt via overdose with medications and alcohol.

Short-Term Goals *Patient will:* (include date for short-term goal to be met)	Intervention *Nurse will:*	Rationale
Be admitted to the behavioral health unit in a voluntary admission.	Facilitate an admission and conduct a comprehensive assessment.	Patient needs to be in a safe milieu with frequent observation.
Be placed on suicidal precautions on the unit, which entails observation to maintain safety.	Conduct a thorough search of Brian's belongings to remove any sharp or dangerous items that could be used in a suicidal gesture.	Prevent suicide by preventing sharp or potentially dangerous items to be with the patient on the hospital unit.
	Place Brian on suicidal precautions, frequent observations to maintain safety.	Close observation reduces isolation and provides therapeutic support to prevent a suicidal gesture.
	Assess level of suicidal thoughts and drive at least daily.	Determine level of needed support and observation based on the patient's risk for suicide.
Seek assistance from staff members if he is experiencing an increase of suicidal thoughts.	The nurse will meet with patient on a one-to-one basis at least 15 minutes per shift.	Initiate a therapeutic relationship with Brian and assess his needs for safety.
	While administering medication, assess Brian for suicidal thoughts.	While giving medications, the nurse can facilitate a quick suicide assessment.
	Encourage Brian to seek assistance from staff by being available when he approaches the nursing station.	The patient will be able to disclose suicidal thoughts if he feels the nurse is open to hearing his needs.
Participate in the groups provided in the milieu to promote problem solving and decrease isolation.	Encourage Brian to participate in the groups on the milieu.	Groups on the unit facilitate problem solving and provide psychoeducation.
	Follow up during the one-to-one daily meeting to determine what Brian learned during the groups.	Reinforce the information obtained during the group experience.
Long-Term Goal Brian will experience a reduction in suicidal drive, as evidenced by patient report and adherence to the treatment regimen.	Prior to discharge, encourage Brian to report triggers and how he managed them to his outpatient therapist.	Promotes autonomy for Brian and instills hope that he can successfully manage future triggers and be able to actively participate in achieving his life goals.

Clinical Reasoning

1. What other nursing diagnoses would be helpful for planning and providing nursing care for Brian?
2. Do you think the selection of Risk for Suicide as the priority diagnosis is appropriate? Why or why not?
3. Are there any other short-term goals that may help Brian become less suicidal? What would be the nursing intervention and the rationale?

Primary, Secondary, and Tertiary Levels of Intervention | table 27-3

Level of Intervention	Teaching Opportunity
Primary intervention	Senior-level nursing students prepare a poster for the college on the symptoms of potential suicide and how to call for help.
Secondary intervention	A nurse assesses a patient who came to the urgent care clinic after her roommate encouraged her to seek help. The patient told her roommate that she was thinking about drinking vodka and taking a handful of medications. The nurse assesses the patient's risk for suicide. The nurse learns that the patient was afraid that she might fail her next test at school and became desperate. The patient has a good relationship with her roommates and a desire to speak to her clergy person. She agrees to seek therapy and can list ways that indicate a level of safety. The nurse uses open-ended questions to help the patient list her internal and external resources that can assist her when she is feeling overwhelmed and afraid of failure. The patient education emphasis is to help the patient seek and use resources to prevent a suicide attempt.
Tertiary intervention	The nurse in a partial hospitalization program co-leads a support group for individuals who have survived a suicide attempt. The group members share with each other how to recognize feelings of hopelessness, fear of failure, and inability to problem-solve as precursors to feeling suicidal. The group focuses on how to use the group members and support systems, such as family and friends, as resources for prevention of another suicide attempt.

Recognition and labeling of the areas of concern and deciding to work on one area or concern at a time can reduce suicidal ideation, particularly when done in the context of a therapeutic relationship. Teaching the patient to outline one problem at a time reduces the feelings of being overwhelmed and hopeless.

It is important to promote hope by employing stress-reducing strategies while working on areas of difficulty. Potential stress busters include exercise, going to the movies, reading an uplifting book if the person is able to concentrate, visiting with friends, and enjoying the company of pets, just to name a few.

Interventions Following Completed Suicide

A nurse sometimes must work with family members and friends who have lost someone to suicide. The initial response often is shock, anger, and guilt. At times, the individual who has died is seen as a hero or in a positive light for having lived with severe physical or mental illness or psychological trauma. Listen without judgment to the reaction of the family and friends. Provide a referral for short-term therapy directed toward assisting the family members in working through the complicated grief that often occurs after a completed suicide. Call the National Suicide Prevention Lifeline to arrange a psychological first aid response for the family, friends, and community.

Evaluation

During the evaluation phase of the nursing process, the patient and nurse examine whether the interventions yielded the expected results. Was the nurse able to facilitate a therapeutic alliance that helped the patient disclose the concerns that contributed to the suicidal drive? Did the patient begin to identify problem areas that can be explored one at a time for possible options to try? Was the patient able to identify the medications that are currently prescribed? Is there a reduction in symptoms of depression and/or anxiety? Can the patient identify when to ask for assistance? Do the patient and family members have knowledge of how to initiate care in the community if there is an increase in suicidal ideation?

It is important to document all the care provided for the patient who is suicidal. The comprehensive assessment, along with the risk factors and protective measures, must be documented to assist the team in determining the appropriate level of care. Document the frequency of observations and a brief description of the patient during each observation. When meeting with the patient for 15 minutes per shift, ask the patient what he or she thinks the chart should reflect about the patient's mood, suicidal drive, and participation in the milieu. This collaboration is very powerful, as it communicates to the patient that the patient is an important participant in his or her own care.

Pause and Reflect

1. *What are your thoughts about a patient who has attempted suicide? If you were working in the emergency department and were assigned to a patient who was brought in due to a suicide attempt, how would you begin to work with that patient?*

2. *Why is it important to assess patients with mental illness, who abuse substances, for suicidal ideation?*

3. *What nursing interventions are appropriate when working with the patient who is at the stage V severity level? Why are these interventions appropriate?*

From Suffering to Hope

Admitting to suicidal ideation is a difficult process. It takes courage to acknowledge this level of psychological pain. Sometimes it also can be painful for the nursing staff to work with patients who are suicidal. Cynicism sometimes occurs, and this can result in nurses labeling patients as just looking for shelter or wanting attention. The nurse misses the patient's suffering, however, when labeling in this manner. Suicidal ideation is a complex problem with many facets. The nurse reaching out and securing a therapeutic alliance is the first step toward helping the patient regain hope. The thorough assessment provides an opportunity for the patient to explore, in depth, some of the causal factors that have been in the background during the patient's struggle with problem areas. Assisting the patient to problem-solve through the use of the therapeutic self, psychoeducational groups, and suggestions of activities to try to promote stress reduction all can help an individual grow from suffering to hope.

critical thinking

Brian Rehabilitation Phase

Jennifer comes to visit Brian on the second day of the hospital stay. Jennifer and Brian have a meeting with the social worker to reflect on their marital issues and to understand Brian's suicide attempt. Jennifer and Brian decide to work together to rebuild their relationship. Brian is discharged the next day, and they drive back to Baltimore and have an opportunity to talk through some of the issues that were bothering them. After Brian returns home and goes back to work, he begins attending weekly individual psychotherapy. He and Jennifer attend couples therapy every other week. Brian begins to understand his reaction to Jennifer's frustration with his traveling. They jointly decide to prepare for his absence the weekend prior to travel, with Brian assisting with some of the household chores. They schedule a family meeting for the Saturday prior to Brian's departure to discuss family issues and to make some decisions, as needed. Jennifer and Brian decide that Brian should continue with his current job and project, but their communication needs to be enhanced while he is away. They decide to use Skype to facilitate better communication. Brian is taking the prescribed medication. His concentration has improved; he has been productive at work. Brian, Jennifer, and their children attend church regularly and use the principles of spirituality in their household. Both Jennifer and Brian feel that they have learned a great deal from this difficult experience.

APPLICATION

1. Describe what Brian demonstrates in the five domains:

   a. Biological

   b. Psychological

   c. Sociological

   d. Cultural

   e. Spiritual

2. What changes can you identify in Jennifer and Brian's relationship?

PERCEPTIONS, THOUGHTS, & FEELINGS: Validating the Needs of a Patient Who Has Attempted Suicide

Brian is brought to the emergency department of the hospital closest to the hotel. He is embarrassed that he was discovered by hotel security and frightened that he was taken to the hospital. He is upset that he survived the suicide attempt, but is open to the evaluation by the psychiatric nurse clinical specialist who is on duty in the emergency department.

Patient's behavior(s)	Nurse's perceptions, thoughts, feelings	Exploration with patient
Brian is lying on a stretcher in the room reserved for psychiatric patients. Brian's head is down and his eyes are closed. When the RN (Diane) walks into the room, Brian looks up as though he is frightened.	*Perceptions:* Brian looks frightened and despondent. *Thoughts:* I wonder how to help him be safe; he took a large overdose and really wanted to die.	**Nurse:** Hello, my name is Diane. I am going to assess you today to determine what care you need to help you stay safe. I understand that you live in Baltimore and came to Boston for work. While you were here you took an overdose in a suicidal attempt. Can you tell me what happened?

VALIDATION By extending herself as an empathic listener, Diane encourages Brian to share his feelings. This will help her assess his suicide potential.

Patient's behavior(s)	Nurse's perceptions, thoughts, feelings	Exploration with patient
Brian: I'm Brian. I come to Boston for work about a week each month. While I was going to the hotel from the airport, my wife called to tell me she is leaving me. I had no idea! I don't know what happened! All I know is I am a failure at home, where it counts, and a failure at work. I don't deserve to live. Now, I am so embarrassed that hotel security found me like that. I don't know what to do now. Jennifer may never want me back. I am a terrible example for our kids.	*Thoughts:* Brian is really distressed. His basic core beliefs are at stake. Seeing himself as a failure is important—it indicates his level of self-loathing. He can really complete suicide. *Feelings:* I hope I can help him.	**Nurse:** I understand that you are feeling embarrassed that the security guard saw you in the hotel after your suicide attempt. It seems to me that if you and I explore some of the issues that went into your taking the overdose, we can begin to understand what happened.

VALIDATION Validating Brian's feelings of embarrassment is an important intervention as it conveys Diane's willingness to listen to him without judgment. Encouraging Brian to explore some of his thoughts about his marriage will assist him to have a better understanding of the issues that caused the suicide attempt.

Patient's behavior(s)	Nurse's perceptions, thoughts, feelings	Exploration with patient
Brian: Okay. Jennifer and I have been arguing a lot recently. She does not understand the demands of my job and resents how much she has to do alone when I'm gone. She says she feels overwhelmed and alone. The research I do here in Boston is tied to my salary, and it is very important work. I look forward to coming up here.	*Thoughts:* I understand some of what is happening in the marriage. Jennifer is feeling overwhelmed when Brian is away. I wonder how he communicates his feelings of pleasure for the research he is doing. I wonder if Jennifer is misreading his enthusiasm for the project as his not caring for her and the kids.	**Nurse:** How were things between you and Jennifer prior to your traveling for the research project?

VALIDATION Diane begins trying to clarify Brian's perception of his marriage.

Patient's behavior(s)	Nurse's perceptions, thoughts, feelings	Exploration with patient
Brian: Jennifer and I were a real team. We understood each other and could even finish each other's sentences. Then, this project began. At first, I brought Jennifer with me to Boston, but she got bored and missed the kids. I would come back to the hotel all jazzed up and she would be down and frustrated.	*Thoughts:* I am beginning to understand some of the marital dynamics. I need to help Brian stabilize in a safe manner. It would help if I can get a sense of Jennifer's needs. This is complex, particularly because Jennifer is in Baltimore and Brian is here.	*Nurse:* Have you spoken to Jennifer since you came to the hospital?

VALIDATION Diane continues to clarify the marital dynamics. This both validates this as a primary concern of Brian's as well as provides important information.

Patient's behavior(s)	Nurse's perceptions, thoughts, feelings	Exploration with patient
Brian: Yes, she is really upset and doesn't know what to do. She says she can't live with herself if I were to die. I don't know what to do. I told her that it is important that we talk this separation through. If I have to stop traveling to save my marriage, I will have to look into that. No project should cost a marriage or my life!	*Thoughts:* I am glad that he is interested in exploring what happened in the marriage. Brian sounds as though he has been thinking about his life priorities of marriage and job. I need to determine his level of safety.	*Nurse:* It sounds as though you are beginning to think through some of the issues that led to your suicide attempt. Are you currently having any thoughts of wanting to die?

VALIDATION Encouraging Brian to talk about the marital dynamics and inviting him to talk further about his suicidal thoughts assists in developing the therapeutic relationship and to gaining important assessment information.

Patient's behavior(s)	Nurse's perceptions, thoughts, feelings	Exploration with patient
Brian: I am not sure. I feel very shaky. I have never felt like this before. I actually was looking forward to dying so that Jennifer and the kids can have a better life. That is something else! I am scared and unsure of myself.	*Thoughts:* I am glad that he is disclosing his thoughts. I can help him determine what to do next when he is open like this. *Feelings:* I hope that Jennifer will talk to him so we can see what work needs to be done in this marriage.	*Nurse:* We need to determine the next step. What level of care do you think you need to stay safe?

VALIDATION Enlisting Brian in the process of getting the level of care that he needs to prevent another suicide attempt.

Patient's behavior(s)	Nurse's perceptions, thoughts, feelings	Exploration with patient
Brian: I was told that if I opened up to you and the doctor, I would be admitted as a voluntary patient. I probably could use a couple of days to sleep, sort out some things, and then talk to Jennifer about whether I can return home.	*Thoughts:* I am glad that Brian is able to see hospitalization as something that may help him. *Feelings:* I feel relieved that Brian will consent to a short-term voluntary hospital stay. He still seems as though he could try another suicidal attempt if he were discharged and Jennifer told him something that upset him, like he cannot come home.	*Nurse:* That sounds like a good plan. During a short-term hospital stay, you can process what happened today as well as looking at what you could do to prevent a suicidal gesture in the future, if you were to become hopeless again.

VALIDATION Empowering Brian by pointing out how he can benefit from a short-term hospital stay.

Patient's behavior(s)	Nurse's perceptions, thoughts, feelings	Exploration with patient

Brian: Okay, please make the arrangements for me to stay here for a couple of days. I still have things in my hotel room; I wonder if someone from work could pick them up for me and bring them here. I will call Jennifer and tell her what I am going to do. I will call my boss and ask him to help me.

Thoughts: A short-term hospital stay is a good choice. I am glad that he is beginning to consider communicating with Jennifer and asking his boss for help. I will need to monitor the marital dynamics, especially Jennifer's reaction to Brian's choice to be hospitalized here in Boston.

Nurse: Okay, I will make the arrangements now. It would be helpful to know what Jennifer says during your call. Helping you explore your marital issues is essential. It is good that you want to call your boss to get your things from the hotel room.

VALIDATION Affirming Brian's choices and determining his protective measure of asking his boss for assistance provides validation and reduces Brian's sense of isolation.

Based on Orlando, I. J. (1972). The Discipline and Teaching of Nursing Process (An Evaluative Study). New York, NY: G. P. Putnam's Sons.

Chapter Highlights

1. The 2010 CDC suicide statistics demonstrate an increase in completed suicides. An increase in suicide has been reported by the military as well as in civilians. The nurse is in a position to assist in suicide prevention in the community as well as in the hospital.

2. A comprehensive assessment for suicidal ideation and possible suicide attempt is very powerful. Assessment questions demonstrate caring to the patient who often has not disclosed the suicidal thoughts to anyone, owing to feelings of guilt and shame. As the patient answers the questions, he or she can begin to understand some of the process that has been happening prior to the attempt. By examining the precipitating factors for the suicide attempt, the nurse and patient can work together on solving some of these problems.

3. Culture and spirituality can act as protective measures that provide comfort to the individual and assist him or her to seek help rather than carry out a suicide plan.

4. Cognitive–behavioral therapy (CBT) and Collaborative Assessment and Management of Suicidality (CAMS) are two

evidenced-based modalities that can help an individual prevent a suicide attempt.

5. Nurses provide safety on an inpatient unit by the use of constant observation. The patient can feel the caring the nurse is providing when the nurse encourages problem-solving strategies while observing the patient.

6. It is important for the patient's family to understand the patient's experience and provide support while the patient is in the initial/relapse and recovery stages.

7. Prior to discharge from an acute setting, the patient should be able to identify the precipitating factor that overwhelmed his or her ability to cope and how the initial attempt at problem solving will begin. The patient should be able to outline a plan for future care, such as obtaining psychotherapy as well as medications, if indicated. The patient should be able to state when to use the National Suicide Prevention Lifeline.

NCLEX®-RN Questions

1. The community health nurse is working on an initiative to decrease the incidence of suicides in a neighborhood. Based on national statistics, which individual would be placed in the highest risk category?
   a. The 25-year-old African American female who is employed and a single parent
   b. The 15-year-old male high school student who volunteers for a hospice organization
   c. The 34-year-old Native American male, who is recently married and has a history of military duty
   d. The 88-year-old Caucasian male who is recently widowed and has chronic congestive heart failure

2. The nurse is participating in a psychological autopsy of a teenager who recently committed suicide. The nurse learns that the teenager immigrated with family from another country, had begun to experience failing grades, had no friends, and was bullied by some classmates. Under which wellness domains would the nurse most likely categorize behaviors and risk factors? Select all that apply.
   a. Biological
   b. Psychological
   c. Sociological
   d. Cultural
   e. Spiritual

3. The nurse is assessing risk factors for suicide. Which would alert the nurse to increased risk? Select all that apply.
   a. Family history of suicide
   b. Strong belief in an afterlife
   c. Unsecured weapons at home
   d. Pregnancy or dependent children
   e. Presence of cardiovascular disease

4. The nurse is using the Level of Suicidal Severity Index to determine the level of risk for a patient. The patient states he often has fantasies about others coming to his funeral and feeling bad about how they have treated him. Although these thoughts make the patient feel better, he has no explicit plan in mind. The nurse determines that the patient is at which stage of suicide severity?
   a. Stage II: mild
   b. Stage III: moderate
   c. Stage IV: advanced
   d. Stage V: severe

5. The nurse in an inpatient unit is caring for a patient who has attempted suicide. Which intervention is consistent with evidence-based practice?
   a. Decreasing monitoring after a patient has completed a written safety agreement
   b. Questioning the patient frequently and explicitly about intent to commit suicide
   c. Providing reassurance that things will get better if the patient holds on and gives it some time
   d. Gently reminding the patient that his behavior has caused pain and suffering

6. The nurse is providing teaching to the family caring for a patient who is at risk for suicide. What should the nurse emphasize? Select all that apply.
   a. Differentiating between real threats and manipulative behavior
   b. Understanding that suicide is usually related to family dysfunction
   c. Encouraging the family to seek counseling and support from professionals
   d. The importance of reaching out to hotlines, crisis care centers, or emergency departments
   e. Recognizing the direct and indirect warning signs that are often present before a suicide attempt

Answers may be found on the Pearson student resource site: nursing.pearsonhighered.com

Pearson Nursing Student Resources Find additional review materials at **nursing.pearsonhighered.com**

References

Aborido, M., Musson, M., & LeGueut, B. (2008). Psychiatric autopsy: Its uses and limits in France. *Encephale, 34*(4), 343–346. Available at http://ncbi.nih.gov/books/NBK7126/

Ackley, B. J., & Ladwig, G. B. (2014). *Nursing Diagnosis Handbook: An Evidence-Based Guide to Planning Care* (10th ed.). St. Louis, MO: Mosby.

American Association of Suicidology (AAS). (2013). Suicide in the USA based on 2010 data. Available at http://www.suicidology.org

American Psychiatric Association (APA). (2010). Practice Guideline for the Assessment and Treatment of Patients with Suicidal Behaviors. Available at http://psychiatryonline.org/data/Books/prac/SuicidalBehavior_4-16-09

Batt, A., Belliver, F., Delatte, B., & Spreux-Varoquaux, O. (2006). Suicide: Psychological autopsy a research tool for prevention. *Expertise Collective 2006.* Available at http://ncbi.nih.gov/books/NBK7126/

Bebbington, P. E., Cooper, C., Minot, S., Brugha, T., Jenkins, R., et al. (2009). Suicide attempts, gender, and sexual abuse: Data from the 2000 British Psychiatric Morbidity Survey. *American Journal of Psychiatry, 166*(10), 1135–1140.

Beck, A. T., Steer, R. A., Kovacs, M., & Garrison, B. (1985). Hopelessness and eventual suicide: A 10-year prospective study of patients hospitalized with suicidal ideation. *American Journal of Psychiatry, 142*(5), 559–563.

Beck, A. T., & Weishaar, M. E. (1990). Suicide risk assessment and prediction. *Crisis, 11*(2), 22–30.

Brent, D. (2009). In search of endophenotypes for suicidal behavior. *American Journal of Psychiatry, 166*(10), 1087–1090.

Calder, J., McVean, A., & Yang, W. (2010). History of abuse and current suicidal ideation: Results from a population based survey. *Journal of Family Violence, 25*, 205–214.

Centers for Disease Control and Prevention (CDC). (2009). National Violent Death Reporting System, 16 states, 2006. CDC *MMWR Surveillance Summaries, 58*(SS01), 1–44. Available at http://www.cdc.gov/mmwr/preview/mmwrhtml/ss5801a1.htm and http://www.cdc.gov/ViolencePrevention/intimatepartnerviolence/consequences.html

Centers for Disease Control and Prevention (CDC). (2012). Intimate partner violence: Consequences. Available at http://www.cdc.gov/violenceprevention/intimatepartnerviolence/consequences.html

Centers for Disease Control and Prevention (CDC). (2013.) Web-based Injury Statistics Query and Reporting System (WISQARS). Available at http://www.cdc.gov/injury/wisqars/index.html

Cornwell, Y. (2009). Suicide prevention in later life: A glass half full, or half empty? *American Journal of Psychiatry, 166*(8), 845–849.

Crosby, A. E., Ortega, L., & Melanson, C. (2011.) Self-directed violence surveillance: Uniform definitions and recommended data elements, version 1.0. Atlanta, GA: Centers for Disease Control and Prevention, National Center for Injury Prevention and Control.

D'Augelli, A. R., Grossman, A. H. Salter, N. P., Vaseym, J. J., et al. (2005). Predicting the suicide attempts of lesbian, gay, and bisexual youth. The American Association of Suicidology. *Suicide and Life-Threatening Behavior, 35*(6), 646–660.

Defense Centers of Excellence for Psychological Health and Traumatic Brain Injury. Available at www.dcoe.health.mil/SuicidePreventionWarriors.aspx

Department of Psychiatry, Penn Behavioral Health. Aaron T. Beck, MD. Beck Scales and Inventories. Available at http://www.med.upenn.edu/suicide/beck/scales.html?6

Durkheim, E. (1951). *Suicide: A Study in Sociology* (Trans. J. Spaulding & G. Simpson). Glencoe, IL: Free Press. Originally published as *Le Suicide: Etude de Sociologie.* (1897). Paris: Alcan. In Shneidman, E. S. (2001). *Comprehending Suicide: Landmarks in 20th-Century Suicidology.* Washington, DC: American Psychological Association, pp. 33–47.

Glover, R. (2012). Proceedings on the state budget crisis and the behavioral health treatment gap: The impact on public substance abuse and mental health treatment systems. National Association of State Mental Health Program Directors Report to Congress, Washington, DC, March 2012. Available at http://www.nasmhpd.org/docs/Summary-Congressional%20Briefing_March%2022_Website.pdf

Grabosky, T. K., Ishii, H., & Mase, S. (2012) The development of the counseling profession in Japan: Past, present and future. *Journal of Counseling and Development, 90*, 221–226.

Green, E., Katz, J., & Marcus, P. E. (1995). Practice guidelines for suicidal/self harm prevention. In E. Green & J. Katz, (Eds.). *Clinical Practice Guidelines for the Adult Patient*. St. Louis, MO: Mosby-Year Book, pp. 250-1–250-21.

Jobes, D. A., & Drozd, J. P. (2004) The CAMS approach to working with suicidal patients. *Journal of Contemporary Psychotherapy, 34*, 73–85.

King, C. A., O'Mara, R. M., Hayward, C. N., & Cunningham, R. M. (2009). Adolescent suicide risk screening in the emergency department. *Academic Emergency Medicine, 16*(11), 1234–1245.

Kjølseth, I., Ekeberg, Ø., & Steihaung, S. (2010). Why suicide? Elderly people who committed suicide and their experience of life in the period before their death. *Psychogeriatics, 22*(2), 209–219.

Lentz, K., Coderre, K., & Watanabe, M. D. (2009). Overview of depression and its management in children and adolescents. *Formulary, 44*(6), 172–181.

Lim, F. A., Brown, D. V., & Jones, H. (2013). Lesbian, gay, bisexual, and transgender health: Fundamentals for nursing education. *Journal of Nursing Education, 52*(4), 198–203.

Meerwijk, E. L., Ford, M., & Weiss, S. J. (2013). Brain regions associated with psychological pain: Implications for a neural network and its relationship to physical pain. *Brain Imaging and Behavior, 7*(1), 1–14.

McGirr, A., Aida, M., Ságuin, M., Cabot, S., Lesage, A., et al. (2009). Familial aggression of suicide explained by Cluster B traits: A three-group family study of suicide controlling for major depressive disorder. *American Journal of Psychiatry, 166*(10), 1124–1134.

Minois, G. (1999). *History of Suicide: Voluntary Death in Western Culture*. (Trans. L. G. Cochrane). Baltimore, MD: Johns Hopkins University Press. Originally published as *Histore de Suicide, Fayard, Libraire Artheme*. (1996). Paris. In Shneidman, E. S. (2001). *Comprehending Suicide: Landmarks in 20th-Century Suicidology*. Washington, DC: American Psychological Association, pp. 13–22.

Orlando, I. J. (1972). *The Discipline and Teaching of Nursing Process (An Evaluative Study)*. New York, NY: G. P. Putnam's Sons.

Shneidman, E. S. (1985). *Ten Commonalities of Suicide and Some Implications for Public Policy*. Washington, DC: ERIC Clearinghouse.

Shneidman, E. (1992). A conspectus for conceptualizing the suicidal scenario. In R. Maris, A. Berman, J. Maltsberger, & R. Yufit, (Eds.). *Assessment and Prediction of Suicide*. New York, NY: Guilford Press, pp. 50–65.

Substance Abuse and Mental Health Services Administration (SAMHSA). (2012). Study Results from the 2010 National Survey on Drug Use and Health, Mental Health Findings. NSDUH series H-42, HHS Publication No (SMA) 11-4667. Rockville, MD: SAMHSA.

Suicide Prevention Resource Center. (2008). Suicide Assessment Five-Step Evaluation and Triage for Mental Health Professionals SAFE-T. Available at http://www.sprc.org/bpr/section-III/suicide-assessment-five-step-evaluation-and-triage-safe-t

Umhau, J. C., George, D. T., Heaney, R. P., Lewis, M. D., Ursano, R. J., et.al. (2013). Low vitamin D status and suicide: A case-control study of active duty military service members. *PLoS One, 8*(1). Available at http://search.proquest.com.exproxy.pgcc.edu/nursing/printviewfile?accountid=13315

U.S. Department of Health and Human Services (DHHS). (2012). Office of the Surgeon General and the National Action Alliance for Suicide Prevention. *National Strategy for Suicide Prevention: Goals and Objectives for Action*. Washington, DC: DHHS. Available at www.surgeongeneral.gov/library/reports/national-strategy-suicide-prevention/index.html

U.S. Preventive Services Task Force. (2013). Screening for suicide risk in adolescents, adults, and older adults: U.S. Preventive Services Task Force recommendation statement. Available at http://www.uspreventiveservicestaskforce.org/draftrec3.htm

Weiyuan, C. (2009). Women and suicide in rural China. *Bulletin of the World Health Organization, Geneva, 87*(12), 888–908.

World Health Organization. (2013). Suicide prevention (SUPRE). Available at http://www.who.int/mental_health/prevention/suicide/suicideprevent/en/index.html

Yellow Horse Brave Heart, M., Elkins, J., Tafiya, G., & Bird, D. (2012). Wicasa Wasáka: Restoring the traditional strength of American Indian boys and men. *American Journal of Public Health, Supplement 2*(102), S117–S183.

Young, A. T., Fuller, J., & Riley, B. (2008). On-scene mental health counseling provided through police departments. *Journal of Mental Health Counseling, 30*, 345–362.

Zlodre, J., & Fazel, S. (2012). All-cause and external mortality in released prisoners: Systematic review and meta-analysis. *American Journal of Public Health. 102*(12), e67–e75.

28

Caring for the Patient Who Is Grieving

Christine L. Williams

Key Terms

Learning Outcomes

1. Identify common situations that lead to loss and grief.

2. Distinguish between grief and depression.

3. Explain critical components of assessment for individuals experiencing loss and grief.

4. Identify assessment information that warrants referral or collaboration.

5. Plan evidence-based care for individuals and families experiencing loss and grief.

6. Apply therapeutic communication strategies to intervene with individuals and families experiencing loss and grief.

7. Evaluate effectiveness of interventions appropriate for individuals and families experiencing loss and grief.

8. Analyze situations in which nurses experience grief related to their work and discuss ways to handle grief responses at work.

Nancy Colton Initial Phase

Nancy Colton is a 35-year-old married woman whose 10-year-old son, Jeffrey, died in a swimming accident in the previous month. She avoids Jeffrey's older brothers, who are 12 and 15, and refuses to go out except to see her primary care provider (PCP). At the appointment with her PCP, the nurse escorts her to the examining room, takes her vital signs, and begins to talk with Mrs. Colton about how she is doing. The nurse learns that Mrs. Colton has been healthy in the past and has no history of mental illness. Her vital signs are: temperature 98.6, pulse 85, respirations 20, and blood pressure 135/80 mmHg. Mrs. Colton says that she has not slept much since the accident and she has no appetite. Although Mrs. Colton was not present at the accident, she states emphatically that it was "all her fault" because she gave him permission to go swimming. She cannot stop thinking about the accident—memories come to mind even when she tries not to think about it.

The nurse learns that Mrs. Colton is a second-generation American, of German descent; she and her family are members of a local Lutheran church that they attend regularly. Mrs. Colton is steadily employed as an office manager and she has completed 1 year of college. Her husband is very concerned about her and is sitting in the waiting area. Mrs. Colton tells the nurse that she has not returned to work because she cannot stop crying, she does not want anyone to see her this way, and she just "cannot think straight." She does not care if she loses her job because "nothing matters anymore." She admits that it is painful to see her other sons because it reminds her that the family is no longer "complete." Mrs. Colton expresses anguish about her prior belief that if she practiced her faith to the best of her ability, she and her family would be safe.

The nurse observes that Mrs. Colton seems restless and anxious, avoids eye contact, and that her eyes are red and puffy from crying. She appears casually dressed and disheveled. Her hair looks unwashed, and she speaks so softly that she is difficult to hear.

APPLICATION

1. Address the five domains for Mrs. Colton:
   a. Biological
   b. Psychological
   c. Sociological
   d. Cultural
   e. Spiritual
2. In what ways do you think Mrs. Colton may be suffering? Why?
3. How you would prioritize Mrs. Colton's needs during this encounter and why?

Introduction

Nurses commonly encounter patients and family members in the midst of loss and grief. **Loss** describes a perceived or real deprivation. Individuals experience loss in a wide variety of situations, including, but not limited to:

- Separation from loved ones due to illness (e.g., Alzheimer disease, coma)
- Loss related to injury (e.g., loss of function, amputation, paralysis)
- Loss as a result of criminal acts (e.g., assault, homicide, missing children)
- Loss related to natural disasters (e.g., loss of home, loss of life)
- Loss as a result of life changes (e.g., aging, immigration, divorce)

Loss may be tangible (for example, the loss of a home or spouse) or intangible, such as the loss of dignity or feeling of security (Table 28-1). The intensity of reaction to loss varies according to the meaning of the loss to the individual (Shear et al., 2011b). *Symbolic meaning of the loss may result in an intense reaction in one person and a mild reaction in another.* Loss of self can occur in relation to anticipating one's own death, losing a body part (for example, from amputation or mastectomy), or following loss of function (as in paralysis). Serious illness may be accompanied by many losses: separation from loved ones (while hospitalized); loss of meaningful roles, such as inability to work or care for family members; loss of income; loss of privacy; and loss of trust in one's body. There are many other forms of loss, including loss of freedom and loss of identity. All loss leads to grief, which is similar in form but differs in intensity and is unique to the individual experiencing it. Loss is generally accompanied by distress and suffering.

Grief

Grief can be defined as the individual's unique response to loss that involves a journey from suffering to healing. Depending on the individual and the significance of the loss, grief may be all-consuming and accompanied by suffering. Grief may result in loss of social and occupational functioning for various amounts of time. Other common responses include disorganization and depression.

Bereavement describes the period of acute sadness or suffering that follows a loss or death. *Bereaved* is a term of respect used to describe individuals who are grieving, which implies that special consideration is necessary to support the individual in the grieving process. The initial phases of grief, during which individuals begin to accept the reality of the loss and experience the suffering associated with grief, may be accompanied by physical symptoms, such as prolonged sleep deprivation, that threaten physical health and contribute to suffering. The recovery phase includes gradual improvement in symptoms as well as the patient's functioning in life roles.

The emotional experience of grief typically occurs in waves, in which the person alternately feels suffering and relief from suffering

---

Common Types of Loss	table 28-1

Tangible Losses	Intangible Losses
Separation from loved ones	Loss of self-esteem
Death of a family member	Loss of memory
Loss of body part or function	Role change
Developmental loss	Loss of income
Loss of property	Loss of privacy
Loss of employment	Loss of freedom
Loss of pet or companion animal	Loss of dignity

(Steeves, 2002). From his research with bereaved spouses, Steeves differentiated between the emotion of grief that is intermittent and the background mood of grief that is constant and filters the patient's way of viewing the world. An intense wave of suffering may occur in intervals of a few minutes, hours, days, or weeks. In time, the intervals get longer, and the suffering diminishes but never disappears completely. In other words, the patient may experience positive emotions but continue to experience sadness in the background. In complicated grief, the individual may not experience any lessening in the intensity of the suffering over time or the suffering may be accompanied by self-destructive feelings of worthlessness and hopelessness. *Patients expressing feelings of worthlessness and hopelessness require evaluation for depression and safety.*

Types of Grief and Loss

Although grief is unique to the individual, nurses learn to recognize certain types or categories of grief that individuals experience to varying degrees (Table 28-2). These include anticipatory grief, ambiguous loss, chronic sorrow, complicated grief, delayed grief, disenfranchised grief, and unresolved grief.

Ambiguous Loss

Ambiguous loss typically is associated with missing family members and is particularly difficult to grieve. In situations in which it is uncertain whether a loved one is alive or not, family members will be likely to experience prolonged and unresolved suffering. Not having the body of the deceased to grieve over can be another source of painful loss. Examples of those suffering ambiguous loss include parents whose child has been kidnapped or the spouse of a service member who is missing in action (Boss & Carnes, 2012). Family members of the missing experience great conflict over whether to maintain or give up hope that they will be reunited with their loved one.

Anticipatory Grief

In **anticipatory grief**, an individual expects the loss before it occurs and has sufficient time to contemplate what it will be like. In some cases, the individual will experience many or all of the emotional, physical, behavioral, and spiritual responses that would be felt after the actual loss. Examples of anticipatory grief may be seen in the wife whose husband is suffering from Alzheimer disease, the family members of a person in the military who have a strong sense of loss at deployment, or the mother whose child is diagnosed with a fatal illness. Unfortunately, anticipatory grief can sometimes lead to withdrawal from the dying person who is in need of support, or withdrawal from other family members. There is conflicting information about whether anticipatory grief lessens the grief that occurs following the actual loss (Kehl, 2005). When patients and family members experience anticipatory grief, they need nonjudgmental support, as with any type of grief.

Chronic Sorrow

Chronic sorrow is grief that is ongoing rather than acute. Chronic sorrow does not decrease in intensity over time. It has been described as "permanent, progressive, recurring and cyclic in nature" (Gordon, 2009, p. 115). The source of the grief is ever-present and unchanging, or may become worse over time. It is not uncommon for parents of children born with congenital anomalies to experience chronic sorrow. The parents grieve the loss of dreams for the future, as well as the child. They suffer as the child suffers. Chronic sorrow may also be observed in parents of children with chronic illness, such as cystic fibrosis, or in spouses caring for partners diagnosed with Alzheimer disease. Nurses can encourage hope in parents by keeping them informed and by offering information about support groups and counseling. Parents and others experiencing chronic sorrow need support as they struggle to find personal meaning in their situation.

Complicated Grief

Complicated grief is a grief response that is outside the ordinary. Complicated grief may be suspected when the intensity of suffering does not diminish over time, the patient does not resume previous roles, or the grief seems out of proportion to the loss, even from the perspective of the bereaved. If the bereaved is surprised by the intensity of the response, this may be an indication that there are previous unresolved losses. When one person survives and another dies, the survivor may experience *survivor guilt*, asking questions such as, "Why not me?" Survivor guilt may contribute to shame and grief (LaTour, 2010; Shear et al., 2011a).

Types of Grief and Loss   table 28-2

Type	Definition
Ambiguous loss	Circumstances surrounding the loss are uncertain, resulting in confusion for the bereaved (e.g., parents whose child is missing may hope for the child's return but also fear the child is dead).
Anticipatory grief	Individuals begin to grieve before the loss occurs as they contemplate what it will be like.
Chronic sorrow	Grief experience that is ongoing and seemingly without end; it may become worse over time.
Complicated grief	Grief is intense, lasts at least 6 months, does not seems to lessen over time, and is accompanied by prolonged feelings of worthlessness, emptiness, or meaninglessness.
Delayed grief	The individual seems to feel no grief for a period of weeks, months, or years. When grief is felt, it may be as intense as would be expected soon after a loss.
Disenfranchised grief	Occurs when individuals hide grief following a loss to which some sort of stigma is or may be attached (e.g., drunk-driving accident, abortion).
Unresolved grief	Ongoing or suppressed grief that affects the individual's response to the current or expected future loss; may result when the individual suppresses grief to make others feel more comfortable or because urgent circumstances delay grieving in the present.

PRACTICE ALERT Not all individuals report distress after a loss; widely varying degrees of distress, even to a similar loss, can be normal. Refer individuals whose grief seems out of proportion to the loss to a mental health specialist for further assessment.

Delayed Grief

When there is a significant period of time between the loss and the individual's grief response, the response is described as **delayed grief**. Delayed grief may persist for months or even years after the loss. In general, delayed grief is likely to occur when the bereaved experiences another loss.

Disenfranchised Grief

Livingston describes **disenfranchised grief** as grief "that is not recognized or socially supported" (2010, p. 205). Some examples of disenfranchised grief include grief following the death of an unmarried partner when the relationship was not publicly acknowledged; grief at the death of a former spouse; grief following an abortion; or grief following the death of a family member who has caused the death of another person, such as in murder or a drunk driving accident. Aspects of disenfranchised grief include grieving alone due to the inability to share the loss with others or to fear of intolerance, and experiencing contempt from others related to stigma associated with the nature of the loss.

Unresolved Grief

Unresolved grief occurs when individuals suppress or avoid grief. After a few weeks or months of mourning, others may pressure the bereaved to "move on," stop grieving, or stop discussing it or showing outward signs of grief. The bereaved may also want to stop grieving because of shame and embarrassment about expressions of emotional pain, particularly in public. Sometimes the person grieving feels the need to be "strong" to support other family members. Suppressing grief can make others feel more comfortable and is common in the workplace. Employers may allow only a few days of bereavement leave, and then the bereaved is expected to resume normal responsibilities. Grieving individuals who are not permitted time to express their grief may experience unexpressed and unresolved grief.

Factors Affecting the Grieving Process

As stated earlier, the significance of the loss is an important factor that affects an individual's grief response. Other factors include expectation, number of losses, whether the loss is cumulative, duration and context of grief, and characteristics of the bereaved.

Expected Versus Unanticipated Loss

In some cases, being able to prepare for a loss may decrease grief intensity. However, even when a death is expected by the family (as in a prolonged illness), the loss of a spouse or child may be just as painful as unexpected death. Grief intensity is not dependent on the length of a relationship. Perinatal loss can be devastating to parents not only for the loss of their child, but also for the loss of their hopes and dreams for that child. Nurses must be prepared to recognize patients' grief, respond appropriately, and prevent or intervene when patients experience unhealthy coping.

Multiple Losses

Multiple losses compound grief and may be overwhelming, leading to despair and hopelessness. For example, when older adults move to a nursing home because of chronic illness and impaired functioning, they face not only loss of independence, but also loss of home, neighbors, and supportive routines, such as religious or social activities. When adolescents lose a parent, they may also lose freedom due to increased responsibilities at home and may even experience loss of hopes and dreams if plans for college are no longer financially feasible. Multiple losses overwhelm usual coping mechanisms and place the individual at risk for depression.

Cumulative Losses

Cumulative losses occur sequentially and can challenge the individual who has not had time to fully grieve one loss before another occurs. Unresolved grief from previous losses can affect the significance of losses that follow. Cumulative loss in aging occurs when an individual outlives spouse, friends, and acquaintances (Gilbert, 2004).

Duration of Grief

Patients may ask how long it will take for them to grieve a loss. It is important that patients and families have realistic expectations about time frames. A patient who experiences a major loss, such as the death of a child or spouse or loss of a limb, may take years to feel ready to resume life with the same enthusiasm felt before the loss. The pain of grief will very likely never go away completely, although it will become less intense and more manageable over time. Periods of time when the patient is free of painful thoughts and feelings will increase in frequency and duration.

Context of Grief

Circumstances surrounding the loss may prolong or decrease suffering. Disenfranchised grief or unacknowledged loss increase feelings of isolation and lack of support. This kind of grief can occur when the loss is associated with shame and guilt (for example, after a rape, when the victim is too ashamed to confide in others). When spouses are in the process of separation or divorce and death of a spouse occurs, the surviving spouse may not be supported by others because family and friends assume that the marriage was not strong enough for a loss to result in suffering. There are many other examples, as well. Consider the example of death of a loved one who caused the death of another (for instance, a drunk-driving fatality or murder–suicide). The network of friends and family may avoid the family of the perpetrator because they disapprove of the crime and feel compassion only for the victim and the victim's family.

When the loss is associated with a crime, the legal ramifications may prolong grief. A trial may include reviewing all the details of a loved one's death. In many states, victims and family members are asked to write an "impact statement" detailing all the ways that the crime has adversely affected them. The extended processes and challenges associated with trials (for example, testifying or making victim impact statements) prolong the length of time that one spends involved with the crime or death, and therefore are likely to prolong the individual's response to the event.

As stated earlier, when an individual dies by suicide, family members may experience shame and guilt, which, in turn, may intensify their grief (Box 28-1). Survivors often blame themselves even when it is clear to everyone else that they are not to blame. Suicide is often described as if it were a crime ("he *committed* suicide"). Family and friends also may believe that the suicide could have been prevented if the bereaved or staff members had been more helpful or vigilant (for instance, "If you had not divorced my son, he would be alive today.").

Grief and Suicide

box 28-1

In some religions, suicide is viewed as a sin. Such beliefs help to explain the stigma associated with suicide in our culture. Nurses can avoid reinforcing these harmful beliefs by referring to the event as death *by* suicide and educating patients about the relationship between mental illness and suicide. Help family members understand that their behavior was not the cause of the suicide.

Nurses experience grief—and, sometimes, guilt—when a patient dies by suicide in the hospital. They may feel responsible for the death because of something they did or did not do. Grief after suicide may impair nurses' morale and lead to blaming one another. Talking to co-workers and a supervisor will help to develop a more realistic perception of the event that could facilitate effective coping. Others can point out the many factors that contribute to suicidal behavior. Nurses also can learn from the death and develop guidelines for future care.

Characteristics of the Bereaved

The way individuals experience grief and express suffering may be affected by their personal characteristics. The individual's emotional expressiveness, prior mental health, coping resources, cultural conditioning, and quality of supportive relationships are important in determining an individual's behavior and resiliency. Prior experience with grief and successful resolution of prior losses contribute to resiliency.

Life Span Considerations

When an older adult dies peacefully, surrounded by loved ones, the family may be comforted that the loss occurred as expected in the life course. Conversely, when a child dies, the family perceives that something is out of order. Children are not expected to die before their parents. Suffering associated with the death of a child is especially intense, and may be more so if parents or other family members believe that they failed in their roles to protect the child and feel that they should have died in the child's place.

Very young children usually are unable to understand death as permanent. As a consequence, their grief may be incomplete until they reach a stage of development at which they are better able to appreciate what they have lost. Children often view the death of a parent as abandonment or punishment. Divorce, especially if it results in separation from a parent, can also initiate significant responses from children. Long-term effects of parental loss, especially death, include depression and behavioral and learning problems. However, some children experience none of these effects. Several factors can mitigate the long-term, adverse effects that significant loss may have on children. Protective factors include a supportive family, the child's development (pre-loss normal functioning being protective), and family stability. In the case of children who lose a parent by suicide, shame and guilt have been reported even after months of grieving. Surviving children, especially younger children, are at increased risk for mental health problems (Hung & Rabin, 2009). Compared to children with two living parents and those whose parent died from another cause, children who lose a parent to suicide are at higher risk for depression and suicidal behavior (Geulayov, Gunnell, Holmen, & Metcalfe, 2011).

Adolescents must deal with conflict about dependence and independence, especially from parents. Death of a family member may result in confusion, as the adolescent does not know whether to remain close to significant others or to create distance in relationships to avoid being hurt. The sense of growing mastery and control normally associated with adolescence can be shaken by loss and grief. Adolescents may feel different or isolated from peers, who are dealing with other issues (Balk, 2011).

Older adults usually have experience with loss of friends, family, function, and roles among others. This experience can be useful when the patient reflects on the use of active coping mechanisms that previously helped them manage distress with prior losses. Despite their experience and learned methods of coping, the loss of a spouse or child is just as devastating to older adults as it is to the young. Grieving a spouse may take many years. During those years, the bereaved is at risk for impaired health.

Pause and Reflect

1. *Do you know anyone who has experienced disenfranchised grief? What kind of support did that person receive?*

2. *Have you experienced any significant losses? What were they, and how did you handle them? Who was helpful to you in your grieving process, and why?*

3. *What factors put individuals at a greater risk for experiencing complicated grief?*

Theoretical Foundations

Patients and family members who are grieving exhibit a variety of responses across the five domains (Table 28-3). Thorough assessment is necessary to determine the nature of an individual's responses as well as the extent to which grief responses may be healthy or unhealthy.

Biological Domain

Intense grief affects individuals in a holistic way and often interferes with physiological functioning, especially in the first days and weeks. Loss and grief can be long-term stressors that heighten sympathetic nervous system activity and subsequently increase stress hormones, such as cortisol (Pierrehumbert et al., 2012; Pruessner et al., 2010). The individual with chronically high levels of stress hormones experiences immediate effects, such as elevated heart rate. When the stressor is prolonged, such as in the loss of a close family member, adverse health conditions (such as hypertension) can occur (Beckie, 2012). The bereaved individual may experience poor appetite and difficulty sleeping. Palpitations, frequent sighing, and feeling short of breath are common. Bereaved individuals report poorer health and visit health care providers more frequently than they did before (Bonnano & Kaltman, 2001). In a 5-year study of widows, Kowalski and Bondmass (2008) found that more than half their subjects

Grief Responses by Domain   table 28-3

Domain	Response
Biological	• Fatigue, exhaustion • Pain • Sleep disturbance • Appetite disturbance • Shortness of breath, tightness in the chest • Increased heart rate or blood pressure • Gastrointestinal distress • Muscle weakness • Hypersensitivity to noise
Psychological	• Shock • Anger, irritability • Sadness • Helplessness • Confusion • Impaired memory • Impaired judgment • Fear, anxiety, panic attacks • Guilt • Numbness • Loneliness, despair • Depression • Forgetfulness • Intrusive thoughts
Sociological	• Withdrawal from activities and others • Impaired functioning affecting work, finances
Cultural/ Spiritual	• Engaging in or withdrawing from traditional cultural and religious practices • Doubting beliefs, values • Finding comfort in beliefs, values • Repeatedly asking "why" • Attributing death to a Higher Power

Based on Bonanno, G. A., & Kaltman, S. (2001). The varieties of grief experience. *Clinical Psychology Review, 21*(5), 705–734; Kowalski, S. D., & Bondmass, M. D. (2008). Physiological and psychological symptoms of grief in widows. *Research in Nursing and Health, 31*(1), 23–30; and Patricelli, K. (2012). Symptoms of grief. Available at http://sevencounties.org/poc/view_doc.php?type=doc&id=12001&cn=174

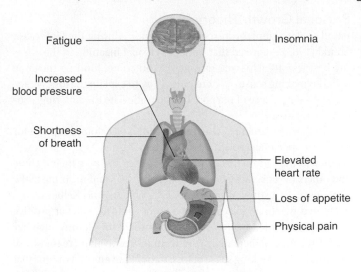

28-1   Common physiological symptoms associated with grief.

reported physiologic symptoms following the death of a spouse, including physical pain (especially musculoskeletal pain), loss of appetite, increased blood pressure, insomnia, and fatigue (Figure 28-1). Symptoms were high in years 1 and 2 following the spouse's death, but gradually decreased in years 3 to 5. This suggests that physical health is impaired long after the death of a spouse. This decline may be exacerbated, at least in part, by unhealthy behavior. Depression and despair may make self-care a low priority. Bereaved individuals may use unhealthy coping strategies, such as alcohol, and may be prone to accidents. When grieving individuals have chronic illnesses that require careful monitoring, they may be less vigilant about self-care. For example, Kowalski and Bondmass's subjects reported increased smoking or resuming smoking if they had quit.

Psychological Domain

Grief responses within the psychological domain also vary. Individuals frequently experience changes in cognition (thinking), affect (emotions), and behavior. Feelings of helplessness, fear, and anxiety may accompany or alternate with feelings of extreme sadness. Some changes are brief; others are long lasting. Most are associated with distress and cause additional suffering. A person may fear "going crazy" and never being "the same person" again. A number of theories help inform understanding of loss and grieving. These theories examine how loss affects individuals and what processes are associated with **grief work**, the responses individuals exhibit following a loss, and their attempts to resolve their grief and return to "normal" after the loss.

Psychoanalytic Theory

Freud wrote about mourning and loss in 1917; his theories continue to influence popular thinking today. He proposed that bereaved individuals would eventually resolve their grief with effort he called *grief work* by detaching from the deceased and reinvesting in a new "love object" (Freud, 1917). The idea of closure resembles Freud's view that mourning comes to a distinct endpoint. *Closure* refers to a point in the grieving process at which it is completed and attachment to the deceased ends (Berns, 2011).

Freud's contention that the bereaved must detach from the lost object has not been supported by current research (Epstein, Kalus, & Berger, 2006). Contemporary researchers and theorists conclude that many people maintain a sense of attachment and can be either comforted or distressed by this perceived involvement. Ongoing "dreaming and yearning" for the deceased was related to distress, whereas others reported a sense of presence that was a source of comfort. Bowlby (1980) further theorized that, when attachments are broken by death, the pair is not separated completely by death. Rather than finding closure, the bereaved finds ways to remain bonded even though the "love object" is not physically present. In a qualitative study of veterans' widows, Wilson and Supiano (2011) described the bereaved spouses' "continuing relationship with the deceased" as "feeling his presence," talking to them, and holding onto belongings. Expecting someone to "detach or to find closure" and to "move on" after the loss of a loved one in order to achieve well-being can inflict further suffering by implying that absence of "closure" is somehow abnormal.

Personal Growth Theory

Based on the traumatic losses he experienced during the Holocaust, Frankl (1963) theorized that finding personal meaning in the loss is the best way to achieve a satisfactory outcome. Finding meaning includes making sense of or creating a way to explain the loss. Meaning and a deep sense of purpose can help alleviate the suffering associated with loss.

In their research, Hogan and Schmidt (2002) found support for a theory of personal growth as an outcome of grief. Although growth is possible, they admit that some individuals grieve over their lifetime and others never achieve better mental health or find meaning in the experience. In a study of caregivers, Ott, Sanders, and Kelber (2007) examined personal growth following loss and found that positive outcomes included becoming closer to the dying family member prior to death and increased self-esteem related to an increased sense of competence. Making sense of loss, rather than amount of time that has passed since the loss, is a predictor of the intensity of grief. For some, being able to make sense of loss may involve turning to spiritual beliefs or resolving to make sure that others do not experience the same pain and suffering in the future. For those grieving a violent death, time and meaning are needed to decrease suffering (Holland & Neimeyer, 2010).

Stage Theory

Several theorists have described predictable stages or tasks that individuals must experience during bereavement to return to previous levels of functioning or to achieve positive outcomes from the experience (Table 28-4). The stages generally begin with disbelief, shock, or numbness and progress from rejecting the loss to finally learning to live with the loss.

John Bowlby (1980) believed that all humans need close relationships with others and that when the attachments are broken, they experience grief by progressing through psychological stages. He identified four stages of grief: numbness/protest, yearning, disorganization and despair, and reorganization. Stages can last from a few hours to years, depending on the strength of the emotional attachment.

According to Bowlby, all humans experience grief when separated from a loved one, even infants as young as 6 months of age. Infants display grief physically with changes in sleep and appetite as well as with behaviors, such as increased crying or apathy (Bowlby, 1961; Hames, 2003).

In her classic book *On Death and Dying*, Elizabeth Kubler-Ross (1969) proposed five stages of grief (see Table 28-4). The stages outlined by Kubler-Ross were originally developed to describe the experience of patients facing their own death, but now they often are applied to any loss. She cautions that everyone is unique and may not experience all five stages. Further, individuals may not experience these stages in the same order, may progress from one stage to the next in widely different periods of time, and may return to a previous stage before moving on.

J. William Worden (1991) outlined five tasks of mourning the loss of a loved one. He believed that the bereaved individual needs to accomplish these tasks to resolve the loss, and not completing the tasks of grieving places the person at risk for future problems with adjustment.

Worden's final stage of withdrawing from the lost relationship is controversial. Current thought is that it is unnecessary to detach in order to move on to new relationships, and the bereaved maintains the attachment to a lost loved one in a number of ways. For instance, the relationship may be maintained though memories and by continuing the deceased's legacy. Examples may include taking flowers to a loved one's grave on her birthday or establishing a foundation to raise money for cancer research in the name of a loved one who has died from cancer.

Evidence Supporting Stage Theory

Holland and Neimeyer (2010) found some support for the stage theory of grief. They found that self-reported disbelief and depression occurred most often in early grief. Anger and depression gradually decreased over time. Acceptance increased at 15 to 17 months following the death, but around the 2-year anniversary of the death, acceptance decreased while depression and yearning increased.

Stage Theories of Grief   table 28-4

Theorist	Stages	Examples of Nursing Interventions
Bowlby	1. Numbness/protest 2. Yearning 3. Disorganization and despair 4. Reorganization	• Be nonjudgmental; avoid arguing. • Use active listening as bereaved talks about the deceased. • Assess for depressed mood and for safety. • Recognize strengths, progress.
Kubler-Ross	1. Denial 2. Anger 3. Bargaining 4. Depression 5. Acceptance	• Avoid contradicting the patient who rejects the loss. • Model calmness, encourage safe expression of anger. • Use active listening. • Refer if symptoms suggest major depression. • Recognize coping efforts.
Worden	1. Accept the reality of the loss. 2. Experience the pain of grief. 3. Adjust to an environment in which the deceased is missing. 4. Withdraw from the lost relationship and reinvest energy in new relationships.	• Confirm the reality of the situation at a pace consistent with awareness of the bereaved. • Show empathy and compassion. • Encourage self-care and problem-solving. • Use active listening.

Based on Bowlby, J. (1980). Attachment and loss. In *The Making and Breaking of Affectional Bonds*, Vol. 3. New York, NY: Tavistock; Kubler-Ross, E. (1969). *On Death and Dying*. New York: Simon & Schuster; Worden, J. W. (1991). *Grief Counseling and Grief Therapy: A Handbook for the Mental Health Practitioner*. London, UK: Routledge.

Evidence Refuting Stage Theory

Stage theory has been criticized because it does not provide a definite path to healthy outcomes. Holman, Perisho, Edwards, and Mlakar (2010) have questioned the relevance of stages of grief when there are so many exceptions to the predictability. Holland and Neimeyer (2010) found that all the emotions associated with stages occurred simultaneously throughout the first 2 years after a death, although the proportions of one emotion or another changed with time. For example, an individual may feel anger at any stage of grief but will probably experience more anger early in grief and less anger 1 year later.

Sometimes, those who are grieving move in and out of stages, seemingly repeating previous reactions to the loss. Although grief generally decreases over time, suffering intensifies when reminders (such as birthdays, anniversaries, and holidays) occur. Reminders serve to focus attention on the loss. The second anniversary of a death is considered particularly difficult for some because the numbness is gone and the support received during the first year may have decreased. Holland and Neimeyer (2010) found that distress peaked at 24 months. By then, supportive persons often assume that the bereaved is feeling better and may worry that to initiate conversation about the deceased will cause suffering rather than comfort the bereaved. Sometimes the bereaved misunderstands the silence and concludes that others have forgotten and no longer care.

Comprehensive Framework

Stroebe, Folkman, Hansson, and Schut (2006) developed a framework to guide research and practice that helps explain why some people have positive outcomes of grief (returning to previous or better physical and mental health and functioning) and others suffer negative consequences, such as prolonged periods of being unable to function or declining physical health. This framework can be used to better predict who is at greatest risk.

Bereavement is characterized by *loss-oriented* and *restoration-oriented* processes (Stroebe, Folkman, Hansson, & Schut, 2006; Hansson & Stroebe, 2007). Loss-oriented processes encompass the psychological responses to loss, such as sadness and suffering, whereas restoration processes involve making accommodations to the new situation. Risk factors increase the likelihood of poor outcomes, whereas other factors are protective.

Loss-Related Risk and Protective Factors

Risk factors that may predict negative outcomes following death include untimely death, violent death, multiple simultaneous losses, and other concurrent stressors such as financial and legal problems. Losses that may accumulate following the death of a loved one include loss of income and loss of independence. Any circumstance that did not include theses additional challenges would be protective.

Interpersonal Risk and Protective Factors

According to Stroebe, Folkman, Hansson, and Schut (2006), relationships play an important role in health outcomes of bereavement. Stressful family dynamics, such as an abusive family dynamic, and lack of social support are risk factors, whereas having sufficient social support is a protective factor.

Intrapersonal Risk and Protective Factors

Characteristics of the individual can increase or decrease grief intensity and its effects on mental and physical health. Examples of intrapersonal risk factors include previous psychiatric diagnosis and current substance abuse. An unrealistic perception of the loss is another example of an intrapersonal risk factor. Distorting the facts of the event may place the individual at risk. An example might be that the bereaved believes that a death resulted from "foul play" when all the evidence supports that it was an accident. Protective factors include a realistic perception of the loss, optimism, intelligence, and resiliency.

Early in bereavement, loss-oriented processes dominate, but with the passage of time restoration processes are more evident. Although this model is comprehensive in that it includes the physical, psychological, and social aspects of the person who is grieving, this model leaves many questions unanswered. For example, it does not address the extent to which age may or may not influence grief outcomes.

Individual Responses to Loss

Both interpersonal and intrapersonal factors help to determine an individual's response to loss. Interpersonal factors include the quality of a person's relationships with others, which helps determine the quality of support available. When the patient has loving relationships, these supportive others may provide practical support (such as relieving the patient of responsibilities), as well as emotional support and/or empathy. Intrapersonal factors involve personal characteristics such as resilience and coping ability. Resilient individuals typically possess a sense of meaning or purpose and active coping skills (Burton, Pakenham, & Brown, 2010). They are also generally able to respond to adversity without compromising mental or physical health.

Cognitive Responses

In the first few hours or days following a significant loss, the individual is forced to begin the process of adjusting to the life-changing event. At first, individuals may report disbelief and no emotional pain. Although this reaction is often referred to as *denial*, it is not a conscious choice to disbelieve. Disbelief is expected to take a few hours or days, but it can take much longer (Bonanno & Kaltman, 2001).

Patients may describe feeling changed in a fundamental way ("part of me is missing") and complain that they are confused, which may manifest in statements such as "I can't think," "I'm having trouble concentrating," and "I can't make decisions." Temporarily, the bereaved individual may not be able to function at work or care for family members as he or she did before the loss. For most people, this confusion improves over the first year of grief. Some individuals will not feel any cognitive changes at all, but there is no evidence that this is unhealthy (Bonanno & Kaltman, 2001).

Emotional Responses

Grief involves a range of emotions (such as ambivalence, anger, loneliness, longing, and despair) (Bonanno & Kaltman, 2001). Grief is part of an active process in which the bereaved copes with the stress of loss, namely grief work (Livingston, 2010). A common feeling in grief is prolonged dysphoria (depressed mood). Most grieving individuals feel some depressed mood in the first year, especially in the first 2 months. The dysphoria may be accompanied by anxiety, anger, and irritability. Some individuals will be at risk for serious depression. In their study of 280 bereaved caregivers 3 months following the loss of a loved one to cancer, Holtslander and McMillan (2011) found that one-third met criteria for clinical depression. About 24% of the caregivers reported significant problems with physical or psychological functioning. Those with previous impaired coping or psychiatric illness were at greater risk of adverse outcomes of grief.

Loneliness (sense of aloneness) and yearning for what or who was lost are also components of early grief. Those who are grieving often feel a sense of isolation or that no one else can completely understand their suffering (Bonanno & Kaltman, 2001). Although yearning cannot bring back the person, it is part of the grief process that can help grieving individuals gain a sense of control over their lives. A sense of control also can be derived from setting goals and making choices (Duggleby, Williams, Wright, & Bollinger, 2009).

Grieving is frequently accompanied by ambivalence or mixed feelings about the deceased or the death itself. Hallberg, Óskarsdóttir, and Klingber (2010) found that parents of a child diagnosed with an anomaly felt both relief and sorrow. They were relieved to discover what was wrong, but sorrowful about their child's condition. A widow also may feel relief that her husband is no longer suffering, along with sadness that his life ended too soon. With more complicated relationships, such as that of a child with an abusive parent, the bereaved may be unsure how to respond or may have conflicting emotional reactions, such as anger and longing concurrently.

Behavioral Responses

A range of behavioral responses is possible during intense grief. Some are common, such as crying, withdrawal, and reaching out for support, whereas others (such as violence) are less common (Bonanno & Kaltman, 2001). Crying is an almost universal response to loss. Many believe that crying is beneficial in resolving grief, but in some cultures people have been taught to avoid crying, especially in public. In other cultures, crying is expected as evidence of the love between the bereaved and the deceased. Nurses should avoid judging others by whether or not they cry after a loss.

Searching for the loved one is not unusual. The bereaved may visit the place where the death occurred or search a crowd for the face of the person they lost. Other ways of dealing with the loss include setting a place at the table for the deceased or "forgetting" that they will not be coming to dinner. Some choose to keep the deceased's room just the way it was before the death occurred. These behaviors do not necessarily indicate a pathological response, but they may need to be examined in relation to the amount of time passed and the degree of the grieving individual's impairment in functioning.

Temporary avoidance coping is not uncommon following a significant loss and may involve suppressing feelings of distress, avoiding reminders of the deceased, and refusing to discuss the loss. Avoiding reminders of the loss is common because they bring the pain of the loss into focus. Some people cannot look at pictures of the deceased or even at family members who look like the deceased. Others refuse to discuss the loss. Giving away the deceased's belongings can be very painful, and the bereaved may delay this for a long period of time. There is no reason to do it quickly, and it may not be advisable for the bereaved to make major decisions while experiencing confusion and bewilderment soon after the death of a close family member. Avoidance coping is not necessarily associated with negative outcomes, especially when used to manage daily challenges soon after death of a loved one. In one study, college students who experienced loss used a variety of coping strategies, including problem-focused, emotion-focused, active, and avoidant methods; the type of coping method was not related to degree of distress (Schnider, Elhai, & Gray, 2007).

Distancing oneself from pain is self-protective and allows the individual some time to take in the events that precipitated the loss. At this stage, it is most helpful to accept the patient's reality and be supportive as gradual awareness increases. It is best if nurses

and other health care professionals avoid trying to influence the bereaved to let go of "denial" and "face" the loss. As discussed earlier, the impact of the loss can be delayed months—and, in some cases, even years. Factors associated with delayed or diminished reactions include urgent responsibilities (for example, pregnancy) that make it difficult to focus on the loss and the need to protect oneself from emotional upheaval. The resilient individual may experience muted feelings of distress because of prior experience with loss, an adequate support system, and healthy pre-loss coping mechanisms.

Extreme anger and despair can lead to violence (either as self-harm or as violence against others). Individuals who blame someone for the death may seek revenge. Those with a history of violence are most at risk for future violence.

Nurses can help the bereaved find hope. Duggleby, Williams, Wright, and Bollinger (2009) conducted a qualitative study of caregivers of patients with dementia and found that hope for a positive future could be found even when a loved one's health is deteriorating. Using interviews, the researchers asked caregivers about their experience of hope. Caregivers remained hopeful about the future but focused attention on specific aspects, such as hope that they would be able to continue care for their family member with dementia. They also looked for positives in their everyday lives such as having someone to call for support, "seeing possibilities," and having choices. They described gradually "coming to terms" with their loss (Duggleby, Williams, Wright, & Bollinger, 2009, pp. 518–519).

Sociocultural Domain

Grief is usually acknowledged by society. Outward manifestations of grief—especially rituals and customs, such as wearing black—are referred to as **mourning**. Rituals or activities of mourning exist to support grieving family members and friends (the mourners) in these difficult times. Rituals and activities that recognize the suffering that follows loss, especially death, include visiting with those who are grieving, organizing religious or nonreligious rituals, and taking on the bereaved's responsibilities (such as driving children to school) temporarily. Grief rituals are determined by culture, religion, and tradition (Figure 28-2). According to Hardy-Bougere (2008), individuals from different cultural groups do not differ in response to grief on

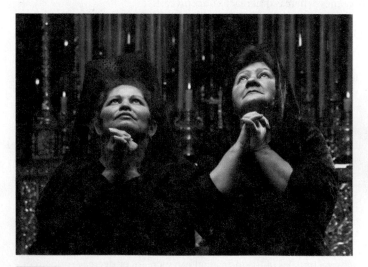

28-2 Mourning practices, including funeral customs and dress, vary among cultures.

Source: Juanmonino/iStock/Getty Images

an emotional level, but they do differ in bereavement practices, traditions, and rituals. Individuals from all cultures can be expected to experience the same suffering and anguish with accompanying psychological and biological responses after a significant loss. Bereavement is influenced by beliefs about death, suffering, and loss. Expression of emotion and interpretation of emotion by others also is affected by culture. Some cultural groups are more expressive, whereas others are taught to be reserved, emphasize the positive, and not to complain.

Cultural traditions determine how the body should be handled after death, whether autopsy is an option, whether the deceased should be buried or cremated, and when this should occur. Social rituals, such as funerals, are part of culture and tradition and help reduce uncertainty and ease the pain of loss. Nurses should be familiar with the cultural practices of groups in their practice environment; however, each person is unique and there may be wide variation between persons within a particular cultural group. *Acculturation*, the adoption of the practices of the prevailing society or culture, is one factor that accounts for differences. For example, an individual from a minority ethnic group may have adopted the traditions and values of the majority culture to the point at which the individual's grief practices are very similar to those of the dominant mainstream culture. Others may retain their cultural grief practices, especially if they continue to live in close contact with members of their cultural or ethnic group.

Grief-Related Cultural Traditions

Most nurses experience the opportunity to work with grieving patients and their family members. In addition to a basic understanding of cultural traditions of grief, as discussed here, nurses should have a more specific understanding of practices that are common in their area. As stated above, individual practices and preferences may vary.

African American Culture

African Americans are those who were born in the United States and trace their heritage to Africa. They share the historical trauma of slavery. African Americans are generally supported by both their nuclear and extended families. Spiritual beliefs are very important, and a spiritual advisor can be a strong source of comfort. Belief in life after death also fosters hope of meeting the loved one again in the future. Communication with health care professionals may be hampered by distrust rooted in the history of racial discrimination and in both real and perceived disparities related to access to quality health care. African American patients and family members may be more expressive when sharing their grief with others of similar cultural backgrounds.

Afro-Caribbeans trace their heritage to the Caribbean Islands and originally to Africa. Although their skin color is similar to that of African Americans, they may not consider themselves African Americans. They are more likely to be immigrants with cultural traditions from their country of origin. Immigrants adopt mainstream American culture to different degrees but many are bicultural, having adopted American culture while retaining the traditions and values of their heritage culture. Family and religion are central to Afro-Caribbean culture. Death traditions in the Caribbean Islands are diverse, influenced by African culture; the religion and culture of the European colonists; and contemporary religions, including Catholicism, Islam, and Hinduism. Decisions about burial or cremation, the length of time before burial, and death rituals are determined by religious traditions. Death is followed by a period of public mourning characterized by surrounding the bereaved with support, including extended community support for the family. Maintaining a relationship with the deceased is advocated, and the relationship continues by treasuring pictures and other reminders (Marshall & Sutherland, 2008).

Asian American Culture

Chinese Americans trace their origins to China or Taiwan. Their cultural beliefs and traditions are influenced by "ancestor worship, Taoism, Confucianism, Buddhism and traditional Chinese medicine" (Hsu, O'Connor, & Lee, 2009, p. 153). Connectedness with nature and the central role of family in all aspects of life are emphasized. Discussing death is considered bad luck, and the Chinese value prolonging life. Dying at home is important to maintain their connection with their ancestors. Behavior is based on values such as *propriety,* meaning loyalty to family and friends while respecting elders and place in society. *Filial piety* means obedience to parents and taking responsibility for the care of aged parents. *Jen* means loving other people. *I* means that individuals should be caring and benevolent to others. *Chun tzu* refers to the value placed on pursuing spiritual development. For many Asian Americans, care of the dying includes "bland food," a peaceful environment, and having freedom from fear and isolation during the dying process (Hsu, O'Connor, & Lee, 2009). Traditional Chinese medicine can be used to provide palliative care. Families will often accept a mixture of Western and Chinese medicine to prolong life.

Hispanic American Culture

Hispanics are a large and diverse group who trace their heritage to Spanish-speaking countries such as Mexico, South and Central America, and Cuba. They share certain values that can guide behavior surrounding bereavement. Those who are more recent immigrants will probably conform to these values more than others who are acculturated. Values and traditions that guide social behavior for Hispanics include the following:

- *Respeto:* Social conventions, respect for authority.
- *Familism:* Valuing the family over individual needs, turning to family, rather than "outsiders," for support.
- *Simpatia:* Maintaining harmonious relationships with others.
- *Hembrism:* Female determination and ability to withstand life challenges.
- *Machismo:* Men are the decision makers who support the family.
- *Personalismo:* Friendly, warm and personal relationships are expected; health care providers who are reserved may seem uncaring.
- *Fatalismo:* Little can be done to change fate.

Examples of how these values can be applied in care of the bereaved include understanding that a woman is likely to defer decisions to the oldest male family member. Aspects of therapeutic communication that may help establish rapport with Hispanic patients include showing friendliness and interest in the family on a personal level. In addition, Hispanic patients may be more comfortable with therapeutic touch than other patients.

Grief Responses and Gender

Men and women often remark that they grieve differently. These differences can lead to misunderstandings and conflict in families when one spouse or family member assumes that the other is not grieving properly or at all. In many societies, men are expected to deny their grief publicly and to be supportive to family members who are grieving. The "breadwinner" may feel an obligation to resume work responsibilities as soon as possible because survival of the family depends on it (McCreight, 2004). Females may also use patterns of grieving that are more often associated with "male" grieving, such as appearing "strong," keeping busy, and using stoicism, whereas men may be very expressive and grieve in ways that are associated with the stereotypical response of women. Americans thought Jackie Kennedy's stoic public response to President Kennedy's assassination was praiseworthy, thus revealing mainstream cultural preferences for emotional reserve in grief.

Women are at higher risk for depression, and girls seem to be affected by loss more than boys (Little et al., 2009). Little et al. studied children (mostly adolescents) who had suffered parental death in the past 9 to 10 months. Girls recovered from feelings of depression and anxiety more slowly than boys, but age did not make a difference. Girls had a greater sense of threat and abandonment and felt the loss of support more acutely than boys. Compared with boys, girls also ruminated about the loss and had more negative thoughts in response to stressors.

Men are deeply affected by loss. Although they may be more apt to intellectualize their grief, return to work early in the grief process, and keep busy, their suffering is no less real. McCreight (2004) studied men who experienced loss related to pregnancy and described the loss as having affected their whole life. They felt unprepared to cope and blamed themselves. They were less likely to receive support and felt the pressure to appear "strong" and to avoid crying in front of their partners.

Expression of grief is influenced by culture, learning, and personality. "Being strong" for others may delay grief reactions but does not eliminate feelings of grief. Some individuals are able to turn their attention away from the loss when necessary in order to carry out essential responsibilities. Nurses must use caution in interpreting patients' behavior.

Spiritual Domain

Spiritual distress is common in those who grieve. Patients and family members may question their beliefs in light of a death or serious illness. Some may reject their previous beliefs, whereas others find strength from religious groups and rituals. Every loss calls for an answer to the question, "Why did this happen?" Other related questions include, "Why did this happen now?" and "Why did it happen to me or to my family member [and not someone else]?" Some question whether the loss was "deserved" or "punishment" for past behavior. Others struggle to understand how something so horrible could happen if there is a loving God. The theme of the "unfairness" of life is common in spiritual distress.

Survivor guilt occurs when one person survives and another dies and the survivor is burdened by guilt about living, asking questions such as "Why not me?" Survivor guilt is a common reaction. In an accident or a disaster, for example, survivors may question whether their actions or the failure to act could have changed the outcome. When a child dies, parents and grandparents may ask themselves why they did not die in place of the child. Nurses can support survivors and educate them that survivor guilt is normal.

Individuals must come to their own explanations and answer the question *Why?* The role of the nurse is to listen and to teach that this questioning is normal. When someone dies by suicide, the bereaved family and friends may experience shame and guilt over what they did or did not do. When the bereaved feels responsible for the loss, whether real or perceived, overwhelming guilt can result in intense suffering. Nurses can ease this suffering by providing patient and family education, listening carefully, promoting communication, and providing referrals for counseling and other resources. See the Nursing Management section for more information on nursing interventions.

Pause and Reflect

1. *What grief responses have you noticed in friends or family? What types of support or activities did they find helpful or comforting?*

2. *If you found yourself working in a community with, say, a large Buddhist population, where would you go to find out more about mourning and funeral practices?*

3. *How do you think you would handle working with a patient experiencing spiritual distress? What is important to keep in mind when caring for patients in spiritual distress?*

Collaborative Care

Nurses work with other health professionals to provide optimal care. In situations of loss related to medical illness or injury, it is common to work with physicians to provide information about the patient and to support the patient and family and to help them understand information and access resources. In addition, clergy may offer comfort and help the patient to find meaning. A referral to a spiritual advisor is indicated if the patient agrees (Rosenbaum, Smith, & Zollfrank, 2011). Communication is essential in understanding what the individual and family know and what their informational needs are. In some cases, social workers, physical therapists, occupational therapists, and other health care providers also will be involved, and a coordinated plan is needed. Social workers have knowledge and experience with counseling, working with families, and linking patients and families to other financial and health resources.

Only a small proportion of bereaved patients will experience clinical depression. Referral to a mental health specialist for antidepressant medication may be warranted when symptoms include prolonged insomnia, severe weight loss, or suicidal ideation (Box 28-2). A referral to a social worker, advanced practice nurse, or clinical psychologist for brief psychotherapy may also offer relief from depression. Patients should be encouraged to make an informed decision about the type of intervention they feel most comfortable with. A combination of antidepressant medication and psychotherapy has been shown to be the most effective treatment for depression.

Nursing Management

The nursing process provides a framework for the nurse to provide comprehensive care to patients experiencing loss and grief.

Assessment

Assessment of the patient experiencing grief and loss is multifaceted. It includes assessing for risk and protective factors, including the

Medication and Grief

box 28-2

Bereaved individuals often seek out health care providers for relief from suffering related to loss. Physical responses to grief, such as lack of appetite, can be a threat to health if significant weight loss (more than 10% weight loss from baseline) results (Rigler et al., 2001). Psychological responses such as anxiety and despair are responsible for much of the suffering that the bereaved experiences. Those who are experiencing persistent depressed mood, self-hatred, or apathy should be evaluated by a mental health specialist for possible treatment of depression. Health care providers who are not mental health specialists may be more likely to prescribe medications that become problematic when overused. Benzodiazepines can bring short-term relief from anxiety but are habit forming, lose effectiveness when used continuously for more than 30 days, and may eventually interfere with normal sleep patterns (Voyer, Roussel, Berbiche, & Preville, 2010). Heavy use of benzodiazepines may block the emotions associated with grief but, when compared with placebo, Warner,

Metcalfe, and King (2001) did not find any relationship between use of benzodiazepines and course of grieving over 6 months following loss.

Antidepressant medication combined with cognitive–behavioral therapy has been found to be very effective in treating depression. Antidepressants relieve symptoms of depression such as hopelessness, helplessness, insomnia, anxiety, and anorexia and do not cause dependence (Widera & Block, 2012). Selective serotonin-reuptake inhibitors (SSRIs) and selective serotonin–norepinephrine-reuptake inhibitors (SNRIs) are also effective in managing chronic anxiety. Bereaved individuals who are depressed may be reluctant to take antidepressant medications because they have been misinformed about their effects. They may have been told that these medications will prolong grief, prevent them from grieving, be addictive, or even block feelings completely. Nurses can educate them about what they can realistically expect. Antidepressants can decrease feelings of despair and apathy, but will not eliminate suffering.

---

patient's perception of the event, coping skills, role functioning, anxiety level, and support system. Listening to the patient's story about the loss will help the nurse obtain information about strengths and vulnerabilities. Strengths include a stable emotional state, social supports, healthy coping skills, and access to health care. Vulnerabilities include previous history of depression, recent situational stressors (for example, job loss, moving), insufficient or unstable support systems, financial constraints and lack of insurance, a history of self-destructive behaviors, and less than a high school education level (Figure 28-3).

Verbal Responses to Loss

By assessing patient statements related to loss and grief, the nurse can gain information about the patient's thought processes and current functioning in social roles (Table 28-5). As in any patient interaction, the nurse uses therapeutic communication to validate the patient's feelings and establish rapport.

Assessment Across the Domains

Assess biological functioning. Ask the patient about biological symptoms, such as loss of appetite and insomnia. Note changes in vital signs (blood pressure, pulse, and respirations) that might indicate anxiety. Ask about constipation, as it may accompany psychomotor retardation.

Assess psychological functioning. Ask the patient about coping strategies and note unhealthy coping, such as alcohol or substance abuse, overspending, gambling, and other addictive behaviors. Assessment should include mood, suicidal ideation, anxiety level, and psychomotor behavior (agitation or retardation). Does the patient display anger or irritation, flat affect, depressed mood, apathy, tearfulness? Determine the patient's general level of functioning.

Assess sociocultural and spiritual functioning. Ascertain the patient and family's beliefs and preferences so that cultural and religious traditions and rituals can be incorporated. Note the presence of

---

Mrs. Colton Recovery Phase

APPLICATION

1. What personal strengths and resources do you notice in Mrs. Colton and her family?

2. Was her grief response unusual? What factors do you think contributed to her grief response?

3. Why do you think Mrs. Colton was placed on citalopram (Celexa)?

4. What is the risk of relapse?

A few weeks later, Mrs. Colton is hospitalized in a psychiatric unit in a general hospital because she has persistent thoughts of suicide and has discussed her suicide plan with her husband. She is placed on suicide precautions and started on the SSRI citalopram (Celexa), 20 mg tablet by mouth daily. After attending daily individual sessions for several days with the psychiatric nurse practitioner and group sessions led by the social worker, Mrs. Colton is no longer suicidal; discharge planning includes a family visit. The psychiatric nurse practitioner meets with the family and Mrs. Colton together. Her sons are distressed at the loss of their mother's involvement in their lives, as well as the loss of their sibling. Her husband remains concerned and supportive while suppressing his own suffering. Plans are made for Mrs. Colton to return home the following day and to continue taking her medicine. Her husband and sons agree to help with responsibilities at home and to hire assistance with housecleaning. Mrs. Colton calls her employer to inform him that she will be returning to work the following week but she will need time off to attend appointments with her therapist.

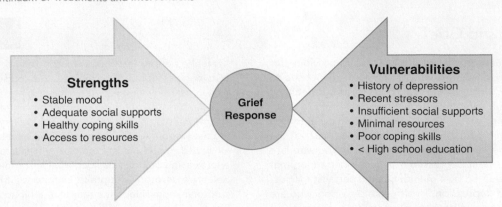

Strengths
- Stable mood
- Adequate social supports
- Healthy coping skills
- Access to resources

Grief Response

Vulnerabilities
- History of depression
- Recent stressors
- Insufficient social supports
- Minimal resources
- Poor coping skills
- < High school education

28-3 An individual's strengths and vulnerabilities may affect the grief response.

guilt, anger at God or a Higher Power, questioning past beliefs, or struggling with the question of "Why?"

Diagnosis and Planning

A number of nursing diagnoses may be relevant when working with patients and families who have experienced significant loss, including, but not limited to:

Sleep Pattern, Disturbed

Sorrow, Chronic

Spiritual Distress (and Risk for Spiritual Distress)

Coping: Family, Compromised

Denial, Ineffective

(NANDA-I © 2014)

Planning effective care for patients and families who are suffering includes eliciting their thoughts and preferences and incorporating cultural and religious preferences. Although it is possible to make some generalizations about prioritizing care, it is important to find out what matters most directly from those involved. A concern such as finding someone to pick up a child at school may be the first priority for the patient at that moment. Provide information as needed, encourage collaboration, come to know the patient as a person, teach the patient and family about the grief process, and support the patient and family in obtaining additional social support and access to clergy or other spiritual resources.

Implementation

Nurses caring for patients and families experiencing loss and grief provide patient and family education and therapeutic communication

Grief Responses and Patient Verbalizations   table 28-5

Common Responses to Loss	Patient Statements	Nurse Responses
Shock, disbelief	• "I can't believe it." • "I don't feel anything." • "Everything seems unreal." • "I am the only one who feels this bad." • "I'm me on the outside, but I'm dying on the inside."	*Validate feelings:* • "It *is* hard to believe."
Anger, irritability, helplessness, rage	• "Get away from me!" • "I don't want your help." • "You don't understand!"	*Provide acceptance:* • "It's understandable to be angry. Many people in your situation would be angry."
Anxiety, worry, panic	• "I'm falling apart." • "I'm going crazy." • "I'm dying." • "Help me!"	*Provide information:* • "Your feelings are normal. I will stay with you until your [mother] arrives."
Guilt, remorse, regrets, survivor guilt	• "I should have called!" • "I should have been there." • "Why didn't I…?" • "I wish it were me."	*Present reality:* • "You did your best at the time. You would have done anything to help, if you knew your [child] needed you."
Spiritual confusion, questioning past beliefs, rejecting religion/God, turning to religion/God	• "Why did this happen to me?" • "How could God let this happen?" • "What does this mean?"	*Encourage meaning-making:* • "What are your beliefs about spirituality?"

Disabling Communication

box 28-3

There are several ways that the nurse can block communication or disable the patient's ability to participate. It is essential that nurses avoid using these strategies, which impede the development of the therapeutic nurse–patient relationship.

Reassuring: "Everything will be OK." Because the nurse cannot know the future, this statement lacks veracity and fails to acknowledge that everything is not "OK" now.

Minimizing: "Everyone goes through this." Such an extreme statement is unlikely to be true, but even if it were true, it does not console the person who is experiencing it now.

Rationalizing: "Your loved one is in a better place." Imposing one's beliefs on the patient blocks further communication and conveys lack of support.

Making false assumptions: "I know just how you feel." Everyone is different, and this assumption is disrespectful of the uniqueness of that person. Another statement that offers a false assumption is "You will get through this." Loss is not "time-bound"; therefore, there will never be a time when the patient is "over it." Grieving is a process that may last a lifetime. The individual may or may not achieve the same level of functioning as before the loss.

Making comparisons: "I've been through this, too; my grandmother died last year." Nurses must avoid comparing their own past losses with the patient's, as the patient may not believe that the losses are equivalent at all. Avoid comparing any loss with any other loss. Sometimes it is assumed that the intensity of grief is related to the length of the relationship, when it is actually unrelated. For example, two parents may each experience the loss of children who were different ages when they died. The parents' grief is not influenced by how long their relationship was or the age of the child. Also, the suddenness of loss does not influence grieving; parents who have had months or years to prepare for the death of a child may experience the same grief intensity as parents whose child died suddenly. Parents whose child was ill may say that they were still shocked when the death finally occurred. Note that their loss involves grieving for the child as well as the loss of their role as caregivers.

---

skills, such as active listening and facilitative communication. Nurses also take care not to communicate in ways that thwart the therapeutic process (Box 28-3). Because patients who experience loss are at higher risk for depression, supportive nursing interventions include offering hope. The nurse has many opportunities to offer hope by challenging patients' negative thinking. Statements by the bereaved such as "It's all my fault" need to be compared to the reality that the patient did the best he or she could under the circumstances. Countering dysfunctional thinking ("I am never going to feel better") with more positive thoughts ("I can feel better if I work at it") is one strategy that nurses can teach patients to practice. Other opportunities include hope that the dying person will receive sufficient pain relief, and the bereaved will be able to find meaning from the loss (Rosenbaum, Smith, & Zollfrank, 2011). Nurses can respect the spiritual beliefs of their patients and families who maintain hope (for example, hope for a miracle, the healing power of prayer, or in life after death) even if they do not share those beliefs.

Patient and Family Education

Patients may have limited knowledge about grief. They may believe that everyone progresses through predictable stages within a certain time frame. Explain that grieving is not always predictable. Patients may be concerned when a family member returns to work soon after a loss and seems to experience less distress than expected. Such behavior may be the cause of concern and presents an opportunity for teaching about individual responses to grief. Another misunderstanding is that emotions must be expressed for healing to take place. Patients may encourage a family member to express grief verbally even when that person may prefer nonverbal expressions or may even continue to deny a loss. Sometimes conflict arises when two members of a family grieve differently and do not understand each other. There is no right or wrong grief response, and there is a lack of research evidence to show an association between lack of expression and negative psychiatric outcomes (Holman, Perisho, Edwards, & Mlakar, 2010).

The patient and supportive others need information about factors that may further strain the bereaved individual's capacity to cope. Teaching about multiple losses and cumulative loss can help the patient and family to better understand why a current loss may have disabling effects. Multiple losses challenge coping abilities because several losses occurring simultaneously may overwhelm coping abilities when any one alone might not. Cumulative loss is challenging because one loss after another occurs sequentially with insufficient time for return to a previous level of functioning between losses.

Commonly, those who have experienced profound loss report increased suffering around anniversary dates. Some may hold memorial events in recognition of the significance of these important dates. For example, memorial services are organized to acknowledge the significance of losses associated with the terrorist attacks of September 11, as well as losses remembered on days such as Veterans Day. Nurses can prepare family members and the patient about the possibility that anniversaries may trigger increased sadness and anxiety. Teach the patient and family to prepare for an anniversary, such as a deceased's birthday or date of death, so they can take an active part in coping with a difficult time. Nurses can teach patients and families that rituals to honor and memorialize the deceased can be helpful in diminishing suffering.

Some patients will express the feeling that they are "going crazy," and statements such as these provide an opportunity to educate about grief and to normalize the experience. Cognitive symptoms that are common but disturbing include feeling confused, indecisive, or preoccupied with some aspect of the loss. Emotions such as profound sadness or rage may be outside the griever's previous experience and may feel pathological. All these experiences may contribute to a sense of being "out of control." Patients who experience severe grief for the first time will benefit from knowing that these feelings are not unusual and do not in themselves indicate an abnormal response. Patients can be taught to direct their attention away from troubling memories with distraction and by substituting problem-solving activities, such as reaching out to teachers, clergy, counselors, friends, and other family members for support.

Information about risk factors, such as lack of support or previous depression, may help family members understand the importance of active involvement at this time. The nurse can offer hope by explaining that for most people, grief becomes less painful with support from family and friends. Giving the patient the chance to share the wisdom and personal meaning that often comes from living with sadness and grief will be a comfort. Encourage the patient and family to think about a way to create a lasting legacy to continue the work or priorities of the person they wish to honor. Common choices include establishing scholarships or awards, planting trees, or establishing fundraising or volunteer activities to honor the person who died. Plans and activities linked to the future are comforting because they keep the memories of that person alive.

Patient and family education includes providing information about and referral to additional resources. Nurses should be aware of community resources, such as grief support groups and grief counselors. Knowing resources that are free of charge is important so patients with limited financial resources and insurance can access community support. Churches, synagogues, and other places of worship often run grief support groups that are open to everyone regardless of religious affiliation.

The Compassionate Friends is a global organization to support bereaved parents, grandparents, and siblings. The Compassionate Friends is made up of local chapters that offer support groups and other community events, such as a candle-lighting ceremony every December to honor the deceased during the holiday season. Another example of grief resources that are available is Grief Share. Patients who are unable to attend a support group in person or who feel uncomfortable in social situations may benefit from blogging or participating in online chats (see Evidence-Based Practice: Programs for Patients Suffering from Loss).

Programs for Patients Suffering from Loss　　　evidence-based practice

Clinical Problem

Individuals in a variety of clinical settings may have insufficient access to support at times of grief. Grief support programs are led by volunteers, staff nurses, specially trained mental health professionals, and others. Nurses are challenged to find creative ways to provide support to patients and to fellow nurses in the fast-paced environment of most health care settings.

Evidence

Aho et al. (2011) tested a program for fathers grieving the death of a young child following hospitalization using a quasi-experimental design. Fathers in the intervention group (n = 62) received peer support and support from a health care professional (usually the nurse) for 2 to 6 weeks in addition to usual care. Those in the control group (n = 41) received the usual care in the form of written educational materials. The intervention group members met with a peer and a health care professional at least once, but many had several meetings. They were educated about grief and coping and encouraged to share their feelings. Those who received support reported greater personal growth than fathers in the usual care group. The intervention group credited contact with nurses as most beneficial.

Smartwood et al. conducted an analysis of an online grief support group using a rating scale that categorized responses into one of four categories "self-disclosure, influence, self-involving, or advice" (2011, p. 161). The researchers wanted to know how participants helped one another online and whether a different type of support was used for specific losses such as sibling or spousal loss. They analyzed 564 postings from a variety of web sites. Most of the postings were about child loss. In all types of loss, most of the postings (66%) consisted of self-disclosure, followed by influence in which the participant tried to change someone's beliefs or attitudes. Next in frequency were self-involving and advice. The researchers also used the qualitative method of constant comparison to analyze themes in the responses. The themes included "telling one's story" (Smartwood et al., 2011, p. 172), in which participants offered hope to others by sharing their personal stories of living through the death of a significant person in their life. The next theme was "validating the grief experience" (p. 172), or using their own experiences with grief to demonstrate to new grievers that they were not alone and their responses were expected. This theme included "giving permission" to do what they needed to do even if it was contrary to the advice of others (p. 173). "Offering resources" was the third theme. This involved sharing information about the grieving process or other sources of help and support online or in the community. The final theme, "offering social support," consisted of participants offering compassionate responses to others who had described their losses.

Using a qualitative design, Michaelson, Blehart, Hochberg, and James (2013) studied the responses of health care professionals (mostly nurses) to a program involving bereavement photography called "memories held," used following the death of 39 children in a pediatric intensive care unit. If parents consented, a professional photographer photographed the children after death so that parents could memorialize their children in a tangible way. Nurses stated that they benefited from the intervention because it provided a way for them to engage with parents in a supportive way and allowed nurses to reflect on their own feelings. Offering the photographs gave them a way to "do" something for the family when care of the child was no longer needed. At a time when nurses often feel helpless and defeated, they had a way to preserve memories and relate to the families on an emotional level.

Implications for Nursing Practice

These studies support the position that a variety of different interventions may offer support to individuals who are grieving, including nurses who experience the death of a patient. Both in-person and online support groups seem to offer helpful support and validation to individuals who are grieving. To help patients access these resources, nurses must be cognizant of the supports available in their area and be aware of current Internet resources for individuals who are grieving.

Critical Thinking Questions

1. Have you ever participated in a support group? In what ways was it helpful? Not helpful?
2. What are the barriers to participation in a support group?
3. What risks might be involved in participating in an online grief support group? What criteria might nurses suggest patients use when seeking resources on the Internet?

Active Listening

Active listening is a skill that is vitally important to facilitate communication with grieving patients. Active listening involves using therapeutic techniques such as encouraging continuation of the conversation with phrases such as "Uh-huh" or "Go on." Reflecting feelings, paraphrasing, and using silence are all part of active listening. By providing support with active listening, nurses are able to hear the patient's story of loss, uncover any cognitive distortions ("This is all my fault") or destructive emotions (self-hatred) and help the patient to examine and question the thoughts and feelings that interfere with coping.

Facilitative Communication

In addition to active listening, facilitative communication is a therapeutic tool that helps nurses communicate and support patients and family members who are grieving. Asking open-ended questions, using therapeutic presence, and other similar interventions can help the bereaved communicate about the loss and will provide a wealth of information for the nurse.

For example, asking general questions such as, "What do you think caused the accident?" is the type of question that encourages elaboration and allows the nurse to listen for cognitive distortions, such as "I shouldn't have gotten angry at him before he left for work." Using therapeutic presence helps the nurse focus calm attention on the patient in the here-and-now rather than on his or her own inner thoughts, with the intention of accepting and being open to the patient (McCollum & Gehart, 2010).

Interactions do not have to be filled with conversation. Waiting quietly in silence encourages the other to talk and conveys caring. Providing therapeutic communication also includes conveying value and respect for those who are grieving. In a study of families following loss of a loved one in intensive care, Lautrette et al. (2007) found that standardized communication could make an important difference in decreasing depression and stress in family members 90 days after the loss. They recommended using the VALUE mnemonic:

Value caregiver and family statements.

Acknowledge emotions.

Listen to family members.

Understand who the patient is as a person.

Elicit questions from family members.

As always, communication must be tailored to the developmental stage of the patient and family members.

No one can easily judge the significance of another person's loss, and significance is important to explaining grief intensity. Even when the nurse has experienced a loss that seems similar, the nurse should avoid claiming, "I know how it feels." Every relationship and circumstance is different and can influence an individual's response to death or any loss. Assuming that you "know" what another is experiencing communicates disrespect for the uniqueness of every person's experience and may result in greater feelings of isolation in the bereaved who does not believe that anyone "understands." It is better for the nurse to convey support and try to understand the loss from the patient's perspective.

Preventing Relapse

Patients who experience depression triggered by loss will need additional interventions. For patients who are hospitalized, the nurse has opportunities for patient and family education to prevent relapse. Topics for education include the importance of continuing to take antidepressants even after the patient feels better, keeping follow-up appointments, the importance of community support groups, and early signs and symptoms of relapse.

Early signs of relapse may include sleep difficulties recurring after improvement, increased anxiety, and withdrawal from relationships and activities that were previously enjoyed. Day programs can help transition the individual from inpatient to outpatient care and provide additional opportunities for nursing interventions. Family meetings are a useful tool to gain insight into patients' ability to resume responsibilities and to interact with family members.

Self-Awareness

Disenfranchised grief often is experienced by health care providers and professional caregivers who are expected to be "strong" and to hide their own distress. Spidell et al. (2011) surveyed 577 chaplains who worked in health care, using quantitative and qualitative questions. All had experience with grief following death of a patient. Their reactions ranged from anger to sadness to social withdrawal and fatigue. Nurses need to examine their own emotional responses to grief. Recent losses, similar experiences, and prolonged care of the patient may all contribute to detrimental responses to loss. Unexamined grief can be detrimental to patient care when it leads to avoidance, emotional distancing, and unmet patient and family needs.

Nurses are exposed to a number of emotional risks when caring for patients who are suffering (Perrin, Sheehan, Potter, & Kazanowski, 2012). Because nursing involves building meaningful relationships with patients, it is understandable for the nurse to grieve when a patient dies. Emotional risks include disappointment or guilt about perceived inadequate care they provided. Nurses expect themselves to project calmness in a crisis, provide errorless care, and to be emotionally available to patients whenever needed. They "bear witness" (p. 249) by fully appreciating the suffering patients experience and acting on that knowledge to reduce suffering. In their review of the literature on nurses' suffering, Perrin et al. wrote that nurses sometimes expressed suffering in the form of complaining or other types of hostility.

McGrath (2011) advises nurses to take steps to deal with emotional suffering, including talking about emotional responses, crying with co-workers, reflecting on the relationship with the patient and the impact of the patient's suffering on the nurse, and, if possible, taking a break from patient care. Reflecting on memories of the patient and family, attending memorial services, and attending a grief support group also may be helpful.

If nurses do not acknowledge and face their painful emotions, they may withdraw emotionally and become less effective, or they may displace their painful emotions, leading to anger at home or in relationships with co-workers. Both in and outside the work environment, nurses can seek support for grief on a one-to-one basis from confidants or professionals. In some cases, support groups may be more helpful. In specialties in which facing death is part of the nurse's role (such as hospice care), it may be very useful to organize a system of peer support.

Pause and Reflect

Ask yourself:

1. *How have I responded to loss in the past? Do I currently have any unresolved losses?*

2. *How do I feel and react when I am around others who are grieving?*

3. *What are some strategies I can use to promote communication with patients who are grieving?*

Mrs. Colton—The Patient Who Is Grieving		NURSING CARE PLAN

Nursing Diagnosis: Risk for complicated grieving related to the loss of her son as evidenced by diminished participation in family life and work symptoms of anxiety and depression, and persistent thoughts of suicide

Short-Term Goals *Patient will:* (include time frame for short-term goal to be met)	Intervention *Nurse will:*	Rationale
Verbalize her understanding and meaning of loss(es) during the first interview.	Use therapeutic communication, such as offering of self and using open-ended questions to help Mrs. Colton articulate the meaning of her losses. Educate the patient about loss and grief.	Clarifying meaning of loss with Mrs. Colton can be helpful as she tries to continue her life without her son Jeff. Helping Mrs. Colton understand that individuals grieve differently can remove expectations she may have about how her grieving "should" take place.
Identify two constructive coping mechanisms by the second meeting.	Ask about previous losses and what helped Mrs. Colton to cope with those losses. Suggest books, journaling, support groups, helping others, and doing special things for herself and with others. Explore Mrs. Colton's belief system and values. Incorporate positive connections into her care.	Using skills that helped in the past can be comforting and provide familiarity. Introducing some new skills may be necessary and healing as well.
Sign a written safety agreement to notify nurse when she experiences thoughts of self-destructive behavior.	While in the hospital, provide protection as necessary, such as 1-to-1 supervision, safety agreements/safety contracts, high visual areas for Mrs. Colton.	Protecting Mrs. Colton during a time of high stress and intense depression may be necessary to prevent self-harm.
Identify two sources of support, such as from family, mental health specialists, faith/religion, and/or grief support groups by second session.	Provide information about resources; work with Mrs. Colton to access resources.	Ensuring that Mrs. Colton stays connected with a support network is one of the most helpful strategies to assist Mrs. Colton to move forward and heal through her loss.
Adhere to medication prescription of citalopram (Celexa) 20 mg PO daily.	Inform Mrs. Colton of indications for medication, side-effect profile, importance of not discontinuing the medication without conferring with her prescriber due to potential worsening of symptoms, and not taking with St. John's wort to prevent serotonin syndrome. Also work with Mrs. Colton on timing of medication, as it affects individuals differently (for example, she may need to take it at night if it makes her sleepy).	Providing patient education about medications may promote adherence and prevent adverse interactions.
Long-Term Goal The patient will return to a more normal level of functioning as evidenced by her return to participation in family and work activities and reduced symptoms of anxiety and depression.	Discuss plans to increase involvement in family and work activities.	Having an objective person to process her plans may help Mrs. Colton return to a more normal routine at home and work.

Clinical Reasoning

1. What other nursing diagnoses might the nurse working with Mrs. Colton consider?
2. What are some additional constructive coping mechanisms that might be helpful to Mrs. Colton? How would you begin to try to discuss those with her?
3. How do you feel about Mrs. Colton's situation? How might you provide hope for Mrs. Colton?

Evaluation

To determine the effectiveness of interventions, nurses can evaluate the patient's affect, physical well-being (for example, sleep and appetite), behavior, verbalizations, role functioning, and family concerns using observation, interviewing, and other clinical assessments. Patients can be asked to evaluate their own progress. If suicidal ideation had been a concern, patients should be asked directly whether they are having thoughts of harming themselves. Outcomes that indicate decreased suffering include decreased anxiety, improved mood, improved sleep quality, improved social and emotional functioning, decreased physical symptoms, strengthening of relationships, finding purpose in the loss, and assigning meaning for the loss. Nurses can use reliable and valid clinical tools to measure symptoms at admission and to monitor progress. For example, sleep quality can be measured at admission and then weekly to note improvement. For more information on assessing sleep, please see Chapter 12.

From Suffering to Hope

A common reaction by those who come in contact with the bereaved person is to decrease the discomfort for nurse and patient as soon as possible with reassurances such as "everything will be OK," which would be premature or untrue. It is important for the nurse to remember that the human response to loss is grief. Suffering is expected and must be acknowledged. Nurses convey hope by acknowledging suffering, providing education about the grieving process, and mobilizing help and support from immediate family and the health care system for those who need it.

Chapter Highlights

1. Grief is a normal human response to loss.
2. Loss occurs in a wide variety of situations, such as separation, injury, illness, and natural disasters, and as a result of life changes.
3. All loss leads to grief that is similar in form but differs in intensity and is unique to the individual.
4. Normal grief may be all-consuming and accompanied by intense suffering.
5. It is important to identify the significance of loss to an individual, as that determines its intensity to the individual.
6. Grief usually becomes more manageable over time.
7. Resolution of loss can lead to personal growth.
8. Patient education, active listening, and facilitative communication are strategies nurses use to provide care for individuals and families who are grieving.

NCLEX®-RN Questions

1. The nurse is assessing a patient for factors contributing to a grief response. Which would the nurse recognize as being an intangible loss?
   a. Marriage ending in divorce
   b. Moving out of a childhood home
   c. Recent unemployment
   d. Feelings of insecurity following a traumatic event

2. The nurse is working with the parent of a child with a disability; the child requires ongoing support and intervention. The parent reveals struggling with anger and sadness that has not decreased in intensity since the child was born several years ago. The nurse understands that the parent is likely to be suffering from which type of grief or sorrow?
   a. Chronic
   b. Ambiguous
   c. Anticipatory
   d. Disenfranchised

3. The nurse is assessing a patient who has just experienced a significant loss. Which question is likely to elicit the best information related to functional status?
   a. "How have you been coping?"
   b. "Are you currently employed?"
   c. "Who do you rely on for help?"
   d. "How do you make sense of this loss?"

4. The nurse is evaluating the progress of a patient who has suffered the loss of a pregnancy. Which finding would be most concerning?
   a. The patient is acting strong to avoid upsetting her spouse.
   b. The patient expresses feeling defective, worthless, and hopeless.
   c. The patient reports that waves of grief occur 1 month after the loss.
   d. The patient is weepy and unable to concentrate 1 week following the loss.

5. The nurse is planning care for the adolescent who has experienced the death of a parent. The nurse recognizes that which aspect of development may complicate the adolescent's grief response?
   a. An exaggerated sense of shame
   b. Feelings of isolation from others
   c. Tendency to view the loss as a punishment
   d. Inability to appreciate the permanence of the loss

6. The nurse is applying techniques of therapeutic communication with the significant other of a patient who has died. The patient is angry and asks the nurse to leave the room, stating, "If you people knew what you were doing, this never would have happened." Which type of nursing response is most appropriate?
   a. Acceptance
   b. Information
   c. Meaning making
   d. Reality orientation

7. The nurse is evaluating the effectiveness of interventions aimed at addressing spiritual distress in a patient who has experienced a significant loss. Which finding best indicates resolution of the distress?
   a. The patient recognizes that she is not to blame.
   b. The patient acknowledges the cause of the distress.
   c. The patient carries out religious activities and rituals.
   d. The patient identifies a positive purpose related to the loss.

8. The nurse is applying principles of grief to build self-awareness of the impact of caring for patients and families experiencing loss. Which does the nurse recognize as having the potential to be detrimental to patients and families?
   a. Expressing feelings to co-workers
   b. Providing uninterrupted care
   c. Examining feelings related to loss
   d. Participating in memorial services

Answers may be found on the Pearson student resource site: nursing.pearsonhighered.com

References

Aho, A. L., Marja-Terttu, T., Astedt-Kurki, P. M., Sorvari, L., & Kaunonen, M. (2011). Evaluating a bereavement follow-up intervention for grieving fathers and their experiences of support after the death of a child-A pilot study. *Death Studies, 35*(10), 879–904.

American Psychiatric Association. (2011). *DSM-5 Development: Adjustment Disorders.* http://www.dsm5.org/ProposedRevisions/Pages/proposedrevision.aspx?rid5367

Balk, D. (2011). Adolescent development and bereavement: An introduction. *The Prevention Researcher, 18*(3), 3–9.

Beckie, T. M. (2012). A systematic review of allostatic load, health, and health disparities. *Biological Research for Nursing, 14*(4), 311–346.

Bennett, K. M., Smith, P. T., & Hughes, G. M. (2005). Coping, depressive feelings and gender differences in late life widowhood. *Aging & Mental Health, 9,* 348–353.

Berns, N. (2011). *Closure: The Rush to End Grief and What It Costs Us.* Philadelphia, PA: Temple University Press.

Bonanno, G. A., & Kaltman, S. (2001). The varieties of grief experience. *Clinical Psychology Review, 21*(5), 705–734.

Boss, P., & Carnes, D. (2012). The myth of closure. *Family Process, 51,* 456–469.

Bowlby, J. (1961). Childhood mourning and its implications for psychiatry. *American Journal of Psychiatry, 18,* 481–498.

Bowlby, J. (1980). Attachment and loss. In *The Making and Breaking of Affectional Bonds,* Vol. 3. New York, NY: Tavistock.

Burton, N. W., Pakenham, K.I., & Brown, W. J. (2010). Feasibility and effectiveness of psychosocial resilience training: A pilot study of the READY program. *Psychology, Health and Medicine, 15*(3), 266–277.

Buysse, D. J., Reynolds, C. F., Monk, T. H., Berman, S. R., & Kupfer, D. J. (1998). The Pittsburgh Sleep Quality Index: A new instrument for psychiatric practice and research. *Psychiatry Research, 28*(2), 193–213.

Coombs, M. A. (2010). The mourning before: Can anticipatory grief theory inform family care in adult ICU? *International Journal of Palliative Nursing, 16*(12), 580–584.

Duggleby, W., Williams, A., Wright, K., & Bollinger, S. (2009). Renewing everyday hope: The hope experience of family caregivers of persons with dementia. *Issues in Mental Health Nursing, 30,* 514–521.

Epstein, R., Kalus, C., & Berger, M. (2006). The continuing bond of the bereaved towards the deceased and adjustment to loss. *Mortality, 11*(3), 253–279.

Frankl, V. E. (1963). *Man's Search For Meaning: An Introduction to Logotherapy.* New York, NY: Simon & Schuster.

Freud, S. (1917). Mourning and melancholia. In J. Strachey, (Ed.). *The Standard Edition of the Complete Psychological Works of Sigmund Freud, 14,* 242–258. London, UK: Hogarth Press.

Freud, S. (1919). On transience. In J. Strachey, (Ed.) *The Standard Edition of the Complete Psychological Works of Sigmund Freud,* Vol. 14. London, UK: Hogarth, 1957.

Freud, S. (1953). Premonitory dreams fulfilled. In J. Strachey, (Ed.). *The Standard Edition of the Complete Psychological Works of Sigmund Freud,* Vol. 5. London, UK: Hogarth, 1957.

Fulton, G., Madden, C., & Minichiello, V. (1996). The social construction of anticipatory grief. *Social Science and Medicine, 43*(9), 1349–1358.

Futterman, E., Hoffman, I., & Sabashin, M. (1972). Parental anticipatory mourning. In B. Schoenberg, A. C. Carr, D. Peretz, & A. H. Kutscher, (Eds.). *Psychosocial Aspects of Terminal Care.* New York, NY: Columbia University Press.

Geulayov, G., Gunnell, D., Holmen, T. L., & Metcalfe, C. (2011). The association of parental fatal and non-fatal suicidal behavior with offspring suicidal behavior and depression: A systematic review and meta-analysis. *Psychological Medicine, 42*(8), 1–14.

Gilbert, R. B. (2004). Aging and loss. *Illness, Crisis & Loss, 12*(3), 199–211.

Goodenough, B., Drew, D., Higgins, S., et al. (2004). Bereavement outcomes for parents who lose a child to cancer: Are place of death and sex of parent associated with differences in psychological functioning? *Psycho-Oncology, 13*(11), 779–791.

Gordon, J. (2009). An evidence-based approach for supporting parents experiencing chronic sorrow. *Pediatric Nursing, 35*(2), 115-119.

Hagman, G. (2001). Beyond decathexis: Towards a new psychoanalytic understanding and treatment of mourning. In R. A. Neimeyer, (Ed.). *Meaning Reconstruction and the Experience of Loss.*Washington, DC: American Psychological Association, pp. 13–31.

Hallberg, U., Óskarsdóttir, S., & Klingber, G. (2010). 22q11 deletion syndrome—the meaning of a diagnosis. A qualitative study on parental perspectives. *Child: Care, Health and Development, 36*(5), 719–725.

Hames, C. C. (2003). Helping infants and toddlers when a family member dies. *Journal of Hospice and Palliative Nursing, 5*(2), 103–112.

Hansson, R. O., & Stroebe, M. S. (2007). *Bereavement in Late Life: Coping, Adaptation, and Developmental Influences.* Washington, DC: American Psychological Association.

Hardy-Bougere, M. (2008). Cultural manifestations of grief and bereavement: A clinical perspective. *Journal of Cultural Diversity, 15*(2), 66–69.

Hogan, N. S., & Schmidt, L. A. (2002). Testing the Grief to Personal Growth Model using structured equation modeling. *Death Studies, 26,* 615–634.

Holland, J., & Neimeyer, R. A. (2010). An examination of stage theory of grief among individuals bereaved by natural and violent causes: A meaning-oriented contribution. *OMEGA, 61*(2), 103–120.

Holman, E. A., Perisho, J., Edwards, A., & Mlakar, N. (2010). The myths of coping with loss in undergraduate psychiatric nursing books. *Research in Nursing and Health, 33*(6), 486–499.

Holtslander, L. F., & McMillan, S. C. (2011). Depressive symptoms, grief, and complicated grief among family caregivers of patients with advanced cancer three months into bereavement. *Oncology Nursing Forum, 38*(1), 60–65.

Hsu, C. Y., O'Connor, M., & Lee, S. (2009). Understandings of death and dying for people of Chinese origin. *Death Studies, 33*(2), 153–174.

Hung, N., & Rabin, L. (2009). Comprehending childhood bereavement by parental suicide: A critical review of research on outcomes, grief processes, and interventions. *Death Studies, 33*(9), 781–814.

Kehl, K. A. (2005). Recognition and support of anticipatory mourning. *Journal of Hospice Palliative Care Nursing, 7*(4), 208–210.

Kowalski, S., & Bondmass, M. (2008). Physiological and psychological symptoms of grief in widows. *Research in Nursing and Health, 31*(1), 23–30.

Kubler-Ross, E. (1969). *On Death and Dying: What the Dying Have to Teach Doctors, Nurses, Clergy, and Their Own Families.* New York, NY: Simon & Schuster.

Kwong, M. J., & Bartholomew, K. (2011). "Not just a dog": An attachment perspective on relationships with assistance dogs. *Attachment and Human Development, 13*(5), 421–436.

Laditka, J. N., & Laditka, S. B. (2003). Increased hospitalization risk for recently widowed older women and protective effects of social contacts. *Journal of Women and Aging, 15*(2–3), 7–28.

LaTour, K. (2010). Getting through survivor guilt. *CURE: Cancer Updates, Research & Education, 9*(3), 58–61.

Lautrette, A., Darmon, M., Megabane, B., Joly, L., et al. (2007). A communication strategy and brochure for relatives of patients dying in the ICU. *New England Journal of Medicine, 356*(5), 469–480.

Lindemann, E. (1976). Grief and grief management: Some reflections. *Journal of Pastoral Care, 30*(3), 198–207.

Little, M., Sandler, I. N., Wolchik, S. A., Tein, J., & Ayers, T. S. (2009). Comparing cognitive, relational and stress mechanisms underlying gender differences in recovery from bereavement-related internalizing problems. *Journal of Clinical Child and Adolescent Psychology, 38*(4), 486–500.

Livingston, K. (2010). Opportunities for mourning when grief is disenfranchised: Descendants of Nazi perpetrators in dialogue with Holocaust survivors. *Omega: Journal of Death and Dying, 61*(3), 205–222.

Marshall, R., & Sutherland, P. (2008). The social relations of bereavement in the Caribbean. *OMEGA, 57*(1), 21–34.

McCollum, E., & Gehart, D. (2010). Using mindfulness meditation to teach beginning therapists therapeutic presence: A qualitative study. *Journal of Marital & Family Therapy, 36*(3), 347–360.

McCreight, B. S. (2004). A grief ignored: Narratives of pregnancy loss from a male perspective. *Sociology of Health and Illness, 26*(3)S, 326–350.

McGrath, J. M. (2011). Neonatal nurses: What about their grief and loss? *Journal of Perinatal and Neonatal Nursing, 25*(1), 8–9.

Michaelson, K. N., Blehart, K., Hochberg, T., & James, K. (2013). Bereavement photography for children: Program development and healthcare professionals' response. *Death Studies, 37*(6), 513–528.

Neimeyer, R. A. (Ed.). (2001). *Meaning Reconstruction and the Experience of Loss.* Washington, DC: American Psychological Association.

Nerken, I. R. (1993). Grief and the reflective self: Toward a clearer model of loss resolution and growth. *Death Studies, 17*(1), 1726.

Ott, C., Kelber, S., & Blaylock, M. (2010). "Easing the way" for spouse caregivers of individuals with dementia: A pilot feasibility study of a grief intervention. *Research in Gerontological Nursing, 3*(2), 89–99.

Ott, C., Sanders, S., & Kelber, S. T. (2007). Grief and personal growth experience of spouses and adult-child caregivers of individuals with Alzheimer's disease and related dementias. *The Gerontologist, 47*(6), 798–809.

Patricelli, K. (2012). Symptoms of grief. Available at http://sevencounties.org/poc/view_doc.php?type=doc&id=12001&cn=174

Perrin, K. O. (2012). The nurse as witness to suffering. In K. O. Perrin, C. A. Sheehan, M. L. Potter, & M. K. Kazanowski, (Eds.). *Palliative Care Nursing: Caring for Suffering Patients.* Sudbury, MA: Jones & Bartlett, pp. 247–275.

Perrin, K. O., Sheehan, C. A., Potter, M. L., & Kazanowski, M. K. (Eds.). (2012). *Palliative Care Nursing: Caring for Suffering Patients.* Sudbury, MA: Jones & Bartlett.

Pierrehumbert, B., Torrisi, R., Ansermet, F., Borghini, A., & Halfon, O. (2012). Adult attachment representations predict cortisol and oxytocin responses to stress. *Attachment and Human Development, 14*(5), 453–476.

Pruessner, J. C., Dedovic, K., Pruessner, M., Lord, C., Buss, C., Collins, L., & Lupien, S.J. (2010). Stress regulation in the central nervous system: Evidence from structural and functional neuroimaging studies in human populations. *Psychoneuroendocrinology, 35,* 171–191.

Rigler, S., Webb, M., Redford, L., Brown, E., Zhou, J., & Wallace, D. (2001). Weight outcomes among antidepressant users in nursing facilities. *Journal of the American Geriatrics Society, 49*(1), 49–55.

Rosenbaum, J. L., Smith, J. R., & Zollfrank, R. (2011). Neonatal end-of-life spiritual support. *Journal of Perinatal & Neonatal Nursing, 25*(1), 61–69.

Sanders, S., Marwit, S. J., Meuser, T. M., & Harrington, P. (2007). Caregiver grief in end-stage dementia: Using the Marwit and Meuser Caregiver Grief Inventory for assessment and intervention in social work practice. *Social Work Health Care, 46*(1), 47–65.

Schnider, K. R., Elhai, J. D., & Gray, M. J. (2007). Coping style use predicts post-traumatic stress and complicated grief symptom severity among college students reporting a traumatic loss. *Journal of Counseling Psychology, 54*(3), 344–350.

Shah, S., & Meeks, S. (2012). Late-life bereavement and complicated grief: A proposed comprehensive framework. *Aging & Mental Health, 16*(1), 39–56.

Shear, M. K., McLaughlin, K. A., Ghesquiere, A., Gruber, M. J., Sampson, N. A., & Kessler, R.C. (2011a). Complicated grief associated with hurricane Katrina. *Depression and Anxiety, 28*(8), 648–657. doi: 10.1002/da.20865

Shear, M. K., Simon, N., Wall, M., Zisook, S., Niemeyer, R., Duan, N., et al. (2011b). Complicated grief and related bereavement issues for DSM-5. *Depression and Anxiety, 28*(2), 103–117.

Smartwood, R. M., Veach, P., Kuhne, J., Lee, H., & Ji, K. (2011). Surviving grief: An analysis of the exchange of hope in online grief communities. *Omega: Journal of Death and Dying, 63*(2), 161–181.

Spidell, S., Wallace, A., Carmack, C. L., Nogueras-Gonzalez, G. M., Parker, C. L., & Cantor, S. B. (2011). Grief in healthcare chaplains: An investigation of the presence of disenfranchised grief. *Journal of Health Care Chaplaincy, 17*(1/2), 75–86.

Steeves, R. H. (2002). The rhythms of bereavement. *Family and Community Health, 25*(1), 1–10.

Stroebe, M., Folkman, S., Hansson, R., & Schut, H. (2006). The prediction of bereavement outcome: Development of an integrative risk factor. *Social Science and Medicine, 63*(9), 2440–2451.

Voyer, P., Roussel, M. E., Berbiche, D., & Preville, M. (2010). Effectively detect dependence on benzodiazepines among community-dwelling seniors by asking only two questions. *Journal of Psychiatric and Mental Health Nursing, 17*(4), 328–334.

Warner, J., Metcalfe, C., & King, M. (2001). Evaluating the use of benzodiazepines following recent bereavement. *British Journal of Psychiatry, 178,* J36–J41.

Widera, E. W., & Block, S.D. (2012). Managing grief and depression at the end of life. *American Family Physician, 86*(3), 259–264.

Wilson, S. C., & Supiano, K. P. (2011). Experiences of veterans' widows following conjugal bereavement: A qualitative analysis. *Journal of Women and Aging, 23*(1), 77–93.

Worden, J. W. (1991). *Grief Counseling and Grief Therapy: A Handbook for the Mental Health Practitioner.* London, UK: Routledge.

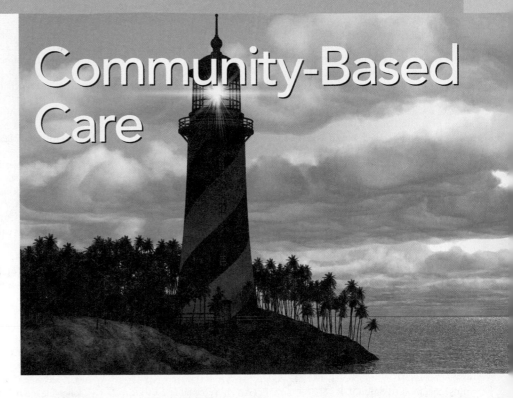

29

Community-Based Care

Mary White Kudless

Key Terms

Learning Outcomes

1. Describe the role of the psychiatric nurse and other members of the community-based interprofessional team in promoting successful person-centered recovery outcomes.

2. Describe community-based, recovery-oriented psychiatric nursing care.

3. Identify specific case management and rehabilitation treatment strategies available in the community.

4. Evaluate case management and rehabilitation treatment strategies in relationship to stages of wellness from initial onset/relapse to recovery and rehabilitation.

5. Create a wellness-focused community nursing plan that incorporates the goals, needs, and preferences of the individual in relation to treatment, housing, employment, access to medical care, and available resources.

Gavin Initial Onset

APPLICATION

1. You are the nurse who interviews Gavin when his parents bring him to the crisis center. Based on the information presented in this scenario, how will you prioritize his care? Why?

2. How will you address the goal of creating a sense of safety and trust for Gavin in your initial assessment?

3. Gavin is from a family of physicians, and his goal of practicing medicine is important to him. How do you think Gavin might view taking a leave of absence from school? What will you say to convey a sense of hopefulness about the future to Gavin?

Gavin Williamston is a 20-year-old man who was an outstanding high school student. He was accepted into the college of his choice with a partial scholarship, and envisioned a career as a pediatrician, joining his father's medical practice in the future. Gavin enrolled in all the required science courses for the pre-medicine track and received good grades in his freshman year. In his sophomore year, Gavin told his parents that he was having difficulty managing his time and found himself up all night, preparing for exams. When he attempted to sleep, he found that he would experience ruminative thoughts that he was not as gifted as his classmates and was bound for failure.

Gavin's roommate, Paul, contacted Gavin's parents before the holiday break, and reported that Gavin was missing class, not eating, and beginning to neglect his personal appearance. Paul told them that Gavin walked the streets for many hours on end and that he recently had been "roughed up" by some young people at a local bar. The police who responded to the bar incident returned Gavin to the dormitory, and expressed concerns that Gavin might be "hearing voices," which led to the misunderstanding at the bar. Paul told the police that he would get in touch with Gavin's parents and try to get him to a mental health evaluation during the semester break, which starts the next day.

Gavin's parents are shocked to see Gavin's unkempt and haggard physical appearance and find that they are unable to calm him or reassure him about his future. Because Gavin's uncle developed schizophrenia in his early 20s and eventually committed suicide, Gavin's parents worry that Gavin may also be developing schizophrenia. On the recommendation of their family doctor, they bring Gavin to the local community mental health center's 24/7 emergency service for an evaluation.

The psychiatric nurse on duty conducts the assessment, gathering information from both Gavin and his parents regarding his symptoms and recent events. As part of this assessment, she conducts a mental status exam and obtains information about Gavin's medical and family history. Gavin tells the nurse that he has been drinking alcohol heavily for the past several months. His parents report that Gavin developed juvenile diabetes at age 11 and that his blood sugar has not been well controlled since he began college. Gavin states that there really is nothing wrong with his thinking. Although he is frightened by the voices he is hearing, he states that he also counts on them for direction about what he should be doing. The nurse concludes that Gavin is experiencing symptoms of a thought disorder, including auditory hallucinations, self-deprecating thoughts, a severe sleep disturbance, weight loss, and anxiety. Gavin denies homicidal or suicidal ideation, but admits to feelings of inadequacy and heavy use of alcohol since the start of the school year. The nurse gives the information to the psychiatrist, who formulates a preliminary diagnosis of schizoaffective disorder (Chapter 17).

Given the severity of Gavin's distress level, the nurse and the consulting psychiatrist recommend that Gavin take a leave of absence from school and enter the adult partial hospitalization program (PHP) that is available at the community mental health center. This recommendation is grounded in the potential of the PHP to offer Gavin daily contact with treatment. The care plan will include cognitive–behavioral treatment through supportive individual and group counseling, family support, medication, and a range of modalities, including educational groups for help with learning about his probable mental health condition and his abuse of alcohol. The initial goal will be to support Gavin in gaining an understanding of his mental health condition and to obtain measurable relief from his symptoms.

This daily level of support is recommended as an alternative to admission to a psychiatric inpatient hospital. The registered nurse knows that a psychiatric hospitalization is an option for Gavin, if his symptoms should worsen and if needed, that can be promptly facilitated by the PHP treatment team. Medication also is prescribed, and Gavin and his family are advised about the intended effects and side effects and potential challenges to adherence. Further, Gavin is provided with educational information about psychiatric illness and his suspected diagnosis of schizoaffective illness, and his parents are referred to the local National Alliance on Mental Illness (NAMI) family support and education group. The nurse initiates recovery-oriented care by offering hope to Gavin and his parents and reassures them that they will obtain the help and information that they need to gain an understanding of the nature of the difficulties that Gavin is experiencing. She explains that they will be asked to participate in a collaboratively developed treatment plan to restore Gavin to an improved level of mental and physical health. She prepares them for some of the challenges that Gavin might anticipate in entering treatment and in learning to manage distressing symptoms.

Introduction

Long-term recovery from mental illness no longer takes place in the hospital setting. Hospitals today provide brief stay environments, used primarily to stabilize acute medical and psychiatric illnesses. The real work of recovery from mental illness occurs in the individual's own community, incorporating the person's natural supports and building on each individual's strengths and assets. The range of mental health resources varies greatly, and the quantity and quality of available services can greatly influence the outcomes for a person with a psychiatric illness. Communities have used private, federal, state, and local resources to build behavioral health outpatient systems of care. These systems focus on the treatment and recovery of persons who experience serious mental illness and substance use disorders. Many also provide the case management and rehabilitation supports needed by another population—those with intellectual disabilities. **Case management** is a process of coordinating and ensuring the provision of a range of services to meet the various and complex needs of individuals with mental illness. There are excellent public and private recovery-oriented systems of care, but funding constraints and high demand can limit timely access to assessments and services.

A critical success factor for individuals with serious mental illness is engagement with providers who support self-determination and the principles of recovery and rehabilitation. This includes the philosophy of a "life like yours and mine"—that is, a life that includes the relief and management of psychiatric symptoms, a desirable living situation, friendships, school or employment, spiritual engagement, access to the arts and entertainment, and financial stability.

Community-based care models are increasingly biological/psychological/sociological/cultural in their orientation. Nurses are key members of interprofessional teams who support the recovery of individuals who experience mental illness and those who struggle with the co-occurring disorders of mental illness and substance abuse. Nurses contribute to recovery-oriented treatment and rehabilitation plans by demonstrating knowledge and the ability to work collaboratively with the individual, attending to cultural differences, and using the evidence-based community practices described in this chapter. Nurses incorporate these approaches into the therapeutic relationships they develop with individuals who are living with and recovering from the symptoms of mental illness and the impairments in role functioning and quality of life that often occur.

Psychiatric nurses bring unique skills to community practice settings, given their focus on patient strengths and their understanding of the biological factors that underlie any illness. They perform in the full role of the psychiatric–mental health nurse in mental health and addiction centers, detoxification units, emergency rooms, day support and rehabilitation programs, residential treatment, correctional settings, public and private outpatient practices, intake and assessment units, and intensive case management teams, such as assertive community treatment (ACT). Psychiatric nurses must acquire knowledge about the range of psychiatric illnesses and mental health disorders that people experience, including biological and neurobiological factors.

Kudless and White (2007) summarized the nursing interventions performed by community mental health nurses across community-based treatment programs:

- Comprehensive psychosocial assessments
- Group, individual, and family treatment (e.g., education, counseling, psychotherapy)
- Monitoring of patients in recovery in residential and acute care settings for safety and response to treatment and medications
- Pharmacotherapy (including medication education and monitoring medication response)
- Physical assessments to evaluate treatment needs of co-morbid physical illnesses
- Psychoeducation services (e.g., wellness groups, lifestyle enhancement groups, dialectic behavior therapy)
- Risk assessments and mental status examinations
- Treatment disposition determinations
- Treatment of individuals with co-occurring disorders
- Treatment planning
- Case management services (including linking clients to benefits and resources)

Community-based practice settings offer excellent opportunities for the use of a nurse's total education and skills. The community itself offers powerful learning environments and the opportunity to journey with the individual from the point when illness is detected to the point when recovery and a personally satisfying life in the community are realized. It is important that nurses note that the experience of the symptoms of mental illness and, in many instances, the exposure to treatments for mental illness can be quite traumatizing for the person. Nurses seek to ensure safety, while at the same time attempting to limit the person's exposure to experiences or treatment settings that compound psychic and physical stress.

There are several typical entry points or doors into community care. Many of these portals to care are far from ideal in terms of helping individuals with serious mental illness obtain what they need quickly and expertly. Nurses are critical providers in these settings, particularly in assisting patients and families to get linked to appropriate treatment that includes evidence-based recovery and rehabilitation practices such as case management and community-based rehabilitation.

Community Mental Health Entry Points

Patients enter community-based mental health care through many different doors (Figure 29-1). The most frequent entry points include emergency rooms in general hospitals, the crisis services of community mental health centers, primary care practices, private and public outpatient psychiatric practices, medical detoxification and substance abuse treatment programs, school-based counseling centers, and homeless, outreach, and jail-based service systems.

Emergency Departments and Intake Services

The portal of entry (or "front door") for many is the emergency department of their local hospital or community mental health center. Some hospitals have designated psychiatric emergency departments or crisis intervention units that are responsible for screening patients for possible admission. Local public community mental health centers typically offer some system of 24-hour emergency services that provide acute assessments and hospital pre-admission screening services. Depending on the needs of the individual, these assessments result in admission to inpatient psychiatric care or referral to community-based treatment options.

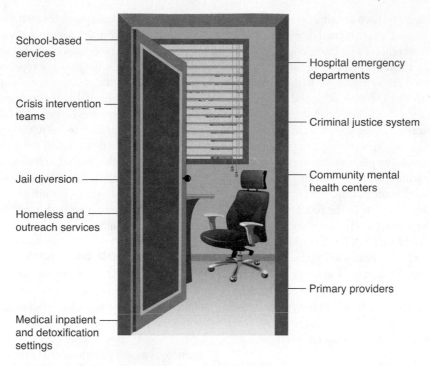

School-based services

Crisis intervention teams

Jail diversion

Homeless and outreach services

Medical inpatient and detoxification settings

Hospital emergency departments

Criminal justice system

Community mental health centers

Primary providers

29-1   Entry points for community mental health intervention and services.

Criminal Justice System

A frequent entry point into community-based treatment is the legal system. This is related to state requirements that dangerousness to self or others is required before an individual can be forced into treatment. Local law enforcement personnel are often called when individuals are experiencing acute mental health symptoms and are in situations in which they are threatening their own life or the safety of others or they may have committed a crime. Recent studies show a very high rate of incarceration for individuals experiencing their first psychiatric illness, especially when that illness manifests in symptoms of mania (Prince, Akincigil, & Bromet, 2007). At least 40% of all psychiatric patients have a history of some form of incarceration related to decreased access to care. When symptoms of mental illness are further exacerbated by substance use disorders, individuals are also more likely to enter through the criminal justice door. Summarizing a multiphase, multiyear research project, Steadman et al. (2009) concluded that the current U.S. rate of serious mental illness for male inmates was 14.5%, and for female inmates it was 31%. A 2006 study by the Bureau of Justice Statistics found that more than half of all jail and prison inmates have mental health issues. Across the United States, approximately 400,000 persons with mental illness are now incarcerated and receiving services in jails and prisons (James & Glaze, 2006).

Many psychiatric nurses are employed as forensic nurses in local jails and state prisons, where they are instrumental in identifying the presence of and the special needs of individuals with mental illness. They work assertively with the judicial system to facilitate proper treatment. Nurses in forensic settings are highly effective in training law enforcement personnel, to recognize mental illness in detention populations, and to make appropriate referrals for evaluation and treatment.

Jail Diversion

The public policy practice of jail diversion is employed by many U.S. communities in an effort to prevent the trauma of incarceration prior

to the diagnosis and treatment of mental illness. **Jail diversion** is a community-based best practice that recognizes the prevalence of symptoms of mental illness in individuals arrested for minor crimes (such as loitering, simple assault, and vagrancy) and seeks to divert them from incarceration to treatment. Often, these crimes occur during a symptomatic episode of illness. Examples of this include the person hearing voices who shouts obscenities on a local bus or the person who carries a knife for fear that others are intent on hurting him.

Jail diversion programs can take many forms, including mental health and alcohol and drug courts, and are outstanding examples of the working partnership among community mental health systems, hospitals, local jails, police and sheriff departments, peer and family advocates, public defenders, judges, and the court system. The goal of these efforts is to limit the potential for persons with mental illness to be jailed for minor offenses and direct or divert them to treatment instead.

The sequential intercept model of jail diversion, as described by Munetz and Griffin (2006), offers a framework for all involved in the intersection of mental illness and criminal justice to help a person get treatment. This approach includes everyone who may possibly interact with the individual, from police to jail personnel, to nurses and mental health providers, to public defenders and judges. Each juncture in the legal process is viewed as a possible "sequential intercept" or intervention point for introducing mental health treatment as an alternative to incarceration. These intercepts start at the point of pre-arrest to booking, to preliminary hearings, to subsequent hearings, and, finally, to planned release.

Crisis Intervention Training for Public Safety Officers

Crisis intervention training, also referred to as crisis intervention teams (CIT), developed initially by the Memphis Police Department in 1988 and adopted by many jurisdictions around the country, is now an internationally regarded approach for improving the success of police interactions with individuals with mental illness. The goal of CIT is to equip law enforcement officers with knowledge about psychiatric disorders and provide them with typical scenarios in which persons who suffer from mental illness may come to their attention. The officers are taught how to best use their skills and authority to assist individuals to obtain mental health assessments and treatment. CIT training programs are excellent examples of the critical nature of collaboration between mental health systems and public safety. Much of the curriculum is taught by peers or consumers (persons with the lived experience of serious mental illness) and family members, in addition to mental health professionals.

A number of high-profile incidents in the past few years have brought increased focus to the interactions between law enforcement personnel and mental illness. NAMI has been working with law enforcement personnel around the country to inform and develop community response protocols through the formation of CIT. This includes rural law enforcement and student resource officers. In addition to providing resources for public safety personnel, NAMI also provides information for individuals with mental illness and their families regarding communicating with law enforcement.

Primary Care Providers

The office of the primary care practitioner (PCP) is another major portal of entry to community-based mental health services. PCPs directly provide approximately 60% of the behavioral health care in our country and are increasingly adding models of collaborative care into their practices, with the hiring of staff with behavioral health expertise.

McDowell, Lineberry, and Bostwick (2011), cite findings from Louoma, Martin, and Pearson (2002), who reported that persons who complete suicide visit primary care physicians more than twice as often as they visit mental health clinicians prior to their death. They summarize numerous research studies that estimate that 45% of persons who ended their life by suicide visited their primary care provider in the month before their death and that internists, pediatricians, and family practice physicians collectively write 62% of the prescriptions for antidepressant medications in our country.

The 2009 U.S. Preventive Services Task Force recommendations no longer promote general depression screening in primary care settings without a collaborative care model in place to support referrals to nurse care managers or other well-trained providers with mental health and addiction treatment expertise who can directly provide or link consumers to needed behavioral health care. The American Academy of Family Physicians (AAFP) has issued a position paper titled "Mental Health Care Services by Family Physicians," which acknowledges the enormous demand for mental health assessment and treatment services in their practices. The AAFP states that "improving the treatment of mental health issues in primary care requires properly organized treatment programs, regular patient follow-up, monitoring of treatment adherence, and the use of mental health specialists for the more severely ill" (AAFP, 2013).

Medical Inpatient and Detoxification Settings

Another common entry point is through referrals from medical–surgical and intensive care units of hospitals when a patient is discovered to have an underlying psychiatric illness during the treatment of the medical condition. If the patient has been admitted to an intensive care unit because of an overdose, nurses will seek an inpatient psychiatric consultation and will work with these recommendations for discharge to appropriate post-hospital treatment. Additionally, medical detoxification units (either free-standing or within a general hospital) are also referral sources to community mental health. The nurses in these units are acutely responsive to the emergence of an underlying psychiatric illness once the offending substance of abuse is detoxified from the patient's body. A careful psychiatric evaluation and referral to community treatment can be a life-saving intervention for individuals who have become medically compromised through a co-morbid medical condition and/or a substance use disorder related to an undiagnosed and untreated underlying psychiatric illness.

School-Based Services

Schools at all grade levels employ various strategies and specialized personnel to identify and treat at-risk youth and young adults. Many of these services are provided by school-based mental health professionals, with high-risk youth typically identified by parents, teachers, and, in some cases, school-based public safety resource officers. Numerous model programs exist across the country that adhere to well-developed assessment and early intervention approaches for identifying students in need of crisis intervention and mental health and substance abuse services. A 2012 survey by the American College Counseling Association found that more than one-third of college students seeking help have severe psychological problems, an increase from 16% in 2000 (Gallagher, 2012). Suicide is the second leading cause of death among college students, according to the Centers for Disease Control and Prevention. Tragic events such as the shootings at Virginia Tech and the movie theater in Aurora, Colorado, have brought national attention to the prevalence of serious psychiatric illness on college campuses and the vital role of student counseling services. Many campuses have developed behavioral intervention teams for early intervention to students at risk, but struggle to keep up with the high demand for services and continue to make many referrals for care to public and private providers in the larger community. It is important to add that only 10% of all homicides in the United States are committed by individuals with mental illness—and the majority of those individuals are off their medications and not engaged in active treatment (Treatment Advocacy Center Backgrounder, 2011).

Homelessness and Outreach Services

Another typical entry point for adults with severe mental illness is through referrals from homeless shelters and outreach programs. Although some of these settings do have mental health expertise on site, most do not and must work diligently to link homeless persons who experience mental illness to treatment and case management.

The National Alliance to End Homelessness (NAEH) reports that some 636,000 people were homeless for some time in 2011 (NAEH, 2012). Numerous forces are at work when an individual or family becomes homeless and ends up living on the street or in a shelter. Since the economic downturn in 2008, unemployment and high rates of home foreclosures have contributed to making a dire situation worse. The Substance Abuse and Mental Health Services Administration (SAMHSA) estimates that 20% to 25% of the homeless population in the United States suffers from some form of severe mental illness. In a 2008 survey of the U.S. Conference of Mayors, the mayors ranked mental illness as the third largest cause of homelessness for single adults in their communities (National Coalition for the Homeless, 2009).

The absence of early and sustained effective treatment and care coordination contributes to the lack of housing for many individuals with mental illness. Psychiatric disorders often appear in young adulthood, when a person's career path and economic security are not yet in place. Poverty levels among persons with psychiatric illness are very high, and even those who qualify for supports, such as Medicaid and Social Security disability, lack sufficient income for even a low-cost rental apartment. Mental illness symptoms can be very debilitating and often undermine the efforts of a person to find, fund, and maintain a safe and stable housing situation. Homelessness is a frequent and tragic outcome of the dual plight of poverty and active symptoms of mental illness.

It is important for nurses to note that it is not necessary for an individual to have good control of the specific symptoms of mental illness to get his or her basic needs met for safety, food, shelter, and income. In the not too distant past, training programs and professional literature suggested that a person should not enter certain programs or housing choices in the absence of sobriety or medication compliance. It is now well understood that these types of exclusionary program criteria can, and do, exacerbate the suffering of people who experience these illnesses. Behavioral and human services professionals must re-examine practices that sustain adverse outcomes (including homelessness) by insisting on treatment compliance or sobriety in the absence of a person's readiness. Consistent with this approach is a nationwide emphasis for "housing first" models in our communities. These programs house people first and build in supports for treatment and recovery in a stage-like manner, as the person demonstrates the readiness to engage.

Ultimately, the preferred approach to initiating community-based treatment and supports starts with a comprehensive assessment at the earliest possible time in the person's experience of symptoms and before longer-term disruption in life functioning can take hold. Homelessness, repeated incarcerations, and hospitalizations are often the result of "too little, too late" responses from the helping community to the magnitude of the needs of persons who present for treatment and support. Nurses need to break down these challenges into manageable pieces with consumers and families by assisting with goal setting, offering sound treatment strategies for the person's consideration, and instilling hope every step of the way.

Pause and Reflect

1. *What would you want police officers and jail personnel to know about serious mental illness? What is the role of law enforcement officers in helping individuals who come to the attention of criminal justice systems to get the care they need?*

2. *What medical detoxification units are available in your area? How are they affiliated with outpatient substance abuse and mental health services?*

3. *What programs in your area serve homeless adults and families? How do they identify persons who need mental health care?*

Evidenced-Based Treatment Strategies

Most communities offer a variety of mental health treatment strategies, based on the concepts of recovery and psychiatric rehabilitation. These interventions are often delivered in the context of programs or services that may include intensive outpatient treatment, PHP or day support and psychosocial rehabilitation programs, case management (CM) services, ACT, peer support services, supported employment, residential and housing supports, and family education. Psychiatric–mental health nurses are involved as mental health service providers in all these programs.

Earlier chapters in this text have described the symptoms and dysfunctions that lead to the psychiatric impairments or disabilities for which a rehabilitation approach can be helpful. The goal of psychiatric rehabilitation is for people to overcome their disabilities so they may achieve their desired goals in life. There is considerable evidence that individuals who experience serious mental illness can and do reach their goals, even while encountering significant symptoms, such as being able to hold down a job while still experiencing auditory hallucinations, taking academic classes while coping with severe levels of anxiety, and maintaining an exercise program in spite of chronic sleep disturbance.

As part of SAMHSA's priority initiative on the behavioral health workforce in primary and specialty care settings, tool kits have been developed that contain information sheets, introductory videos, practice demonstration videos, and training manuals. Currently, five tool kits are available: Assertive Community Treatment, Integrated Treatment for Co-Occurring Disorders (see Evidence-Based Practice: Integrated Treatment for Dual Diagnosis), Supported Employment, Family Psychoeducation, and Illness Management and Recovery. These five practices are core to the skills of the psychiatric nurse in the community. They have demonstrated significant value in supporting the efforts of individuals to gain mastery over the challenges of their mental health conditions and to experience the risks and rewards of moving forward with their personal version of mental health recovery. These programs are available on the SAMHSA website and include manualized programs that registered nurses can implement. The American Psychiatric Nurses Association received a grant from the SAMHSA Recovery to Practice initiative and developed a series of webinars to teach registered nurses the basic concepts of psychiatric recovery and rehabilitation.

Partial Hospitalization Programs

Partial hospitalization programs (PHPs) are intensive, time-limited outpatient programs intended to provide a daily level of support and treatment. PHPs, when they are available, are often used to support a person's mastery over acute symptoms and serve as an alternative to a psychiatric hospitalization or as a "step down" level of treatment following a psychiatric admission. The PHP typically offers cognitive–behavioral treatment in individual and group formats, medications and medication adherence support, social skills training, and symptom management support. There are two common ways to access a PHP. The first occurs in conjunction with discharge from an acute inpatient hospitalization in which it has been determined that the patient needs ongoing support to be able to sustain functioning in the community. The second is by referral from the case manager and

Integrated Treatment for Dual Diagnoses

Clinical Question

Why is it important for communities to offer integrated treatment for the dual diagnoses of mental illness and substance abuse?

Evidence

There is considerable evidence that the addition of a substance use disorder for a person already struggling with symptoms of serious mental illness is a factor that often slows progress and recovery. The National Co-Morbidity Study (Kessler et al., 1996) estimated that as many as 50% of persons who experience serious mental illness also report sufficient symptoms to establish a concurrent, diagnosable substance use disorder. Essentially, all community-based mental health programs and community-based psychiatric nurses must be skilled in assessing and treating these two conditions in an integrated manner. This aspect of treatment is endorsed by SAMHSA (2009).

Corrigan et al. (2008) identified five principles of dual diagnosis care. The first principle is the provision of integrated treatment that combines and individually tailors the mental health and substance abuse interventions for each client. Second is the development of stage-wise treatments that match treatments to the client's level of motivation and stage of recovery. Next is the principle of long-term retention that keeps treatment, rehabilitation, and support available and easily accessible for as long as needed. The fourth principle is the provision of comprehensive services that address all biological, psychological, sociological, cultural, and spiritual areas of the individual's personal recovery. Last is the provision of interventions for people who are not responding to current treatment that provide different approaches for clients who are not making progress toward recovery.

Initial phases of integrated services are geared to client engagement and education regarding the interactive nature of mental illness and substance use/abuse. Integrated dual disorders treatment offers a coherent and helpful framework for treating the "whole person." Integrated treatment should be available in any service arena in the behavioral health system, from the inpatient setting to outpatient care. This framework offers all clients and their service providers concrete tools to move toward recovery, while taking into account the individual's level of motivation and readiness for change. This approach has proven to be the most effective in assisting a person to make the necessary lifestyle modifications, developing an understanding of the potentially dangerous interaction of the two conditions, and learning the new skills needed for a recovery-oriented lifestyle.

Implications for Nursing

Lack of access to integrated services can result in poor treatment outcomes, such as continuing abuse of drugs and alcohol with vulnerability to criminal charges, homelessness, and medical illnesses, including acquired infections, such as HIV and hepatitis C. Psychiatric nurses must be leaders and advocates in assuring that integrated services are in place in their practice settings, relying on the plethora of outstanding training and best-practice materials that are readily available.

Critical Thinking Questions

You are the nurse case manager in a day support program in which 10 of the 16 enrolled patients are struggling with symptoms of both serious mental illness and substance use disorder. You are asked by the team leader to evaluate the program's dual diagnosis treatment capability and to determine whether the program is providing the correct group treatment "menu" to ensure positive outcomes for all participants.

1. How do you go about determining which treatment or educational groups should be offered on the spectrum from early engagement to treatment to relapse prevention?

2. Where would you go to identify evidence-based practices related to group treatment services for individuals with co-occurring serious mental illness and substance use disorder?

3. What client-specific outcomes would inform you that the integrated treatment design is achieving positive recovery outcomes?

---

treatment team when the individual is showing an increase in symptoms and/or a decrease in the ability to function and seeks to avoid a hospitalization. Guidelines for PHPs are provided by the American Association of Ambulatory Care.

Many types of intensive day services, such as PHPs, use the Illness Management and Recovery (IMR) best-practice model (Mueser et al., 2006). IMR is a rehabilitation practice that supports the person with information about his or her illness and recovery process, so the person may manage more effectively. This program was also adopted by SAMHSA as a best-practices tool kit. IMR approaches are emphasized in day support mental health programs, relying on a cognitive–behavioral approach and often delivered through group education. Nine topic areas are typically covered:

- Learning recovery strategies
- Practical facts about mental illness
- Stress vulnerability model and treatment strategies
- Building social support and reducing relapses
- Using medications effectively

- Coping with stress
- Coping with problems and symptoms
- Meeting one's needs in the mental health service system
- Addressing drug and alcohol use

The overall goal is to involve individuals fully in their own recovery and support their efforts to develop their own tailored coping strategies and, most of all, to promote their role in decision making about their own treatment and rehabilitation plans.

Case Management Services

All mental health service providers must become effective case managers. The recognized need for case management services goes back to the early 1970s with the advent of the deinstitutionalization movement, when persons were discharged into the community from long-term psychiatric hospitalizations in state hospitals. Historically, state hospitals were organized to meet all the person's basic needs for treatment, food, clothing, and shelter. The deinstitutionalization effort quickly demonstrated the community's lack of readiness and capability. There were no jobs or housing options for persons leaving long-term hospitalization. Families were completely unprepared for the return of their loved one and many persons ended up on the street or in jail or quickly returned to the hospital. With support from the National Institute of Mental Health and its establishment of the Community Support Program, a new framework emerged that recognized that individuals with serious mental illness were also coping with a multitude of impairments that hindered their ability to function successfully in the community. Providers noted that discharged patients needed basic supports, such as housing, medical services, transportation, and financial benefits, to live outside the hospital. Case management rapidly evolved to become well understood as the common sense, core service that people with serious mental illness needed.

Nurse case managers learn the resources that are available for accessing public supports, locating subsidized housing, securing employment, and obtaining primary health care. They must be highly skilled in assessing the person's total care coordination needs, introducing options such as access to Social Security disability income or affordable apartments and facilitating the person's movement toward them. The more active the debilitating symptoms of a person's illness, the greater the need for the nurse case manager to be active and assertive in gathering, organizing, coordinating. and assuring these supports.

Assertive Community Treatment

Of the various models of case management, **assertive community treatment** (sometimes referred to as Program for Assertive Community Treatment, or PACT) has been extensively researched. It is an evidence-based practice that is most successfully employed with individuals who have the greatest need for intensive community support as the best foundation for their recovery. Marx, Test, and Stein (1973) devised the ACT approach in Madison, Wisconsin. Their goal was to offer a comprehensive, community-based alternative model to the state hospitals that were discharging very large numbers of persons to the community. They conceptualized a "hospital without walls" approach; the pioneer ACT service providers were inpatient staff who shifted their service focus from the hospital to the community, working with individuals at home, on the job, and in their neighborhood.

Over the past 40 years, many communities replicated the ACT approach and, over time, it became clear that it worked best with adherence to certain fidelity measures, such as a high staff-to-client ratio of 1:10 and the 24/7 availability of team support. The team is multidisciplinary, employing mental health and substance use disorder specialists, employment experts, nurses, peers (persons with the lived experience of mental illness), and psychiatrists. The team works in a very individualized manner with each person, focusing on a comprehensive recovery plan, to include a focus on overall mental and physical health, effective medication treatment, and access to financial entitlements, housing, and employment.

In recognition of the growing body of research evidence regarding the effectiveness of the ACT approach, the NAMI sponsored the development of a training manual, called *The PACT Model of Community Based Treatment for Persons with Severe and Persistent Mental Illnesses: A Manual for PACT Start-up* (1999), and established a technical assistance center. This manual became one of the most helpful publications available to professionals and to mental health systems, committed to establishing effective ACT services. ACT has been

further refined with its inclusion in the SAMHSA Evidenced-Based Practices Kit on Assertive Community Treatment, available in a free digital version from the SAMHSA website.

ACT produces significant outcomes by successfully engaging persons in mental health treatment and case management. It has been shown to be effective in reducing hospitalizations, increasing housing retention, reducing incarceration, and demonstrating high levels of client and family satisfaction. Individuals receive all needed services from the treatment team while they require the intensive ACT level of support. All staff members of the ACT team work together to help patients achieve their recovery goals. Although tailored specifically for the individual, all treatment plans incorporate the evidence-based practices that are associated with psychiatric rehabilitation.

Peer Support

Peer specialists are individuals who are in recovery from a serious and persistent mental illness and/or dual mental illness and substance use disorder. Well-trained peer specialists work in many different settings and roles in the community. A growing body of knowledge supports the positive impact of consumer or peer-operated services on the recovery of individuals who experience mental illness. There are many excellent peer-directed programs across the country. These include drop-in support centers, homeless outreach teams, and housing and employment programs. Many peer-driven programs are nonprofit agencies, funded by state, federal, and local governments and by private grants. Distinctive from peer-only provided programming, many peers are behavioral health agency direct service employees, working on ACT teams, on jail diversion teams, in detoxification settings, and the like. Many communities and states have developed rigorous peer specialist certification programs as a prerequisite for this type of employment.

To date, there have been few formal evaluations of peer-operated services. There is a great need for controlled research studies on the impact of peer-driven services on recovery outcomes. As part of the Consumer Operated Services Program (COSP), SAMHSA is promoting such research with the goal of moving best practice peer-driven programs into the Evidence-Based Practices Tool Kit.

Supported Employment

Supported employment (SE) programs help individuals with mental illness find and maintain employment. Employment specialists work with the individual and other members of the treatment team to help the individual identify interests and strengths and to focus on areas for training and education as well (Figure 29-2). The research on supported employment is extensive and supports the belief that competitive jobs are a helpful pathway to recovery. SE recognizes that many persons who experience mental illness want to work. The practice, as described by Cook et al. (2008), is based on six principles: (1) everyone is eligible who is interested in working; (2) employment is integrated with treatment; (3) competitive employment is the goal; (4) the job search starts soon after a client expresses interest in working with no prerequisites, such as job readiness classes or special training; (5) follow-along supports are continuously provided; and (6) consumer preferences drive the decisions about the type of work and the type of follow along support that is desired.

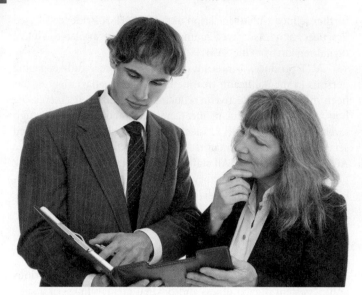

29-2 Supported employment programs link individuals with serious mental illness with employment specialists who help them identify strengths and weaknesses and focus on areas for education and job training.

Source: Lisa F. Young/Fotolia

Family Education and Engagement

Family education is also one of the SAMHSA evidenced-based practices with its own customized tool kit. This approach recognizes the healing power of an effective partnership among consumers, families, and practitioners. Families are informed about mental illness and substance use disorders. They are supported in developing their coping skills for responding empathically and knowledgably to the family member who is struggling with these conditions.

NAMI has played a major leadership role in advocating for awareness, funding, legislation, and services across our nation. It has worked with the provider community and through the political advocacy process to greatly improve service quality and endeavor, as do many consumer leadership groups, to eliminate stigma. Stigma speaks to the community's lack of understanding about mental health conditions and is often the basis for the individual's reluctance to seek treatment. NAMI has partnered with psychiatric nurses on numerous recovery initiatives and offers a platform for everyone,

including providers, to get involved in advocacy and legislative efforts to reduce stigma and improve mental health care for everyone. The NAMI Family to Family Education program, which is provided by family members for family members, is an outstanding example of this best practice.

In addition to NAMI, there are important consumer or peer-led organizations that advocate for the rights of those who experience mental illness and that inform the public about mental illness and the positive message of recovery. They offer a national and statewide network of information, technical support, and affiliation for persons who experience mental illness and provide leadership at the state and national level on public policy and legislative development. These organizations are led by persons with the lived experience of mental illness and are giving a voice and an opportunity for inclusion and leadership to all and are developing best practices, improving policy, and eliminating stigma and discrimination. Key organizations include the National Coalition for Mental Health Recovery, the National Empowerment Center, and the National Mental Health Consumer Self Help Clearinghouse.

Pause and Reflect

1. *Why do you think the multidisciplinary approach that is a cornerstone of ACT programs is so successful in helping persons reach their recovery goals?*
2. *What distinct skills do nurse case managers bring to the person served by an ACT team?*
3. *What do you believe about the potential effectiveness of peer-provided services?*

Community Mental Health Nursing Care

The nurse working as a member of the interprofessional team will bring all skills and experience to the relationship with the individual. The nurse is not there to do "for the person," but rather to find out what the individual would like to accomplish. Together, they develop a plan of care, aimed toward recovery and based on the person's needs, strengths, and preferences.

To illustrate this point, Gavin would like to use his time at home to gain some work experiences. Gavin works with his ACT team, and together they develop a care plan (see Community Mental Health Care

---

critical thinking

Gavin Recovery Stage

Gavin is discharged from the PHP to the ACT team because he is interested in adding a focus to his recovery plan on alcohol use/abuse and has expressed an interest in working before he returns to college. Gavin is feeling very anxious about his future and continues to deal with intrusive thoughts that he is unworthy and a failure. He believes that he needs fairly intensive support to maintain the progress he has made.

The ACT team assigns a nurse case manager to work with Gavin; she immediately helps him link with the team's employment specialist to discuss his goals for work. Gavin is still on a leave of absence from school and is considering whether he should transfer to a college closer to home. Regardless of his pending decision, Gavin indicates that he desires to work at least 20 hours per week. The employment specialist gathers information about Gavin's employment history and his preferences for the type of work he would like to do. With this support, Gavin finds a part-time job as a billing clerk in a primary care office and begins working. He continues frequent contact with the ACT team, particularly with his nurse case manager and with the employment specialist, for help with managing the stressors associated with his new job.

APPLICATION

1. How do you think regular employment might benefit Gavin's recovery?
2. What stressors are likely to be associated with Gavin starting a job?
3. What might be the risks and benefits of Gavin returning to school?

Gavin	COMMUNITY MENTAL HEALTH CARE PLAN

Diagnoses: Schizoaffective disorder, type 1 diabetes

Concerns identified by team: History of sleep disturbance, heavy drinking; symptoms associated with schizoaffective disorder include self-neglect, wandering, rumination, hearing voices. family history (uncle) of suicide.

Concerns identified by client: Alcohol use, need to find employment while pending decision about return to school

Care plan priorities:
- Continue medication regimen; anticipate and discuss concerns or challenges with adherence
- Identify triggers for alcohol use and psychiatric relapse
- Identify employment strengths and goals
- Engage in active symptom management strategies, e.g., sleep hygiene plan
- Re-engage with community and educational activities.

Short-Term Goals	Intervention/Treatment Activity
Gavin will participate in the therapeutic elements of his ACT care plan, to include medications and therapy appointments	<ul><li>Be present for contacts with ACT team providers.</li><li>Discuss his understanding for the reason he is taking medications, desired therapeutic effects and potential side effects, and any adherence concerns he has.</li><li>Engage in CBT strategies to develop effective symptom management techniques.</li></ul>
Gavin will refrain from alcohol use.	<ul><li>Work with team to identify triggers for alcohol use.</li><li>Identify activities that help relieve feelings of anxiety associated with triggers that prompt alcohol use.</li><li>Attend dual diagnosis recovery groups and maintain connection with recovery sponsor.</li></ul>
Gavin will find employment.	Work with employment specialist to:<ul><li>Identify interests and strengths</li><li>Develop resume</li><li>Practice interviewing skills</li></ul>While working, attend follow-along support group and problem-solve work concerns.

Long-Term Goals	Intervention/Treatment Activity
Gavin will return to school at least part-time.	<ul><li>When he is ready, contact the college office on disabilities to facilitate necessary academic accomodations.</li></ul>
Gavin will maintain engagement with the community care and college-based care system.	<ul><li>Assign a case manager that will assist in navigating between the community and the college.</li></ul>
Gavin will develop an advanced directive and engage in symptom self-management strategies.	<ul><li>Create a relapse prevention plan that includes symptom self-management and provide detailed instructions on how Gavin would like to manage relapse.</li></ul>

Clinical Reasoning

1. What additional interventions or treatment activities are likely to support Gavin in his long-term goals?
2. What additional concerns would you have if you were the nurse working with Gavin on his recovery?

Plan). He decides what type of employment he would like to pursue. The nurse is ready to help him explore the risks and benefits of his choices and is available to anticipate stressors, analyze certain approaches over others, problem solve recurring symptoms, fine-tune medications, or do whatever else is needed. The nurse's actions are grounded in the evidence-based practices used in psychiatric rehabilitation. Corrigan et al. (2008) describe the principles of rehabilitation that underlie these practices and guide the nursing care plan: (1) self-determination; (2) focused attention to the individual's strengths, goals, and preferences; (3) real-world focus; (4) skills training; (5) environmental modifications and supports; (6) integration of rehabilitation and treatment; (7) use of multidisciplinary teams; (8) continuity of services; (9) community integration; and (10) recovery orientation.

Promotion and Prevention Programs

Along with providing direct care psychiatric services, most communities offer mental health promotion and mental illness prevention programs. These programs are designed for early case finding and crisis intervention to prevent acute illnesses, and include such efforts as mental health first aid, disaster nursing, and rural mental health outreach and intervention programs.

Mental Health First Aid

The sometimes tragic outcomes of untreated mental illness or substance use disorders has shaped a growing national awareness of the importance of recognizing the early signs, symptoms, and distress levels of persons in our communities who are suffering from these illnesses. Events such as the shootings at Sandy Hook and Virginia Tech and the devastating losses related to shootings at the public appearance of a U.S. Congresswoman in her own district highlight the need for a more comprehensive system of preventive mental health services. A proactive, prevention-oriented, nationwide effort is under way to promote **mental health first aid** programs. Developed initially in Australia, the mental health first aid curriculum is based on the familiar life-saving principles of first aid: preserve life; prevent further harm; promote recovery; and provide comfort to the person who is ill or injured. Mental health first aid is help that is offered to an individual who may be developing a mental health condition or experiencing a mental health crisis and has four major aims: preserve life when a person may be a danger to self or others; provide help to prevent the problem from becoming more serious; promote and enhance recovery; and provide comfort and support

The mental health first aid curriculum currently in use was a joint effort in 2008 by the Maryland Department of Health and Mental Hygiene, the Missouri Department of Mental Health, and the National Council for Community Behavioral Health Care (Mental Health First Aid USA, 2013). The curriculum teaches the general public how to recognize the symptoms of mental health problems and how to actively help and guide an affected person or family member toward treatment and support. Communities benefit greatly from mental health first aid for several reasons, because mental health problems are quite common and people are not well informed about how to actually recognize mental health problems. Additionally, many people with mental health problems do not seek help or delay seeking help, often letting years go by as their condition worsens. Furthermore, the stigma associated with mental health problems causes people to feel ashamed or reluctant to share information about their suffering for fear of rejection or lack of understanding. Another reason for mental health first aid is that people with mental health problems may not have an awareness that they need help, as a result of the thinking and decision-making deficits that can be characteristic of various mental health conditions. Finally, professionals and other support services are not always immediately available when mental health problems arise and it helps for lay persons to be able to take action.

The mental health first aid action plan is based on the mnemonic ALGEE:

Assess for the risk of suicide or harm to others

Listen nonjudgmentally

Give reassurance and information

Encourage appropriate professional help

Encourage self-help and other support strategies

Disaster Nursing

In 2011, the National Oceanic and Atmospheric Administration (NOAA) reported that the United States experienced 12 weather-related events that cost at least $1 billion each, with a death toll of 646 persons and thousands who were displaced. The lesson learned from 2011 is that our nation must be ready—and, sadly, we are not. Veenema (2009) reports that globally there is at least one massive disaster per week that requires international assistance. This documented increase in the sheer numbers of disasters is attributed to a number of factors, including shifting climates, rising sea levels, and the incidence of war and terrorism.

Psychological casualties from a given disaster can far outnumber physical casualties. Nurses, who represent the largest number of members of the health care workforce, are critical disaster response professionals with a professional mandate to participate in the five foci germane to emergency and disaster preparedness, regardless of type: preparedness, mitigation, response, recovery, and evaluation.

Nurses serve on response teams with public safety, health departments, the American Red Cross, school personnel, family services, and other organizations, so they may contribute their particular expertise to the disaster response in their communities. A disaster response or **disaster plan** refers to a community-wide effort to respond to a crisis or disaster with the goals of caring for those who need treatment and restoring a sense of normalcy and well-being to the community as soon as possible. Many communities have developed disaster plans to cope with the range of catastrophic events that can, and do, occur. These plans range from responses to dramatic weather events, such as hurricanes, tornadoes, and earthquakes, to unexpected "person driven" catastrophes, such as sniper incidents with mass causalities or acts of terrorism. The psychiatric nurse is often called on as a member of first-responder teams to crisis events that, though not at disaster level, do disrupt the well-being and safety of the community, often creating long-term disruption (Box 29-1).

Many psychiatric nurses who work in community-based settings receive disaster preparedness, crisis intervention, or incident management training in their work settings and do contribute positively to improving the community's response to critical events. Veenema (2009) has developed a curriculum in partnership with the American Red Cross, called Ready RN: Disaster Nursing and Emergency Preparedness, which is an excellent foundation for the contributions that any community can expect from its nurses. All 50 states have published disaster plans developed and executed by public health and behavioral health agencies.

Rural Mental Health Services

Hauenstein (2008) reported that 20% of Americans live in rural areas. Rural communities, like urban communities, work to establish a system of health care that includes behavioral health services. However, there are often challenges in access to mental health care in rural states. These include the size of the geographic area to be served and the often disproportionate lower ratio of service providers to population. This is especially true in the limited availability of licensed and highly skilled providers, such as psychiatrists and psychiatric nurses. Transportation also tends to be a major barrier. Other potential limitations include the absence of specialized services, such as ACT teams, crisis stabilization programs, and the like. Rural residents are more likely to receive their mental health care in a primary care practice.

A defining feature of rural communities may be the large number of municipalities or jurisdictions within the service area and the potential need for collaborative partnerships, and even contractual relationships to ensure that service levels are actually available, such as 24-hour psychiatric emergency services. The sheer number of agencies involved and the limited resources rural agencies typically possess can make establishing and maintaining such collaborations challenging. On the plus side, rural communities can be very creative in their deployment of limited resources and often serve as models for the use of outreach and telemedicine approaches to ensure assessment and treatment services.

Disaster and Crisis Nursing: Three Scenarios

box 29-1

Review these examples and consider the questions that follow.

1. You are a psychiatric nurse in the local mental health center's crisis services unit. You are asked to "debrief" with a team of firefighters who responded to a house fire that resulted in the deaths of a young mother and her two children. Several of the firefighters have young children of their own and are distraught.

2. You are a psychiatric nurse who is a highly trained member of the local police department's hostage negotiation team. You respond on the scene with the police to a private home where a man with a known history of mental illness is holding his wife at gunpoint and threatening to end both her life and his.

3. You are a psychiatric nurse who lives in an agricultural community in the Midwest. A tornado sweeps through the community in the early morning hours while residents are sleeping.

There is limited time to respond to warning sirens; 40 homes, a church, and an elementary school in a three-block area are destroyed. Two hours after the event, many residents remain unaccounted for. The roof of the elementary school has been torn off and several walls have collapsed. As a member of the disaster response team, you report to the aid and recovery center.

Critical Thinking Questions

1. In the first scenario, what are the initial nursing priorities?

2. In the second scenario, what is the primary goal of the intervention?

3. In the last scenario, what initial contributions might the nurse make at the tornado aid and recovery center?

Psychiatric nurses are in high demand in rural communities, and there is a great demand for nurses who possess advanced preparation as psychiatric nurse practitioners and clinical nurse specialists. There are many opportunities for nurses to practice in more autonomous roles in communities with limited numbers of licensed professionals, given their holistic training, their licensure, and their clinical expertise. Peer specialists are also often trained to extend the impact of the small cadre of licensed professionals who may be available.

Behavioral health professionals, with skills in public policy and with knowledge of community-based systems, including the primary care community and hospitals, can have enormous impact on the quality and accessibility of care. They use their skills in networking, developing memoranda of agreements, building integrated electronic health records, and coalition building to get the job done. They also encourage local academic institutions to create targeted curricula to train the types of health and behavioral health providers that the rural community requires.

Nurses have produced significant research on rural mental health services and systems. Prominent findings from rural nursing researchers, Fox, Blank, and Rovnyak (1999), as summarized by Hauenstein (2008), report disparities in access to behavioral health care in rural states, as compared with urban areas. They have also highlighted the presence of "gateway" providers in rural areas who may or may not facilitate access to evidence-based services. The "gatekeepers" can be primary care physicians, concerned family members, and/or clergy. Rural primary care providers, in the absence of behavioral health colleagues, do assume responsibility for the treatment of a broad range of mental health and addiction disorders. They should be supported in this effort through consistent consultation with behavioral health providers or through their participation in collaborative care arrangements, through university linkages, and through the application of telemedicine technologies to improve the efficacy of services and positive patient outcomes.

Pause and Reflect

1. *Do you see yourself as an effective provider of mental health services in a disaster circumstance? What specific skills do nurses bring to these interventions?*

2. *As a nurse in a rural community, how might you influence primary care physicians and primary care nurse practitioners in expanding their practices to include behavioral health services?*

From Suffering to Hope

The SAMHSA National Survey on Drug Use and Health (2010) found that 11.4 million adults (5% of the adult population) suffered from serious mental illness in the past year. The report indicates that only about 4 in 10 persons experiencing any form of mental illness received mental health treatment in the past year. Rates for treatment among those experiencing serious mental illness were higher, at almost 61%. There is no question that mental illness is a very serious and prevalent public health concern in our country.

Psychiatric nurses will encounter young adults such as Gavin, for whom the correct behavioral health services were effectively mobilized early. However, they will also meet many more people who have lived with the functional impairments and symptoms of their illnesses for many years because they have not received effective treatment, rehabilitation, and case management services and supports. Their suffering is seen through the lens of their poor physical health, lack of sustained housing, lack of access to primary care, estrangement from families, the absence of simple pleasures such as social events and friendships, limited employment opportunities, and frequent encounters with jails, hospitals, and homeless shelters. These individuals need the skills and empathy of knowledgeable nurses.

At whatever stage of health and well-being the individual is, the nurse has the opportunity to instill hope and to ensure that proven and effective services and supports are provided. Adults who experience a serious cardiovascular event, such as a myocardial infarction, are not treated with the protocols of the 1990s. Serious mental illness does not differ from biological illness in the patient's need to receive the very best standard of care. Promoting recovery is about assisting individuals in pursuing their goals and becoming a nurse who is active and informed and skilled at building a trusting relationship. The nurse shares evidence-based knowledge and expertise with individuals at the earliest possible time in their illness. Early, expert intervention is the gold standard of care, but it is never too late for the community mental health nurse to intervene in people's suffering and help them gather their energies to find their own path to recovery.

Gavin Rehabilitation Phase

After 9 months of engaging in services with the ACT team and working part-time at the medical office, Gavin decides that he is ready to resume college. He hopes to succeed in his goal to attend medical school, but is also open to considering other health-oriented career pathways. His nurse case manager partners with him to identify a mental health clinician at the university's counseling center who will provide individual treatment while Gavin is at school and a psychiatrist who will monitor his medications and overall health status, including his diabetes. Gavin learns that there is a sober (substance-free) living dormitory on campus, applies for housing there, and is approved to receive it.

Prior to his return to school, Gavin and his nurse case manager work on a psychiatric advance directive, which will allow him to define what treatment he wants to receive if he should relapse and lose the capacity to make decisions for himself (see Chapter 10). Gavin writes his directive to give permission to his family to make treatment decisions for him should he become incapacitated by psychiatric symptoms. Gavin makes very clear that he would like to avoid hospitalization and substantial changes in the primary medication he is receiving. He further details that he is open to intensive services, such as ACT or entry into a crisis stabilization unit, if needed.

Gavin works with his nurse case manager to identify relapse triggers for both his mental health and substance abuse symptoms so that he and others are well prepared to intervene early in any possible setbacks. Knowing that there will be high levels of stress in returning to school, he identifies the risk factors that he must be aware of and verbally details the strategies that he could employ to deal with these. He develops a sleep hygiene approach and a plan for mapping out his coursework, and sets a goal of attending AA at least twice per week. His visits with the university's counseling center clinician will be weekly and his visits with the psychiatrist will start out on a biweekly schedule. He will be seeking an AA sponsor on campus, but until this is in place, he intends to maintain contact with his recovery sponsor via telephone. He and his nurse case manager will maintain regular phone contact until the new relationships are firmly in place at the counseling center; they also plan to have regular contact during school semester breaks.

APPLICATION

1. Why is it important for Gavin to work with his nurse case manager on a relapse prevention plan as he returns to college?

2. Do you think Gavin's plan is comprehensive? If yes, why? If not, what elements are missing?

3. What skills are crucial for Gavin to possess at this point in his recovery? How could you help him further develop these skills?

Chapter Highlights

1. The real work of recovery from any illness takes place within the community. The specific resources available in communities greatly influence the level of care individuals with psychiatric illness can access.

2. Community entry points to mental health care include emergency departments, primary care, school-based counseling centers, the legal system, inpatient and medical detoxification units, and homeless shelters.

3. Partial hospitalization programs (PHPs) are designed to provide a level of support and treatment that will meet the needs of an individual who does not require the structure, intensity, or safety focus of an inpatient setting. Psychosocial rehabilitation and crisis stabilization programs also offer intensive outpatient care.

4. Case management services are designed to help individuals coordinate their mental health care and gain access to a range of basic services needed to return to optimal functioning.

5. Assertive community treatment services incorporate a multidisciplinary team, typically employing mental health and dual disorder specialists, employment experts, nurses, peers, and psychiatrists. The team assists individuals with the work of recovery, including overall health management and effective medication treatment, and access to financial entitlements, housing, and employment.

6. Peer specialists are individuals who are in recovery from a serious and persistent mental illness and employed in a variety of positions throughout the behavioral health system, from inpatient to ACT teams.

7. Supported employment services help individuals with mental illness find and maintain employment.

8. Family members are supported in developing their own coping skills for responding in a healthy and compassionate manner to the family member with mental illness and/or a substance use disorder.

9. Nurses are key members of interprofessional teams who support the recovery of individuals who experience mental illness and those who struggle with the co-occurring disorders of mental illness and substance use.

10. Key nursing interventions performed by nurses in community mental health settings include comprehensive assessment, building trusting therapeutic relationships, monitoring patients for safety and response to treatments and medications, care and treatment planning, and case management services.

11. As one of the largest groups of health care professionals, nurses participate in care of individuals following disasters and critical incidents to help restore a sense of normalcy and well-being to the community as soon as possible, including addressing prevention and readiness for future events.

NCLEX®-RN Questions

1. The psychiatric mental health nurse has just accepted a position working in the community mental health clinic. Which activities is the nurse likely to carry out in this role? Select all that apply.
   a. Conduct therapeutic groups with patients.
   b. Monitor the progress of patients in residential settings.
   c. Limit community exposure to the individuals being treated.
   d. Evaluate the needs of patients with co-morbid physical illness.
   e. Prevent hospitalization of patients who are a danger to self or others.

2. The nurse working in the community mental health setting is evaluating the progress of a patient with a serious mental illness. Which patient response best indicates that a recovery and rehabilitation goal has been met?
   a. Engages in activities that provide enjoyment.
   b. Recognizes a need for financial assistance.
   c. Begins to identify with others with the same diagnosis.
   d. Defers to the nurse before making important decisions.

3. The nurse is completing an intake on an individual presenting for community mental health services. The individual states that while living in a different area, he was hospitalized and then attended a group day program that emphasized a number of areas, including practical strategies to cope with mental illness and meeting his own needs. The nurse recognizes that the patient most likely participated in a partial hospital treatment center using which model?
   a. Community support
   b. Peer-supported treatment
   c. Assertive community treatment
   d. Illness management and recovery

4. The nurse is working with a patient with a dual diagnosis who is receiving integrated community health services geared toward promoting recovery and wellness. Which evaluation finding indicates progress toward initial treatment goals?
   a. The patient returns to work.
   b. The patient maintains sobriety.
   c. The patient attends treatment sessions.
   d. The patient engages in symptom self-management.

5. The community mental health nurse is addressing concerns presented by the school committee related to the safety of students and school personnel following media reports of school shootings across the country. Which approaches are consistent with the mental health first aid model? Select all that apply.
   a. Providing education to reduce the stigma of mental illness
   b. Reviewing measures to promote the safety and security of anyone at risk
   c. Discussing the impact of the shootings on the emotional well-being of the community
   d. Promoting early identification and treatment of mental illness in the community
   e. Discussing the importance of more restrictive treatment for individuals with mental illness

Answers may be found on the Pearson student resource site: nursing.pearsonhighered.com

Pearson Nursing Student Resources Find additional review materials at **nursing.pearsonhighered.com**

References

American Academy of Family Physicians (AAFP). (2013). *Mental Health Care Services for Family Physicians: A Position Paper.* Available at http://www.aafp.org/about/policies/all/mental-services.html

Association for Ambulatory Behavioral Health Care. (2010). *Facts on partial hospitalization programs.* Available at www.aabh.org

Bureau of Justice Statistics. (2006). *Study finds more than half of all prison and jail inmates have mental health problems.* Available at http://www.bjs.gov/content/pub/press/mhppjipr.cfm

Cook, J. A., Blyler, C. R., Leff, H. S., McFarlane, W. R., Goldberg, R. W., Gold, P. B., … Razzano, L. A. (2008). The employment intervention demonstration program: Major findings and policy implications. *Psychiatric Rehabilitation Journal, 31*(4), 291–295.

Corrigan, P. W., Mueser K. T., Bond, G. R., Drake, R. E., & Solomon, P. (2008). *Principles and Practice of Psychiatric Rehabilitation.* New York, NY: Guilford Press.

Domonell, K. (2013). Sound mind: Sound student body. *University Business Magazine.* 26–30. Available at http://kristendomonell.files.wordpress.com/2013/05/pages.pdf

Fox, J. C., Blank, M., & Rovnyak, V. G. (1999). Mental disorders and help seeking in a rural impoverished population. *International Journal of Psychiatry in Medicine, 29,* 181–195.

Gallagher, R. P. (2012). National survey of college counseling by the American College Counseling Association. The International Association of Counseling Services, Inc., Monograph Series #9–10. Available at http://www.collegecounseling.org/wp-content/uploads/NSCCD_Survey_2012.pdf

Georgia Certified Peer Specialist Project. (2003). Available at www.gacps.org

Hauenstein, E. J. (2008). Building the rural mental health system: From de facto system to quality care. *Annual Review of Nursing Research, 26,* 143–173.

James, D. J. & Glaze, L. E. (2006). *Mental health problems of prison and jail inmates.* Washington, DC: U.S. Department of Justice, Office of Justice Programs. Bureau of Justice Statistics. Available at http://www.bjs.gov/content/pub/pdf/mhppji.pdf

Kessler, R. C., Nelson, C. B., McGonagle, K. A., Edlund, M. J., Frank, R. G., & Leaf, P. J. (1996). The epidemiology of co-occurring addictive and mental disorders: Implications for prevention and service utilization. *American Journal of Orthopsychiatry, 66*(1), 17–31.

Kudless, M., & White, J. (2007). Competencies and roles of community mental health nurses. *Journal of Psychosocial Nursing, 45*(5), 36–44.

Luoma, J. B., Martin, C. E., & Pearson, J. L. (2002). Contact with mental health and primary care providers before suicide: A review of the evidence. *American Journal of Psychiatry, 159,* 909–916.

Marx, A. J., Test, M. A., & Stein, L. (1973). Extra-hospital management of severe mental illness. *Archives of General Psychiatry, 29,* 505–511.

McDowell, A. K., Lineberry, T. W., & Bostwick, J. M. (2011). Practical suicide risk management for the busy primary care physician. *Mayo Clinic Proceedings, 86*(8), 792–800.

McGovern, M. (2009). *Living with Co-Occurring Addiction and Mental Health Disorders: A Handbook for Recovery.* Minneapolis, MN: Hazelden Press.

Memphis Police Department. (2011). *Crisis Intervention Team: The "Memphis Model."* Available at http://www.memphispolice.org/crisis%20intervention.htm

Mental Health First Aid USA. (2013). Available at http://www.mentalhealthfirstaid.org/cs/

Mueser, K. T., Meyer, P. S., Penn, D. L., Clancy, R., Clancy, D. M., & Salyers, M. P. (2006). The illness management and recovery program: Rationale, development, and preliminary findings. *Schizophrenia Bulletin, 32*(Suppl 1), S32–S43.

Munetz, M. R., & Griffin, P. A. (2006). Use of the sequential intercept model as an approach to decriminalization of people with serious mental illnesses. *Psychiatric Services, 57*, 544–549.

National Alliance to End Homelessness. (2012). State of Homelessness 2012: Chapter One, Homelessness Counts. Available at http://www.endhomelessness.org/library/entry/soh-2012-chapter-one-homelessness-counts

National Association on Mental Illness (NAMI). (1999). *The PACT Model of Community Based Treatment for Persons with Severe and Persistent Mental Illnesses: A Manual for PACT Start-up.* Available at http://www.nami.org/Template.cfm?Section=ACT-TA_Center&template=/ContentManagement/ContentDisplay.cfm&ContentID=132547

National Coalition for the Homeless. (2009). *Mental Illness and Homelessness.* Available at http://www.nationalhomeless.org/factsheets/Mental_Illness.html

Prince, J. D., Akincigil, A., & Bromet, E. (2007). Incarceration rates of persons with first-admission psychosis. *Psychiatric Services, 58*(9), 1173–1180.

Steadman, H., Osher, F., Robbins, P. C., Case, B., & Samuels, S. (2009). Prevalence of serious mental illness among jail inmates. *Psychiatric Services, 60*, 761–765.

Substance Abuse and Mental Health Services Administration (SAMHSA). (2009). *Integrated Treatment for Co-Occurring Disorders: Getting Started with Evidence-Based Practices.* DHHS Pub. No. SMA-08-4366. Rockville, MD: Center for Mental Health Services, Substance Abuse and Mental Health Services Administration, U.S. Department of Health and Human Services. Available at http://store.samhsa.gov/shin/content/SMA08-4367/GettingStarted-ITC.pdf

Substance Abuse and Mental Health Services Administration (SAMHSA). (2010). *National Survey on Drug Use and Health.* Available at http://www.samhsa.gov/data/NSDUH/2k10NSDUH/2k10Results.pdf

Treatment Advocacy Center Backgrounder. (2011). *Violent behavior: One of the consequences of failing to treat individuals with severe mental illnesses.* Available at http://treatmentadvocacycenter.org/storage/documents/violent-behavior-backgrounder.pdf

U.S. Conference of Mayors. (2011). *Hunger and homelessness survey: A status report on hunger and homelessness in America's cities.* Available at http://usmayors.org/pressreleases/uploads/2011

U.S. Department of Justice. (1999). *Mental Health and Treatment of Inmates and Probationers.* Pub. No. NCJ 174463. Washington, DC: Department of Justice, Office of Justice Programs, Bureau of Justice Assistance.

U.S. Preventive Health Services Task Force Screening for Depression in Adults. (2009). U.S. Preventive Services Task Force Recommendation Statement. *Annals of Internal Medicine, 151*, 784–792.

Veneema, T. G. (2013). *Disaster Nursing and Emergency Preparedness.* New York, NY: Springer Publishing.

Veneema, T. G., in collaboration with the American Red Cross. (2009). *Disaster Nursing and Emergency Preparedness.* Available at www.ReadyRN.com

Disorders of Childhood and Adolescence

30

Julie Carbray

Learning Outcomes

1. Understand the biological, developmental, sociological, spiritual, and cultural context of psychiatric disorders in children and adolescents.

2. Examine the epidemiology and symptom criteria for psychiatric and mental health disorders in children and adolescents.

3. Discuss the effects of abuse and trauma on child and adolescent mental health.

4. Evaluate systems (family, school, community) that promote wellness, recovery, and mental health among child and adolescent populations.

5. Contrast differences in perceptions, thoughts, and feelings of the nurse and patient during care delivery (patient/other awareness).

6. Understand how developmentally based psychotherapies assist children and their families to manage psychiatric and mental health concerns.

7. Summarize different pharmacologic and nonpharmacologic therapies used in the treatment of childhood psychiatric disorders.

8. Plan evidence-based nursing care for children and adolescents diagnosed with psychiatric disorders.

Key Terms

attachment, 653
attention-deficit/hyperactivity
  disorder (ADHD), 656
brain plasticity, 651
child abuse, 668
conduct disorder, 657
disruptive mood dysregulation
  disorder, 660
neglect, 668
oppositional defiant disorder, 656
posttraumatic growth (PTG), 658
resilience, 655
selective mutism, 659
self injury, 660
separation anxiety, 659
Tourette syndrome, 657

Darius Initial Onset

Darius Smith is an 8-year-old African American boy who is a frequent visitor to the school nurse due to disruptive behaviors, problems with peers, and struggles with social interaction in the classroom. Today, Joanna, a registered nurse working at Darius's elementary school, is called to his classroom at the beginning of school. His teacher asks Joanna to help him manage his anxiety and intense rocking behavior. Joanna talks with Darius and gives him time to sit in her quiet office and rock. Once he is calm and collected, she assists him in returning to class.

An hour or so later, Darius's teacher calls for help again when he gets upset at being asked to return a toy train that he snatched from another student. Darius's teacher shares with Joanna her concerns that Darius is blurting out answers in class and getting out of his seat to wander around the room. She voices her frustration with managing Darius's needs along with those of her other students. She is worried that he is not socializing with his peer group.

Joanna and Darius's teachers meet after school and agree that Darius is a very bright student who is capable of doing excellent work, but that his distractibility interferes with his performance and his ability to get along with other students. The team agrees that Joanna will lead a meeting with Darius's family to explore whether a psychiatric evaluation might help everyone better understand Darius's developmental and behavioral challenges.

Joanna meets with Darius's mother, Cheryl, and reviews his developmental and medical history. Joanna asks Darius to sit and draw at a nearby table while she speaks quietly with his mother. Cheryl has been worried about Darius for some time and welcomes Joanna's expressions of concern. Cheryl reports that she lost connection with his biological father about four years earlier because of his ongoing struggle with alcohol abuse; they were never married. She shares that Darius has always been hyperactive, has had sleep problems since infancy, and has always been difficult to soothe. Cheryl is not aware that Darius was ever exposed to trauma or abuse, but several family members have struggled with depressive and bipolar disorders, as well as substance use disorders. Cheryl shares that she has been taking an antidepressant since the birth of her last child 2 years ago. She reiterates that Darius has always been an active boy, even as a toddler, but had some early difficulties with speech and that he seems to have a hard time playing with other children. Also, when Darius is frustrated, he either rocks until he feels comfortable or spins a toy in front of his eyes until he is able to relax. Cheryl notes that her brother, Robert, had similar challenges as a child, and that he "grew out of it." She also comments that Darius is smart, and that he loves trains and can name every detail of any given steam engine.

While taking the history, Joanna notes that Darius is extremely active, that his mother's attempts to contain his behavior are ineffective, and that Darius often does not look at adults when speaking to them. While Joanna and Cheryl talk, Darius colors, singing and rocking while doing so. Joanna asks Darius, "What did you draw for us, Darius?" and he replies, "A train—you can't tell?" Joanna notes the lack of developmentally appropriate skill and detail in his drawing of a circle as well as lack of connection with his mother throughout the interview, something his teachers have also reported observing.

As they complete the interview, Joanna asks Cheryl if she would feel comfortable having Darius see one of her colleagues, who is an Advanced Practice Registered Nurse, for a more complete psychiatric evaluation; Joanna also asks for consent to share information with the school team.

Joanna observes that Darius's symptoms include the following:

- Poor social communication
- Disturbed sleep patterns
- Hyperactivity, distractibility, and inattention
- Self-stimulating behaviors
- Developmental delays

APPLICATION

1. In what ways do you think Darius may be suffering? Why? How may his mother be suffering?

2. How you would prioritize Darius's needs during this encounter and why?

3. How could Joanna consider Darius's family system while planning her interventions?

4. In what ways does Joanna convey hope to Darius or Cheryl? What might you have done differently?

Introduction

For most families, childhood and adolescence is a time of play, growth, and discovery. In any given year, though, 13% to 20% of children and adolescents suffer from a mental health disorder (Centers for Disease Control and Prevention [CDC], 2013). Despite the presence of well-established criteria for the diagnoses of children's psychiatric disorders, parents and teachers often fail to recognize children suffering from these disorders. Common misconceptions that children are simply small versions of adults, that childhood offers protection from stress, and that abnormal behaviors can be explained by misconceptions of normal development have resulted in children who are in need of mental health services not getting the services they need. In addition, even when children are identified as being symptomatic, they often are not seen by any type of mental health provider to address symptom control (Jensen et al., 2011). Therefore, connecting children in need of mental health care with appropriate service providers

Critical Pediatric Symptoms Indicating Need for Assessment and Possible Intervention

box 30-1

- Sudden and dramatic changes in personality or behavior occurring over time
- Suicide attempt or suicidal ideation
- Temper tantrums accompanied by rage and physical aggression
- Recurrent fighting, wanting to harm others
- Vomiting, starvation, or use of laxatives to achieve substantial weight loss

- Sudden, panic level anxiety or fear without a precipitant
- Anxious distress, excessive worry, or severe sadness that impairs participation in daily activities
- Impairment in concentration to the extent that the child's success at school or physical safety is threatened
- Repeated use of drugs or alcohol

is critical to providing effective assistance (Jensen et al., 2011). Nurses working with children need to be knowledgeable of critical psychiatric symptoms that warrant further mental health attention (Box 30-1).

Once identified as at risk, children and adolescents with psychiatric disorders are treated most often in their community settings by their pediatrician, primary care provider, or school or church staff (Lenardson et al., 2010). In both urban and rural areas, access to child and adolescent mental health professionals is limited due to the high demand for services, as well as to an inadequate number of trained providers. Therefore, nursing care for children and adolescents with psychiatric disorders will be provided mostly in "nontraditional" mental health settings. The largest focus of care, because of the obstacles already discussed, is preventive in nature. However, when children are identified as psychiatrically ill, they typically are served across a continuum of care (Figure 30-1), from the least restrictive settings (such as pastoral care or service with their school counselor) to those with more service and oversight (such as an outpatient or inpatient service).

Theoretical Foundations

Early childhood experiences, brain circuitry development, and their combined effect on the child's developing central nervous system have been linked to both risk and resiliency for psychopathology in adulthood. A growing body of evidence indicates that environmental factors, such as toxins, early childhood maltreatment, diet, and stress, can change gene activity and increase the risk for developing psychopathology later in life (Roth & Sweatt, 2011).

Approximately 75% of adult psychiatric disorders have their onset in childhood and adolescence (McGorry, Purcell, Goldstone, &

Amminger, 2011). Early mental health promotion interventions that target these factors can change the course of development for children at risk for psychiatric disorders and alter the course of development along the psychological, biological, sociological, cultural, and spiritual domains (Table 30-1).

Biological Domain

Family history of a psychiatric disorder increases the likelihood that a child will also suffer from the disorder. Advances in genetic technology have implicated genetic associations in attention-deficit/hyperactivity disorder (ADHD), autism, Tourette syndrome, and schizophrenia in childhood and adolescence. However, the impact of environmental effects, heterogeneity, and other factors complicate what this means for diagnosis and treatment of children with these disorders (Addington & Rapoport, 2011). It is becoming clear that biological risk for these and potentially other disorders may be identified and, in the future, will help to inform prevention, diagnosis, and treatment targets for illness.

Brain plasticity refers to the development and strengthening of neural connections in response to environmental stimuli, resulting in the creation and enhancement of various neural pathways ("cells that fire together, wire together") and the "growth" of brain regions associated with specific functions (such as larger cortical representation for unique components of motor movement). Certain areas of the brain also develop sooner than others; evidence exists that adult levels of dorsolateral prefrontal cortex thickness that control impulses, judgment, and decision making are not yet developed in the brains of children and adolescents. Because of the still developing prefrontal cortex, children and adolescents may show poor impulse control, judgment, and decision making merely because their brains are not fully developed. The implications of late maturation of this

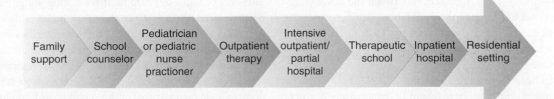

30-1   Continuum of care for children and adolescents.

Factors Influencing Development Across the Wellness Domains — table 30-1

Domain	Responses
Biological	• Developing language skills • Development of bowel and bladder control • Brain development • Genetic makeup • Temperament
Psychological	• Attachment • Morality • Identity formation • Intellectual growth • Character
Sociological	• Attachment • Family ecology • Child-rearing practices • Gender roles • Gender identity
Cultural	• Connectedness or sense of belonging to others from the same race, religion, or culture • Connectedness to those with similar values, shared language, or experiences • Access to services due to language or other cultural barriers
Spiritual	• Connectedness with God or higher power and/or with others of like-minded beliefs • Learning about one's faith • Adopting faith beliefs that are the same or different from those of the family • Struggling with meaning and purpose • Expressing feelings of guilt related to symptoms

area have entered educational, social, political, and judicial arenas in matters ranging from whether minors are cognitively mature enough to qualify for the death penalty to the age at which teenagers should be allowed to drive.

More than 12.8% of children born in the United States are born prematurely (March of Dimes, 2011). Increased survival rates of premature infants, neurodevelopmental issues, family stress, and medical illness may also contribute to mental illness in the infant's lifetime. The earlier the preterm birth, the higher the risk for developing mental illness; overall, preterm infants are at a higher risk than infants carried to term for attention-deficit/hyperactivity disorder, cognitive impairment and learning disabilities, and other psychiatric illness (Vanderbilt & Gleason, 2011). Interaction between the developing premature infant and the parent appears to have a significant role in building resilience to these potential consequences of prematurity. Early supportive and educational interventions designed for the neonatal intensive care unit (NICU) result in positive outcomes for the long-term mental health of children born preterm.

Brain imaging studies also have begun to demonstrate distinct biological underpinnings of psychiatric illness in childhood psychiatric disorders, implicating developmental trajectories for those affected by illness that are different from normally developing children (Maddison, Clarke, & Kutcher, 2011). In particular, evidence is growing that certain brain circuits are implicated in symptoms. For example, overactivation of the amygdala has been implicated in mood dysregulation disorders, and newer evidence suggests that the neural systems involved in impulsivity, reward systems, and executive function engage differently in pediatric bipolar disorder and ADHD (Mayanil, Wegbreit, Fitzgerald, & Pavuluri, 2011; Passerotti & Pavuluri, 2011). These studies offer a window into the brain of normally developing and psychiatrically ill children, promising hope for new understanding of illness effects and treatment possibilities.

Medically ill children also may be at risk for developing psychiatric disorders. Children with chronic illnesses, such as diabetes or asthma, may struggle with coping with the effects of managing their illness, and children with physical disabilities may struggle with coping with the limitations their physical challenges present. It is also possible that children with medical illness are genetically inclined to have psychiatric disorders. In addition, acute infections of *Streptococcus pyogenes* or viral infection have resulted in a syndrome called pediatric autoimmune neuropsychiatric disorder associated with streptococcus (PANDAS). Children with PANDAS have had exposure to or partially treated streptococcus infections. An enzyme produced by the strep bacteria can affect the basal ganglia, creating symptoms of obsessive–compulsive disorder (OCD) or a tic disorder. Affected children can also demonstrate neurological abnormalities in the context of their symptoms (such as abnormal movements) and have an acute onset of illness that remits (Williams, 2011). Although studies of PANDAS have revealed possible mechanism and treatment outcomes, consensus about PANDAS in the scientific literature is still forthcoming.

Child temperament is thought to be inherited, or genetically determined, and interfaces with the child's environment, resulting in reactivity or self-regulation behaviors that are thought to be neurobiologically driven (Lemery-Chalfant, Kao, Swann, & Goldsmith, 2013). A child who tends to be easygoing and nonreactive in temperament style may adjust successfully to a loud school environment. A child who tends to be sensitive and reactive in temperament style, however, may start to cry in the same environment and run out of the room. Temperament traits are neurobiologically driven and will shape how the child manages stress and distress and ultimately contributes to the child's illness experience.

Psychological Domain

A number of factors other than biology influence a child's development. The ways in which a child progresses through developmental milestones, acquires social skills and abilities, responds to parenting influences, interacts with family relationships, and develops cognitive function all play a role in the development of mental health in children.

Developmental Theories

Theories of child development have long sought to understand what children do, and why, as they grow into adulthood (Chapter 4). Although each developmental theory describes its own distinct developmental challenge, these theories highlight the overall tasks of childhood that are essential to healthy development and eventual independent living and strong social relationships. There is seldom a single cause or reason for a childhood psychiatric disorder. Although these theories offer guidelines for resolution of common developmental tasks, it is important to recognize that the combination of the child's own biological and psychological growth, that of the family, and the interactions among them and their environment

Developmental Theories of Childhood and Adolescence

table 30-2

Developmental Theory	Theorist	Stages
Sexual and aggressive development	**Freud** *Birth–2 yrs:* oral phase *2–3 yrs:* anal phase *3–6 yrs:* phallic phase *6–12 yrs:* sexual motivation takes back seat to development of skills *Puberty:* heterosexual relations	• Children shift impulses from oral to anal regions. • Parents help child find balance between delayed and instant need gratification.
Social process	**Erikson** *Birth–1 yr:* trust vs. mistrust *1–3 yrs:* autonomy vs. shame and doubt *3–6 yrs:* initiative vs. guilt *Adolescence:* identity vs. identity diffusion	• Ego as a positive force in development. • Resolution of conflicts in each phase determines adjustment/maladjustment.
Attachment	**Bowlby** **Mahler**	• If attachment does not take place, the parent–child relationship will always be vulnerable. • Missteps in the progression from dependence to independence can lead to psychological problems.
Behavioral theories	**Seligman**	• Behavior develops when desired behavior is rewarded and unwanted behavior is ignored or punished. • Behavior is learned from modeling that of others, and shaped through experience.
Child in system	**Bronfenbrenner**	• Children develop in relation to their environmental context.
Cognitive, intellectual competence	**Piaget** *Birth–2 yrs:* sensorimotor *2–7 yrs:* preoperational *7–11 yrs:* concrete operational *11yrs and beyond:* formal operations	• Children construct cognitive development actively. • Thinking moves from sensory based, to use of language and symbols, to logical reasoning ending in abstract thinking.

and culture all contribute to the child's development into an adult. Understanding normal development by encompassing the biological, psychological, sociological, cultural, and spiritual context of the child will help the nurse to better distinguish illness from normal developmental or social and environmental effects (Table 30-2).

Parenting

For many years, childhood mental illness was blamed on "bad" parents, or parents who "did" something to raise children who later were diagnosed with mental illness. It is now understood that children grow, are nurtured, and interact within their family system. Biological makeup, temperament, and personality, as well as how the child fits with the rest of the family and environment, combine to shape a child's development. These factors also affect outcomes for children with psychiatric disorders. **Attachment** is a concept first identified in the 1940s by John Bowlby, a British researcher who studied children who were orphaned as a result of World War II. Bowlby identified four distinguishing characteristics of attachment:

1. *Proximity maintenance:* The desire to be near the people we are attached to.

2. *Safe haven:* Returning to the attachment figure for comfort and safety in the face of a fear or threat.

3. *Secure base:* The attachment figure acts as a base of security from which the child can explore the surrounding environment.

4. *Separation distress:* Anxiety that occurs in the absence of the attachment figure. (Bowlby, 1953)

Based on the responses observed, Canadian researcher Mary Ainsworth, who studied with Bowlby, described three major styles of attachment: secure attachment, ambivalent–insecure attachment, and avoidant–insecure attachment (Ainsworth, Blehar, Waters & Wall, 1978). Later, researchers Main and Solomon (1990) added a fourth attachment style, disorganized–insecure attachment, based on their own research.

Bowlby made three key propositions about attachment theory (Bowlby, 1969, 1973). First, he suggested that when children are raised with confidence, their primary caregiver will be available to them, and they are less likely to experience fear than those who are raised without such conviction. Second, he believed that this confidence is forged during a critical period of development—during the years of infancy, childhood, and adolescence—and that the expectations that are formed during that period tend to remain relatively unchanged for the rest of the person's life. Finally, Bowlby suggested that these expectations that are formed are directly tied to actual experience. In other words, children develop expectations that their caregivers will be responsive to their needs because, in their experience, their caregivers have been responsive in the past.

When children do not form significant and stable emotional connections with the significant people in their lives, many relationship problems can occur. Troubled attachment relationships have been linked with developmental psychopathology. Insecure attachments in infancy have been linked with a higher incidence of emotional problems, including anxiety, depression, conduct problems, suicidality, drug use, aggressive and antisocial behaviors, and ADHD in childhood and adolescence (Keskin & Cam, 2010). Secure attachment relationships constitute healthy relationships, so children with poor attachments early in life (those who are neglected, orphaned, or have numerous foster caregivers) may lack the healthy psychological foundation to foster self-confidence and calm to minimize fears and rejection. Thus, early attachment relationships appear to help shape early mental health in children and adolescents.

Decades of research into attachment theory by Bowlby have identified that attachment between a child and caregiver lays the foundation for future relationships with others and their surroundings (Bowlby & Fry, 1953; Bowlby, 1969, 1973). For patterns of attachment to remain intact and functioning, the individual must be able to synthesize experiences and new information about the self and the environment (Bowlby, 1973). A number of negative experiences (such as parental divorce or childhood experience of physical or sexual abuse) can negatively influence attachment stability (Bowlby & Fry, 1953).

In the famous "strange situation" study, researchers observed 26 mother–infant pairs in a room where the child was briefly left alone and in the company of a stranger before the mother returned to comfort the distressed child (Ainsworth, Blehar, Waters, & Wall, 1978). It was from this study that the categories of secure and insecure attachment were more clearly developed and defined, with specific categories of ambivalent–insecure and avoidant–insecure. Main and Solomon added the disorganized–insecure attachment style in which the infant displayed "bouts or sequences of behavior which seemed to lack a readily observable goal, intention or explanation" (1990, p. 122).

Life events can shape the dynamics of the whole family as well as that of the child. Stable and warm influences in the home environment help protect the child from the stresses of the outside world. In addition, parents' own fears, sadness, and emotional regulation can shape the child's developing sense of self. Outcomes of illness are more positive if children have protective factors in place (Table 30-3) and more negative with accumulative risks. Therefore, work with children and adolescents should always include work with their families.

Cognitive Function

Psychological risk factors such as personality and cognitive function (including early information processing, attention, and aspects of memory and executive function) have been examined for posing risk for vulnerability to childhood psychiatric disorders. Subtle dysfunction in elements of social cognition (including affect recognition, empathy, and theory of mind) may also increase risk for psychiatric illness (Hassel, McKinnon, Kusi, & MacQueen, 2011). For example, children with early negative experiences with peers may have chronic patterns of hopelessness and low self-esteem that affect their ability to manage stress and painful emotion beyond childhood. As another example, a child with limited intellectual functioning, or an inability to see things from the standpoint of others (theory of mind), may not fully understand the content or context of social interactions with normally developing peers. For that child, the experience of social interactions becomes one of social isolation rather than inclusion.

Sociocultural Domain

Much of a child's day is spent with family, in school, or with peers. The social domain of a child refers to relationships and social interactions within relationships. Building relationships and significant attachments, and forming the foundation of social support, are

Protective and Risk Factors for Psychiatric Disorders in Childhood	table 30-3

Protective Factors	Risk Factors
Consistency of caregivers, especially in early childhood	Frequent changes in caregivers
	Low socioeconomic status
Exercise	Domestic violence
Diet	Exposure to trauma
Time in nature	Drugs
Improved relationships	Parental divorce
Recreation/enjoyable activities	Child abuse and neglect
Relaxation	
Stress management	
Service to others	
Stable family life	
High IQ	
High socioeconomic status	
Faith base	

developmental goals of childhood that help protect a child from illness. The stronger the family support, school environment, and peer group, the more resilient a child will be when confronted with life stressors. Stressors such as divorce, bullying, child abuse and neglect, community violence, or negative peer influences can be mediated by protective factors such as strong family and extended support or connection with religious activities or strong teacher mentors (Box 30-2). Building strong social networks is critical for protecting children and adolescents from distress that can contribute to psychiatric disorders.

Although psychiatric disorders and syndromes are universal and have core symptoms, how these symptoms manifest may vary across cultures or subgroups within a culture (Canino & Allegria, 2008). Thus, the same internal disorder can manifest differently in different cultures, but the underlying psychopathology is the same across cultures (Chapter 5). In addition, deprived environments may cause enduring biological dysfunctions in empathy and impulse control characteristic of conduct disorders, but the same environment may also cause nondisordered youth to react in socially undesirable ways out of motives of self-protection or social conformity. This may be illustrated by presenting two examples of the same behavior with differing biological components but the same environmental context.

Community Violence	box 30-2

Community violence is any act of interpersonal violence toward an individual by another individual who has no relationship to the victim (National Center for Children Exposed to Violence, 2006).

Common forms of community violence include physical and sexual assault, shootings, gang violence, drugs, and burglary (Kelly, 2010). Exposure to community violence has been linked to violent behavior, symptoms of anxiety and depression, participation in gangs, feelings of hopelessness, posttraumatic stress, drug and alcohol use, and risky behaviors.

In one example, an adolescent who becomes tired of not having money or social opportunities chooses to start selling drugs, even though neither he nor anyone in his family uses drugs. The converse example would be the adolescent who grows up in a home where drug use is common in his family, and he starts using with his family at an early age as a way of life. Both these adolescents live in an impoverished environment, but one sees drug use as a means of self-protection and social conformity, whereas the other likely has a strong biological and familial predisposition for substance use.

The influence of culture on the incidence and features of psychiatric diagnoses in childhood and adolescence also appears to differ according to diagnoses. Data for child and adolescent ADHD seems to point consistently toward a universal syndrome across culture and gender related to these attentional disorders, but the data on cross-cultural validity for conduct disorder and oppositional defiant disorders seem to be less clear and possibly more subject to variation across cultures (Canino & Allegria, 2008). Gender effects on illness, however, appear to be more universal, with ADHD being more common with boys and depressive disorders more common in adolescent girls. Another universal finding is that co-occurring psychiatric disorders appear across cultures, with the most common being major depression with anxiety disorders and conduct disorders with ADHD. Clarification of symptoms and their cultural impact for children and adolescents is an important tool for deciphering the impact of social and cultural effects on their psychiatric illness (Lutz & Warren, 2007).

Spiritual Domain

Spiritual practices, faith-based communities, and spiritual growth have been linked to resiliency in childhood. **Resilience** is an individual's ability to cope with stress and adversity. As a protective factor and strength-based practice, practicing their religious faith appears to give children and adolescents meaning and purpose in their lives (Briggs, Akos, Czyszczon, & Eldridge, 2011). This seems to be true particularly as children gain independence and adolescents determine their individuality and life goals. Spiritual practice can provide structure, routine, and a source of hope and meaning as children and adolescents encounter stress in their lives. For adolescents, encountering their faith and determining its relevance in their lives while taking perspective with others helps them to rely less on the authority of others while establishing more of their core identity (Garcia, 2010). Participating in youth activities or worship helps to build a sense of support and connection to others with similar goals and foundation, and has a positive impact on coping and academic performance, as well as peer relationships (Regnerus & Elder, 2003). Spirituality can serve as a protective factor, giving meaning and hope to life experiences of children, adolescents, and their families as they manage their psychiatric illness.

Pause and Reflect

1. *What techniques could be used with a child who has a reactive temperament style and is being told for the first time that she has a chronic illness?*
2. *When assessing pain response, how can the nurse understand whether temperament is affecting the child's pain experience?*
3. *Are parents typically good reporters of their child's temperament? What may influence their views?*

Child and Adolescent Psychiatric Disorders

For a child or adolescent, a psychiatric disorder can influence daily functioning at home and at school. Relationships with family members, adults, and peers are affected. The child may find the impairment particularly frustrating when others respond inappropriately as a result of their failure to understand or sympathize with the child's responses. Nurses working with children and adolescents need to be aware of the psychiatric disorders that affect this age group and how to help these patients and their families move beyond suffering into improved daily functioning, wellness, and hope for the future. Nurses may participate in mental health promotion activities in their communities. These activities often provide protective measures and lower children's risk for mental health problems (Box 30-3).

Mental Health Promotion | box 30-3

Mental health promotion activities help maximize protective factors and minimize risk among families with children who could be at risk for illness due to genetics, environment, or exposure to stressful events. Two such programs, the Nurse Family Partnership Program and Early Head Start, use home visits to foster healthy development and family coping in populations at risk for illness, and have been shown to prevent child maltreatment and associated outcomes such as injuries (MacMillan et al., 2009). In the Nurse Family Partnership Program, nurses visit the homes of expecting parents and develop trusting relationships aimed at strengthening families and providing education about effective parenting. In Early Head Start programs, similar in-home early support and learning are put into place for families of young children at risk of stress or difficulties. These programs help families to strengthen skills and build support for their children before they reach school age.

A study by Beeber et al. found that short-term, in-home psychotherapy provided to low-income Latina mothers experiencing depression resulted in a decrease in depressive symptoms and fewer reports of aggressive behavior among their children when compared with mothers who did not receive this treatment (Beeber et al., 2010). Supporting families with in-home nursing intervention appears to have a protective effect on the development of mental illness in children, as well as addressing problematic parenting. The Safe Schools/Healthy Students initiative, a federally funded but state-run program, provides grants that fund local mental health promotion activities, especially those aimed at reducing the number of children who are exposed to violence (Substance Abuse and Mental Health Services Administration [SAMHSA], 2013). Mindfulness-based therapies have also helped to reduce these risk factors among urban youth (Sibinga et al., 2011), providing a tool for managing stress using meditation and mindfulness techniques. Such promising outcomes for these and other prevention efforts help mental health professionals reach larger groups of children who may otherwise suffer.

Neurodevelopmental Disorders

Neurodevelopmental disorders include intellectual disability; global developmental delay; language, speech, and communication disorders; autism spectrum disorder (ASD); and ADHD. These disorders are characterized by developmental deficits that impair functioning in multiple areas and usually manifest before a child begins school. Nurses in all settings that serve children and adolescents will encounter children with any of these disorders, but nurses will most frequently be involved in the assessment and care of children with ASD and ADHD.

Autism Spectrum Disorders

The core symptoms of ASDs are impairment of social interactions and communication, and restricted, repetitive behaviors and interests (Nazeer, 2011) (Figure 30-2). With the publication of the DSM-5, ASD now covers disorders previously identified separately, including Asperger syndrome, pervasive developmental disorder not otherwise specified, high-functioning autism, and childhood disintegrative disorder (APA, 2013).

Children with ASDs struggle with making and keeping friends, and they often do not understand why others do not befriend or understand them. The challenges of social interaction can isolate these children, who feel as if the world does not understand them, and they get confused by the world as well. Levels of severity are recognized by the degree to which the child or adolescent needs assistance. For example, some children may be able to use complete sentences and communicate with others but be unable to maintain a conversation, whereas others have difficulty forming intelligible words and are unable to respond to communication from others.

Co-morbidity with other disorders has a 9% to 10% prevalence rate, with some studies showing up to a 70% rate of co-morbidity (Nazeer, 2011; Simonoff et al., 2008). Often, children are misdiagnosed due to the overlap of ASD with symptoms of other disorders (such as ADHD or anxiety); African American children experience even greater delay in diagnosis (Mandell, Ittenback, Levy, & Pinto-Martin, 2007). Intellectual impairment is associated with 70% to 80% of ASD cases, further adding complexity to children and adolescents with the disorder. In addition, parenting a child with an ASD results in low adaptive behaviors for the child, high stress levels for parents,

increased need for family support, and coping difficulties for parents (Hall & Graf, 2011).

Psychosocial therapies that address communication, daily living skills, socialization, and offer support to families are best practices when developing nursing care for the child with an ASD (Bekhet, Johnson, & Zauszniewski, 2012; Johnson, Frenn, Feetham, & Simpson, 2011). In addition, psychopharmacologic interventions to address key symptoms of irritability, aggression, and aberrant behaviors (Robb, 2010) offer further care to children as they work toward minimizing the functional impairment of these disorders on their lives.

Attention-Deficit/Hyperactivity Disorder

Attention-deficit/hyperactivity disorder (ADHD) is the most common psychiatric disorder in childhood and adolescence, affecting an estimated 3% to 7% of school-age children, although findings from one study suggests as many as 11% may be affected (Visser et al., 2014). The core symptoms of ADHD affect the child in school, home, and social settings. ADHD may be diagnosed when symptoms persist for more than 6 months across a minimum of two separate settings (for example, school and home). Core symptoms fall into three categories: inattention, hyperactivity, and impulsivity (APA, 2013; National Institute of Mental Health [NIMH], 2012).

- *Symptoms of inattention:* making careless mistakes, not listening when spoken to directly, difficulty organizing tasks or focusing attention, becoming distracted or bored easily, and difficulty following directions.

- *Symptoms of hyperactivity:* fidgeting, squirming, nonstop talking, difficulty playing quietly, inappropriate activity (for instance, climbing on furniture), excessive talking.

- *Symptoms of impulsivity:* difficulty waiting in line or in turn, frequently interrupting others, blurting inappropriate comments, acting without regard for consequences.

Children with ADHD may present with a primarily hyperactive/impulsive type of ADHD; a primarily inattentive type (in which children have difficulty with concentration, organization, and distractibility); or a combined type (a combination of inattention and hyperactivity and impulsiveness). The primarily inattentive type is more prevalent among girls and may go undiagnosed for years, whereas the combined type is seen more in boys and typically is associated with more school and social problems, along with greater parental stress, generally prompting earlier diagnosis (Tzang, Chang, & Liu, 2009). Symptoms of ADHD are effectively relieved with a combination of psychosocial and medication treatments (Poncin, Sukhodolsky, McGuire, & Scahill, 2007).

Disruptive, Impulse Control, and Conduct Disorders

Disruptive behavior disorders include oppositional defiant disorder (ODD), intermittent explosive disorder (IED), and conduct disorder (CD). These disorders can not only impair functioning of the individual child, but they also can disrupt the environments in which the child interacts, especially home and classroom environments.

Oppositional Defiant Disorder

Oppositional defiant disorder (ODD) is defined by symptoms of irritability and defiance of adult authorities. Prevalence rates range

---

Social Deficits
- Responses often inconsistent to situation
- Lack of engagement in family or group activity
- Lack of attention to social cues

Language Deficits
- Slow to respond to verbal communication from others
- Delayed or impaired language development
- Communicates using visual cues, pictures
- Uses words in ways that have meaning only within the family

Repetitive Behaviors
- Preoccupation with specific objects (e.g., trains, buses)
- Stereotypical or repetitive movements or behaviors
- Comforted by routine activities and surroundings

30-2 Autism spectrum disorder is characterized by social and communication deficits, restricted interests, and repetitive behaviors.

from 1% to 13% of school-age children; symptoms typically include persistent resistance to authority and anger and aggression that disrupt daily functioning and relationships with others (APA, 2013). The clinician is more likely to suspect ODD when the child exhibits oppositional, vindictive, negativistic, and hostile behavior that creates a disturbance in social, academic, or occupational functioning (American Academy of Child and Adolescent Psychiatry, 2007). Evidence suggests that without early intervention, behavioral problems such as aggression, oppositional behavior, or conduct problems in young children may become crystallized patterns of behavior by age 8, beginning a trajectory of escalating academic problems, dropping out of school, substance abuse, delinquency, and violence (Sourander et al., 2012). Treatment of ODD often is complicated and requires multimodal approaches such as psychosocial interventions, parent coaching, and, occasionally, medication management (American Academy of Child and Adolescent Psychiatry, 2007; Dunsmore, Booker, & Ollendick, 2012).

Intermittent Explosive Disorder

Intermittent explosive disorder may be diagnosed in children older than age 6 who exhibit recurrent outbursts and inability to control aggressive impulses. Aggressive behaviors may manifest as temper tantrums, arguments, or physical aggression toward property or others. Notable characteristics for diagnosis include aggressive behaviors that are out of proportion to the stressor; behaviors that are not premeditated; and distress or impairment in functioning related to the behaviors (APA, 2013).

Conduct Disorder

Conduct disorder (CD) is a prevalent syndrome, recognized in both DSM-5 and the International Standard Classification of Diseases (ICD-10). It is defined by a relatively persistent pattern of multiple antisocial behaviors during childhood and adolescence, including fighting, bullying, stealing, vandalism, and lying for personal gain. Evidence suggests that deficits in inhibitory behavioral control, poor verbal abilities, family histories of antisocial behavior, callous–unemotional traits, severe anger dysregulation, and poor parental monitoring may be underlying developmental pathways that lead to conduct disorder among youth (Pardini & Frick, 2013). These and other CD traits harm victims in physical and psychological ways. Furthermore, children and adolescents who meet diagnostic criteria for CD are themselves at substantially increased risk for incarceration, depression, substance use disorders, and suicide (Lahey & Walman, 2012).

Without intervention, children and adolescents with ODD or CD are likely to have a poor prognosis. Promising work using early parent and child training programs have improved social competence and minimized effects of these disorders as children grow (Webster-Stratton, Reid, & Beauchaine, 2011). Nurses who are able to recognize common examples and patterns of problematic behavior in childhood will be able to help parents and clinicians identify issues for treatment earlier, thus hopefully increasing a child's chances of appropriate early intervention (Box 30-4).

Tic Disorders and Tourette Syndrome

Tourette syndrome is a neurologic disorder with childhood onset that is defined by an enduring pattern of motor and phonic tics, whereas *tic disorders* involve tics that do not meet the required pattern of motor and phonic tics. Tics are sudden, purposeless, repetitive, stereotyped movements (such as eye blinking, facial grimacing, or head jerking) or vocalizations (such as throat clearing, grunting, snoring, swearing, or repeating short phrases) (Chao et al., 2010). Tics can be mild to severe and have a varied course, with most cases declining in severity by late adolescence. In fact, most cases of Tourette syndrome resolve by early adulthood, with only 20% of cases remaining symptomatic in adulthood (Swain et al., 2007). Tourette syndrome affects 1 to 10 children in 1,000; 80% of children with Tourette syndrome have a co-occurring disruptive behavior disorder (Conelea et al., 2011; Specht et al., 2011). Patients with Tourette syndrome are sensitive to stress, and the frequency and intensity of tics are worse during periods of excitement and fatigue (Leckman, Bloch, Scahill, & King, 2006). Educational interventions, psychotherapy to help with coping and stress management, and medication management are necessary components of treatment for children with a tic disorder or Tourette syndrome. In addition, recent evidence suggests that a comprehensive behavioral intervention for tics (CBIT) is an effective and promising therapy that helps children and families to reverse tic habits, identify and mitigate triggers, and ultimately change the severity and social impact of tics on the lives of children suffering from these disorders (Scahill et al., 2013).

Feeding and Eating Disorders

Eating disturbances can be transient and common among developing children and adolescents, and one in four girls considers themselves as fat regardless of their weight; almost half of all girls have

---

Common Examples and Patterns of Problematic Behavior in Childhood

box 30-4

The following are common examples or patterns of problematic behaviors in children that require further evaluation and possible intervention:

- Withdrawal: child will not participate in life of family or attend school
- Tantrums or rages: emotional outbursts in which the child struggles to gain control over emotional experience
- Problematic sleep behaviors
- Oppositional behavior: child does not follow directions or defies authority

- Altered eating behaviors: stealing food; refusing to eat; eating excessively; eating odd or nonfood items
- Reactivity: excessive emotional response to condition or situation
- Toileting: soiling clothes, eliminating in unusual places
- Lying
- Stealing
- Aggression toward self or others

attempted to lose weight (Hautala et al., 2008, 2011). In some cases, these attempts lead to prolonged problematic eating patterns, which can result in binge eating, obesity, anorexia, or bulimia. Risks factors for feeding and eating disorders include depression, anxiety, perceived stress, and dissatisfaction with appearance. Prevention programs aimed at preventing self-dissatisfaction, increasing self-esteem, and promoting diversity in appearance between individuals may help decrease the incidence of these disorders among growing girls. Care for the patient with an eating disorder is focused on (1) relearning normal patterns of eating and exercise, (2) restoring social relationships and community participation, and (3) generalizing new eating patterns within the community (van Ommen et al., 2009). Family therapy, psychoeducation, medication management, and cognitive–behavioral therapy are among interventions that may be helpful to adolescents with feeding and eating disorders. Nurses help patients initially with decision making about eating, serve as coaches and role models, then become a "fall back" support as individuals gain more skill in healthy eating behaviors (Chapter 15, Feeding and Eating Disorders).

Substance-Related and Addictive Disorders

Co-morbid substance use is common among children and adolescents with psychiatric disorders. Outpatient and residential drug treatment for children and adolescents can be effective, and the longer the treatment, generally the more effective it is (Chapter 20). Adolescents appear to stay with drug abuse programs if they have internal motivation to stop using and an expectation that treatment will work, have a past or current legal charge, or are in a youth detention center (Pagey, Deering, & Sellman, 2010). Adolescents who use substances often are viewed as having the ability to exercise personal control over their use, and therefore are seen as weak or at blame for their illness (Livingston, Milne, Fang, & Amari, 2012). This stigma can get in the way of families seeking care or support for the illness. Acceptance and commitment therapy groups, vocational training, and motivational interviewing have been found to decrease stigma associated with individuals with substance use disorders (Jackman, 2012). In addition, parents of children with substance use disorders need their own support as they set limits, deal with the consequences, grieve their pre-using children and try to keep them safe,

find appropriate services, live with the blame and shame commonly experienced, and attempt self-preservation (Usher, Jackson, & O'Brien, 2007).

Childhood Trauma

In a national study, 905,000 children were found to be maltreated. Some 16% were physically abused, 8.8% sexually abused, and 6.6% psychologically or emotionally abused (U.S. Department of Health and Human Services, Administration for Children and Families, 2010). Although most children do not develop long-term problems secondary to abuse, some continue to respond to their environment in ways that have a long-lasting impact on their functioning. The frequency and number of abusive events influences the severity of psychological distress. Emotional experiences of trauma can be overwhelming for children, who depend on adults to help them cope. If the home environment is the source of maltreatment, trauma can result in more significant consequences due to the lack of supports. In these cases, foster care or alternative family environments can ensure the safety of the child during the healing process, and stop the pattern of abuse.

Trauma- and stressor-related disorders seen most frequently in children include reactive attachment disorder, disinhibited social disengagement disorder, and posttraumatic stress disorder (PTSD) (Chapter 13). PTSD may look different in children and adolescents than in adults. Symptoms characteristic of children and adolescents affected by the disorder are outlined in Box 30-5.

A high percentage of children in residential facilities have reported being victims of violence or witnesses to violence in their home or communities (Singer, 2007). Caregivers of children who suspect that a child has been the victim of physical, emotional, or sexual abuse or neglect are mandated reporters of abuse. Nurses who have any evidence of abuse of a child are mandated by law to contact their state's department of child protective services to report concerns; if they do not do so, they risk losing their nursing license. Reporting laws exist to protect and provide services to child victims and their families. Stress and trauma research traditionally has focused on negative consequences of trauma. Recently, research has begun to focus on positive outcomes, specifically **posttraumatic growth** (PTG), defined as positive changes resulting from the process of overcoming trauma. PTG theory emphasizes the transformative

---

Common PTSD Symptoms in Children and Adolescents   box 30-5

- Recurring, distressing dreams related to the event
- Re-experiencing through flashbacks
- Hyperarousal
- Avoidant, numb, or dissociative behavior when in stress
- Memory impairment, impaired information processing, difficulty concentrating
- Impaired attachment
- Difficulties with self-monitoring, behavioral control, limit setting, interpersonal awareness

- Possible impact on immunity and neurologic development
- Low level of interest or participation in activities, play
- Revisiting trauma through play
- Withdrawal
- Impulsive or aggressive behaviors
- Mood swings
- Somatic symptoms such as headache or stomachache
- Regressive language or behaviors (language or behaviors younger than age)

Based on American Psychiatric Association. (2013). *Diagnostic and Statistical Manual of Mental Disorders* (5th ed.). Washington, DC: American Psychiatric Publishers; U.S. Department of Veterans Affairs. (2007). PTSD in Children and Teens. Available at http://www.ptsd.va.gov/public/pages/ptsd-children-adolescents.asp; American Academy of Child and Adolescent Psychiatry. (2011). Posttraumatic Stress Disorder (PTSD). Available at http://www.aacap.org/AACAP/Families_and_Youth/Facts_for_Families/Facts_for_Families_Pages/Posttraumatic_Stress_Disorder_70.aspx

potential of one's experiences with highly stressful events and circumstances. The positive changes of PTG are generally thought to occur in five areas: new possibilities, relating to others, personal strength, appreciation of life, and spiritual change. In a meta-analysis of studies examining positive growth (or postraumatic positive growth), Meyerson, Grant, Carter, and Kilmer (2011) found that childhood victims of trauma who are of younger age and have less trauma severity, less subjective stress, and more social support and more religious involvement have more positive growth than others. In addition, the researchers noted that positive growth experiences may be optimal during late adolescence and when posttraumatic stress is moderate. This research offers hope to families of children who have experienced trauma.

Elimination Disorders

Elimination disorders are common disturbances of childhood. Of all 7-year-olds, 10% wet at night, 2% to 3% wet during the daytime, and 1% to 3% soil. Often, these disorders coexist. Despite a high remission rate, 1% to 2% of all adolescents are affected by nocturnal enuresis and 1% by either daytime wetting or encopresis. More than 90% of elimination disorders are not due to a medical cause. A diagnosis of enuresis is made if a child continues to be enuretic from the age of 5 years, and encopresis may be diagnosed if the child continues to soil from 4 years onward, after ruling out organic causes (von Gontard, 2011). Criteria for diagnosis of encopresis include repeated passage of feces into inappropriate places (such as clothing or floor), whether involuntary or intentional; at least one event a month for a minimum of 3 months; chronological age or equivalent developmental level of at least 4 years of age; and ruling out potential causative factors, such as laxative use or a general medical condition (APA, 2013).

Stress can affect the ability a child has to control elimination patterns, as can a short attention span, resulting in a child who urinates or defecates outside the typical routine. Children and adolescents with encopresis or enuresis often feel ashamed and may avoid situations that might lead to embarrassment or shame (such as sleepovers or camp). Treatment typically will include psychoeducation, nutritional changes, behavioral therapy that is positively focused, family support, and medication management (Coelho, 2011).

Anxiety Disorders

Approximately 8% to 10% of youth suffer from anxiety disorders (Degnan, Almas, & Fox, 2010). Symptoms of stress and anxiety in children and adolescents include recurrent fears and worries; sleep disturbances and nightmares; extreme difficulty separating from parents; fear of going to school; discomfort in social situations (school, parties, mealtimes); irritability, crying, or tantrums; and/or inability to recover after a stressor.

Separation anxiety occurs when a child exhibits great fear and distress when separated from parents or home. Generalized anxiety disorder is more a chronic state of worry over unrealistic stressors. Specific phobias can also happen in childhood; for example, children can be afraid of social situations or of storms. Avoidance behaviors such as school refusal or refusing to leave the house when it rains may be an indication of a specific fear. Although now in a separate category from the anxiety disorders, obsessive–compulsive disorder (OCD) is diagnosed in children and adolescents when compulsive actions develop as a mechanism for relieving obsessive worrying. A

child with a fear of germs, for example, will avoid sitting on public seating and carry a tissue in her hand at all times to avoid touching a possible germ. Nursing care of children with anxiety involves helping them with cognitive and behavioral strategies to relieve anxiety, using the mnemonic CHAT:

> Check how my body is feeling
>
> Having bad thoughts?
>
> Attitudes and actions that can help
>
> Time for a reward

More information on anxiety disorders can be found in Chapter 13.

A specific condition related to anxiety that may be seen in children is **selective mutism**, a rare childhood disorder that occurs in 0.47% to 0.76% of the general population. Children with selective mutism are fully capable of speech in some settings, but fail to speak in selected social situations (APA, 2013). Typically, children will speak in their own homes but not at school or in more social environments. Selective mutism usually is first detected when the child begins attending school and can be severe enough severe enough to impair academic and social functioning. Common associated features of selective mutism include shyness, anxiety, withdrawal, compulsivity, and oppositional defiant behavior, particularly at home. Previous definitions operated under assumption that selective mutism was characterized by oppositionality and manipulative withholding of speech; however, newer definitions include the possibility that children are reacting anxiously in response to a threatening environment—they are "scared speechless." A combination of family, school, and individual cognitive–behavioral therapies (CBTs) have been shown to be most effective in helping selectively mute children find their voice. Specific therapies that have met with some success include augmented self-modeling (in which the child videotapes himself or herself while speaking, then models in new settings) and the Meeky Mouse Therapy Manual, a CBT program for children with selective mutism developed by Fung and Mendlowitz (Kehle et al., 2011; Viana, Beidel, & Rabian, 2009). From some children, use of selective serotonin-reuptake inhibitors (SSRIs) may also be indicated.

Mood Disorders

The ways in which children manifest mood disorders can differ from the ways in which the disorders are manifested by adults. Nurses working with children and adolescents must be aware of manifestations in children and adolescents associated with mood disorders such as depression and pediatric bipolar disorder. Nurses must also understand the issues surrounding self-injury and suicide among children and adolescents.

Depression

Depression is common among children and adolescents and can result in risky behaviors such as self-injury, substance abuse, loss of functioning, and suicide. Approximately 5% of children and adolescents experience depression at some point (American Academy of Child and Adolescent Psychiatry, 2013). Children who are depressed typically cannot communicate their sadness with words, but instead communicate to others with their withdrawn, sad, and/or irritable mood states. A child who is depressed may mope about the house, refuse to play with friends, and sleep more than usual (Hamrin, Antenucci, & Magorno, 2012). A teen who is depressed may stop doing schoolwork, get into frequent conflicts with peers, or begin to stay in his or her room all the time. Other symptoms of depression in children and adolescents may include the following:

- Depressed or irritable mood
- Low frustration level
- Changes in appetite and sleep
- Physical complaints such as stomachaches, headaches, or getting tired easily
- Depressive or morbid themes in play or dreams
- Intense anger or rage
- Loss of pleasure in activities
- Impaired concentration
- Thoughts of death, self-harm, or suicide

The criteria for diagnosis of a major depressive episode or dysthymia in this age group are similar to the criteria used with adults; however, the way the symptoms look and how long they last are more developmentally based with children and adolescents. A hallmark study of teens with depression found that the most effective treatment was combination treatment of medication management with CBT. When children and adolescents with depression are treated, the prognosis is excellent. There is increasing evidence that depression prevention programs may help to decrease the development of depressive symptoms in childhood (Hamrin, Antenucci, & Magorno, 2012; Merry et al., 2011). Such programs typically are based in educational or family group formats, with the content focus being CBT with psychoeducation.

Pediatric Bipolar Disorder

Pediatric bipolar disorder (PBD) is characterized by significant mood disturbances, including elated or irritable mood; cycling mood episodes; episodes of rage, grandiosity, or inflated self-esteem; hypersexual behavior; decreased need for sleep; and poor judgment (West & Pavuluri, 2009). The DSM-5 does not recognize PBD because it is very hard to diagnose accurately in children. Therefore, the criteria used for adults are used in a developmental context, with elation, irritability, and cycling of mood being the most evident symptoms of illness in the pediatric type. Published reports have indicated that children as young as age 3 can manifest symptoms of PBD; rage episodes can be the most common complaint with younger children diagnosed with PBD (Luby, Tandon, & Belden, 2009). The DSM-5 notes that chronic, severe irritability in children, especially in the absence of elation or cycling, may fit more closely with a diagnosis of disruptive mood dysregulation disorder (APA, 2013).

Disruptive Mood Dysregulation Disorder

Because not all children who rage have symptoms of mania, a new diagnosis of **disruptive mood dysregulation disorder** was proposed to best capture children who have severe mood dysregulation without distinct symptoms of mania or cycling (APA, 2013; Carlson et al., 2009). Characterized by recurrent, frequent outbursts inconsistent with the child's developmental level and occurring for a year or more, this disorder may be diagnosed provided that the behaviors are not better explained by another diagnosis (such as PTSD or ASD) (APA, 2013). The symptoms of this disorder—in particular, chronic, extreme irritability—generally result in significant impairment in function in a variety of settings and in relationships with others. Disruptive mood dysregulation disorder can be particularly challenging

to family members, and nurses are well advised to assess both patient and family functioning at each health care interaction.

Psychosis

Psychosis in childhood can occur within the context of depression, PBD, or anxiety. In addition, psychosis can also indicate a prodromal or beginning onset of schizophrenia. Symptoms of psychosis in childhood are similar to those seen in adult populations, although they are complicated by developmental challenges (limited language and differentiation of play and reality) as well as severity (younger children exhibit less symptom severity upon intake). Differentiation between what is the child's imagination and what are delusions, hallucinations, or disruptions in thought can be difficult. It often depends on parental input in combination with an extensive assessment of symptoms and the child's environment. Although rare, early onset schizophrenia (before the age of 10) has been thought to result in a poor prognosis over the life span. However, recent data have shown better prognosis and more hope for children affected by psychosis at a young age (Amminger et al., 2011). Early diagnosis and intervention that includes developmentally oriented psychoeducation and psychosocial interventions using a recovery approach will decrease the duration of untreated psychosis, result in more favorable outcomes, and provide hope for children and adolescents suffering from psychosis (Ruiz-Veguilla et al., 2012).

Self Injury

Self injury in children and adolescents is associated with poor coping, interpersonal conflict, academic problems, and risk for suicide (Crowell et al., 2012). Children or adolescents may cut or scratch themselves when frustrated, angry, or experiencing mood dysregulation. Some adolescents will express relief with self-injurious behavior, as if they felt an itch and scratched it. Others will self injure in response to arguments with friends or parents, or when they feel stressed or overwhelmed. Regardless of the trigger, nursing care of the self-injurious child or adolescent is to ensure safety first, and then to help the adolescent develop new skills for problem solving and managing difficult emotions and interpersonal conflicts. Increasingly, more evidence is growing to support the idea that adolescents who self injure are very different from adolescents who are depressed (Crowell et al., 2012). Adolescents who self injure differ from those with depression in delinquent behavior, PTSD symptoms, reports of substance and tobacco use, greater degree of hopelessness, higher impulsivity, and suicidal ideation. Therefore, treatments for youth who engage in self harm should be tailored differently from those with depression alone. Dialectical behavior therapy is a treatment that has been modified for adolescents and teaches these new skills and behaviors.

Suicide

Suicide is the third leading cause of death among adolescents in the United States (NIMH, 2010). Risk factors for suicide include depression, media-reported suicide, academic problems, and impulsivity (Box 30-6). Protective factors include having a sense of belonging and purpose, self-esteem, and family cohesion and support (Sharaf, Thompson, & Walsh, 2009; Shimshock, Williams, & Sullivan, 2011). Since the 1990s, national surveys of high school youth show that Latinos attempt suicide at higher rates than their African American and White peers, and that, in this population, familialism is a mediating protective factor against parent–child conflict (Kuhlberg, Pena, &

Risk Factors for Suicide among Children and Adolescents	box 30-6

Academic problems	Being a gay male teenager
Depression	Impulsivity
Media reports of suicide	Substance abuse
Exposure to trauma	Exposure to trauma
Family conflicts	Family history of mental illness, substance abuse, suicide
Access to means	Family violence (including physical or sexual abuse)

Based on Dickens, G. (2010). Imitative suicide: An issue for psychiatric and mental health nursing? *Journal of Psychiatric and Mental Health Nursing, 17*(8), 741–749; National Institute of Mental Health. (2010). Suicide in the U.S. Statistics and Prevention. Available at http://www.nimh.nih.gov/health/publications/suicide-in-the-us-statistics-and-prevention/index.shtml#factors; Russell, S. T., & Toomey, R. B. (2012). Men's sexual orientation and suicide: Evidence for U.S. adolescent specific risk. *Social Science and Medicine, 74*(4), 523–529.

Zayas, 2010). Enhancing communication between Latino adolescents and their parents may reduce conflict and the risk of suicidal actions by enhancing familialism, thus enhancing support and warmth for adolescents at risk. Suicide prevention in children and adolescents is best accomplished by identifying those at risk and mediating risk with appropriate treatment.

Pause and Reflect

1. *How does trauma affect a developing child? How can a family minimize these effects?*

2. *How can the school nurse help children with psychiatric disorders? What is considered abuse or an event that warrants a report to the department of child and family services?*

3. *Why do you think a combination of therapies may be helpful in treating children and adolescents with psychiatric disorders? How do you feel personally about children receiving medication for a psychiatric disorder?*

Special Considerations

Children and adolescents face challenges differently than do adults. An increasing number of children in the United States are homeless, a situation that jeopardizes their ability to learn and interact with their environment. Lesbian, gay, bisexual, and transgender youth (LGBTY) face challenges not experienced by their heterosexual peers. Bullying, a phenomenon approaching epidemic proportions in children and adolescents, and violence are all contributing to new and increasing concerns for those working with this population.

Homeless Youth

The recent international recession has brought more faces to the issues of poverty and homeless youth across the world. On any given night, between 1.6 and 2 million homeless youth live on the street, in shelters, or other temporary accommodations (Edidin, Ganim, Hunter, & Karnik, 2012). Most young people who leave home do so because of family violence, intolerable conditions, or poverty (Hughes et al., 2010). Precarious living conditions, lack of access to education, malnutrition, violence, family stress, and substance use all can overwhelm the child without a safe place to call home. At least 50% of homeless youth are thought to have a serious mental illness

and/or substance use disorder, placing them at risk for suicide and other high risk behaviors (Edidin, Ganim, Hunter, & Karnik, 2012; Hughes et al., 2010). In addition, homeless youth have poor access to health and mental health care, which can contribute to a sense of hopelessness and further compromise their ability to manage their illness. Instilling hope, fostering motivation, advocating for external supports such as housing, and building internal support (resiliency) can help children manage their illness despite their homelessness. The first step toward building hope in homeless youth is building trust with a child who will likely have a hard time discerning who is "trustworthy" (Hughes et al., 2010). In doing so, the nurse will be able to find relevant and sustainable ways to help the child as the child moves toward recovery.

Lesbian, Gay, Bisexual, and Transgender Youth

More lesbian and gay young people are coming out in adolescence at an earlier age and with earlier sexual experiences (Society for Adolescent Health and Medicine, 2013). Although development of sexual orientation and identity starts in early childhood, the process of consolidating a child's identity as gay or lesbian often includes increased disclosure to family, peers, and community, or staying quiet (or closeted). Nursing care of lesbian, gay, bisexual, and transgender youth (LGBTY) requires knowledge about the LGBTY culture, the social challenges of coming out and navigating the heterosexually oriented world, attending to associated health care concerns, and sensitivity to stressors such as bullying, isolation, and rejection (Dysart-Gale, 2010). Suicide risk and suicidal behavior are almost four times higher in LGBTY than heterosexual youth, and evidence indicates that suicidality, anxiety, substance use, risky behaviors such as unsafe sex practices, and depression *accompany* the social experience (stigma, prejudice, discrimination) of LGBTY rather than *characterize* this group (Haas et al., 2011).

Protective factors such as family connectedness, perceived caring from other adults, and school safety have been identified as being helpful in protecting youth from suicidality and other risk behaviors. In addition, advocacy efforts to protect LGBTY from harmful or ineffective therapies (including "reparative therapy") will help the child find effective and sensitive care providers for supporting his or her growth and continued building of strengths (Hein & Matthews, 2010). The nurse can offer hope to LGBTY by working to better understand their experience, minimizing risk for suicidality and other risk behaviors, and providing education and support using culturally appropriate and sensitive interventions for LGBTY and their families. In addition, maintaining confidentiality and understanding the process of "coming out" for both the child and family will help establish a trusting and supportive environment for navigating this developmental step (Riley, 2010).

Bullying

Bullying is a form of aggressive behavior in which (1) the behavior is intended to harm or hurt another; (2) the behavior occurs repeatedly over time; and (3) there is an imbalance of power, with the more powerful individual or group attacking a less powerful one (Liu & Graves, 2011). Approximately 30% to 40% of children and adolescents are bullied or bully others in their school years. Bullying may take place in person or in the form of cyberbullying—electronic bullying that takes place through text messaging or social media (Figure 30-3). There are repercussions of both bullying behavior and being bullied that warrant nursing interventions that take into consideration the biopsychosocial underpinnings of both sides of bullying behavior (Warren, 2011). A comprehensive review of anti-bullying efforts by Carter (2012) found that anti-bullying efforts in schools may be of limited benefit for students who bully others. A proactive, collaborative approach that includes peer nominations, engaging parents in the process, and training educators about mental health disorders of childhood and adolescence appears to have the greatest outcomes on changing bullying behaviors. Collaboration among nurses, parents, and teachers in developing a strong alliance to prevent and respond to bullying can also result in better outcomes for victims of bullying (Blaney & Chiocca, 2011). Associated features of bullies and children who are bullied are presented in Table 30-4, which also highlights potential treatment targets for nursing interventions aimed at preventing or changing the course of bullying.

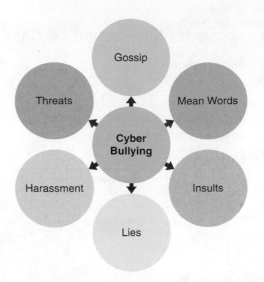

30-3 Cyberbullying is a form of bullying that takes place through text messaging or social media.

Violence

As stated earlier, exposure to violence increases a child's or adolescent's risk for mental illness. Gang violence and dating violence are two forms of violence of which nurses working in pediatric settings should be aware.

Gang violence is an escalating problem in American society with common forms of associated violence that can include physical and sexual assaults, shootings, acts of violence committed by gang members, drugs, and burglary (Kelly, 2010). Gang violence affects mostly African American and Latino adolescent males ages 12 to 18; however, as gang violence has increased, more children and adolescents outside gangs have been witnesses to or victims of gang activity. In addition, adolescent girls also may find affiliation with gangs either

Bullying		table 30-4
Characteristics of Person Who Bullies	**Victims of Bullying**	**Interventions**
• Peaks during grades 6–8 and declines through high school • Lack of self-confidence, helplessness, and past experience as a victim of bullying • Emotional processing dysregulation, impulsivity, exposure to community violence • Desire to be accepted by antisocial peers, low expectations of adults about school performance, unsupportive school environments, smoking and alcohol/drug use • Poor parental communication • Increased risk for mental illness/suicide	*Males:* experience more direct and physical forms of bullying, externalize bullying experience (act aggressive, act out) *Females:* less direct and more verbal forms of bullying—internalize bullying experience (feel anxious or depressed) • Risk factors include: shyness, anxiety, depression low self-regard, reduced assertiveness, early aggressive behaviors • Family characteristics: violence in the home, parental depression, harsh and reactive parenting, low socioeconomic status • Increased risk for mental illness/suicide	• Adopt policies against bullying. • Early intervention: decreases risk of adverse emotional/psycholgical effects. • Educate about bullying behaviors. • Actively respond to bullying behaviors (parents, teachers, peers). • Preventively offer anger management, social skills groups. • Promote family interventions aimed at reducing violence, controlling television watching, supporting positive parenting. • Focus on academic achievement. • Encourage parents to meet their child's friends; this may help reduce incidence of bullying behavior.

Based on Arsenault, L., Bowes, L., & Shakoor, S. (2010). Bullying victimization in youth and Mental health problems: "Much ado" about nothing. *Psychological Medicine, 40,* 717–729; Liu, J. & Graves, N. (2011). Childhood bullying: A review of constructs, concepts, and nursing implications. *Public Health Nursing, 28*(6), 556–568; Shetgiri, R., Hua, L., Avila, R., & Flores, G. (2012.) Parental characteristics associated with bullying perpetration in US children aged 10 to 17 years. *American Journal of Public Health, 102*(12), 2280–2286.

through their own actions or in dating relationships. In some communities, participation in gangs offers a sense of community and protection from violence from other gangs. Exposure to gang violence has been associated with disruptive behaviors and violence, as well as more internalizing behaviors such as anxiety and depression (Kelly, 2010). Parental support and involvement appear to be a positive mediator in the effect of violence on long-term outcomes for children and adolescents exposed to gang violence. Nurses can play an active role in understanding the context of gang affiliation and violence, as well as educating children and adolescents and their families about signs and symptoms of traumatic stress and strategies for avoiding potentially violent situations.

Dating violence in adolescence is associated with mental health concerns, academic problems, substance use and abuse, problematic eating behaviors, injury, and sexual risk behaviors (Centers for Disease Control and Prevention [CDC], 2012). Approximately 10% of adolescents reported being physically harmed by a girlfriend or boyfriend in the past 12 months (CDC, 2012). A study by Drauker, Martsolf, and Shokey (2012) sheds light on the interpersonal, cognitive, and developmental underpinnings of violent dating behavior, which can lead to effective primary, secondary, and tertiary nursing interventions. Views of relationships and expectations based on primary family attachments, developing expectations of what dating relationships are while continuing to develop one's own identity, and ambiguity in relationships all pose developmental, cognitive, and interpersonal challenges unique to adolescent dating relationships (Drauker, Martsolf, & Shokey, 2012). Victims of dating violence report extreme difficulties with navigating these issues in their relationships. The nurse can explore these typical challenges with patients to help gain understanding and empower toward self-care.

Interventions that can help children who have witnessed violence include:

- Peer support and education about violence
- Mentoring, anger management, and conflict resolution programs
- Involvement of community (schools, churches, day care centers) in nonviolence efforts
- Early intervention and outreach to exposed or at-risk children
- Stress reduction and fun activities
- Referral of high-risk children (children with incarcerated parents, those exposed to domestic violence, those seen in emergency departments after violence exposure) to mental health services (Willis et al., 2010)

Collaborative Care

Collaborative care of children and adolescents experiencing mental illness or in need of intervention may include milieu management, pharmacotherapy, and psychotherapy. When caring for this population, it is essential for parents to support, and even participate in, the plan of care.

Milieu Management

One of the most important components of care for children and adolescents is milieu therapy or management. Whether it be in a therapeutic school (a special school licensed by the state to provide an integrated educational milieu that addresses and promotes emotional, behavioral, familial, and academic development) or an

inpatient setting, the nurse interacts with child and adolescent patients and shapes and models the ways in which the child or adolescent interacts with others.

Practice parameters for milieu management of children and adolescents with mental illness have been developed that outline best practices for inpatient nurses working with children and adolescents in the milieu (International Society of Psychiatric Nurses [ISPN], 2010). Interventions include activities that promote self-efficacy and problem solving, such as teaching about affect and how to manage it, interrupting patterned behavior, and using reinforcement techniques (Delaney, 2006, 2009). Milieu therapy interventions have been tailored to meet the needs of children and adolescents with specific disorders as well. For example, milieu interventions for young children with ASD in natural settings resulted in increased communication skills, decreasing dependence on prompts, and decreasing aberrant behaviors (Mancil, Conroy, & Haydon, 2009).

Psychopharmacology

Medications can help minimize symptoms of child and adolescent psychiatric disorders. They are increasingly being used as evidence grows to support their efficacy and safety. The most commonly used medications are stimulants, antidepressants, and atypical antipsychotics.

Parents may have difficulty deciding to use medications for their child's symptoms because of the child's age and development. Education and support for families, along with continued monitoring of effects, side effects, and adherence, help families make informed decisions about choosing medications to help their child with symptoms. These efforts also help parents address their expectations and fears surrounding use of medication to treat their child's illness (Cormier, 2012). Off-label prescribing is common in child and adolescent psychiatry. Estimates indicate that 50% to 75% of pediatric medication use is off-label and is typically based on extrapolation of efficacy, dosing, administration, and side effect profiles from adult studies (Harrison, Cluxton Keller, & Gross, 2012; Patten, Waheed, & Bresee, 2012). The Medications feature outlines the most commonly used FDA approved (on-label) medications for treating children and adolescents diagnosed with psychiatric disorders.

Clinical trials have yet to establish safety and efficacy for commonly used off-label medications in youth populations. Because of possible risk, monitoring conducted before and throughout medication therapy with children and adolescents includes the following:

- Physical assessment: pulse, respiration rate, blood pressure, height and weight (using standardized growth charts), and body mass index (BMI).
- Lab panels, such as a complete blood count, urinalysis, blood urea nitrogen, serum electrolyte, and liver function tests to establish a baseline and assist with monitoring of emergent adverse drug events.
- A baseline electrocardiogram may be appropriate for stimulants and other drugs that may cause cardiac changes, particularly if the child has a family history of cardiac events.

PRACTICE ALERT   Selective serotonin-reuptake inhibitors (SSRIs) carry a black box warning that they may cause suicidal ideation or behavior. Parents whose children are prescribed SSRIs should work with their child's mental health provider to develop a safety plan to follow in the event that their child exhibits suicidal ideation.

Children and Adolescents

medications commonly used to treat

Drug Class/Drug	FDA-Approved Age	Dosing Range (dose per day)	Common Side Effects
Antidepressants			
fluoxetine (Prozac)	• 8 and older	2.5–20 mg	• Headache
sertraline (Zoloft)	• 6 and older (for OCD only)	2.5–10 mg	• GI distress
escitalopram (Lexapro)	• 12–17 for major depressive disorder	25–100 mg	• Agitation
			• Anxiety
fluvoxamine (Luvox)	• 8 and older for OCD only	100–250 mg	• Insomnia
clomipramine (Anafranil)	• 10 and older for OCD only	25–200 mg	
Mood stabilizers			
valproic acid (Depakote)	• 2 and older for seizures	125–1800 mg	• Weight gain
carbamazepine (Tegretol)	• Any age for seizures	200–1800 mg	• Hair loss
oxcarbazepine (Trileptal)	• 4 and older	150–1200 mg	• GI distress, toxicity
lithium carbonate (Eskalith, Lithobid)	• 12 and older	50 mg–1800 mg (up to lithium level of 0.6 mEq/L–1.2 mEq/L)	• Rash, thrombocytopenia
			• Cognitive dulling
Stimulants			
methylphenidate (Ritalin, Concerta, Metadate ER, Metadate CD, Methylin, Daytrana, Focalin, Focalin XR, Ritalin SR and LA)	• 6 and older	2.5–20 mg (Ritalin) 18–72 mg (Concerta) 5–30 mg (Metadate ER/CD) 5–40 mg (Focalin, Focalin XR)	• GI distress • Poor appetite • Headache • Agitation
dextroamphetamine (Dexedrine, Dextrostat)	• 3 and older	2.5–20 mg	• Sleep disruption (if taken too late in the day)
amphetamines (Adderall)	• 3 and older	5 mg–30 mg	
lisdexamfetamine dimesylate (Vyvanse)	• 6 and older	10–70 mg	
Non-stimulants			
• atomexetine (Strattera)	• 6 and older	10–80 mg	• Sedation
			• Dizziness
			• GI distress
			• Agitation
			• Urinary retention
Alpha agonists			
clonidine (Kapvay)	• 6 and older	0.1 mg–0.4 mg (Kapvay) 1–4 mg (Intuniv)	• Sedation
guanfacine (Intuniv)			• Dizziness
			• Hypotension
Atypicals			
risperidone (Risperal)	• 6 and older	0.25–3 mg	• Weight gain • Tiredness • Prolactin elevation • Headache
aripriprazole (Abilify)	• 13 and older for schizophrenia; 10 and older for bipolar mania and mixed episodes; 5 to 16 for irritability associated with autism	2.5–30 mg	• Weight gain • Akathesia • Sedation • Headache
ziprasidone (Geodon)	• 10 and older for bipolar disorder, manic or mixed episodes; 13–17 for schizophrenia and bipolar disorder	20–80 mg	• Sedation • Dizziness • Headache
quetiepine (Seroquel)	• 13 and older for schizophrenia; 18 and older for bipolar disorder; 10–17 for treatment of manic and mixed episodes of bipolar disorder	25–200 mg	• Sedation • Dizziness • Headache • Weight gain
olanzapine (Zyprexa)	• 18 and older; ages 13–17 as second-line treatment for manic or mixed episodes of bipolar disorder and schizophrenia	2.5–10 mg	• Sedation • Dizziness • Headache • Weight gain
haloperidol (Haldol)	• Ages 3 and older for psychosis	0.5–2 mg	• Sedation • Extrapyramidal symptoms

Drug Class/Drug	FDA-Approved Age	Dosing Range (dose per day)	Common Side Effects
Others			• Hypotension
pimozide (Orap)	• Tourette syndrome 12 and older	0.25–10 mg	• QT prolongation
			• Tachycardia
			• Prolactin elevation
desmopressin (DDAVP)	• Nocturesis/enuresis 6 and older	0.1–0.4 mg	• Headaches, dizziness
			• Nausea
			• Cramps
			• Nasal congestion

Based on National Institute of Mental Health. (2011). Mental health medications: Alphabetical list of medications. Available at http://www.nimh.nih.gov/health/publications/mental-health-medications/alphabetical-list-of-medications.shtml; Leahy, L.G., & Kohler, C. (2013). *Manual of Clinical Psychopharmacology for Nurses.* Arlington, VA: American Psychiatric Publishers; Janiciak, P., Marder, S. R., & Pavuluri, M. (2011). *Principles and Practice of Psychopharmacotherapy.* Philadelphia, PA: Lippincott Williams & Wilkins.

Psychotherapy

Psychotherapy with children and adolescents is an important part of their treatment. The most important goals of therapy are to establish a therapeutic relationship in which the child can trust the nurse or therapist to help the child build new understanding and skills. Specific skills can be mastered depending on the context of the therapy. Psychotherapy with children and adolescents often needs to be active, given the level of activity that is common to growing children. Drawings, journaling, role playing, and play are commonly used to help build these skills in the context of a safe and helpful therapeutic relationship (Figure 30-4). Effective therapies have been developed for specific disorders as well. For example, exposure response prevention is an effective type of CBT that helps children overcome their fears and symptoms of OCD (Olino et al., 2011). Increasingly, therapies tailored to children and adolescents with combined approaches of psychoeducation with

CBT are being tested and show positive outcomes for minimizing suffering and instilling hope (West & Pavuluri, 2009; West et al., 2009). Appropriate types of individual therapy may include CBT, brief therapy, interpersonal psychotherapy, dialectical behavior therapy, mindfulness therapy, and therapies that use art, music, and dance to help patients express their feelings and learn new coping skills.

Play Therapy

Play therapy helps children and adolescents, especially younger children, to express feelings and work through conflicts and stress in

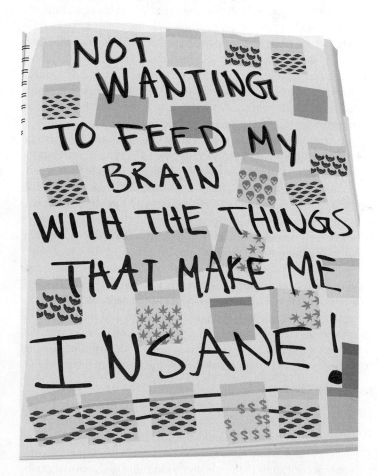

30-4 (A) Drawing from a 5-year-old who has been more withdrawn and agitated, and shutting down in school. She draws a horse and talks with the nurse about how busy the horse is and how he wants to run and play in the sun. The nurse talks more with her about what would help the horse feel more comfortable and who might be able to help the horse. (B) Illustration of a journal page of a 16-year-old struggling with addiction to marijuana. The teen made the journal page with old dime bags from drugs she had used in the past.

Source: Pearson Education

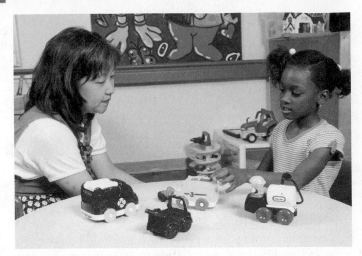

30-5 Children often need to play or fidget when talking about difficult emotions. Play is an area of competence for them, so it offers a comfortable avenue to share more about their experiences.

Source: George Dodson/Pearson Education

their play. The therapist will use play scenarios to script a problem, allow expression of feelings, and to facilitate new solutions. For example, a child with anxiety may play with dolls who meet each other for the first time and try to play together. The therapist helps the "patient" doll to master this situation with the other doll. The child then sees the scenario played out with success in the play. Play therapy may include using toys to get children comfortable talking about issues, and using role playing and physical activity to help manage symptoms (Figure 30-5). An example of this might be using the game "red light, green light" to demonstrate to a child that he or she has control over stopping and going with behaviors.

Another example is the Creating Opportunities for Personal Empowerment (COPE) program, developed by nurse researchers for use in a community mental health practice to provide treatment to teenagers with depression (Lusk & Melnyk, 2011). COPE is a CBT-based intervention that can be delivered in 30 minutes to teens suffering from depression. The focus is on practical strategies to improve problem solving and the ability to cope with stress through healthy behaviors and positive thinking. Researchers used the COPE intervention with 15 depressed teens and recorded their depressive symptoms before and after the intervention using the Beck Youth Inventory scale, which measures symptoms of depression. Researchers found that the teens appreciated the therapy and felt it was useful to them, and that depressive symptoms improved post-intervention. Symptom improvement was seen in teens with both internalizing and externalizing symptoms of depression (Lusk & Melnyk, 2011).

Family Therapy

Family therapy is always an important component of care for any child or adolescent suffering with a psychiatric disorder (Chapter 24). Family therapy helps the family to provide structure, support, and education, and to help minimize the stress and conflicts that can commonly occur. Family therapy is always individualized according to the needs of each family, but newer models of family therapy combine common skills such as education, cognitive–behavioral techniques, and conflict resolution of collaborative problem solving techniques. Collaborative problem solving occurs when two or more family members come together to solve the problem at hand. For example, an

adolescent might want to get his driver's license, but his parents may fear that his past use of substances poses too much of a safety risk for them to feel comfortable with him behind the wheel. He shares that he has been sober for 4 months and wants the chance to show them he is dependable and should be allowed to drive. His parents acknowledge this need, and pose a solution that he will begin to work toward his license with their oversight, so he will be behind the wheel only with them and while sober for a 2-month period. If he continues to do well, and stays sober, they will sit down again to discuss expectations for his driving independently and consequences if this trust is thwarted.

Complementary Therapies

Complementary therapies provide relief from suffering in children and adolescents with psychiatric disorders. Addressing dietary quality by eliminating food artificial flavorings and minimizing food additives, increasing essential fatty acids, maintaining low carbohydrate/high protein diets, and minimizing use time for electronic devices have resulted in positive influences on symptoms among youth (Pellow, Solomon, & Barnard, 2011). Melatonin, a hormone produced by the pineal gland, has been shown to help alleviate insomnia, which is common to many disorders among children and adolescents. Relaxation techniques, exercise, sunlight, and nutritional supplements also may provide relief.

An adapted form of Hatha yoga was incorporated into a trauma-sensitive intervention for use with complexly traumatized youth exhibiting chronic affective and somatic dysregulation. (Spinazzola et al., 2011). Yoga was an effective adjunctive treatment that helped with three components: breathing, meditation, and rhythmic movement. The effect of yoga may be activation of the parasympathetic nervous system. This activation enhances one's capacity to feel safe and grounded. Cultivation of safe, healthy relationships with their bodies helps adolescents with the body healing process and has been found to show a positive impact on survivors through gentle breath and movement, easing stress. Through gentle breath and movement, trauma-sensitive yoga offers a means by which children can cultivate a more positive relationship to their bodies and ease symptoms of traumatic stress (Emerson, Sharma, Chaudhry, & Turner, 2009).

Pause and Reflect

1. *What do parents need to know about their child's medications? What does the child need to know?*
2. *Are there any concerns about medicating children in varied cultures? What might be some cultural considerations?*
3. *What are the goals of play therapy? Family therapy?*

Nursing Management

Nursing care of children and their families can pose unique opportunities for the nurse to use his or her own interpersonal growth, reflection, and knowledge of development and family systems to plan and implement care. When caring for a child or adolescent with psychiatric disorders, the nurse must be careful to understand and mediate his or her own experiences as a child and as an adult, and to engage the perspectives of both the child and their families when planning care. In a family system, each member has a unique perspective about similar interpersonal events, and the nurse must take these into account when appraising treatment needs and implementing interventions. Keeping the family view at all times and checking with oneself about current and past experiences and how they may affect nursing care will help the nurse to stay family focused and client

Darius Recovery Phase

Cheryl takes Darius to see Cindy, the PMH-APRN. Cindy spends time with Darius, asking him about his thoughts and feelings and, with Cheryl, completing questionnaires about his development and symptoms. Prior to the visit with the family, she spoke with Darius's teacher and with Joanna, and they completed rating scales to evaluate his behavior in class as well as his attention and stress. She goes over this information with Darius's mother, and asks Darius to tell her about his day. Darius plays while they speak, and becomes more agitated and frustrated as the interview progresses. Cindy recognizes that Darius may need more breaks, and has him play with a box of toys in her room while she takes turns asking him and his mother questions.

Cindy discusses with Cheryl her preliminary diagnosis of autism spectrum disorder and shares how Darius's problems with social relatedness, his developmental delays in interactions and motor skill development, and his restricted interests are beyond those of the neurotypically developing child. She talks about how anxiety, hyperactivity, and distractibility are often co-morbid with ASD, and how Darius has symptoms of both ADHD and ASD. She takes time to answer Cheryl's questions about Darius's development, and then they discuss their plan of care, including meeting with the school, starting family therapy, and connecting Darius with a social skills group in the community for children with ASD. They discuss Darius's frequent problems at school with irritability, agitation, and anxiety, as well as reviewing his problems with sleep. Cindy encourages Cheryl to try some new routines to help with his sleep, and discusses starting a low dose of sertraline to help decrease Darius's irritability and anxiety, and potentially lessen his repeated behavior of rocking and twirling. Cheryl agrees to the plan, and Darius agrees also to try to take a new medicine to help with his frustrations. He also agrees to come back. Cindy asks that he bring one of his trains with him when he comes next time.

APPLICATION

1. Address the five domains for Darius.

2. What are the criteria for ASD? What symptoms of ASD does Darius exhibit?

3. How does Cindy help Cheryl become involved in the development of Darius's care plan?

4. Why is sertraline (Zoloft) an appropriate medication recommendation for Darius?

---

centered. An example of an interaction between Joanna and Darius, the nurse at the school, is given in the Perceptions, Thoughts, and Feelings feature near the end of this chapter.

Assessment

Because children and adolescents may not yet have the skills to effectively communicate their feelings and experiences to others, the nurse needs keen observation and communication skills to help assess the domains of the patient. The nurse should use all sources of information possible, such as teacher reports and observation of the child alone and with his or her parents, as well as collecting information about the child's developmental stages. During the assessment, this information will help the nurse to plan developmentally tailored care to match the expectations and needs that both the family and child identify.

Observation and Physical Assessment

Physical assessment of children and adolescents helps ensure that information gathered about the patient is comprehensive. For example, medication side effects such as hyperprolactinemia, which results in enlarged breast tissue, may not be discussed by an adolescent male but can be detected by observation or physical exam. Other symptoms, such as poor hygiene or a decrease in weight, also can be assessed by physical assessment and observation. The nurse should use all senses to observe and complete a thorough assessment of the child's physical development and symptoms of concern.

Assessment of behavior and emotion should include observations of the child or adolescent's level of activity, emotionality, aggression, ability to relate to the nurse, speech and language, and affect. Interactions with parents, as well as information the child or adolescent shares about self-concept, image, and competence, are important to gather while inquiring about symptoms and the view of the child or adolescent's life. The use of clinician, patient, or parent rating scales can also help collect more both objective and subjective information about symptoms and stressors.

Patient Interview

Interviewing children and adolescents requires patience and the use of developmentally appropriate language. The nurse should attempt to engage children's interest and make an attempt to meet children on their level, either by sitting in a place where eye contact can occur and allowing them to fidget or play while the interview takes place. Questions that can be answered with a simple yes or no should be avoided, with the nurse instead using open-ended questions that will help children to speak in their own terms. Pertinent open-ended questions may include the following:

- "Tell me about why you are here. And why now?"
- "Tell me what worries you about this. How does it worry your parents?"
- "How long has this been going on? Has anything helped?"
- "How was this different before? When did it change?"
- "How were things when you were younger?"
- "How has this affected your family? How has this affected things at school?"
- "What are you hoping will happen from coming here today?"

If a child uses certain language to describe a feeling or experience, the nurse should attempt to use that language in further understanding the child's experience, as in the following example:

Child: "My mom made me come today because I've been bad at school."

Nurse: "Tell me how you have been bad at school."

A balance between obtaining information from parents and the child, in their own language of experiences, will provide the nurse with a solid view of the family's struggles and how they manifest in their environments.

Child Abuse and Neglect Assessment

As stated throughout this text, **child abuse,** the physical, emotional, or sexual harm of a child or adolescent, and **neglect,** the failure to provide for a child or adolescent's basic needs, are risk factors for mental illness (Figure 30-6). Nurses in all settings are required to report suspected child abuse or neglect following their agency's protocols and state regulations. Key to this is being able to recognize indicators of abuse and neglect. Indicators of physical abuse include the following:

- Frequent injuries that do not fit the child's or parent's explanations or for which conflicting explanations are given
- Guarding, awkward movements that indicate pain
- Wearing clothes inappropriate to the weather (to hide evidence of injury)
- Recurrent absence from or lateness to school without credible explanation (to give child time to heal from injuries)

Sexual abuse includes any type of direct sexual contact as well as non-contact activities, such as exposing children to sex or pornography. Indicators of sexual abuse vary by the age of the child. Behaviors common across the age spectrum include regression to earlier behaviors, nightmares, sleep disturbances, withdrawal, feeding or eating problems, and poor school performance. Adolescents may also engage in substance abuse, sexual promiscuity, and suicidal ideation or gestures.

Neglect encompasses a variety of areas and may vary according to state laws. Physical neglect includes failure to provide proper nourishment and safe living quarters. Medical neglect may arise when a parent or caregiver fails to ensure proper medical care for a sick or injured child.

Child abuse and neglect may be difficult to prove until a pattern establishes itself, especially without cooperation from the child. Children and adolescents may fear that information and feelings they share about their parents or friends may be repeated to them. The nurse must clarify at the outset that information and sharing of feelings is for use only in treatment and will be kept confidential. Clarify that information that implies the child or adolescent is being harmed or harming another will be the only information that may be shared, and that the purpose for sharing that information is to keep the child safe.

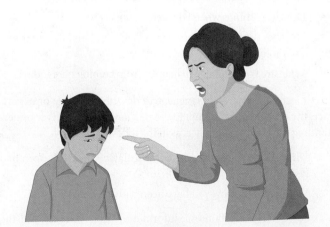

30-6 Emotional abuse includes yelling, shaming, and belittling. Nurses must be able to recognize and report all types of child abuse.

Diagnosis and Planning

Common nursing diagnoses for children and adolescents experiencing mental health challenges and disorders may include any of the following:

- Injury, Risk for
- Violence, Self-Directed, Risk for
- Suicide, Risk for
- Spiritual Distress, Risk for
- Social Isolation
- Social Interaction, Impaired
- Sleep Deprivation
- Self-Esteem, Chronic Low
- Body Image, Disturbed
- Hopelessness
- Anxiety
- Post-Trauma Syndrome, Risk for

Nursing diagnoses that may apply to families include:

- Role Conflict, Parental
- Parenting, Risk for Impaired
- Family Processes, Interrupted
- Coping: Family, Compromised
- Coping, Ineffective
- Caregiver Role Strain
- Attachment, Risk for Impaired

    (NANDA-I © 2014)

Working together with the patient and family to establish nursing diagnoses not only ensures that everyone is in agreement with the plan, but also helps the nurse to understand the patient's and family's priorities for symptom control.

As the nurse develops plans and goals within the nursing care plan, the nurse keeps the patient involved as much as possible. When asking whether the patient is capable of developing and following a care plan, the child or adolescent's developmental level is an important consideration. The nurse must also determine what the most distressing symptoms are from the child's perspective, as well as which symptoms are most distressing to the family and other caregivers.

When developing the plan, the nurse focuses on how patient needs can be articulated and addressed as *specific, realistic,* and *measurable* goals for the patient's care. For example, if the patient has difficulty with aggression, the nurse might state the following specific, measurable, and realistic goals:

- The patient will decrease incidence of yelling, throwing items, or physical aggression by 50%.
- The patient will demonstrate use of collaborative problem solving strategies when triggers for aggressive behavior occur.
- The patient will report feeling more confident in using problem solving to manage difficult feelings.

In developing the plan of care, the nurse will consider with the patient how the five domains are involved. Asking targeted questions may

Primary, Secondary, & Tertiary Levels of Intervention

table 30-5

Level of Intervention	Teaching Opportunity
Primary intervention	Nursing students enrolled in a public health nursing course implement a parenting class for parents at a local elementary school. The course content covers nutrition, exercise, general health management, and stress management techniques for parents and children.
Secondary intervention	A school nurse sees a child who has been inattentive and impulsive in his classroom setting. The nurse administers the patient's stimulant medication per instructions, and talks with the student about techniques to help him focus throughout his school day (sitting close to the teacher, doodling when his mind wanders, using a small item in his pocket to fidget with when he feels fidgety).
Tertiary intervention	The nurse in an inpatient setting co-leads a cognitive–behavioral therapy group for helping children with managing anger. The content of the group includes encouraging the children to use collaborative problem-solving strategies with adults in their lives to help with coping and managing frustrating interactions.

help elicit information that will help inform the care plan. For children and adolescents, it is particularly important to consider family relationships and stressors and school stressors and peer relationships in addition to biological, cultural, and spiritual considerations.

Revising the Care Plan During Recovery and Rehabilitation

Ongoing review of the care plan is necessary to keep the patient engaged in treatment, and must be revised to reflect the patient's growth and progress in reaching treatment goals. For instance, a child might become less aggressive but continue to struggle with irritability (a precursor to aggression). The care plan will shift to managing triggers for irritability and promoting relaxation rather than on managing conflict. As the child continues in recovery and rehabilitation, the nurse, family, and child should revisit the plan of care to determine whether the goals and plan are still meaningful and appropriate for the symptoms and circumstances. If the child's symptoms have warranted a higher level of care or service, the plan should reflect this change so the child and family understand what has driven the changes (for instance, the child is seeing a prescriber due to continued lack of response in therapy, or therapy is occurring twice weekly because of recent re-experiencing of symptoms of trauma). Without these revisions, and a review with the child and family, the family and child will not understand what the treatment is for, what problems are being addressed, and how problems will be addressed.

Factors to consider when working on minimizing relapses include events or situations that trigger symptoms in the patient, the state of the family system, how things are going at school, supports currently in place for the patient, and how the child or adolescent patient can ask for help.

Implementation

When a patient and family experience a high level of suffering, hope may seem impossible to reach. The nurse must first understand how the family has suffered before he or she can help offer hope for the end of suffering. Joining with the family in active listening, understanding, and planning care helps the family be able to sense hope. The nurse helps both the patient and family find hope, and to expect that by working together, the plan of care will bring relief.

Primary, Secondary, and Tertiary Interventions

Nursing interventions may be made on the primary, secondary, or tertiary level with children and adolescents (Table 30-5). The main focus in primary intervention of child or adolescent psychiatric disorders is to reduce risk factors. Involvement in community activities can be considered potential primary intervention. These include school programs that help students boost their self-esteem by teaching recreational and personal skills, physical activity programs and sports activities, and "mothers' morning out" groups for mothers of small children to build support networks (Figure 30-7). Other examples of primary interventions include prevention programs that aim to educate mothers about the risks of drug and alcohol use during pregnancy, or those that provide support to teen parents.

Secondary intervention involves early intervention and treatment. An example of a secondary level of intervention would involve providing play therapy for a child who has been the victim of trauma. Patient education is focused on developing coping skills

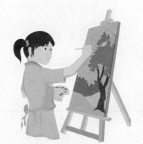
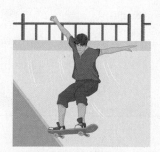
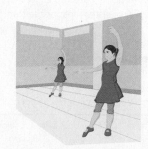

30-7   School programs and activities that teach children and adolescents personal, social, and physical or artistic skills can enhance self-esteem and feelings of belonging.

when flashbacks or occur. The nurse would help the child incorporate these skills when anxiety increases. Another example of a secondary intervention would be for the nurse to help a family who is experiencing a high level of conflict, yelling, and emotion at home to learn more effective communication skills. Helping the family members to better advocate and communicate within the family would help to decrease the high emotion at home, improve social support, and help provide a backdrop for more effective problem solving in the home.

Tertiary intervention involves post-intervention with an established unhealthy behavior or risk of recurrence of an unhealthy behavior. The goal is to restore and rehabilitate children and adolescents whose functioning has been impaired by their psychiatric disorder. Education is directed toward reducing established behavior (such as aggression) or the risk of recurrence and promoting restoration and functioning of the individual to a healthier state. An example of a tertiary intervention would be for the nurse to help the child with encopresis with establishing toileting behaviors, coping strategies, and educating the family about effective responses to anxiety around these behaviors, and about diet and behaviors surrounding episodes of encopresis.

Patient Education

Education about symptoms, the impact on functioning, and therapies should include both the patient and family. Visual aids such as mood charts and slides using examples, stories, and metaphors will best help younger children relate to the content. Capturing the attention of children or adolescents while teaching information may be a challenge for the nurse, so reinforcing material that has already been taught is an important component of each therapeutic interaction. Empowering patients to have a good understanding of their illness, its effect on their life, and how their treatment helps them to recover gives hope and control over aspects of their life that seemed outside their control prior to treatment.

Targeted Interventions

Most children will benefit from interventions targeted to their specific disorder. Many of these have already been mentioned. Two areas

of particular note to nurses are interventions aimed at reducing mood dysregulation and those aimed at reducing disruptive behaviors (Box 30-7).

Interventions that may be helpful in working with youth experiencing dysregulation include the following:

- Maintain a positive tone during interactions.
- Reduce threats by using sensible rules that elicit cooperation and facilitate children's sense of control.
- Increasing structure and buffering the unexpected may help reduce frustration.
- Consider the child's attention control and processing abilities when setting expectations.
- Be attuned to the child/adolescent's feelings (empathic attunement) (Delaney, 2009).

Evaluation

Evaluation of treatment interventions should be done in all environments of care for the child. Questionnaires such as the Connors Behavior Rating Scale, which rates symptoms of ADHD; report cards; notes from school; and behavior charts or calendars will help with measuring progress of treatment goals. In addition, feedback from the patient and the family about ongoing struggles, successes, and their experiences with helpful and unhelpful interventions will offer more information for evaluation.

Pause and Reflect

1. *What tools or strategies would you recommend for Darius and his family to use to track his progress toward recovery and rehabilitation? How do you see these as being helpful?*

2. *What aspects of therapeutic communication do you see as being most helpful when meeting with a patient to evaluate the plan of care?*

3. *Understanding that development of independence is a developmental goal for all children and adolescents, how would the nurse incorporate this goal into planning care for the child/adolescent patient?*

Interventions to Reduce Disruptive Behaviors   box 30-7

Children with disruptive behaviors often benefit from interventions specifically targeted to these behaviors. Appropriate interventions include:

1. Increase parent attention to desired child behaviors.
2. Reduce harsh and inconsistent responses to problematic child behaviors.
3. Educate parents about the:
   - Concept of child-centered time.
   - Importance of family routines and traditions.
   - Value of praise and encouragement.
   - Role of rewards for reducing challenging behavior.

- Importance of setting clear limits on behavior and of following through on limit setting.
- Need to establish consequences in response to misbehavior parents want stopped.
- Use of specific parenting strategies, such as ignore, distract, and time out.

4. Teach stress management and problem-solving skills to parents and children.
5. Incorporate culturally relevant models in family education to promote constructive behaviors.

Based on Webster-Stratton, C., Reid, M. J., & Beauchaine, T. (2011). Combining parent and child training for young children with ADHD. *Journal of Clinical Child and Adolescent Psychology, 40*(2), 191–203.; Gross, D., Garvey, C., Wrenetha, J., Fogg, L., Tucke, S., & Mokros, H. (2009). Efficacy of the Chicago Parent Program with low-income African American and Latino parents of young children. *Prevention Science, 10*(1), 54; Breitenstein, S. M., Gross, D., Fogg, L., Ridge, A., Garvey, C., Julion, W., & Tucker, S. (2012). The Chicago Parent Program: Comparing 1-year outcomes for African American and Latino parents of young children. *Research in Nursing and Health, 35*(5), 475–489.

Social Networking

Clinical Problem

Social networking sites have become a common place for children and adolescents to communicate with peers, share ideas, and express themselves. For many children, social networking serves as a sounding board for their experiences of their growing self in the larger world. However, risky online behaviors (including sharing personal information, cyber bullying, lying, accessing sex sites, or participating in developmentally inappropriate forums) can pose potential threats to children and adolescents in venues both public and at the same time secret from the view of family. What is the prevalence of child and adolescent unsafe use of social networking?

Evidence

To gain more information about use of social networking sites by children and adolescents, Dowdell, Burgess, and Flores (2011) conducted a survey of 404 middle school students, 2,077 high school students, and 466 adult sex offenders to obtain information that nurses could use to better focus education and prevention efforts regarding safe use of social networks. Of middle school students, 27% to 29.5% reported they had posted a "rude or nasty comment" online about someone they knew; and 11% to 17% reported they had talked with someone they did not know through the online sites. Among high schoolers, 50% knew someone who had been "sexted," and 15.2% reported they had been sexted. In addition, chat rooms where students talked with others to share ideas and meet strangers were reportedly used by one-third to half of the students sampled.

In the survey of sex offenders, the same social networks used by children included in the study were also commonly used to engage children in sexual behaviors.

Implications for Nursing

Because social networks are increasingly being used by children and adolescents for social interaction, primary prevention efforts educating children and families about these risks will help protect them from threatening behavior, victimization, and sexual abuse. In addition, helping parents and children navigate this venue for opportunity with safety and privacy is an important family intervention that will protect the entire family from potential harm.

Critical Thinking Questions

1. Do you know what protections are available from social network sites commonly used by children and adolescents? How would you go about learning more about this?

2. How could you incorporate issues related to social networking into the nursing assessment? Into the plan of care?

Darius—A Child with ADHD and ASD

Nursing Diagnosis: Deficient family and patient knowledge about ADHD as manifested by his family's lack of understanding about the illness, its consequences, and how the illness symptoms exceed the "normal" limits of a developing child's behavior.

Short-Term Goals *Patient will:* (include date for short-term goal to be met)	Intervention *Nurse will:*	Rationale
Darius's family will learn about the core features of autism spectrum disorder (ASD) and attention-deficit/hyperactivity disorder (ADHD) during the first interview.	Ask Darius and his mother to describe core symptom complaints.	Determine treatment targets with the family.
Darius's family will learn about the biological foundation of ASD and ADHD during the first interview.	Discuss the biologic foundation of ASDs with family and with Darius.	Clarify with the family Darius's symptoms and family responses.
Darius will exhibit reduced frustration at home within one week.	Help family to reward Darius's positive behaviors.	Use behavior therapy techniques to increase positive behaviors.
Darius's family will voice understanding normal and abnormal developmental milestones within one month.	Provide family education about development and coach family in promoting optimal developmental growth for Darius.	Education will assist Darius's family with understanding his strengths and limitations.
Darius's family will articulate an understanding of medication effects and side effects at the end of the first interview.	Provide teaching related to medications used to treat ADHD and ASD, and their effects, side effects.	Understanding expected effects and potential adverse effects. Pharmacologic therapy will assist Darius and his family with managing expectations and outcomes.

(Continued)

Short-Term Goals *Patient will:* (include date for short-term goal to be met)	Intervention *Nurse will:*	Rationale
Long-Term Goal Darius's self-control will improve, resulting in: • Less than one report of problematic school behavior per week • Grades B or above • Less than one visit to the school nurse per week • Sustained peer relationships (invite one friend over a week)	Support, educate, and provide collaborative problem solving to Darius and his family.	Darius will feel safe and competent at school, home, and with friends.

Clinical Reasoning

1. What other nursing diagnoses might the nurse working with Darius consider?

2. Do you think Darius will be able to make a friend? Why or why not?

3. In addition to deficient knowledge, what other nursing diagnoses might be appropriate for Darius's family? Why? What else might help Darius to build self-esteem?

From Suffering to Hope

When a child experiences mental illness, the entire family suffers. Parents wonder why the illness occurred, what they can do to help their child heal, what the future holds for their child who is struggling, and how they can minimize the impact of the illness symptoms on their other children. Children and adolescents can feel ashamed, isolated, afraid, blamed, and frustrated with adults in their lives who may not understand how to help. Adding to the complexity of individual and family suffering, stigma associated with mental illness may keep families from reaching out to friends, family, and professionals who can help the family get to the path of healing and hope. As an important start, the nurse can extend a caring hand to the child and family, acknowledging their suffering and establishing themselves as a bridge to healing and hope.

The nurse can help families by listening and understanding how the child's illness has affected the child's functioning and that of the family, and by working with the family to understand how the child and family understand each other and generally solve problems together. This is a critical step that helps the nurse understand the family's culture, strengths, and history of problem solving so the nurse can build on their strengths and identify challenges unique to each child and family. Collectively identifying symptoms and challenges, developing a family plan to address problems, helping provide resources for healing, and clarifying the plan with the family will help draw the child and family away from the chaos and fear that illness can bring and move toward clarity and a plan of action. In addition, the nurse can discuss evidence-based treatment options and speak specifically about how the strengths of the child and family can help improve healing and prognosis. For example, the nurse can help the child who enjoys drawing to start using a "drawing journal" to discuss difficult feelings. Or the nurse might suggest that a family's "TV time" together no longer include violent

Darius Rehabilitation Phase

Darius is starting a new school year, and has finished almost 6 months of treatment. He is comfortable in his new classroom and sits next to his friend Scott, a shy boy who is patient and kind to Darius. Darius's teacher understands that he will need frequent breaks through his school day, and that he learns best when he sits closer to her. He regularly attends a social group in his school setting and works with Cindy, his mental health APRN, to manage his behavior and anxiety through a combination of cognitive–behavioral therapy techniques and management of his Zoloft. Cheryl has been receiving support from this therapy as well, and has also been attending a group for parents of children with developmental disabilities. From this group she has learned successful sleep routines for Darius, which have resulted in better sleep for them both and, as a result, less irritability as well. Incidentally, she and Darius have also begun to attend church functions at the church where the parent support group is held, and have experienced even more support from new friendships there.

Cheryl and Joanna talk regularly to ensure that Darius continues to have success at home and at school, and that they all maintain the gains they have made in the past 6 months. Darius's extended family still does not understand his needs, but their comments about how much calmer he seems have helped Cheryl to feel that they will understand at some point. Cheryl has expressed hope that Darius will complete school and live a happy successful life, though perhaps different from the life she originally dreamed for him. Darius also has been talking about his future goals of working for the local museum he still visits with his Grandpa, and hopes to volunteer there when he is a teenager.

critical thinking

APPLICATION

1. Does Darius's current functioning mean he is no longer ill?

2. What are his current needs for treatment? What are Cheryl's?

3. What steps has Darius taken to gain confidence and skill in managing his symptoms? What steps has Cheryl taken to help Darius and herself manage these symptoms?

or disturbing content that might activate their child's symptoms. Providing information on sources of both web-based and personal support can also help families to connect with others who have traveled the same illness path and can provide additional resources for families. Sharing the nurse's own experience of seeing children with mental illness recover also helps children and families in meaningful ways.

Often the biggest fear the child and family may have is the question, "Will he always struggle with mental illness in his lifetime?" There are no answers for this question, as we are still learning about illness trajectories across the life span. However, the nurse can reassure families that early treatment, a supportive family and social environment, and access to evidence-based treatment result in the best outcomes for mentally ill children. Hope will come to families

with children suffering from mental illness, and the nurse is an important conduit for helping families navigate their illness experience with compassion and a plan.

Pause and Reflect

1. *How might the nurse convey empathy toward the adolescent patient who comes to the clinic with a parent? How will the nurse share the perspectives of both child and parent while completing the assessment?*
2. *How might obtaining a patient's height and weight inform assessment and care planning for the child or adolescent patient?*
3. *What types of questions would you ask to collect information about a child's stressors? An adolescent's?*

PERCEPTIONS, THOUGHTS, & FEELINGS: Validating the Needs of a Child With Symptoms of Anxiety and Irritability

Patient's behavior(s)	Nurse's perceptions, thoughts, feelings	Exploration with patient
Darius comes into the school nurse's office and begins to pace back and forth. He does not look at Joanna, the nurse, until she validates his presence.	*Thoughts:* He seems agitated and anxious. I wonder what's going on.	*Nurse:* Hello, Darius. I see you're pacing. What can I do to help?

VALIDATION Joanna senses that Darius is agitated and may need assistance. By acknowledging his pacing, Joanna validates that she sees he is in some sort of distress.

Patient's behavior(s)	Nurse's perceptions, thoughts, feelings	Exploration with patient
Darius: I just need to take a walk. I feel like getting out of here.	*Thoughts:* I wonder if there was a particular stress for Darius in class today, and if this is one we have worked on before or something new. He seems irritated and anxious, and I wonder if he tried to use one of his tools in class before he came to the office.	*Nurse:* What happened to make you feel the need to get out and take a walk?

VALIDATION Joanna responds by acknowledging Darius's expressed need. Asking an open-ended question is more likely to elicit a meaningful response from Darius and helps Joanna avoid making assumptions about what is prompting Darius's response.

Patient's behavior(s)	Nurse's perceptions, thoughts, feelings	Exploration with patient
Darius: I can't believe that Tommy thinks they still have steam trains. I told him everything went to diesel in the '50s and he says no!	*Thoughts:* Trains are really his domain, and it sounds like he is struggling with moving forward in his day with Tommy with this "error." His need for accuracy and sameness seems to be colliding with his need for friends.	*Nurse:* You know a lot about trains. Tell me when steam engines stopped making their way across America.

VALIDATION Affirming Darius's knowledge base and strengths promotes therapeutic communication.

Patient's behavior(s)	Nurse's perceptions, thoughts, feelings	Exploration with patient
Darius stops pacing and instead stands in front of Joanna and rocks from one leg to the next. *Darius:* They basically disappeared in the 1950s, so you won't see them except for in museums.	*Thoughts:* Darius has stopped his pacing and is more engaged with me as he recounts his knowledge of trains. I wonder if he had the opportunity to share this with his classmate.	*Nurse:* Wow, yes, Darius, I knew you would know about steam trains. Have you ever had the chance to see a steam train yourself at a museum?

VALIDATION Affirming to Darius that he holds knowledge and further engaging him in the interaction rather than in his emotion.

(Continued)

Patient's behavior(s)	Nurse's perceptions, thoughts, feelings	Exploration with patient
Darius: Yeah, my Grandpa takes me to see the steam engines at the museum a couple of times a year. Last time I went he got me one of my trains too, it's a replica. It's in my desk. Darius takes a breath and looks at Joanna for the first time.	*Thoughts:* He is disengaging from his need for accuracy and sameness and has shared more about his experiences. I know that Darius relaxes with his trains, but we cannot disrupt the class to go get it now. Maybe planning ahead for Darius to share the train later with Tommy will help Darius to have a productive discussion about their disagreement.	*Nurse:* Darius, it is wonderful that your Grandpa takes you to the museum, and that you even have a steam engine here! I wonder if Tommy would like to see it later today, maybe at recess, and I would be glad to help you share what you know about steam engines with him then.

VALIDATION Joanna invites Darius to begin some collaborative problem solving about the interpersonal conflict.

Patient's behavior(s)	Nurse's perceptions, thoughts, feelings	Exploration with patient
Darius: Maybe. I am not sure he will listen though. Sometimes I talk to Tommy and he is not listening. It always has to be his way, and I don't know why I had to leave class and he didn't. He sits down and begins to twirl a pencil from Joanna's desk.	*Feelings:* Poor guy. Things do not go his way and I feel sorry that Darius seems to always struggle with friends. *Thoughts:* He is calming down, using his twirling along with following our conversation, I think he might see me as someone who can help. *Feelings:* I want to help him. *Thoughts:* Let's see if I can transition him back to class with a plan. Maybe he will agree if I help.	*Nurse:* Darius, what do you think about waiting to talk more to Tommy about this until recess today, when I might help? You can go back to class now, and at the end of recess I will come bring you your train. Together we can show it to Tommy and answer any questions he may have about steam engines. What do you think?

VALIDATION Continuing to enlist Darius in the process of problem solving.

Patient's behavior(s)	Nurse's perceptions, thoughts, feelings	Exploration with patient
Darius: But he doesn't listen!	*Thoughts:* I am sure he has had negative experiences with peers and may feel hopeless about trying. *Feelings:* I am worried about what will happen if Tommy is not receptive. *Thoughts:* I know Tommy and Darius, and Tommy will be receptive to this. He is usually a very cooperative child.	*Nurse:* I think he will want to know more about your trains, and he will appreciate hearing what you may know about steam engines, but at a time where you both can share. I think today in class, it was hard to do it, because in class you need to learn what the class is learning. This will give you a special time for this learning.

VALIDATION Giving Darius language about boundaries, and empowering his role in sharing information with others.

Patient's behavior(s)	Nurse's perceptions, thoughts, feelings	Exploration with patient
Darius: OK, can I go back to class?	*Thoughts:* He seems to be calmer now that he knows this may be resolved. I will help him get back to class and tell him specifically when I will come to help him with the conversation. I will bring his train and remind him I have it, so he does not worry about it.	*Nurse:* Yes, Darius. Remember, I will hold onto your train until I see you on the playground. When I give it to you, I will also bring Tommy with me and we can talk more about steam engines. I will help you both to have a turn so you can share together.

VALIDATION Restating plans and validating Darius's role in problem solving. Assuring support.

Patient's behavior(s)	Nurse's perceptions, thoughts, feelings	Exploration with patient
Darius: OK, let's go now.	*Thoughts:* I think Darius's attention is dropping; it's time to move on. He seems to have a good grasp of what is next and understands the plan. He seems calm now too, and ready to return to class now that his frustration and anxiety have been addressed.	*Nurse:* Great, Darius. Let me walk you back to class and I will see you soon.

VALIDATION Empathizing with Darius's limited attention and continued need for support.

Based on Orlando, I. J. (1972). The Discipline and Teaching of Nursing Process (An Evaluative Study). New York, NY: G. P. Putnam's Sons.

Chapter Highlights

1. Child and adolescent psychiatric disorders affect 13% to 20% of the U.S. population.

2. Co-morbidity of disorders is common in children and adolescents; affected children are treated more in non-mental health settings than in specialized settings.

3. Normal development and symptoms of psychiatric disorders interface, with each affecting the other.

4. Tourette syndrome, selective mutism, separation anxiety disorder, ADHD, and ODD are disorders first seen in childhood.

5. Symptoms of psychiatric disorders seen in adult populations may look different from those seen in childhood and adolescence.

6. Family work is extremely important for relieving distress and building hope for children and adolescents with psychiatric disorders.

7. Nursing interventions must be active and engaging for children and adolescents and incorporate familiar avenues of expression (play, journaling).

8. Nursing diagnosis and care will always consider the child's environments of family, peers, and school.

NCLEX®-RN Questions

1. The nurse is addressing health promotion activities across wellness domains that may reduce the incidence of childhood psychopathology. Which areas of focus are most appropriate? Select all that apply.
   a. Diet
   b. Prenatal care
   c. Stress reduction
   d. Parenting support
   e. Milieu management

2. The nurse is providing teaching to school personnel related to the need to recognize and respond to children with mental health needs. Which statement by school personnel requires follow up?
   a. "The presentation of mental illness in children is similar to that observed in adults."
   b. "Most mental health care for children and adolescents occurs in nontraditional settings."
   c. "Mental health disorders affect as many as one in five children and adolescents in any given year."
   d. "It is easy for parents and teachers to fail to recognize symptoms of mental illness due to common misconceptions. "

3. The pediatric nurse is working with children with a variety of emotional and neurodevelopmental issues. Which disorders does the nurse recognize as indicative of maltreatment and/or a response to an overwhelming stressor? Select all that apply.
   a. Anxiety disorder
   b. Attachment disorder
   c. Posttraumatic stress disorder
   d. Pervasive developmental disorder
   e. Disinhibited social engagement disorder

4. The nurse is evaluating the classroom setting for modifications used to support a group of children with reactive temperament style. Which finding would be of most concern?
   a. Advance notice of fire drills is provided.
   b. Open-ended activities are kept to a minimum.
   c. Children are asked to raise their hands before speaking.
   d. Highly stimulating activities are used to promote engagement.

5. The nurse is working with a child who has been bullied at school. The nurse understands that which variable has the greatest potential to negatively affect the quality of care the nurse provides?
   a. The nurse has a child who is being bullied at school.
   b. The nurse had few experiences with bullying as a child.
   c. The nurse recently attended a conference that addressed bullying.
   d. The nurse has worked with a number of children affected by bullying.

6. The parents of a 4-year-old child receiving treatment for mental health issues ask the nurse, "What good is it doing our child to spend all this time playing with the therapist?" Which response by the nurse is most appropriate?
   a. "It is difficult to comment on activity that is not within my area of nursing expertise."
   b. "Play helps your child to see the therapist as a friend so your child will open up and talk freely."
   c. "Play is a developmental activity that is used to help children learn to solve problems and cope with difficult experiences."
   d. "If you don't feel this type of therapy is a good fit for your child, you should request a different type of therapist."

7. The nurse is providing teaching to the parents of a child receiving medication to treat a mental health disorder. The parents state that they found an article online stating the drug had not been approved for use in children. What common variable related to psychopharmacology with children should the nurse explain at this time?
   a. Black box warnings
   b. Off-label prescribing
   c. Medical incompetence
   d. Nonpharmacologic alternatives

8. The nurse is considering evidence-based interventions with teenagers suffering from depression. The nurse is considering using Creating Opportunities for Personal Empowerment (COPE) as an intervention model. Which would be most appropriate for the nurse to identify as an expected outcome?
   a. Participants explore traumatic events that may have contributed to mental health issues.
   b. Participants recognize the importance of adhering to pharmacologic therapies to treat depression.
   c. Participants identify and utilize adaptive strategies to cope with situations that are causing stress.
   d. Participants use hourly sessions to talk about feelings and provide emotional support to one another.

Answers may be found on the Pearson student resource site: nursing.pearsonhighered.com

References

Addington, A., & Rapoport, J. L. (2011). Annual research review: Impact of advances in genetics in understanding developmental psychopathology. *Journal of Child Psychology and Psychiatry*, 53(5), 510–518.

Ainsworth, M. D. S., Blehar, M. C., Waters, E., & Wall, S. (1978). *Patterns of Attachment: A Psychological Study of the Strange Situation*. Hillsdale, NJ: Erlbaum.

American Academy of Child and Adolescent Psychiatry. (2007). Practice parameter for the assessment and treatment of children and adolescents with oppositional defiant disorder. *Journal of the American Academy of Child and Adolescent Psychiatry*, 46(1), 126–141.

American Academy of Child and Adolescent Psychiatry. (2011). *Posttraumatic Stress Disorder (PTSD)*. Available at http://www.aacap.org/AACAP/Families_and_Youth/Facts_for_Families/Facts_for_Families_Pages/Posttraumatic_Stress_Disorder_70.aspx

American Academy of Child and Adolescent Psychiatry. (2012). *A Guide for Community Child Serving Agencies on Psychotropic Medications for Children and Adolescents*. Available at http://www.aacap.org/App_Themes/AACAP/docs/press/guide_for_community_child_serving_agencies_on_psychotropic_medications_for_children_and_adolescents_2012.pdf

American Academy of Child and Adolescent Psychiatry. (2013). *The depressed child*. Available at http://www.aacap.org/AACAP/Families_and_Youth/Facts_for_Families/Facts_for_Families_Pages/The_Depressed_Child_04.aspx

American Psychiatric Association (APA). (2013). *Diagnostic and Statistical Manual of Psychiatric Disorders* (5th ed.). Washington, DC: American Psychiatric Publishers.

Amminger, G. P., Henry, L. P., Harrigan, S. M., Harris, M. G., Alvarez-Jimenez, M., … McGorry, P. D. (2011). Outcome in early-onset schizophrenia revisited: Findings from the Early Psychosis Prevention Centre long-term follow up study. *Schizophrenia Research*, 131, 112–119.

Arseneault, L., Bowes, L., & Shakoor, S. (2010). Bullying victimization in youth and mental health problems: "Much ado" about nothing. *Psychological Medicine*, 40, 717–729.

Barrish, H. H., Saunders, M., & Wolf, M. M. (1969). Good behavior game: Effects of individual contingencies for group consequences on disruptive behavior in a classroom. *Journal of Applied Behavioral Analysis*, 2(2), 119–124.

Beeber, L. S., Holditch-Davis, D., Perreira, K., Schwartz, T., Lewis, V., Blanchard, H., Canuso, R., & Goldman, B. D. (2010). Short-term in-home intervention reduces depressive symptoms in Early Head Start Latina mothers of infants and toddlers. *Research in Nursing and Health*, 33(1), 60–76.

Bekhet, A. K., Johnson, N. L., & Zauszniewski, J. A. (2012). Effects on resilience of caregivers of persons with autism spectrum disorder: The role of positive cognitions. *Journal of the American Psychiatric Nurses Association*, 18(6), 337–344.

Birmaher, B., Arbelaez, C., & Brent, D. (2002). Course and outcome of child and adolescent major depressive disorder. *Child and Adolescent Psychiatric Clinics of North America*, 11(3), 619–637.

Blaney, B. K., & Chiocca, E. M. (2011). Has your patient been bullied? *The Nurse Practitioner*, 36(11), 41–47.

Bowlby, J. (1953). *Child Care and the Growth of Love: A Summary of a Report Prepared under the Auspices of the World Health Organization on the Importance of Mother-Love in the Development of the Child's Character and Personality and the Problem of the Motherless Child* (abridged and edited by M. Fry). Harmondsworth, UK: Penguin Books.

Bowlby, J. (1969). *Attachment and Loss* (Vol. 1). New York: Basic Books.

Bowlby, J. (1973). *Attachment and Loss* (Vol. 2). New York: Basic Books.

Breitenstein, S. M., Gross, D., Fogg, L., Ridge, A., Garvey, C., Julion, W., & Tucker, S. (2012). The Chicago Parent Program: Comparing 1-year outcomes for African American and Latino parents of young children. *Research in Nursing and Health*, 35(5), 475–489.

Briggs, M. K., Akos, P., Czyszczon, G., & Eldridge, A. (2011). Assessing and promoting spiritual wellness as a protective factor in secondary schools. *Counseling and Values*, 55(2), 171–184.

Bronfenbrenner, U. (1995). The bioecological model from a life course perspective reflections of a participant observer. In P. Moen, H. Elder, Jr. & K. Lusher, (Eds.). *Examining Lives in Context*. Washington, DC: American Psychological Association, pp. 599–618.

Canino, G., & Alegria, M. (2008). Psychiatric diagnosis—is it universal or relative to culture? *Journal of Psychology and Psychiatry*, 49(3), 237–250.

Carlson, G. A., Potegal, M., Margulies, D., Gutkovich, Z., & Basile, J. (2009). Rages—what are they and who has them? *Journal of Child and Adolescent Psychopharmacolgy*, 19(3), 281–288.

Carter, S. (2012). The bully at school: An interdisciplinary approach. *Issues in Comprehensive Pediatric Nursing*, 35(3–4), 153–162.

Centers for Disease Control and Prevention (CDC). (2012).Understanding teen dating violence fact sheet. Available at http://www.cdc.gov/Violence Prevention/pdf/TeenDatingViolence2012-a.pdf

Centers for Disease Control and Prevention (CDC). (2013). Mental health surveillance among children—U.S. 2005–2011. *Morbidity and Mortality Weekly Report*, 62(2), 1–35. Available at http://www.cdc.gov/mmwr/preview/mmwrhtml/su6202a1.htm?s_cid=su6202a1_w

Chao, K.Y., Wang, H. S., Chang, H. L., Wang, Y. W., & See, L. C. (2010). Establishment of the reliability and validity of the stress index for children or adolescents with tourette syndrome (SICATS). *Journal of Clinical Nursing*, 19(3–4), 332–340.

Coelho, D. P. (2011). Encopresis: A medical and family approach. (2011). *Pediatric Nursing*, 37(3), 107–112.

Conelea, C. A., Woods, D. W., Zinner, S. H., Budman, C., Murphy, T., Scahill, L. D., Compton, S. N., & Walkup, J. (2011). Exploring the impact of chronic tic disorders on youth: Results from the Tourette syndrome impact survey. *Child Psychiatry and Human Development*, 42(2), 219–242.

Cormier, E. (2012). How parents make decisions to use medication to treat their child's ADHD: A grounded theory study. *Journal of the American Psychiatric Nurses Association*, 18(6), 345–356.

Crowell, S. E., Beauchaine, T. P., Hsiao, R. C., Vasilev, C. A., Yaptango, M., Linehan, M., & McCauley, E. (2012). Differentiating adolescent self-injury from adolescent depression: Possible implications for borderline personality development. *Journal of Abnormal Child Psychology*, 40, 45–57.

Degnan, K. A., Almas, A. N., & Fox, N. A. (2010). Temperament and the environment in the etiology of childhood anxiety. *Journal Of Child Psychology and Psychiatry*, 51(4), 497–517.

Delaney, K. R. (2006). Top 10 milieu interventions for inpatient child/adolescent treatment. *Journal of Child and Adolescent Psychiatric Nursing*, 19(4), 203–214.

Delaney, K. (2009). Reducing reactive aggression by lowering coping demands and boosting regulation: Five key staff behaviors. *Journal of Child and Adolescent Psychiatric Nursing*, 22(4), 211–219.

Dickens, G. (2010). Imitative suicide: An issue for psychiatric and mental health nursing? *Journal of Psychiatric and Mental Health Nursing*, 17(8), 741–749.

Dowdell, E. B., Burgess, A. W., & Flores, J. R. (2011). Original research: Online social networking patterns among adolescents, young adults, and sexual offenders. *American Journal of Nursing*, 111(7), 28–36.

Drauker, C. B., Martsolf, D., & Shokey, P. (2012). Ambiguity and violence in adolescent dating relationships. *Journal of Child and Adolescent Psychiatric Nursing*, 25(3), 149–157.

Dunsmore, J. C., Booker, J. A., & Ollendick, T. H. (2012). Parental emotion coaching and child emotion regulation as protective factors for children with oppositional defiant disorder. *Social Development*, 22(3), 444–466.

Dysart-Gale, D. (2010). Social justice and social determinants of health: Lesbian, gay, bisexual, transgendered, intersexed, and queer youth in Canada. *Journal of Child and Adolescent Psychiatric Nursing*, 23(1), 23–28.

Edidin, J., Ganim, Z., Hunter, S. J., & Karnik, N. S. (2012). The mental and physical health of homeless youth: A literature review. *Child Psychiatry and Human Development, 43*(3), 354–375.

Emerson, D., Sharma, R., Chaudhry, S., & Turner, J. (2009). Trauma-sensitive yoga: Principles, practice, and research. *International Journal of Yoga Therapy, 19*, 123–128.

Erikson, E. (1950). *Childhood and Society.* New York, NY: W.W. Norton.

Ferguson, C. J. (2011). The influence of television and video game use on attention and school problems: a multivariate analysis with other risk factors controlled. *Journal of Psychiatric Research, 45*(6), 808–813.

Garcia, C. (2010). Conceptualization and measurement of coping during adolescence: A review of the literature. *Journal of Nursing Scholarship, 42*(2), 166–185.

Gross, D., Garvey, C., Wrenetha, J., Fogg, L., Tucke, S., & Mokros, H. (2009). Efficacy of the Chicago Parent Program with low-income African American and Latino parents of young children. *Prevention Science, 10*(1), 54.

Haas, A. P., Eliason, M., Mays, V. M., Mathy, R. B., Cochran, S. D., D'Augelli, A. R., ... Clayton, P. J. (2011). Suicide and suicide risk in lesbian, gay, bisexual, and transgender populations: Review and recommendations. *Journal of Homosexuality, 58*(1), 10–51.

Hall, H. R., & Graff, J. C. (2011). The relationships among adaptive behaviors and children with autism, family support, parenting stress, and coping. *Issues in Comprehensive Pediatric Nursing, 34*(1), 4–25.

Hamrin, V., Antenucci, M., & Magorno, M. (2012). Evaluation and management of pediatric and adolescent depression. *The Nurse Practitioner, 37*(3), 22–30.

Harrison, J. N., Cluxton Keller, F., & Gross, D. (2012). Antipsychotic medication prescribing trends in children and adolescents. *Journal of Pediatric Health Care, 26*(2), 139–145.

Hassel, S., McKinnon, M. C., Cusi, A. M., & MacQueen, G. (2011). An overview of psychological and neurobiological mechanisms by which early negative experiences increase risk of mood disorders. *Journal of the Canadian Academy of Child and Adolescent Psychiatry, 20*(4), 277–288.

Hastings, E. C., Karas, T. L., Winsler, A., Way, E., Madigan, A., & Tyler, S. (2009). Young children's video/computer game use: Relations with school performance and behavior. *Issues in Mental Health Nursing, 30*(10), 638–649.

Hautala, L., Helenius, H., Karukivi, M., Maunula, A. M., Nieminen, J., Aromaa, M., ... Saarijarvi, S. (2011). The role of gender, affectivity and parenting in the course of disordered eating: A 4-year prospective case-control study among adolescents. *International Journal of Nursing Studies, 48*(8), 959–972.

Hautala, L. A., Junnila, J., Helenius, H., Vaananen, A. M., Liuksila, P. R., Raiha, H., Valimaki, M., & Saarijarvi, S. (2008). Towards understanding gender differences in disordered eating among adolescents. *Journal of Clinical Nursing, 17*(13), 1803–1813.

Hein, L. C., & Matthews, A. K. (2010). Reparative therapy: The adolescent, the psych nurse, and the issues. *Journal of Child and Adolescent Psychiatric Nursing, 23*(1), 29–35.

Hughes, J. R., Clark, S. E., Wood, W., Cakmak, S., Cox, A., MacInnis, M., ... Broom, B. (2010). Youth homelessness: The relationships among mental health, hope, and service satisfaction. *Journal of Child and Adolescent Psychiatry, 19*(4), 274–283.

International Society of Psychiatric Nurses (ISPN). (2010). *Practice parameters: Child and adolescent inpatient psychiatric treatment.* Available at http://www.ispn-psych.org/docs/PracticeParameters.pdf

Jackman, K. (2012). Motivational interviewing with adolescents: An advanced practice nursing intervention for psychiatric settings. *Journal of Child and Adolescent Psychiatric Nursing, 25*(1), 4–8.

Janiciak, P., Marder, S. R., & Pavuluri, M. (2011). *Principles and Practice of Psychopharmacotherapy.* Philadelphia, PA: Lippincott Williams & Wilkins.

Jensen, P. S., Goldman, E., Offord, D., Costello, E. J., Friedman, R., Huff, B., ... Roberts, R. (2011). Overlooked and underserved: "Action signs" for identifying children with unmet mental health needs. *Pediatrics, 128*(5), 970–979.

Johnson, N., Frenn, M., Feetham, S., & Simpson, P. (2011). Autism spectrum disorder: Parenting stress, family functioning and health-related quality of life. *Families, Systems, and Health, 29*(3), 232–252.

Kehle, T. J., Bray, M. A., Byer-Alcorace, G. F., Theodore, L. A., & Kovac, L. M. (2011). Augmented self-modeling as an intervention for selective mutism. *Psychology in the Schools, 49*(1), 93–103.

Kellam, S. G., Brown, C. H., Poduska, J. M., Ialongo, N. S., Wang, W., Toyinbo, P., ... Wilcox, H. C. (2008). Effects of a universal classroom behavior management program in first and second grades on young adult behavioral, psychiatric, and social outcomes. *Drug and Alcohol Dependence, 95*(Suppl 1), S5–S28.

Kelly, S. (2010). The psychological consequences to adolescents of exposure to gang violence in the community: An integrated review of the literature. *Journal of Child and Adolescent Psychiatric Nursing, 23*(2), 61–73.

Keskin, G., & Cam, O. (2010). Adolescents' strengths and difficulties: approach to attachment styles. *Journal of Psychiatric and Mental Health Nursing, 17*(5), 433–441.

Kuhlberg, J. A., Pena, J. B., & Zayas, L. H. (2010). Familism, parent-adolescent conflict, self-esteem, internalizing behaviors and suicide attempts among adolescent Latinas. *Child Psychiatry and Human Development, 41*(4), 425–440.

Lahey, B. B., & Waldman, I. (2012). Annual research review: Phenotypic and causal structure of conduct disorder in the broader context of prevalent forms of psychopathology. *Journal of Child Psychology and Psychiatry, 53*(5), 536–557.

Leahy, L. G., & Kohler, C. (2013). *Manual of Clinical Psychopharmacology for Nurses.* Arlington, VA: American Psychiatric Publishers.

Leckman, J. F., Bloch, M. H., Scahill, L., & King, R. (2006). Tourette syndrome: The self under siege. *Journal of Child Neurology, 21*(8), 642–649.

Lemery-Chalfant, K., Kao, K., Swann, G., & Goldsmith, H. H. (2013). Childhood temperament: Passive gene-environment correlation, gene-environment interaction, and the hidden importance of the family environment. *Developmental Psychopathology, 25*(1), 51–63.

Lenardson, J. D., Ziller, E. C., Lambert, D., Race, M., & Yousefian, A. (2010). Access to mental health services and family impact of rural children with mental illness. *Rural Health Research and Policy Centers.* Available at http://muskie.usm.maine.edu/Publications/rural/WP45/mental-health-access-rural-children-family-impact.pdf

Liu, J., & Graves, N. (2011). Childhood bullying: A review of constructs, concepts, and nursing implications. *Public Health Nursing, 28*(6), 556–568.

Livingston, J. D., Milne, T., Fang, M. L., & Amari, E. (2012). The effectiveness of interventions for reducing stigma related to substance use disorders: A systematic review. *Addiction, 107*, 39–50.

Luby, J. L., Tandon, M., & Belden, A. (2009). Preschool bipolar disorder. *Child and Adolescent Psychiatry Clinics of North America, 18*(2), 391–403.

Lusk, P., & Melnyk, B. M. (2011). COPE for the treatment of depressed adolescents: Lessons learned from implementing an evidence-based practice change. *Journal of the American Psychiatric Nurses Association, 17*(4), 297–309.

Lutz, W. J., & Warren, B. J. (2007). The state of nursing science—cultural and lifespan issues in depression: Part II: Focus on children and adolescents. *Issues in Mental Health Nursing, 28*(7), 749–764.

MacDonald, H. Z., Beeghly, M., Grant Knight, W., Augustyn, M., Woods, R. W., Cabral, H., ... Frank, D. A. (2008). Longitudinal association between infant disorganized attachment and childhood posttraumatic stress symptoms. *Development and Psychopathology, 20*(4), 493–508.

MacMillan, H. L., Wathen, C. N., Barlow, J., Fergusson, D. M., Leventhal, J. M., & Taussig, H. N. (2009). Interventions designed to prevent child maltreatment and associated impairment. *Lancet, 373*(9659), 250–266.

Maddison, M. A., Clarke, M. E., & Kutcher, S. (2011). The science of brain and biological development: Implications for mental health research, practice and policy. *Journal of the Canadian Academy of Child and Adolescent Psychiatry, 20*(4), 298–304.

Main, M., & Solomon, J. (1990). *Procedures for Identifying Infants as Disorganized/Disoriented during the Ainsworth Strange Situation. Attachment in the Preschool Years.* Chicago, IL: University of Chicago Press.

Mancil, G., Conroy, M. A., & Haydon, T. F. (2009). Effects of a modified milieu therapy intervention on the social communicative behaviors of young children with autism spectrum disorders. *Journal of Autism and Developmental Disorders, 39*(1), 149–163.

Mandell, D. S., Ittenbach, R. F., Levy, S. E., and Pinto-Martin, J. A. (2007). Disparities in diagnoses received prior to a diagnosis of autism. *Journal of Autism and Developmental Disorders, 37*(9), 1795–1802.

March of Dimes. (2011). *Peristats.* Available at http://www.marchofdimes.com/prematurity

Mayanil, T., Wegbreit, E., Fitzgerald, J., & Pavuluri, M. (2011). Emerging biosignature of brain function and intervention in pediatric bipolar disorder. *Minerva Pediatrica, 63*(3), 183–200.

McGorry, P. D., Purcell, R., Goldstone, S., & Amminger, G. P. (2011). Age of onset and timing of treatment for mental and substance use disorders: Implications for preventive intervention strategies and models of care current opinion in psychiatry. *Current Opinions in Psychiatry, 24*(4), 301–306.

Merry, S. N., Hetrick, S. E., Cox, G. R., Brudevold-Iversen, T., Bir, J. J., & McDowell, H. (2011). Psychological and educational interventions for preventing depression in children and adolescents (review). *Cochrane Database of Systematic Reviews, 12*, 1–209, article CD003380.

Meyerson, D. A., Grant, K. A, Carter, J. S., & Kilmer, R. P. (2011). Posttraumatic growth among children and adolescents: A systematic review. *Clinical Psychology Review, 31*(6), 949–964.

Morstein, J. (2009). Assessing behavior and social competence of severely emotionally disturbed youth admitted to psychiatric residential treatment. *Journal of Child and Adolescent Psychiatric Nursing, 22*(3), 143–149.

National Center for Children Exposed to Violence. (2006). *Community violence.* Available at http://www.nccev.org/violence

National Institute of Mental Health. (2010). *Suicide in the U.S. Statistics and prevention.* Available at http://www.nimh.nih.gov/health/publications/suicide-in-the-us-statistics-and-prevention/index.shtml#factors

National Institute of Mental Health. (2011). *Mental health medications.* Alphabetical list of medications. Available at http://www.nimh.nih.gov/health/publications/mental-health-medications/alphabetical-list-of-medications.shtml

National Institute of Mental Health. (2012). *Attention deficit hyperactivity disorder.* Available at http://www.nimh.nih.gov/health/publications/attention-deficit-Hyperactivity-disorder/index.shtml

Nazeer, A. (2011). Psychopharmacology of autistic spectrum disorders in children and adolescents. *Pediatric Clinics of North America, 58*(1), 85–97.

North American Nursing Diagnosis Association. (2008). *NANDA Nursing Diagnoses: Definitions and Classification, 2007–2008.* Philadelphia, PA: North American Nursing Diagnosis Association.

O'Connell, M. E., Boat, T., & Warner, K. E. (Eds.). (2009). *Institute of Medicine report: Preventing mental, emotional, and behavioral disorders among young people: Progress and possibilities.* Committee on the Prevention of Mental Disorders and Substance Abuse Among Children, Youth and Young Adults: Research Advances and Promising Interventions; Institute of Medicine; National Research Council.

Olino, T. M., Gillo, S., Rowe, D., Palermo, S., Nuhfer, E. C., Birmaher, B., & Gilbert, A. R. (2011). Evidence for successful implementation of exposure and response prevention in a naturalistic group format for pediatric OCD. *Depression and Anxiety, 28*, 342–348.

O'Loughlin, E. K., Dugas, E. N., Sabiston, C. M., & O'Loughlin, J. L. (2012). Prevalence and correlates of exergaming in youth. *Pediatrics, 130*(5), 806–814.

Orlando, I. J. (1972). *The Discipline and Teaching of Nursing Process (An Evaluative Study).* New York, NY: G. P. Putnam's Sons.

Pagey, B., Deering, D., & Sellman, D. (2010). Retention of adolescents with substance dependence and coexisting mental health disorders in outpatient alcohol and drug group therapy. *International Journal of Mental Health Nursing, 19*(6), 437–444.

Pappadopoulous, E., Rosato, N. S., Correll, C. U., Findling, R. L., Lucas, J., Crystal, S., & Jensen, P. (2011). Expert recommendations for treating maladaptive aggression in youth. *Journal of Child and Adolescent Psychopharmacology, 21*(6), 505–515.

Pardini, D., & Frick, P. J. (2013). Multiple developmental pathways to conduct disorder: Current conceptualizations and clinical implications. *Journal of the Canadian Academy of Child and Adolescent Psychiatry, 22*(1), 20–25.

Passarotti, A. M., & Pavuluri, M. N. (2011). Brain functional domains inform therapeutic interventions in attention-deficit/hyperactivity disorder and pediatric bipolar disorder. *Expert Review of Neurotherapeutics, 11*(6), 897–914.

Patten, S. B., Waheed, W., & Bresee, L. (2012). A review of pharmacoepidemiologic studies of antipsychotic use in children and adolescents. *Canadian Journal of Psychiatry, 57*(12), 717–721.

Pellow, J., Solomon, E. M., & Barnard, C.N. (2011). Complementary and alternative medical therapies for children with attention-deficit/hyperactivity disorder (ADHD). *Alternative Medicine Review, 16*(4), 323–337.

Pine, D. S., Costello, J., Dahl, R., James, R., Leckman, J., Leibenluft, E., … Zeanah, C. (2010). Increasing the developmental focus in DSM-V: Broad issues and specific potential applications in anxiety. In American Psychiatric Association. (2013). *The Conceptual Evolution of DSM-5.* Arlington, VA: American Psychiatric Publishers, pp. 305–321.

Poncin, Y., Sukhodolsky, D. G., McGuire, J., & Scahill, L. (2007). Drug and non-drug treatments of children with ADHD and tic disorders. *European Child and Adolescent Psychiatry, 16*(1), 78–88.

Regnerus, M. D., & Elder, G. H. (2003). Staying on track in school: Religious influences in high- and low-risk settings. *Journal for the Scientific Study of Religion, 42*(4), 633–649.

Riley, B. H. (2010). GLB adolescent's "coming out." *Journal of Child and Adolescent Psychiatric Nursing, 23*(1), 3–10.

Robb, A. S. (2010). Managing irritability and aggression in autism spectrum disorders in children and adolescents. *Developmental Disabilities Research Reviews, 16*(3), 258–264.

Roth, T. L., & Sweatt, J. D. (2011). Annual research review: Epigenetic mechanisms and environmental shaping of the brain during sensitive periods of development. *Journal of Child Psychology and Psychiatry, 52*(4), 398–408.

Rowe, J. (2010). Dealing with psychiatric disabilities in schools: A description of symptoms and coping strategies for dealing with them. *Preventing School Failure, 54*(3), 190–198.

Ruiz-Veguilla, M., Barrign, M., Diaz, F. J., Ferrin, M., Morano-Granados, J., Salcedo, M., Cervilla, J., & Gurpegui, M. (2012). The duration of untreated psychosis is associated with social support and temperament. *Psychiatry Research, 200*(2,3), 687–692.

Russell, S. T., & Toomey, R. B. (2012). Men's sexual orientation and suicide: Evidence for U.S. adolescent specific risk. *Social Science and Medicine, 74*(4), 523–529.

Ryan, C., Futterman, D., & Stine, K. (1998). Helping our hidden youth. *American Journal of Nursing, 98*, 37–41.

Scahill, L., Sukhodolsky, D. G., Bearss, K., Findley, D., Hamrin, V., Carroll, D. H., & Rains, A. L. (2006). A randomized trial of parent training in children with tic disorders and disruptive behavior. *Journal of Child Neurology, 21*(8), 650–656.

Scahill, L., Woods, D. W., Himie, M. B., Peterson, A. L., Wilhelm, S., Piacentini, J. C., … Mink, J. W. (2013). Current controversies on the role of behavior therapy in Tourette syndrome. *Movement Disorders, 28*(9), 1179–1183.

Sharaf, A. Y., Thompson, E. A., & Walsh, E. (2009). Protective effects of self-esteem and family support on suicide behaviors among at risk adolescents. *Journal of Child and Adolescent Psychiatric Nursing, 22*(3), 160–168.

Shetgiri, R., Hua, L., Avila, R., & Flores, G. (2012). Parental characteristics associated with bullying perpetration in US children aged 10 to 17 years. *American Journal of Public Health, 102*(12), 2280–2286.

Shimshock, C. M., Williams, R. A., & Sullivan, B. J. (2011). Suicidal thought in the adolescent: Exploring the relationship between known risk factors and the presence of suicidal thought. *Journal of Child and Adolescent Psychiatric Nursing, 24*(4), 237–240.

Sibinga, E. M., Kerrigan, D., Stewart, M., Johnson, K., Magyari, T., & Ellen, J. (2011). Mindfulness-based stress reduction for urban youth. *Journal of Alternative and Conplementary Medicine, 17*(3), 213–218.

Simonoff, E., Pickles, A., Charman, T., Chandler, S., Loucas, T., & Baird, G. (2008). Psychiatric disorders in children with autism spectrum disorders: Prevalence, comorbidity, and associated factors in a population-derived sample. *Journal of the American Academy of Child and Adolescent Psychiatry, 47*(8), 921–929.

Singer, M. I. (2007). Assessment of violence exposure among residential children and adolescents. *Residential Treatment for Children and Youth, 24*(1–2), 159–174.

Smith, A. T., Kelly-Weeder, S., Engel, J., McGowan, K., Anderson, B., &Wolfe, B. E. (2011). Quality of eating disorders websites: What adolescents and their families need to know. *Journal of Child and Adolescent Psychiatric Nursing, 24*(1), 33–37.

Society for Adolescent Health and Medicine. (2013). Recommendations for promoting the health and well-being of lesbian, gay, bisexual, and transgender adolescents: A position paper of the Society for Adolescent Health and Medicine. *Journal of Adolescent Health, 52*(4), 506–510.

Sourander, A., Fossum, S., Ronning, J. A., Elonheimo, H., Ristkari, T., Kumpulainen, K., … Almqvist, F. (2012). What is the long-term outcome of boys who steal at age eight? Findings from the Finnish nationwide "from a boy to a man" birth cohort study. *Social Psychiatry and Psychiatric Epidemiology, 47*(9), 1391–1400.

Specht, M. W., Woods, D. W., Piacentini, J., Schhill, L., Wilhelm, S., Peterson, A. L., … Walkup, J. T. (2011). Clinical characteristics of children and adolescents with a primary tic disorder. *Journal of Developmental and Physical Disabilities, 23*, 15–31.

Spinazzola, J., Rhodes, A. M., Emerson, D., Earle, E., & Monroe, K. (2011). Application of yoga in residential treatment of traumatized youth. *Journal of the American Psychiatric Nurses Association, 17*(6), 431–444.

Substance Abuse and Mental Health Services Administration (SAMHSA). (2013). *SAMHSA news release: SAMHSA awards up to $56.9 million in grants over four years in FY 13 to support safe schools and healthy students.* Available at http://www.samhsa.gov/newsroom/advisories/1310230410.aspx

Swain, J. E., Scahill, L., Lombroso, P. J., King, R. A., & Leckman, J. F. (2007). Tourette syndrome and tic disorders: A decade of progress. *Journal of the American Academy of Child and Adolescent Psychiatry, 46*(8), 947–968.

Taylor, J. Y., Caldwell, C. H., Baser, R. E., Fasion, R., & Jackson, J. S. (2007). Prevalence of eating disorders among blacks in the National Survey of American Life. *International Journal of Eating Disorders, 40,* 10–14.

Tzang, R-F., Chang, Y-C., & Liu, S-I. (2009). The association between children's ADHD subtype and parenting stress and parental symptoms. *FollowInternational Journal of Psychiatry in Clinical Practice, 13*(4), 318–325.

U.S. Department of Health and Human Services, Administration for Children and Families, Administration on Children, Youth, and Families, Children's Bureau. (2010). Child maltreatment, 2009. Available at http://www.acf.hhs.gov/programs/cb/resource/child-maltreatment-2009

U.S. Department of Veterans Affairs. (2007). PTSD in children and teens. Available at http://www.ptsd.va.gov/public/pages/ptsd-children-adolescents.asp

Usher, K., Jackson, D., & O'Brien, L. (2007). Shattered dreams: Parental experiences of adolescent substance abuse. *International Journal of Mental Health Nursing, 16,* 422–430.

Vanderbilt, D., & Gleason, M. M. (2011). Mental health concerns of the premature infant through the lifespan. *Pediatric Clinics of North America, 58*(4), 815–832.

van Ommen, J., Meerwijk, E., Kars, M., van Elburg, A., & van Meijel, B. (2009). Effective nursing care of adolescents diagnosed with anorexia nervosa: The patients' perspective. *Journal of Clinical Nursing, 18*(20), 2801–2808.

Viana, A. G., Beidel, D. C., & Rabian, B. (2009). Selective mutism: A review and integration of the last 15 years. *Clinical Psychology Review, 29,* 57–67.

Visser, S. N., Danielson, M. L., Bitsko, R. H., Holbrook, J. R., Kogan, M. D., Ghandour, R. M., Perou, R., & Blumberg, S. J. (2014). Trends in the parent-report of health care provider-diagnosed and medicated attention-deficit/hyperactivity disorder: United States, 2003–2011. *Journal of the American Academy of Child and Adolescent Psychiatry, 53*(1), 34–46.

von Gontard, A. (2011). Elimination disorders: A critical comment on DSM-5 proposals. *European Child and Adolescent Psychiatry, 20*(2), 83–88.

Warren, B. J. (2011). Two sides of the coin: The bully and the bullied. *Journal of Psychosocial Nursing and Mental Health Services, 49*(10), 22–29.

Webster-Stratton, C., Reid, M. J., & Beauchaine, T. (2011). Combining parent and child training for young children with ADHD. *Journal of Clinical Child and Adolescent Psychology, 40*(2), 191–203.

Webster-Stratton, C., Reid, M. J., & Stoolmiller, M. (2008). Preventing conduct problems and improving school readiness: Evaluation of the Incredible Years teacher and child training programs in high-risk schools. *Journal of Child Psychology and Psychiatry, 49*(5), 471–488.

West, A. E., & Pavuluri, M. N. (2009). Psychosocial treatment for childhood and adolescent bipolar disorder. *Child and Adolescent Psychiatric Clinics of North America, 18,* 471–482.

West, A., Jacobs, R. H., Westerholm, R., Lee, A., Carbray, J., Heidenreich, J., & Pavuluri, M. (2009). Child and family-focused cognitive-behavioral therapy for pediatric bipolar disorder: Pilot study of group treatment format. *Journal of the Canadian Academy of Child and Adolescent Psychiatry, 18*(3), 239–246.

Williams, K. (2011). Pediatric autoimmune neuropsychiatric disorder associated with streptococcus (PANDAS): An update on diagnosis and treatment. *Current Medical Literature—Psychiatry, 22*(3), 81–88.

Williamson, E. D., & Martin, A. (2010). Psychotropic medications in autism: Practical considerations for parents. *Journal of Autism and Developmental Disorders, 0162-3257,* 1–7.

Willis, D., Hawkins, J., Pearce, C., Phalen, J., Keet, M., & Singer, C. (2010). Children who witness violence: What services do they need to heal? *Issues in Mental Health Nursing, 31*(9), 552–560.

31

Adult Transitions

J. Goodlett McDaniel
Lora Peppard

Key Terms

genetics, 687
genomics, 687
resilience, 688
sandwich generation, 685
sickness behavior, 682

Learning Outcomes

1. Contrast events during adulthood that may contribute to mental illness.

2. Describe how co-morbid medical conditions complicate treatment.

3. Relate the influence of a patient's stage of life to the nursing assessment and treatment.

4. Explain risks associated with use of psychotropic medications in patients who are pregnant.

5. Summarize the role of genetics in mental health nursing.

6. Compare two theoretical frameworks that can assist nurses in providing appropriate care to adult patients.

7. Describe interventions that support resilience in adult patients.

Timothy Barksdale Relapse Stage

APPLICATION

1. Based on this information, what are the priority nursing interventions for this patient?

2. To what extent is what you are seeing a psychiatric emergency as well as a medical emergency?

3. What additional information about Mr. Barksdale do you think would be helpful in planning nursing care for him?

You have just received the 7 a.m. to 7 p.m. shift change report on a 30-bed, adult, inpatient psychiatric unit that is part of a medical school teaching hospital. You are a part-time nurse on the unit, making rounds on seven patients. Although the staffing pattern for the unit usually is appropriate to the number and acuity of patients, the RN scheduled to come on duty at 10:00 p.m. has called in sick. Currently, the charge nurse is on the telephone with a physician regarding an anticipated involuntary admission to the intensive care unit of a patient described as combative and actively hallucinating.

During report, you heard that the evening hospital supervisor will work on getting some "help," in response to the need for an additional nurse. The 7 a.m. to 7 p.m. staff members have left the unit. The charge nurse from the day shift reported that "things were quiet" on the psychiatric unit for most of the shift.

The census is full on hall B, where you are rounding. As you walk down the hall, you hear a gurgling noise and enter the room of Timothy Barksdale, a 50-year-old married White man with recurrent major depression and a history of "heart problems," diabetes, and chronic pain related to peripheral neuropathy of the feet.

Mr. Barksdale is lying flat in a hospital bed, diaphoretic, with visible neck veins and circumoral cyanosis. His vital signs are: pulse 110 and thready, BP 144/50 mmHg, and respirations 34 and shallow. Mr. Barksdale's hands and ankles are swollen and his abdomen appears distended. As you approach the patient, he looks panic stricken, and his color is ashen.

You remember from report that Mr. Barksdale had made a suicide attempt prior to this hospitalization by overdosing on "sleeping pills" while drinking. He and his wife of 30 years are estranged, and he has two adult daughters living in the area who "do not visit." Mr. Barksdale's history indicates that one daughter suffers from major depression, the other with obesity and marijuana abuse. Mr. Barksdale has a sister with whom he talks on occasion, but she does not live in the area. His sister suffers from generalized anxiety disorder and has great difficulty traveling. Mr. Barksdale's parents are both deceased. His father died at age 85 from a "heart attack"; his mother died as a result of complications from diabetes. You remain calm and perform a quick physical assessment while clicking the call bell and requesting assistance.

You learn that Mr. Barksdale has been given the following diagnoses: major depression, dependent personality disorder, hypertension, diabetes, hypercholesterolemia, sleep apnea, chronic pain, and a history of suspected myocardial infarction.

Introduction

Mental health care in the United States is defined, legislated, funded, and consumed in large part by adults. The processes and products of this work have been discussed in previous chapters. What makes the role of the adult unique in mental health is that this is often where both consumers and caregivers are related in ways that imply differing levels of power, responsibility, and accountability. In many psychiatric nursing texts, for instance, indexes have dozens of references to child, adolescent, and geriatric patients. Look under "adult," however, and you are likely to find far fewer references.

The purpose of this chapter is to introduce the nursing student to major concepts and practices unique to the care of adult psychiatric patients. Understanding the evidence that supports the need for psychiatric nursing skills in all areas of nursing can lead to a lifetime of successful practice in the care and well-being of all adult patients.

Specific Issues in Adult Mental Health

Although the adult experience can vary considerably among individuals, two issues that affect mental health and treatment, co-morbidity and widespread anxiety, are prevalent in the adult population.

Co-Morbidity

The interaction between medical and psychiatric conditions is complex. Individuals with serious mental illness are at increased risk for acute and chronic medical illnesses and reduced life expectancy. The National Association of State Mental Health Program Directors (NASMHPD) reports that the average life expectancy for people with serious mental illness is 25 years less than that of the general population (Parks et al., 2006).

It is estimated that three of five individuals with serious mental illness die as a result of preventable health conditions such as cancer, cardiovascular disease, and diabetes. Moreover, modifiable risk factors (such as smoking, drinking, drug abuse/misuse, poor nutrition, obesity, and lack of exercise) place people with serious mental illness at higher risk for morbidity and mortality (Parks et al., 2006; Colton & Manderscheid, 2006). Gastrointestinal disorders also have both psychiatric and physical causes and consequences. Factors such as onset, severity, and outcome of many gastrointestinal disorders (including irritable bowel syndrome, celiac disease, and less severe forms of gastritis) may be exacerbated by psychiatric illness (Gautam, 2010). Increasingly, care of patients with mental illness requires collaboration with clinicians and other professionals providing care for patients' biophysical illnesses (see Evidence-Based Practice: Integrative Strategies for Care).

The body's ability to recover from both acute and debilitating threats depends on a complex set of chemical reactions. Mind, body, and spirit influence one another. Gautam (2010) has discussed bio-chemical studies and the effects on neurochemical, immune, and endocrine responses to stress as part of a growing body of nursing literature. Gautam states that the catabolism of tryptophan is stimulated under the influence of stress and hormone release. Tryptophan is an amino acid that is a precursor to the formation of serotonin in the brain. According to Gautam, impairment in tryptophan production results in impairment of serotonin synthesis in the brain. A recent study by Kurz (2011) found that a buildup of neurotoxic metabolites in the brain may result in depression. Kurz attributed this buildup to immune-mediated tryptophan degradation. The importance of tryptophan depletion, whether the cause or the result of depression, is most likely related directly to both physical and mental illnesses.

Cardiac illnesses associated with psychiatric disorders include congestive heart failure, a diagnosis described in the case study. As many as 20% of congestive heart failure patients meet the criteria for a diagnosis of major depressive episode, and some 16% meet the criteria for unspecified depressive disorder. According to Gautam (2010), 51% of patients with congestive heart failure were determined to have depression using the Beck Depression Inventory.

The fact that a patient has a history of medical illness as well as mental illness may lead to the logical next question: Which came first? That question, however, may not be the correct one to ask. The more important questions when treating psychiatric or medical patients may be "What do I know?" and "What do I need to know to better help my patient?"

The way a nurse views the patient's condition may be influenced by the setting in which the nurse cares for the patient. For example, on a cardiac rehabilitation unit, a patient such as Mr. Barksdale (featured in the case study) would be monitored, have an IV or port in place, and have his vital signs assessed frequently. The oncoming nurse would complete a head-to-toe physical assessment, looking especially for signs of cardiac distress. If that same nurse were to see Mr. Barksdale on an inpatient psychiatric unit, the nurse may take vital signs daily, expect the patient to ambulate and participate in groups, and may focus on signs, verbal or otherwise, that Mr. Barksdale is having suicidal thoughts and is taking his medications as prescribed.

Cardiac disease is common in psychiatric patients, but diabetes is reported as more common. The Centers for Disease Control and Prevention (CDC) reports that individuals with diabetes are more likely to suffer from depression (CDC, 2011). Adults with depression have poorer glycemic control, and those with depression are at increased risk of developing diabetes (Gautam, 2010).

Research has suggested that high levels of depression and anxiety observed in Parkinson disease, for instance, are a primary consequence of brain changes found in the disease. Similarly, depression has been reported in 10% to 20% of cancer patients (Gautam, 2010). Cancer patients with depression have been reported to have higher plasma concentrations of certain interleukin levels than do patients without cancer (Gautam, 2010). Higher than normal plasma interleukin levels may contribute to sickness behavior that has overlapping symptoms with major depression (Musselman et al., 2001). **Sickness behavior** refers to a group of symptoms that act to conserve energy in the presence of acute inflammatory response. Many symptoms of sickness behavior, such as anorexia, fatigue, withdrawal, and aching, are also common symptoms of depression (Figure 31-1) (Maes et al., 2012).

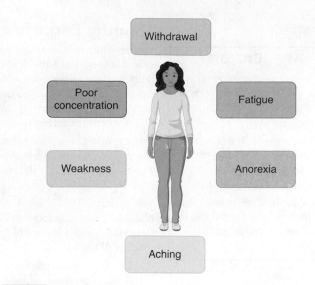

31-1 Patients with acute inflammatory illness may exhibit sickness behavior, a constellation of symptoms similar to those of depression.

In all cases, the nurse remains the caregiver who assesses, plans for, and treats patients in a holistic manner. The importance of understanding the current and emerging body of evidence that supports the complex biological and psychological relationships that affect disease and recovery cannot be overstated.

Widespread Anxiety

Anxiety is prevalent among adults, with anxiety disorders affecting nearly 40 million adults in the United States. Sadly, two-thirds of those affected do not receive treatment. Anxiety disorders cost $42 billion a year in lost productivity, treatment, and human suffering (Anxiety and Depression Association of America [ADAA], 2012). For patients in the workplace, anxiety disorders also can result in increased accidents and errors, higher absenteeism, and violence.

In caring for adult patients, it often is useful to think of the cumulative and clustering effects of anxiety. When clustered together, otherwise manageable stressors, such as a flat tire or a minor illness, may result in feeling loss of control or overwhelming anxiety. At times, adults do not recognize that the smaller stressors of life have the power to overwhelm coping mechanisms if not acknowledged and addressed. Patients with chronic or severe mental illness experience even greater challenges in this area and may lack the cognitive functioning necessary to prevent, remove, or limit those stressors.

Critical changes that occur in adults are particularly relevant when caring for patients with mental illness. Important facts regarding adults experiencing multiple life changes, whether these changes are positive or negative, include the following: (1) Stressors may have the power to overwhelm coping mechanisms rapidly and profoundly; (2) stressors may complicate other illnesses; and (3) stressors may not be apparent to the patient, but may be discovered only through a process that includes systematic patient evaluation. In addition to recognizing these changes as they occur for patients, nurses will find it helpful to recognize and address changes that may result in stress for themselves (Box 31-1).

Integrative Strategies for Care

Clinical Problem

As stated throughout this text, patients with co-morbid illnesses or severe physical illness are at greater risk for experiencing mental illness, and psychiatric patients are at greater risk for co-morbid physical illness. Patients with co-occurring illness experience the most debilitating and dangerous symptoms, and therefore incur greater expenses related to treatment. Additionally, Americans are becoming more interested in nonpharmacologic therapies and more involved and informed in the costs of their treatment. Does integrating different types of therapies (including mental health care) reduce the cost of treatment and provide other benefits?

Evidence

A recent international study exploring the cost of co-morbid, chronic conditions and mental health provides a comprehensive review of how patients with such health needs can be supported in a more integrated way (Naylor et al., 2012). The researchers documented the necessity of the study by citing findings that support the complexity and costs associated with co-morbid illness, including the following: (1) Depression is two to three times more common in patients with cardiovascular disease and/or diabetes than in patients who have only one diagnosis; (2) patients with chronic obstructive pulmonary disease are two to three times more likely to have mental illness than are other patients; (3) one-third of female patients with chronic musculoskeletal disorders suffer from depression; and (4) mental health problems increased the costs of care for long-term conditions by at least 45% after controlling for severity of physical illness.

In addition, a number of studies have reported the costs of co-morbid illness. In a study of cardiovascular patients in Germany, psychiatric co-morbidity increased the average length of inpatient stays by 4 days, resulting in an increased cost of care of nearly 50% (Hochlehnert et al., 2011). Another study found that treatment costs for patients with co-morbid depression and diabetes may be as much as 4.5 times greater than treatment costs for patients with diabetes alone (Katon, 2008).

Naylor et al. (2012) examined integrative strategies, such as screening patients with co-occurring illness for mental health problems and using multiple technologies to assist patients with information and support. They discovered that understanding and practicing models of integrated health care may be useful as health care systems continue to look for ways to support quality, access, and cost containment for patients. Intermountain Health, a program

providing mental and physical care to patients in Utah and Idaho, was cited as a model of a nonprofit clinic whose mission is to provide care to patients with mental health concerns. Intermountain Health employed a team approach, using both mental health and primary care professionals. The researchers found that by integrating patient care to address both physical and mental health issues, patients experienced better outcomes at lower costs than more traditional care models. The practices that were successfully used to achieve positive outcomes included the following:

1. Effective use of electronic health records
2. Routine screenings of patients at risk for mental health problems using standardized tools
3. Application of web-based and other technologies that provide patients with follow-up information and support resources between visits
4. Integration of peer support and community care as part of a comprehensive treatment plan
5. Use of evidence-based guidelines and disease registries as a routine part of treatment (Naylor et al., 2012)

Naylor et al. reported that in the Intermountain program, medical costs following a diagnosis of depression were as much as 48% lower per patient than costs for those receiving care at other treatment clinics. They cited the work of Reiss-Brennan et al., who concluded that the savings included reduced medical inpatient and a greater than 50% decrease in emergency room visits (Reiss-Brennan et al., 2010).

Implications for Nursing

Models such as the Intermountain program offer valuable insight for nurses into effective ways of improving quality and reducing costs based on specific evidence-based practice guidelines. As members of one of the most highly regarded professions (Gallup, 2013), nurses are in a unique position to offer guidance on the appropriate use a variety of therapies.

Critical Thinking Questions

1. What is your opinion about the costs of health care?
2. What do you think about the approach of organizations such as Intermountain Health that promote mental health care in addition to offering physical care to their patients?
3. What organizations in your area offer this type of care?

Nurses and Stress

box 31-1

Nurses are not immune to stress. Like other professionals, nurses have both professional and life responsibilities, are required to manage multiple roles, and experience both acute and chronic stressors. The same is true for nursing students, most of whom manage multiple roles as they negotiate the college environment. Preparing for exams and participating in simulations and clinical rotations represent new stressors that require planning, careful study, and learning new skills.

As in most clinical rotations, it is normal for students to imagine that they have the illness that they are studying. Examination of personal behavior and the opportunity that nurses have to reflect on their strengths and talents are useful activities. Understanding the power that nurses have to heal and provide hope through therapeutic use of self can be a profound discovery that provides relief of human suffering (Perrin, 2012).

Pause and Reflect

1. *Do you know anyone who has become overwhelmed by a positive life change? What happened? How can positive life changes create stress?*

2. *How do prevalent issues such as co-morbidity and widespread anxiety among adults affect nursing practice?*

Transitions in Adulthood

Adulthood is a time of transitions. Going to and graduating from college, selecting a career, experiencing a promotion, initiating long-term relationships and/or marriage, starting a family, and facing retirement are just a few of the transitions adults encounter.

Nursing students also experience transitions as they gain knowledge and skills necessary to enter their profession. Some skills, such as competency in starting IVs or palpating a lump, can seem of little value to nursing students when the door of the psychiatric unit locks behind them. With psychiatric patients, therapeutic interventions include providing support, being genuine, demonstrating understanding and empathy, and showing respect. Becoming expert in demonstrating these qualities may seem hard to measure. However, the work done by nurses when completing a process recording, reflecting on responses to behavior, or practicing empathy and providing hope is key to successful patient care in any setting.

The most serious mental health disorders often have onset in early adulthood (De Hert et al., 2011). Schizophrenia, bipolar disorder, and a number of the most burdensome anxiety disorders may have their most negative consequences on a patient's well-being, family, work life, and ability to successfully negotiate his or her world during adulthood. Working with patients who may not look physically ill yet are incapable of reality testing or engaging in a coherent conversation can be both surprising and overwhelming for students and new nurses.

From a purely developmental standpoint, the first five stages of Erikson's psychosocial model help explain a path for healthy transition from infancy to late adolescence (Chapter 4). However, only three remaining stages cover an ever increasing time period during which most of the care of psychiatric patients occurs—adulthood. According to Erikson, humans confront and master new life challenges during each stage. Furthermore, each stage builds on the successful completion of earlier stages. Developmental models help nurses track whether patients have successfully mastered important developmental tasks while, at the same time, challenging them to review their own growth.

Americans are living longer. Those born in 1900 could expect to live until approximately age 50, whereas the U.S. Centers for Disease Control and Prevention reports life expectancy at birth in the United States now averages beyond age 70 (Figure 31-2) (Hoyert & Xu, 2012). As a result, the challenges and complexities of adulthood last far longer than they did a century ago, and the variety of experiences that adults face changes over time as well. Today, adults entering older adulthood at age 60 years now may have almost a third of their life ahead of them. Nurses who are able to provide support during transitions and who understand the issues associated with specific transitions will be in a better position to provide individualized care.

Single Adulthood

For many individuals, single adulthood represents the first stage of adult life. Being a single adult has benefits and liabilities in society. Questions such as, "Table for one?" and "Are you married?," whether an individual is single by choice, death, or circumstance, can be difficult to answer. Cultural norms in most societies favor couples over singles. If adults are not in acceptable relationships, they may be perceived as a threat to the ability of the group (tribe) to survive: Families can protect and prosper only by bonding and procreating. Although many adults might not consider this cultural norm as a source of anxiety or depression, there is some evidence to support this. For example, a meta-analysis of 25 epidemiological studies found a 12% prevalence of depression correlated with being female, young, unmarried, and having less than a college education (Gaderman et al., 2012).

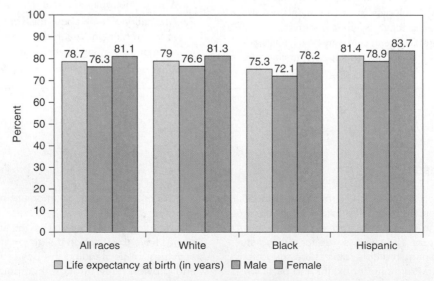

31-2   Life expectancy at birth (in years) by race in the United States—preliminary figures for 2011.

Data from Hoyert, D. L., & Xu J. Q. (2012). Deaths: Preliminary data for 2011. *National Vital Statistics Reports, 61*(6). Hyattsville, MD: National Center for Health Statistics.

The fact that adults enter and exit life alone and live in a space and time bounded by oneness is something that tribes cannot prevent, control, or change. The expectation is that the individual will stand alone (as evidenced by familiar statements such as "It's time that you take responsibility for your own life" or "Give her some space") during periods of strong emotion, developmental change, or when there are inadequate fiscal or emotional resources within families, for instance. Being single may or may not be a choice in adult life; however, single patients have unique needs that require consideration by nurses charged with their care. Some may not have support systems available to them, which could magnify the impact of simple challenges.

Pregnancy and the Postpartum Period

Research indicates that 3% to 6% of women will develop major depression or anxiety during pregnancy or the postpartum period (American Psychiatric Association [APA], 2013), and women with chronic mental illness are at high risk for both pregnancy and delivery complications (Jablensky et al., 2005). Nursing management of a pregnant patient requires an understanding of (1) the hormonal influence on a woman's mental status during pregnancy and the postpartum period; (2) the psychological changes encountered during pregnancy, and additionally, for the patient with a psychiatric diagnosis; and (3) knowledge of the risks to both the mother and the fetus when psychotropic intervention is either administered or discontinued or when the mental illness is left untreated during pregnancy (Chapter 16, Mood Disorders).

Biological Changes

During pregnancy, estrogen and progesterone levels fluctuate, causing blood sugar levels to shift rapidly. Pregnancy affects every woman differently. Some may struggle with negative mood symptoms as the physical changes their bodies take a toll or elevated stress hormones (for example, high basal cortisol) contribute to mood changes such as melancholic depression (Kammerer, Taylor, & Glover, 2006).

Psychological and Social Changes

Motherhood adds a new dimension to a woman's identity and role within her family. A pregnant woman may begin thinking about what kind of parent she wants to be and begin to evaluate the parenting she received. Memories of past traumas, anxieties, or disappointments may be reactivated (Frayne, Nguyen, Allen, & Rampono, 2009). Current relationships with partners or spouses may improve or worsen, and domestic violence may begin or cease. It is important for nurses to understand how family dynamics may change during a pregnancy and to always consider these changes when assessing a pregnant client experiencing symptoms of mental illness.

Medications and Pregnancy

All medications are assigned a level of risk by the U.S. Food and Drug Administration (FDA) for use in pregnancy. The levels are lettered A, B, C, D, and X. A medication categorized as level X is contraindicated in pregnancy, but a medication categorized as level A may be an option, as controlled studies have not shown any risk to the fetus (U.S. FDA, 2012). Considering the risks associated with use of psychotropic medication during pregnancy, many pregnant women may choose to discontinue or avoid pharmacologic treatment (Table 31-1). A careful risk–benefit analysis must always be performed, as psychiatric illness in the mother can significantly affect morbidity for both the mother and child. Nurses are responsible for understanding the risks involved for either option, taking into account the specific diagnosis and recommendations of the woman's health care provider.

Risks of Refusing Treatment

The fear or guilt experienced when taking medication or listening to others' warnings about the risks involved may cause a woman to abruptly discontinue her medication when she learns she is pregnant. Discontinuation of treatment during pregnancy has been shown to increase rates of relapse (Jablensky et al., 2005; Viguera et al., 2000). In addition, untreated or inadequately treated depression or anxiety can have a negative impact on the neurodevelopment of the fetus, along with pregnancy and delivery outcomes (Bonari et al., 2004; O'Connor, Heron, Golding, Beveridge, & Glover, 2002). A comprehensive risk–benefit analysis for both the mother and the fetus should be performed with the patient's provider. The patient's decision should be supported by the nursing staff.

Divorce or Death of a Spouse

Divorce or death of a spouse may return an adult to the single life. Each has profound consequences on the life of an adult. Income, friendships, housing, effects of divorce or death, and children and the parent–child relationship (if the couple has children) are all affected. Changes in these areas can affect the adult's sense of self. That being said, the number of never-married adults in the United States has been increasing over the past decade (Population Reference Bureau, 2012). Although more couples are choosing not to marry, many couples choose to live in a long-term commitment without the formality of marriage. For these couples, separation or death can be as significant as it is for a couple legally married. Nurses must assess patients' relationship status and be aware of how their spousal or personal relationships affect their daily lives.

The Sandwich Generation

Changes in resources, forced dependence, loss of function, and the mobility of families are all concerns faced by adults who care for both children and aging parents, sometimes termed the **sandwich generation**. The responsibilities of caring for both children and aging parents have contributed to a new set of stressors seen in adult patients (Figure 31-3). Knowing the challenges faced by these adults can help in planning for a more meaningful exchange, supporting newly affected patients, and becoming more empathetic to the needs of adult patients.

The Adult Orphan

Although many adult orphans (those who have experienced the loss of both parents) successfully adapt to loss, others exhibit adverse outcomes, including complicated grief, depression, and anxiety. For children who were primary caregivers of a parent, high levels of reported caregiver burden, physical exhaustion, and lack of social support—along with more commonly associated predictors, such as pre-bereavement anxiety and depression and being female—all are associated with poor post-bereavement outcomes (APA, 2013; Schulz, Hebert, & Boerner, 2008). As increasing numbers of adults become adult orphans, nurses, social workers, and other health care workers would benefit from a better understanding of the important role they can play in identifying individuals at risk, providing anticipatory guidance, and making appropriate referrals for those who need them.

Effects of Psychotropic Medications during Pregnancy   table 31-1

Medication	Effects
Antidepressants	• General: Adverse pregnancy and neonatal outcomes including spontaneous abortion, neonatal serotonin discontinuation symptoms, prematurity, small for gestational age, low birth weight and persistent pulmonary hypertension of the newborn (Udechuku, Nguyen, Hill, & Szego, 2010). • Tricyclics: No association with malformations; however, there is evidence that infants have a risk of poorer neurobehavioral adaptation at birth, similar to the discontinuation symptoms seen with selective serotonin-reuptake inhibitors (SSRIs) (Yonkers et al., 2009). • Monoamine oxidase inhibitors: Contraindicated in pregnancy; increased rates of congential abnormalities based on animal studies (Altshuler et al., 1996). • Newer antidepressants (selective noradrenaline or norepinephrine reuptake inhibitors [SNRIs], noradrenergic and specific serotonergic antidepressants, and others): Limited data are available on the use of these medications during pregnancy. None have shown an association with malformations. SNRIs have been associated with neonatal discontinuation symptoms similar to the SSRIs (Yonkers et al., 2009). Data from longer-term follow-up are not currently available.
Antipsychotics	• Limited evidence on malformation risks related to antipsychotic exposure during pregnancy (Gentile, 2010). • Increased risk of neonatal complications including large-for-date and low-birth-weight babies (Babu, Desai, Tippeswamy, & Chandra, 2010; Newham et al., 2008). • Many atypical antipsychotics can induce metabolic syndrome, increasing the risk for gestational diabetes in the mother, which increases the overall pregnancy risk and requires close monitoring throughout the pregnancy (U.S. FDA, 2011). • Low-potency typical antipsychotics (e.g., thioridazine [Mellaril]) are associated with increased risk of mild malformations. High-potency typical antipsychotics (e.g., haloperidol [Haldol]) are not associated with increased risk (Patton et al., 2002).
Benzodiazepines	• Increased risk for preterm birth and low birth weight during first trimester exposure, but no increased risk for orofacial clefts or other major malformations (Wikner et al., 2007). • No increase in the rate of any specific congenital malformation type during exposure in early pregnancy (Czeizel, Rockenbauer, Sorensen, & Olsen, 2004). • Significant increased risk for major malformations or oral cleft alone (Dolovitch et al., 1998).
Mood stabilizers (including lithium carbonate and antiepileptic drugs such as sodium valproate, carbamazepine, lamotrigine)	• Increased teratogenic risk compounded by polypharmacy (Galbally, Roberts, & Buist, 2010; Walker, Permezel, & Berkovic, 2009). • Sodium valproate (Depakote) and carbamazepine (Tegretol) have been associated with an increased risk of neural tube defects and fetal anticonvulsant syndromes, whereas lithium has been associated with the cardiac defect Ebstein's anomaly (Galbally, Roberts, & Buist, 2010). • Associated with a range of pregnancy and neonatal complications such as gestational diabetes, polyhydramnios, and neonatal hypothyroidism (Galbally, Roberts, & Buist, 2010). • Increased risk of poor long-term child developmental outcomes with doses above 1000 mg of sodium valproate (Cummings et al., 2011; Galbally, Roberts, & Buist, 2010; Walker, Permezel, & Berkovic, 2009). • Risk for fetal valproate syndrome consisting of cardiac, facial and central nervous system anomalies and intrauterine growth restriction with use of sodium valproate (Galbally, Snellen, Walker, & Permezel, 2010; Walker, Permezel, & Berkovic, 2009).

Retirement

Retirement can add stressors to adults not found in any other stage of life. Carolyn Myss, a five-time *New York Times* bestselling author and internationally renowned speaker in the field of human consciousness, addresses retirement by asking the question, "What makes you lose your power as an older adult?" In, *The Call to Live a Symbolic Life*, Myss describes the retired adult in Western culture as living on the "pension of purpose" (Myss, 2004). Myss describes a culture found in the United States that may reduce adults' highest potential to the work that they do. Americans may have the reputation of being human *doers* rather than human *beings*. Myss theorizes that unless one's purpose in life leads to a job that brings financial gain and status, a sense of failure may result. This type of perceived failure, as well as the many other stressors faced by adults of all ages, adds to the growing number of Americans facing mental illness.

Nurses may help adult patients approaching retirement define their ways of *being* rather than *doing*. Understanding what the patient believes he or she has contributed, and what resources may exist to support a full and meaningful retirement, may allow a shift of perspective. Certainly it is not unusual for older adults to continue working, develop new interests, and continue to engage in activities and actions that they identify as important. Encouraging adults who are transitioning into retirement to pursue their passions and stay active may help promote a healthier period of older adulthood.

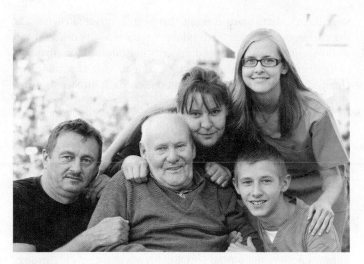

More adults are caring for both parents and children. This sandwich generation faces special challenges, especially for the caregiver with mental illness or for the caregiver of a family member with mental illness.

Source: Barabas Attila/Fotolia

Pause and Reflect

1. *How can nurses help patients focus on being rather than doing?*

2. *How might you respond to a patient with depression who is pregnant and tells you she no longer wants to continue taking her antidepressant? What considerations will be important to this patient?*

3. *Do you know people who are taking care of both their own children and their own parent(s)? How do they handle it? What difficulties do they face?*

The Role of Genetics and Genomics

Understanding the interplay of genetics and genomics with environmental factors in mental health is crucial to grasping a better understanding of mental illness. **Genetics** refers to the study of heredity and variation in gene expression; **genomics** refers to the study of gene function related to health and illness. Genes may influence the development of mental disorders by governing the organic causes of disorders, such as schizophrenia and Alzheimer disease; these influences may produce abnormalities in individual development, or

influence an individual's vulnerability to disorders such as major depression and generalized anxiety (APA, 2013). In addition, with a 50% risk of heritability in offspring, an adult having Huntington disease may be quite challenged trying to decide whether or not to bear children. The American Nurses Association (ANA) has published competencies for genetic and genomic nursing, assisting nurses in incorporating genetic and genomic knowledge and skills into their practice (ANA, 2008).

Although genetics and genomics application transcends all areas of nursing practice, as essentially all illnesses have a genetic link, this section takes a closer look at the influence of genetics and genomics on mental health. As an example, genetic bases have been found for bipolar disorder, schizophrenia, and attention deficit/hyperactivity disorder (Conley, Steele, & Puskar, 2004), psychosis, panic disorder, suicidal behavior (Cheng et al., 2006), and most other mental health disorders. Therefore, familiarity with the risks of inheriting major mental health disorders such as schizophrenia and bipolar disorder is important when considering the pathogenesis of mental illnesses. Important factors to integrate into a nursing assessment include the following:

- Eliciting information from three generations of the family health history and constructing a pedigree from the information collected using standardized symbols and terminology (Chapter 24 Group and Family Therapy).

- Conducting comprehensive health and physical assessments that incorporate knowledge about genetic, environmental, and genomic influences and risk factors.

- Analyzing the history and physical assessment findings for genetic, environmental, and genomic influences and risk factors.

- Assessing clients' knowledge, perceptions, and responses to genetic and genomic information (ANA, 2008).

As discussed in Chapter 3, genotyping for cytochrome P450 variations carries implications for mental health and illness. Because many adults with mental illness have tried several medications and remain symptomatic, cytochrome P450 testing can assist in determining which psychotropic medications might be more beneficial for an individual. Medications that may be analyzed are those metabolized by cytochrome P450 enzymes such as CYP2D6 and CYP2C19 (Pestka et al., 2007). Even though cytochrome P450 testing is not a common intervention yet, when gathering a family history it is important for nurses to develop a list of medications family members

Mr. Barksdale Recovery Phase

APPLICATION

1. What are your concerns about Mr. Barksdale as he is discharged to home?

2. What would you include in Mr. Barksdale's discharge plan if you were working with him?

Mr. Barksdale's inpatient treatment was successful, and he is discharged home with the following goals:

- Return home and resume work.

- Attend intensive outpatient group therapy three times per week for two weeks.

- Attend his follow-up appointment with the cardiologist that is scheduled for 1 week after discharge.

The overall goal of a comprehensive treatment plan for Mr. Barksdale is to help him safely return to the highest level of functioning that he can, given his psychiatric and medical diagnoses and his personal and professional resources.

have tried, as the likelihood of positive effect from a medication choice increases if a family member has tried it and received a positive response.

Nursing Care

Nursing care for adults experiencing transition focuses on responding to the individual's presenting symptoms and frustrations, but also requires thorough assessment to identify any underlying disorders or risks for harm or injury. For patients experiencing increased anxiety or exacerbation of co-morbid conditions related to stress, interventions to promote change and resilience may be sufficient to help patients identify successful coping strategies and manage through the current period of stress. Other patients, however, may need additional interventions, as outlined in other chapters in this text.

Promote Successful Change

Supportive change may be considered as patients with chronic or serious illness make small improvements by helping promote realistic and achievable gains. To illustrate supportive change, Guillot, Kilpatrick, Herbert, & Hollander (2004) adapted Prochaska's model of change to suggest techniques that support the change process. This

stage theory offers many insights that help the psychiatric nursing student hoping to understand and support the recovery process of an adult psychiatric patient. Appropriate nursing interventions that promote change range from validating a patient's lack of readiness to change to encouraging and providing feedback on steps toward change (Table 31-2).

The concepts of developmental stage models describe actions that adults take when contemplating change, especially when that change involves unwanted behaviors such as smoking or lack of exercise. Stage models address the fact that patients move among the various stages on a timeline that is unique to their individual circumstances. Prochaska's model, in particular, can help nurses identify language and behavior that may indicate that the patient is in a change process, which can be useful for new nurses who may feel the need to "do something" to help. Unlike changing a dressing, practicing self-restraint is an important nursing intervention to avoid getting in the way of the patient's involvement in and ownership of the change process.

Promote Resilience

The ability to support patients in transition may be enhanced by an understanding of the concepts related to resilience. **Resilience** can be defined as an ability to bounce back from potentially debilitating

Nursing Interventions and Prochaska's Stages of Change   table 31-2

Stage of Change	Characteristics	Nursing Interventions
Precontemplation	Not currently considering change. Patient prefers to remain uninformed.	• Validate the patient's lack of readiness. • Clarify that the decision belongs to the patient. • Encourage re-evaluation of current behavior (e.g., smoking). • Encourage self-exploration rather than action. • Explain and provide examples of how risk can affect a person.
Contemplation	Patient may be ambivalent about change. Not considering change within a fixed period of time (e.g., until summer).	• Validate lack of readiness. • Clarify that the decision belongs to the patient. • Encourage evaluation pros and cons of behavior (e.g., unsafe sex). • Identify and promote new, positive outcome expectations (e.g., testing may relieve anxiety and safe sex practices may significantly reduce feelings of guilt and shame).
Preparation	Some experience with change and trying to change. Plan to act within a month.	• Identify and assist in problem solving (e.g., helping patient identify primary obstacle to making change). • Help the patient identify social support for the change (e.g., support groups). • Verify skills the patient possesses to assist the patient in making a change. • Encourage and provide feedback on small steps toward change.
Action	Practicing new behavior for a fixed period of time (3–6 months).	• Focus on restructuring cues and how social support is helping. • Bolster the patient's self-efficacy for managing barriers to change. • Help the patient identify feelings of loss and contrast with long-term benefits.
Maintenance	Support the patient's commitment and success in sustaining behavior (6 months or longer, as necessary).	• Plan for follow-up support. • Reinforce internal rewards that the patient has identified. • Discuss relapse prevention and coping strategies that have been developed or may need to be used.
Relapse	Resumption of unwanted and/or harmful behavior.	• Evaluate possible triggers leading to relapse. • Reassess patient's motivation and barriers. • Plan other coping strategies together.

Adapted from Guillot, J., Kilpatrick, M., Herbert, E., & Hollander, D. (2004). Applying the trans theoretical model to exercise adherence in clinical settings. *American Journal of Health Studies, 19*(1). Available at http://www.thefreelibrary.com/Applying+the+transtheoretical+model+to+exercise+adherence+in+clinical...-a0115495857

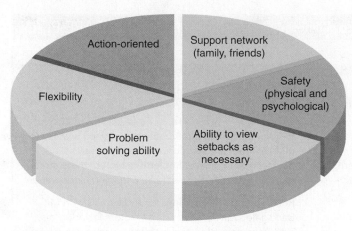

31-4 Characteristics and attributes that support resiliency in adults.

Differences among Initial/Relapse, Recovery, Rehabilitation Phases

Following assessment of the patient, feedback from the treatment team, and reviewing care records, the nurse creates or follows an initial plan of care that promotes the patient's mental and physical wellness (see the Nursing Care Plan that follows).

The patient experiencing recurring symptoms of mental illness may understand how these symptoms are manifested and what treatments are most likely to be successful. The patient may or may not, however, recognize what happened to exacerbate the illness. Helping the patient understand the disease concept through interaction, information, and example will assist the patient in gaining an increased understanding of the illness and reduce the potential for guilt related to a sense of "losing control" over the illness.

The patient in recovery may be able to take medications as prescribed, practice therapeutic techniques to interrupt negative thinking, find someone to confide in, avoid isolation when early symptoms occur, and review a plan that will help avoid relapse. With patience, support, and time, the patient may be able to help prevent relapses and reduce human suffering.

The patient who has reached the rehabilitation phase may recognize early signs of symptom onset and use individualized disease management strategies to help prevent acute exacerbation. Rehabilitation strategies will vary among patients, who may rely on trusted others, including nurses, counselors, and family members. The use of biological, psychosocial, cultural, and spiritual resources to avoid more debilitating illness are indicators of a patient's level of rehabilitation.

Pause and Reflect

1. *What questions would you ask to help evaluate behaviors such as smoking, heavy drinking, and unsafe sex? Would you make any referrals?*
2. *How do you think promoting physical activity and appropriate nutrition would be helpful in promoting patient resilience?*

From Suffering to Hope

Adult psychiatric patients have unique needs. A comprehensive assessment includes reviewing psychosocial and medical factors that contribute to thoughts, behaviors, and symptoms. It is important to remember that, in some cases, the nurse may be the adult patient's only advocate. Psychiatry is not a distinct and separate science. The future of caring for adult patients

circumstances to regain balance (Dyer & McGuinness, 1996). Some commonalities seen in resilience literature describe social, cognitive, and contextual attributes that underlie resilience. These include attributes such as having a network of supportive friends or family, viewing setbacks as temporary, and feeling safe at work and at home (Figure 31-4).

Dr. Mark J. Bates and other military clinicians are using resilience data to develop programs and research outcomes on how building well-being models in military leaders can reduce the risk of suicide and other serious mental illnesses (Bates & Bowles, 2011). As an example of a current use of resilience training to help reduce suicide in members of the armed forces, Bates has been working with groups of military leaders who influence their units. Training leaders in using actions to reinforce healthy behaviors and discourage unhealthy behaviors may have applicability in mental health settings.

Although protective factors for adults suffering from mental illness are not specific, resilient adults have some qualities in common. They include factors such as flexibility, seeing setbacks as temporary, nurturing an attitude of gratitude, calling on unique personal resources, and being action oriented (Polk, 1997). Characteristics of resilience reported by Bates that provide a basis for nursing actions to enhance patient resilience are described in Box 31-2.

Nursing Interventions to Promote Resilience   box 31-2

- Help patients identify what provides them with a sense of well-being related to their state of mind to reduce the effect that external circumstances have on well-being. In this way, nurses help patients to engage in intentional activities.
- Identify patients' strengths through assessment and nurture these strengths by aligning them with patients' goals, which will help patients develop intrinsic motivation.
- Encourage patients to help others, when appropriate, to increase their feelings of control and self-worth. This helps patients develop altruism.
- Give patients choices in task completion in a safe environment with minimal oversight to promote autonomy and, therefore, resilience.

- Encourage patients to develop and maintain relationships with family and friends and value social support.
- Give patients opportunities and encourage them to participate in pleasant activities together. This also helps patients value relationships and social support.
- Encourage patients to identify personal successes and positive events that support a sense of resilience.
- Assist patients with regular physical activity, appropriate nutrition, and developing a sleep schedule to promote self-care and thereby enhance resilience.

Mr. Barksdale—The Patient with Depression and Co-Morbid Illness — NURSING CARE PLAN

Nursing Diagnosis: Readiness for Enhanced Resilience

Short-Term Goals Patient will: (include date for short-term goal to be met)	Intervention Nurse will:	Rationale
Participate in treatment designed to address his depression and co-morbid cardiac illness within 48 hours of admission.	Coordinate or provide therapies, including psychoeducation, psychotherapy, and medication administration, weight management, and lifestyle. Administer screenings or rating scales as appropriate to measure progress and adjust treatment plan.	Psycho- and pharmacotherapies combined with lifestyle modifications are most often recommended as evidence-based practice. Implementation of these strategies will assist Mr. Barksdale in managing his condition. Recommended screenings for individuals with Mr. Barksdale's diagnoses and risk factors include waist circumference, BMI, and weights measured at all visits, and Hamilton Depression Scale administered every 6 months or as needed.
State several warning signs of exacerbated depressive or medical symptoms prior to discharge.	Provide Mr. Barksdale education in relation to symptom exacerbation, including lifestyle modifications and adherence to treatment plan, and ask him to reflect his understanding of the plan.	Mr. Barksdale's understanding of the full extent of his illness and how to prevent exacerbations is critical to his recovery.
Discuss and participate in discharge plans.	Plan discharge process, provide referrals and linkages with support services and providers, and arrange follow-up appointments. Confirm and document Mr. Barksdale's understanding of teaching. With Mr. Barksdale, develop a crisis management and safety plan for depression and worsening cardiac symptoms.	Patients who engage in their treatment plan are more likely to engage in resilience promoting behaviors. A comprehensive discharge plan including direct connections with outpatient services enhances Mr. Barksdale's ability to care for himself.
Long-Term Goal Resume pre-hospital level of functioning at home and work within 6 to 8 weeks.	Determine a realistic wellness plan that incorporates a realistic work schedule to minimize stress associated with returning to work.	Promotes autonomy and strengthens resilience.

Clinical Reasoning

1. How might treatment of Mr. Barksdale's sleep apnea assist in improving his symptoms of depression?
2. Given that Mr. Barksdale is estranged from his family at this time, what nursing interventions might help promote his sense of connectedness to others?

depends on nurses understanding the interactive forces that, although influenced by factors in all the domains, all are framed by interrelated developmental changes and cut across professional disciplines.

Suffering can be witnessed and more easily understood when nurses fight to save a middle-aged mother of four who dies from a heart attack, while the frenzy of the resuscitation team fades into the solitude of a family helplessly holding onto the life that was. Hope comes through well-understood, evidence-based, and developmentally predictable processes, unique to the human spirit. Adults who suffer from mental illness, however, may suffer both from the real pain of perceived death of self as well as from the lack of understanding and support of others. Nurses hold hope clearly within the patient's sight by offering appropriate care and deep empathy, allowing the patient to embrace and live with that same hope.

Mr. Barksdale Rehabilitation Phase

Mr. Barksdale has been home for 4 weeks. His depression is in partial remission. He goes for a follow-up appointment with his primary care provider (PCP) and sees you, the RN, prior to the PCP. He tells you his "lady friend" is not happy with his slow recovery. She is wondering when and if he will be able to return to his job at the post office. You were not aware that Mr. Barksdale was in a relationship. Somewhat embarrassed, Mr. Barksdale asks when he and his "lady friend" can resume sexual relations.

APPLICATION

1. What are the priority nursing care issues at this time for Mr. Barksdale?
2. In what ways do you think it is important to clarify to Mr. Barksdale that the decision to return to work belongs to him?

Chapter Highlights

1. Adults experience milestones that both affect and are affected by adult mental health and illness.
2. Nurses working with adults with mental illness must be alert to the potential or presence of co-morbid illness.
3. Anxiety is widespread among the adult population in the United States.
4. Adult transitions such as divorce, pregnancy, and caring for children and aging parents can affect adults across the domains.
5. Nurses can help adults manage life transitions by engaging in nursing interventions that promote change and resilience.

NCLEX®-RN Questions

1. The nurse has just started a job working in the psychiatric emergency department. Based on an understanding of psychosocial and developmental factors contributing to mental illness, the nurse expects which age group to most likely present with recent onset of serious mental illness?
   a. Youth ages 10–16
   b. Adults ages 18–30
   c. Adults ages 30–55
   d. Adults ages 55–85

2. The nurse is caring for a middle-aged adult presenting with hypertension. The patient also has a history of major mental illness. The nurse understands that which of the following are true about nursing role and health outcomes for adults with mental illness? Select all that apply.
   a. Most patients with mental illness have limited interest in improving their health.
   b. Health promotion activities may have a positive impact on physical and emotional well-being.
   c. Genetic and neurobiological factors make it difficult to prevent many associated health problems.
   d. The patient would be better served by nursing care provided by an experienced psychiatric nurse.
   e. Lifestyle factors may require additional attention and support in adult patients with mental illness.

3. The nurse is caring for a patient with a previous history of depression who has just learned that she is expecting her first child. The patient asks the nurse what she can expect in terms of illness management. Which statement by the nurse is accurate?
   a. "Your mood should improve during the pregnancy."
   b. "The risks of medications in pregnancy always outweigh the benefits."
   c. "Memories of anxieties, disappointments, or trauma may be reactivated."
   d. "Your risk for medical complications is about the same as any other woman's."

4. The maternal–child nurse is providing care to the postpartum mother and her newborn. The nurse notes that the mother took a selective norepinephrine-reuptake inhibitor (SNRI) to manage depression during pregnancy. Based on an understanding of the effects of this medication, which neonatal assessment finding is the nurse likely to encounter?
   a. Irritability
   b. Hyperglycemia
   c. Heart murmurs
   d. Hypothyroidism

5. The nurse is caring for a patient with serious mental illness who has been not responded to treatment and remains symptomatic. The provider orders genotyping for cytochrome P450 variations. Which best describes the rationale for this test?
   a. To determine whether there is a medical condition responsible for the mental illness
   b. To assist in determining whether different medications might be more beneficial for the patient
   c. To determine the likelihood that the condition will be passed on to other generations
   d. To determine whether the patient is hiding the fact that he is taking a medication metabolized by the same enzymes

6. The nurse is attempting to assist a patient with serious mental illness to make realistic gains toward recovery. Which intervention is most consistent with the model of supportive change?
   a. Encouraging the patient to help others
   b. Assessing the individual for protective factors
   c. Providing pleasant rewarding activities for the patient
   d. Identifying and promoting new outcome expectations

7. The nurse is evaluating outcomes for a patient with depression who has a co-morbid illness. Which best demonstrates that interventions focused on promoting resilience have been effective?
   a. The patient resolves to take responsibility for managing her affairs without assistance from others.
   b. The patient provides a detailed history of traumatic events that have contributed to the current situation.
   c. The patient maintains a regular schedule that includes physical activity, adequate sleep, and appropriate nutrition.
   d. The patient acknowledges that she needs help and will defer to the plan implemented by the nurse.

Answers may be found on the Pearson student resource site: nursing.pearsonhighered.com

References

Altshuler, L. L., Cohen, L., Szuba, M. P., Burt, V. K., Gitlin, M., & Mintz, J. (1996). Pharmacologic management of psychiatric illness during pregnancy: Dilemmas and guidelines. *American Journal of Psychiatry, 153*(5), 592–606.

American Nurses Association. (2008). *Essentials of Genetic and Genomic Nursing: Competencies, Curricula Guidelines, and Outcome Indicators* (2nd ed.). Silver Spring, MD: American Nurses Association.

American Psychiatric Association. (2013). *Diagnostic and Statistical Manual of Mental Disorders* (5th ed.). Washington, DC: American Psychiatric Publishers.

Anxiety and Depression Association of America [comment]. (2012). *Facts and statistics.* Available at www.adaa.org/about-adaa/press-room/facts-statistics

Babu, G. N., Desai, G., Tippeswamy, H., & Chandra, P. S. (2010). Birth weight and use of olanzapine in pregnancy: A prospective comparative study. *Journal of Clinical Psychopharmacology, 30*(3), 331–332.

Barlow, S. K. (2007). *Mental illness and inherited predisposition—schizophrenia and bipolar disorder.* Centre for Genetics Education. Available at http://www.genetics.edu.au/Publications-and-Resources/Genetics-Fact-Sheets/Fact%20Sheet%2058

Barnes, C., Bergant, A., Hummer, M., Saria, A., & Fleischhacker, W. (1994). Clozapine concentration in maternal and fetal plasma, amniotic fluid, and breast milk. *American Journal of Psychiatry, 151*(6), 945.

Bates, M. J., & Bowles, S. V. (2011). *Mental Health and Well-Being across the Military Spectrum* (pp. 29-1–29-35). Presented at the RTO Human Factors and Medicine Panel (HFM) Symposium, Bergen, Norway: NATO Science and Technology Organization. Available at https://www.cso.nato.int/pubs/rdp.asp?RDP=RTO-MP-HFM-205

Bonari, L., Pinto, N., Ahn, E., Einarson, A., Steiner, M., & Koren, G. (2004). Perinatal risks of untreated depression during pregnancy. *Canadian Journal of Psychiatry, 49*(11), 726–735.

Caley, C. F. (2011). Interpreting and applying CYP450 genomic test results to psychotropic medications. *Journal of Pharmacy Practice, 24*(5), 439–446.

Centers for Disease Control and Prevention (CDC). (2011). *National Diabetes Fact Sheet 2011.* Available at http://www.cdc.gov/diabetes/pubs/pdf/ndfs_2011.pdf

Cheng, R., Juos, H., Loth, J. E., Nee, J., Iossifov, I., Blumenthal, R., Sharpe, L., et al. (2006). Genome-wide linkage scan in a large bipolar disorder sample from the National Institute of Mental Health Genetics Initiative suggests putative loci for bipolar disorder, psychosis, suicide, and panic disorder. *Molecular Psychiatry, 11*(3), 252–260.

Cohen, L. S., Altshuler, L. L., Harlow, B. L., Nonacs, R., Newport, D. J., Viguera, A. C., Suri, R., et al. (2006). Relapse of major depression during pregnancy in women who maintain or discontinue antidepressant treatment. *Journal of the American Medical Association, 295*(5), 499–507.

Colton, C. W., & Manderscheid, R. W. (2006). Congruencies in increased mortality rates, years of potential life lost, and causes of death among public mental health clients in eight states. *Preventing Chronic Disease, 3*(2), A42.

Conley, Y. P., Steele, A. M., & Puskar, K. R. (2004). Genetic susceptibility to psychiatric disorders. *Medsurg Nursing, 13*(5), 319–325.

Cummings, C., Stewart, M., Stevenson, M., Morrow, J., & Nelson, J. (2011). Neurodevelopment of children exposed in utero to lamotrigine, sodium valproate and carbamazepine. *Archives of Disease in Childhood, 96*(7), 643–647.

Czeizel, A. E., Rockenbauer, M., Sorensen, H. T., & Olsen, J. (2004). A population-based case-control study of oral chlordiazepoxide use during pregnancy and risk of congenital abnormalities. *Neurotoxicology and Teratology, 26*(4), 593–598.

De Hert, M., Correll, C., Bobes, J., Cetokovich-Bakmas, M., Cohen, D., Asai, I., et al. (2011). Physical illness in patients with severe mental disorders: I. Prevalence, impact of medications and disparities in health care. *World Psychiatry, 10*(1), 52–77.

Dolovich, L. R., Addis, A., Vaillancourt, J. M., Power, J. D., Koren, G. & Einarson, T. R. (1998). Benzodiazepine use in pregnancy and major malformations or oral cleft: meta-analysis of cohort and case-control studies. *British Medical Journal, 317*(7162), 839–843.

Dyer, J. G., & McGuinness, T. M. (1996). Resilience: Analysis of the concept. *Archives of Psychiatric Nursing, 10*(5), 276–282.

Flynn, H. A., Blow, F. C., & Marcus, S. M. (2006). Rates and predictors of depression treatment among pregnant women in hospital-affiliated obstetrics practices. *General Hospital Psychiatry, 28*(4), 289–295.

Frayne, J., Nguyen, T., Allen, S., & Rampono, J. (2009). Motherhood and mental illness. *Australian Family Physician, 38*(8), 594–600.

Gaderman, A. M., Engel, C. C., Naifeh, J. A., Nock, M. K., Peukhova, M., Santiago, P. N., … Kessler, R.C. (2012). Prevalence of DSM-IV major depression among U.S. military personnel: Meta-analysis and simulation. *Military Medicine, 177*(8), 47–59.

Galbally, M., Roberts, M., & Buist, A. (2010). Mood stabilizers in pregnancy: A systematic review. *Australia and New Zealand Journal of Psychiatry, 44*(1), 967–977. doi: 10.3109/00048674.2010.506637

Galbally, M., Snellen, M., Walker, S., & Permezel, M. (2010). Management of antipsychotic and mood stabilizer medication in pregnancy: Recommendations for antenatal care. *Australia and New Zealand Journal of Psychiatry, 44*(2), 99–108.

Gallup. (2013). *Honesty/Ethics in Professions.* Available at http://www.gallup.com/poll/1654/honesty-ethics-professions.aspx

Gautam, S. (2010). Fourth revolution in psychiatry—addressing comorbidity with chronic physical disorders. *Indian Journal of Psychiatry, 52*(3), 213–219.

Gentile, S. (2010). Antipsychotic therapy during early and late pregnancy. A systematic review. *Schizophrenia Bulletin, 36*(3), 518–544. doi: 10.1093/schbul/sbn107

Glisson, C., Landsverk, J., Schoenwald, S., Kelleher, K., Hoagwood, K., Mayberg, S., & Green, P. (2008). Assessing the organizational social context (OSC) of mental health services: Implications for research and practice. *Administration and Policy in Mental Health and Mental Health Services Research, 35*(1), 98–113.

Golstein, D. J., Corbin, L. A., & Fung, M. C. (2000). Olanzapine exposed pregnancies and lactation: early experience. *Journal of Clinical Psychopharmacology, 20*(4), 399–403.

Guillot, J., Kilpatrick, M., Herbert, E., & Hollander, D. (2004). Applying the transtheoretical model to exercise adherence in clinical settings. *American Journal of Health Studies, 19,* 1–10. Available at http://www.thefreelibrary.com/Applying+the+transtheoretical+model+to+exercise+adherence+in+clinical...-a0115495857

Guttmacher, A., & Collins, F. (2002). Genomic medicine: A primer. *New England Journal of Medicine, 347*(19), 1512–1520.

Hickie, I. B., & McGorry, P. D. (2007). Increased access to evidence-based primary mental health care: Will the implementation match the rhetoric? *Medical Journal of Australia, 187*(2), 100–103. Available at https://www.mja.com.au/journal/2007/187/2/increased-access-evidence-based-primary-mental-health-care-will-implementation

Hochlenert, A., Niehoff, P., Wild, B., Junger, J., Herzog, W., & Lowe, B. (2011). Psychiatric comorbidity in cardiovascular inpatients: Costs, net gains, and length of hospitalization. *Journal of Psychosomatic Research, 70*(2), 135–139.

Hoyert, D. L., & Xu, J. Q. (2012). Deaths: Preliminary data for 2011. *National Vital Statistics Reports, 61*(6). Hyattsville, MD: National Center for Health Statistics.

Jablensky, A. V., Morgan, V., Zubrick, S. R., Bower, C., & Yellachich, L. (2005). Pregnancy, delivery and neonatal complications in a population cohort of women with schizophrenia and major affective disorders. *American Journal of Psychiatry, 162*(1), 79–91.

Kammerer, M., Taylor, A., & Glover, V. (2006). The HPA axis and perinatal depression: A hypothesis. *Archives of Women's Mental Health, 9*(4), 187–196.

Katon, W. J. (2008). The comorbidity of diabetes mellitus and depression. *American Journal of Medicine, 121*(11 Suppl 2), S8–S15.

Kruger, S., Alda, M., Trevor Young, L., & Goldapple, K. (2006). Risk and resilience markers in bipolar disorder: Brain responses to emotional challenge in bipolar patients and their siblings. *American Journal of Psychiatry, 163*(2), 257–264.

Kurz, K. (2011). Association between increased tryptophan degradation and depression in cancer patients. *Current Opinion in Clinical Nutrition and Medical Care, 14*(1), 49–56.

Maes, M., Berk, M., Goehler, L., Song, C., Anderson, G., Galecki, P., & Leonard, B. (2012). Depression and sickness behavior are Janus-faced responses to shared inflammatory pathways. *BMC Medicine 10*(66). Available at http://www.biomedcentral.com/1741-7015/10/66

Mental Health America. (2012). *Co-occurring disorders and depression.* Available at http://www.mentalhealthamerica.net/conditions/co-occurring-disorders-and-depression

Musselman, D. L., Miller, A. H., Porter, M. R., Manatunga, A., Gao, F., Penna, S., et al. (2001). Higher than normal plasma interleukin-6 concentrations in cancer patients with depression: Preliminary findings. *American Journal of Psychiatry, 158*(8), 1252–1257.

Myss, C. M. (2004). *The Call to Live a Symbolic Life*. Carlsbad, CA: Hay House Audio.

Naylor, C., Parsonage, M., McDaid, D., Knapp, M., Fossey, M., & Galea, A. (2012). *Long-Term Conditions and Mental Health: The Cost of Co-Morbidities*. London, UK: The King's Fund and Centre for Mental Health. Available at http://www.kingsfund.org.uk/publications/long-term-conditions-and-mental-health

Newham, J. J., Thomas, S. H., MacRitchie, K., McElhatton, P. R., & McAllister-Williams, R. H. (2008). Birth weight of infants after maternal exposure to typical and atypical antipsychotics: Prospective comparison study. *British Journal of Psychiatry, 192*(5), 333–337.

O'Connor, T. G., Heron, J., Golding, J., Beveridge, M., & Glover, V. (2002). Maternal antenatal anxiety and children's behavioral/emotional problems at 4 years. *British Journal of Psychiatry, 180*, 502–508.

Parks, J., Svendsen, D., Singer, P., Foti, M. E., & Mauer, B. (2006). Morbidity and mortality in people with serious mental illness. National Association of State Mental Health Program Directors (NASMHPD). *Medical Directors Council*. Available at http://www.nasmhpd.org/docs/publications/MDCdocs/Mortality%20and%20Morbidity%20Final%20Report%208.18.08.pdf

Patton, S. W., Misri, S., Corral, M. R., Perry, K. F., & Kuan, A. J. (2002). Antipsychotic medication during pregnancy and lactation in women with schizophrenia: Evaluating the risk. *Canadian Journal of Psychiatry, 47*(10), 959–965.

Perrin, K. O. (2012). The nurse as witness to suffering. In K. O. Perrin, C. A. Sheehan, M. L. Potter, & M. K. Kazanowski, (Eds.). *Palliative Care Nursing: Caring for Suffering Patients*. Sudbury, MA: Jones & Bartlett Learning, pp. 247–276.

Pestka, E. L., Hale, A. M., Johnson, B. L., Lee, J. L., & Poppe, K. A. (2007). Cytochrome P450 testing for better psychiatric care. *Journal of Psychosocial Nursing, 45*(10), 15–18.

Polk, L. V. (1997). Toward a middle-range theory of resilience. *Advances in Nursing Science, 19*(3), 1–13.

Population Reference Bureau. (2012). Household Change in the United States. Available at http://www.prb.org/Publications/Reports/2012/us-household-change.aspx

Reiss-Brennan, B., Briot, P. C., Savitz, L. A., Cannon, W., & Staheli, R. (2010). Cost and quality impact of Intermountain's mental health integration program. *Journal of Healthcare Management, 55*(2), 97–113.

Schulz, R., Hebert, R., & Boerner, K. (2008). Bereavement after caregiving. *Geriatrics, 63*(1), 20–22. Available at http://www.ncbi.nlm.nih.gov/pmc/articles/PMC2790185/

Udechuku, A., Nguyen, T., Hill, R., & Szego, K. (2010). Antidepressants in pregnancy: A systematic review. *Australia and New Zealand Journal of Psychiatry, 44*(1), 978–996.

U.S. Food and Drug Administration (FDA). (2011). *A drug safety communication: Antipsychotic drug labels updated on use during pregnancy and risk of abnormal muscle movements and withdrawal symptoms in newborns*. Available at https://www.fda.gov/Drugs/DrugSafety/ucm243903.htm

U.S. Food and Drug Administration (FDA). (2012). Drug safety and availability. Available at http://www.fda.gov/Drugs/DrugSafety/default.htm

Viguera, A., Nonacs, R., Cohen, L. S., Tondo, L., Murray, A., & Baldassarini, R. J. (2000). Risk of recurrence of bipolar disorder in pregnant and nonpregnant women after discontinuing lithium maintenance. *American Journal of Psychiatry, 157*(2), 179–184.

Walker, S. P., Permezel, M., & Berkovic, S. F. (2009). The management of epilepsy in pregnancy. *BJOG: An International Journal of Obstetrics and Gynaecology, 116*(6), 758–767.

Wikner, B. N., Stiller, C. O., Bergman, U., Asker, C., & Kallen, B. (2007). Use of benzodiazepines and benzodiazepine receptor agonists during pregnancy: Neonatal outcome and congenital malformations. *Pharmacoepidemiology Drug Safety, 16*(11), 1203–1210.

Yonkers, K. A., Wisner, K. L., Stewart, D. E., Oberlander, T. F., Dell, D. L., Stotland, N., Ramin, S., et al. (2009). The management of depression during pregnancy: A report from the American Psychiatric Association and the American College of Obstetricians and Gynaecologists. *Obstetrics and Gynecology, 114*(3), 703–713.

32

Older Adults

Brendan P. Wynne
Mertie L. Potter
Patrick Gagnon

Key words

Learning Outcomes

1. Discuss the impact of mental illness on older adults.

2. Summarize the impact of biological, psychological, sociological, cultural, and spiritual domains on older adults.

3. Examine the unique role of accumulated losses in older adults.

4. Differentiate among delirium, depression, and dementia in older adults.

5. Distinguish pharmacologic issues specific to older adults being treated for psychiatric disorders.

6. Describe risks for and types of elder abuse.

7. Plan evidence-based nursing care for older adult patients with psychiatric disorders.

8. Explain end-of-life concerns for older adults.

Celia Taylor Initial Onset

APPLICATION

1. What do you anticipate will be the priorities of care for Mrs. Taylor?

2. What do you suspect is going on with Mrs. Taylor?

3. How can you assess the relationship between Mrs. Taylor and her daughter Carolyn?

You are a registered nurse working at a nursing center that offers three levels of care: assisted living, skilled nursing, and dementia care. It is just after 7 p.m. when Celia Taylor, a widow, age 77, arrives by private ambulance. She has been discharged from a large hospital 2 hours away to skilled nursing care following surgery for a hip fracture. Mrs. Taylor has advanced chronic obstructive pulmonary disease (COPD) and a history of depression. She had limited mobility prior to the fall in which she broke her hip.

On arrival, Mrs. Taylor says very little, offering only "yes" and "no" answers to intake and assessment questions. She is quite "weepy." Approximately 20 minutes later, Mrs. Taylor's adult daughter, Carolyn, arrives. When Mrs. Taylor sees Carolyn, she asks, "Why did you bring me here? When can I go home?"

Mrs. Taylor is admitted to the skilled nursing care unit for rehabilitaton following her hip surgery and to rule out dementia.

Introduction

Worldwide, more and more people are living longer. This trend reflects improvements in health, nutrition, and medical care for older adults (Cremens & Wiechers, 2010). However, there is great variation in life expectancy. An individual living in Chad, for example, has a life expectancy of 49 years (the lowest worldwide), whereas adults in the United States have a life expectancy of 78 years, and those living in Monaco have a life expectancy of 90 years (the highest worldwide) (Central Intelligence Agency, 2013). In the United States, the number of people living to the age of 100 in 2010 was 71,991—almost double the number recorded in 1990 (Werner, 2011). Although old age should not be viewed as a disease state, it is important to note that as the number of older adults increases, so too does their risk for psychiatric and medical illnesses (Cremens & Wiechers, 2010).

Defining old age is complex. It is affected by both biological and sociocultural factors. Individuals between and within different cultures have different capabilities. For example, a 65-year-old man in a Western country may be very fit, possess a great amount of energy, and not be ready to retire nor need to do so, whereas another may be physically challenged and ready to retire at a much earlier age. For the most part, the definition of old age depends on the government-defined age for retirement, which thrusts a change of roles on an individual. For the purposes of this chapter, **older adult** refers to individuals 60 years of age and older (World Health Organization [WHO], 2014).

As the population ages, it is becoming increasingly important for the nurse to be aware of the unique physical, psychological, sociological, cultural, and spiritual issues faced by older adults. Although more individuals are living longer, more also are living with chronic disease or disability, such as cardiovascular disease, chronic back pain, and depression (Gulland, 2012). Some become overwhelmed by the many changes associated with aging, including declining physical health, financial stresses, multiple losses, isolation, and mobility issues. Many older adults, however, live full lives, working or volunteering well into old age, traveling, or enjoying family time.

Older adults who are overwhelmed by the challenges associated with aging may develop mental illness, especially if they have additional risk factors. Those who were diagnosed with mental illness when they were younger face the challenge of living with mental illness while navigating the changes of aging. Nurses working with older patients must address acute and time-limited stressors, such as acute illness; long-term changes, such as development of chronic illness (for example, chronic obstructive pulmonary disease or dementia) or the death of a spouse; and multiple stressors, such as a hip fracture that requires relocation to a nursing facility.

Challenges in Older Adulthood

The challenges of aging may occur in one or more of the domains in wellness and may fluctuate over time.

Biological

Most older adults will experience some number of age-related changes. In many cases, these changes may result in only minimal impairment of function and require only slight modification—for example, the need to use reading glasses. Other changes common in older adults may require further intervention. These include sensory losses, musculoskeletal changes, changes in sleep patterns, and changes that occur with the development of chronic illness.

Sensory Changes

Many older adults experience some diminishing of the senses. Hearing loss is the most common, affecting between 30% and 47% of older adults (National Institute on Deafness and Other Communication Disorders, 2010). Vision changes—ranging from slight changes in visual acuity to glaucoma, cataracts, or macular degeneration—also are common. Olfactory senses may be affected by illness, vascular changes, or decrease in neural function. Smell affects the ability to taste, and older adults may experience decline in this important sense, which, in turn, can result in diminished eating habits and altered nutritional status. Reduction in the amount of saliva produced, tooth decay, and dentures can all affect the ability to taste. Because taste sensation may be linked to illness affecting the olfactory sense, older adults reporting diminished ability to taste should be evaluated for the presence of an illness, such as a sinus infection, or another contributing factor (Boyce & Shone, 2006).

Musculoskeletal Changes

Musculoskeletal decline is an important topic in the health of the older adult. Loss of muscle that occurs normally with aging may result in decreased balance and stability. Musculoskeletal decline places older adults at greater risk for falls.

Falls are a leading cause of accidental deaths in adults over age 65; in 2009, some 20,400 adults died from injuries sustained in falls (Centers for Disease Control and Prevention [CDC], 2012a). The

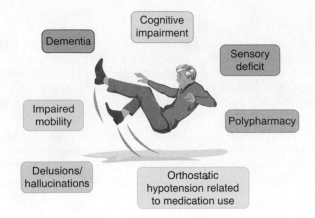

32-1   Factors that increase risk of falls in older adults.

mortality rate related to falls increases dramatically with age (Figure 32-1). In addition, falls can be markers of poor health and declining function. Most hip fractures in older adults occur as a result of falls. Cognitive impairment, sensory deficits, and medication use all increase the risk for falls (CDC, 2012a). Diminished motor ability in the older adult can be due to musculoskeletal decline or may be associated with injury or disease processes developed earlier in life. For example, aging athletes who experienced injuries earlier in life may experience arthritis, back pain, and orthopedic problems.

In addition to increased musculoskeletal decline, diseases such as diabetes, Alzheimer disease, and Parkinson disease impair mobility as they progress. Interestingly, muscle strength in the older adult is a protective factor from death—not only related to falls, but also from all causes, including heart disease and cancer (Ruiz et al., 2008). This supports the recommendation that older adults engage in regular exercise, particularly weight-bearing exercise (CDC, 2012a).

Multiple Illnesses

As the likelihood of developing a chronic condition increases with age, so, too, does the likelihood of developing multiple chronic conditions. Approximately 75% of adults older than age 65 have multiple chronic illnesses (Anderson, 2010). As the number of chronic conditions an individual has increases, the individual's risk for mortality, poor function, adverse drug events, and unnecessary hospitalizations also increases. Mental health issues are known to co-occur with other chronic illnesses, and the combination produces poor outcomes for the individual (U.S. Department of Health and Human Services [DHHS], 2010).

One of the risks of treating two or more chronic conditions is the use of multiple medications. Adults over age 65 use the greatest number of medications of any age group (Sadock & Sadock, 2007). Many older adults may experience **polypharmacy**, in which multiple medications are prescribed (typically by more than one provider) and interact poorly with one another. Polypharmacy in older adults often is associated with increased morbidity and mortality, impaired cognition, decreased mobility, and poor quality of life (Hajjar, Cafiero, & Hanlon, 2007).

PRACTICE ALERT Nurses working with older adults should carefully assess use of both prescribed and over-the-counter medications, as well as herbal supplements, at each visit. Encourage the patient to use the same pharmacy for prescriptions so the pharmacist can alert the patient and providers when a new prescription is likely to conflict with an existing one.

Sleep

More than 50% of the population over age 60 report some difficulty with sleep (Aging and Sleep, 2013). Some individuals do not require as much sleep as others do. Typically, if the individual feels awake and energetic during the day, the individual is receiving enough sleep. Causes of poor sleep in older adults include medications, stress, physical and mental illnesses, retirement, sleep disorders, and poor sleep hygiene (Chapter 12).

Major Organ Changes

Age-related reduction in liver, kidney, and digestive function can cause difficulty in the older adult's ability to metabolize medications (Cremens & Wiechers, 2010). This can be particularly dangerous when the patient is prescribed a psychoactive medication. Because toxicity can occur in individuals who do not metabolize medications efficiently, older adults often are prescribed half the normal dose of some antipsychotics. Given the anticholinergic nature of many of the psychotropic medications, caution should be taken to avoid dry skin, dry mouth, blurred vision, and constipation.

Urinary tract infections (UTIs) can cause major problems for older adults. UTIs can occur anywhere in the urinary tract (kidneys, ureters, bladder, or urethra). Women tend to acquire UTIs more frequently than men, owing to their short urethra and its proximity to the anus. Confusion often is the only symptom observed in the older adult with a UTI and may be confused with dementia (Zieve & Eltz, 2012).

Psychological

Older adults often experience changes in two areas within the psychological domain: cognitive changes and caregiver burden. It is important to understand that cognitive changes that impair function are *not* a normal part of aging and should be investigated. Older adults and family members caring for a loved one with mental illness may experience a number of stressors that become burdensome, creating new worries and challenges.

Cognitive Changes

The structure of the brain is constantly changing. With aging, a normal brain shrinks in volume and the ventricles enlarge. Changes to the blood vessels within the brain also occur. These structural changes likely are responsible for reductions in certain cognitive abilities (for instance, processing speed, executive function, and episodic memory) experienced by many older adults (Cutilli, 2008; Fjell & Walhovd, 2010).

As discussed in Chapter 21, dementia is a progressive decline in cognitive functioning that usually develops over a period of months or years. More than 50 disorders can cause dementia. The most common symptom of dementia is memory loss, but other symptoms must also be present. These include difficulty expressing or understanding speech (**aphasia**); problems recognizing objects (**agnosia**); difficulty performing motor tasks, despite intact motor function (**apraxia**); and disturbances in executive function, such as the ability to think abstractly, organize thoughts, and make plans or carry out complex behaviors. Other symptoms can include personality changes, behavioral problems, psychiatric symptoms (such as paranoia or hallucinations), and poor judgment (Falk & Wiechers, 2010; National Institute of Neurological Disorders and Stroke, 2013).

Approximately 13% of people over age 65 are diagnosed with some form of dementia (Alzheimer's Association, 2011). Currently, there is no cure for dementia; however, medications are now available that, in some cases, can slow the progression of cognitive decline.

Comparison of Delirium, Depression, and Dementia table 32-1

	Delirium	Depression	Dementia
Onset of symptoms	Rapid (hours to days)	Variable	Slow (months to years)
Initial symptoms	Difficulty with attention or disturbed consciousness	Dysphoric mood or lack of pleasure	Memory deficits
Course	Fluctuating over days to weeks	Persistent—usually lasting months if untreated	Gradually progressive over years
Sleep	Disturbed, but with no set pattern	Disturbed, with early morning awakening or hypersomnia	May be disturbed with an individual pattern occurring most nights
Family history	Not contributory	Positive association	Positive association
Memory problems	Poor registration—recording new memories	Patchy or inconsistent	Progressive decline, with greater problems with recent memories
Mood disturbance	Labile	Depressed or irritable	Variable—may be normal
Screening	Confusion Assessment Method (CAM) Assessment for underlying causes	Geriatric Depression Scale Other standardized depression screenings	Mini Mental Status Exam Mini-Cog Dementia Screening

Based on Falk, W., & Wiechers, I. (2010). Demented patients. In T. A. Stern, G. L. Fricchione, N. H. Cassem, M. S. Jellinek, & J. F. Rosenbaum. (Eds.). *Massachusetts General Hospital Handbook of General Psychiatry* (6th ed.). St. Louis, MO: Mosby; Registered Nurses' Association of Ontario. (n.d.). Best Practices Toolkit. *Recognizing Delirium, Depression, and Dementia (3D's) Comparison Chart*. Available at http://ltctoolkit.rnao.ca/sites/ltc/files/resources/3Ds/EducationResources/3DComparisonFinal.pdf; American Psychiatric Association. (2013). *Diagnostic and Statistical Manual of Mental Disorders* (5th ed.). Washington, DC: American Psychiatric Publishers; Downing, L. J., Caprio, T. V., & Lyness, J. M. (2013). Geriatric psychiatry review: Differential diagnosis and treatment of 3 D's: Delirium, dementia, and depression. *Current Psychiatry Reports, 15,* 365.

Delirium is an acute confusional state. It is characterized by rapid onset (hours to days), disturbance in consciousness, fluctuation of attention, memory deficits, disorientation, language disturbances, and perceptual disturbances (APA, 2013). Delirium can often be misdiagnosed as dementia, depression, or other psychiatric disorders (Table 32-1). Delirium is not a psychiatric disorder, but an urgent medical situation. Some of the many causes of delirium include infection, hypoxia, increased intracranial pressure, metabolic imbalances, drug interaction, toxicity, drug or alcohol withdrawal, vitamin deficiencies, traumas, and acute vascular changes (Falk & Wiechers, 2010; Somes, Donatelli, &

Barrett, 2010). The treatment for delirium is the identification and correction of the underlying medical problem.

Caregiver Burden

Those caring for older adults with mental illness—whether a spouse, an adult child, or another caregiver—may experience caregiver burden. **Caregiver burden** is the extent to which caregivers feel that their emotional or physical health, social life, and financial status are suffering as a result of caring for their relatives (Bevens & Sternberg, 2012; Zarit, Reever, & Bach-Peterson, 1980) (Figure 32-2). Risk for caregiver

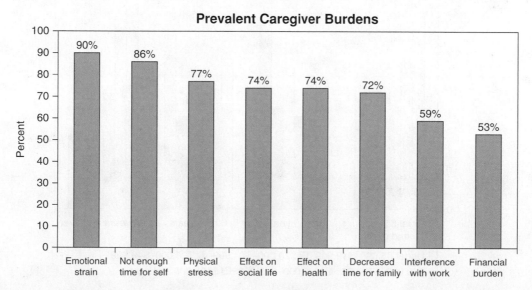

Prevalent Caregiver Burdens

32-2 Prevalence of caregiver burdens as reported by survey participants.

Data from New York State Office for the Aging. (2009). *Sustaining informal caregivers: New York state caregiver support programs participants survey.* Available at http://www.aging.ny.gov/ReportsAndData/CaregiverReports/index.cfm

burden becomes greater as the need for care increases. In particular, patients whose care is limited by financial constraints, patients with dementia, patients who are combative or delusional, and those who require assistance with activities of daily living present challenges to family members and caregivers. Futeran and Draper (2012) found that the most frequent diagnosis among older adults with chronic mental illness was schizophrenia, with 66% of their sample having a diagnosis of schizophrenia. Bipolar disorder was next, at 16%, with schizoaffective and depressive disorder representing 11% and 7%, respectively. Caring for an older adult who displays symptoms of psychosis, mania, or depression can be challenging for even the most able caregiver.

Caregiver burden also may be seen in the older adult who is caring for an adult child with serious mental illness. The aging parent may experience distress related to planning future provision of care for an adult child, as well as the distress associated with actual provision of care.

For many families, assistance with patient care may be necessary, especially if the caregiver is an aging spouse or relative. Many communities have organizations that provide some level of respite care to give caregivers a short break. By being aware of services available in their communities, nurses can offer greatly needed support to refer patients and their caregivers.

Sociological

In the sociological domain, older adults with mental illness often face a number of unique challenges. Among them are ageism, financial stressors, and accumulated losses.

Ageism

Ageism refers to negative stereotyping of or discrimination against older adults. Ageism is pervasive, affecting many parts of society. For example, older adults often are viewed less positively as job applicants than younger people, despite research that job performance does not decline with age (North & Fiske, 2012). In health care, older adults often receive less aggressive treatments for common ailments as a result of providers minimizing the complaints or dismissing them as a normal part of aging.

Ageism includes three domains. The first is cognitive and relates to beliefs and stereotypes about older adults. The second is emotional, related to prejudicial attitudes. The third is behavioral, which includes direct or indirect discrimination and, in some cases, abuse. The psychological impact of ageism on older adults can lead to feelings of being isolated, devalued, and dehumanized (Phelan, 2011).

Financial Stressors

Many older adults, especially those diagnosed with mental illness, experience challenges related to the cost of health care. Retirement plans may include reduced health insurance coverage, and most individuals experience a reduction in income on retirement (Figure 32-3). Nurses working with older adults must be aware of financial resources related to nutrition support (for example, Meals on Wheels), income support (such as Social Security), and transportation services available in the area.

Accumulated Losses

Older adults often experience multiple losses. These losses may include death of loved ones, such as spouses, caregivers, siblings, and friends. Losses may include home, health, mobility, roles, cognitive functions, and economic status (Potter, 2012). One loss may lead to others. For example, if a caregiver dies, the older adult may no longer

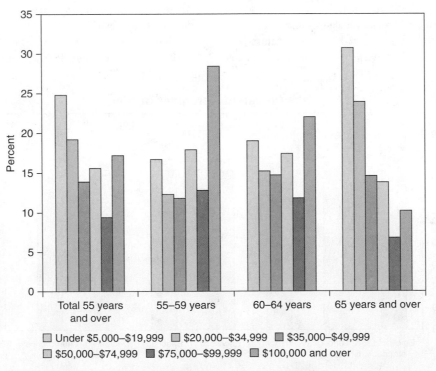

32-3 Household income declines with age.

Data from U.S. Census Bureau. (2011). Current Population Survey, Annual Social and Economic Supplement. Available at http://www.census.gov/population/age/data/2011.html

be able to remain in the house, causing the individual to simultaneously grieve both the loss of the caregiver and the loss of home. Accumulated losses can lead to overwhelming feelings of grieving as well as a sense of disconnection from a familiar life and identity. As losses mount, the older adult's support systems may shrink (Victoria Hospital Bereavement Services, n.d.).

Cultural

As with all nursing care, care of the older adult occurs within a cultural context. Factors such as language, ethnicity, gender, and support systems can have a unique impact on adjustment and mental health (Neimeyer et al., 2011). Unfortunately, disparities in mental health care exist along both age and cultural lines. Older adults, in general, are less likely to receive mental health care than younger adults and children; older African-American, Hispanic, and Asian adults have far less access to mental health services than older White Americans (Arean, n.d.). Providing mental health care to patients from different cultures and to patients who speak different languages presents challenges to nurses. It is important to assess the patient's cultural context and ensure provision of culturally competent care.

Spiritual

Religion and spirituality are important factors in the lives of many older adults. Newport (2006) reported that of individuals age 65 or older, 72% said that religion was very important in their lives. Research has associated spirituality with health and wellness, life satisfaction, self-esteem, and the ability to cope with issues faced by the older adult, such as fear of falling, vision loss, and lifetime trauma (Hodge, Bonifas, & Chou, 2010). For example, in an analysis of the impact of spiritual and other factors on attitudes about the end of life, Neimeyer et al. (2011) found that patients with an internalized religious world view had less emotional suffering and greater acceptance of death than those without this world view. As with culturally competent care, it is important that the nurse recognize, assess, and provide spiritually competent care to the older adult.

Pause and Reflect

1. *What changes common in older adults are likely to affect the older adult's safety?*
2. *How can the nurse distinguish between delirium and dementia? Between delirium and depression?*
3. *What types of ageism have you witnessed in U.S. culture? As a nurse, what could you do to prevent ageism in care settings?*

Special Issues in Care

Providing care for older adults involves a number of special considerations. Some key areas to be addressed include safety, advance directives, options for care, elder abuse, transfer trauma, and restraints.

Safety

Maintaining the safety of individuals with mental health issues is one of the core components of psychiatric nursing. Fall risks, the risk for suicide, cognitive decline, sensory changes, and polypharmacy are just a few of the safety concerns that require special attention in the older adult. Initial nursing interventions focus on engaging the patient in treatment and attaining and maintaining a safe and therapeutic environment. Reducing risk for suicide or accidental injury is a key

element. The nurse should assess for the presence of suicidal ideation as well as for the presence of guns, drugs, or other potentially harmful objects in the home. Other factors to assess include patients' ability to care for themselves (both cognitively and physically); medications prescribed; adherence to prescribed medications and use of over-the-counter medications, as well as herbs and supplements; and risk factors for adverse effects of medications. Some medications carry greater risk for adverse effects in older adults than in the general population. The American Geriatric Society publishes the Beers Criteria for Potentially Inappropriate Medication Use in Older Adults to guide prescribers in the use of these medications with older adults

Advance Directives

Individuals who were diagnosed with a psychiatric disorder as adults and who were able to manage it appropriately may experience increased difficulty in older adulthood. This may occur with onset of co-occurring illness, change in living or financial circumstances, or other considerations. It is important for these patients to establish advance directives, including a psychiatric advance directive that details the patient's preferences related to psychiatric care (Chapter 10).

Options for Care

Many older adults live independently. However, when living at home is no longer an option, relocation to community settings may become necessary. The senior living spectrum is broad. There are numerous levels of care, ranging from independent living to end-of-life hospice care, as well as varying levels of expense for services provided.

Independent living facilities offer independent living in an apartment setting. The older adult may live alone or with a roommate or spouse in a small apartment. Onsite services provided typically include a cafeteria, hair salon, and planned activities. Many facilities offer transportation to medical appointments and recreational events and activities.

Assisted living centers offer some opportunity for independence, with additional, but limited, support of nursing staff. Professional staff may assist with medication reminders or distribution (depending on the facility), and rooms and apartments typically have call bells to summon staff in the event of an emergency.

Skilled nursing facilities offer a higher level of nursing care, and typically have a physician on call. These facilities often offer collaborative care with a team consisting of a geriatrician, nurses, a social worker, and a dietician. The team generally meets monthly or as needed with the patient or a family member to discuss the treatment plan. Onsite care provided at skilled nursing facilities may include individual and family therapy; physical, occupational, and speech therapy; and physician consults. These facilities arrange transportation for patients who need to consult with specialists. Both assisted living centers and skilled nursing facilities typically offer onsite recreational activities and related services.

Additionally, there are memory care facilities or communities that are specially designed to care for patients with advanced dementia. Hospice care is discussed under "end-of-life issues" later in this chapter.

Elder Abuse

Elder abuse is the physical, emotional, sexual, or financial abuse of an older adult. Neglect also is a form of elder abuse. Because older adults most at risk for abuse are those suffering from dementia and mental illness, some experts suggest that all older patients diagnosed with mental illness and dementia should be screened for elder abuse (Pisani & Walsh, 2012). Signs and symptoms of elder abuse include the following:

- *Physical abuse:* inadequately explained injuries (fractures, sores, bruises, burns); delay in seeking medical attention
- *Emotional abuse:* unexplained changes in behavior (depression, withdrawal, or altered mental status); isolation from family and friends; a caregiver who appears to be controlling, demeaning, or aggressive toward the older adult
- *Financial abuse:* excessive gifts or compensation for providing companionship; lack of amenities that the older adult should be able to afford; suspicious transactions (ATM withdrawals when the older adult is hospitalized)
- *Sexual abuse:* bruising around the breasts or genitals; unexplained bleeding from the genitals or anus; unexplained sexually transmitted infections
- *Neglect:* lack of necessary supervision; unexplained weight loss; unsanitary living conditions; clothing inappropriate for the weather (Bond & Butler, 2013; Yaffe & Tazkarji, 2012)

The nurse's duty to protect the health, safety, and rights of the patient is critical. The nurse has both an ethical and a legal obligation to ensure that older adults are safe from abuse and neglect. In addition to the moral obligation to protect vulnerable patients, in many states the nurse is legally required to report abuse of older adults to protective agencies. Any nurse who suspects that a patient is being abused or neglected is to follow the reporting procedures outlined by both the employing organization and state regulations.

Transfer Trauma

Changing living environments can be stressful to anyone. Older adults are at increased risk of developing symptoms related to relocations and housing transitions. This is especially true when the older adult moves from a private residence to a nursing home or assisted living facility. Termed **transfer trauma** or **relocation stress syndrome**, this phenomenon comprises the physiological and psychosocial disturbances that result after transfer from one environment to another (Walker, Curry, & Hogstel, 2007).

Characteristics of transfer trauma can include withdrawal, anxiety, confusion, fear, helplessness, hopelessness, loneliness, suspicion, and suicidal ideation. There is controversy as to whether transfer trauma is a discrete phenomenon or if, in fact, the patient had a preexisting, undiagnosed depression that was triggered by the stress of relocation (Walker, Curry, & Hogstel, 2007). Regardless of the cause, nurses should be cognizant of the possibility of older adults developing symptoms as a result of environmental transition and complete a thorough assessment that includes a depression screening at the time of relocation.

Nurses can help decrease the stress of transition by helping the older adult develop a sense of control and familiarity over the new environment. Interventions include the following:

- Involving the older adult in decision making
- Accommodating the older adult's preferences and routines
- Facilitating communication with the older adult's social network
- Providing open communication about the older adult's relocation experience (Kao, Travis, & Acton, 2004; Walker, Curry, & Hogstel, 2007)

Restraints

As discussed in Chapter 25, a **restraint**, either chemical or physical, is any device that restricts freedom and mobility. Chemical restraints include medications, especially antipsychotics, that restrict an individual's freedom. Physical restraints include bedrails, limb or trunk belts, vests, and reclining chairs. With older adults, these devices often are used for fall prevention or for the management of challenging behaviors, despite accumulating evidence indicating that restraints are ineffective at preventing falls or for ensuring safety in older patients (Gulpers et al., 2012; Meyer, Kopke, Haastert, & Muhlhauser, 2009).

Restraints may cause negative physical, psychological, and social consequences for older adults. Both short- and long-term restraint use are associated with pressure ulcers, loss of muscle strength, joint contractures, incontinence, demoralization, poor self-esteem, impaired social functioning, depression, and aggression (Gulpers et al., 2010). Nurses treating older adults must be aware that restraints should be used only in an emergency, after all less-restrictive alternatives have been exhausted, and for as brief a period of time as possible. Each state, as well as Medicare and the Joint Commission, has strict regulations governing the use of restraints. Nurses should be fully familiar with these regulations before using restraints in the older patient.

Pause and Reflect

1. *Why do you think financial abuse is included as a category of elder abuse? What indicators might suggest to a nurse that an older patient is the victim of financial abuse?*
2. *Why do you think older adults who move from one environment to another are at risk for transfer trauma?*
3. *What would you include in a plan of care for an older adult who transfers from his or her own home to a skilled nursing facility?*

Mental Illness and Older Adults

In the United States, older adults compose more than 13% of the population—more than 41 million people. As stated earlier, more Americans are living longer, and many of them will suffer from multiple chronic illnesses—including mental illnesses (Administration on Aging, 2012). The current mental health system is poorly prepared for this influx of new patients. For example, currently there are 5.6 million to 8 million older adults with mental health disorders in the United States. By 2030, this number is estimated to be 10 million to 14.4 million. By that time, there will only be about 1650 geriatric psychiatrists—less than one psychiatrist per 6,000 older adults with a mental illness (Bartles & Naslund, 2013). It is likely that, in the coming years, older adults with mental health issues will rely increasingly on nurse clinicians to provide their mental health care.

For patients who have been living with a chronic mental illness, aging presents unique problems. Coping and support systems are tested, and may even deteriorate, when patients experience death of a spouse or caregiver or diagnosis of a serious illness. For example, when an individual caring for a patient with dementia receives a diagnosis of a terminal illness, or experiences a major illness or injury, both the patient and caregiver will experience increased stress, which may complicate both physical and mental health. For older parents,

Celia Taylor Recovery Phase

APPLICATION

1. How would you address Mrs. Taylor's desire to return home?

2. What nursing care concerns are present at this time?

3. How can you assist Carolyn to express her thoughts and feelings in relation to Mrs. Taylor's treatment at this point?

Two days after her admission, Mrs. Taylor develops intermittent confusion, including difficulty paying attention and recognizing familiar objects. One of her nurses suspects that Mrs. Taylor may have a urinary tract infection. Testing confirms that she does, and Mrs. Taylor is started on sulfamethoxazole and trimethoprim (Bactrim), 2 tablets every 12 hours for 10 days. A few days later, Mrs. Taylor's confusion begins to resolve, but the staff observes that her weepiness has increased. Her care team initiates a consultation with a geriatric psychiatrist, who diagnoses Mrs. Taylor with major depressive disorder, recurrent, moderate. Mrs. Taylor's daughter, Carolyn, tells the nurse that sertraline (Zoloft) 50 mg daily helped Mrs. Taylor in the past. Carolyn admits that she also takes it and finds it helpful. Mrs. Taylor is started on sertraline 25 mg PO every morning for one week, to increase to 50 mg PO thereafter.

After a couple of weeks, the nurse notices that Mrs. Taylor's mood has improved: She is expressing interest in her physical therapy and is seen talking with her roommate more frequently. At the end of the third week, Mrs. Taylor's gait is improving but still somewhat unsteady. Carolyn tells the nurse that she is exhausted from trying to accommodate her mother's requests for special items to be brought in, such as particular foods, clean clothes, and various other items. The treatment team meets with Mrs. Taylor and Carolyn to plan the next steps of her care. Mrs. Taylor indicates that she still wishes to go home and stresses that her daughter Carolyn lives nearby and can come to her house daily to help. Carolyn appears hesitant to speak at the meeting.

---

especially those diagnosed with a serious chronic or terminal illness who are taking care of adult children with mental illness, the fear of leaving their ill adult child alone often is overwhelming.

Mental illness secondary to aging also is a growing problem. Examples of disorders that may appear for the first time in older adults include cognitive decline, dementia, addiction disorders, anxiety disorders, and depression. In some cases these disorders are primary, whereas in others they are secondary due to a developed medical illness such as hypothyroidism, anemia, multiple sclerosis, or vitamin B_{12} deficiency.

Schizophrenia

The older patient with schizophrenia often has issues specific to the aging process. These may include onset of additional illnesses, change in ability to metabolize medication, and decline in cognitive function as a result of medications used to control the symptoms of schizophrenia.

Nurses working with older adults diagnosed with schizophrenia should be especially alert to the risk for injury related to orthostatic hypotension in patients taking antipsychotics. Confusion, delusions, hallucinations, fatigue, and unsteadiness also may be seen in these patients, and all increase patient risk for injury.

First-generation antipsychotics should be avoided in older adults because of the risks for tardive dyskinesia, cardiac complications, and falls. Anticholinergic and antipsychotic agents that are highly dopamine blocking should also be avoided. Benzodiazepines increase risk for cognitive impairment and significantly increase fall risk (American Geriatrics Society, 2012).

Nursing strategies to help older adults cope with schizophrenia should address needs for socialization, activity, physical health promotion, and medication collaboration, as well as screening for possible abuse, such as neglect or exploitation (Chapter 17).

Depression

Recognition of the problem of depression in older adults has increased in recent years. Unlike schizophrenia, which usually manifests itself early in a patient's life, depression may develop at any age. Therefore, in addition to taking a full history to screen for a previous diagnosis of depression, it is important to use screening tools that are validated for use with new-onset depression (see the section on assessment). Depression in older adults may often exist in association with physical illness (Melillo & Houde, 2011). Most research supports the hypothesis that depression is still underdiagnosed in the elderly.

Co-morbidity of physical illness and depression in older adults may explain why depression has been referred to as a "fatal illness" in this population (Melillo & Houde, 2011). Untreated depression contributes to higher medical costs and higher use of medical care services. Patients who are untreated make frequent visits to their primary care providers and to emergency departments. Nurses working in these settings should be alert to screen older adult patients with repeated visits for depression.

Initial nursing interventions for the older adult patient with depression should focus on screening for suicidality, decreasing isolation, providing education about depression, increasing exercise, encouraging proper rest and nutrition, and ensuring that the patient is evaluated for potential medication treatment.

Medication strategies for older adults include avoiding medications such as tricyclic antidepressants that can cause significant cardiac side effects, including postural hypotension or QT prolongation. Although SSRIs are generally well tolerated, they can have significant GI side effects and also are implicated in causing hyponatremia.

Suicide

Suicide in the elderly is a major public health concern. Individuals 65 years of age and older are at highest risk for committing suicides (Garand et al., 2006). Individuals between 45 and 65 years of age made up the highest rate (18.6%) of suicide attempts in 2010; the second-highest rate occurred in the over-85-year age bracket (17.6%) (American Foundation for Suicide Prevention, 2013). Unlike the case with younger adults and adolescents, suicide in the older adult is often linked to co-occurring mental health issues (especially depression), medical conditions, and social functioning. Additional risk factors include previous suicide attempts and social isolation. The nurse must be diligent in screening older adults at risk for suicide. Assessment tools and techniques helpful in patients at risk for suicide or who have made a suicidal gesture are discussed in detail in Chapter 27.

Bipolar Disorder

Bipolar illness has increased among older adults, and a large percentage of acute inpatient psychiatric admissions of older patients are to treat mania. There is considerable debate, however, as to whether mania in the older adult is due to bipolar illness or is, in fact, related to delirium, dementia, or other cognitive impairment (Dorey et al., 2008). Older adults with cognitive impairment may experience periods of agitation and psychosis, which may be mistaken for bipolar illness. The important factor for the nurse to consider is that bipolar disorder is treated with mood stabilizers and antipsychotics, but these medications are not the treatment of choice for delirium, which is treated by correcting the precipitating factor.

Nursing assessment of the patient with bipolar disorder should focus on identifying the degree of mania or depression, as well as looking for potential physical causes of mania or delirium. Patients should also be assessed for safety. Manic behaviors that are potentially harmful (such as drug use, hypersexuality, and unsafe sex) should be brought to the attention of the patient's provider. Community-dwelling patients may need to be stabilized in an inpatient environment if they are truly manic.

Pharmacologic therapy of bipolar disease in older adults includes use of mood stabilizers as the basis of treatment; however, dosage reduction may be necessary to minimize side effects. Furthermore, the use of lithium may be contraindicated in older adult patients owing to the presence of increased side effects associated with aging. Older adults may not need blood levels as high as those associated with treatment success in younger clients (Stahl, 2009).

Anxiety and Trauma-Related Disorders

Generalized anxiety disorder is the most common anxiety disorder experienced by older adults (Kaiser et al., 2013). Older adults who experience sudden or life-altering changes associated with aging (for instance, death of a spouse, retirement, or multiple losses) may have difficulty coping with memories of trauma. It is estimated that between 70% and 90% of older adults have experienced at least one traumatic event. Prevalence of posttraumatic stress disorder (PTSD) among older adults may be as high as 4%. Among older veterans seeking treatment for mental health issues, the lifetime exposure rate to traumatic events is 85% (Kaiser et al., 2013).

Older adults are less likely to receive treatment for anxiety disorders. Those who have lived with anxiety for years may view their symptoms as normal. Others may be distrusting of seeking treatment or may not recognize that they have a problem. Anxiety is often underdiagnosed due to the presence of co-morbid illness and/or being attributed to side effects of medication (American Geriatrics Society, 2009). If left untreated, anxiety can lead to decreased quality of life, cognitive impairments, and increased utilization of public health services.

Nursing interventions for older adults with anxiety or trauma-related disorders include interventions appropriate for adults generally (see Chapter 13). Relaxation techniques, exercise, and diversion may be helpful for many patients. Assess for factors that may serve as barriers to activities that promote engagement; transportation,

incontinence, and fear may all prevent the older client from accessing activities that reduce anxiety.

Long-term management of anxiety is usually best achieved using medications other than benzodiazepines. Appropriate options include trazodone (Desyrel), a tricyclic antidepressant, and buspirone (BuSpar), a nonbenzodiazepine anxiolytic. Benzodiazepines carry additional risks for older clients, increasing risks for falls and cognitive impairment. For some patients, they may result in paradoxical agitation and acting out, especially if the patient has a preexisting mental illness or cognitive impairment (Wilson, Shannon, & Shields, 2012).

Substance Abuse

Although the standards for diagnosis of addiction in older adults do not differ from those for the general population, a simple definition for the practicing clinician is a harmful pattern of use of any substance despite negative consequences. This allows the clinician to avoid overdiagnosing typical behavior such as social use of alcohol. This definition also is easily explained to patients and can help reassure cancer patients that correct use of pain medications, even when physiologic dependence is present, is not an addiction disorder. Although dependency may be a component of addiction, it is neither a necessary component (as in gambling) nor a sufficient component (as in opiate use in end of life) for diagnosing addiction.

Substance abuse among older adults is believed to be on the rise (Dowling, Weiss, & Condon, 2008). It is important for clinicians to routinely screen for substance abuse and not to rely solely on reported history of substance abuse or stereotypical signs of substance abuse. Although certain medical conditions, such as liver disease or hepatitis C, may trigger the clinician to inquire about substance abuse, many older adults will show no sequelae of substance abuse. Families are often instrumental in providing information about reality-based use.

Alcohol is widely regarded as the most common substance abused by older adults in the United States (Dowling, Weiss, & Condon, 2008). In addition to alcohol, the clinician should be alert for the abuse of other drugs, especially prescription medications. Abuse of prescription medications can be difficult to track when the patient has multiple prescribers. This may be discovered by asking the patient to bring all medications to the appointment for review, including over-the-counter (OTC) and herbal products, although some patients may avoid this.

Screening for substance abuse can be accomplished through the use of screening tests, including the use of the CAGE questionnaire (Chapter 20). Initial nursing interventions should focus on ensuring prevention of withdrawal or delirium tremens. Carefully monitor vital signs. Follow clinician orders regarding the use of detoxification medications. Lorazepam (Ativan), oxazepam (Serax), and chlordiazepoxide (Librium) are commonly used medications in the treatment of alcohol and benzodiazepine withdrawal, whereas buprenorphine/naloxone (Suboxone) and methadone are used in the treatment of opioid addiction.

Following detoxification, the nurse should engage the older adult in strategies to help abstain from relapsing. The type of care provided should be individualized to the patient's preferences. For example, some patients prefer the social interaction and support provided by Alcoholics Anonymous, whereas others prefer one-on-one therapy by a trained addiction specialist. Some patients may require a combination of interventions and strategies.

Assessment

Assessment of older adults with mental health concerns begins with the understanding that these patients are at higher risk for medical illness and may have medical co-morbidities that are presenting as primary psychiatric problems (Figure 32-4). Standard nursing assessment of physical health, vital signs, overall presentation, grooming, hygiene, and presence of medical illness should always be included in the comprehensive nursing assessment. In addition, a home safety assessment may be necessary for patients with limited mobility. Assessment of the patient's ability to adhere to the therapeutic regimen may also be necessary. For example, the patient with dementia will need increasing levels of care, starting with assistance with taking medications, preparing food, and transportation.

First, the basic neurologic assessment should include whether the patient is alert and the patient's level of orientation and overall mood (for instance, depressed, flat, or bright). Next, assess for signs of neurologic diseases that affect movement (such as Parkinson or Huntington disease) by noting the presence or absence of tremor, the quality of the tremor, and whether it is seen most at rest (as in Parkinson disease) or when using the extremity (as seen in essential tremor). Assess for hypothyroidism, an often overlooked cause of depression. Left untreated, severe hypothyroidism can lead to psychosis and cognitive impairment. Signs of hypothyroidism include dry skin, weight gain, cold intolerance, and thinning hair. Women are most at risk for hypothyroidism.

Assessment of cognitive impairment is especially important and requires the use of standardized testing, such as the Mini Mental Status Exam (Chapter 9). The clinician should be familiar with the exam, and should have at least 10 to 15 minutes available for screening in an area free of distractions. A score of 25 or less should be considered indicative of possible dementia; if the patient has not had a previous diagnosis of dementia, referral should be made for further evaluation.

Likewise, when seeing an older adult for a physical complaint, assessment should always include opportunities to assess mental health as well as physical health. Use of validated, standardized assessment may help rapidly screen seniors for mental health issues. Two critical areas of assessment are depression and pain.

Depression

Standard tools that can be used include the Geriatric Depression Scale and the Cornell Scale for Depression in Dementia. The Geriatric Depression Scale asks direct questions of the patient that assess for mood and affect, level of satisfaction with life, and feelings of hope or hopelessness. The Cornell Scale for Depression in Dementia is used with a patient's primary caregiver. This screening tool assesses a patient's mood state, behavioral disturbances, physical symptoms (such as appetite and energy), cyclic functions (such as sleep and wake habits), and ideational disturbances.

In addition to standardized tools, it is also important for the clinician to look for signs of chronic mental illness as well as co-morbid illness during the physical assessment. When screening for depression, nurses must be alert to the possibility for depression or dementia. As stated earlier, these can be mistaken with delirium. See Chapter 21 for a more complete discussion of the differences among delirium, depression, and dementia.

Pain

Pain is a common problem in older adults. The increased prevalence of chronic diseases, such as osteoarthritis, puts older adults at greater risk for pain (Flaherty, 2012). It is estimated that between 50% and 86% of older adults experience a level of pain that interferes with their quality of life (Pautex & Gold, 2006). Half of all adults 65 years of age or older have experienced pain within the past month (U.S. DHHS, 2006).

Despite being a common problem, pain is undertreated in older adults. Older adults present special challenges with pain. Some may experience a higher pain threshold, and physiological changes modify absorption, bioavailability, and transport of medications within the body (Fine, 2009). Older adults with cognitive impairment may not be able to verbalize their pain level. Other factors contributing to the undertreatment of pain in older adults include the belief that pain is an inevitable part of aging, fear of becoming addicted to pain medications, and lack of routine pain assessment on the part of health care providers (Flaherty, 2012). Appropriate treatment of pain in older adults is critical: Chronic or poorly treated pain is associated with a number of adverse outcomes, including functional impairments, falls, slow rehabilitation, depression, anxiety, sleep impairments, decreased socialization, and poor quality of life (American Geriatrics Society, 2009).

Assessment of pain in the older adult begins with asking whether the patient is experiencing any pain. Be alert to common barriers to communicating pain, including language issues, sensory deficits (such as hearing loss), and cognitive issues (such as dementia). With these barriers in mind, assess the patient using simple questions. Even patients with mild to moderate dementia are usually able to answer simple questions about their pain. When patients report pain, use a standardized tool to assess pain severity. This may include using a verbal rating scale from 0 to 10, with 0 being "no pain" to 10 being the "worst pain," or using a more formalized descriptor scale. When a patient's dementia is advanced to the point at which accurate pain communication is impaired, the nurse can use a standardized scale, such as the Pain Assessment in Advanced Dementia (PAINAD) scale. This scale uses categories of behavior observed by the nurse

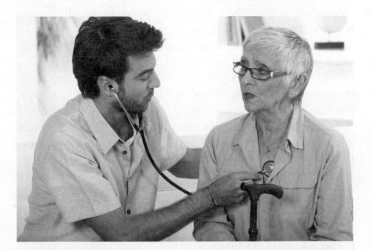

32-4 Older adults are at higher risk for medical illnesses related to psychiatric symptoms. A thorough assessment of the older adult that includes physical assessment and screening for depression is necessary regardless of setting.

Source: Barabas Attila/Fotolia

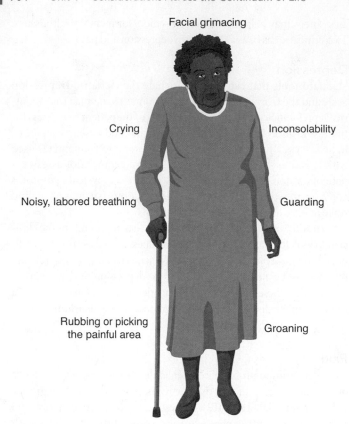

Facial grimacing

Crying

Inconsolability

Noisy, labored breathing

Guarding

Rubbing or picking
the painful area

Groaning

32-5 Behavioral indicators of pain in older adults.

(breathing, negative vocalization, facial expressions, body language, and consolability) to rate the patient's pain (Flaherty, 2012; Horgas, 2012). These behavioral indicators include noisy, labored breathing; crying; inconsolability; and facial grimacing, among others (Figure 32-5). Although no single indicator is sufficient to determine pain, the presence of multiple indicators as identified through the PAINAD scale will help determine the level of pain the patient is experiencing. A patient may also express pain by guarding, rubbing, groaning, or picking at a painful area.

Pause and Reflect

1. *What considerations are important when providing nursing care to older adults with mental illness?*
2. *Why is it important to include screenings for depression and pain in comprehensive assessments of older adults regardless of the care setting?*

End-of-Life Issues

Nursing assessment for end-of-life issues is patient specific. Patients with advanced metastatic cancer, for instance, may have quite different needs from patients with end-stage lung disease. The presence of acute or chronic mental illness greatly affects the nursing care plan.

Initial end-of-life nursing assessment focuses on meeting immediate needs. Many patients may not present until late in the end-of-life process and may need immediate referral to hospice or palliative care. Other patients may present early after diagnosis of a terminal illness for advanced planning.

Hospice and Palliative Care

Although many clinicians still view hospice as a physical place of care, hospice is best thought of as a philosophy. **Palliative care** attempts to improve quality of life and emphasizes pain management and holistic care of terminally ill patients, as well as caring for the patient's identified family. Palliative care may be provided to a patient regardless of setting and with or without the added benefits of hospice care. At its core, **hospice care** embraces the belief that quality of life is as important as quantity of life. Hospice provides terminally ill patients with caregivers who address all aspects of their care. Spiritual, emotional, and physical needs are addressed in hospice. As such, nurses must work as members of a strong interdisciplinary team with the patient at its center.

Nursing Care at End of Life

Nursing care at end of life should address the following core components: pain and stress management, physical needs, and spiritual needs, and an assessment of the patient's need for completion of life tasks. These tasks may include resolution of relationship issues with loved ones, telling loved ones and others things that the patient may need to share, and opportunities to complete final tasks, such as leaving a favorite belonging to a grandchild (see the Nursing Care Plan that follows). Other needs at the end of life include pain management needs and the need for elimination. Hospice nurses and mental health providers should collaborate to provide comfort. As in all aspects of nursing care, patient preferences related to pain management and medication use must be assessed and taken into consideration. In addition, if a patient had been prescribed antidepressant or antipsychotic medication, discontinuing these medications at the initiation of hospice care might be counterproductive and create unneeded emotional distress.

From Suffering to Hope

A major advantage of working with older adults is drawing upon their stories and experiences. Older adults often have lived full lives and witnessed diverse aspects of history and family life. Encouraging older adults to share their stories is a way to provide affirmation. Some of the stories may be painful to share, but providing older adults opportunities to share assists in validating them as individuals and helping them recognize survival skills and moments of success.

There is great variation in capabilities among older adults across the age spectrum from age 60 (or, in some situations, 50) to 90+ years. For example, some 60-year-olds are more impaired in functioning than some 85-year-olds. It is important to avoid stereotyping older adults. Helping older adults recognize their strengths and abilities will be more helpful than focusing on what they cannot do any more. In addition, valuing them as the individuals they *are* rather than for what they can *do* may convey hope to those who are grieving loss of independence or of role function.

Pause and Reflect

1. *What are some factors that can affect an older adult's risk for unrecognized or undertreated pain?*
2. *What are some life tasks that may be important for older adults to complete as they near the end of their lives?*
3. *What are your thoughts on assisted suicide?*

Celia Taylor Rehabilitation Phase

The treatment team, Mrs. Taylor, and her daughter Carolyn agreed that Mrs. Taylor would try the assisted living unit at the facility. Mrs. Taylor has been there for 4 weeks, and it is time for another treatment team meeting. There has been no evidence of any recurring urinary tract infection. Her mood has stabilized further. Her gait continues to be unsteady unless she uses a walker. Mrs. Taylor is ambivalent about going home or staying longer at the facility in the assisted living unit. She states that everyone has treated her nicely, but she thinks she needs to get back into her routine at home and let people who need "such a place as this" have her bed.

Carolyn shares with the team that her favorite uncle, Mrs. Taylor's 83-year-old brother, has cancer and is in a nearby hospice, in and out of consciousness. She would like to arrange for her mother to visit him. Carolyn's eyes fill with tears as she shares this information. Mrs. Taylor comments that he also is her favorite sibling, and she begins to cry.

APPLICATION

1. What do you anticipate are priority concerns for Mrs. Taylor at this time?

2. How can you use Mrs. Taylor's ambivalence to help her in deciding what is best for her?

3. How can you help both Mrs. Taylor and Carolyn in relation to the anticipated loss of this favorite family member?

Mrs. Taylor—A Patient With Co-Morbid Disorders | NURSING CARE PLAN

Nursing Diagnosis: Grieving related to anticipated loss of brother, loss of independence, reduced mobility (status post left hip surgery)

Short-Term Goals Patient will: (Include date for short-term goal to be met)	Interventions Nurse will:	Rationale
Maintain as much as possible her current level of functioning after hearing news about anticipated loss of brother.	Assess Mrs. Taylor for symptoms of grief, such as verbalizations of loss, crying, looking downcast, decreased/increased appetite, insomnia, depression. Also assess all levels of functioning, including mobility and fall risk.	It is important to determine Mrs. Taylor's responses to news about the anticipated loss of her brother, as well as how Mrs. Taylor (and her daughter Carolyn) might need assistance in processing this grief and be supported during it.
	Assess if her current medications are appropriate at this time but avoid medicating to "numb" suffering.	Patients may need medications during a time of grief if depression is severe. However, medications should not be used to "numb" or delay suffering.
	Identify strategies and barriers to moving forward in grief process and functioning.	Unresolved or ambiguous relationships impede grieving. Strong relationships and support people can facilitate the grieving process.
	Provide empathy and concern.	Patients may share more readily in an environment of empathy and concern.
Discuss feelings about anticipated loss of brother on first day of hearing news.	Explore with Mrs. Taylor her relationship with brother. Help her express her feelings of grief.	Grieving is unique to each person. Individuals in early stages of dementia, like Mrs. Taylor, generally have better long-term memory than short-term memory but may need assistance remembering people or circumstances related to the loss.
	Enlist her daughter's assistance in remembering times past about the brother/uncle if Mrs. Taylor struggles. Enlist the daughter's support in keeping Mrs. Taylor active.	Carolyn is a key support person for Mrs. Taylor but also is grieving for this relative while Mrs. Taylor is grieving.
Make a plan related to reaching out to brother with her daughter and the nurse on day 2 after hearing the news about her brother.	Consider options that may help Mrs. Taylor and her daughter connect with Mrs. Taylor's brother, such as a phone call, a visit to the facility where the brother is, write a note, share a memory and write it down, send a taped voice message over Carolyn's cell phone, etc.	Mrs. Taylor needs to connect with her dying brother in the best possible way for her, her brother, and her daughter. Her daughter Carolyn needs to be involved in whatever plans are made.
	Ask Mrs. Taylor and Carolyn if they would like a visit with a clergy member or someone else whom they identify as being helpful. If they would like, make arrangements for this person to visit Mrs. Taylor.	Many individuals find comfort in spiritual practices, which may include meeting with clergy or other individuals of their choice when experiencing grief.

(continued)

Short-Term Goals *Patient will:* *(Include date for short-term goal to be met)*	Interventions *Nurse will:*	Rationale
Express decreased distress and symptoms (as determined in first goal).	Determine if Mrs. Taylor is feeling less distressed and demonstrating decreased symptoms once a plan is in place in relation to her connecting with her brother.	Having something concrete and constructive to do when one is feeling stressed and grieving often brings a sense of relief.
	Continue to have Mrs. Taylor share stories about her brother.	Giving Mrs. Taylor time to reminisce is important in the grieving process.
	Educate Mrs. Taylor and Carolyn about grieving and grief work, including the uniqueness of each individual's response to grief.	Individuals grieve in different ways and on different time tables.
Long-Term Goal Mrs. Taylor will successfully grieve the loss of her brother and continue activities that bring her enjoyment, such as outings with her daughter.	Assess Mrs. Taylor's progress, provide additional grief support as determined helpful, and keep Carolyn as involved as possible.	Keeping Mrs. Taylor involved with her family and in activities she enjoys should help her maintaining functioning and navigate the grieving process.

Clinical Reasoning

1. What other nursing diagnoses might the nurse working with Mrs. Taylor and her daughter Carolyn consider?
2. How do you think Mrs. Taylor's diagnosis of dementia and depression will impact her grief work?
3. How might this latest news of Mrs. Taylor's brother's anticipated death affect her current decision to reside in the assisted living facility?

Chapter Highlights

1. Older age increases risk for chronic disease and disability.
2. Common physical changes that occur with aging include sensory losses, musculoskeletal changes, multiple illnesses, sleep disturbances, and changes in functioning of major organs.
3. Although minor cognitive changes are expected in older adults, cognitive changes that impair function are not a normal part of aging and should be investigated.
4. Delirium is an acute state of confusion marked by rapid onset. Delirium signals an underlying medical condition that requires rapid treatment.
5. Ageism, financial stressors, and accumulated losses are among the factors that affect patient wellness in the sociological domain.
6. Polypharmacy puts the older adult at risk for many problems when multiple medications are prescribed by multiple providers.
7. Elder abuse includes physical, emotional, sexual, or financial abuse or neglect of an older adult.
8. Older adults who relocate from one environment to another may experience transfer trauma; nurses working with older adults who relocate should screen for and be prepared to provide interventions to older adults experiencing transfer trauma.
9. Pain and depression screenings should be included as part of the comprehensive assessment of the older adult.

NCLEX®-RN Questions

1. The nurse is working with an older adult patient presenting for the first time for mental health services. The patient's family expresses concern because the patient has no previous history of mental illness. Which response is most appropriate?
   a. "It is possible that the family is not providing an adequate level of support at this time."
   b. "Decline in cognition is part of the aging process and is typical in the older adult population."
   c. "We are better at keeping people alive longer, but unfortunately, quality of life continues to be poor."
   d. "Some older adults may have difficulty coping with changes that can occur with aging, leading to mental health issues."

2. The nurse is completing an assessment of an older adult that incorporates the biological, psychological, sociological, cultural, and spiritual domains affecting mental health. Which does the nurse recognize as alterations? Select all that apply.
   a. The patient declines any spiritual interventions.
   b. The patient elects to forgo a life-sustaining treatment.
   c. The patient is unable to afford nutritious foods on a fixed income.
   d. The patient experiences a progressive decline in cognitive function.
   e. The patient is overwhelmed by multiple chronic, disabling physical problems.

3. The nurse is evaluating an older adult patient who has just experienced the loss of a spouse. The nurse understands that which factor is most likely to complicate the grief process and is associated with accumulated losses?
   a. The patient does not have any children.
   b. The patient has a lifelong chronic health condition.
   c. The patient was the primary caregiver for the spouse.
   d. The patient is legally blind and was dependent on the spouse to drive.

4. The nurse is assessing the patient presenting to the mental health clinic with cognitive symptoms. Which finding is most likely to suggest depression rather than delirium?
   a. A history of labile mood
   b. Rapid onset of cognitive changes
   c. Disturbed sleep with no set patterns
   d. Patchy or inconsistent memory problems

5. The nurse is providing teaching to an older adult about to begin treatment with a selective serotonin-reuptake inhibitor (SSRI). The patient states that he took a tricyclic antidepressant many years ago and asks why the same medication is not being prescribed now. The nurse would explain that tricyclic antidepressants are associated with which adverse effect in older adults?
   a. EKG changes
   b. Hypertension
   c. Hyponatremia
   d. Gastrointestinal distress

6. The nurse is participating in a community health screening program aimed at preventing elder abuse. Which finding does the nurse recognize as placing the patient at increased risk of abuse?
   a. The patient has a history of mental illness.
   b. The patient is taking multiple medications.
   c. The patient lives in an assisted care facility.
   d. The patient has not established advance directives.

7. The nurse is caring for an older adult with schizophrenia. The patient has started to experience problems with an antipsychotic medication that was previously well tolerated. The nurse recognizes that this is most likely due to which nonmodifiable factor associated with aging?
   a. Poor adherence
   b. Lifestyle changes
   c. Metabolic changes
   d. Polypharmacy

8. The hospice nurse is initiating end-of-life care for an older adult patient who suffers from a co-morbid major mental illness. Which essential component of care would the nurse anticipate carrying out?
   a. Assisting the patient to identify issues that need to be resolved
   b. Ensuring that only nonpharmacologic pain management is used
   c. Weaning the patient off any prescribed psychotropic medications
   d. Deferring to a more competent individual on health care decisions

Answers may be found on the Pearson student resource site: nursing.pearsonhighered.com

---

Pearson Nursing Student Resources Find additional review materials at **nursing.pearsonhighered.com**

References

Administration on Aging. (2012). *Profile of older Americans.* Available at http://www.aoa.gov/AoARoot/(S(2ch32qw55k1qylo45dbihar2u))/Aging_Statistics/Profile/index.aspx

Aging and Sleep. (2013). Available at http://www.webmd.com/sleep-disorders/guide/aging-affects-sleep

Alzheimer's Association. (2011). *2011 Alzheimer's Disease Facts and Figures.* Available at http://www.alz.org/downloads/facts_figures_2011.pdf

American Foundation for Suicide Prevention. (2013). *Facts and figures: Suicide deaths.* Available at http://www.afsp.org/understanding-suicide/facts-and-figures

American Geriatrics Society. (2009) Pharmacological management of persistent pain in older persons. *Journal of the American Geriatrics Society, 57*(8), 1331–1346.

American Geriatrics Society. (2012). Updated Beers criteria for potentially inappropriate medication use in older adults. *Journal of the American Geriatrics Society, 60*(4), 616–631.

American Psychiatric Association. (2013). *Diagnostic and Statistical Manual of Mental Disorders* (5th ed.). Washington, DC: American Psychiatric Publishers.

Anderson, G. (2010). *Chronic care: Making the case for ongoing care.* Robert Wood Johnson Foundation. Available at http://www.rwjf.org/en/research-publications/find-rwjf-research/2010/01/chronic-care.html

Anxiety and Depression Association of America (ADAA). (2012). *Older adults.* Available at http://www.adaa.org/living-with-anxiety/older-adults

Arean, P. (n.d.). *Mental health service use disparities in low-income, ethnic-minority older adults.* American Psychological Association. Available at http://www.apa.org/about/gr/issues/aging/arean-briefing.pdf

Bartles, S., & Naslund, A. (2013). The underside of the silver tsunami: Older adults and mental health care. *New England journal of Medicine, 368,* 493–496.

Bevens, M. F., & Sternberg, E. M. (2012). Caregiving burden, stress, and health effects among family caregivers of adult cancer patients. *Journal of the American Medical Association, 307*(4), 398–403. Available at http://www.ncbi.nlm.nih.gov/pmc/articles/PMC3304539/

Bond, M., & Butler, K. (2013) Elder abuse and neglect: Definitions, epidemiology and approaches to emergency department screening. *Clinical Geriatric Medicine, 29*(1), 257–273.

Boyce, J. M., & Shone, G. R. (2006). Effects of ageing on smell and taste. *Postgraduate Medical Journal, 82*(966), 239–241.

Centers for Disease Control and Prevention (CDC). (2012a). *Falls among older adults: An overview.* Available at http://www.cdc.gov/homeandrecreationalsafety/falls/adultfalls.html

Centers for Disease Control and Prevention (CDC). (2012b). *National suicide statistics at a glance.* Available at http://www.cdc.gov/ViolencePrevention/Suicide/statistics/index.html

Central Intelligence Agency. (2013). *The World Factbook.* Available at https://www.cia.gov/library/publications/the-world-factbook/.

Cremens, M., & Wiechers, I. (2010). Care of the geriatric patient. In T. A. Stern, G. L. Fricchione, N. H. Cassem, M. S. Jellinek, & J. F. Rosenbaum, (Eds.). *Massachusetts General Hospital Handbook of General Psychiatry* (6th ed.). St. Louis, MO: Mosby, pp. 593–600.

Cutilli, C. C. (2008). Teaching the geriatric patient: Making the most of "cognitive resources" and "gains." *Orthopedic Nursing, 27*(3), 195–198.

Dorey, J., Beauchet, O., Anterion, C., Rouch, I., Krolak-Salmon, P., Gaucher, J., Gonthier, R., & Akiskal, H. (2008). Symptoms of dementia and bipolar spectrum disorders: Relationship and treatment. *CNS Spectrum, 13*(9), 796–803.

Dowling, G., Weiss, S., & Condon, T. (2008). Drugs of abuse and the aging brain. *Neuropsychopharmacology, 33*(2), 209–218.

Downing, L. J., Caprio, T. V., & Lyness, J. M. (2013). Geriatric psychiatry review: Differential diagnosis and treatment of 3 D's: delirium, dementia, and depression. *Current Psychiatry Reports, 15,* 365.

Falk, W., & Wiechers, I. (2010). Demented patients. In T. A. Stern, G. L. Fricchione, N.H. Cassem, M. S. Jellinek & J. F. Rosenbaum, (Eds.). *Massachusetts General Hospital Handbook of General Psychiatry* (6th ed.). St. Louis, MO: Mosby, pp. 105–118.

Fjell, A., & Walhovd, K. (2010). Structural brain changes in aging: Courses, causes and cognitive consequences. *Reviews in Neuroscience, 21*(3), 187–221.

Fine, P. G. (2009). Chronic pain management in older adults: Special considerations. *Journal of Pain Symptom Management, 38*(2 Suppl), S4–S14. Available at http://www.ncbi.nlm.nih.gov/pubmed/19671470

Flaherty, E. (2012). Pain assessment in older adults. *Best Practices in Nursing Care to Older Adults.* Available at http://consultgerirn.org/topics/pain/want_to_know_more

Fuller, G. (2000). Falls in the elderly. *American Family Physician, 61,* 2159–2168.

Futeran, S., & Draper, B. M. (2012). An examination of the needs of older patients with chronic mental illness in public mental health services. *Aging and Mental Health, 16*(3), 327–334.

Garand, L., Mitchell, A., Dietrick, A., Hijjawi, S., & Pan, D. (2006). Suicide in older adults: Nursing assessment of suicide risk. *Issues in Mental Health Nursing, 27*(4), 355–370.

Gulland, A. (2012). People are living longer but are not in best health, global study finds. *British Medical Journal, 345,* e8511.

Gulpers, M., Bleijlevens, M., Capezuti, E., van Rossum, E., Ambergen, T., & Hamers, J. (2012). Preventing belt restraint use in newly admitted residents in nursing homes: A quasi-experimental study. *International Journal of Nursing Studies, 49*(12), 1473–1479.

Gulpers, M., Bleijlevens, M., van Rossum, E., Capezuti, E., & Hamers, J. (2010). Belt restraint reduction in nursing homes: Design of a quasi-experimental study. *BMC Geriatrics, 10*(11). Available at http://www.biomedcentral.com/1471-2318/10/11

Hajjar, E., Cafiero, A., & Hanlon, J. (2007). Polypharmacy in elderly patients. *American Journal of Geriatric Pharmacotherapy, 5*(4), 345–351.

Hodge, D., Bonifas, R., & Chou, R. (2010). Spirituality and older adults: Ethical guidelines to enhance service provision. *Advances in Social Work, 11*(1), 1–16.

Horgas, A. (2012). Assessing pain in older adults with dementia. *Best Practices in Nursing Care to Older Adults.* Available at http://consultgerirn.org/topics/pain/want_to_know_more

Kaiser, A. P., Schuster, J. W., Potter, C., Moye, J., & Davison, E. (2013). Posttraumatic stress symptoms among older adults: A review. Available at http://www.adaa.org/living-with-anxiety/older-adults

Kao, H., Travis, S., & Acton, G. (2004). Relocation to a long-term care facility: Working with patients and families before, during, and after. *Journal of Psychosocial Nursing, 42*(3), 10–16.

Melillo, K. D., & Houde, S. C. (2011). *Geropsychiatric and Mental Health Nursing* (2nd ed.). Sudbury, MA: Jones & Bartlett.

Meyer, G., Kopke, S., Haastert, B., & Muhlhauser, I. (2009). Restraint use among nursing home residents: Cross-sectional study and prospective cohort study. *Journal of Clinical Nursing, 18*(7), 981–990.

Mohler, R., Richter, T., Kopke, S., & Meyer, G. (2012). Interventions for preventing and reducing the use of physical restraints in long term geriatric care: A Cochrane review. *Journal of Clinical Nursing, 21,* 3070–3081.

National Institute on Deafness and Other Communication Disorders, National Institutes of Health. (2010). *Quick Statistics.* Available at http://www.nidcd.nih.gov/health/statistics/Pages/quick.aspx

National Institute of Neurological Disorders and Stroke. (2013). *Alzheimer's disease related dementias: Research challenges and opportunities.* Available at http://www.ninds.nih.gov/disorders/dementias/dementia.htm

Neimeyer, R., Currier, J., Coleman, R., Tomer, A., & Samuel, E. (2011). Confronting suffering and death at the end of life: The impact of religiosity, psychosocial factors, and life regret among hospice patients. *Death Studies, 35*(9), 777–800.

Nelson, H. D., Nygren, P., McInerney, Y., & Klein, J. (2004). *Screening Women and Elderly Adults for Family and Intimate Partner Violence: A Review of the Evidence for the U.S. Preventive Services Task Force.* (Originally in *Annals of Internal Medicine, 140*(5), 387–396.) Rockville, MD: Agency for Healthcare Research and Quality. Available at https://www.pmrts.samhsa.gov/Prev-Courses/ViewFile.aspx?filename

Newport, F. (2006). *Religion most important to Blacks, women, and older Americans.* Available at http://www.gallup.com/poll/25585/religion-most-important-blacks-women-older-americans.aspx

New York State Office for the Aging. (2009). *Sustaining informal caregivers: New York state caregiver support programs participants survey.* Available at http://www.aging.ny.gov/ReportsAndData/CaregiverReports/index.cfm

North, M., & Fiske, S. (2012). An inconvenienced youth? Ageism and its potential intergenerational roots. *Psychological Bulletin, 138*(5), 982–997.

Pautex, S., & Gold, G. (2006). Assessing pain intensity in older adults. *Geriatrics and Aging 9*(6), 399–402.

Phelan, A. (2011). Socially constructing older people: Examining discourses which can shape nurses' understanding and practice. *Journal of Advanced Nursing, 67*(4), 893–903.

Pisani, L., & Walsh, C. (2012). Screening for elder abuse in hospitalized older adults with dementia. *Journal of Elder Abuse and Neglect, 24*(3), 195–215.

Potter, M. L. (2012). Grieving and suffering. In K. O. Perrin, C. A. Sheehan, M. L. Potter, & M. K. Kazanowski, (Eds.). *Palliative Care Nursing: Caring for Suffering Patients.* Sudbury, MA: Jones and Bartlett Learning, pp. 53–76.

Registered Nurses' Association of Ontario. (n.d.). Best Practices Toolkit. *Recognizing Delirium, Depression, and Dementia (3D's) Comparison Chart.* Available at http://ltctoolkit.rnao.ca/sites/ltc/files/resources/3Ds/EducationResources/3DComparisonFinal.pdf

Ruiz, J., Sui, X., Lobelo, F., Morrow, J., Jackson, A., Sjostrom, M., & Blair, S. (2008). Association between muscular strength and mortality in men: Prospective cohort study. *British Medical Journal, 337*(7661), 92–95.

Sadock, B. J., & Sadock, V. A. (2007). *Kaplan & Sadock's Synopsis of Psychiatry* (10th ed.) Philadelphia, PA: Lippincott Williams & Wilkins.

Sheikh, J. I., Yesavage, J. A., Brooks, J. O. III, Friedman, L. F., Gratzinger, P., Hill, R. D., et al. (1991). Proposed factor structure of the Geriatric Depression Scale. *International Psychogeriatrics 3,* 23–28.

Somes, J., Donatelli, N., & Barrett, J. (2010). Sudden confusion and agitation: Causes to investigate! Delirium, dementia, depression. *Journal of Emergency Nursing, 36,* 486–488.

Stahl, S. (2009). *The Prescriber's Guide: Stahl's Essential Psychopharmacology.* New York, NY: Cambridge University Press.

Substance Abuse and Mental Health Services Administration (SAMHSA). (2003a). Seclusion and restraint: Breaking the bonds. *SAMHSA News.* Available at http://www.samhsa.gov/samhsa_news/VolumeXI_2/text_only/article6txt.htm

Substance Abuse and Mental Health Services Administration (SAMHSA) (2003b). *Seclusion and restraint.* Available at http://www.samhsa.gov/seclusion/sr_handout.aspx

U.S. Census Bureau. (2011.) *Current Population Survey, Annual Social and Economic Supplement.* Available at http://www.census.gov/population/age/data/2011.html

U.S. Department of Health and Human Services (DHHS), National Center for Health Statistics. (2006). *Chartbook on Trends in the Health of Americans 2006, Special Feature: Pain.* Available at http://www.cdc.gov/nchs/data/hus/hus06.pdf

U.S. Department of Health and Human Services (DHHS). (2010). *Multiple chronic conditions: A strategic framework: optimum health and quality of life for individuals with multiple chronic conditions.* Available at http://www.hhs.gov/ash/initiatives/mcc/mcc_framework.pdf

Victoria Hospice Bereavement Services. (n.d.). *Difficult grief and multiple losses.* Available at http://www.victoriahospice.org/sites/default/files/imce/VicHospDifficultGrief.pdf

Walker, C., Curry, L., & Hogstel, M. (2007). Relocation stress syndrome in older adults transitioning from home to a long-term care facility: Myth or reality? *Journal of Psychosocial Nursing, 45*(1), 38–45.

Werner, C. (2011). *The older population: 2010.* Available at http://www.census.gov/prod/cen2010/briefs/c2010br-09.pdf

Wilson, B. A., Shannon, M. T., & Shields, K. M. (2012). *Pearson Nurse's Drug Guide 2012.* Upper Saddle River, NJ: Pearson Education.

World Health Organization (WHO). (2014). Definition of an older or elderly person. Retrieved from: http://www.who.int/healthinfo/survey/ageingdefnolder/en/

Yaffe, M., & Tazkarji, B. (2012). Understanding elder abuse in family practice. *Canadian Family Physician, 58,* 1336–1340.

Zarit, S. H., Reever, K. E., & Bach-Peterson, J. (1980). Relatives of the impaired elderly: Correlates of feelings of burden. *Gerontologist, 20*(6), 649–655.

Zieve, D., & Eltz, D. R. (2012). *Urinary tract infection—adults.* Available at http://www.nlm.nih.gov/medlineplus/ency/article/000521.htm

WELLNESS DOMAINS: A QUICK GUIDE FOR PATIENTS

Health (ENERGIES)

Exercise: The goal is one consecutive hour of exercise a day. Build up gradually rather than getting too tired and giving up.

Nutrition: Maintain nutritional balance. Eat fruits and vegetables each day. Eliminate aspartame and monosodium glutamate from the foods and beverages you consume.

Each body system in balance: Do not overdo in one area and forget about the others.

Rest: Balance a healthy sleep/wake cycle in daily activities. The body repairs itself better if you are asleep by 11:00 pm.

Good Health Habits: Eliminate caffeine, alcohol, street drugs, nicotine, and nitrates. Decrease fat intake to less than 30% of daily intake.

Information Processing: Validate all information you receive. Use strategies to improve memory and problem solving.

Endocrine/Immune system: Avoid contact with infectious disease. Seek medical attention for infections. Seek medical attention for endocrine and immune system disorders. Know what your thyroid levels and blood glucose levels are.

Sensory Function: Obtain needed help such as reading glasses, contacts, hearing aids, and learn to compensate for difficulties.

Attitudes/Behavior (EMPOWERS)

Enjoy Life: Find something to do each day that brings pleasure, i.e., view the sunset, read, listen to music.

Manage Wellness: Learning how to care for and manage your disorders in ways that decrease interference with life.

Pain/Pleasure: Allow self to feel both physical and emotional pain and pleasure. Pain is a warning signal that needs a response.

Outlook: Focus on the positive aspects of life rather than feel self pity. Life is hard. Enjoy the progress you make as it occurs.

Worthwhile: Seek those things about you that are worthwhile

Elect to love: Love others and self. Learn to express your love in appropriate ways.

Responsible For Own Behavior: Obey the four no harm rules—No harm to self, others, animals, or property.

Success Takes Action: Make step wise plans for success and do them in small increments.

Environment/Interpersonal Relationships (SERVICES)

School/Work: Learn new skills and information to help preserve and increase brain function. Feeling *pressure to perform* will decrease your ability to function.

Enjoy nature: Do things that will help health in general and stimulate brain function.

Resources/residence: Find a suitable place to live. Learn to access resources important to wellness.

Value life skills: Appreciate the skills you have and identify new ones to learn. What we learn depends on what we value.

Interpersonal. relationships: Establish relationships with people who are positive, limit contact with negative people. Do not harm others or allow others to harm you.

Communication skills: Learn to negotiate, to ask for clarification, and correct misunderstandings. Learn to process sensory information to determine if a situation is dangerous or not.

Economics: Obtain resources to insure having income for basic necessities.

Service: Obtain appropriate services for needs and give service to others.

Spiritual (PEACEFUL)

Positive attitude: Try to find the positive in every life situation.

Embrace truth: Seek after and use truth to improve your life.

Accept forgiveness: Learn to give and accept forgiveness.

Clarify values: Identify what is important to you in life. Change your social group if their values are different from yours.

Express gratitude: Tell others thank-you for what they do for you. Do something nice for someone each day in gratitude for that person.

Friendship with self and others: Spend time meditating on what motivates you and what causes you to feel good about yourself and others.

Understanding heart: Try to understand and appreciate others instead of being judgmental.

Learn to develop insight: Keep a journal about what you learn about yourself each day.

Cultural (CULTURES)

Customs and actions: Share the traditions and activities of your cultural group with your health care provider. Maintain your family traditions.

Understand speech and communication: If you do not speak or understand English, seek a clinic that provides translators. Enroll in a class to learn English as a second language.

Language: Tell your health care provider that you can't understand what is being said or explained. Ask for instructions that use pictures.

Thoughts and beliefs: Share your thoughts and beliefs when they are different from the new culture. Seek understanding of the new cultural beliefs you are learning.

Understand values: Do not be afraid to discuss values that are different from the dominant culture. Ask others to help you understand the different values that you are observing.

Race and religion: Find a religious group that is compatible with your beliefs and practices.

Ethnicity: Join a group that shares your ethnic beliefs and practices.

Social groupings: Go to various neighborhood activities that are culturally compatible with experiences that you are familiar with.

NANDA-APPROVED NURSING DIAGNOSES 2015–2017

Activity, Deficient Diversional

Activity Intolerance

Activity Intolerance, Risk for

Activity Planning, Ineffective

Activity Planning, Risk for Ineffective

Adaptive Capacity: Intracranial, Decreased

Adverse Reaction to Iodinated Contrast Media, Risk for

Airway Clearance, Ineffective

Allergy Response, Risk for

Allergy Response, Latex

Allergy Response, Latex, Risk for

Anxiety

Anxiety, Death

Aspiration, Risk for

Attachment, Risk for Impaired

Bleeding, Risk for

Blood Glucose Level, Risk for Unstable

Body Image, Disturbed

Body Temperature: Imbalanced, Risk for

Bowel Incontinence

Breast Milk, Insufficient

Breastfeeding, Ineffective

Breastfeeding, Interrupted

Breastfeeding, Readiness for Enhanced

Breathing Pattern, Ineffective

Cardiac Output, Decreased

Cardiac Output, Decreased, Risk for

Cardiovascular Function, Impaired, Risk for

Caregiver Role Strain

Caregiver Role Strain, Risk for

Childbearing Process, Ineffective

Childbearing Process, Readiness for Enhanced

Childbearing Process, Risk for Ineffective

Chronic Pain Syndrome

Comfort, Impaired

Comfort, Readiness for Enhanced

Communication, Readiness for Enhanced

Communication: Verbal, Impaired

Confusion, Acute

Confusion, Chronic

Confusion, Risk for Acute

Constipation

Constipation, Perceived

Constipation, Risk for

Contamination

Contamination, Risk for

Coping: Community, Ineffective

Coping: Community, Readiness for Enhanced

Coping, Defensive

Coping: Family, Compromised

Coping: Family, Disabled

Coping: Family, Readiness for Enhanced

Coping: Readiness for Enhanced

Coping, Ineffective

Corneal Injury, Risk for

Decision Making, Readiness for Enhanced

Decisional Conflict (Specify)

Denial, Ineffective

Dentition, Impaired

Development: Delayed, Risk for

Diarrhea

Disuse Syndrome, Risk for

Dry Eye, Risk for

Dysreflexia, Autonomic

Dysreflexia, Autonomic, Risk for

Electrolyte Imbalance, Risk for

Emancipated Decision-Making, Impaired

Emancipated Decision-Making, Impaired, Risk for

Emancipated Decision-Making, Readiness for Enhanced

Emotional Control, Labile

Falls, Risk for

Family Processes, Dysfunctional

Family Processes, Interrupted

Family Processes, Readiness for Enhanced

Fatigue

Fear

Fluid Balance, Readiness for Enhanced

Fluid Volume: Deficient

Fluid Volume: Deficient, Risk for

Fluid Volume: Excess

Fluid Volume: Imbalanced, Risk for

Frail Elderly Syndrome

Frail Elderly Syndrome, Risk for

Functional Constipation, Chronic

Gas Exchange, Impaired

Gastrointestinal Motility, Risk for Dysfunctional

Gastrointestinal Motility, Dysfunctional

Grieving

Grieving, Complicated

Grieving, Risk for Complicated

Growth: Disproportionate, Risk for

Health: Community, Deficient

Health Behavior, Risk-Prone

Health Maintenance, Ineffective

Health Management, Family, Ineffective

Health Management, Ineffective

Health Management, Readiness for Enhanced

Home Maintenance, Impaired

Hope, Readiness for Enhanced

Hopelessness

Human Dignity, Risk for Compromised

Hyperthermia

Hypothermia

Hypothermia, Risk for

Impulse Control, Ineffective

Infant Behavior: Disorganized

Infant Behavior: Disorganized, Risk for

Infant Behavior: Organized, Readiness for Enhanced

Infant Feeding Pattern, Ineffective

Infection, Risk for

Injury, Risk for

Insomnia

Jaundice, Neonatal

Jaundice, Neonatal, Risk for

Knowledge, Deficient

Knowledge, Readiness for Enhanced

Labor Pain

Lifestyle, Sedentary

Liver Function, Risk for Impaired

Loneliness, Risk for

Maternal/Fetal Dyad, Risk for Disturbed

Memory, Impaired

Mobility: Bed, Impaired

Mobility: Physical, Impaired

Mobility: Wheelchair, Impaired

Mood Regulation, Impaired

Moral Distress

Nausea

Neglect, Unilateral

Neurovascular Dysfunction: Peripheral, Risk for

Noncompliance

Nutrition, Imbalanced: Less than Body Requirements

Nutrition, Readiness for Enhanced

Mucous Membrane: Oral, Impaired

Mucus Membrane: Oral, Impaired, Risk for

Obesity

Overweight

Overweight, Risk for

Pain, Acute

Pain, Chronic

Parenting, Impaired

Parenting, Readiness for Enhanced

Parenting, Risk for Impaired

Perfusion: Gastrointestinal, Risk for Ineffective

Perfusion: Renal, Risk for Ineffective

Perioperative Hypothermia, Risk for

Perioperative Positioning Injury, Risk for

Personal Identity: Disturbed

Personal Identity: Disturbed, Risk for

Poisoning, Risk for

Post-Trauma Syndrome

Post-Trauma Syndrome, Risk for

Power, Readiness for Enhanced

Powerlessness

Powerlessness, Risk for

Pressure Ulcer, Risk for

Protection, Ineffective

Rape-Trauma Syndrome

Relationship, Ineffective

Relationship, Risk for Ineffective

Relationship, Readiness for Enhanced

Religiosity, Impaired

Religiosity, Readiness for Enhanced

Religiosity, Risk for Impaired

Relocation Stress Syndrome

Relocation Stress Syndrome, Risk for

Resilience, Impaired

Resilience, Readiness for Enhanced

Resilience, Risk for Impaired

Role Conflict, Parental

Role Performance, Ineffective

Self-care, Readiness for Enhanced

Self-care Deficit: Bathing

Self-care Deficit: Dressing

Self-care Deficit: Feeding

Self-care Deficit: Toileting

Self-Concept, Readiness for Enhanced

Self-Esteem, Chronic Low

Self-Esteem, Chronic Low, Risk for

Self-Esteem, Situational Low

Self-Esteem, Situational Low, Risk for

Self-Mutilation

Self-Mutilation, Risk for

Self Neglect

Sexual Dysfunction

Sexuality Pattern, Ineffective

Shock, Risk for

Sitting, Impaired

Skin Integrity, Impaired

Skin Integrity, Risk for Impaired

Sleep Deprivation

Sleep Pattern, Disturbed

Sleep, Readiness for Enhanced

Social Interaction, Impaired

Social Isolation

Sorrow, Chronic

Spiritual Distress

Spiritual Distress, Risk for

Spiritual Well-Being, Readiness for Enhanced

Standing, Impaired

Sudden Infant Death Syndrome, Risk for

Stress Overload

Suffocation, Risk for

Suicide, Risk for

Surgical Recovery, Delayed

Surgical Recovery, Delayed, Risk for

Swallowing, Impaired

Thermal Injury, Risk for

Thermoregulation, Ineffective

Tissue Integrity, Impaired

Tissue Integrity, Impaired, Risk for

Tissue Perfusion: Cardiac, Risk for Decreased

Tissue Perfusion: Cerebral, Risk for Ineffective

Tissue Perfusion: Peripheral, Ineffective

Tissue Perfusion: Peripheral, Risk for Ineffective

Transfer Ability, Impaired

Trauma, Risk for

Trauma: Vascular, Risk for

Urinary Elimination, Impaired

Urinary Elimination, Readiness for Enhanced

Urinary Incontinence, Functional

Urinary Incontinence, Overflow

Urinary Incontinence, Reflex

Urinary Incontinence, Stress

Urinary Incontinence, Urge

Urinary Incontinence, Urge, Risk for

Urinary Retention

Urinary Tract Injury, Risk for

Ventilation: Spontaneous, Impaired

Ventilatory Weaning Response, Dysfunctional

Violence: Other-Directed, Risk for

Violence: Self-Directed, Risk for

Walking, Impaired

Wandering

GLOSSARY

abstinence Refraining from use of drugs, alcohol, or other substances of addiction.

accommodation Changing schemas to meet life realities.

acetylcholine A neurotransmitter essential to memory, concentration, and attention.

acquaintance rape Forcible sexual intercourse committed by someone the victim knows.

active listening Carefully attending to the patient during an interaction, including being alert to patient cues and demonstrating interest in what the patient communicates, both verbally and nonverbally.

actualization Establishing desired life goals and actually engaging in goal-directed activities that were common pre-illness.

acupuncture A traditional Eastern practice involving stimulation of specific points on the body and using a variety of techniques to restore balance and maintain health.

adaptation The modification of behaviors to meet environmental needs.

addiction The repetitive use of a substance despite negative consequences to the user.

addictive disorder A clinical problem of addiction, including specific symptoms, which can be identified as a specific disorder.

advance directive A legal document that specifies health care instructions or identifies a proxy (surrogate decision maker) for making health care decisions.

adventitious crisis A type of **crisis** that may arise from traumatic events that are well beyond the expected scope of normal human experience, such as violent crime, natural disasters, war, and terrorism.

adverse effects Uncomfortable, harmful, unexpected, or emergent reactions to a drug.

affinity The strength of interest or attraction a drug has for a particular receptor.

ageism Negative stereotyping of or discrimination against older adults.

aggression Any type of behavior intended to intimidate, harm, or injure another.

agonist A drug that combines with a specific receptor to initiate the same reaction as that of a naturally occurring substance.

agnosia Difficulty recognizing familiar objects.

agoraphobia Significant fear or anxiety about situations from which escape could be difficult or help not immediately accessible, leading to avoidance or enduring with distress.

akathisia Sensations of restlessness, pacing, and an inability to sit still.

alexithymia The inability to label feelings with words.

allopathic medicine Conventional, or traditional, medicine.

alternative medicine The use of herbs, supplements, or various therapies in place of traditional medicine.

Alzheimer disease A neurocognitive disorder characterized by progressive dementia leading to inability to maintain activities of daily living, recognize familiar individuals and surroundings, and inevitable loss of functions leading to death; the most common form of dementia.

ambiguous loss Loss associated with uncertain circumstances that result in confusion for those experiencing the loss (e.g., parents whose child is missing may experience ambiguous loss while not knowing whether the child will return).

amnesia Loss of recent or remote memory.

amnestic disorder A type of neurocognitive disorder characterized by the inability to learn new information and the inability to retrieve information previously learned.

anal stage One of the stages of psychosexual development proposed by Freud, encompassing ages 18 months to three years and involving the anus, rectum, and bladder zones.

anhedonia Loss of interest or pleasure in nearly all activities.

anorexia nervosa A **feeding and eating disorder** that is characterized by unrelenting fear of weight gain in association with extreme distortions of body image, preoccupation with food, and refusal to eat in pursuit of thinness.

antagonist A drug that combines with a specific receptor to inhibit or block a biochemical response.

anticipatory grief Grief that occurs in anticipation of impending loss.

anxiety A generally normal, healthy response to stress that may present as unidentified worry that may or may not relate to a specific circumstance; may exhibit as feelings of apprehension, as an initial response to threat, or as feelings of uneasiness and dread; may also occur as a response to a specific stressor.

anxiety disorders Disorders of mental health characterized by psychological (fear, anxiety) and somatic (e.g., panic attacks) manifestations of anxiety.

aphasia Difficulty or loss of ability to express or understand speech.

apraxia Loss or impairment of purposeful movement.

assault The threat of harm from unauthorized touching.

assertive community treatment (ACT) An evidence-based practice that provides intensive community support to individuals in recovery from mental illness.

assessment The first step of the nursing process, involving the collection of information about the patient across the wellness domains that includes, but is not limited to, data gained through observation, patient interviews, and assessment tools such as vital signs measurements and mental status examinations.

assimilation Taking new information and interpreting it to conform to already existing information.

asterognosis The inability to recognize objects by touch.

asylum Historically, a point of residential care for those with mental illness, particularly patients who exhibited violence.

attachment A concept of child development that describes the desire of the individual to be with an attachment figure; the need to seek comfort and safety from the attachment figure; and the use of the attachment figure as a secure base from which to explore the world.

attention-deficit/hyperactivity disorder The most common psychiatric disorder of childhood and adolescence, characterized by symptoms of inattention, hyperactivity, and impulsivity.

authenticity The nurse's awareness of genuine personality, character, and values, as well as the nurse's demonstrated behavior that is consistent with that awareness despite pressures to behave otherwise.

automatic obedience An exaggerated, robotic cooperation with requests.

autonomy An individual's right to self-determination; the right of patients to make their own decisions about their care consistent with their personal values.

avoidant/restrictive food intake disorder A lack of interest in food and eating food (when food is available) as supported by weight loss and nutritional deficiencies.

avolition Lack of motivation.

axon A separate structure of the neuron that is composed of white matter; the main signal conducting unit of the neuron cell, whose responsibility is to transmit information away from the cell body.

battery Unlawfully touching another individual.

behavior modification A technique that can be used to facilitate changes in an individual's behavior patterns—for example, adding something desired to encourage positive behavior.

behavioral theory Theory that focuses on elements that reinforce and maintain maladaptive behaviors.

beneficence The nurse's moral obligation to do good.

bereavement The period of acute sadness or suffering following a loss.

binge drinking The consumption of five or more drinks for men or four or more drinks for women within a 2-hour period.

binge-eating disorder A **feeding and eating disorder** characterized by recurrent episodes of binge eating in the absence of extreme weight-control behavior accompanied by a sense of lack of control.

biofeedback A technique that uses instruments that measure body function and provide sensory feedback (e.g., blood pressure, heart rate) to train patients to control certain bodily functions voluntarily

blood–brain barrier (BBB) A three-wall barrier that serves to isolate brain circulation from systemic circulation and governs the quality of and rapidity with which substances in the blood penetrate into the brain.

body dysmorphic disorder (BDD) Repetitive behaviors or mental acts in response to preoccupation with perceived deficits or flaws in physical appearance that are not observable or appear slight to others.

body image An aspect of **self-concept**, how an individual views his or her own body in relation to one's own perceptions of what is beautiful as well as in relation to how the individual views others' perceptions.

body mass index (BMI) Measurement of body fat based on comparison of weight to height.

body space The amount of distance that provides a sense of comfort in social situations.

boundary crossings Decisions to deviate from a boundary for a therapeutic purpose, such as appointment changes, disclosing personal bits of information, or exchanging small gifts.

boundary violations Decisions to deviate from a boundary for a purpose that is other than therapeutic; this might include holding dual roles with a patient, inappropriate self-disclosure or touching, or sexual misconduct.

bracket A technique nurses use to acknowledge a feeling or reaction that is occurring and to set aside the reaction for examination and reflection on how it might be interfering with the actual relationship developed with the patient.

bulimia nervosa A **feeding and eating disorder** that is characterized by repeated binge-eating episodes and inappropriate compensatory behaviors (e.g., food restriction, dieting, and repeated episodes of binging and purging) aimed at controlling weight gain.

bullying Repeated events or a pattern of behavior involving abuse or misuse of power.

burnout A state of physical and emotional exhaustion that nurses experience during times of unrelenting stress when they fail to or are unable to renew and conserve energy.

cachexia Muscle wasting associated with severe illness.

caregiver burden The extent to which caregivers feel that their emotional or physical health, social life, and financial status are suffering as a result of caring for their relatives.

case management The process of accessing, coordinating, and ensuring the receipt of services for individuals with mental illness to meet their complex needs in an effective and efficient manner.

catatonia The total absence of movement—the individual's muscles are waxy and semi-rigid; mutism, negativism, echolalia, or echopraxia may be present in individuals experiencing catatonia.

centering A technique that involves attending to the events of the day and identifying the feelings associated with them; it allows nurses to acknowledge their feelings and set them aside to concentrate on the work of patient care.

central nervous system (CNS) System consisting of the brain and spinal cord, responsible for integrating, processing, and coordinating sensory data and motor commands; decides how to respond to what happens in the world based on the information that is provided by the **peripheral nervous system** (PNS) and further relies on the PNS to send appropriate responses to the various parts of the body.

cerebrum The largest portion of the brain, controlling intelligence, motor, and sensory functions.

chemical restraint The use of medications to subdue or restrain a patient

child abuse Physical assault or violence, mental abuse (including intimidation and verbal threats), or sexual abuse perpetrated against a child or adolescent

cholinesterase inhibitors (ChEIs) Neurotransmitters that act by slowing the degradation of acetylcholine, thereby increasing concentration of the neurotransmitter in the cerebral cortex.

chronic sorrow Sorrow or grief that is ongoing rather than acute.

circadian rhythm Biochemical, physiological, and behavioral processes that are driven endogenously, spanning a 24-hour cycle.

classic neurotransmission The fastest and most predominant method of neurotransmission; in classic neurotransmission, signals travel from one neuron directly to the next neuron.

classical response A conditioned response to a recurrent stimulus.

Code of Ethics for Nurses Developed by the ANA, a code that mandates every professional nurse's obligations and commitment to society.

codependency Phenomenon that occurs when family members fail to address the behavior of a family member who is using substances.

coercion, or undue influence The power of one person to affect the decision of another; includes persuasion and manipulation.

cognition (or thought) The complex process of creating order and meaning from experiences; describes a relatively high level of intellectual processing in which perceptions and information are acquired, used, or manipulated.

cognitive–behavioral therapy (CBT) One of the most effective psychotherapies; may be used to treat a wide variety of mental disorders.

collaboration skills Skills for working with and alongside other professionals that include the ability to form interpersonal relationships and foster effective communication, to use formal and informal power to gain access to information, and to support and opportunities for professional growth and development.

co-morbidity A coexisting or co-occurring medical condition.

compassion fatigue A sense of exhaustion that can develop secondary to providing clinical crisis care repetitively over long periods of time.

compassion satisfaction A sense of fulfillment, value, and joy derived from helping others.

complementary and alternative medicine A group of diverse medical and health care systems, practices, and products that are not generally considered part of **allopathic,** or conventional, medicine.

complementary health approaches *See* complementary and alternative medicine.

complementary medicine The use of herbs, supplements, and/or mind–body therapies in conjunction with conventional medicine.

complicated grief Grief that is intense, lasts at least 6 months, does not seem to lessen over time, and is accompanied by prolonged feelings of worthlessness, emptiness, or meaninglessness.

compromise A balance between unattractive alternatives.

compulsions Repetitive behaviors or mental acts that the individual feels driven to perform in response to an obsession or according to rules that must be applied rigidly.

compulsivity The reinitiation of habitual acts that continue despite the potential for adverse consequences.

conduct disorder A relatively persistent pattern of multiple antisocial behaviors during childhood and adolescence, including fighting, bullying, stealing, vandalism, and lying for personal gain.

confabulation The creation of imaginary events to fill in memory gaps.

confidentiality The obligation not to disclose private information.

conversion disorder (functional neurological symptom disorder) A somatic-related disorder in which patients experience one or more changes in the performance of a voluntary motor or sensory function; patients with symptoms of abnormal voluntary motor function may present with a weakness or a paralysis, abnormal movements, and abnormal extremity functioning or positions.

countertransference Phenomenon that occurs when the nurse attributes feelings regarding someone within the nurse's life to the patient and responds unconsciously based on these feelings.

craving A compelling desire for previously experienced positive or euphoric effects of a psychoactive substance; can increase in the presence of both internal and external cues (e.g., stressors), particularly with perceived substance availability.

crisis A state of disequilibrium having three characteristics: (1) a perceived threat or danger; (2) an imbalance or disturbance in psychological functioning; and (3) no ready or feasible solution.

critical incident Any sudden, unexpected event that has an emotional impact sufficient to overwhelm the usual effective coping skills of an individual or group.

cultural awareness The nurse's self-examination and continual reflection on his or her own roots, biases, and prejudices.

cultural competence The capacity to function effectively as an individual and an organization within the context of the cultural beliefs, behaviors, and needs of consumers and communities.

cultural desire A personal motivation to be culturally competent and not just meet some external requirement.

cultural encounters Conversations and exchanges with individuals of other cultures that help nurses validate and refine their own beliefs and values about other cultures.

cultural humility The ability to recognize the limitations of one's own culture and be motivated to learn about other cultures.

cultural knowledge Information about other cultures and ethnic groups.

cultural pain Incongruence between the patient's cultural needs and the nurse's inappropriate response or lack of response.

cultural skill The ability to assess others and provide care that incorporates cultural knowledge.

culture The set of distinctive, spiritual, material, intellectual, and emotional features of society or a social group; encompasses art and literature, lifestyles, ways of living together, value systems, traditions, and beliefs.

culture-bound syndromes Disorders found among specific cultural groups that typically are seen only in individuals from that culture.

curative point The point of view that a patient can be treated as if he or she can be cured (as opposed to palliative care).

cyberbullying Bullying via text messaging or the Internet.

cytochrome P450 system System that contains metabolic liver enzymes that greatly influence how the body responds to medication, medication sensitivity, drug–drug or drug–food interaction, and how much of a medication the body receives.

defense mechanisms Strategies used by the individual when experiencing a threat to the ego that the ego cannot handle through regular problem-solving strategies.

delayed grief Grief that occurs months or years after a loss; feelings may be as intense as if the loss has just happened.

delirium A typically abrupt, short-term change in mental state marked by confused thinking, disorientation, perceptual disturbances, agitation, and mood swings; results from an underlying medical condition, substance intoxication or withdrawal, exposure to a toxin, or other etiology.

delirium tremens Temporary visual, auditory, or tactile hallucinations characteristic of abrupt withdrawal from alcohol, typically developing 48 to 72 hours after withdrawal begins.

delusions False beliefs based on incorrect inference or perception.

dementia A progressive disorder characterized by gradual loss of cognitive functioning (including memory, language, and executive function).

denial A behavior often seen in patients with substance abuse in which the patient denies use of any substance or problems/consequences associated with it.

deontology Ethical behavior characterized by unchanging, self-evident moral duty; "rule-based" ethics.

dependence The body's physical need for a specific substance; cessation (abruptly stopping) use of a substance can result in specific withdrawal syndrome.

depersonalization The experience of unreality or detachment from the individual's mind, sense of self, and/or physical body.

depression Clinical depression involves a change from previous functioning and involves five or more symptoms listed in DSM-5 that last for 2 or more weeks.

derealization The experience of unreality or detachment from the person's surroundings.

designer drugs Synthetic substances that are considered extremely dangerous to physical, as well as mental, health.

detoxification The process of safely and effectively withdrawing an individual from an addictive substance.

dialectical behavior therapy (DBT) A form of cognitive–behavioral therapy introduced by Marsha Linehan that employs a unique blend of psychotherapy and skills training; instead of the change focus of cognitive–behavioral therapy, DBT stresses a balance of acceptance and change that is derived from the mindfulness and judgment avoidance of Zen meditation.

diathesis–stress model Theory that individuals inherit tendencies to express certain traits or behaviors when exposed to the right conditions or stressors.

disaster plan A community-wide effort to respond to a crisis or disaster with the goals of caring for those who need treatment and restoring a sense of normalcy and well-being to the community as soon as possible.

disenfranchised grief Grief that occurs when individuals hide grief following a loss to which some sort of stigma is or may be attached (e.g., drunk driving accident, abortion).

disequilibrium Physical and/or emotional symptoms that occur when an individual's coping response is insufficient to meet stress or demand.

disruptive mood dysregulation disorder Disorder characterized by recurrent, frequent outbursts inconsistent with a child's developmental level and occurring for a year or more; may be diagnosed only if other disorders (e.g., PTSD) do not better explain the symptoms and presentation.

dissociation Disruption and/or discontinuity of the individual's normal sense of memory, emotions, perception, motor control, behavior, and sense of identity. Patients have described dissociation as a sense of the body being present with an absent mind. This disruption causes difficulty in day-to-day functioning.

dissociative fugues Episodes of travel with no memory of how the individual reached the location.

dissociative identity disorder (DID) Disorder that may occur in individuals who have sustained horrific physical and psychological abuse over time—usually in early childhood—that is characterized by dissociation from the trauma, which may result in a fragmented personality. The dissociated fragment of memory may be identified with a personality and may be labeled with a name or act in a different manner than the individual's usual behavior.

distress An individual's response to anxiety-provoking circumstances that results in unmet needs.

domains Areas of wellness (biological, psychological, sociological, cultural, and spiritual) that affect an individual's ability to respond to stressors and achieve quality of life.

drug abuse The use of illicit drugs or the abuse of prescription or over-the-counter drugs for purposes other than those for which they are indicated or in a manner or in quantities other than directed.

duty to warn Duty of a clinician to warn an individual of foreseeable harm when a patient threatens the safety of that individual.

dysphoric mood An unpleasant mood state, such as sadness, anxiety, or irritability.

dystonia Spastic contractions of muscle groups.

echolalia The repetition of words spoken by another.

echopraxia The compulsive imitation of another's actions.

efficacy The ability of a drug to produce the desired response.

ego One of three states of being posited by Freud, serving as the referee between the **id** and the **superego**.

ego dystonic Aspects of an individual's thoughts and behaviors that are incongruent or uncomfortable with the individual's sense or idea of self.

ego syntonic Aspects of an individual's thoughts or behaviors that are congruent or comfortable with the individual's sense or idea of self.

elder abuse The physical, emotional, sexual, or financial abuse of an older adult; neglect also is a form of elder abuse.

electroconvulsive therapy (ECT) Unilateral or bilateral electrical stimulation under general anesthesia for a total of 6 to 12 treatments; commonly used for individuals with severe mood disorders, including severe mania, for both acute treatment and maintenance treatment.

emotional dysregulation Emotional responses that fall outside the realm of accepted responses or are out of control.

emotional intelligence A measurement of interpersonal phenomena that includes accurate, conscious perception and monitoring of one's own emotions and modification of those emotions into appropriate expression; includes the ability to manage one's own anxiety and sustain hope in the face of adversity.

emotional regulation Ability to regulate or control emotions and the expression of emotions.

empathy Understanding and experiencing the feelings, thoughts, and experience of another from the other's perspective—feeling what the other person is feeling.

empowered nurses Nurses who experience full empowerment in the workplace, including experiencing congruence between their own values and the requirements of their role and having a sense of being able to influence patient outcomes and provide optimal patient care.

empowerment Individuals' power in relationship to their position in the organization.

enabling Family members engaging in behaviors that support the continued use or abuse of substances by another family member.

enacted stigma Actual discrimination or mistreatment related to having a stigmatizing condition.

endophenotype A genetic concept that takes into consideration the complexity, heterogeneity, and multigenetic disorders that make up psychiatric illnesses.

equilibrium The balance between taking in new information (assimilation) and changing schemas to meet life reality (accommodation).

ethical dilemma Circumstance in which moral obligations demand or appear to demand that a person adopt each of two (or more) alternative but incompatible actions, such that the person cannot perform all the required actions.

ethics Moral tenets that characterize conduct as right or wrong and reflects individual or societal values.

ethics of care Identifying empathy and emotional connectedness as dictating moral behavior.

ethnicity Description of how a group of people share common characteristics such as race, nationality, religion, language, and cultural heritage.

euthymic mood A mood in the "normal" range.

evaluation Process by which the nurse determines progress that has been made relevant to the plan of care.

excessive daytime sleepiness Inability to maintain wakefulness during the day; a score greater than 10 on the Epworth Sleepiness Scale.

executive functioning The ability to order sequential behaviors, establish goal-directed plans, and monitor personal behavior.

external locus of control The attribution of control of control of one's life to other people and on circumstances outside the self.

extrapyramidal side effects (EPS) Common side effects in patients treated with antipsychotic medications: Acute EPSs include medication-induced Parkinsonism (e.g., muscle rigidity, tremors), dystonia, akathisia, and neuroleptic malignant syndrome. These side effects are dose dependent and reversible if medication is reduced or discontinued. The primary chronic EPS is tardive dyskinesia (TD), which occurs after months or years of medication exposure and may be irreversible.

factitious disorder Disorder that may be diagnosed when the clinician can demonstrate that the individual is taking steps to fabricate an illness.

false imprisonment Unlawful confinement of a patient against his or her will.

fatigue A state of physical and/or mental weakness, lethargy.

fear Worry about a specific and identified threatening event or issue.

feeding and eating disorders Disorders characterized by alterations in normal eating patterns that are marked by distinct and persistent disturbances in eating behaviors, weight regulation, and perceptions toward body weight and shape.

female circumcision (genital mutilation) Any procedure involving partial or total removal of the external female genitalia, or other injury to the female genital organs, for nonmedical reasons.

fidelity The nurse's obligation to be dedicated to patients and faithful in the performance of his or her duties.

flashbacks Dissociative reactions in which the individual feels or acts as if a traumatic event is recurring; hallucinations or alterations in perception that may occur as a result of substance use.

flight of ideas Rapid speech that involves ideas that jump from topic to topic and may be loosely associated.

formal power Power that results from a person's role title and position description and articulates what accountabilities and authority are commensurate with that position.

formal thought disorder (FTD) Often referred to as symptoms of disorganization, FTD describes a lack of progressive goal-directed thought processes (related to the severity of neurobiological deficits) that manifest in abnormal/odd speech, affecting overall communication; symptoms include loose associations, tangentiality, incoherence/word salad/neologism, illogicality, circumstantiality, pressured/distractible speech, and poverty of speech.

front line The environment or space where nurses and patients interact directly on a daily basis.

frontline nursing leadership The process by which nurses at the unit level motivate themselves and their nursing staff colleagues to engage in professional practice behaviors to accomplish the goal of a safe and healing environment.

frontal lobe Lobe of the brain that is responsible for executive function and personality; it maintains focused attention, organizes thinking, planning, speech, and motor activities.

functional neurological symptom disorder (conversion disorder) A somatic-related disorder in which patients experience one or more changes in the performance of a voluntary motor or sensory function; patients with symptoms of abnormal voluntary motor function may present with a weakness or a paralysis, abnormal movements, and abnormal extremity functioning or positions.

gender An individual's personal, social, and legal status as a male or female.

gender dysphoria Distress associated with psychosocial incongruence between an individual's assigned gender and the gender with which the individual more clearly identifies.

General Adaptation Syndrome A pscychophysiologic response to stress with three distinct levels of response: alarm reaction, stage of resistance, and stage of exhaustion.

generalized anxiety disorder (GAD) Type of anxiety disorder characterized by excessive anxiety and worry about multiple domains or events that occurs more days than not during a period of at least 3 months.

genetics The study of heredity and variation in gene expression.

genital mutilation (female circumcision) Any procedure involving partial or total removal of the external female genitalia, or other injury to the female genital organs, for nonmedical reasons.

genital period The stage of psychosexual development proposed by Freud in which sexual needs re-emerge due to puberty; characterized by emotional turmoil, infatuation, and the need to development satisfying sexual associations.

genomics The study of gene function related to health and illness.

Glasgow coma scale The universally accepted method for assessing a patient's level of consciousness and to measure or predict the progression of the patient's condition.

gray matter The working area of the brain containing synapses and neuronal connections, consisting of nerve cell bodies and dendrites.

grief An individual's unique response to loss.

grief work The responses individuals exhibit following a loss and their attempts to resolve their grief and return to "normal" after the loss.

half-life The time it takes a drug to journey from metabolism to excretion, eliminating 50% of the drug from the body.

hallucinations Abnormal perceptual (visual, auditory, olfactory, gustatory, and tactile) experiences that occur without external stimuli.

hard signs Neurological signs or symptoms that indicate impaired reflex, sensory, or motor functioning and are localized to a particular brain region; include hypoalgesia, impaired olfactory functioning, and oculomotor abnormalities.

hardiness A group of characteristics that helps provide resistance to stressful life events; include commitment to oneself and work, feeling control over events and outcomes, and viewing change as challenge.

heavy drinking A pattern of drinking that consists of more than two drinks per day for men and more than one drink per day for women.

history The record of human behavior over time.

hoarding disorder A disorder related to obsessive–compulsive disorder that is characterized by continued difficulty discarding or parting with possessions due to a perceived need to save the items and distress associated with discarding them.

homeostasis A state of equilibrium demonstrated when the magnitude of stressors an individual experiences is matched by that of the coping response, and the individual's coping response is sufficient to resolve the stressors.

homosexuality Sexual attraction to individuals of the same gender.

hope A feeling that something an individual wants or longs for has a good chance of coming to pass.

hospice care Care that embraces the belief that quality of life is as important as quantity of life, providing terminally ill patients with caregivers who address all aspects of their care.

humane treatment Respectful treatment of patients that conveys dignity and worth, such as patients receiving the same food as staff.

hydrotherapy Therapy using the application of water.

hypomania A persistently elevated, expansive, irritable mood state that does not impair functioning.

hypoxyphilia The use of oxygen deprivation to enhance sexual arousal and orgasm (also called *autoerotic asphyxiation* or *asphyxiophilia*).

id One of three states of being posited by Freud, the id seeks self-gratification.

ideal self The self that one should or would like to be.

illness anxiety disorder A somatic-related disorder characterized by preoccupation with having an illness, even though typically there are no physical symptoms of an illness.

impact The nurse's sense that he or she can influence important outcomes.

impulsive aggression Aggressive activity during which the individual is in a state of emotional arousal. This form of aggression is overt and reactive, and it may involve self-protection.

impulsivity A predisposition toward rapid, unplanned reactions to internal and external stimuli without regard for negative consequences.

informal power Type of power that emerges from an individual's network of relationships with colleagues within an organization.

information Formal and informal knowledge needed to be effective in the workplace.

informed consent The permission that a patient, or the patient's representative, grants a clinician to provide medical treatment.

insomnia The most common sleep disorder in adults; characterized by repeated difficulty with sleep initiation, duration, consolidation, and/or quality that occurs despite adequate time and opportunity for sleep and results in some form of daytime impairment.

integrative medicine The combining of conventional medicine with complementary and alternative medicine therapies for which there is scientific evidence of safety and effectiveness.

integrity The ability to consistently adhere to character-resonating values.

integrity-preserving compromises Positions or actions that simultaneously account for potentially conflicting alternatives.

internal locus of control Attributing control of one's life to one's own actions and motivations.

internalized stigma The individual's accepting the stigma as a characteristic of self that contributes to self-hatred.

interneurons Connectors of sensory and motor (afferent and efferent) neurons in the CNS that exchange messages, interpret, communicate, and play a role in thought process, learning, perception, and memory.

interpersonal relations theory Theory developed by Hildegard Peplau that helped define psychiatric nursing; tenets of the theory include that who the nurse is as a person affects what the patient learns and that fostering personality development is a function of nursing and nursing education.

interpersonal violence The physical, sexual, or psychological harm of a current or former intimate partner by another; includes physical aggression, sexual coercion, psychological abuse, and controlling behaviors; also called **intimate partner violence**.

intersex (formerly known as hermaphroditism) A group of conditions resulting from hormonal errors during fetal development in which internal genitalia differ from external genitalia.

interventions Activities that nurses employ during the implementation phase of the nursing process to achieve the goals established in the planning phase

intimate partner violence The physical, sexual, or psychological harm of a current or former intimate partner by another; includes physical aggression, sexual coercion, psychological abuse and controlling behaviors. Also called **interpersonal violence**.

intrinsic motivation Doing something because it is inherently interesting or enjoyable rather than doing something to attain an unrelated goal, such as pay or prestige.

involuntary commitment Admission to treatment of an individual against his or her will.

jail diversion A community-based best practice that recognizes the prevalence of symptoms of mental illness in individuals arrested for minor crimes and seeks to divert them from incarceration to treatment.

Johari window A visual model that describes the process of interaction and the relationship of self-awareness to interaction.

justice The fair and equal treatment of patients and others.

kindling A process in which cerebral voltage channels become overexcited and overfire, resulting in excesses of neurotransmission.

kinship Safe and comfortable relationships with people (not necessarily relatives) who will reach out to the patient and be available for help in a time of need as well as for social and supportive interactions.

labile Changeable, unregulated; typically used to refer to a mood state.

latency period One of the stages of psychosexual development proposed by Freud, this stage occurs during middle childhood. During this period, sexuality is suppressed and play is associated with either female or male perspectives.

laws Rules that organize society and regulate behavior.

ligand The drug molecule that binds to the receptor.

limbic system The hypothalamus, thalamus, hippocampus, and amygdala; essential to the regulation and modulation of emotions and memory.

loss A real or perceived deprivation; loss may be tangible (as in the loss of a spouse or home) or intangible (as in the loss of dignity).

malpractice Professional negligence.

management skills The ability to mobilize the human and material resources required to meet the organization's goals, which include patient and staff safety and satisfaction and positive care outcomes at the unit level.

mania An abnormally elevated or irritable mood characterized by high levels of arousal and energy that cause significant social, vocational, or academic impairment.

Maslow's hierarchy of needs Abraham Maslow asserted that individuals prioritize needs in five areas: physiological needs, requirements for safety and security, needs for love and belonging, self-esteem, and self-actualization. Individuals must meet their basic physiologic needs for food, water, and shelter before they can progress to higher-order needs.

masochism Sexual pleasure or arousal derived from receiving physical or mental abuse or humiliation.

maturational crisis Crisis that arises when an individual has difficulty achieving developmental tasks using available resources and coping strategies. Maturational crises may occur during milestones or developmental tasks.

meaning One of the domains of **psychological empowerment**; reflects a congruence between a nurse's beliefs and values and his or her work requirements.

meditation A practice that cultivates internal awareness through contemplation, concentration or attention to thoughts, feelings, and sensations of the mind and body.

melancholia A group of features associated with depression, including early morning awakening, anhedonia, vegetative symptoms, and symptoms worse in morning.

memory The ability to recall or reproduce what has been learned or experienced.

mental health A state of emotional and psychological well-being in which an individual is able to use his or her cognitive and emotional capabilities, function in society, and meet the ordinary demands of everyday life.

mental health first aid Help that is offered to an individual who may be developing a mental health condition or experiencing a mental health crisis. It has four major aims: preserve life when a person may be a danger to self or others; provide help to prevent the problem from becoming more serious; promote and enhance recovery; and provide comfort and support.

mental illness Any of various conditions characterized by impairment of an individual's normal cognitive, emotional, or behavioral functioning, and caused by social, psychological, biochemical, genetic, or other factors.

meta communication The context in which communication occurs, including those involved in the interaction (e.g., who is sending the message and who is receiving it), how the message is sent (e.g., in person, over the telephone, or through email), the context of the message (e.g., nurse and patient in a clinical setting, supervisor and employee in a workplace, friends in a restaurant), and other factors.

metabolites The products of the enzymatic breakdown of medications; typically far less chemically potent than the original drug.

mind and body practices Complementary health approaches that require a certified practitioner or teacher.

mind–body therapies Therapies that attempt to improve functioning and promote health by incorporating behaviors (e.g., deep breathing, progressive relaxation, or stretching) that require interactions between the mind and body.

mindfulness A form of self-awareness described as a state of being in the present moment and accepting things for what they are, without judgment.

mixed episode Depression plus mania/hypomania.

mood An internal personal barometer that can be defined as a pervasive emotional tone that profoundly influences one's outlook and perception of self, others, and the environment.

mood disorders Sustained emotional states that are a departure from the individual's usual functioning and that cause significant impairment in social or vocational functioning.

moral therapy A system of care that stresses kindness to patients and employment of patient in meaningful activity.

moribund On the verge of death.

motivational interviewing (MI) A collaborative, person-centered prescribed set of interviewing strategies used to help patients identify their readiness for change and to facilitate change in health-related behaviors.

motor neurons Also called *efferent neurons*, nerve cells that carry neural signal messages from inside the brain, the CNS, back out to the PNS, again through the spinal nerves.

mourning Outward manifestations of grief, especially rituals and customs, such as wearing black.

narcissism Excessive interest in or preoccupation with the self, which is often illustrated in manipulative or demanding behaviors and a lack of empathy for others.

narcolepsy A disorder of the wakefulness system, whose key symptom is excessive daytime sleepiness/sleep attacks caused by the intrusion of REM sleep into wakefulness.

negative symptoms Affects and behaviors that are diminished or absent in patients with schizophrenic spectrum disorders; these include having a flat or blunted affect, thought blocking, poverty of speech (alogia), avolition, and social withdrawal.

neuroleptic malignant syndrome A rare but potentially life-threatening neurological response to medications that can occur at any point in treatment; symptoms include an alteration in sensory process, cognitive changes that may look like delirium, hyperthermia, hyperreflexia, muscle rigidity, autonomic instability, hypotension, tachycardia, tachypnea, diaphoresis, and sialorrhea.

neuron A single nerve cell.

neuroplasticity The ability of the brain to change structurally and functionally as a result of input from the environment.

neurotransmitter A chemical substance that transmits nerve impulses across a synapse.

night eating syndrome A pattern of excessive eating after the evening meal or after awakening from sleep.

nonmaleficence The obligation to do no harm.

nonverbal communication Gestures, posture, appearance and other types of personal communication other than verbal.

North American Nursing Diagnosis Association—International (NANDA-I) A professional organization that provides oversight of the development and standardization of nursing diagnoses.

nursing diagnosis The second step of the **nursing process**, in which the nurse synthesizes the information gathered and identifies and categorizes the presenting needs of the patient in a salient way, following both nursing diagnosis and psychiatric diagnostic criteria.

nursing ethics Codes or rules that address how nurses determine the appropriate course of action in day-to-day clinical practice.

Nursing Interventions Classification (NIC) A method of classifying nursing interventions according to the **North American Nursing Diagnosis Association—International**.

Nursing Outcomes Classification (NOC) A method of classifying outcomes according to the **North American Nursing Diagnosis Association—International**.

nursing process The steps nurses use to identify needs for care; analyze, prioritize, and plan for intervention; and evaluate the nursing care that is delivered to patients.

nursing theory Theory or theories that focuses on aspects of nursing care, helping explain behavior and nursing roles by identifying and defining components that are relevant.

obsessions Recurrent and persistent thoughts, urges, or images that cause significant anxiety or distress.

obsessive–compulsive disorder (OCD) A disorder characterized by recurring obsessions or compulsions that are so persistent that they take up an unreasonable amount of time or cause severe distress or impairment.

occipital lobe Area of the brain primarily responsible for vision and visual memory, as well as reading, language formation, and reception of vestibular, acoustic, and tactile stimuli.

older adult A term used to refer to individuals 60 years old or older.

opioid peptide receptors (OP) Neuromodulators that modify the action of neurotransmitters and are naturally designed by the body to relieve pain, affect perception of pain, enhance feelings of well-being, produce pleasurable feelings, lift mood, promote tissue regeneration, and enhance the immune system.

oppositional defiant disorder A pediatric disorder characterized by symptoms of irritability and defiance of adult authorities, as well as anger and aggression that disrupt daily functioning.

oral stage One of the stages of psychosexual development proposed by Freud, occurring between birth and 18 months and emphasizing sensitivity and pleasurable achievement of sucking and biting within the mouth, lips, and tongue zones.

orientation phase The phase of the **therapeutic relationship** that corresponds with the initial meeting of the patient and the nurse.

other specified feeding or eating disorder A type of **feeding and eating disorder** characterized by symptoms of a feeding or eating disorder that cause clinically significant impairment or distress but that do not meet the full diagnostic criteria for a particular disorder.

palliative care Care that attempts to improve quality of life and emphasizes pain management and holistic care of terminally ill patients, as well as caring for the patient's identified family.

panic attack A period of intense fear or discomfort in which the individual senses impending doom and experiences physiologic symptoms such as palpitations and sweating.

panic disorder A form of anxiety disorder characterized by recurrent, unexpected **panic attacks** that are accompanied by a significant change in behavior.

paraphilic disorders A classification of disorders that are characterized by overwhelming sexual arousal and/or behaviors related to unusual objects or activities and that result in significant distress and impairment in functioning.

parasympathetic nervous system Portion of the nervous system that innervates the cranial nerves III, VII, IX, and X, regulates automatic functions, and is responsible for "resetting" the autonomic nervous system after activation.

parietal lobe Lobe of the brain that regulates primary sensory areas, including pain, taste, touch, proprioception (location of the body in space), and the sensation of temperature. The processes for reading and writing also occur in the parietal lobe, which also helps maintain focused attention and processes certain motor activities, including attention and perception of spatial relations and registration of acts of aggression.

paternalism The intentional overriding of another's preferences with the intent to do good.

patient-centered care A way of caring for patients in which patients determine the direction of their treatment and goal identification starts with the individual patient.

pedophilia Sexual activity with a prepubescent child.

peer specialists Individuals who are in recovery from a serious and persistent mental illness and employed in a variety of positions throughout the behavioral health system, from inpatient to assertive community treatment (ACT) teams.

perception The primary cognitive process by which an individual collects sensory data (via the five senses) and clusters it into a pattern.

peripheral nervous system (PNS) The nerves and ganglia located outside the central nervous system; also includes the cranial nerves just outside the brainstem. The PNS acts as a relay communication network, bringing sensory information to the body.

perseverance The ability to persist despite opposition or discouragement.

personality A distinctive set of traits, behavior styles, and patterns that make up one's character.

personality disorder A persistent, maladaptive pattern of thinking, coping, and relating to others.

phallic stage One of the stages of psychosexual development proposed by Freud, taking place between ages 3 and 7 years, involving the sensitivity area of the genitals and pleasure associated with masturbation.

pharmacodynamics The way medications affect the body.

pharmacokinetics The way the body processes medications.

pharmacotherapeutics The clinical application of medications to brain circuit and neurotransmitter–receptor dysfunction.

physical restraint The immobilization of a patient either by staff (a physical hold) or by mechanical restraint using locked restraints.

pica The persistent eating of nonnutritive, nonfood substances (e.g., soap, cloth, dirt, pebbles).

point of service The relationship between nurse and patients; the place where safety and healing can be nurtured.

polypharmacy Condition that occurs when multiple medications are prescribed and interact poorly with each other.

positive symptoms Typically associated with schizophrenic spectrum disorders, symptoms that involve additions to normal experiences and include **hallucinations** and **delusions** as well as abnormal movements and problems with speech (**formal thought disorder**).

positivism Theory that the only real "truth" is found in observable, scientific facts, and that rejects the transcendent and religion as sources of truth.

positron emission tomography (PET) scan A radioactive, computer-imaged scan of the brain, breast, heart, or lung that produces a 3D image of the glucose uptake of the tissue area scanned; often done in conjunction with a CT scan.

postmodernism Era of ideas and beliefs that began in the early 20th century and is characterized by many ideas, including an affirmation of diverse perspectives and a rejection of the idea of absolute truth or broad explanations about the nature of reality, such as those contained in both science and religion.

posttraumatic stress disorder (PTSD) A disorder consisting of a group of characteristic symptoms that occur following exposure to traumatic events, experienced either directly or through witnessing trauma to others.

potency The amount (dose) of the drug necessary to produce the desired response.

pre-orientation phase Initial phase of the nursing relationship that occurs prior to the first meeting of the patient and nurse, in which the patient and nurse may have some information about each other (e.g., prehospital report, observations) but have not yet met.

predatory aggression Aggressive activity that is premeditated or planned, with the aggressor usually being calm, unemotional, and controlled, and having a goal.

premorbid Prior to onset of symptoms.

presence Being with and attending to the patient in a way that promotes a level of human engagement and interchange between the nurse and patient that is meaningful to the patient; may also be described as a condition in which all the nurse's attention and energy are focused *in the moment on* the purpose of that moment.

primary appraisal A stage of coping during which an individual determines whether or not a stressor has an impact on the person's well-being.

primary gain Gain that results from an immediate benefit to the individual; specifically, relief from anxiety.

privileged communications Confidential communications, usually between two individuals recognized as having a unique professional relationship (e.g., patient and health care provider).

process recording A written record of an interaction between two or more individuals.

prodrome (or prodromal period) A symptomatic period prior to the diagnosis of SSDs that represents a definite change from premorbid functioning, is clearly identified as problematic, and continues until the emergence of psychotic symptoms.

projection The transfer of blame to another person to avoid the feelings that would be experienced by blaming oneself.

projective identification Experiencing the emotions of another.

protective measures Factors that can assist the individual to feel hopeful and worthy enough to begin problem solving; factors that reduce risk for physical or mental illness.

proxemics The way in which body space is used.

pseudodementia Cognitive changes that arise secondary to depression.

psychiatric advance directive (PAD) A specific type of advance directive that permits individuals to specify treatment options should they become incapacitated due to mental illness (e.g., psychosis).

psychiatric–mental health nursing The nursing specialty in which nurses care for patients with mental illnesses, and their family members.

psychiatric nursing theory A type of **theory** that systematically identifies, assesses, and solves issues within areas that are uniquely related to psychiatric–mental health nursing.

psychiatry Broad discipline of medicine that encompasses the diagnosis and treatment of individuals with mental illnesses.

psychoanalytic theory A **theory** that proposes that personality develops in a progressive manner grounded in psychosexual stages.

psychological debriefing Brief, one-time interventions conducted within 72 hours of crisis onset.

psychological empowerment An interpersonal process that is shaped by an individual's personal experiences and belief about his or her work role.

psychological first aid A brief and practical intervention that is often used in the immediate aftermath of disasters and other large-scale trauma experiences.

psychopharmacology The study of the use of medications in the treatment of psychiatric–mental health disorders and conditions.

psychosis A symptom of mental illness characterized by distorted perceptions of reality, marked changes in personality, and greatly impaired functioning.

psychosocial theory A **theory**, proposed by Erik Erikson, that focuses on the achievement and mastery of life challenges that occur within certain time periods, as opposed to Freud's focus on pathology in developmental stages. The expected outcome for mastery of the stages is a healthy personality.

psychotomimetic Producing a condition resembling psychosis.

purging disorder A pattern of purging to influence weight or shape.

race Genetically determined and geographically based characteristics.

rape Forced sexual intercourse (using a body part or object).

reality orientation Conversational aid designed to help orient the patient with dementia.

reasonable doubt A method of questioning another's perceptions without arguing.

receptor A protein molecule (on the postsynaptic neuron) that receives and responds to a neurotransmitter ligand, a drug ligand (or medication), or other substances such as hormones and antigens.

recovery Period following illness in which symptoms are under control and the individual is able to perform basic self-care; the level of wellness is defined as stable.

refeeding syndrome A potentially fatal condition that can occur when severely malnourished patients begin the refeeding process.

reflection The thinking and feeling behaviors that are used to both create and clarify the meaning of an event.

relapse Return of symptoms after stabilization.

religion A formalized and often structured way of answering questions about the nature of life. This formalization may include structured ways of worship or spiritual practices, such as specific prayers said for specific purposes; sacred texts that outline instructions for daily living; and/or a hierarchy of leadership.

relocation stress syndrome Physiological and psychosocial disturbances that result of transfer from one environment to another; also known as **transfer trauma.**

reminiscence therapy Therapy that helps patients with dementia access older memories as a means or promoting self-esteem and identity in older adults and to stimulate communication with patients.

resilience The capacity to adapt successfully to adversity.

resolution phase The phase of the **therapeutic relationship** in which the goals that could be attained in the setting have been met and, and as the patient moves forward toward discharge or the next stage of care, the relationship with the nurse comes to an end.

restraint The physical, mechanical, or chemical involuntary constraint or restriction of a patient's freedom, including restriction or constraint of movement.

retrograde neurotransmission A method of neurotransmission in which the postsynaptic cell communicates with the presynaptic neuron.

right to privacy The patient's prerogative to be left alone, free from intrusion, and in command of personal information.

rumination disorder Repeated regurgitation of food.

sadism Sexual arousal associated with causing mental or physical suffering to another person.

schemas Cognitive ways of dealing with the environment.

schizoaffective disorder Disorder characterized by major mood symptoms (depression, mania, or both) occurring during most of the same period of illness as delusions or hallucinations and lasting at least 2 weeks.

schizophrenia A disturbance lasting at least 6 months (if untreated) that consists of at least two major positive or negative symptoms; one of the cardinal symptoms must be either **delusions**, **hallucinations**, or disorganized speech.

seclusion The placing of a patient in a locked room; may be used if the patient requires a place where there is low stimulation and when it is not safe for the patient to be on the regular unit.

secondary appraisal The stage of coping following primary appraisal. During secondary appraisal, the individual considers how to respond to a threat with the resources currently available.

secondary gain A type of gain or benefit that occurs when an individual experiences indirect benefit from having a disorder or condition; indirect benefits may include financial compensation, disability benefits, personal services and attention, and/or escape from work or a difficult responsibility.

selective mutism A rare childhood disorder in which children fully capable of speech in some settings fail to speak in selected social situations.

self The union of elements (body, emotion, thoughts, and sensations) that constitute the individuality of a being, as well as the consciousness of one's own being.

self-awareness The capacity to become the object of one's own attention and actively identify, process, and collect information about one's internal mental state and public behaviors, including general physical appearance.

self-concept The part of self that lies within the conscious awareness; self-concept encompasses perceptions, thoughts, and feelings as well as values and ideals that are part of the self.

self-efficacy Ability to adapt and reinforce positive, healthier responses to a stimulus; confidence in one's ability to perform a behavior combined with expectations of benefits from the behavior.

self-esteem A personal judgment of self-worth, based on the amount of overlap that exists between **ideal self**—"the self one should or would like to be"—and what one believes to be true about the actual self.

self-help groups Wellness support groups composed of and led by individuals who share the same or similar illness or addiction.

self-injurious behaviors Behaviors individuals engage in to cause harm to themselves, including cutting, abrading, hair pulling, biting, burning, or scratching, without the overt purpose to end life.

self-medicating Use of substances to blunt or negate challenging or painful symptoms or feelings.

self-reflection The process of examining one's own actions and motivations and feelings.

sensory neuron (or afferent neuron) A type of nerve cell that carries neural signal information from the periphery (outside the body through the peripheral nervous system) up to the CNS through the spinal nerves.

separation anxiety disorder A disorder of mental health characterized by a developmentally innappropriate and excessive fear or anxiety concerning separation from those to whom the individual is attached; children will experience great fear or distress when separated from parents or home.

serious mental illness A diagnosable mental, behavioral, or emotional disorder resulting in substantial impairment in carrying out major life activities.

serotonin syndrome A constellation of symptoms caused by an excess of serotonin; symptoms include agitation, sweating, fever, tachycardia, hypotension, rigidity, and/or hyperreflexia.

sex Biological indicators of an individual's sexuality, including sex chromosomes, hormones, and genitalia; also, sexual intercourse.

sexual dysfunction Interruption or impairment of the **sexual response cycle** or pain associated with intercourse.

sexual orientation Description that refers to the object of the individual's sexual attraction.

sexual response cycle The cycle of human sexual response, which occurs in a predictable cycle with five distinct phases: desire, excitement, plateau, orgasm, and resolution.

sexual violence Any unwanted sexual contact, ranging from unwanted kissing or touching to rape.

sexuality The manifestation of several psychosexual factors: sexual identity, gender identity, and sexual orientation.

side effects Symptoms that occur when a medication produces additional actions by interacting with neurotransmitters other than those at the target site.

simple assault A physical attack by one individual on another, without the use of or display of a weapon and without any resulting serious or aggravated injury.

situational crises A type of **crisis** that develops in response to sudden, unexpected traumatic life events, and often are beyond the established coping capabilities of the individuals experiencing them.

sleep architecture The structure of stages (1, 2, 3) and phases (REM and NREM) of sleep.

sleep continuity Measure that includes **sleep latency** (minutes to get to sleep), minutes awake during the night, sleep efficiency (total sleep time/minutes in bed × 100), and number of awakenings from sleep.

sleep-disordered breathing The presence of partial or complete airway obstruction or dysfunction of the central drive to breath that occurs during sleep.

sleep latency Length of time it takes an individual to fall asleep.

sleepiness Difficulty maintaining wakefulness.

sobriety Complete abstinence from alcohol or other drugs of abuse in conjunction with a satisfactory quality of life.

social cognitive theory Proposed by Albert Bandura, a **theory** that indicates that a level of **self-efficacy** is a critical component for individuals' ability to effectively manage occurrences within their everyday functioning.

social roles Roles individuals choose or establish within a group or society. Roles can be chosen or acquired without voluntary decision making. Leader, follower, boss, and employee are all social roles that could be described as chosen.

soft signs Neurological deficits that do not implicate a specific brain area. Soft signs include grimacing, increased blink rates, problems sequencing motor tasks, and **asterognosis**.

somatic symptom disorder Disorder in which patients express symptoms through their body, feeling pain and other somatic sensations that others may not experience. These sensations become the individual's focus and concern, often to the exclusion of other areas of life and resulting in functional impairment.

somatization The process by which psychological distress is expressed in physical symptoms.

spirituality The inherent quality of all humans that activates and drives the search for meaning and purpose in life.

splitting A behavior in which the individual divides and plays one person or group against another.

stalking Harassment or other unwanted communication or contact (including following, phone calls, messages, and vandalizing property).

steady state State achieved in about five half-lives of a medication, when the amount of a medication being taken equals the amount leaving the body.

stereotyping Overgeneralizing group characteristics that reinforce societal biases and distort individual characteristics.

stigma The discrimination or social rejection of individuals diagnosed with mental illness.

stress An individual's perception of demands and the perception of his or her ability to meet those demands.

structural empowerment theory Theory that asserts that when workplace situations are structured in such a way that employees feel empowered, employees will respond accordingly and rise to the challenges present in their work environment.

substance abuse A pattern of harmful use of any substance for mood-altering purposes.

suicidal ideation Thoughts about committing suicide.

suicide Death as a result of self-inflicted injury accompanied by an intent to die from the injury.

superego One of three states of being posited by Freud, which functions as a moral compass.

support Regular feedback and guidance to individual nurses to promote optimal nursing professional performance.

supported employment Services to help individuals with mental illness find and maintain employment.

survivor guilt Feelings of guilt that occur when one person survives and another dies and the survivor is burdened by guilt about living, asking questions such as "Why not me?"

sympathetic nervous system System that innervates the thoracolumbar spine and rapidly mobilizes body systems during activity (most especially during stress), acting in sympathy with the body.

synapse The junction where one bulb of the presynaptic axon terminal makes contact with the post synaptic dendrite receptor membrane site of another nerve.

tai chi Eastern mind–body practice that focuses on gentle, linked movements.

tardive dyskinesia (TD) A movement disorder characterized by involuntary, repetitive movements, often associated with neuroleptic therapy and advanced age.

target effects Changes in symptoms that occur when a medication reaches the target site and produces the desired effect or expected or intended response.

telescoping A quick progression from the start of substance use to dependence and problematic use, requiring treatment.

temporal lobes Lobes of the brain located just above the ears, which process auditory and olfactory senses. Emotion, learning, and memory circuits are here as well. This area gives emotional tone to memories and is involved in making moral judgments.

teratogenic effect An extreme adverse effect that disturbs the development of an embryo or fetus.

tertiary gain A gain or benefit achieved by someone other than the patient as a result of the patient's illness.

theory A group of interconnected concepts, definitions, and/or models that help explain why a series of incidents occur.

therapeutic alliance Alliance achieved when the patient is able to freely discuss concerns and needs and work to achieve goals. This alliance develops from the safe, neutral space provided through the successful development of the therapeutic relationship and is based on the trust that the nurse establishes with the patient over time.

therapeutic communication The communication that takes place between patient and nurse; the primary tool used by clinicians to help clients in the mental health setting.

therapeutic neutrality An aspect of the therapeutic relationship in which the nurse allows the patient exposure to experiences and emotions without imposing judgment or sharing the nurse's own views or emotions.

therapeutic range the range at which therapeutic efficacy can be achieved without risking harm to the patient.

therapeutic relationship A planned, goal-directed relationship that exists for the purpose of the nurse to assist the patient to progress toward goal attainment.

tolerance Occurs when increasing amounts of the substance are required to achieve the same effect.

tort law A category of law that deals with harmful or wrongful acts resulting in injury to either another person or another person's property.

Tourette syndrome A neurologic disorder with childhood onset that is defined by an enduring pattern of motor and phonic tics.

toxicity The concentration of the amount of drug in the body that is harmful to an individual.

transcendent Referring to the belief that something (e.g., nature) or someone (e.g., a supreme being) that goes beyond the physical and material and beyond that which can be understood by human knowledge.

transcultural nursing The caring practice of helping individuals achieve and maintain health or reach death in a culturally relevant way.

transfer trauma Physiological and psychosocial disturbances that result of transfer from one environment to another; also known as **relocation stress syndrome**.

transference Phenomenon that occurs when the patient attributes feelings to the therapist regarding another person in the patient's life.

transitional objects Objects, such as blankets or stuffed animals, that patients can carry from setting to setting to help maintain a sense of security and comfort.

type I trauma A one-time, limited experience that causes trauma to an individual.

type II trauma A recurring or chronic experience that causes trauma to an individual (e.g., military deployment, child abuse).

unconditional positive regard A positive, accepting manner that supports nurses in treating patients with respect and dignity.

unresolved grief Ongoing or suppressed grief that affects the individual's response to the current or expected future loss; may result when individual suppresses grief to make others feel more comfortable or because urgent circumstances delay grieving in the present.

unspecified feeding or eating disorder A type of **feeding and eating disorder** in which symptoms do not meet the full diagnostic criteria for a specific disorder, and the clinician chooses *not* to specify which specific order the presentation resembles.

utilitarianism Ethics based on the consequences of an action, with good or pleasure as the ethical imperative.

validation therapy An approach that involves searching for the emotion and meaning in the patient's disoriented or confused words and behavior (such as wandering) and validating them verbally; used with patients with dementia.

values Ideals that assign meaning to individuals' decisions.

values clarification A process that involves identifying and prioritizing the unarticulated beliefs that drive decision making.

vascular dementia A form of dementia that results from decreased blood supply to the brain and is characterized by progressive decline in cognitive function, weakness of the limbs, small-stepped gait, and difficulty with speech.

vegetative symptoms the corporeal manifestations of depression, including sleep and appetite disturbance, decreased energy, psychomotor symptoms (agitation or retardation), sexual dysfunction, and the neurocognitive symptoms of decreased concentration or cognition, lack of pleasure, guilty ruminations, and suicidal ideation.

verbal communication The words that people use when they speak.

Vermont study Study said to be one of the longest-running studies in American clinical medical research, involving the deinstitutionalization and rehabilitation of clients with schizophrenia in their communities.

violence The purposeful use of force, resulting in physical or psychological injuries or death.

volume neurotransmission Neurotransmission occurring (without a synapse) to an adjacent neuron by process of diffusion; occurs when nearby receptors pick up the neurotransmitter and perform a weaker signal.

voluntary admission Admission that occurs when a patient voluntarily consents to treatment, particularly admission into a residential treatment facility.

waxy flexibility A tendency to remain immobile.

wellness The interaction of biological and environmental factors, such as interpersonal relationships, spirituality, attitudes, and behaviors, in a way that enables individuals to attain a satisfactory quality of life as they define it.

white matter The myelinated axons of neurons.

withdrawal An array of negative psychological and physiological symptoms experienced when individuals who use a substance consistently stop abruptly.

working phase The phase of the therapeutic nurse–patient relationship in which the nurse and patient identify problems and develop trust.

workplace bullying Deliberate, repeated, mistreatment of a worker over time by another worker, involving negative and aggressive behaviors such as harassment, social exclusion, or interference with job performance.

world view The cognitive map or view of the world that is developed in childhood and adolescence, which includes all the learning that shapes one's beliefs and feelings about the world.

yoga A mind–body practice based on ancient Indian philosophy that incorporates physical postures, breathing techniques, meditation, and relaxation.

INDEX

SPECIAL FEATURES